THE ESSENTIAL GUIDE TO PRESCRIPTION DRUGS

1998 EDITION

James J. Rybacki, Pharm. D.
James W. Long, M.D.

HarperPerennial

A Division of HarperCollins *Publishers*

HarperCollins books may be purchased for educational, business, or sales promotional use. For information please write: Special Markets Department, HarperCollins Publishers Inc., 10 East 53rd Street, New York, NY 10022.

Designed by C. Linda Dingler

Library of Congress Catalog Card Number 87–657561

ISSN 0894–7058
ISBN 0–06–271606–9   97 98 99 RRD 10 9 8 7 6 5 4 3 2 1
ISBN 0–06–273506–3 (pbk.) 97 98 99 RRD 10 9 8 7 6 5 4 3 2 1

Contents

Author's Note
for the 1998 Edition

Once again, many HMOs and health care in general seem to have lost track of you, the patient—the life which should be the focus of care. For example, chronic diseases presently account for a large portion of the U.S. health care budget, but few HMOs are held accountable for tracking outcomes or maintaining strong disease prevention, management, or outcomes management systems. Many HMOs even have "gag orders" on their physician providers that preclude them from telling you about ALL available options in treating a condition you may be facing. Sadly, adverse drug reactions and problems from people failing to take their medicines correctly also continue to have a huge impact on our lives.

The most recent estimate of the cost of problems caused by medicines was in the *Journal of the American Medical Association* (JAMA) in an article by Dr. Classen. It's impossible to place a value on the human aspect, but the current estimate of the financial toll is now **136 billion dollars a year**. This means that problems with medicines cause a financial and human toll **greater than** the cost of *diabetes or cardiovascular care* in the United States. My own father had a serious reaction to one of his heart medications, and all of his doctors missed it—I know enough to prevent that now, but it's too late for him. When I read about reactions other families have suffered, I find myself taking them personally, wondering if I could prevented the problem if I had only been there. Remember, the decision to use **every** prescription and nonprescription medicine is based on a balance between benefit and risk. Please, please take the time to know your medicines. **Always** ask your doctor or pharmacist **BEFORE** you combine **any** prescription, nonprescription, or herbal medicines.

I believe that the best colleague any physician, pharmacist, nurse practitioner, or physician's assistant can have is a fully informed patient. Protect yourself and your loved ones with the power of this book. If you ever think you may be having a reaction to your medicines, call your doctor or pharmacist immediately. Some adverse reactions to medicines can actually be stopped if they are caught early. **Insist** that your medicines are arranged on a **medication map** for you. I have pioneered this concept. Many errors happen because the information for each prescription is treated as though the medicine will be taken by itself. In reality the medicines all go into the same body, and those over 60 years old often take more than six medicines AT THE SAME TIME. Prescription labels **always** tell how many times a day to take the drug—for example, three times a day—but a physician or pharmacy **never** gives you a single piece of paper that outlines how and with what all of your medicines should be taken. The current system also usually fails to organize all of your medicines into a schedule that makes sense for you. When several medicines must be taken throughout the day, I think it is unconscionable that patients are left on their own to figure out when to take them and which medicines should be combined.

Today, many of us get our care through HMOs. This has been a phenomenon purported to save money while getting results equal to other providers. It is time to question these results. The power of your choice is great. When considering an HMO, ask exactly how **their results** or outcomes compare with **other** providers of the same care. Ask if theirs is a restricted formulary and whether prescriptions must be filled through a mail-order pharmacy, versus your local pharmacy. If mail order is to be used, ask how you will be able to ask questions of a pharmacist, and who will review all of your medicines on a regular basis. It is one thing to merely cut costs; it is very different to be able to contain costs while maintaining the same results or outcomes! The National Committee for Quality Assurance (NCQA) is attempting to set uniform standards, but it has a long way to go in national implementation. It is also critical for consumers to ask if physician providers have any kind of gag order in their contracts with the HMO. A physician who is restricted from telling you about ALL available options may be of limited benefit to you.

The NCQA has developed the Health Plan Employer Data and Information Set (HEDIS) in order to help tell how effective physicians are and how they compare to one another. It is perfectly acceptable for you to ask your doctor if they have been assessed using this measure, and how they compare to their colleagues. Senators Lieberman and Chafee introduced legislation that would require competition for federal health care provision to be based on quality. Ganske and Markey have reintroduced a bill to ban restriction of medical communication. Don't hesitate to contact your congressman or the president to ask how outcomes management and legislation preventing gag orders is being integrated into our health care system. A health care system without a total plan for checking results is like a factory that never looks at the product it makes. Washington needs to wake up, and you can help them with your letters.

Like the systems today that actually deliver health care, research, science, and available medicines are constantly changing. My "True Breakthroughs in Medicines" section brings you the newest information about products that are truly novel approaches to helping the human condition. So too have the tables and profiles been updated with the latest FDA approvals, as well as current research on unlabeled uses for medicines that may make the difference for you.

I've gotten many letters praising "The Leading Edge" section of this book. I'm pleased to be able to bring you news of medicines just over the next horizon, as well as information which may lead to new medicines. Many of the medicines from last year's section have since gained FDA approval and are covered in detail in their own drug profiles. Several readers also wrote about profile information on adjusting medicine dosing to chronic conditions. Remember, as we age our kidneys undergo a "natural" decline, and this is commonly missed. Since many medicines are removed from the body by the kidneys, make certain you ask your doctor to adjust doses of medicines for kidney function if you are over 60 years old.

Never let health care be something that is done *to* you. Be an active participant in your health care. Rybacki's first recommendation: "It's always better to prevent a disease or condition than to have to treat it." Ask about nutrients (such as calcium supplements in osteoporosis) that can help prevent disease; aspirin (which can help prevent first heart attacks, strokes, and perhaps even intestinal cancer); as well as available vaccines to prevent illnesses you may be prone to. I know it is difficult to give up any habit that you enjoy, but try to decrease ongoing risk. For example, **there are virtually no data to show that smoking is good for you**. That double or triple cheeseburger can add a lot of cholesterol. Limit how much fat you eat, and you may add years to your life. Many hospitals and clinics now have complementary care programs, systems that combine medicines with holistic and nontraditional approaches to helping prevent or cure diseases. These programs can help you get the benefit of a combination of different approaches, and return to health faster and remain healthy. Work with your doctor as a partner in health care, your nurse practitioner to keep and maintain your health, your pharmacist to make certain you have the right medicine in the right dose at the right time, and **ALWAYS** use the knowledge in this book to help protect you and your loved ones. Human errors take a terrible toll every year. Don't become a statistic—become an informed consumer.

As noted in each previous edition, no claim is made that *all* known actions, uses, side effects, adverse effects, precautions, interactions, etc., for a drug are included in the information provided in the sections that constitute this book. Although diligent care has been taken to ensure the accuracy of the information provided during the preparation of this revision, the continued accuracy and currentness are ever subject to change relative to the dissemination of new information derived from drug research, development, and general usage.

James Joseph Rybacki, Pharm. D.

Points for Consideration by the Patient

Research on medicine usage performed over the past 15 years have shown that more than half of patients take their prescription drugs incorrectly. Study after study finds similar results. Dr. Lucian L. Leape of Harvard found 334 drug errors in 6 months at two major teaching hospitals in the United States. Fourteen of these errors were life-threatening. A U.S. and Canadian study placed the financial cost at more than **9 billion dollars** in each country. A more recent study by Dr. Classen published in the *Journal of the American Medical Association* (JAMA) placed the expense at 136 billion dollars a year. The human cost cannot be calculated. Of course we must **do** something, rather than simply record an ever-increasing toll.

If you are being treated for a recurrent or chronic disorder, such as asthma or diabetes, **learn as much as you can** about the nature and medical management of your condition. Dr. James Long's book, *The Essential Guide to Chronic Illness*, is a superb resource. Ask your doctor and pharmacist for written information, visit your local libraries for pertinent publications, and call local chapters of national organizations. The more you know about your disorder and its treatment, the more you'll be able to use your prescribed medications safely and effectively. Never be afraid to ask your doctor or pharmacist questions—you help them when you help yourself. Any competent physician or pharmacist will welcome the chance to help you understand, regardless of how busy they may be. If they won't give you this critical time, find another physician or pharmacist.

Cooperate fully with your physician and pharmacist to ensure that the treatment prescribed is the most appropriate for you. It is incumbent upon you to **share the responsibility** for obtaining safe and effective drug treatment. Be certain every prescriber and pharmacist who helps provide your health care knows **all** of the medicines you are taking, including prescription, nonprescription, and any herbal or nutritional support you take.

Television, newspaper, and radio ads can be seductive, but try not to be unduly influenced. Ask your doctor and pharmacist for **printed information sheets** that provide unbiased information about the drug's benefits and risks—and its appropriateness for you. Drug therapy **MUST** be individualized, and based on current research and studies. **NEVER** take someone else's medicine because your symptoms sound just like theirs.

When Your Physician Prescribes a Drug for You

- Ask your doctor to fill out the medication map from the back of this book for you. This will help you organize all of your medicines to avoid adverse effects and get the most from your health care dollars.
- Tell your doctor about any known drug allergies and of any prior drug-induced adverse effects.
- Always honestly talk about **all other drugs** (prescription, nonprescription, herbal or nutritional) that you are taking currently. Include alcohol and marijuana. Also remember that some herbal extracts contain the same ingredients found in a prescription product. Make certain you include these in your medication history.
- Many medicines **require** special precautions such as avoidance of certain foods, interaction with alcohol, exposure to sun, interaction with other drugs, or hazardous activities.
- Be sure you understand how long to take a medicine. Talk with your prescriber about this and, if applicable, when and how to stop it.
- ALWAYS ask the person writing the prescription to include on the prescription label both the **name of the drug** and the **disorder** for which the drug is taken. For example: Fosamax for osteoporosis. This helps avoid "sound-alike" errors.
- Ask your doctor to give you a **written summary** of appropriate information about the drug prescribed. It is not surprising that you have difficulty remembering all of the information and instructions that have been talked about. A concept I have pioneered is the **medication map.** Many medicine errors are made because people forget, make incorrect combinations of medicines, or take medicine with food when it should not be. A medication map organizes all the medicines you are taking, and tells you how much, when, and with what the medicines should be taken. Take the blank form from this book to your doctor or pharmacist and ask them to fill in the form for you. This will help you to clarify and verify pertinent information while taking the medicine itself in the best possible way.
- ALWAYS ask your doctor if the medicine prescribed offers the best balance of price and outcomes for you. This simple question will help focus a busy practitioner on his or her available choices. Remember

to ask whether the dosing has been adjusted for any compromise in kidney or liver function or other chronic condition that you may have.

- Many HMOs or health care insurers may not pay for some medicines. This can impact your doctor's prescribing authority and the pharmacist's ability to fill your prescription. Write the payer to complain.
- Tell your doctor if new symptoms develop after you start taking the drug(s) prescribed.
- Keep follow-up appointments with your physician; many drugs must be monitored closely.
- If you go to any other health care provider, tell him or her of all medications you are taking currently—prescription and nonprescription. Remember any herbal remedies.
- Ask your doctor if there is a gag rule he or she is working under which restricts him or her to a limited formulary and lower-cost medicines. There may be a conflict of interest in the advice he or she is giving you.

When You Obtain Your Prescription Drug(s) From Your Pharmacist

- Read your prescription carefully. Check that both the **name of the drug** and the **disorder** are specified. If these are missing, ask your pharmacist to call your doctor for permission to add them.
- If your prescription is a refill, verify that the drug issued is the same as the drug in your original supply. If it is not the same, ask your pharmacist to explain the difference. (Generic drug products from different manufacturers often vary in size, shape, color, etc.)
- There are more than 1,000 drug names that "look alike" in print or "sound alike" in speech. Examples: Acutrim–Accutane, cyclosporine–cycloserine, Prilosec–Prozac, Xanax–Zantac. Mistaking one drug for the other can lead to serious dispensing errors. "Sound-alikes" cause problems when a prescription is given by telephone. Since sound-alike medicines are used to treat different conditions, listing the **disorder** on the prescription will help the pharmacist realize the mistake. Many of the most-often prescribed drugs are pictured in the Color Chart insert in this book.
- Ask the pharmacist to give you **printed information sheets** that provide specific information about the drug(s) prescribed for you. The information on these sheets is similar to that presented in the Drug Profiles found in Section Two of this book, but usually is less comprehensive and less detailed. Ask the pharmacist to fill out the **medication map** from the back of this book for you.
- Read each warning label that the pharmacist attaches to the container as well as the main prescription label. They serve to distinguish between eyedrops and ear drops, identify dosage forms that

should not be altered (opened, crushed, or chewed), and provide numerous precautions that improve the effectiveness of your medicine.

- Most pharmacies have a computer system that records and analyzes each patient's drug history. Take advantage of this excellent tool to prevent serious allergic reactions and significant drug interactions. Tell your pharmacist of all drugs (remember to include herbal remedies, megavitamins, alcohol, and nonprescription agents) you are currently taking. Take a further step and ask them to fill out a medication map for you. This is a single sheet of paper that organizes all of the medicines you take into a schedule of times which seeks to avoid drug interactions, works within the real aspects of your day, and helps get the best results from your medicines.

Your Responsibilities—to Yourself—as a Patient

- Know both the generic and brand name of all drugs prescribed for you.
- If you are taking more than one drug, be sure that the label of **each** container includes the **name of the drug** and the **condition it treats**.
- Remember that foods can react with medicines. Something as simple as grapefruit juice is now known to interact with some high blood pressure medicines. The best liquid to take with most medicines is water, but not for all. Be aware.
- If you do not clearly understand the directions for using a drug, ask your physician or pharmacist **before** taking it.
- Remember that many nonprescription medicines were once available only with a prescription. Talk with your pharmacist or physician **BEFORE** combining any nonprescription or prescription medicines.
- Follow all dosing instructions carefully and completely. For example, **DO NOT** stop an antibiotic 7 days into a 10-day prescription because you feel better. This can lead to serious treatment failure and resistant bacteria. If you have trouble remembering to take your medications on schedule, ask your pharmacist for a dosing calendar or a weekly medication box.
- If you are taking medications prescribed by more than one physician, check the **generic names** of all prescriptions for duplicate drugs with different brand names. This could cause serious overdosage.
- Ask your doctor or pharmacist if they offer "brown-bag sessions" for your medicines. These consist of filling a bag with the medicines you currently take, and having the pharmacist review the medicines for potency, appropriateness, and dating.
- When considering an insurance plan or HMO, ask if there is a required formulary. Find out if a mail-order pharmacy must be used. Finally, ask who will regularly review your medicines and how you will be able to contact a pharmacist with your questions if a mail-order pharmacy must be used.

- Be certain all drugs you take are "in date" (have not expired).
- View effective and timely control of pain as a basic right to which you are entitled. The Agency for Health Care Policy and Research has released *Clinical Practice Guidelines* which clearly outline the management of cancer pain, but also broadly apply to the management of pain in general. Demand that your pain is responded to with as much care and attention as a high fever (it should be considered a vital sign).
- If you are facing a terminal illness, ask whether the hospital you are considering has a palliative care program as well as a hospice program.

Suggestions for Containing the Costs of Drug Therapy

- Cooperate fully with your physician to ensure accurate diagnosis so that the initial selection of drugs will be as safe and effective as possible.
- Ask your doctor to prescribe the drug that is most appropriate for you, selecting the product which offers the best balance of price and outcomes. For example, if you are have several chronic diseases at the same time, what appears to be a more expensive antibiotic may have a better **outcome** for you than a less costly one. For someone facing a single infection unchallenged by other chronic diseases, a less costly, very specific antibiotic may offer an equal outcome and decreased expense.
- Ask your physician whether the drug prescribed is available as an acceptable generic product that is less expensive than the brand-name product.
- Ask your doctor if there are any vitamins or minerals (such as folic acid for some heart attacks or calcium for osteoporosis) that you should be taking to **PREVENT** a disease or condition for which your physician thinks you may be at risk.
- Follow your doctor and pharmacist's advice about your prescriptions.
- Many HMOs and physician groups use a concept called dual-product substitution to help contain costs. This is a measure that I agree with. For example: some prescription products are merely different names for **the same** medicine (Vanceril or Beclovent; Normodyne or Trandate). It makes perfect sense that the lowest-priced brand be freely substituted for a particular prescription. Ask your doctor about this idea when he or she is writing a prescription for you.
- Ask how the HMO or physician group who provides care for you and your loved ones measures against other groups in your area. Remember, many groups are benchmarked or measured by groups such as the NCQA. It is perfectly acceptable to ask how your physician, HMO, or medical group compares.

Points for Consideration by the Pharmacist

Pharmacists are in a unique position to help people get the most from their medicines. Remember, the current estimate is that adverse drug events cost 136 billion dollars a year. Be a part of the solution! Many pharmacists are being paid for their expertise in medicines (cognitive services), and in many instances, such as in Veterans Administration hospitals, are even prescribing medicines via guidelines. Many states have given pharmacists the opportunity to provide vaccinations, and large numbers of you are starting to offer them. In a setting where the pressure of time is somewhat less restrictive, the pharmacist is able to focus more on helping the patient with their medicines.

Accept the FDA initiative to define your role and responsibility as counselor to consumers regarding the proper use of medicinal drugs. The FDA's position is that the patient has a right to demand and receive essential drug information, and that the pharmacist should offer it. The FDA recommends that **printed information** be dispensed with medicines to reinforce what the pharmacist says. The combined use of talking about prescriptions and giving printed materials gets the best results.

In community pharmacies and outpatient hospital or clinic sites, **you** are the final check before a patient gets a medicine. **Guard and value this role** above any distraction or volume of prescriptions that must be filled. I've often told patients that "we're always there for you" on the *Pharmacist Minute* radio series. Be there for your patients and make a difference.

The outcomes or results from medicines will be the hallmark of the use of medicines for the future. Pharmacists need to understand outcomes research; the FDA will be applying them to patient-directed advertising, xvi   Points for Consideration by the Pharmacist

physicians will be facing questions about who gets better on what medicine, and you will have a role in retrospective and potentially concurrent drug use review. Disease management and pharmacoeconomic principles will be widely applied.

Some pharmacists have made great inroads in clinical service by helping manage medicines for asthmatics, providing vaccines (where state law allows), offering smoking cessation groups, and helping monitor anticoagulation. Contact your state board of pharmacy for more information. Many pharmacists are now accepting appointments and charging a fee for cognitive services, and I advise consumers to take the fullest advantage of their pharmacist's training and experience.

Pharmacists should have a copy of the *Agency for Health Care Policy and Research Clinical Practice Guidelines Number 9* on the management of cancer pain, as well as copies of the patient guide on cancer pain. The Agency for Health Care Policy and Research is advocating effective and timely control of pain as a basic human right. This is a clear opportunity for you to help in offering effective therapeutic options and superb pharmaceutical care. Call 1–800–422–6237 for more information.

When You Fill a Prescription

- Clarify with the prescriber any prescription information that is illegible, uncertain, or a potential source for erroneous interpretation—by you or the patient.
- Be alert to "look-alike" and "sound-alike" drug names. This is a significant cause of dispensing error. In accepting prescriptions by telephone, ask the caller to spell the name of the drug, as appropriate.
- As the situation warrants (multiple drugs taken concurrently, the older patient, etc.), include both the **name of the drug** and the **disorder** on the label (for example: Fosamax for osteoporosis) if the patient does not object, and consult with the prescribing physician when necessary. The inclusion of the **disorder** on the label will serve to (1) reduce dispensing errors caused by "look-alike" and "sound-alike" drug names; and (2) prevent confusion during concurrent use of multiple drugs: mistaken identity of drug and purpose, mistakenly altered dosing schedules, etc.
- Use all of the appropriate instructional add-on labels designed to enhance compliance and drug performance. Even though people seem to understand while you are counseling them, they may forget once they return home.
- Check the stock bottle for accurate identification and appropriate dating. If a technician fills the prescription, be certain you open the dispensing container as well as the completed prescription and check the drug personally.

When You Counsel the Patient as You Dispense the Filled Prescription

- If it seems advisable, ask the patient to read all of the labeling on the container. Clarify any points of confusion or misunderstanding.
- Verify that the patient recognizes the **name of the drug** and the **disorder being treated**. Explain what the drug is supposed to do.
- Review the details of dosing instructions: how much to take, when to take it, and for how long. It doesn't do them any good if it stays in the bottle. See if your computer vendor has a module for medication maps. If not, use the map provided in this book. Advising patients about how to organize their medicines over their day can be critical.
- Talk about possible side effects or adverse effects that may occur. Tell the patient about what to do if any of these occur. Encourage the patient to call his or her physician if new symptoms develop while taking the medication.
- As appropriate, tell the patient of any precautions to observe while taking the drug. This includes possible interactions with foods, beverages, or other drugs. Specify any activities that should be avoided or modified.
- Provide **written information** about the drug(s) dispensed and the patient's **disorder** (if available).
- Be sure your patient knows how to store their medicine. This not only includes refrigeration, but avoiding the humidity of a medicine chest. If any patient requests a non-childproof lid, remind him or her to keep the drug out of reach whenever children are visiting.
- Remind the patient that nonprescription (over-the-counter) drugs can alter the effects of prescription drugs. Be certain to ask about any herbal remedies or megavitamins the patient may take. Encourage them to call your pharmacy or their physician if help is needed before combining medicines.
- If your pharmacy has a computerized information system, always take a good medication history, and invite the patient to participate in this program.
- Encourage the patient to ask questions—at the time of dispensing and later—whenever the need arises.

Suggestions for Containing the Costs of Drug Therapy

- As judgment dictates, fill the prescription with the most reasonably priced drug available—within legally possible and appropriate guidelines. Consult with the prescribing physician regarding generic substitution when feasible.

- If the patient is taking other drugs (prescribed by other physicians), explore the possibility of drug duplication—taking the same generic drug under more than one brand name. Offer "brown-bag sessions" where patients can bring in all their medicines and get your help regarding possible problems.

Points for Consideration by the Physician

Critical paths, outcomes tracking and management, and closed formulary considerations have significantly changed the thinking and basic approach to many therapeutic decisions. I believe that a renewed focus on outcomes simply creates an atmosphere of continuous improvement and is just good medicine. One of the best colleagues to have in attaining the best outcomes from any medicine is a fully informed patient. Michael Weintraub, M.D., recognized this in 1991, when in his introduction to the *Yearbook of Drug Therapy* he stated, "In looking for trends in the medical literature, it is apparent that the need for the physician to be an educator of patients and their families is becoming greater and greater." In addition, citing an increased need for patient education, he summarized with the following opinion: "Treatment principles correctly applied by patients educated about their condition and involved in its management seem to be the wave of the future." More than ever before, the volume and characteristics of the drugs in use today require deliberate individualization of treatment. The overall effectiveness of any drug therapy depends on how carefully the drug is selected, dispensed, and administered. Responsible communication between physician, pharmacist, nurse, and patient must be achieved to the greatest extent possible. This process begins with the physician. It is absolutely unacceptable that current estimates of the expense of adverse drug events cost some 136 billion dollars a year . . . more is spent on diabetes or cardiovascular care.

When You Evaluate a Patient for Drug Therapy

- Review the patient's drug history for known drug allergies and prior drug-induced adverse reactions.

- Ask if the patient is currently under treatment by other health care providers.
- Ask about all drugs used currently—prescription and over-the-counter. Remember that many over-the-counter agents were once prescription medicines. Make certain that you do not gloss over this aspect of the medicines they can take without ever obtaining your guidance.
- Remember the prevalence of herbal remedy and nutriceutical use. Include these substances in your questions.
- Consider a patient's history and lifestyle, think about diseases or conditions for which the patient is at risk, and vitamins (such as folic acid for heart disease) or minerals (calcium to prevent osteoporosis) that may be used to prevent the process. Rybacki's first recommendation: It is always better to prevent a disease or condition than to have to treat it.
- Make certain that you are absolutely current. Many daily fax services are available which can be individualized to your practice and can easily be read after your morning rounds.
- Establish the nature and severity of the disorder under consideration for drug treatment.
- Elicit significant coexisting disorders—possible absolute contraindications for certain drugs.
- Evaluate any suspected or obvious organ dysfunction—possible relative contraindications for certain drugs. When creatinine values are available, take the time to calculate creatinine clearance. Many drugs have break points for adjustment of dosage at various levels of renal impairment. Even though an older patient's creatinine is within the "normal limits," their clearance will not be. For example, a 72-year-old, 70-kg man with a 1.4 creatinine will have a creatinine clearance of about 48.6 ml/min. This is **below the level where doses or intervals of renally eliminated medicines must be adjusted.** Hepatic disease will also impact doses or intervals for many drugs, particularly those which are highly protein-bound or heavily metabolized.
- Assess the patient's potential for compliance or noncompliance with drug therapy. Remember the expense that a given prescription presents. The most brilliant prescription choice is totally ineffective if financial considerations prevent compliance. Once-a-day dosing is much easier for patients to remember and, combined with a dosing calendar, gets excellent results. See if the patient's pharmacist offers a medication mapping service. If not, map your patient's medicines yourself.

When Selecting Drugs for Therapy

- Try to match the drug's power to the patient's problem. Avoid overprescribing—medicinal "overkill." For example: mild to moderate stress reactions (situational anxiety–tension states) respond well to antianxiety drugs; they do not require antipsychotic medication. An uncomplicated urinary tract infection with a broadly sensitive single organism does not require a broad spectrum anti-infective drug.

- Obtain a copy of the *Agency for Health Care Policy and Research Clinical Practice Guidelines Number 9*. The AHCPR is advocating effective and timely pain control as a basic human right. Increase your awareness of the World Health Organization Pain Ladder and the use of the agents that are primary analgesics and adjuvants. AHCPR publications are great tools to help your patients understand their medicine and their disease. Push to make pain the fifth vital sign in your hospital.
- Always check for drug–drug, drug–food, and drug–disease interactions. Remember to take a "new" drug history periodically.
- Many new oral anti-infectives are effective against pathogens which historically required intravenous therapy. Although this allows you to avoid hospitalization, it makes the patient's compliance more critical.
- Consider the desired onset of drug action (immediate versus delayed) and the consequences or benefits of that effect.
- Choose the drug with the most favorable benefit-to-risk ratio: the best clinical effects with the least adverse reactions.
- When you prescribe narrow-therapeutic-window drugs that require periodic blood level determinations, be certain that blood sampling is done after the drug has reached its steady state (usually 5 half-lives). Understand which level is preferable to measure: "peak" level (as for theophylline), "trough" level (as for digoxin), and "peak and trough" for aminoglycosides (such as tobramycin). Many clinical pharmacists (the author included) will willingly calculate the best dose and interval for you, and make a consultative recommendation.
- Give due consideration to the patient's prior experience with other drugs similar to the one you are considering and prescribe accordingly. Prescribing a second drug from the same drug class from which a patient already had an allergic or adverse drug effect that required discontinuation of therapy or provided no therapeutic benefit is not prudent.
- Remember individual patient factors such as age, education, and cultural factors (including genetic effects on medication elimination).
- Think about the desired extent of effect (systemic or local).
- If drug treatment fails after a reasonable trial with good compliance, change to a drug of another chemical class, or consider combination therapy with two medicines with different mechanisms of action. For example: if viral load decreases for a time, then increases in an AIDS patient, you MUST change treatment.
- Select the drugs you prescribe critically, utilizing independent, objec-

tive reviews of available information. The "most frequently pre-scribed" drug is not necessarily the best drug within its class. Slick, glossy detail pieces should always be confirmed by primary litera-ture.

- Even "drugs of choice" in objective reviews can be poor choices when you consider the characteristics of individual patients. A renally com-promised patient may better tolerate an "alternate drug" with dual elimination (hepatic and renal) than a "drug of choice" that is limited to renal elimination.
- Remember the pharmacokinetic and pharmacodynamic changes that occur in those over 65 can lead to accumulation and excessive responses to "normal" doses and dosing intervals.
- Be objective and discerning as you review the claims made for a newly released drug within a sizable class of drugs already available. Only 20% of newly approved drugs each year are classified by FDA as truly innovative or more advantageous than similar drugs in current use. The remaining 80% are largely "me too" drugs with a limited history of use and a potential for "surprises" after a period of general use. It is best to select drugs with established records showing them to be the best in their class.

When You Issue Prescriptions in Writing or by Telephone

- When prescribing for outpatient use, consider the advantage of in-cluding both the **name of the drug** and the **therapeutic indication** (the patient's disorder) on the prescription label. For example: Sine-met CR for Parkinson's. Putting the disorder on the label will help (1) reduce dispensing errors caused by "look-alike" and "sound-alike" drug names, and (2) prevent confusion that often occurs during con-current use of multiple drugs, especially among the elderly: mistaken identity of drug and purpose, mistakenly altered dosing schedules, etc.
- Respect your patients' wishes as to whether or not they *want* the name of the disorder written on the prescription label. If they prefer you not include it, recommend that they write it on the label them-selves *after* the prescription is filled.
- Keep dosing schedules as simple as possible. Once-a-day dosing im-proves compliance.
- Alert the pharmacist to "look-alike" and "sound-alike" drug names. Print the drug name on written prescriptions. Spell the drug name when prescribing by telephone.

When Counseling Patients About Drug Therapy

- Briefly explain the nature of the patient's disorder and its treatment. Use language that is readily understood by the average person.
- Provide written information or references for educational material about the disorder. If the disorder is chronic in nature (diabetes, hy-

pertension), explain the need to continue drug therapy indefinitely, possibly for life.

- Briefly explain the name and nature of the drugs you are prescribing. Stress the importance of strict compliance with the medicine. It is wise to tell the patient—in advance—about potential adverse effects. The patient who has such effects is more likely to be understanding and forgiving if they do not come as a surprise to them.
- To supplement your discussion, **provide a printed document** that summarizes the essential information the patient needs to use the drug(s) safely and effectively. This is comforting and will save you an amazing number of telephone calls. Be sure the patient knows what to do if a dose is missed. Look at an add-on program to your office management program that prints out relevant information for your patients to take home. Such services can provide detailed descriptions of drugs, general guidelines for drug use, and personalized instructions.
- Explain the need for follow-up visits to monitor the effects of drug treatment and the course of the disorder.
- Explain that drugs may not work in practice exactly as expected. Tell the patient to be alert to the possibility that a new symptom or sign *may* be drug related. If one of your patients does experience a novel adverse drug reaction, it is critical that you (or your designate) call the FDA MedWatch at 1–800–332–1088. This fulfills your obligation to phase four reporting and makes medication use safer for everyone. Encourage the patient to call as needed regarding any aspect of drug treatment. Recognize the need to adjust drug selection and/or dosage regimens to accommodate individual variability.
- Give special attention to the older patient on drug therapy. The elderly (1) generally use multiple drugs concurrently, and (2) are more prone to experience adverse drug effects.
- If you refer any of your patients to a specialist, be certain to take a repeat medication history when they are returned to your care. Check for duplications in medicines by cross-referencing brand or generic names.
- Every 6 months, ask your patients to bring in all the prescription, nonprescription, and herbal medicines that they routinely take. This kind of "brown bag session" can help you best understand all of the potential or actual interactions of therapies your patient is or will be taking.

Remember: An informed patient can be your greatest ally in optimal therapeutics!

Suggestions for Containing the Costs of Drug Therapy

- When you have selected the most appropriate drug, consider its cost. If the patient requests an available generic product, direct the pharmacist to dispense one with certified bioequivalence. Because of s neric product variability, caution the patient to have the prescription refilled with the identical generic (same manufacturer) each time.

- Avoid polypharmacy whenever possible. Limit the number of drugs that the patient is taking concurrently to the fewest required. Do not let the cure become the disease. Medicate serious, significant disorders; discourage the use of drugs for minor, transient complaints.
- Consider carefully any requests from patients for a prescription drug they have learned about through direct-to-consumer advertising. Explain to your patients the profit motive of the producer and assure them that you will prescribe the drug that, in your judgment, is the most appropriate for them.
- When circumstances permit, use home intravenous drug therapy in preference to hospitalization.
- The move toward managed care and other health care reform initiatives brings increased scrutiny to the outcomes of your therapeutic and clinical decisions. Become more familiar with the expense of various medicinal options, as well as the specific patient populations where the benefit-to-risk and cost-to-outcome ratios make the most sense. Pharmacoeconomic and disease management approaches will bring the best balance of cost and outcome.

1

HOW TO USE THIS BOOK

2

GUIDELINES FOR SAFE AND EFFECTIVE DRUG USE

3

TRUE BREAKTHROUGHS IN MEDICINES

1

How to Use This Book

A visit to your doctor's office can be at best a disconcerting experience. Many physicians face severe time constraints brought on by HMOs, managed care, and the realities of medical practice today. Most of us have had the sense of our doctor needing, but not wanting, to hurry out of the exam room to see the next patient—this can be especially true in emergency departments in hospitals. You may be left with a prescription for yourself or a loved one. The problem lies in the fact that you may have been told very little about the medicines prescribed. In any case, even in the best circumstances, it certainly will never be possible or practical for the physician or other prescriber to provide you with *all* the information that could be considered appropriate and useful, or whatever information is given may be provided in complicated medical terms and will be difficult for you to remember.

Unfortunately, medical technology and medical research have advanced much more rapidly than our social ability to realize that there is such a thing as a good death. Comfort and palliation will need to replace extraordinary means and the huge expense and measures which actually become cruel when used to "help" the dying patient. In reality, few patients die at home and many die in pain. We should be shocked that there is a program called Project Death In America . . . yet it is a start to make some needed changes. My own stepfather looked back at me from his deathbed and said, "Make a difference in people's pain." I've rewritten this book again with the intent to make a difference in health care, and to bring you current and important information to protect yourself and your family.

The goal of this book is to give you the kind of information presented in easy-to-understand words that you can use to supplement the direction and guidance you receive from your doctor. Your resource is arranged into six sections. The first section will help you to better understand the

1

modern drug therapy, give you some helpful tips on taking medicines safely, and even tell how to prevent some adverse drug reactions. Once again, "True Breakthroughs in Medicines" will help identify completely new medicines that have gained FDA approval and offer a novel drug molecule or completely new drug package, or are the first new agents in many years to help treat an existing disease or condition.

Section Two gives you detailed Drug Profiles covering more than 2,000 brand-name prescription drugs and nearly 400 generic medicines used widely in the United States and Canada. The selection of each drug is based upon three considerations: the extent of its use, the urgency of the conditions for which it is prescribed, and the volume and complexity of the information essential to its proper use. Profiles are arranged alphabetically by generic name. Read carefully to be sure you have the correct generic name.

Each Profile is presented in the same way. When you become familiar with the format, you'll be able to quickly find specific information on any drug, without having to read the entire Profile. Each Drug Profile contains at least 45 helpful categories of information, including:

Year Introduced

This tells you how long the drug has been in general use. Remember, the longer the drug has been in general use, the more likely its full spectrum of actions is known and the less likely its continued use will produce new surprises.

Drug Class

The class is important because many actions, reactions, and interactions with other drugs are often shared by drugs of the same class. For example, *if you are allergic to one medicine in a class, you most likely will be allergic to a second medicine from the same class.*

Prescription Required

This tells whether a drug is a prescription or a nonprescription (over-the-counter) purchase. Just because a medicine does not require a prescription does not mean the medicine is unimportant. Remember, over the last 10 years there has been a great shift in medicines from prescription to nonprescription. Current examples include medicines for yeast infections, patches and gum to help you stop smoking, as well as histamine blockers for heartburn. Virtually all of these medicines were previously available only by prescription. If you have questions about combining any of these medicines with other medicines you may already be taking, your pharmacist can be a readily available resource. Be certain to mention nonprescription medicine use when asked about the "medicines" you take.

Controlled Drug

Drugs subject to regulation under the Controlled Substances Act of 1970 (those with abuse potential) are assigned to a specific schedule in the United States. A Canadian schedule is also given when applicable. A description of the schedules of controlled drugs is found at the back of this guide.

Available for Purchase by Generic Name

In general, costs can be greatly reduced by buying a generic equivalent of a brand-name product. The key word is "equivalent." It is important to make sure that "bioavailability and bioequivalence"—the comparative composition, quality, and effectiveness of the generic versus the brand-name drug product—is the same if a substitution is made. Further discussion of bioavailability and bioequivalence will be found in the Glossary, Section Five.

Brand Names

These names help you recognize a brand name that may have caused problems for you. Brand names are listed for the United States and for Canada (✦). A combination drug (one with more than one active ingredient) is identified by [CD] following the brand name. In some cases a name used in both the United States and Canada will represent entirely different generic drugs (in a single drug product), or a significantly different mixture of generic medicines. The generic composition of such brand-name products is identified by country in the index. If you travel between the two countries, verify that the drug contains the same generic medicine(s).

Benefits versus Risks

This section summarizes the "pros" and "cons" for each drug. The Profiles use capital letters to emphasize the drug's principal benefits and risks, while lowercase letters are used for less critical benefits and risks. One look reveals the "comparative weights" of the two columns and gives an initial impression as to how a drug's benefits relate to its potential risks. This is meant to help you become more circumspect in your use of medicines and is not intended to be the sole basis for deciding whether or not to use the drug. **Failure to individualize drug selection and dose is probably the greatest weakness in current drug therapy.**

Principal Uses

A drug may be available as a single drug product or in combination with other drugs. "As a Single Drug Product" tells the primary use(s) of the drug when used alone. The "As a Combination Drug Product [CD]" gives the primary use(s) when combined with other drugs in the same "pill." The uses stated are a consensus in the medical community and substantiated by current research. Where appropriate, the therapeutic logic for combining certain drugs is explained.

How This Drug Works

This section tells what a drug does to have its effect(s). If a specific method of action has not been established, I tell you about the currently held theory.

Available Dosage Forms and Strengths

This gives you available manufacturers' dosage forms (tablets, capsules, elixirs, etc.) and strengths, without company identification. Included are those dosage forms appropriate for use by outpatients and in extended care facilities and nursing homes. Dosage forms limited to hospital use are often not included. The section on Dosage Forms and Strengths in the Glossary can help with those few abbreviations used to describe strengths of each dosage form.

Usual Adult Dosage Range

Dosage information given represents a carefully derived consensus by appropriate authorities and is the currently recommended standard. It is provided as a guide showing how much of the drug can reasonably be expected to be both effective and safe. Under certain circumstances, your doctor may decide to modify this "standard" dose. Some dosage forms not covered (for example, extemporaneously made suppositories) may require different doses than those listed.

Conditions Requiring Dosing Adjustments

Medical conditions can actually change the effect a medicine has on your body. This is a fact that is **often missed** in selecting a dose or dosing interval and can lead to serious injury and hospitalization. People over 60 years old often have a decline in their kidney function, which can mean that drugs stay in their bodies longer than younger patients. **It is critical to ask your doctor if any prescribed medicine dose has been adjusted for this age-related decline in how well your kidneys work.**

Dosing Instructions

Some medicines are affected by food—this section tells you about them. There are also occasions when a patient finds it difficult or impossible to swallow a tablet or capsule, and the drug is not available in a liquid dosage form. If the medicine is urgently needed, you may want to crush the tablet or open the capsule and mix the contents with a food or beverage. Some medicines should **NEVER** be crushed or altered in order to give them. This information category identifies those dosage forms of each drug that may and those that should not be changed. Your pharmacist can once again be a great resource.

Usual Duration of Use

Many factors determine how long a medicine must be taken: the nature and severity of your symptoms, formulation and strength of the drug, ability of the patient to respond, and use of other drugs, among others. The focus here is to help keep you from stopping a medicine in treatment situations where it may seem to you that it is taking too long to get better. Where appropriate, limitations in how long a medicine should be taken are given.

This Drug Should Not Be Taken If

These are the *absolute* contraindications to the use of the drug (see Contraindication in the Glossary). By consensus, these are circumstances where the medicine should NEVER be taken. Tell your physician or other prescriber **immediately** if any information in this category applies to you.

Inform Your Physician Before Taking This Drug If

This category lists the *relative* contraindications to the use of the drug. One way to think of this information is as a relative benefit-to-risk decision. Here again, it is important that you tell your physician or other prescriber if these factors apply to you.

Possible Side Effects

This category tells the natural, expected, and usually unavoidable actions of the drug—the normal and anticipated consequences of taking it. It gives a realistic perspective balancing occurrence of side effects and the goals of treatment.

Possible Adverse Effects

This category details unusual, unexpected, and infrequent drug effects, commonly referred to as adverse drug reactions. These are classified as mild or serious in nature. I am often asked how often these effects will happen. In the past, I've attempted to give set percentages to help you. These were often derived from Phase Three studies or current research. In order to more accurately define how often these effects happen, I've developed a new system for you:

- Possible: An effect that has been documented for other drugs in the same family, but not the profiled drug. Also assigned when the effect occurs in some limited patient populations and not in others.
- Case Reports: This means that an effect has been documented to happen, but only has been seen in isolated cases.
- Rare: This means that an effect is seen in less than 2% of patients. Another way to look at this is that 98% of people will take the medicine and NOT have the effect.
- Infrequent: An effect that is seen in 2 to 10% of patients.
- Frequent: These effects happen in more than 10% of patients.

Tell your doctor if you suspect you may be having an adverse drug effect. Serious adverse reactions may start with mild, unthreatening symptoms. It is also possible to have an adverse reaction that has not yet been reported. Don't discount an adverse effect just because it is not listed. It's important that you recognize and understand that *a properly selected drug usually has a comparatively small chance of producing serious harm*. Most of the drugs included in this book rarely produce serious adverse effects. Knowledge that a drug is capable of causing a serious adverse reaction should not deter you from using it when it has been properly selected and its use will be carefully supervised.

Possible Effects on Sexual Function

This information is often NOT something people want to discuss, or something that patients are told about.

Currently available information (often inadequate and vague) from all reliable sources is presented. Both physician and patient are well advised to discuss frankly any potential effect that drug therapy could have on sexual expression.

Adverse Effects That May Appear Similar to Natural Diseases or Disorders

Medicines can actually cause effects similar to widely diagnosed diseases or disorders. Quite often this inadvertent error is compounded by prescribing another drug to relieve the "symptoms" of the first. For milder symptoms (e.g., nasal congestion or diarrhea from reserpine), the oversight may not be too serious. But in the case of Parkinson-like effects of some drugs, the mistake can be devastating. This section tells you about this common flaw in the management of drug therapy.

Natural Diseases or Disorders That May Be Activated by This Drug

Many drugs can "activate" latent disorders that may not be recognized as drug induced. If a new and seemingly unrelated disorder starts during the course of treatment with any new medicine, ask your doctor if it may be drug related.

Possible Effects on Laboratory Tests

Most drugs have significant effects on body chemistry and organ systems. Some effects are intended and beneficial (therapeutic); others are unintended, unavoidable, and potentially harmful. Timely use of laboratory tests lets us check how well a drug is working and the course of the condition being treated. Knowledge of selected test results can greatly increase your understanding and skill in the proper use of medicines.

Caution

This category gives you information on aspects of drug action and/or drug use that require special emphasis. Occasionally these warnings may relate to information provided in other categories. When included here, such entries warrant being repeated.

Precautions for Use by Infants and Children

Doses often MUST be changed for infants and children under 12 years of age, and some drugs and/or treatment situations call for special precautions. When administering *any* prescription or over-the-counter drug, it is best to ask your doctor or pharmacist about needed precautions.

Precautions for Use by Those Over 60 Years of Age

Our bodies change as we age, and people age at different rates and in different ways. Assessment of "age" must be based upon individual mental and physical condition, and never upon years alone. In general, changes that accompany aging may affect the actions of the body on the drug, as well as actions of the drug on the body. Appropriate precautions are outlined in this category.

Advisability of Use During Pregnancy: Pregnancy Category

Information about safe use of a particular drug during pregnancy was one of the most forceful concerns that led to the formal petitioning of the Food and Drug Administration in 1975 to make sure that information was disclosed to the public. The FDA definitions of the five pregnancy categories are listed at the back of this book. The FDA does not make the initial category assignment; this is the responsibility of the manufacturer that markets the drug. The initial designation is then subject to review and modification by the FDA. The "Pregnancy Category" designations presented in each Profile were determined after thorough review of pertinent literature and consultation with appropriate authorities. They are offered at this time for initial guidance only. They are in no sense "official" and do not have the endorsement of either the manufacturer or the FDA.

Advisability of Use If Breast-Feeding

This section tells you about effects of the drug on milk production, if the drug goes into human milk, and the possible effects of the drug on the nursing infant. Prudent recommendations are given where appropriate. Also included are impacts of disease where appropriate.

Suggested Periodic Examinations While Taking This Drug

Getting the best results from your medicines often means that your doctor may ask you to get periodic examinations while taking the drug(s) he or she has prescribed. Which examinations and when they are made depends: your past and present medical history, the nature of the condition being treated, the dose and duration of drug use, and your doctor's observations of your response. There may be many occasions when he or she will feel no examinations are necessary. Always tell your doctor about all developments you think may be drug related.

While Taking This Drug, Observe the Following: Marijuana Smoking

The widespread "social" use of marijuana by virtually all age groups and the approval of medicinal smoking of marijuana in two states has led to inquiries about interactions between the active chemicals in marijuana smoke and medicines in common use. Currently available literature on the health aspects of marijuana use contains very little practical information concerning the potential for drug interactions. The limited information presented in this category of selected Drug Profiles represents those *possible interactions* considered likely to occur in view of the known pharmacological effects of the principal components of marijuana and of the medicine reviewed in the Profile. In most instances, the interaction statements are not based on documented evidence since very little is available. However, the conclusions stated—derived by logical inductive reasoning—represent the concurrence of authorities with expertise in this field.

While Taking This Drug, Observe the Following: Other Drugs

This confusing and often controversial area of drug information is divided into five subcategories of possible interactions between drugs. Look carefully at the wording of each subcategory heading (see also Interaction in Glossary). Some of the drugs listed do not have a representative Profile. If you are using one of these drugs, ask your doctor or pharmacist for help about potential interactions. A brand name (or names) that follows the generic name of an interacting drug is given as an example only. It is not intended to mean that the particular brand(s) named have interactions that are different from other brands of the same generic drug. If you are taking the generic drug, *all* brand names under which it is marketed

MUST be considered as possible interactants. Medicines in the same or similar families may also interact.

Driving, Hazardous Activities

Clearly, medicines can change coordination and alertness. In addition to driving motor vehicles, the information in this category applies to any activity of a dangerous nature, such as operating machinery, working on ladders, using power tools, and handling weapons. Your individual response and degree of reaction may vary from others. Talk with your doctor or pharmacist if you take a medicine which may impair your abilities.

Aviation Note

Military pilots enjoy the expert guidance and surveillance provided by the flight surgeon, but no tightly structured control system exists for their civilian counterparts. However, the need for practical information regarding the possible effects of medicinal drugs on flight performance is the same for pilots in all settings. This section can tell civilian pilots how a particular drug may affect his or her eligibility to fly and when it is advisable or necessary to consult a designated Aviation Medical Examiner or an FAA medical officer.

Occurrence of Unrelated Illness

Some medicines such as "blood thinners" or anticoagulants require careful regulation of daily doses to maintain a constant drug effect within critical limits. In this section of your book, emphasis is given to those illnesses that might affect drug use.

Discontinuation

How and when to stop is often as important as ever starting a medicine in the first place. Unfortunately, this aspect of drug use is often overlooked when a medicine is first discussed. Often, it is mandatory that the patient be fully informed on *when* to discontinue, when *not* to discontinue, and precisely *how* to stop use of the drug. When one medicine is stopped, other drugs being taken at the same time may also need to be adjusted. The doctor who is primarily responsible for your overall management must be kept informed of *all* the drugs you are taking at a given time.

I believe that the remaining information categories in the Drug Profiles are self-explanatory, but I always welcome your letters and questions. I have also started a Web site called **medinfo** and can be reached at http://www.medinfo.com. Section Three is a section called "The Leading Edge," which offers what are, in my opinion, medicines that show great promise and are just over the horizon from FDA approval. Some of these medicines may not actually be approved, but they give such significant hope that they're worth consideration. The information may actually let patients facing serious diseases ask to be included in scientific studies and get the medicine prior to actual approval. I've also included some particularly newsworthy research on some nonprescription medicines and one medicinal plant.

Section Four is a presentation of Drug Classes arranged alphabetically by their chemical or therapeutic (generic) class. Because of chemical composition and biological activities, some drugs appear in two or more classes. For example, the drug product with the brand name Diuril will be represented by its generic name, chlorothiazide, in three drug classes: the Thiazide Diuretics (a chemical classification), the Diuretics (a drug action classification), and the Antihypertensives (a disease-oriented classification).

Frequently in the Drug Profiles in Section Two you are advised to "see (a particular) Drug Class." This alerts you to a possible drug contraindication, or to possible interactions with certain foods, alcohol, or other drugs. In each case, you can find the more readily recognized brand names for each drug listed generically within a drug class by looking at the appropriate Drug Profile. Timely use of these references can help you to avoid many possible hazards of medication.

Section Five is a glossary of drug-related terms used throughout the book. The preferred use of each term is explained. Frequent references to the Glossary are made in the Drug Profiles. Use of the Glossary will help you understand how to recognize and interpret significant drug effects.

Section Six offers tables of drug information. The title and introductory material explains the content and purpose of each table. The information emphasizes pertinent aspects of drug behavior. The tables give you another source of ready reference. The Medication Map in this section is a way for you to use your doctor or pharmacist's expertise to arrange all of the medicines you take into a reasonable schedule. Take the time to have them help you get the most from your medicines.

The index of brand and generic names in the back of the book is a single alphabetical listing that provides page references to the appropriate Drug Profile(s) for all drugs found in this book. It will be more useful if you first read the introductory explanation of the special features of this combined index.

2

Guidelines for Safe and Effective Drug Use

DO NOT

- pressure your doctor to prescribe drugs that, in his or her judgment, you do not need. A pill is not always the answer.
- blindly accept care from any provider. Ask your HMO or medical group how their results or outcomes compare to other groups in the area and the country.
- assume that all doctors know all the drugs you take. Always ask your doctor or pharmacist BEFORE combining any other medicine with medicines already prescribed.
- take prescription drugs on your own or on the advice of friends and neighbors because your symptoms are "just like theirs." Drug therapy must be individualized, based on liver and/or kidney function, medicines you currently take, and many other factors.
- offer drugs prescribed for you to anyone else without a physician's guidance.
- change the dose or timing of any drug without the advice of your physician (except when the drug appears to be causing adverse effects).
- leave it to a guess that you've taken your medicine. ALWAYS get a dosing calendar or make one so that you can check off **each dose** as you take it.
- continue to take a drug that you feel is causing problems, until you are able to talk with your doctor.
- store your medicines in a bathroom medicine cabinet. This is often an area of high humidity which can (even though the bottle is closed) enter the medicine and degrade the active drug. Select a lockable kitchen cabinet out of reach of children.

- take *any* drug (prescription or nonprescription) while pregnant or nursing an infant until you talk to your doctor or pharmacist. Many herbal combinations may have active ingredients similar to those found in prescription medicines.
- take any more medicines than are absolutely necessary. (The greater the number of drugs taken at the same time, the greater the likelihood of adverse effects.)
- withhold from your doctor information about previous prescription or nonprescription drug use. He or she will want to know what has helped and what has caused problems.
- take any drug in the dark. Identify every dose of medicine carefully in adequate light to be certain you are taking the intended drug.
- keep drugs on a bedside table. Drugs for emergency use, such as nitroglycerin, are an exception. It is best to have only one such drug at the bedside for use during the night.

DO

- talk with your doctor about the results or outcomes expected from any medicine being considered.
- talk with your HMO or medical group every year about how their results or outcomes compare to other providers of health care in the area and in the country. This is especially important for businesses since the preferred provider they choose impacts the health of many people.
- ask your HMO or medical group what their disease management programs are, and how any specific disease or condition that you may have is addressed within the scope of their disease management plan. Find out how the results or outcomes of the program compare with other programs in the area or the country.
- know the name (and correct spelling) of the drug(s) you are taking. It is best to know both the brand name and the generic name.
- read the package labels of all nonprescription drugs so you know what is in them.
- follow the prescribed dosing schedules as closely as possible. Tell your doctor if it becomes necessary to make major changes in your treatment routine.
- thoroughly shake all liquid suspensions of drugs to ensure uniform distribution of ingredients.
- use a standardized measuring device for giving liquid medicines by mouth. The household "teaspoon" varies greatly in size.
- follow your doctor's advice on dietary or other measures designed to help the prescribed drugs work their best. For example, decreasing or eliminating salt when taking high blood pressure medicines may help achieve desired drug effects with smaller doses.
- tell your anesthesiologist, surgeon, and dentist of *all* drugs you are taking, before any surgery.

- tell your doctor if you become pregnant while you are taking any drugs from any source.
- keep a written record of *all* drugs (prescription and nonprescription), vaccines, and herbal remedies you take during your entire pregnancy— name, dose, dates taken, and reasons for use.
- keep a written record of *all* drugs (and vaccines) to which you become allergic or have an adverse reaction to. This should be done for each member of the family, especially the elderly or infirm.
- keep a written record of *all* drugs (and vaccines) to which *your children* become allergic or experience an adverse reaction.
- fill out "Your Personal Drug Profile" (Table 14). Get the number of your Poison Control Center **today** and post it by your telephone. The worst time to try to find an emergency number is while there is a dire need for it. Fill in the Medication Map, and ask your doctor if the times selected and combinations of medicines are appropriate.
- tell your doctor of all known or suspected allergies, especially allergies to drugs. Be sure that allergies are a part of your medical record. People with allergies are four times more prone to drug reactions.
- call your doctor immediately if you think you are having an overdose, side effect, or an adverse effect from a drug.
- ask if it is safe to drive a car, operate machinery, or engage in other hazardous activities while taking the drug(s) prescribed.
- ask if it is safe to drink alcoholic beverages while taking the drug(s) prescribed. We often forget that alcohol is a drug with its own pharmacology and drug–drug interactions.
- determine if any particular foods, beverages, or other prescription or nonprescription medicines should be avoided while taking the drug(s) prescribed.
- keep all appointments for follow-up examinations or laboratory tests.
- ask for help to understand any point that confuses you. If you are concerned about remembering information or instructions for use, ask for written materials.
- throw away all outdated drugs.
- ask your doctor if a prescribed medicine offers the best balance of cost and outcomes for you.
- store all drugs for intermittent use out of the reach of children. This is critical for those of you with grandchildren who visit infrequently.

PREVENTING ADVERSE DRUG REACTIONS

For the most part, we cannot identify people who are at greater risk of having a true adverse effect. Tests for the early detection of toxicity are of definite value, but do not provide complete protection. As our understanding of drug actions and reactions has expanded, we learned that many adverse effects are, to some extent, predictable and preventable.

Several contributing factors are now well recognized, and specific recommendations exist to guide both physician and patient. These fall into 11 categories.

Previous Adverse Reaction to a Drug

Patients who have had an adverse drug reaction in the past are more likely to have adverse reactions to other drugs, even though the drugs are unrelated. This suggests that some people may have a genetic (inborn) predisposition to unusual or abnormal drug responses. *Always tell your doctor about any history of prior adverse drug experiences.*

Allergies

Some people are allergic by nature (have hay fever, asthma, eczema, hives) and are more likely to develop allergies to drugs. The allergic patient must be watched very closely when medicines are used. Known drug allergies must be written in the medical record. Patients must tell every health care provider that he or she is allergic by nature and is allergic to specific drugs. *Provide this information without waiting to be asked.* Your doctor will then be able to avoid prescribing those drugs that could provoke an allergic reaction, as well as related (cross sensitivity) drugs.

Contraindications

Both patient and physician must strictly observe contraindications to any drug under consideration. *Absolute contraindications* include those conditions and situations that prohibit the use of the drug for any reason. *Relative contraindications* are those conditions that, in the judgment of the physician, do not preclude the use of the drug, but make it essential that special care be given to its use. Often, dosing adjustments, additional supportive measures, and close supervision are needed.

Precautions in Use

Patients should know any special precautions needed while taking a drug. This includes advisability of use during pregnancy or while nursing; precautions on sun exposure (or ultraviolet lamps); avoidance of extreme heat or cold, heavy physical exertion (such as with fluoroquinolone antibiotics), etc.

Dosage

It is important to take any medicine exactly as prescribed. *This is most important with those drugs that have narrow margins of safety.* Even once-a-day medications should be taken at the same time of day or night to ensure the most constant blood levels. Call your doctor if nausea, vomiting, diarrhea, or other problems interfere with taking your medicine as prescribed.

Interactions

Some drugs can interact with foods (including vitamins and some herbal remedies), alcohol, and other drugs (prescription and nonprescription) to cause serious adverse effects. *The patient must be told about all likely interactants*. If, during the course of treatment, you feel you have discovered a new interaction, tell your doctor so that its full significance can be determined.

Warning Symptoms

Many drugs will cause symptoms that are early warnings of a developing adverse effect: for example, severe headaches or visual disturbances *before* a stroke in a woman taking oral contraceptives. *It is imperative that you know symptoms and signs that could be early warnings of adverse reactions*. The patient is then empowered to act in his or her own behalf by calling their doctor **before** taking another dose of their medicine.

Examinations to Monitor Drug Effects

Many drugs in common use can damage vital body tissues (such as bone marrow, liver, kidney, eye structures, etc.)—especially when these drugs are used for a long time or in high doses. Sometimes these adverse effects are not discovered until a newly approved drug has been in wide use for a long time. This damage may be reversible if found quickly. *Cooperate fully with your doctor when he or she asks for periodic exams to check for adverse drug effects*.

Advanced Age and Debility

When we age or as some disease processes progress, vital organs may not work as well, and can greatly influence the body's response to drugs. These patients often poorly tolerate drugs with inherent toxic potential and frequently need smaller doses at longer intervals. *The effects of drugs on the elderly and severely ill are often unpredictable*. Great care must be taken to prevent or minimize adverse effects.

Appropriate Drug Choice

The use of any medicine is always a benefit-to-risk decision. The medication used should offer the best balance of overall cost (including lab tests) and outcomes (including quality of life). Many adverse reactions can be prevented if both physician and patient exercise good judgment and restraint.

Polypharmacy

Unfortunately, the cure can become the disease. Patients who are cared for by several physicians may end up with several drugs prescribed separately by more than one physician for different disorders—often without appropriate communication between patient and prescriber. This frequent practice can lead to serious drug–drug interactions. *The patient should routinely talk to* **each** *health care provider about all the drugs—prescription and nonprescription—that he or she may be taking.* It is **mandatory** that each prescriber has this information before prescribing additional drugs.

DRUGS AND THE ELDERLY

Advancing age brings changes that can alter how you react to medicines. An impaired digestive system may interfere with drug absorption. Declines in liver and kidney ability to metabolize and remove drugs may lead to toxic drug levels. We slowly lose the ability to maintain "steady state" (or homeostasis), and face increased sensitivity of many tissues to the actions of drugs, even in "normal" drug doses. If aging causes a decline in understanding, memory, vision, or coordination, these patients may not always use drugs safely and effectively. Adverse reactions to drugs occur three times more frequently in the older population. An unwanted drug response can change an independent older person into a confused or helpless patient. For these reasons, drug treatment in the elderly must **always** be accompanied by the most careful consideration of the individual health and tolerances. Once-daily dosing may be the only viable option.

Guidelines for the Use of Drugs by the Elderly

- Be certain that drug treatment is necessary. Many health problems of the elderly can be managed **without** the use of drugs.
- Avoid (if possible) the use of many drugs at one time.
- Dosing schedules should be as simple as possible. Once a medicine is selected, ask your doctor if a once- or twice-a-day formulation is available and appropriate.
- Treatment with most drugs is often best started by using less-than-standard doses. Maintenance doses should also be individualized and are often smaller for those over 60 years of age.
- Avoid large tablets and capsules if other dosage forms are available. Liquid forms are easier for the elderly or debilitated to swallow.
- Have all drug containers labeled with the drug name and directions for use in large, easy-to-read letters.
- Ask the pharmacist to package drugs in easy-to-open containers. Avoid childproof caps and stoppers.

- Do not take any drug in the dark. Identify each dose of medicine carefully in adequate light to be certain you are taking the intended drug.
- To avoid taking the wrong drug or an extra dose, do not routinely leave medicines on a bedside table. Drugs for emergency use, such as nitroglycerin, are an exception. It is best to have only one such drug at the bedside for use during the night.
- Drug use by older people may require supervision; watch constantly to ensure safe and effective use.
- Remember the adage: "Start low, go slow, and (when appropriate) learn to say no."

Drugs Best Avoided by the Elderly Because of Increased Possibility of Adverse Reactions

antacids (high sodium)*
barbiturates*
benzodiazepines
 (long-acting)
cyclophosphamide

diethylstilbestrol
estrogens
indomethacin
monoamine oxidase
 (MAO) inhibitors*

oxyphenbutazone
phenacetin
phenylbutazone
tetracyclines*

Drugs That Should Be Used by the Elderly in Reduced Dosages Until Full Effect Has Been Determined

anticoagulants (oral)*
antidepressants*
antidiabetic drugs*
antihistamines*
antihypertensives*
anti-inflammatory drugs*
barbiturates*
beta-blockers*
colchicine

cortisonelike drugs*
digitalis preparations*
diuretics* (all types)
ephedrine
epinephrine
haloperidol
isoetharine
nalidixic acid

narcotic drugs
prazosin
pseudoephedrine
quinidine
sleep inducers
 (hypnotics)*
terbutaline
thyroid preparations

Drugs That May Cause Confusion and Behavioral Disturbances in the Elderly

acyclovir
albuterol
amantadine
anticholinergics*
antidepressants*
antidiabetic drugs*
antihistamines*
anti-inflammatory drugs*
asparaginase
atropine* (and drugs
 containing belladonna)
barbiturates*
benzodiazepines*
beta-blockers*

bromocriptine
carbamazepine
cimetidine
digitalis preparations*
diuretics*
ergoloid mesylates
famotidine
haloperidol
levodopa
meprobamate
methocarbamol
methyldopa
narcotic drugs

nizatidine
pentazocine
phenytoin
primidone
quinidine
ranitidine
reserpine
sedatives
sleep inducers
 (hypnotics)*
thiothixene
tranquilizers (mild)*
trihexyphenidyl

Drugs That May Cause Orthostatic Hypotension in the Elderly

antidepressants*   neuroleptics*   selegiline
antihypertensives*   phenothiazines*   tranquilizers (mild)*
diuretics* (all types)   sedatives   vasodilators*

Drugs That May Cause Sluggishness, Unsteadiness, and Falling in the Elderly

barbiturates*   diazepam   methyldopa
beta-blockers*   diphenhydramine   prazepam
chlordiazepoxide   flurazepam   sleep inducers
clorazepate   halazepam   (hypnotics)*

Drugs That May Cause Constipation and/or Retention of Urine in the Elderly

acebutolol   calcium   ketorolac
amantadine   cholestyramine   metoclopramide
amiodarone   epinephrine   narcotic drugs
androgens   ergoloid mesylates   phenothiazines*
anticholinergics*   famotidine   ranitidine
antidepressants*   iron (some forms)   sucralfate
anti-parkinsonism drugs* isoetharine   terbutaline
atropinelike drugs*

Drugs That May Cause Loss of Bladder Control (Urinary Incontinence) in the Elderly

diuretics* (all types)   tacrine   tranquilizers (mild)*
sedatives   thioridazine
sleep inducers
  (hypnotics)*

THERAPEUTIC DRUG MONITORING
Measuring Drug Levels in Blood

The ability to accurately measure how much medicine is in your blood has evolved since the early 1970s. People vary greatly in nature and degree of their responses to drugs, and blood levels can help find the best dose. For many drugs, the clinical response clearly shows that the drug is working as intended. However, for some drugs—especially those with narrow safety margins—toxic reactions may closely resemble the symptoms being treated. In many cases, the patient's expected response is not in keeping with his or her clinical condition. By measuring blood levels at appropriate times, the physician or clinical pharmacist can adjust dosing schedules more accurately, reduce the risk of toxicity, and achieve the best results or outcomes.

*See Drug Classes, Section Four.

Some medications require both a peak and trough level to ensure best results, and timing of blood sampling is critical. Sampling should be avoided during the two hours after an oral dose because during this absorption period, blood levels do not represent tissue levels of the drug, and the tissue is where many medicines actually work. The peak, or highest, level of the drug can measure several things: how effectively bacteria are killed or toxic levels within the body, for instance. The trough, or lowest, level tells how effectively a medicine is cleared from the body between doses. This can also be important because if too much drug remains toxicity can result, and if too little, it may not work well. The following drugs are those most suitable for therapeutic drug monitoring. If you are using any of these on a regular basis, ask your doctor about checking blood levels. These numbers are ranges where effects are *usually* seen, but people react differently. Therapeutic ranges listed are not absolute fixed levels where lack of effect or toxicity definitely occur. Some have a therapeutic response at a level lower than the low end of the range. Generally in this case, the level should be followed closely and left alone. A blood level higher than the high end of the range is not always toxic, but is a level higher than desirable, and dosing changes should be made. Fortunately most physicians "treat the patient, not the level."

Generic Name/Brand Name	*Blood Level Range*
acetaminophen/Tylenol, etc.	10–20 mcg/ml
amikacin/Amikin	12–25 mcg/ml (peak)
	5–10 mcg/ml (trough)
amitriptyline/Elavil, etc.	120–250 ng/ml
(combined with nortriptyline)	
amoxapine/Asendin	200–500 ng/ml
aspirin (other salicylates)	100–250 mcg/ml
carbamazepine/Tegretol	5–10 mcg/ml
chloramphenicol/Chloromycetin	10–25 mcg/ml
chlorpromazine/Thorazine	50–300 ng/ml
ciprofloxacin/Cipro	0.94–3.4 mcg/ml
clonazepam/Klonopin	10–50 ng/ml
cyclosporine/Sandimmune	100–150 ng/ml
desipramine/Norpramin, Pertofrane	150–300 ng/ml
digitoxin/Crystodigin	15–30 ng/ml
digoxin/Lanoxin	0.5–2.0 ng/ml
diltiazem/Cardizem	100–200 ng/ml
disopyramide/Norpace	2.0–4.5 mcg/ml
doxepin/Adapin, Sinequan	100–275 ng/ml
ethosuximide/Zarontin	40–100 mcg/ml
flecainide/Tambocor	0.2–1.0 mcg/ml
flucytosine/Ancobon	50–100 mcg/ml
gentamicin/Garamycin	4.0–10 mcg/ml (peak)
	less than 2 mcg/ml (trough)
gold salts/Auranofin, etc.	1.0–2.0 mcg/ml

Generic Name/Brand Name	*Blood Level Range*
imipramine/Janimine, Tofranil, etc.	150–300 ng/ml
kanamycin/Kantrex	25–35 mcg/ml
lidocaine/Xylocaine, etc.	2.0–5.0 mcg/ml
lithium/Lithobid, Lithotabs, etc.	0.3–1.3 mEq/L
mephobarbital/Mebaral	1–7 mcg/ml
methotrexate/Mexate	up to 0.1 mcmol/L
methsuximide/Celontin	up to 1.0 mcg/ml
metoprolol/Lopressor	20–200 ng/ml
mexiletine/Mexitil	0.75–2.0 mcg/ml
nifedipine/Procardia	25–100 ng/ml
nortriptyline/Aventyl, Pamelor	50–150 ng/ml
combined with amitriptyline	125–250 ng/ml
phenobarbital/Luminal, etc.	10–25 mcg/ml
phenytoin/Dilantin	10–20 mcg/ml
primidone/Mysoline	6–12 mcg/ml
procainamide/Pronestyl	4–10 mcg/ml
(NAPA metabolite)	4–10 mcg/ml
propranolol/Inderal	50–100 ng/ml
protriptyline/Vivactil	70–250 ng/ml
quinidine/Quinaglute, etc.	1.0–4.0 mcg/ml
(specific to quinidine test method)	
sulfadiazine/Microsulfon	100–120 mcg/ml
sulfamethoxazole/Gantanol	90–100 mcg/ml
theophylline/Aminophylline, etc.	10–20 mcg/ml
thioridazine/Mellaril	50–300 ng/ml
tobramycin/Nebcin	4.0–10 mcg/ml (peak)
	less than 2 mcg/ml (trough)
tocainide/Tonocard	5–12 mcg/ml
trimethadione/Tridione	10–30 mcg/ml
trimethoprim/Proloprim	1–3 mcg/ml
valproic acid/Depakene	50–100 mcg/ml
vancomycin/Vancocin	30–40 mcg/ml (peak)
	5–10 mcg/ml (trough)
verapamil/Calan	50–200 ng/ml

3

True Breakthroughs in Medicines

Constant advances are being made in available medicines. This section tells you about some of the best medicines that have recently been FDA approved or offer novel approaches to treatment, or truly new uses of existing medicine are covered. I want to distinguish here between the "me too" products, which may be simply be a broader product line, from forward-looking advances that help make certain you are getting the latest treatment.

ALENDRONATE (FOSAMAX)

This bisphosphonate was featured in last year's "True Breakthroughs" section, and has since gained FDA approval for **prevention** of post-menopausal osteoporosis. It is always better to prevent a disease or condition than to have to treat it.

ANTI-LEUKOTRIENE DRUGS

Zafirlukast (Accolate) is a leukotriene receptor antagonist that blocks the action of leukotrienes. It belongs to a completely new type of chemical family and may be especially useful in mild to moderate asthma where patients are aspirin sensitive. Zileuton (Zyflo) is the latest anti-leukotriene to be approved, and prevents the formation of leukotrienes.

ASPIRIN

I include aspirin once again in this section, because the indications for using this very old medicine have been broadened. It appears to prevent first heart attacks, limit damage from heart attacks that happen, have a role in preventing strokes, and may also help prevent bowel cancer. Talk to your doctor to see if regular use of aspirin makes sense for you.

ATORVASTATIN CALCIUM (LIPITOR)

The newest HMG-CoA reductase inhibitor to be approved. This medicine is now the most potent drug in lowering LDL cholesterol. The added benefit that atorvastatin offers is that it also lowers triglyceride levels as well!

HYDROCHLOROTHIAZIDE (ESIDRIX)

This thiazide diuretic has been available for many years. The breakthrough aspect of it is a large Veterans Hospital study that showed it delivered (in low dose use) the same outcomes as beta-blockers or ACE inhibitors in mild to moderate hypertension. This medicine costs pennies to use while the other medicines cost 70 to more than 100 dollars per month.

INSULIN LISPRO (HUMALOG)

This is the first new insulin to be approved since 1982. It works more quickly than currently available insulins. This may be of benefit for patients who have blood sugar that rises very quickly in response to food. Insulin lispro also appears to be more like naturally occurring insulin.

MIRTAZAPINE (REMERON)

The first in a new class of medicines for depression called noradrenergic and selective serotonin reuptake inhibitors. This medicine works to increase both norepinephrine and serotonin.

OLANZAPINE (ZYPREXA)

This new treatment for schizophrenia is a thienobenzodiazepine. It is effective in treating psychosis, and may work where other agents have failed.

PROTEASE INHIBITORS

This new class of medicines now includes four FDA-approved members. They have made the losing effort in treating AIDS into a battle once again. Combination therapy including a protease inhibitor actually started discussions of **eradication** potential in HIV-infected patients. In any case, they have shown significant decreases in viral load and recovery of CD4 counts.

TROGLITAZONE (REZULIN)

This medicine is the first to be approved that belong to a new class of medicines for diabetes. This medicine works to decrease serum blood sugar, plasma insulin, and hemoglobin A1C. I have also included troglitazone in a profile in the main text of this edition of the book.

DRUG PROFILES

Drugs Reviewed in This Section

I've presented detailed Drug Profiles for you of more than 300 drugs of major importance. This medicines met the following criteria:

1. The drug is used to treat or prevent a prevalent, relatively serious or significant disease or disorder.

2. The drug is recognized by experts to be among the "best choices" in its class.

3. The drug has a current benefit-to-risk ratio that compares favorably with those in its class.

4. The safe and effective use of the drug requires special information and guidance for both the health care practitioner (physician, dentist, pharmacist, nurse) and the health care consumer (patient and family).

5. The drug is suitable (safe and practical) for use in an outpatient setting (home, work site, school, etc.). It can be self-administered, or may require administration by trained medical personnel (as with home intravenous therapy, or freestanding cancer, emergency, or pain centers).

ACARBOSE (a KAR boz)

Introduced: 1996   **Class:** Antidiabetes agent, oral; alpha glucosidase inhibitor   **Prescription:** USA: Yes   **Controlled Drug:** USA: No; Canada: No
Available as Generic: No
Brand Name: Precose

BENEFITS versus RISKS

Possible Benefits	*Possible Risks*
EFFECTIVE LOWERING OF BLOOD SUGAR	Gas and abdominal pain (often decreases over time)
DECREASED RISK OF HIGH BLOOD PRESSURE, HEART DISEASE, AND OTHER LONG-TERM EFFECTS OF ELEVATED BLOOD SUGAR (WITH TIGHTER SUGAR CONTROL)	Mild possible decreases in hematocrit (was only seen in clinical trials)
MAY BE COMBINED TREATMENT WITH A SULFONYLUREA FOR BETTER SUGAR CONTROL	

▷ **Principal Uses**

As a Single Drug Product: Uses currently included in FDA-approved labeling: (1) Used with diet in patients with diabetes who do not require insulin injections, yet do not have sufficient blood sugar control with diet alone; (2) used in combination with a sulfonylurea (see Drug Classes) if diet plus acarbose or diet and sulfonylurea do not acceptably control blood sugar.
Other (unlabeled) generally accepted uses: None at present.

How This Drug Works: By blocking the enzymes intestinal alpha glucosidase and pancreatic alpha amylase, this medicine impairs sugar digestion, and actually keeps sugar low after meals.

Available Dosage Forms and Strengths
Tablets — 50 mg, 100 mg

▷ **Recommended Dosage Ranges:** (Actual dosage and administration schedule must be determined for each patient individually.)

Infants and Children: Safety and effectiveness have not been established in those less than 18 years old.

18 to 65 Years of Age: Initially 25 mg three times daily, taken at the start of each meal (after first bite). Any needed dose increases are made at 4- to 8-week intervals in order to achieve needed blood sugar control while minimizing intestinal side effects. This is done using 50 mg three times daily taken at the start of each meal. If the response still is not acceptable, patients weighing more than 132 pounds (60 kg) may be given doses up to 100 mg three times daily. Those weighing less than 60 kg should NOT be given be given more than 50 mg three times daily. If a given dose increase does not result in better sugar control, consideration should be given to decreasing the dose.

Over 65 Years of Age: No specific recommendations at present.

Conditions Requiring Dosing Adjustments

Liver Function: Specific dosing changes do not appear to be needed.

Kidney Function: Increases in blood levels occur. Dose decreases may be needed, but specific guidelines are not available. Only about 2% of a given oral dose is usually absorbed.

▷ **Dosing Instructions:**   This medicine should be taken after starting breakfast, lunch, and dinner—after the first bite of a meal has been eaten. Gas (flatulence) or diarrhea are common side effects. These problems can be decreased by limiting sucrose in the diet. In general, diarrhea and gas decrease over time. Dosing changes are usually made at 4- to 8-week intervals. This helps find the best dose and blood sugar response, while minimizing the potential gas (flatulence) or diarrhea. Usually, the blood sugar is checked one hour after a meal (1 hr postprandial) and the dose adjusted to obtain the best balance of blood sugar and side effects.

Usual Duration of Use: Dosing must be individualized, and dose changes are made at 4- to 8-week intervals if needed. Regular use is required to realize tighter blood glucose control. Since noninsulin-dependent diabetes is a chronic condition, use of acarbose will be ongoing. Periodic hemoglobin A1C (glycosylated hemoglobin) tests and physician follow-up are needed. Keeping the sugar close to normal minimizes effects of diabetes over time.

Possible Advantages of This Drug

May be used in combination with sulfonylurea oral hypoglycemics (see Drug Classes) to get the best control of blood sugar. Works using a different (novel) mechanism than other oral hypoglycemic agents.

▷ **This Drug Should Not Be Taken If**

- you have had an allergic reaction to it previously.
- you are in diabetic ketoacidosis.
- you have a tendency to develop intestinal obstruction or have a partial obstruction of the intestine.
- you have inflammatory bowel disease or ulceration of the colon.
- your serum creatinine is greater than 2 mg/dl (talk with your doctor).
- you have cirrhosis of the liver.
- you have an intestinal condition that may worsen (such as a megacolon or bowel obstruction) if there is increased gas (flatus) formed in the intestine.
- you have a long-standing (chronic) intestinal disease that alters digestion or your ability to absorb materials from the intestine.
- you are pregnant or are breast-feeding your infant (no data exists on use in pregnancy or breast-feeding).

▷ **Inform Your Physician Before Taking This Drug If**

- you do not know what the symptoms of hypoglycemia are.
- you have a history of kidney or liver disease.
- you plan to have surgery under general anesthesia in the near future.
- you take other prescription or nonprescription medications that were not discussed.
- you are unsure of how much to take or how often to take acarbose.

Possible Side Effects (natural, expected, and unavoidable drug actions)

Gas (flatulence) or diarrhea results from bacterial action on sugars in the intestine, and tends to decrease over time.

> **Possible Adverse Effects** (unusual, unexpected, and infrequent reactions)
>> **If any of the following develop, consult your physician promptly for guidance.**
>> *Mild Adverse Effects*
>> Allergic reactions: skin rash, itching.
>> Sleepiness, headache, dizziness—of questionable causation.
>> Pain or swelling of the belly (abdomen)—frequent.
>> Gas (flatulence) or diarrhea—frequent.
>> Very rare increased liver enzymes (in clinical trials with greater than 100 mg three times a day).
>> *Serious Adverse Effects*
>> May make other allergic reactions less responsive to treatment and more severe.
>> Low blood sugar if combined with sulfonylureas—possible.
>> Anemia—rare and occurred in some studies and not in others.

▷ **Possible Effects on Sexual Function:**   None reported.

Possible Effects on Laboratory Tests
Hemoglobin A1C: trending more toward normal.
Blood sugar one hour after eating (postprandial): decreased.
Serum lipids: variable effect.

CAUTION
1. This medicine itself does not cause hypoglycemia, but hypoglycemia may result if it is combined with insulin or sulfonylureas.
2. Infections may cause loss of glucose control and require temporary insulin use.
3. This medicine is only one part of the total program for managing your diabetes. A properly prescribed (and followed) diet and regular exercise are also still required for the best control of blood sugar.
4. If you develop kidney failure while taking this medicine, be certain to tell your doctor. This medicine should not be used if your serum creatinine is greater than 2 mg/dl.

Precautions for Use
By Infants and Children: Safety and effectiveness for use by those under 18 years of age have not been established.
By Those Over 60 Years of Age: Specific recommendations are not made at this time.

▷ **Advisability of Use During Pregnancy**
Pregnancy Category: B. See Pregnancy Risk Categories at the back of this book.
Animal studies: No significant increase in birth defects in rats or rabbits.
Human studies: Adequate studies of pregnant women are not available.
Most clinicians use insulin as the drug of first choice for controlling blood sugar in pregnancy. Use of acarbose drug during pregnancy should occur only if clearly needed. Ask your doctor for help.

Advisability of Use If Breast-Feeding
Presence of this drug in breast milk: Yes, in rats. No human data available.
Avoid drug or refrain from nursing.

Habit-Forming Potential: None.

Effects of Overdosage: Temporary increase in gas (flatus), abdominal discomfort and diarrhea.

Possible Effects of Long-Term Use: None reported in humans.

Suggested Periodic Examinations While Taking This Drug (at physician's discretion)

Periodic blood sugar tests one hour after eating. Tests of hemoglobin A1C levels are helpful. Liver function tests (serum transaminases) should be obtained every 3 months during the first year of treatment and periodically thereafter. Serum iron or iron-binding capacity may be prudent if anemia develops while taking this medicine.

▷ **While Taking This Drug, Observe the Following**

Foods: Follow the diet your doctor has prescribed for you closely.

Tight blood sugar control will help you avoid or delay long-term effects of your diabetes!

Beverages: No restrictions. May be taken with milk.

▷ *Alcohol:* An interaction is not expected with acarbose; however, if you are also taking a sulfonylurea (see Drug Classes), alcohol may exaggerate that drug's ability to lower the blood sugar, and can cause a disulfiramlike (see Glossary) reaction with some sulfonylureas.

Tobacco Smoking: No interactions expected; however, there are no studies that show smoking is good for you. Discuss ways to stop smoking with your doctor or pharmacist.

▷ *Other Drugs*

Acarbose may *increase* the effects of

- sulfonylureas (see Drug Classes) and result in excessive lowering of blood sugar. This is not an effect of acarbose on the sulfonylurea, but a result of its beneficial effect on blood sugar after meals. This may be used for therapeutic benefit.

Acarbose *taken concurrently* with

- clofibrate (Atromid-S) may result in hypoglycemia.
- digestive enzyme products that contain amylase or lipase may result in loss of blood sugar control.
- digoxin (Lanoxin) may cause lower (subtherapeutic) blood levels of digoxin and loss of benefits.
- disopyramide (Norpace) may result in hypoglycemia.
- high-dose aspirin or other salicylates and some NSAIDs (see Drug Classes) may result in hypoglycemia.
- insulin (see profile) poses an increased risk of hypoglycemia.
- sulfonamide antibiotics (see Drug Classes) may pose an increased risk for hypoglycemia.

The following drugs may *decrease* the effects of acarbose:

- adrenocorticosteroids (see Drug Classes).
- beta-blockers (see Drug Classes).
- calcium channel blockers (see Drug Classes).
- furosemide (Lasix) and bumetanide (Bumex).
- isoniazid (INH).
- nicotinic acid.
- phenytoin (Dilantin).
- rifampin (Rifadin, others).

- theophylline (Theo-Dur, others).
- thiazide diuretics (see Drug Classes).
- thyroid hormones (see Drug Classes).

> *Driving, Hazardous Activities:* Use caution until you see how drowsy and lethargic you may become.

Aviation Note: Diabetes *is a disqualification* for piloting. Consult a designated Aviation Medical Examiner.

Exposure to Sun: No restrictions.

Heavy Exercise or Exertion: Because this drug can lower the peak in blood sugar seen after meals, caution is advised. Discuss dosing changes with your doctor.

Occurrence of Unrelated Illness: Illness can change blood sugar control, and temporary use of insulin may be required.

Discontinuation: Talk with your doctor **before** stopping acarbose if you are considering stopping this medicine.

ACEBUTOLOL (a se BYU toh lohl)

Introduced: 1973   **Class:** Antihypertensive, heart rhythm regulator, beta-adrenergic blocker   **Prescription:** USA: Yes   **Controlled Drug:** USA: No; Canada: No   **Available as Generic:** Yes

Brand Names: Sectral, ✦Monitan, ✦Rhotral

BENEFITS versus RISKS	
Possible Benefits	*Possible Risks*
EFFECTIVE ANTIHYPERTENSIVE in mild to moderate high blood pressure	CONGESTIVE HEART FAILURE in advanced heart disease
MAY DECREASE the number of deaths that occur after a heart attack	Worsening of angina in coronary heart disease (abrupt withdrawal)
CAN DECREASE DEATH AND INCIDENCE OF HEART PROBLEMS WITH LONG-TERM USE	Masking of low blood sugar (hypoglycemia) in drug-treated diabetes
	Rare lupus erythematosus syndrome

▷ **Principal Uses**

As a Single Drug Product: Uses currently included in FDA-approved labeling: (1) Treats mild to moderate high blood pressure alone or combined with other drugs; (2) used to prevent premature ventricular heartbeats.

Other (unlabeled) generally accepted uses: (1) Stablizes angina pectoris; (2) used after a heart attack to help prolong life; (3) may have a role in easing the symptoms of panic attacks.

How This Drug Works: By blocking the sympathetic nervous system, this drug slows the rate and force of the heart. This reduces the extent of blood vessel contraction, expanding the walls and lowering blood pressure. It also slows the speed of nerve impulses through the heart, which helps ease some heart rhythm disorders.

Available Dosage Forms and Strengths
Capsules — 100 mg (in Canada), 200 mg, 400 mg

▷ **Recommended Dosage Ranges:** (Actual dosage and administration schedule must be determined for each patient individually.)
Infants and Children: Not indicated.
18 to 65 Years of Age: High blood pressure: Some patients may benefit from 200 mg per day, but most require 400 to 800 mg once daily. Selectivity for the heart decreases as doses increase.
   Arrhythmias: 400 mg daily, as 200 mg taken morning and evening (12 hours apart). Doses are increased as needed and tolerated. Total dose should not exceed 1200 mg every 24 hours, given as 600 mg twice daily.
   Angina: 600 to 1600 mg are divided into two or three equal doses spaced 8 to 12 hours apart.
Over 65 Years of Age: Bioavailability (amount taken into your body) doubles. Lower maintenance doses are needed. **Maximum** daily dose is 800 mg per day.

Conditions Requiring Dosing Adjustments
Liver Function: Extensively metabolized in the liver. Use with caution in compromised liver function.
Kidney Function: Dose must be decreased by up to 75% in severe kidney failure.

▷ **Dosing Instructions:**   May be taken without regard to eating. Capsule may be opened when taken. NEVER stop this drug abruptly.

Usual Duration of Use: Use on a regular schedule for 5 to 10 days may be required to see drug peak benefits in lowering blood pressure or stopping premature heartbeats. Long-term use is determined by sustained benefit and patient response to a combined program (weight reduction, salt restriction, smoking cessation, etc.). See your doctor regularly.

Possible Advantages of This Drug
Slows the heart less than most other beta-blocker drugs, and less likely to cause asthma (in susceptible patients) when used in low doses.

▷ **This Drug Should Not Be Taken If**
• you have had an allergic reaction to it previously.
• you are in heart failure (overt).
• you have a severely slow (bradycardia) heart rate or serious heart block (second or third degree).
• you are taking, or took within the past 14 days, any monoamine oxidase (MAO) type A inhibitor drug (see Drug Classes).

▷ **Inform Your Physician Before Taking This Drug If**
• you have had an adverse reaction to any beta-blocker (see Drug Classes).
• you have serious heart disease or episodes of heart failure (this drug may aggravate it).
• you have hay fever (allergic rhinitis), asthma, chronic bronchitis, or emphysema. Some drugs in this class should not be taken if you have asthma.
• you have an overactive thyroid function (hyperthyroidism).
• you have problems with circulation to your arms and legs (peripheral vascular disease or intermittent claudication).
• you have a history of low blood sugar (hypoglycemia).
• you have impaired liver or kidney function.
• you have diabetes or myasthenia gravis.

- you take digitalis, quinidine, or reserpine, or any calcium blocker (see Drug Classes).
- you plan to have surgery under general anesthesia in the near future.
- you are unsure of how much to take or how often to take acebutolol.
- you have not asked if the dose prescribed was adjusted for your age-related kidney decline.

Possible Side Effects (natural, expected, and unavoidable drug actions)

Lethargy and fatigability, cold extremities—rare; slow heart rate, light-headedness in upright position (see Orthostatic Hypotension in Glossary).

▷ **Possible Adverse Effects** (unusual, unexpected, and infrequent reactions)

If any of the following develop, consult your physician promptly for guidance.

Mild Adverse Effects

Allergic reactions: skin rash, itching.

Headache, dizziness, insomnia, fatigue, or abnormal dreams—infrequent.

Indigestion, nausea, constipation, diarrhea—infrequent.

Decreased tearing with long-term use—case reports.

Increased frequency and painful or nighttime urination—infrequent.

Joint and muscle discomfort, fluid retention (edema)—infrequent.

Serious Adverse Effects

May make other allergic reactions less responsive to treatment and more severe.

Mental depression or low blood sugar—rare.

Liver toxicity—rare.

Chest pain, shortness of breath, precipitation of congestive heart failure—rare.

Induction of bronchial asthma (in people with asthma)—possible.

Positive ANA and lupus erythematosus—infrequent to frequent, up to 33%.

▷ **Possible Effects on Sexual Function:**   Impotence—rare; decreased libido, Peyronie's disease (see Glossary).

Possible Effects on Laboratory Tests

Antinuclear antibodies (ANA) and LE cells: often positive after 3 to 6 months.

Free fatty acids (FFA): decreased.

Glucose tolerance test (GTT): decreased; abnormal tests at 60 and 120 minutes.

Potassium: mild increases.

CAUTION

1. ***Do not stop this drug suddenly*** without the knowledge and help from your physician. Carry a note which says that you take this drug.
2. Call your physician or pharmacist before using nasal decongestants. These can cause sudden increases in blood pressure if taken with beta-blockers.
3. Report the development of any tendency to emotional depression.
4. This medicine may worsen preexisting kidney insufficiency.

Precautions for Use

By Infants and Children: Safety and effectiveness for use by those under 12 years of age have not been established. If this drug is used, watch for fainting as a sign of low blood sugar (hypoglycemia) if a meal is skipped.

By Those Over 60 Years of Age: All antihypertensive drugs should be used ***cautiously***. High blood pressure should be lowered slowly, avoiding the risks (such as stroke or heart attack) of excessively low blood pressure. Small doses and frequent blood pressure checks are indicated. Total daily dosage should not exceed 800 mg. Watch for dizziness, unsteadiness, tendency to fall, confusion, hallucinations, depression, or urinary frequency.

▷ **Advisability of Use During Pregnancy**
Pregnancy Category: B. See Pregnancy Risk Categories at the back of this book.
Animal studies: No significant increase in birth defects in rats or rabbits.
Human studies: Adequate studies of pregnant women are not available.
Use this drug only if clearly needed. Ask your doctor for help.

Advisability of Use If Breast-Feeding
Presence of this drug in breast milk: Yes, and it is concentrated there.
Avoid drug or refrain from nursing.

Habit-Forming Potential: None.

Effects of Overdosage: Weakness, slow pulse, low blood pressure, fainting, cold and sweaty skin, congestive heart failure, possible coma, and convulsions.

Possible Effects of Long-Term Use: Decreased heart reserve and heart failure in some people with advanced heart disease.

Suggested Periodic Examinations While Taking This Drug (at physician's discretion)
Measurements of blood pressure, evaluation of heart function.

▷ **While Taking This Drug, Observe the Following**
Foods: No restrictions. Avoid excessive salt intake.
Beverages: No restrictions. May be taken with milk.
▷   *Alcohol:* Alcohol may exaggerate lowering of blood pressure and may increase its mild sedative effect.
Tobacco Smoking: Nicotine may reduce this drug's effectiveness in treating high blood pressure. May increase the closing of bronchial tubes seen in regular smokers. I advise everyone to quit smoking.
▷   *Other Drugs*
Acebutolol may *increase* the effects of
- other antihypertensive drugs and excessively lower the blood pressure. Dosage adjustments may be necessary.
- reserpine (Ser-Ap-Es, etc.) and cause sedation, depression, slow heart rate, and low blood pressure.

Acebutolol *taken concurrently* with
- amiodarone (Cordarone) may result in severe slowing of the heart leading to sinus arrest. Use with great caution.
- clonidine (Catapres) may cause rebound high blood pressure if clonidine is withdrawn while acebutolol is still being taken.
- fluoxetine (Prozac), fluvoxamine (Luvox), paroxetine (Paxil), or venlafaxine (Effexor) may decrease the rate or removal of acebutolol from the body (not reported as yet). Caution is advised.
- insulin may cause low blood sugar (hypoglycemia).
- nilvadipine (Escor) may pose a rare risk of heart failure (cardiac failure).
- NSAIDs (see Drug Classes) may result in decreased lowering of blood pressure.

- oral antidiabetic drugs (see Drug Classes) may result in slow recovery from low blood sugar.
- ritonavir (Norvir) and perhaps other protease inhibitors may increase the metabolism of this medicine and blunt therapeutic benefits of acebutolol. The following drugs may *decrease* the effects of acebutolol:
- indomethacin (Indocin) and some other "aspirin substitutes" (NSAIDs) can blunt acebutolol's antihypertensive effect.

Driving, Hazardous Activities: Use caution until you see how drowsy and lethargic you may become.

Aviation Note: The use of this drug *is a disqualification* for piloting. Consult a designated Aviation Medical Examiner.

Exposure to Sun: No restrictions.

Exposure to Heat: Hot environments can exaggerate the effects of this drug.

Exposure to Cold: The elderly must be careful in preventing hypothermia (see Glossary).

Heavy Exercise or Exertion: This drug can intensify the increased blood pressure (hypertensive) response to isometric exercise. Avoid exertion causing dizziness, excessive fatigue, or muscle cramps.

Occurrence of Unrelated Illness: Fevers can lower blood pressure and require decreased doses. Nausea or vomiting may interrupt the dosing schedule. Ask your doctor for help.

Discontinuation: Avoid stopping the drug suddenly. Slow reduction of dose over a period of 2 to 3 weeks is recommended. Ask your physician for guidance.

ACETAZOLAMIDE (a set a ZOHL a mide)

Introduced: 1953 **Class:** Anticonvulsant, antiglaucoma, diuretic, sulfonamides **Prescription:** USA: Yes **Controlled Drug:** USA: No; Canada: No **Available as Generic:** USA: Yes; Canada: No

Brand Names: ✦Acetazolam, Ak-Zol, ✦Apo-Acetazolamide, Dazamide, Diamox, Diamox Sustained release, Diamox Sequles, Storzolamide

BENEFITS versus RISKS	
Possible Benefits	*Possible Risks*
REDUCTION OF INTERNAL EYE PRESSURE in selected cases of glaucoma	Rare bone marrow, liver, or kidney injury
CONTROL OF ABSENCE (PETIT MAL) SEIZURES	Acidosis with long-term use
	Increased risk of kidney stones
TREATMENT OF PERIODIC PARALYSIS	Tingling in the arms and legs (paresthesia)
REDUCTION OF FLUID IN CONGESTIVE HEART FAILURE OR DRUG-INDUCED EDEMA	Paralysis (rare)
	Bone weakening (with long-term use)
PREVENTION OR LESSENING OF SYMPTOMS OF ACUTE MOUNTAIN SICKNESS	

▷ **Principal Uses**

As a Single Drug Product: Uses currently included in FDA-approved labeling: (1) Treatment of some kinds of glaucoma—especially in combination with other agents; (2) used with other drugs to manage petit mal epilepsy; (3) treats familial periodic paralysis and prevents altitude (acute mountain) sickness; (4) can be used to show how much blood flow (cerebrovascular reserve) patients have in their brains; (5) used to correct metabolic problems (acid–base) in people with chronic obstructive pulmonary disease (COPD).

Other (unlabeled) generally accepted uses: (1) Taken orally as a urine alkalinizing agent in patients who have had uric acid kidney stones; (2) given intravenously to increase elimination of some drugs in overdoses; (3) helps patients on ventilators by correcting chemical imbalances; (3) may have a role in easing both kinetic and postural tremor in combination with other agents.

How This Drug Works: By blocking the enzyme carbonic anhydrase, it slows the formation of fluid (the aqueous humor) in the eye and increases the volume of urine. It causes fluid loss by lowering the hydrogen ion concentration in the kidney and increasing elimination of bicarbonate (a basic chemical), potassium, sodium, and water.

Available Dosage Forms and Strengths

Capsules, prolonged action (sustained release) — 500 mg

Injection — 500 mg per vial

Tablets — 125 mg, 250 mg

▷ **Recommended Dosage Ranges (Actual dosage and administration schedule must be determined for each patient individually.)**

Infants and Children: Not indicated in infants.

Acute glaucoma in children: Give 5–10 mg per kg of body mass intramuscularly (IM) or intravenously (IV) every 6 hours.

Children with glaucoma: Give 8–30 mg per kg of body mass per day in three divided doses.

Epilepsy in children: Give 8–30 mg per kg of body mass per day in one to four divided doses. Lower the doses used if drug is combined with other medications (250 mg per day).

Diuretic in children: Give 5 mg per kg of body mass IV or orally once daily in the morning.

18 to 65 Years of Age: For glaucoma: 250 to 1000 mg every 24 hours, in two or three doses (often used by vein [intravenously] in acute or sudden cases).

For epilepsy: 250 to 1000 mg every 24 hours.

As a diuretic: 250 to 375 mg every 24 hours, in one morning dose for 1 or 2 days.

Mountain sickness: 250 mg every 8 to 12 hours for prevention; 500 to 1000 mg daily in divided doses is used with dosing started 1 to 2 days before climbing.

Over 65 Years of Age: Most of a given dose is eliminated via the kidneys. Use with caution in this age group, and start with the lower end of the dosage range.

Conditions Requiring Dosing Adjustments

Liver Function: Use with extreme caution in patients with liver problems, as it may lead to a coma.

Kidney Function: Use with extreme caution in kidney compromise: mild kidney failure requires dosing every 6 hours; every 12 hours is used with moderate failure. This drug may not work in severe failure.

> **Dosing Instructions:** Best taken with food or milk to prevent stomach irritation. Tablet may be crushed. Diamox Sequels may be opened, but do not chew or crush contents.

Usual Duration of Use: Treatment of glaucoma and epilepsy require long-term use. If taken to control seizures, do not stop this drug abruptly. See your doctor regularly.

> **This Drug Should Not Be Taken If**
> • you have had an allergic reaction to any form of it previously.
> • you have serious liver or kidney disease.
> • you have Addison's disease.
> • your adrenal gland has failed.
> • you have low blood sodium or potassium (electrolyte problems).
> • you have some types of glaucoma (chronic noncongestive angle-closure).

▷ **Inform Your Physician Before Taking This Drug If**
> • you have had an allergic reaction to any "sulfa" drug.
> • you have gout or lupus erythematosus.
> • you have emphysema or blockages of your lungs.
> • you have a history of low blood platelets or bone marrow problems.

Possible Side Effects (natural, expected, and unavoidable drug actions)
Drowsiness, temporary nearsightedness.

▷ **Possible Adverse Effects** (unusual, unexpected, and infrequent reactions)
If any of the following develop, consult your physician promptly for guidance.
Mild Adverse Effects
Allergic reactions: skin rash, hives, drug fever.
Reduced appetite, indigestion, nausea—infrequent.
Taste disturbance—possible.
Confusion, fatigue; weakness; dizziness; tingling of face, arms, or legs—infrequent. Tingling effect may be from lowering of blood potassium, which often eases with time.
Excessive growth of hair in females—case reports.
Serious Adverse Effects
Allergic reactions: hemolytic anemia (see Glossary), spontaneous bruising (reduced blood platelet count; see Glossary).
Bone marrow depression (see Glossary): fatigue, weakness, fever, sore throat, abnormal bleeding or bruising—case reports.
Metabolic changes (acidosis)—possible and more likely in patients with kidney problems or the elderly.
Hepatitis (see Glossary): yellow eyes/skin, dark-colored urine, light stools—case reports.
Severe muscle weakness leading to paralysis—rare.
Weakness of the bones with long-term use (osteomalacia)—case reports.

▷ **Possible Effects on Sexual Function:** Decreased libido (male and female)—infrequent; impotence—case reports. Effects may begin after 2 weeks of use and subside when drug is stopped.

Adverse Effects That May Mimic Natural Diseases or Disorders

Toxic liver reaction may suggest viral hepatitis.

Lupus erythematosuslike syndrome—case reports.

Natural Diseases or Disorders That May Be Activated by This Drug

Gout, acidosis caused by chronic obstructive lung disease—asthma, bronchitis, emphysema.

Possible Effects on Laboratory Tests

Complete blood counts: decreased red cells, hemoglobin, white cells, and platelets.

Blood chloride level: increased.

Blood potassium and possibly magnesium: decreased.

Blood glucose level: increased in prediabetics and with use of oral antidiabetic drugs (see Drug Classes).

Blood lupus erythematosus (LE) cells: positive.

Blood theophylline tests: may be falsely increased.

Blood uric acid level: increased.

CAUTION

1. Watch for loss of diuretic (fluid) or seizure control effect.
2. Emotional depression can be an adverse effect of this drug.
3. May cause excessive loss of potassium. Ask your doctor about a high potassium diet or potassium supplements.

Precautions for Use

By Infants and Children: Excess dose may cause drowsiness or numbness of the face or extremities. Not recommended for use as a diuretic in children.

By Those Over 60 Years of Age: Do not exceed recommended doses. Increased dose may lead to weakness, confusion, numbness in the extremities, and nausea. If taking a digitalis preparation (digitoxin, digoxin), you may need a high potassium diet or potassium supplements. Ask your doctor for advice.

▷ **Advisability of Use During Pregnancy**

Pregnancy Category: C. See Pregnancy Risk Categories at the back of this book.

Animal studies: Limb and skeletal defects reported in mice and rats.

Human studies: Adequate studies of pregnant women not available.

Avoid completely during the first 3 months and during labor and delivery.

Advisability of Use if Breast-Feeding

Presence of this drug in breast milk: Yes.

May temporarily impair milk production. Watch nursing infant closely and stop drug or nursing if adverse effects develop.

Habit-Forming Potential: None.

Effects of Overdosage: Drowsiness, numbness and tingling, thirst, nausea, vomiting, confusion, excitement, convulsions, coma.

Possible Effects of Long-Term Use: The development of low blood potassium (first few weeks) and/or acidosis. Weakening of bones (osteomalacia).

Suggested Periodic Examinations While Taking This Drug (at physician's discretion)

Complete blood cell counts, measurements of blood sodium, potassium, and uric acid levels, liver and kidney function tests.

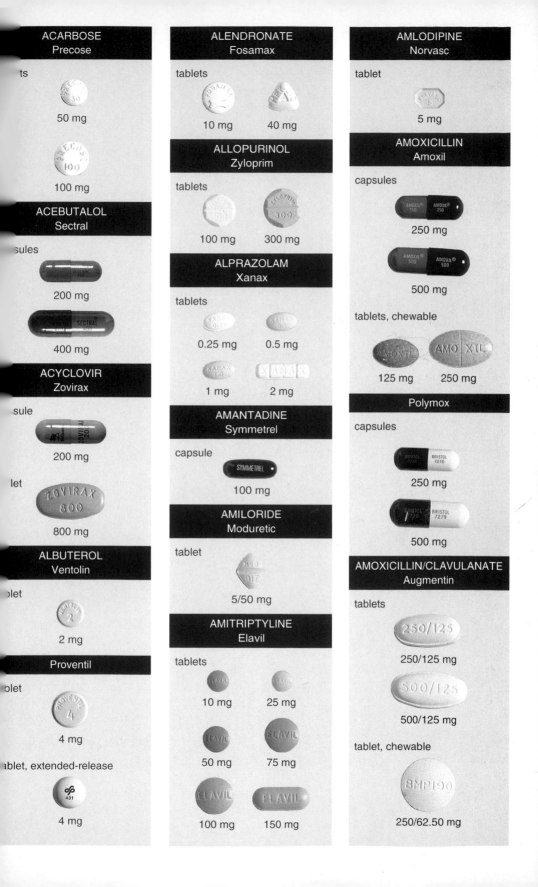

ACARBOSE
Precose

ts

50 mg

100 mg

ACEBUTALOL
Sectral

sules

200 mg

400 mg

ACYCLOVIR
Zovirax

sule

200 mg

let

800 mg

ALBUTEROL
Ventolin

let

2 mg

Proventil

let

4 mg

ablet, extended-release

4 mg

ALENDRONATE
Fosamax

tablets

10 mg   40 mg

ALLOPURINOL
Zyloprim

tablets

100 mg   300 mg

ALPRAZOLAM
Xanax

tablets

0.25 mg   0.5 mg

1 mg   2 mg

AMANTADINE
Symmetrel

capsule

100 mg

AMILORIDE
Moduretic

tablet

5/50 mg

AMITRIPTYLINE
Elavil

tablets

10 mg   25 mg

50 mg   75 mg

100 mg   150 mg

AMLODIPINE
Norvasc

tablet

5 mg

AMOXICILLIN
Amoxil

capsules

250 mg

500 mg

tablets, chewable

125 mg   250 mg

Polymox

capsules

250 mg

500 mg

AMOXICILLIN/CLAVULANATE
Augmentin

tablets

250/125 mg

500/125 mg

tablet, chewable

250/62.50 mg

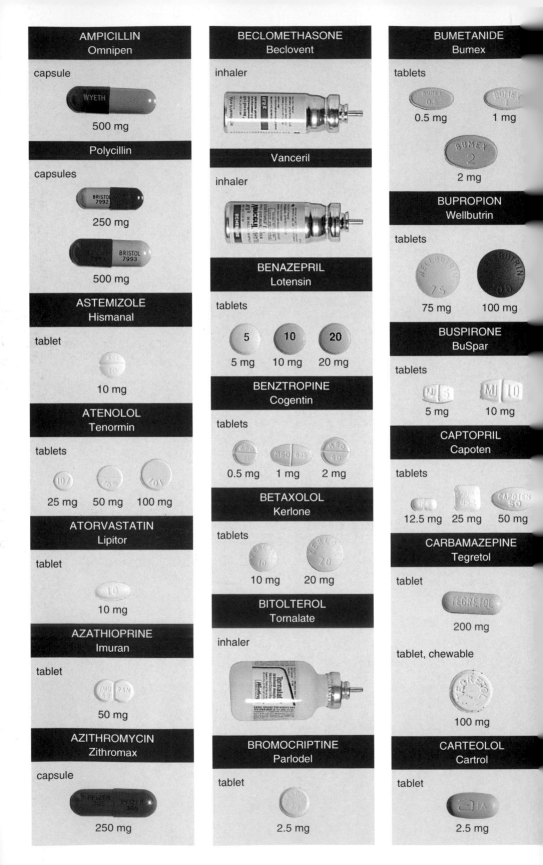

AMPICILLIN
Omnipen
capsule

500 mg

Polycillin
capsules

250 mg

500 mg

ASTEMIZOLE
Hismanal
tablet

10 mg

ATENOLOL
Tenormin
tablets

25 mg   50 mg   100 mg

ATORVASTATIN
Lipitor
tablet

10 mg

AZATHIOPRINE
Imuran
tablet

50 mg

AZITHROMYCIN
Zithromax
capsule

250 mg

BECLOMETHASONE
Beclovent
inhaler

Vanceril
inhaler

BENAZEPRIL
Lotensin
tablets

5 mg   10 mg   20 mg

BENZTROPINE
Cogentin
tablets

0.5 mg   1 mg   2 mg

BETAXOLOL
Kerlone
tablets

10 mg   20 mg

BITOLTEROL
Tornalate
inhaler

BROMOCRIPTINE
Parlodel
tablet

2.5 mg

BUMETANIDE
Bumex
tablets

0.5 mg   1 mg

2 mg

BUPROPION
Wellbutrin
tablets

75 mg   100 mg

BUSPIRONE
BuSpar
tablets

5 mg   10 mg

CAPTOPRIL
Capoten
tablets

12.5 mg   25 mg   50 mg

CARBAMAZEPINE
Tegretol
tablet

200 mg

tablet, chewable

100 mg

CARTEOLOL
Cartrol
tablet

2.5 mg

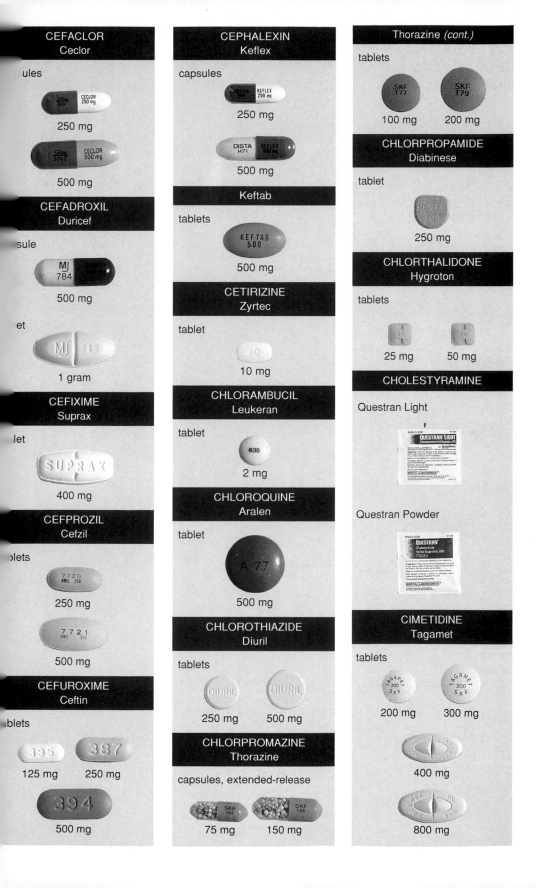

CEFACLOR
Ceclor

ules

250 mg

500 mg

CEFADROXIL
Duricef

sule

500 mg

et

1 gram

CEFIXIME
Suprax

let

SUPRAX

400 mg

CEFPROZIL
Cefzil

blets

7720
BMS 250

250 mg

7721
BMS 500

500 mg

CEFUROXIME
Ceftin

blets

395

125 mg

387

250 mg

394

500 mg

CEPHALEXIN
Keflex

capsules

DISTA | KEFLEX
250 mg

250 mg

DISTA
H71 | KEFLEX
500 mg

500 mg

Keftab

tablets

KEFTAB
500

500 mg

CETIRIZINE
Zyrtec

tablet

10

10 mg

CHLORAMBUCIL
Leukeran

tablet

635

2 mg

CHLOROQUINE
Aralen

tablet

A 77

500 mg

CHLOROTHIAZIDE
Diuril

tablets

DIURIL

250 mg

DIURIL

500 mg

CHLORPROMAZINE
Thorazine

capsules, extended-release

SKF
164

75 mg

SKF
166

150 mg

Thorazine *(cont.)*

tablets

SKF
T77

100 mg

SKF
T79

200 mg

CHLORPROPAMIDE
Diabinese

tablet

PFIZER
394

250 mg

CHLORTHALIDONE
Hygroton

tablets

22

25 mg

30

50 mg

CHOLESTYRAMINE

Questran Light

QUESTRAN LIGHT

Questran Powder

QUESTRAN
POWDER

CIMETIDINE
Tagamet

tablets

TAGAMET
200
S K F

200 mg

TAGAMET
300
S K F

300 mg

400 mg

800 mg

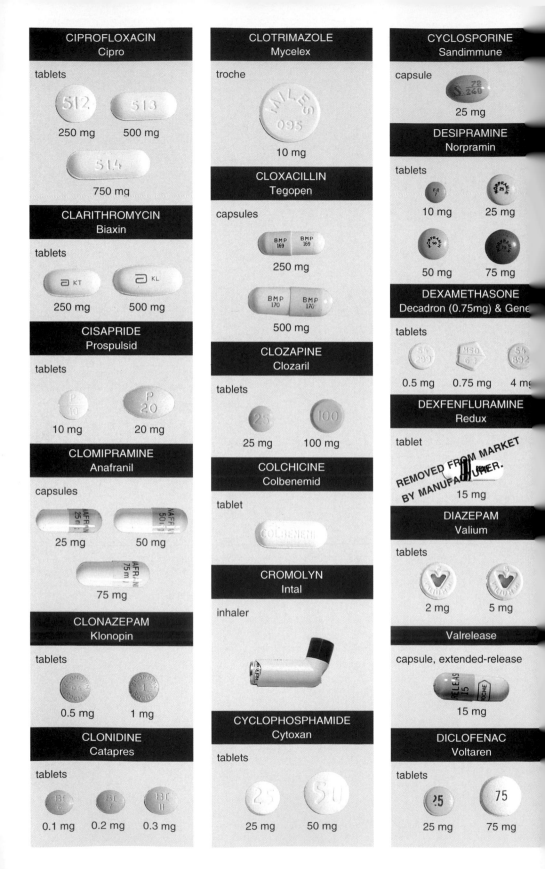

CIPROFLOXACIN
Cipro
tablets

512 — 250 mg
513 — 500 mg
514 — 750 mg

CLARITHROMYCIN
Biaxin
tablets

a KT — 250 mg
a KL — 500 mg

CISAPRIDE
Prospulsid
tablets

P 10 — 10 mg
P 20 — 20 mg

CLOMIPRAMINE
Anafranil
capsules

ANAFRANIL 25 m — 25 mg
ANAFRANIL 50 m — 50 mg
ANAFRANIL 75 m — 75 mg

CLONAZEPAM
Klonopin
tablets

CLONOPIN 0.5 ROCHE — 0.5 mg
CLONOPIN 1 ROCHE — 1 mg

CLONIDINE
Catapres
tablets

BI 6 — 0.1 mg
BI 7 — 0.2 mg
BI 11 — 0.3 mg

CLOTRIMAZOLE
Mycelex
troche

MILES 095 — 10 mg

CLOXACILLIN
Tegopen
capsules

BMP 169 — 250 mg
BMP 170 — 500 mg

CLOZAPINE
Clozaril
tablets

25 — 25 mg
100 — 100 mg

COLCHICINE
Colbenemid
tablet

COLBENEMID

CROMOLYN
Intal
inhaler

CYCLOPHOSPHAMIDE
Cytoxan
tablets

25 — 25 mg
50 — 50 mg

CYCLOSPORINE
Sandimmune
capsule

78 240 — 25 mg

DESIPRAMINE
Norpramin
tablets

68 7 — 10 mg
NORPRAMIN — 25 mg
NORPRAMIN 8 — 50 mg
NORPRAMIN — 75 mg

DEXAMETHASONE
Decadron (0.75mg) & Gene
tablets

54 299 — 0.5 mg
MSD 63 — 0.75 mg
54 892 — 4 mg

DEXFENFLURAMINE
Redux
tablet

REMOVED FROM MARKET BY MANUFACTURER.

REDUX — 15 mg

DIAZEPAM
Valium
tablets

VALIUM — 2 mg
5 VALIUM — 5 mg

Valrelease
capsule, extended-release

RELEASE 15 ROCHE — 15 mg

DICLOFENAC
Voltaren
tablets

25 — 25 mg
75 — 75 mg

DIDANOSINE
Videx

...et

VIDEX
BL.

25 mg

DIFLUNISAL
Dolobid

...lets

DOLOBID — DOLOBID

250 mg   500 mg

DIGOXIN
Lanoxicaps

...sules

0.1 mg   0.2 mg

Lanoxin

...lets

...125 mg   0.25 mg   0.5 mg

DILTIAZEM
Cardizem

...blets

177   17

30 mg   60 mg

90 mg

120 mg

Cardizem CD

capsules

180 mg

Cardizem CD
capsules *(cont.)*

240 mg

300 mg

Cardizem SR

capsules

60 mg   90 mg

120 mg

DIPHENHYDRAMINE
Benadryl

capsules

PD
471

25 mg   50 mg

DISOPYRAMIDE
Norpace

capsules

SEARLE   NORPACE
2752   100 MG.
SEARLE   NORPACE
2762   150 MG.

100 mg   150 mg

Norpace CR

capsules, extended-release

RPACE C
00 m
EARLE
2732

100 mg

PACE
0 m

150 mg

DISULFIRAM
Antabuse

tablets

ANTABUSE
250

500
ANTABUSE

250 mg   500 mg

DONEPEZIL
Aricept

tablet

5

5 mg

DOXAZOSIN
Cardura

tablets

1 mg   2 mg

4 mg   8 mg

DOXEPIN
Sinequan

capsules

10 mg   25 mg

50 mg

DOXYCYCLINE
Zenith generic

tablet

3626

100 mg

ENALAPRIL
Vasotec

tablet

2.5 mg

ERGOTAMINE
Ergostat

tablet

2 mg

ERYTHROMYCIN
Ery-Tab

tablet, delayed-release

a EH

333 mg

E-Mycin
tablets, delayed-release

250 mg   333 mg

Eryc
capsule, delayed-release

250 mg

Erythrocin
tablets

250 mg   500 mg

ESTROGENS
Estrace

tablets

1 mg   2 mg

Ogen
tablets

0.625 mg   1.5 mg

Premarin
tablets

0.3 mg   0.625 mg

0.9 mg   1.25 mg

2.5 mg

ETHAMBUTOL
Myambutol

tablet

400 mg

ETHOSUXIMIDE
Zarontin

capsule

250 mg

ETRETINATE
Tegison

capsules

10 mg

25 mg

FAMOTIDINE
Pepcid

tablets

20 mg   40 mg

FELODIPINE
Plendil

tablets

5 mg   10 mg

FENOPROFEN
Nalfon

capsule

200 mg

FEXOFENADINE
Allegra

capsule

60 mg

FINASTERIDE
Proscar

tablet

5 mg

FLUCONAZOLE
Diflucan

tablets

50 mg   100 mg

FLUCYTOSINE
Ancobon

capsule

500 mg

FLUOXETINE
Prozac

capsule

20 mg

FLUPHENAZINE
Prolixin

tablets

1 mg   5 mg

FLURAZEPAM
Dalmane

capsules

15 mg   30 mg

FLURBIPROFEN
Ansaid

tablets

ANSAID 50 mg — 50 mg
ANSAID 100 mg — 100 mg

FLUTAMIDE
Eulexin

capsule

SCHERING 525 | SCHERING 525 — 125 mg

FOSINOPRIL
Monopril

tablets

SQUIBB 158 — 10 mg
MI 609 — 20 mg

FUROSEMIDE
Lasix

tablets

LASIX — 20 mg
LASIX 40 — 40 mg
LASIX 80 — 80 mg

GABAPENTIN
Neurontin

capsule

Neurontin 100 mg — 100 mg

GEMFIBROZIL
Lopid

tablet

Lopid — 600 mg

GLIPIZIDE
Glucotrol

tablets

PFIZER 411 — 5 mg
PFIZER 412 — 10 mg

GLYBURIDE
DiaBeta

tablets

Dia β — 1.25 mg
Dia β — 2.5 mg
Dia β — 5 mg

Micronase

tablets

MICRONASE 1.25 — 1.25 mg
MICRONASE 2.5 — 2.5 mg
MICRONASE 5 — 5 mg

GUANFACINE
Tenex

tablets

TENEX — 1 mg
TENEX — 2 mg

HALOPERIDOL
Haldol

tablets

HALDOL — 0.5 mg
HALDOL — 1 mg
HALDOL — 2 mg
HALDOL 5 — 5 mg
HALDOL 10 — 10 mg

HYDRALAZINE
Apresoline

tablets

101 — 100 mg

HYDROCHLOROTHIAZIDE
Esidrix

tablets

22 — 25 mg
46 — 50 mg

HYDROCODONE
(& acetaminophen)
Vicodin

tablet

VICODIN — 5/500 mg

Vicodin ES

tablet

VICODIN ES — 7.5/750 mg

HYDROXYCHLOROQUINE
Plaquenil

tablet

PLAQUENIL — 200 mg

IBUPROFEN
Motrin

tablets

MOTRIN 400 mg — 400 mg
MOTRIN 600 mg — 600 mg
MOTRIN 800 mg — 800 mg

IMIPRAMINE
Tofranil

tablets

32 — 10 mg
140 — 25 mg
136 — 50 mg

Tofranil-PM

capsule

Geigy 45 — 125 mg

INDAPAMIDE
Lozol

tablet

— 2.5 mg

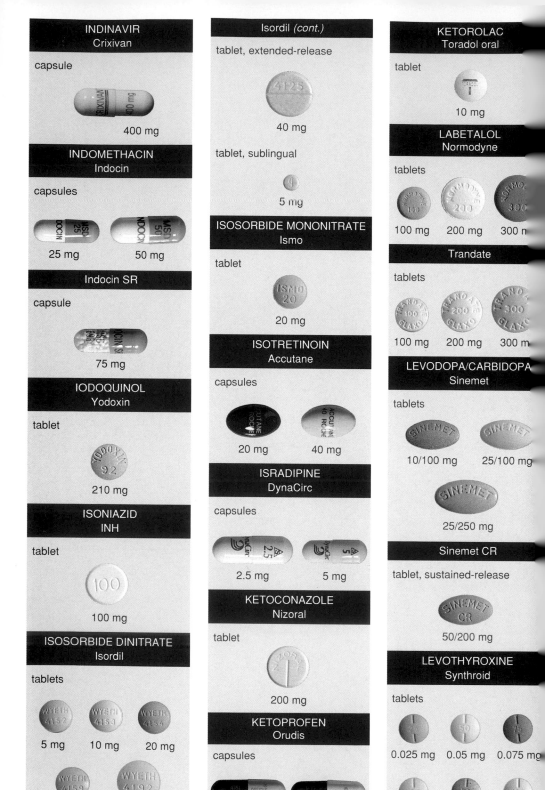

INDINAVIR
Crixivan

capsule

400 mg

INDOMETHACIN
Indocin

capsules

25 mg   50 mg

Indocin SR

capsule

75 mg

IODOQUINOL
Yodoxin

tablet

210 mg

ISONIAZID
INH

tablet

100 mg

ISOSORBIDE DINITRATE
Isordil

tablets

5 mg   10 mg   20 mg

30 mg   40 mg

Isordil *(cont.)*

tablet, extended-release

40 mg

tablet, sublingual

5 mg

ISOSORBIDE MONONITRATE
Ismo

tablet

20 mg

ISOTRETINOIN
Accutane

capsules

20 mg   40 mg

ISRADIPINE
DynaCirc

capsules

2.5 mg   5 mg

KETOCONAZOLE
Nizoral

tablet

200 mg

KETOPROFEN
Orudis

capsules

50 mg   75 mg

KETOROLAC
Toradol oral

tablet

10 mg

LABETALOL
Normodyne

tablets

100 mg   200 mg   300 mg

Trandate

tablets

100 mg   200 mg   300 mg

LEVODOPA/CARBIDOPA
Sinemet

tablets

10/100 mg   25/100 mg

25/250 mg

Sinemet CR

tablet, sustained-release

50/200 mg

LEVOTHYROXINE
Synthroid

tablets

0.025 mg   0.05 mg   0.075 mg

0.1 mg   0.112 mg   0.125 mg

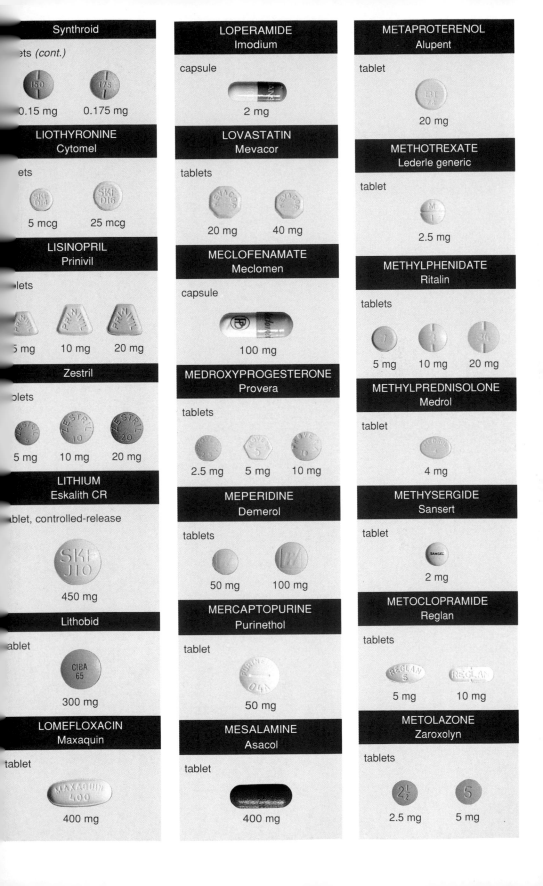

Synthroid
lets *(cont.)*

0.15 mg 0.175 mg

LIOTHYRONINE
Cytomel

ets

5 mcg 25 mcg

LISINOPRIL
Prinivil

lets

5 mg 10 mg 20 mg

Zestril

olets

5 mg 10 mg 20 mg

LITHIUM
Eskalith CR

ablet, controlled-release

450 mg

Lithobid

ablet

300 mg

LOMEFLOXACIN
Maxaquin

tablet

400 mg

LOPERAMIDE
Imodium

capsule

2 mg

LOVASTATIN
Mevacor

tablets

20 mg 40 mg

MECLOFENAMATE
Meclomen

capsule

100 mg

MEDROXYPROGESTERONE
Provera

tablets

2.5 mg 5 mg 10 mg

MEPERIDINE
Demerol

tablets

50 mg 100 mg

MERCAPTOPURINE
Purinethol

tablet

50 mg

MESALAMINE
Asacol

tablet

400 mg

METAPROTERENOL
Alupent

tablet

20 mg

METHOTREXATE
Lederle generic

tablet

2.5 mg

METHYLPHENIDATE
Ritalin

tablets

5 mg 10 mg 20 mg

METHYLPREDNISOLONE
Medrol

tablet

4 mg

METHYSERGIDE
Sansert

tablet

2 mg

METOCLOPRAMIDE
Reglan

tablets

5 mg 10 mg

METOLAZONE
Zaroxolyn

tablets

2.5 mg 5 mg

METOPROLOL
Lopressor

tablets

50 mg

100 mg

Toprol XL

tablets, extended-release

50 mg   100 mg

METRONIDAZOLE
Flagyl

tablets

250 mg   500 mg

MEXILETINE
Mexitil

capsules

150 mg

200 mg

MIBEFRADIL
Posicor

tablet

50 mg

MINOXIDIL
Loniten

tablet

2.5 mg

MIRTAZAPINE
Remeron

tablet

15 mg

MISOPROSTOL
Cytotec

tablets

0.1 mg   0.2 mg

MOLINDONE
Moban

tablets

10 mg   25 mg   100 mg

MORPHINE
MS Contin

tablets

15 mg   30 mg

60 mg   100 mg

NABUMETONE
Relafen

tablets

500 mg

750 mg

NADOLOL
Corgard

tablets

20 mg   40 mg   80 mg

NALTREXONE
ReVia

tablet

50 mg

NAPROXEN
Naprosyn

tablets

250 mg   375 mg

500 mg

NEOSTIGMINE
Prostigmin

tablet

15 mg

NIACIN
Nicobid

capsules, extended-release

250 mg

Slo-Niacin

tablets, extended-release

500 mg

NICARDIPINE
Cardene

capsules

20 mg   30 mg

NICOTINE
Nicorette

chewing gum

2 mg

4 mg

NIFEDIPINE
Adalat

capsules

ADALAT
Miles 811

ADALAT
Miles 821

10 mg   20 mg

Procardia

capsules

PROCARDIA
PFIZER 260

10 mg

PROCARDIA 2
PFIZER 261

20 mg

Procardia XL

tablets, extended-release

PROCARDIA XL
30

PROCARDIA XL
60

30 mg   60 mg

PROCARDIA XL
90

90 mg

NITROFURANTOIN
Furadantin

tablet

50 mg

Macrodantin

capsules

MACRO
50 mg

MACRO
100 mg

50 mg   100 mg

NITROGLYCERIN
Nitrostat

tablets, sublingual

0.4 mg

NIZATIDINE
Axid

capsules

Lilly
3144

AXID
150mg

Lilly
3145

AXID
300mg

150 mg   300 mg

NORFLOXACIN
Noroxin

tablet

MSD
705

400 mg

NORTRIPTYLINE
Pamelor

capsules

10 mg   25 mg

50 mg   75 mg

OFLOXACIN
Floxin

tablets

FLOXIN 200 mg

FLOXIN 300 mg

200 mg   300 mg

FLOXIN 400 mg

400 mg

OLANZAPINE
Zyprexa

tablet

LILLY
4115

5 mg

OLSALAZINE
Dipentum

capsule

PENTUM
250 mg

250 mg

OMEPRAZOLE
Prilosec

capsule

20 mg

OXTRIPHYLLINE
Choledyl SA

tablet, sustained-action

PD   214

400 mg

OXYCODONE
Roxicodone

tablet

54
582

5 mg

OXYCODONE
(& acetaminophen)
Percocet

tablet

PERCOCET

5/325 mg

PAROXETINE
Paxil

tablet

PAXIL   PAXIL

20 mg   30 mg

PENCICLOVIR
Denavir

cream

1% 10 mg tube

PENICILLAMINE
Depen

tablet

37   4401

250 mg

PENICILLIN V
Beepen VK

tablets

185   186

250 mg   500 mg

Pen-Vee-K

tablets

WYETH

250 mg

V-Cillin K

tablets

V-CILLIN K 250 Lilly   V-CILLIN K 500 Lilly

250 mg   500 mg

PENTAZOCINE/NALOXONE
Talwin Nx

tablet

T 51

50/0.5 mg

PENTOXIFYLLINE
Trental

tablet

TRENTAL

400 mg

PERGOLIDE
Permax

tablets

Lilly 4131   Lilly 4135

0.05 mg   1 mg

PERPHENAZINE
Trilafon

tablets

705   9x0

2 mg   4 mg

PHENOBARBITAL
Warner Chilcott generic

tablets

WC 698   WC 700

15 mg   30 mg

WC 607   WC 693

60 mg   100 mg

PHENYTOIN
Dilantin

capsules

P-D 362   P-D 362

100 mg

tablet, chewable

P-D 007

50 mg

PINDOLOL
Visken

tablets

25   3.5   410   3.5

5 mg   10 mg

PIROXICAM
Feldene

capsules

FELDENE   PFIZER 322

10 mg

FELDENE   PFIZER 323

20 mg

PRAVASTATIN
Pravachol

tablets

10   20

10 mg   20 mg

PRAZOSIN
Minipress

capsules

MINIPRESS   PFIZER 431

1 mg

MINIPRESS   PFIZER 437

2 mg

MINIPRESS   PFIZER 438

5 mg

PREDNISONE
Deltasone

tablets

5   DELTASONE 10

5 mg   10 mg

DELTASONE 20

20 mg

PRIMIDONE
Mysoline

tablets

50   250 MYSOLINE

50 mg   250 mg

PROBENECID
Benemid

...et

500 mg

PROBUCOL
Lorelco

...ets

LORELCO
250

250 mg

LORELCO
500

500 mg

PROCAINAMIDE
Pronestyl

...sules

PPP
757   PPP
757

500 mg

Procan-SR

...blet, extended-release

PD | 204

500 mg

PD | 205

750 mg

PROCHLORPERAZINE
Compazine

...apsules

SKF
C44

10 mg

SKF
C46

15 mg

...ablets

SKF
C66

5 mg

PROPRANOLOL
Inderal

tablets

INDERAL
10

INDERAL
20

INDERAL
40

10 mg   20 mg   40 mg

INDERAL
60

INDERAL
80

60 mg   80 mg

Inderal LA

capsules, extended-release

LA 60

60 mg   80 mg

121

120 mg

16...

160 mg

PYRAZINAMIDE
Lederle generic

tablet

P
36

500 mg

PYRIDOSTIGMINE
Mestinon

tablet

MESTINON
60

60 mg

PYRIMETHAMINE
Daraprim

tablet

DARAPRIM
A 3 A

25 mg

QUINAPRIL
Accupril

tablets

5   10

5 mg   10 mg

20   40

20 mg   40 mg

QUINIDINE
Quinaglute

tablet

324 mg

Quinidex

tablet

QUINIDEX
AHR

300 mg

RAMIPRIL
Altace

capsules

2.5 mg   5 mg

10 mg

RANITIDINE
Zantac

tablets

ZANTAC
150

ZANTAC
300

150 mg   300 mg

RIFABUTIN
Mycobutin

capsule

COB...

150 mg

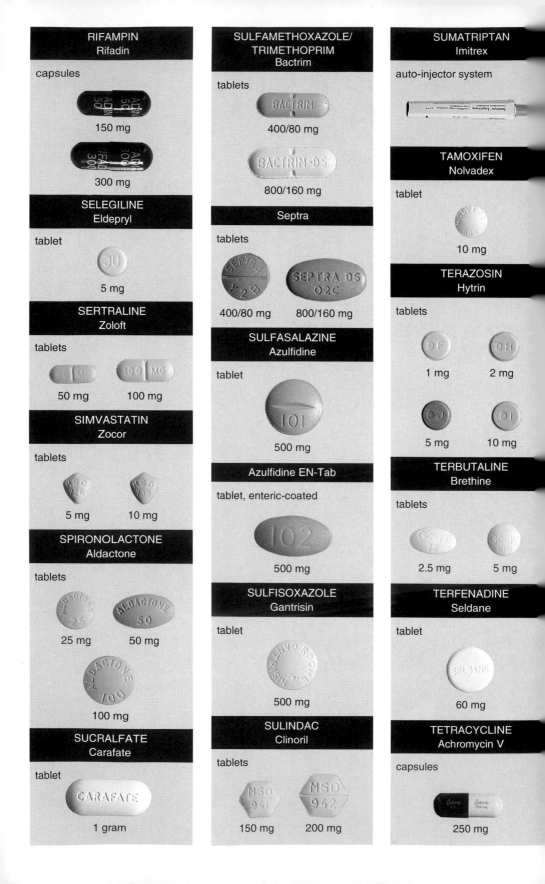

RIFAMPIN
Rifadin

capsules

150 mg

300 mg

SELEGILINE
Eldepryl

tablet

5 mg

SERTRALINE
Zoloft

tablets

50 mg   100 mg

SIMVASTATIN
Zocor

tablets

5 mg   10 mg

SPIRONOLACTONE
Aldactone

tablets

25 mg   50 mg

100 mg

SUCRALFATE
Carafate

tablet

1 gram

SULFAMETHOXAZOLE/
TRIMETHOPRIM
Bactrim

tablets

400/80 mg

800/160 mg

Septra

tablets

400/80 mg   800/160 mg

SULFASALAZINE
Azulfidine

tablet

500 mg

Azulfidine EN-Tab

tablet, enteric-coated

500 mg

SULFISOXAZOLE
Gantrisin

tablet

500 mg

SULINDAC
Clinoril

tablets

150 mg   200 mg

SUMATRIPTAN
Imitrex

auto-injector system

TAMOXIFEN
Nolvadex

tablet

10 mg

TERAZOSIN
Hytrin

tablets

1 mg   2 mg

5 mg   10 mg

TERBUTALINE
Brethine

tablets

2.5 mg   5 mg

TERFENADINE
Seldane

tablet

60 mg

TETRACYCLINE
Achromycin V

capsules

250 mg

Sumycin

capsules

250 mg

SQUIBB 763 / SQUIBB 763
500 mg

THEOPHYLLINE
Quibron-T/SR Dividose

tablet

300 mg

Slo-bid

capsules

WHR 50 mg
50 mg

WHR 100 / WHR 100
100 mg

Slo-bid 200 / RORER
200 mg

Slo-bid 300 mg
300 mg

Slo-Phyllin

capsules

WHR 1355 / WHR 1355
125 mg

WHR 1356 / WHR 1356
250 mg

tablets

WHR 952
200 mg

Theo-Dur

capsules

THEO-DUR SPRINKLE 50 mg
50 mg

75 mg

Theo-Dur

capsules (cont.)

THEO-DUR SPRINKLE 125 mg THIS END UP
125 mg

THEO-DUR SPRINKLE 200 mg
200 mg

tablets

THEO DUR 100
100 mg

THEO DUR 200
200 mg

THEO-DUR 300
300 mg

THEO-DUR 450
450 mg

Theo-24

capsule

SEARLE 2852
300 mg

THIORIDAZINE
Mellaril

tablets

10 mg

MELLARIL 25
25 mg

MELLARIL 50
50 mg

MELLARIL 100
100 mg

THIOTHIXENE
Navane

capsules

NAVANE ROERIG 571
1 mg

NAVANE ROERIG 572
2 mg

NAVANE ROERIG 573
5 mg

NAVANE ROERIG 574
10 mg

NAVANE ROERIG 577
20 mg

TICLOPIDINE
Ticlid

tablet

250
250 mg

TIMOLOL
Blocadren

tablets

MSD 59
5 mg

MSD 136
10 mg

MSD 437
20 mg

TOLAZAMIDE
Tolinase

tablets

TOLINASE 250
250 mg

TOLINASE 500
500 mg

TOLBUTAMIDE
Orinase

tablet

ORINASE 500
500 mg

TOLMETIN
Tolectin

tablet

TOLECTIN 600 McNEIL
600 mg

Tolectin DS

capsule

McNEIL
400 mg

TRAMADOL
Ultram

tablet

451
50 mg

TRAZODONE
Desyrel

tablets

50 mg 100 mg

150 mg

TRIAMTERENE/ HYDROCHLOROTHIAZIDE
Dyazide

capsule

50/25 mg

Maxzide

tablets

37.5/25 mg 75/50 mg

TRIFLUOPERAZINE
Stelazine

tablets

SKF 503 — 1 mg SKF 504 — 2 mg SKF 506 — 5 mg

TRIMETHOPRIM
Trimpex

tablet

100 mg

TROGLITAZONE
Rezulin

tablet

200 mg

VALACYCLOVIR
Valtrex

tablet

500 mg

VALPROIC ACID
Depakote Sprinkle

capsule

125 mg

Depakote

tablets

125 mg 250 mg

500 mg

VENLAFAXINE
Effexor

tablet

25 mg

VERAPAMIL
Calan

tablets

80 mg 120 mg

Calan SR

tablets, extended-release

120 mg 180 mg

240 mg

Verelan

capsules, extended-release

120 mg

Verelan
capsules, extended-release (cont.)

180 mg

240 mg

WARFARIN
Coumadin

tablets

1 mg 2 mg 2.5 mg

5 mg 7.5 mg 10 mg

ZAFIRLUKAST
Accolate

tablet

20 mg

ZALCITABINE
Hivid

tablets

HIVID 0.375 — 0.375 mg HIVID 0.750 — 0.750 mg

ZIDOVUDINE
Retrovir

capsule

100 mg

ZILEUTON
Zyflo

tablet

600 mg

> **While Taking This Drug, Observe the Following**
>> *Foods:* A high potassium diet may be advisable early in therapy. See Section Six for Table 13, "High Potassium Foods." Talk with your doctor before making any diet changes.
>> *Beverages:* No restrictions. May be taken with milk.
>> *Alcohol:* Alcohol can blunt the anticonvulsant effect of this drug and reduce seizure control.
>> *Tobacco Smoking:* No interactions expected, but I advise everyone to quit smoking.
>> *Other Drugs*
>>> Acetazolamide may *increase* the effects of
>>> • quinidine (Quinaglute, others).
>>> Acetazolamide may *decrease* the effects of
>>> • lithium (Lithobid, others).
>>> • oral antidiabetic drugs (see Drug Classes).
>>> Acetazolamide *taken concurrently* with
>>> • amphetamines may result in amphetamine toxicity. Amphetamine dose must be decreased.
>>> • anesthetic agents such as halothane may lead to metabolic problems (hypokalemia), which lead to heart and lung difficulties during surgery.
>>> • aspirin may result in aspirin toxicity. Watch for ringing in the ears, confusion, rapid heartbeat.
>>> • cyclosporine (Sandimmune) may lead to cyclosporine toxicity. Avoid combining where possible.
>>> • diflunisal (and perhaps other NSAIDs; see Drug Classes) may decrease elimination of acetazolamide and result in increased effects or toxicity.
>>> • phenytoin (Dilantin) may lead to bone problems (osteomalacia).
>>> • primidone (Mysoline) can decrease primidone blood levels and therapeutic effects. More frequent blood levels are needed.
>>> • theophylline (Theo-Dur, others) may increase the amount of fluid (diuresis) that is removed.
>>> • timolol (Timoptic) can help lower eye pressure more successfully than either agent alone.
>> *Driving, Hazardous Activities:* Drowsiness or dizziness may occur. Talk with your doctor about the individual effect of this medicine on your ability to perform such activities.
>> *Aviation Note:* The use of this drug *may be a disqualification* for piloting. Consult a designated Aviation Medical Examiner.
>> *Exposure to Sun:* No restrictions.

ACETIC ACIDS
(Nonsteroidal Anti-Inflammatory Drugs)

Diclofenac (di KLOH fen ak)   **Etodolac** (e TOE doh lak)   **Indomethacin** (in doh META a sin)   **Ketorolac** (KEY tor o lak)   **Nabumetone** (na BYU me tohn)   **Sulindac** (sul IN dak)   **Tolmetin** (TOHL met in)

Introduced: 1976, 1986, 1963, 1991, 1984, 1976, 1976, respectively   **Class:** NSAID, mild analgesic   **Prescription:** USA: Yes   **Controlled Drug:** USA:

No; Canada: No   **Available as Generic:**   USA: Yes: indomethacin, sulindac, tolmetin.; Canada: No

Brand Names: Indomethacin: ✦Apo-Indomethacin, Indameth, ✦Indocid, ✦Indocid-SR, ✦Indocid PDA, Indocin, Indocin-SR, ✦Novomethacin, ✦Nu-Indo, Zendole; Diclofenac: ✦Apo-Diclo, Cataflam, ✦Novo-Difenac, ✦Nu-Diclo, Voltaren, Voltaren SR, Voltaren Ophthalmic; Etodolac: Lodine, Lodine XL; Ketorolac: Toradol, Acular (ketorolac ophthalmic); Nabumetone: Relafen; Sulindac: ✦Apo-Sulin, Clinoril, ✦Novo-Sundac; Tolmetin: Tolectin, Tolectin DS, Tolectin 600

BENEFITS versus RISKS	
Possible Benefits	*Possible Risks*
EFFECTIVE RELIEF OF MILD TO MODERATE PAIN AND INFLAMMATION	Gastrointestinal pain, ulceration, bleeding
Easy change from the IM or IV form to the oral form (ketorolac)	Liver or kidney damage
Decreased stomach (GI) problems (etodolac)	Fluid retention
	Bone marrow depression
	Pneumonitis (sulindac)
	Aseptic meningitis (diclofenac)
	Possible severe skin reactions (diclofenac, etodolac, ketorolac, and sulindac)

▷ **Principal Uses**

As a Single Drug Product: Uses currently included in FDA-approved labeling: (1) All of the drugs in this class except ketorolac are approved to treat osteoarthritis; (2) all of the drugs in this class except ketorolac and etodolac are approved to relieve rheumatoid arthritis; (3) etodolac and ketorolac are used to treat mild to moderate pain; (4) diclofenac and sulindac are useful in ankylosing spondylitis; (5) sustained-release form of indomethacin as well as the immediate-release form of sulindac help symptoms of tendonitis, bursitis, and acute painful shoulder; (6) tolmetin eases symptoms of juvenile rheumatoid arthritis; (7) sulindac therapy is useful in acute gout; (8) ophthalmic form of diclofenac is useful after cataract surgery; (9) ketorolac ophthalmic dosing has been changed to open-ended status.

Other (unlabeled) generally accepted uses: (1) Diclofenac used intramuscularly is effective in acute migraine headache and kidney colic; (2) indomethacin helps reduce systemic reactions in kidney transplants, and addresses low-grade neonatal intraventricular hemorrhage; (3) ketorolac has been helpful in reducing swelling after cataract surgery and treating reflex sympathetic dystrophy by injection; (4) sulindac is effective in treating colon polyps (Gardner's syndrome) and easing diabetic neuropathic pain.

How These Drugs Work: It is thought that these drugs reduce tissue concentrations of prostaglandins (and related compounds), chemicals involved in the production of inflammation and pain.

Available Dosage Forms and Strengths

Indomethacin:

Capsules — 25 mg, 50 mg, 75 mg
Gelatin capsule (Canada) — 25 mg, 50 mg
Capsules, SR (prolonged action) — 75 mg

Oral suspension — 25 mg/ 5 ml
Suppositories — 50 mg, 100 mg
Diclofenac sodium:
Suppositories — 50 mg, 100 mg (Canada)
Tablets — 25 mg, 50 mg
Tablets, prolonged action — 50 mg, 75 mg, 100 mg (Canada)
Ophthalmic solution — 1 mg/ 1 ml
Etodolac:
Capsules — 200 mg, 300 mg
Tablets, extended-release form — 400 mg, 600 mg
Ketorolac:
Tablets — 10 mg
Ophthalmic solution — 3 ml, 5 ml and 10 ml (0.5%)
Injection — 15 mg, 30 mg
Nabumetone:
Tablets — 500 mg, 750 mg
Sulindac:
Tablets — 150 mg, 200 mg
Tolmetin:
Capsules — 400 mg, 492 mg
Gelatin capsules — 400 mg (Canada)
Tablets — 200 mg, 600 mg

▷ **Usual Adult Dosage Range:**   Indomethacin: For arthritis and related conditions: 25 to 50 mg two to four times daily. If needed and tolerated, dose may
be increased by 25 or 50 mg per day at intervals of 1 week. For acute gout:
100 mg initially; then 50 mg three times per day until pain is relieved. Maximum daily dose is 200 mg.
SR form: 75 mg daily for ankylosing spondylitis or rheumatoid arthritis.
Diclofenac potassium: Maximum daily dose is 200 mg.
Diclofenac sodium: 100 to 200 mg daily to start in two to five divided doses.
Reduction to the minimum effective dose is advisable. Maximum daily dose
is 225 mg.
Etodolac: For osteoarthritis: A starting dose of 800 to 1200 mg is given in
divided doses. The lowest effective dose is advisable, and effective treat-
ment has been accomplished with 200 to 400 mg daily.
Etodolac is available in an extended release form (Lodine XL), which
allows once-a-day dosing for many patients. Dosing range is 400 to 1000
mg daily. Maximum dose is 1000 mg daily.
Ketorolac: 10 mg is used every 4 to 6 hours for short-term treatment of pain.
Maximum daily dose is 40 mg orally. Ophthalmic dosing has been left open
ended in time frame.
Nabumentone: 1000 mg daily as a single dose is given. Dosage is increased as
needed and tolerated to 1500 mg daily. The lowest effective daily dose is
advisable. Maximum daily dose is 2000 mg.
Sulindac: Therapy is started with 150 to 200 mg twice daily taken 12 hours
apart. Maximum daily dose is 400 mg.
Tolmetin: 400 mg three times daily is started, with usual ongoing doses of 600
to 1600 mg as needed and tolerated. Total daily dose should not exceed
1600 mg for osteoarthritis or 2000 mg for rheumatoid arthritis.

Children 2 years of age or older may be given 20 mg per kg of body mass orally, divided into three or four doses daily. The dose may be increased as needed and tolerated to a maximum daily dose of 30 mg per kg of body mass.

Note: Actual dose and dosing schedule must be determined for each patient individually.

Conditions Requiring Dosing Adjustments

Liver Function: These drugs are extensively metabolized in the liver. They should be used with caution in patients with liver compromise.

Kidney Function: All nonsteroidal anti-inflammatory drugs may inhibit prostaglandins and alter kidney blood flow in patients with kidney (renal) compromise. Use with caution or not at all in patients with kidney compromise.

▷ **Dosing Instructions:**   Take with or following food to prevent stomach irritation. Take with a full glass of water and remain upright (do not lie down) for 30 minutes. Regular-release tablets may be crushed, but not extended-release forms. The regular capsules may be opened for administration, but not the prolonged-action capsules. Food actually increases absorption of nabumetone. Ketorolac ophthalmic should NOT be used while soft contacts are worn.

Usual Duration of Use: Continual use on a regular schedule for 1 to 2 weeks is usually necessary to determine drug benefit in relieving arthritic discomfort. The usual length of treatment for bursitis or tendonitis for indomethacin or sulindac is 7 to 14 days. Ketorolac oral or IV is used for short-term pain treatment, while ophthalmic dosing is open ended. Long-term use of the other agents in this class requires physician supervision and periodic evaluation.

These Drugs Should Not Be Taken If

- you have had an allergic reaction to them previously.
- you are subject to asthma or nasal polyps caused by aspirin.
- you are pregnant (all NSAIDs during the last 3 months of pregnancy) or you are breast-feeding.
- you have active peptic ulcer disease or any form of gastrointestinal ulceration or bleeding.
- you have active liver disease.
- you have a bleeding disorder or a blood cell disorder.
- you have severe impairment of kidney function.
- you have a history (indomethacin suppositories) of rectal bleeding or proctitis.
- you have porphyria (diclofenac, indomethacin).

▷ **Inform Your Physician Before Taking This Drug If**

- you are allergic to aspirin or to other aspirin substitutes.
- you have a history of peptic ulcer disease, Crohn's disease, ulcerative colitis, or any type of bleeding disorder.
- you have a history of epilepsy, Parkinson's disease, or mental illness (psychosis).
- you have impaired liver or kidney function.
- you have high blood pressure or a history of heart failure.
- you are taking acetaminophen, aspirin, or other aspirin substitutes or anticoagulants.

Possible Side Effects (natural, expected, and unavoidable drug actions)
Drowsiness, ringing in ears, fluid retention.

> **Possible Adverse Effects** (unusual, unexpected, and infrequent reactions)
If any of the following develop, consult your physician promptly for guidance.
Mild Adverse Effects
Allergic reactions: skin rash, hives, itching, localized swellings of face and/or extremities.
Headache—infrequent to frequent (indomethacin); dizziness, feelings of detachment—infrequent.
Mouth sores, indigestion, nausea, vomiting, diarrhea—infrequent.
Ringing in the ears—possible.
Temporary loss of hair (indomethacin)—case reports.
Serious Adverse Effects
Allergic reactions: worsening of asthma, difficult breathing, mouth irritation.
Blurred vision, confusion, depression—rare.
Active peptic ulcer, with or without bleeding—possible.
Liver damage with jaundice (see Glossary)—case reports.
Kidney damage with painful urination, bloody urine, reduced urine formation—rare.
Bone marrow depression (see Glossary): fatigue, fever, sore throat, bleeding, or bruising—case reports.
Severe skin rash (Stevens-Johnson syndrome—diclofenac, ketorolac, etodolac, sulindac)—case reports.
Fluid retention, increased blood pressure, or edema—possible with all.
Congestive heart failure (indomethacin)—case reports.
Peripheral neuritis (see Glossary): numbness, pain in extremities (indomethacin)—rare.
Lung fibrosis (nabumetone)—case reports.
Pancreatitis (sulindac)—rare; (indomethacin)—case reports.
Pneumonitis (sulindac)—rare.
Aseptic meningitis (diclofenac)—rare.
Seizures (indomethacin only)—case reports.

▷ **Possible Effects on Sexual Function**
Enlargement and tenderness of both male and female breasts (indomethacin, sulindac)—rare.
Nonmenstrual vaginal bleeding (indomethacin)—rare.
Impotence (indomethacin, diclofenac, nabumetone)—rare. Decreased libido (indomethacin)—rare.
Uterine bleeding (etodolac, sulindac)—rare.

Possible Delayed Adverse Effects: Mild anemia due to "silent" blood loss from the stomach.

Adverse Effects That May Mimic Natural Diseases or Disorders
Liver reactions may suggest viral hepatitis. Pancreatitis has occurred with sulindac.

Natural Diseases or Disorders That May Be Activated by These Drugs
Peptic ulcer disease, ulcerative colitis.

Possible Effects on Laboratory Tests
> Complete blood cell counts: decreased red cells, hemoglobin, white cells, and platelets—rare.
> INR (prothrombin time): increased.
> Blood lithium level: increased.
> Liver function tests: increased liver enzymes (ALT/GPT, AST/GOT and alkaline phosphatase), increased bilirubin.
> Blood sugar (glucose): increased (indomethacin only)—rare.
> Kidney function tests: increased blood creatinine and urea nitrogen (BUN) levels (kidney damage).
> Fecal occult blood test: positive.
> Urine protein: tolmetin only: may be falsely positive.

CAUTION
1. Dose should be limited to the smallest amount that produces reasonable improvement.
2. These drugs may mask early signs of infection. Tell your doctor if you think you are developing an infection of any kind.

Precautions for Use
> *By Infants and Children:* Indomethacin: This drug frequently impairs kidney function in infants. Fatal liver reactions are possible in children between 6 and 12 years of age; avoid the use of this drug in this age group. Note: This medicine is used in infants (patent ductus arteriosus intravenously).
> Diclofenac, etodolac, ketorolac, nabumetone, sulindac: Safety and efficacy for those under 12 years of age not established.
> Tolmetin: Safety and efficacy for those under 2 years of age not established.
> *By Those Over 60 Years of Age:* Small doses are advisable until tolerance is determined. Watch for any signs of liver or kidney toxicity, fluid retention, dizziness, confusion, impaired memory, depression, peptic ulcer, or diarrhea, often with rectal bleeding.

▷ **Advisability of Use During Pregnancy**
> *Pregnancy Category:* Indomethacin, diclofenac, tolmetin: B. Indomethacin, etodolac, ketorolac, nabumetone, and sulindac: D. (Indomethacin is category D if used after 34 weeks or for more than 48 hours); See Pregnancy Risk Categories at the back of this book.
> Animal studies: Indomethacin: significant toxicity and birth defects reported in mice and rats.
> Diclofenac: Mouse, rat, and rabbit studies reveal toxic effects on the embryo but no birth defects.
> Ketorolac: Rat and rabbit studies did not reveal teratogenicity, however, oral dosing after the 17th day of pregnancy caused increased pup mortality.
> Nabumetone, tolmetin: Rat and rabbit studies revealed no defects.
> Human studies: Indomethacin: adequate studies of pregnant women are not available. However, birth defects have been attributed to the use of this drug during pregnancy.
>> The manufacturer recommends that indomethacin not be taken during pregnancy.
> Diclofenac, nabumetone, sulindac, tolmetin: Adequate studies of pregnant women are not available. Avoid this drug completely during the last 3 months of pregnancy. Use it during the first 6 months only if clearly needed. Ask your doctor for guidance.

Ketorolac: Adequate studies of pregnant women are not available. Ask your doctor for guidance.

Etodolac: Adequate studies of pregnant women not available. The manufacturer advises that this drug be avoided during pregnancy.

Advisability of Use If Breast-Feeding
Presence of these drugs in breast milk: Yes (all)

Avoid drugs or refrain from nursing (may have bad effects on infant's nervous system).

Habit-Forming Potential: None.

Effects of Overdosage: Drowsiness, agitation, confusion, nausea, vomiting, diarrhea, disorientation, seizures, coma.

Possible Effects of Long-Term Use: Indomethacin and tolmetin: eye changes—deposits in the cornea, alterations in the retina.

Suggested Periodic Examinations While Taking These Drugs (at physician's discretion)
Complete blood cell counts, liver and kidney function tests, complete eye examinations if vision is altered in any way.

While Taking These Drugs, Observe the Following
Foods: No restrictions. These medicines are taken with food to decrease stomach irritation.

Nutritional Support: Indomethacin: Take 50 mg of vitamin C (ascorbic acid) daily.

Beverages: No restrictions. May be taken with milk.

▷   *Alcohol:* Use with caution. Alcohol can irritate the stomach lining, and when this is added to irritation from these drugs, can increase the risk of stomach ulceration and/or bleeding.

Tobacco Smoking: No interactions expected, but I advise everyone to quit smoking.

▷   *Other Drugs*

Medications in this class may ***increase*** the effects of
- acetaminophen (Tylenol, etc.), and increase the risk of kidney damage; avoid prolonged use of this combination (no indomethacin data).
- aminoglycoside antibiotics (amikacin, others see Drug Classes) by increasing blood levels.
- anticoagulants such as warfarin (Coumadin), and increase the risk of bleeding; monitor INR (prothrombin time), adjust dose accordingly.
- cyclosporine (Sandimmune) and cause toxicity.
- digoxin (Lanoxin)—indomethacin only.
- lithium, and cause lithium toxicity (except sulindac, which may decrease lithium levels).
- methotrexate (Mexate, others) and cause toxic levels.
- phenytoin (Dilantin) because of increased phenytoin blood levels.
- thrombolytics such as streptokinase or TPA.
- zidovudine (AZT) and lead to toxicity of either medicine (indomethacin).

Medications in this class may ***decrease*** the effects of
- ACE inhibitors (see Drug Classes).
- beta-blocker drugs (see Drug Classes), and reduce their antihypertensive effectiveness.

- bumetanide (Bumex).
- captopril (Capoten).
- ethacrynic acid (Edecrin).
- furosemide (Lasix) and other loop diuretics.
- thiazide diuretics (see Drug Classes).

Medications in this class *taken concurrently* with the following drugs may increase the risk of bleeding or serious side effects; avoid these combinations:

- aspirin or other NSAIDs.
- dicumarol.
- diflunisal (Dolobid).
- dipyridamole (Persantine).
- probenecid (Pro-Biosan, others).
- sulfinpyrazone (Anturane).
- valproic acid (Depakene).
- warfarin (Coumadin).

▷ *Driving, Hazardous Activities:* These drugs may cause drowsiness, dizziness, or impaired vision. Restrict activities as necessary.

Aviation Note: The use of these drugs *may be a disqualification* for piloting. Consult a designated Aviation Medical Examiner.

Exposure to Sun: Use caution. Several of the medicines in this class have caused increased sensitivity (photosensitivity—see Glossary) to the sun.

ACYCLOVIR (ay SI kloh ver)

Other Name: Acycloguanosine   **Introduced:** 1979   **Class:** Antiviral
Prescription: USA: Yes   **Controlled Drug:** USA: No; Canada: No   **Available as Generic:** Yes (capsule, suspension, and tablets)
Brand Name: Zovirax

BENEFITS versus RISKS	
Possible Benefits	*Possible Risks*
FASTER RECOVERY FROM INITIAL EPISODE OF GENITAL HERPES	Nausea, vomiting, diarrhea
Prevention of recurrence of genital herpes	Joint and muscle pain
Lessens the severity of chickenpox in some children	Seizures or coma with IV use (rare)
May reduce acute pain in herpes zoster	

Author's Note: This medication was rejected by the FDA for a change to nonprescription "over-the-counter" (OTC) status. This was based on fear of development of viral resistance—NOT safety issues.

▷ **Principal Uses**

As a Single Drug Product: Uses currently included in FDA-approved labeling: (1) Treats or helps prevent genital herpes; (2) used to lessen the severity of chickenpox in children using inhaled steroids or who have a lung disease or who are otherwise healthy; (3) treats shingles (herpes zoster); (4) treats skin and mucous infections (mucocutaneous) caused by herpes simplex in patients with immune problems; (5) used to treat brain infections caused by herpes simplex; (6) used to prevent herpes simplex virus infections in bone marrow transplant patients; (6) treats varicella (chickenpox) in children over a year old who have a chronic pulmonary condition or a chronic skin condition, children receiving short courses of corticosteroids via the lungs, or children who are over 13 years old and are otherwise healthy.

Other (unlabeled) generally accepted uses: (1) Acyclovir helps treat herpes simplex infections of the eye and rectum, and pneumonia caused by the chickenpox (varicella) virus; (2) some data support its use in nonmalignant skin growths in the throat (laryngeal papillomatosis); (3) it is a trial (in combination) AIDS treatment; (4) can prevent recurrent erythema multiforme that may occur with herpes simplex infections.

How This Drug Works: By blocking genetic material formation of the herpes simplex virus, this drug stops viral multiplication and spread, reducing severity and duration of the herpes infection.

Available Dosage Forms and Strengths
>
      Capsules — 200 mg
      Intravenous — 500 mg, 1 g
Oral suspension — 200 mg/5 ml
            Tablets — 200 mg (Canada only), 400 mg and 800 mg
      Ointment — 5%, 50 mg/g (Canada)

▷ **Recommended Dosage Ranges** (Actual dosage and administration schedule must be determined for each patient individually.)

Infants and Children: Safety and efficacy of oral use in children younger than 6 weeks of age has NOT been established. Topical acyclovir use data in children less than 10 is lacking; however, the drug would be expected to follow the same patterns of side effects and risk-to-benefit decisions as the oral formulation.

18 to 65 Years of Age: For initial episode of genital herpes: 200 mg every 4 hours for a total of five capsules daily for 7 to 10 days (or until what your doctor describes as "clinical resolution" happens). Some clinicians use 400 mg three times a day for 7 to 10 days. For intermittent recurrence: 200 mg every 4 hours for a total of five capsules daily for 5 consecutive days (total dose of 25 capsules) or 400 mg three times a day for 5 days. Start treatment at the earliest sign of recurrence. For prevention of frequent recurrence: 400 mg taken twice daily for up to 12 months, and then evaluation of ongoing need for this medicine. For the ointment form: Cover all infected areas every 3 hours for a total of six times daily for 7 consecutive days. Start treatment at the **earliest sign** of infection.

In attempting to decrease the pain of herpes zoster: 800 mg five times daily for 7–10 days.

Treatment of chickenpox (for those 2 or older): 20 mg per kg of body mass (do not exceed 800 mg) orally, four times a day for 5 days. If over 40 kg: 800 mg four times daily for 5 days. Start treatment at the first symptom or sign.

Over 65 Years of Age: The dose **must** be adjusted if the kidneys are impaired.

Conditions Requiring Dosing Adjustments

Liver Function: Specific adjustment in liver dysfunction is not defined.

Kidney Function: The dose MUST be adjusted in people with compromised kidney function. For example: creatinine clearance of 25–50 ml/min gets usual dose every 12 hours; 10–25 ml/min gets usual dose once daily.

Obesity: Dosing here (intravenous form) should be made on ideal body weight and given as 10 mg per kg of body mass. Maximum dose is 500 mg per square meter every 8 hours.

▷ **Dosing Instructions:**   May be taken without regard to food. Capsule may be opened to take it. The maker of this medicine recommends drinking 1 liter of fluid for each gram (1000 mg) of this medicine that is taken. Take the full course of the exact dose prescribed. Use a finger cot or rubber glove to apply the ointment.

Usual Duration of Use: Use on a regular schedule for 10 days is usually needed to see this drug's effect in reducing the severity and duration of the initial infection. Continual use for 6 months may be needed to prevent frequent recurrence of herpes eruptions.

▷ **This Drug Should Not Be Taken If**
  • you have had an allergic reaction to it previously.

▷ **Inform Your Physician Before Taking This Drug If**
  • you have impaired liver or kidney function.
  • you are taking any other drugs at this time.
  • you think you are dehydrated and can't or will not drink water.
  • you are unsure of how much or how often to take acyclovir.

Possible Side Effects (natural, expected, and unavoidable drug actions)
  With use of capsules—none.
  With use of ointment—mild pain or stinging at site of application.

▷ **Possible Adverse Effects** (unusual, unexpected, and infrequent reactions)
  If any of the following develop, consult your physician promptly for guidance.
  Mild Adverse Effects
  Allergic reaction: skin rash.
  Headache, dizziness, nervousness, confusion, insomnia, depression, fatigue—rare.
  Nausea, vomiting, diarrhea—infrequent with IV form.
  Joint pains, muscle cramps—rare.
  Acne, hair loss—rare.
  Serious Adverse Effects
  Superficial thrombophlebitis—infrequent with IV form.
  Seizures or coma with IV use—rare.
  Kidney problems—rare.
  Lowered red or white blood cells or platelets—rare.
  Colitis—case reports.

▷ **Possible Effects on Sexual Function:**   Altered timing and pattern of menstruation—case reports.

Possible Effects on Laboratory Tests
  Complete blood cell counts: decreased red cells , white cells, or hemoglobin—rare.
  Blood urea nitrogen (BUN) or creatinine: increased—rare.
  Liver function tests: increased—rare.

CAUTION
1. This drug does **not** eliminate all herpes virus and is **not a cure**. Recurrence is possible. Resume treatment at the earliest sign of infection.
2. Avoid sexual intercourse if herpes blisters and swelling are present.
3. Do not exceed the prescribed dosage.
4. Tell your doctor if frequency or severity of infections don't improve.
5. The maker of this medicine recommends 1 liter (1000 ml) of fluid for each gram (1000 mg) of the oral or intravenous form of this medicine taken.

Precautions for Use
By Infants and Children: Specific dosing is required for children and fluid intake must be adequate.
By Those Over 60 Years of Age: Avoid dehydration. Drink 2 to 3 quarts of liquids daily.

▷ **Advisability of Use During Pregnancy**
Pregnancy Category: C. See Pregnancy Risk Categories at the back of this book. The company has a pregnancy registry at 1–800–722–9292.
Animal studies: No birth defects found in mouse, rat, or rabbit studies.
Human studies: The pregnancy registry has followed more than 400 cases to date. There was no consistent pattern of birth defects, and the number of patients (sample size) is still too small to detect small increases in risk. Avoid use if possible. Use only if clearly needed.

Advisability of Use If Breast-Feeding
Presence of this drug in breast milk: Yes.
Ask your physician for guidance.

Habit-Forming Potential: None.

Effects of Overdosage: Possible impairment of kidney function, increased occurrence of existing possible adverse effects.

Possible Effects of Long-Term Use: Development of acyclovir-resistant strains of herpes virus. Treatment will fail if this occurs.

Suggested Periodic Examinations While Taking This Drug (at physician's discretion)
Kidney function tests.

▷ **While Taking This Drug, Observe the Following**
Foods: No restrictions.
Beverages: No restrictions. May be taken with milk. **Drink 2 to 3 quarts of liquids** (if not contraindicated for you) **daily.**
▷ *Alcohol:* Use caution; dizziness or fatigue may be accentuated.
Tobacco Smoking: No interactions expected, but I advise everyone to quit smoking.
▷ *Other Drugs*
The following drugs may *increase* the effects of acyclovir:
- cyclosporine (Sandimmune): Use may result in increased risk of kidney toxicity.
- probenecid (Benemid): May delay acyclovir elimination.
Acyclovir *taken concurrently* with
- meperidine (Demerol) may result in neurologic problems.

- varicella vaccine (Varivax) will blunt the vaccine effectiveness.
- zidovudine (AZT) may result in severe fatigue and lethargy.

▷ *Driving, Hazardous Activities:* Use caution if dizziness or fatigue occurs.

Aviation Note: The use of this drug **may be a disqualification** for piloting. Consult a designated Aviation Medical Examiner.

Exposure to Sun: No restrictions; however, some data indicates that sun exposure may trigger release of herpes simplex from its dormant state (from the optic nerve).

ALBUTEROL (al BYU ter ohl)

Other Name: Salbutamol

Introduced: 1968   **Class:** Antiasthmatic, bronchodilator   **Prescription:** USA: Yes   **Controlled Drug:** USA: No; Canada: No   **Available as Generic:** Yes

Brand Names: ✦Apo-Salvent, ✦Novo-Salmol, Proventil HFA, Proventil Inhaler, Proventil Repetabs, Proventil Tablets, ✦Salbutamol, ✦Ventodisk, Ventolin Inhaler, Ventolin Nebules, Ventolin Rotacaps, Ventolin Syrup, Ventolin Tablets, ✦Volmax Controlled-Release Tablets, Volmax Extended-Release Tablets

BENEFITS versus RISKS	
Possible Benefits	*Possible Risks*
VERY EFFECTIVE RELIEF OF BRONCHOSPASM	Increased blood pressure Fine hand tremor Irregular heart rhythm and fatalities (with excessive use)

▷ **Principal Uses**

As a Single Drug Product: Uses currently included in FDA-approved labeling: (1) Relieves acute bronchial asthma and reduces frequency and severity of chronic, recurrent asthmatic attacks; (2) helps prevent exercise-induced bronchospasm.

Other (unlabeled) generally accepted uses: May have a role (nebulized route) in some cases where blood potassium is too high.

How This Drug Works: By increasing cyclic AMP, this drug relaxes constricted bronchial muscles to relieve asthmatic wheezing.

Available Dosage Forms and Strengths

Aerosol — 90 mcg per actuation
Capsules for inhalation — 200 mcg, 400 mcg (Canada)
Nasal inhaler (Canada) — 100 mcg/dose
Solution for inhalation — 0.83 mg/ml and 5 mg/ml
Syrup — 2 mg/5 ml
— 2.4 mg/5 ml
Rotacaps — 200 mcg
Tablets — 2 mg, 4 mg
— 2.4 mg, 4.8 mg (Canada)
Tablets, controlled release (Canada) — 4 mg, 8 mg

Tablets, extended release — 4 mg, 8 mg, 9 mg
Ventodisk (Canada) — 200 mcg and 400 mcg per disk

▷ **Recommended Dosage Ranges** (Actual dosage and administration schedule must be determined for each patient individually.)
Inhaler—Adults and children 12 or older: Two inhalations repeated every 4 to 6 hours. For some patients, one inhalation every 4 hours may be enough. Taking a larger number of inhalations is **not** recommended. If the dose that previously worked does not provide relief, call your doctor **immediately**, as the status of your asthma must be examined. Tablets (immediate release)—2 to 4 mg three to four times daily, every 4 to 6 hours; (sustained release)—1 or 2 tablets every 12 hours. **Do not exceed** eight inhalations (720 mcg) every 24 hours, or 32 mg (tablet form) every 24 hours.
Author's Note: Proventil FHA was recently FDA approved, and dosing is still pending.

Conditions Requiring Dosing Adjustments
Liver Function: Use with caution and in low doses in people with liver compromise.
Kidney Function: No specific changes in dosing are available.
Coronary Artery Disease: A maximum starting dose should be 1 mg in order to avoid chest pain (angina).
Thyroid Disease: People with low (hypoactive) thyroids may require increased doses.

▷ **Dosing Instructions:** May be taken on empty stomach or with food or milk. Nonsustained-release tablets may be crushed. Sustained-release forms should NEVER be crushed. For inhaler, follow the written instructions carefully. Do not use excessively.

Usual Duration of Use: Do not use beyond the time necessary to stop episodes of asthma.

▷ **This Drug Should Not Be Taken If**
- you have had an allergic reaction to any dosage form of it.
- you have an irregular heart rhythm.
- you are taking, or took within the past 2 weeks, any monoamine oxidase (MAO) type A inhibitor drug (see Drug Classes).

▷ **Inform Your Physician Before Taking This Drug If**
- you have a heart or circulatory disorder, especially high blood pressure or coronary heart disease.
- you have diabetes.
- you have an overactive thyroid (hyperthyroid).
- you are taking any form of digitalis or any stimulant drug.
- you take other prescription or nonprescription medications that were not discussed when albuterol was prescribed for you.
- you are going to have a baby (this medicine may make contractions difficult to have).
- you are unsure how much to take or how often to take albuterol.

Possible Side Effects (natural, expected, and unavoidable drug actions)
Aerosol: dryness or irritation of mouth or throat, altered taste.
Tablet: nervousness, palpitation, fast heart rate (tachycardia)—infrequent.

▷ **Possible Adverse Effects** (unusual, unexpected, and infrequent reactions)
　　If any of the following develop, consult your physician promptly for guidance.

Mild Adverse Effects
　　Itching—rare.
　　Headache, dizziness, restlessness, insomnia—infrequent.
　　Fine hand tremor—frequent.
　　Nausea—rare.
　　Leg cramps, flushing of skin—rare.
　　Difficulty urinating—rare.
　　Rapid heart rate—infrequent.
　　Decreased platelets—possible, but not clinically significant.

Serious Adverse Effects
　　Heart attack—case reports after intravenous use.
　　Chest pain—possible with higher doses in patients with coronary artery disease.
　　Hallucinations or convulsions (with excessive dosing)—possible.
　　Decreased blood potassium (hypokalemia)—possible and dose related.
　　High blood sugar (hyperglycemia)—possible and more likely with intravenous use.

▷ **Possible Effects on Sexual Function:**　None reported.

Natural Diseases or Disorders That May Be Activated by This Drug
　　Latent coronary artery disease, diabetes, or high blood pressure.

Possible Effects on Laboratory Tests
　　Blood aldosterone: increased.
　　Blood HDL cholesterol level: increased.
　　Blood glucose level: increased.
　　Blood potassium: decreased.
　　Blood platelets: decreased (with high doses).

CAUTION
　　1. This drug may be dangerous if patients increase their dose and/or frequency, as it may result in rapid or irregular heart rhythm and fatalities with overuse.
　　2. Use of this drug by inhalation with beclomethasone aerosol (Beclovent, Vanceril) may increase the risk of fluorocarbon propellant toxicity. Use albuterol aerosol 20 to 30 minutes *before* beclomethasone aerosol to reduce toxicity and enhance the penetration of beclomethasone.
　　3. Serious heart rhythm problems or cardiac arrest can result from excessive or prolonged inhalation.
　　4. Call your doctor if you begin to increase the number of times you use this drug on a daily basis.

Precautions for Use
　By Infants and Children: Used to help prevent bronchospasm caused by exercise in children ages 4–11.
　By Those Over 60 Years of Age: Avoid excessive and continual use. If asthma is not relieved promptly, other drugs will have to be tried. Watch for nervousness, palpitations, irregular heart rhythm, and muscle tremors.

▷ **Advisability of Use During Pregnancy**
　Pregnancy Category: C. See Pregnancy Risk Categories at the back of this book.

Animal studies: Cleft palate reported in mice.
Human studies: Adequate studies of pregnant women are not available.
Avoid use during first 3 months if possible.

Advisability of Use If Breast-Feeding
Presence of this drug in breast milk: Unknown.
Avoid drug or refrain from nursing.

Habit-Forming Potential: A few cases of dependency and abuse have been described. These may be cases of use for the effect of the propellants or the drug itself.

Effects of Overdosage: Nervousness, palpitation, rapid heart rate, life-threatening arrhythmias, sweating, headache, tremor, vomiting, chest pain.

Possible Effects of Long-Term Use: Loss of effectiveness.

Suggested Periodic Examinations While Taking This Drug (at physician's discretion)
Blood pressure measurements, evaluation of heart status.

▷ **While Taking This Drug, Observe the Following**
Foods: No restrictions.
Beverages: Avoid excessive caffeine as found in coffee, tea, cola, chocolate.
▷ *Alcohol:* No interactions expected.
Tobacco Smoking: No interactions expected; however, smoking may cause problems with other medications used to treat asthma. I advise everyone to quit smoking.
▷ *Other Drugs*
Albuterol *taken concurrently* with
- amphetamines may result in worsening of cardiovascular side effects.
- bendroflumethiazide (Corzide, Naturetin) and other thiazide and loop diuretics (see Drug Classes) may result in additive lowering of blood potassium.
- beta-blockers such as propranolol (Inderal) results in loss of effect of both medications.
- dopamine (Intropin) may worsen adverse effects on the heart. Avoid this combination.
- ephedrine (Bronkaid, Tedrigen) excessive heart effects.
- ipratropium (Atrovent) can result in better (longer time) opening of the bronchi (beneficial interaction).
- isoproterenol (Isuprel) may result in worsening of heart (cardiac) side effects.
- monoamine oxidase (MAO) type A inhibitor drugs can cause very high blood pressure and undesirable heart stimulation.
- phenylpropanolamine (Acutrim, Alka-Seltzer Plus, Contac, others) may worsen bad effects on the heart (adverse reaction). Do not combine.
- pseudoephedrine (Sudafed, others) may worsen adverse heart effects. DO NOT COMBINE.
- theophylline (Theo-Dur, others) may result in rapid removal of theophylline and loss of therapeutic theophylline effect.
- tricyclic antidepressants (see Drug Classes) may cause a severe increase in blood pressure.
▷ *Driving, Hazardous Activities:* Use caution if excessive nervousness or dizziness occurs.

Aviation Note: The use of this drug *is a disqualification* for piloting. Consult a designated Aviation Medical Examiner.

Exposure to Sun: No restrictions.

Heavy Exercise or Exertion: Use caution. Excessive exercise can cause (induce) asthma in some asthmatics.

ALENDRONATE (a LEN druh nate)

Introduced: 1996   **Class:** Aminobisphosphonate   **Prescription:** USA: Yes   **Controlled Drug:** USA: No   **Available as Generic:** No   **Brand Name:** Fosamax

BENEFITS versus RISKS	
Possible Benefits	*Possible Risks*
EFFECTIVE TREATMENT OF OSTEOPOROSIS	Esophageal irritation
INCREASE IN BONE MASS	Minor muscle pain
EXPECTED PREVENTION OF OSTEOPOROSIS	
DECREASED RISK OF BONE FRACTURES	
SYMPTOM RELIEF IN PAGET'S DISEASE	
PREVENTION OF POSTMENOPAUSAL OSTEOPOROSIS (new indication)	

▷ **Principal Uses**

As a Single Drug Product: Uses currently included in FDA-approved labeling: (1) Treatment of postmenopausal osteoporosis; (2) treatment of Paget's disease; (3) prevention of postmenopausal osteoporosis.

Other (unlabeled) generally accepted uses: Expected to work in the prevention and treatment of male osteoporosis.

How This Drug Works: This medicine works at the brush border of the osteoclast cell. This effectively prevents this cell from resorbing bone while letting the osteoblast or bone-building cell continue to work. The net benefit is stronger bone and decreased risk of fractures.

Available Dosage Forms and Strengths

Tablets — 5 mg, 10 mg, and 40 mg

▷ **Recommended Dosage Ranges:** (Actual dosage and administration schedule must be determined for each patient individually.)

Infants and Children: Efficacy and safety are not established.

18 to 65 Years of Age: In female postmenopausal osteoporosis: 10 mg taken once daily.

Osteoporosis prevention: 5 mg once daily.

I strongly recommend an appropriate amount of dietary calcium and/or calcium supplementation to ensure adequate calcium intake *every day*. Discuss the need for vitamin D with your doctor. Calcium and vitamin D are critical in osteoporosis prevention and treatment.

Paget's disease: 40 mg once daily for 6 months.

Over 65 Years of Age: Same as in those 18 to 65 years old.

Conditions Requiring Dosing Adjustments

Liver Function: The liver is not involved in the elimination of this medicine. No changes needed.

Kidney Function: Lower doses are needed for patients with kidney compromise. Patients with creatinine clearances (see Glossary) of less than 35 ml/min **should not** be given this medicine.

▷ **Dosing Instructions:**   TAKE THIS MEDICINE WITH 6 TO 8 OUNCES OF TAP WATER TO GET THE BEST RESULTS. DO NOT take this medicine with food or other medicines as the therapeutic benefit will be decreased. Take it at least half an hour before the first food or liquids (other than plain water) of the day. Waiting longer than 30 minutes to eat or drink will further improve the absorption of alendronate. In order to decrease the risk of irritation or ulceration of the esophagus, DO NOT lie down for at least 30 minutes (preferably an hour) after taking this medication.

Usual Duration of Use: In Paget's disease, this medicine is used once daily for 6 months, with reassessment after that course of therapy. In treating osteoporosis in postmenopausal women, many physicians will obtain a bone mineral density test (DEXA is presently the most widely used) to help in the decision to start treatment, and then get a second measurement 1 to 2 years later in order to assess the outcome of therapy. Further study is needed to identify the best dosing strategies in long-term (greater than 3 years) use of alendronate. Prevention of postmenopausal osteoporosis involves assessment and appropriate follow-up.

Possible Advantages of This Drug

This drug increases bone mass to a greater extent than other (anti-resorptive) therapies, which then decreases the risk of fractures.

This medicine also helps form bone of normal form (microarchitecture).

Better side-effect profile than earlier bisphosphonates.

▷ **This Drug Should Not Be Taken If**
  - you are allergic to the drug or any of the components of the tablets.
  - you have a low blood calcium (hypocalcemia). Talk with your doctor.
  - you have a significant kidney disease (this medicine should NOT be taken if creatinine clearance is less than 35 ml/min, because of lack of data in this population).
  - you are unable to sit or stand for 30 minutes after taking this medicine (can increase risk of esophageal problems).
  - you are pregnant or are nursing your infant.
  - you have esophageal disease (abnormal esophagus) or difficulty emptying the esophagus.

▷ **Inform Your Physician Before Taking This Drug If**
  - you have ulcers or inflammation of the duodenum.
  - you have difficulty swallowing.
  - you have a vitamin D deficiency.
  - you have a diet poor in calcium (low calcium diet).

Possible Side Effects (natural, expected, and unavoidable drug actions)
Irritation of the esophagus and potential ulceration—rare. This effect may be worsened if patients lie down soon after taking this medicine.

▷ **Possible Adverse Effects** (unusual, unexpected, and infrequent reactions)
If any of the following develop, consult your physician promptly for guidance.

Mild Adverse Effects
Allergic reactions: rare skin rash or redness.
Headache—infrequent.
Gas (flatulence), diarrhea, or constipation—infrequent.
Pain in the muscles or skeleton (musculoskeletal)—infrequent.
Mild decrease in calcium—2% decrease in some patients taking 10 mg daily.
Mild decrease in phosphorous—up to 6%.
Mild muscle pain—infrequent with the 10-mg dose.
Fever (drug fever) with intravenous use—rare.

Serious Adverse Effects
Allergic reactions: none reported.
Esophageal ulceration—rare. (May be worsened if you lie down immediately after taking this medicine. It is best NOT to lie down for at least half an hour after taking this medicine.)
One case report of a patient with a history of peptic ulcer disease who had stomach surgery and who was also taking aspirin developed an ulcer (anastomotic) and had mild hemorrhaging.

▷ **Possible Effects on Sexual Function:**   None reported.

Possible Effects on Laboratory Tests
Serum calcium: lowered.
Liver function tests: rarely increased in patients given the intravenous form (asymptomatic and transient).

CAUTION
1. A "dear doctor" letter was sent out by the FDA warning of increased occurrence of esophageal ulceration. This may have been caused by patients taking the medicine with less water than directed. It is also advisable NOT TO LIE DOWN for 30 minutes after taking this medicine; and patients should eat BEFORE they lie down.
2. Patients who take more than 10 mg of alendronate a day should avoid aspirin and aspirin-containing compounds because upper gastrointestinal adverse effects may be increased in this situation if the medicines are combined.
3. Other causes of osteoporosis besides estrogen or aging (secondary osteoporosis) must be ruled out.
4. Depression was recently found to be a risk factor for osteoporosis. Talk with your doctor if depression is a problem for you.

Precautions for Use
By Infants and Children: Safety and efficacy in this age group have not been established.
By Those Over 60 Years of Age: The amount that goes into the body (bioavailability) and the places alendronate goes to (disposition) are similar as for those less than 60. No specific dosing changes are needed for those in this age group.

Advisability of Use During Pregnancy

Pregnancy Category: C. See Pregnancy Risk Categories at the back of this book. Studies in rats have shown toxicity to the mother as well as neonatal death following dosing of alendronate during pregnancy. Adequate studies of pregnant women are not available. Avoid this medicine during pregnancy.

Advisability of Use If Breast-Feeding

Presence of this drug in breast milk: Yes in rats; unknown in humans. Avoid drug or refrain from nursing.

Habit-Forming Potential: None.

Effects of Overdosage: Nausea, vomiting, hypocalcemia, and hypophosphatemia. Heartburn, ulceration of the upper gastrointestinal tract.

Possible Effects of Long-Term Use: Increased bone density and decreased fracture risk (beneficial).

Suggested Periodic Examinations While Taking This Drug (at physician's discretion)

Measurement of bone mineral density.
Blood calcium. Measurement of height.

▷ **While Taking This Drug, Observe the Following**

Foods: Intake of adequate elemental calcium is needed; however, calcium supplements (classified as a food) should be taken at least half an hour after taking alendronate.

Beverages: Any liquid other than water will decrease the amount of alendronate that gets into your body to help you. It is critical that this medicine only be taken with 6 to 8 ounces of water.

▷ *Alcohol:* Alcohol (especially in high doses) may act as a bone-forming cell (osteoblast) poison and excessive use is a risk factor for osteoporosis. Alcohol may also irritate the stomach lining.

Tobacco Smoking: Tobacco may act to increase the elimination of estrogen and is a risk factor for osteoporosis. Smoking is never advisable.

▷ *Other Drugs*

Alendronate *taken concurrently* with

- antacids may decrease the total absorption of alendronate and decrease its therapeutic benefit.
- aspirin or aspirin-containing products or salicylates may pose an increased risk of upper gastrointestinal adverse effects if more than 10 mg of alendronate is taken daily. Although other NSAIDs (see Drug Classes) were not presented as potential problems with alendronate doses greater than 10 mg, caution is advised.
- estrogens (various) were taken by a small number of women in the clinical trials of this medicine without any adverse effects. The combination is not presently recommended because of lack of specific data.
- foscarnet (Foscavir) may result in an additive decrease in calcium.
- medicines in general should NOT be taken at the same time as alendronate. The most prudent approach is to separate any dose of alendronate and any other medicine by at least half an hour.
- ranitidine (Zantac) (intravenous form and perhaps oral form) may double how much alendronate gets into your body. The clinical importance of this is not yet known.

The following drugs may *decrease* the effects of alendronate:
- Once again, because a small amount of alendronate gets into the body under the best conditions, it is prudent to only take alendronate with a full 6 to 8 ounces of water, and to take any other needed medicines at least half an hour after alendronate.

▷ *Driving, Hazardous Activities:* No specific limitations.

Aviation Note: The use of this drug *is probably not a disqualification* for piloting. Consult a designated Aviation Medical Examiner.

Exposure to Sun: No restrictions.

Heavy Exercise or Exertion: If your bone density is low, heavy aerobic exercise may not be a good idea. Discuss this with your doctor. In general, weight-bearing exercise stimulates receptors (mechanoreceptors) to release factors that result in increased bone strength.

Discontinuation: Talk with your doctor **before** stopping this medicine.

ALLOPURINOL (al oh PURE i nohl)

Introduced: 1963   **Class:** Antigout   **Prescription:** USA: Yes   **Controlled Drug:** USA: No; Canada: No   **Available as Generic:** USA: Yes; Canada: No

Brand Names: ✦Alloprin, ✦Apo-Allopurinol, Lopurin, ✦Novopurol, ✦Purinol, Zurinol, Zyloprim

BENEFITS versus RISKS	
Possible Benefits	*Possible Risks*
EFFECTIVE CONTROL OF GOUT CONTROL OF HIGH BLOOD URIC ACID due to polycythemia, leukemia, cancer, and chemotherapy	Increased frequency of acute gout initially Peripheral neuritis Allergic reactions in skin, lung, blood vessels, and liver Bone marrow depression Kidney toxicity

▷ **Principal Uses**

As a Single Drug Product: Uses currently included in FDA-approved labeling: (1) Used in long-term management of gout to *prevent* episodes of acute gout (does not relieve acute gout attacks); (2) helps prevent excessive blood levels of uric acid in people who have recurrent uric acid kidney stones, those who are receiving chemotherapy or radiation therapy for cancer, or people taking thiazide diuretics (see Drug Classes).

Other (unlabeled) generally accepted uses: (1) May be a great benefit in decreasing pain and occurrence of mouth sores in people receiving 5-fluorouracil chemotherapy; (2) could be of use for people who have swelling of the prostate (nonbacterial prostatitis) not caused by bacteria.

How This Drug Works: By blocking the enzyme xanthine oxidase, it decreases uric acid formation.

Available Dosage Forms and Strengths

Tablets — 100 mg, 300 mg (and 200 mg in Canada)

▷ **Usual Adult Dosage Range:**   Initially 100 mg every 24 hours. Increase by 100 mg every 24 hours (1 week apart) until uric acid blood level is 6 mg/dl or less. Usual dose is 200 to 300 mg every 24 hours for mild gout, and 400 to 600 mg every 24 hours for moderate to severe gout. Daily doses of 300 mg or less may be taken as a single dose. Doses exceeding 300 mg daily should be divided into two or three equal portions; for the high uric acid levels associated with cancer, 600 to 800 mg every 24 hours, divided into three equal portions.

Kidney stone (calcium oxalate) recurrence prevention: 100–300 mg per day.

Note: Actual dosage and administration schedule must be determined for each patient individually.

Conditions Requiring Dosing Adjustments

Liver Function: Need for dose adjustment in liver compromise is not documented.

Kidney Function: Allopurinol dosing **must** be adjusted in renal compromise.

Malnutrition: Patients who are malnourished or who have been placed on low protein diets will not eliminate allopurinol normally and are at risk for toxicity. Doses **must** be decreased.

▷ **Dosing Instructions:**   Best taken with food or milk to reduce stomach irritation. Tablet may be crushed. Drink 2 to 3 quarts of liquids daily.

Usual Duration of Use: Blood uric acid levels often begin to decrease in 48 to 72 hours and may reach a normal range in 1 to 3 weeks. Regular use for several months may be needed to prevent attacks of acute gout. Continual use for many years may be needed for adequate control. See your doctor regularly.

▷ **This Drug Should Not Be Taken If**
  • you have had an allergic reaction to it previously.
  • you are experiencing an acute attack of gout at the present time.

▷ **Inform Your Physician Before Taking This Drug If**
  • you have a personal or family history of hemochromatosis.
  • you have a history of liver or kidney disease.
  • you have had a blood cell or bone marrow disorder.
  • you have any type of seizure or convulsive disorder (epilepsy).
  • you take other prescription or nonprescription medications that were not discussed when allopurinol was prescribed for you.
  • you are unsure of how much to take or how often to take allopurinol.
  • you are on a low protein diet.
  • you are pregnant.

Possible Side Effects (natural, expected, and unavoidable drug actions)

Frequency and severity of episodes of acute gout may occur during the first several weeks of drug use. Ask your doctor about the need for other drugs during this period.

▷ **Possible Adverse Effects** (unusual, unexpected, and infrequent reactions)

If any of the following develop, consult your physician promptly for guidance.

Mild Adverse Effects

Allergic reactions: skin rash, hives, itching—frequent; drug fever.

Confusion, headache, dizziness, drowsiness—rare.

Nausea, vomiting, diarrhea, stomach cramps—rare.

Taste disturbance—possible.

Loss of scalp hair—rare.

Serious Adverse Effects

Allergic reactions: severe skin reactions, high fever, chills, joint pains, swollen glands, kidney damage.

Hepatitis with or without jaundice (see Glossary): yellow eyes and skin, dark-colored urine, light-colored stools (may be part of allergy)—rare.

Bone marrow depression (see Glossary)—rare.

Peripheral neuritis—rare.

Bronchospasm (part of hypersensitivity)—rare.

Eye damage (macular), cataract formation—rare.

▷ **Possible Effects on Sexual Function:**   Less than 1% and questionable cause: male infertility, male breast enlargement, impotence.

Adverse Effects That May Mimic Natural Diseases or Disorders

Toxic liver reaction may suggest viral hepatitis.

Severe skin reactions may resemble the Stevens-Johnson syndrome (erythema multiforme).

Possible Effects on Laboratory Tests

Complete blood cell counts: decreased red cells, hemoglobin, and platelets; increased eosinophils.

Liver function tests: increased ALT/GPT, AST/GOT, and alkaline phosphatase.

CAUTION

1. Early in treatment (first few weeks) the frequency of acute attacks of gout may increase. These subside with continuation of therapy.
2. This drug should not be started if acute gout symptoms are present, as it will not help.
3. Vitamin C in doses of 2 g or more daily can increase the risk of kidney stone formation during the use of allopurinol.
4. Frequency of rash may be increased in patients also taking a penicillin.
5. Allergic-type kidney damage can result if thiazide diuretics (see Drug Classes) are taken with allopurinol. Avoid this combination.
6. Patients on low protein diets will not eliminate allopurinol normally. Doses must be decreased.

Precautions for Use

By Infants and Children: Not used in children except for increased uric acid caused by malignant growths. Watch closely for allergic skin reactions and blood cell disorders. The toxicity of azathioprine (Imuran) or mercaptopurine (Purinethol) may be increased in children receiving chemotherapy.

By Those Over 60 Years of Age: Smaller initial and maintenance doses of this drug must be used.

▷ **Advisability of Use During Pregnancy**

Pregnancy Category: C. See Pregnancy Risk Categories at the back of this book.

Animal studies: Results are conflicting and inconclusive.

Human studies: Adequate studies of pregnant women are not available.

Avoid use of drug during the first 3 months. Use during the last 6 months only if clearly needed.

Advisability of Use If Breast-Feeding
Presence of this drug in breast milk: Yes.
Avoid drug or refrain from nursing.

Habit-Forming Potential: None.

Effects of Overdosage: Nausea, vomiting, or diarrhea. Hypersensitivity reactions, kidney and liver function decline.

Possible Effects of Long-Term Use: None identified.

Suggested Periodic Examinations While Taking This Drug (at physician's discretion)
Blood uric acid levels, complete blood cell counts, liver and kidney function tests. If appropriate, eye examinations (possible cataract formation or macular damage). Complete blood counts.

▷ **While Taking This Drug, Observe the Following**
Foods: Follow physician's advice regarding the need for a low-purine diet.
Beverages: No restrictions. May be taken with milk.
▷ *Alcohol:* No interactions expected.
Tobacco Smoking: No interactions expected, but I advise everyone to quit smoking.
▷ *Other Drugs*
Allopurinol may ***increase*** the effects of
- azathioprine (Imuran) and mercaptopurine (Purinethol), making dose decreases necessary.
- oral anticoagulants (see Drug Classes) such as warfarin (Coumadin).
- theophylline (aminophylline, Elixophyllin, Theo-Dur, etc.).
Allopurinol ***taken concurrently*** with
- ampicillin (and perhaps other penicillins) may increase the incidence of skin rash.
- antacids containing aluminum will decrease the therapeutic effect of allopurinol.
- captopril (Capoten) or other ACE inhibitors (see Drug Classes) can increase the likelihood of allergic reactions.
- cyclophosphamide (Cytoxan, Neosar) may result in cyclophosphamide toxicity.
- cyclosporine (Sandimmune) can result in cyclosporine toxicity.
- iron salts may result in undesirable reactions (avoid this combination).
- mercaptopurine (Purinethol) can lead to increased mercaptopurine toxicity.
- tamoxifen (Nolvadex) may result in increased allopurinol levels and increased risk of liver toxicity.
- thiazide diuretics (see Drug Classes) may lead to decreased kidney function.
- theophylline (Theo-Dur, various) may increase theophylline to toxic levels.
- vidarabine (Vira-A) may increase risk of neurotoxicity.
▷ *Driving, Hazardous Activities:* Drowsiness may occur in some people. Use caution.
Aviation Note: The use of this drug ***may be a disqualification*** for piloting. Consult a designated Aviation Medical Examiner.
Exposure to Sun: No restrictions.

Discontinuation: If you have a seizure disorder, this medicine dose should be slowly decreased and then stopped.

ALPRAZOLAM (al PRAY zoh lam)

Introduced: 1973   **Class:** Antianxiety drug, benzodiazepines   **Prescription:** USA: Yes   **Controlled Drug:** USA: C-IV*; Canada: No   **Available as Generic:** Yes

Brand Names: Alprazolam Intensol, ✦Apo-Alpraz, Novo-Alprazol, Nu-Alpraz, Xanax

Warning: The brand names Xanax and Zantac are similar and can lead to **serious** medication errors. These names represent very different drugs. Xanax is the mild tranquilizer alprazolam. Zantac is ranitidine, used to treat peptic ulcer disease. Make sure your prescription was filled correctly.

BENEFITS versus RISKS	
Possible Benefits	*Possible Risks*
RELIEF OF ANXIETY AND NERVOUS TENSION	Habit-forming potential with prolonged use
EFFECTIVE TREATMENT OF PANIC DISORDER	Minor impairment of mental functions with therapeutic doses
Wide margin of safety with therapeutic doses	Tachycardia and palpitations
May have some antidepressant activity	

▷ **Principal Uses**

As a Single Drug Product: Uses currently included in FDA-approved labeling: (1) Used for the short-term relief of mild to moderate anxiety and nervous tension; (2) helps relieve anxiety associated with neurosis; (3) eases irritable bowel syndrome; (4) decreases the frequency and severity of panic disorder.

Other (unlabeled) generally accepted uses: (1) May have a role in helping control extreme PMS symptoms; (2) can lessen a variety of types of cancer pain when given with various narcotics; (3) eases agoraphobia; (4) can decrease symptoms in essential tremor; (5) decreases the loudness of the sensation of ear ringing in tinnitus; (6) can be helpful in alcohol withdrawal.

How This Drug Works: Produces a calming effect by enhancing the action of the nerve transmitter gamma-aminobutyric acid (GABA), which in turn blocks higher brain centers.

Available Dosage Forms and Strengths

Tablets — 0.25 mg, 0.5 mg, 1 mg, 2 mg
Oral solution — 0.25 mg, 0.5 mg, 1 mg/5 ml
— 0.25 mg/2.5 ml

*See Schedules of Controlled Drugs at the back of this book.

▷ **Usual Adult Dosage Range:**   For anxiety and nervous tension: 0.25 mg to 0.5 mg three times daily. Maximum dose is 4 mg every 24 hours, taken in divided doses.

For panic disorder: Initially 0.5 mg three times daily; increase dose by 1 mg every 3 to 4 days as needed and tolerated. Some patients stopped having panic attacks with 6 mg a day. Maximum daily dose is 10 mg. **Note: Actual dosage and administration schedule must be determined for each patient individually.**

Conditions Requiring Dosing Adjustments

Liver Function: Manufacturer recommends a starting dose of 0.25 mg in patients with advanced liver disease, with slow increase in dose only if needed.

Kidney Function: Specific dosage reductions are not defined by the manufacturer.

Obesity: Takes a longer time to reach final concentrations in obese people. Doses should be calculated based on ideal rather than actual body weight.

▷ *Alcoholism:* Because of some of the physiological and liver changes that can occur in alcoholism, the removal of this drug from the body may be delayed. Lower doses or longer times (intervals) between doses are needed.

▷ **Dosing Instructions:**   May be taken on empty stomach or with food or milk. Tablet may be crushed. Do not stop this drug abruptly if taken for more than 4 weeks (stop slowly by decreasing 0.5 mg every 3 days or longer).

Usual Duration of Use: Several days to several weeks. Avoid prolonged and uninterrupted use. Continual use should not exceed 8 weeks without evaluation by your doctor.

▷ **This Drug Should Not Be Taken If**

- you have had an allergic reaction to it previously.
- you are pregnant (first 3 months).
- you have acute narrow-angle glaucoma.
- you have myasthenia gravis.

▷ **Inform Your Physician Before Taking This Drug If**

- you have a history of palpitations and tachycardia (may be worsened).
- you are allergic to benzodiazepines (see Drug Classes).
- you are pregnant (last 6 months) or planning pregnancy.
- you are breast-feeding your infant.
- you have a history of depression or serious mental illness (psychosis).
- you have a history of alcoholism or drug abuse.
- you have impaired liver or kidney function.
- you have open-angle glaucoma.
- you have a seizure disorder (epilepsy).
- you have severe chronic lung disease.
- you take other prescription or nonprescription medications that were not discussed when alprazolam was prescribed for you.
- you are unsure of how much alprazolam to take or how often to take it.

Possible Side Effects (natural, expected, and unavoidable drug actions)

Drowsiness, light-headedness.

▷ **Possible Adverse Effects** (unusual, unexpected, and infrequent reactions)
  If any of the following develop, consult your physician promptly for guidance.

  Mild Adverse Effects
  Allergic Reactions: skin rash, hives.
  Headache, dizziness, fatigue, blurred vision, dry mouth—infrequent.
  Drowsiness—frequent, up to 50%.
  Nausea, vomiting, constipation—infrequent.
  Increased salivation—infrequent.

  Serious Adverse Effects
  Confusion, hallucinations, depression, excitement, agitation (paradoxical reaction)—rare.
  Tachycardia and palpitations—infrequent.
  Increased liver enzymes—rare.
  Low blood pressure (hypotension)—case report.

▷ **Possible Effects on Sexual Function:**   Rare but documented: inhibited female orgasm (5 mg/day); impaired ejaculation (3.5 mg/day); decreased libido, impaired erection (4.5 mg/day); altered timing and pattern of menstruation (0.75–4 mg/day).

Possible Effects on Laboratory Tests
  Liver function tests: increased ALT/GPT, AST/GOT—rare and insignificant.
  Urine screening tests for drug abuse: may be **positive** (depends upon amount of drug taken and testing method).

CAUTION
  1. **Do not** stop taking this drug abruptly if it has been taken continually for more than 4 weeks.
  2. Some nonprescription products have antihistamines (allergy and cold preparations, sleep aids) and can cause excessive sedation.

Precautions for Use
  By Infants and Children: Safety and effectiveness for use by those under 18 not established.
  By Those Over 60 Years of Age: Starting dose should be 0.25 mg two or three times daily. Watch for excessive drowsiness, dizziness, unsteadiness, and incoordination (possible low blood pressure).

▷ **Advisability of Use During Pregnancy**
  Pregnancy Category: D. See Pregnancy Risk Categories at the back of this book.
  Animal studies: Diazepam (a closely related benzodiazepine) can cause cleft palate in mice and skeletal defects in rats. No data on alprazolam.
  Human studies: Some studies suggest an association between diazepam use and cleft lip and heart deformities. Adequate studies on the use of alprazolam by pregnant women are not available.
  Avoid use during entire pregnancy if possible.

Advisability of Use If Breast-Feeding
  Presence of this drug in breast milk: Yes.
  Avoid drug or refrain from nursing.

Habit-Forming Potential: This drug can cause psychological and/or physical dependence (see Glossary), especially if used in large doses for an extended period of time.

Effects of Overdosage: Marked drowsiness, weakness, feeling of drunkenness, staggering gait, tremor, stupor progressing to deep sleep or coma.

Possible Effects of Long-Term Use: Psychological and/or physical dependence.

Suggested Periodic Examinations While Taking This Drug (at physician's discretion)
None required for short-term use.

▷ **While Taking This Drug, Observe the Following**
Foods: No restrictions.
Beverages: Avoid excessive intake of caffeine-containing beverages: coffee, tea, cola. This drug may be taken with milk.
▷   *Alcohol:* Use with extreme caution. Alcohol may increase the sedative effects of alprazolam. Alprazolam may increase the intoxicating effects of alcohol. Avoid alcohol completely—throughout the day and night—if you find it necessary to drive or engage in *any* hazardous activity.
Tobacco Smoking: Heavy smoking may reduce the calming action of alprazolam. I advise everyone to quit smoking.
Marijuana Smoking: Occasional (once or twice weekly): Mild increase in the sedative effect.
Daily: Marked increase in the sedative effect of this drug.
▷   *Other Drugs*
Alprazolam may *increase* the effects of
• digoxin (Lanoxin), and cause digoxin toxicity.
Alprazolam may *decrease* the effects of
• levodopa (Sinemet, etc.), and reduce its effect in treating Parkinson's disease.
The following drugs may *increase* the effects of alprazolam:
• azole antifungals, such as itraconazole (Sporanox) or ketoconazole (Nizoral).
• cimetidine (Tagamet).
• disulfiram (Antabuse).
• fluoxetine (Prozac).
• fluvoxamine (Luvox).
• isoniazid (INH, Rifamate, etc.).
• macrolide antibiotics (such as erythromycin or azithromycin—see Drug Classes).
• omeprazole (Prilosec).
• oral contraceptives (various).
• ritonavir (Norvir) and perhaps other protease inhibitors (see Drug Classes).
• valproic acid (Depakene).
The following drugs may *decrease* the effects of alprazolam:
• carbamazepine (Tegretol).
• rifampin (Rimactane, etc.).
• theophylline (aminophylline, Theo-Dur, etc.).
Alprazolam *taken concurrently* with
• alcohol (ethanol) will worsen coordination and mental abilities.
• benzodiazepines (see Drug Classes) can cause increased central nervous system (CNS) depression.
• buspirone (Buspar) can result in additive CNS depression.

- central nervous system active agents (see Antihistamine and Antipsychotic Drug Classes) can cause increased central nervous system (CNS) depression.
- narcotics (morphine, meperidine, and others) will result in additive CNS depression.
- tricyclic and other kinds of antidepressants (see Drug Classes) results in additional CNS depression.

▷ *Driving, Hazardous Activities:* This drug can impair mental alertness, judgment, physical coordination, and reaction time. Avoid hazardous activities accordingly.

Aviation Note: The use of this drug *is a disqualification* for piloting. Consult a designated Aviation Medical Examiner.

Exposure to Sun: Use caution; rare photosensitivity reports (see Glossary).

Discontinuation: If this drug has been taken for an extended period of time, do not stop it abruptly. Slowly reduce dose by 1 mg per week until a total daily dose of 4 mg is reached; by 0.5 mg per week until a total daily dose of 2 mg is reached; then by 0.25 mg per week thereafter. Ask your doctor for help.

AMANTADINE (a MAN ta deen)

Introduced: 1966   **Class:** Anti-parkinsonism, antiviral   **Prescription:** USA: Yes   **Controlled Drug:** USA: No; Canada: No   **Available as Generic:** USA: Yes; Canada: No

Brand Names: Symadine, Symmetrel

BENEFITS versus RISKS	
Possible Benefits	*Possible Risks*
Partial relief of rigidity, tremor, and impaired motion in all forms of parkinsonism	Skin rashes, mild to severe
	Confusion, hallucinations
	Congestive heart failure
Prevention and treatment of respiratory infections caused by influenza type A viruses*	Increased prostatism (see Glossary)
	Abnormally low white blood cell counts

▷ **Principal Uses**

As a Single Drug Product: Uses currently included in FDA-approved labeling: (1) Treats all forms of parkinsonism; (2) prevents or treats respiratory tract infections caused by influenza type A virus (although rimantadine is currently the drug of first choice because of amantadine's higher occurrence of CNS side effects); (3) treatment of drug-induced extrapyramidal symptoms.

Other (unlabeled) generally accepted uses: (1) May have a small role in helping manage behavioral problems that can happen after some brain injuries; (2) has had some success in reversing symptoms of mild dementia; (3) can ease some resistant myoclonic or absence seizures; (4) may help bedwetting (enuresis) in children; (5) eases fatigue in multiple sclerosis (MS)

*Does **NOT** prevent or treat viral infections other than those caused by influenza type A viruses.

and may be of use in MS patients who experience fatigue that keeps them from living normally.

How This Drug Works: By increasing the nerve transmitter known as dopamine in some nerve centers, this drug reduces muscular rigidity, tremor, and impaired movement associated with parkinsonism. By blocking penetration of infectious material from viruses into cells, this drug prevents development of influenza.

Available Dosage Forms and Strengths

Capsules (gelatin and softgel) — 100 mg

Syrup — 50 mg/5 ml

▷ **Usual Adult Dosage Range:** Anti-parkinsonism: 100 mg once or twice daily. The total daily dose should not exceed 300 mg.

Antiviral: 200 mg once daily; or 100 mg every 12 hours.

Children 1 to 9 years old: For treatment of type A flu: 4.4 to 8.8 mg per kg of body mass per day, up to a maximum of 150 mg once daily. **Note: Actual dosage and administration schedule must be determined for each patient individually.**

Conditions Requiring Dosing Adjustments

Liver Function: The liver is not known to be involved in the elimination of amantadine.

Kidney Function: Must be carefully adjusted to blood levels in patients with kidney problems. Those with creatinine clearances of 30–50 ml/min should receive 100 mg daily. Those with 15–29 clearance should receive 100 mg every other day. Those with clearances less than 15 should receive 200 mg once a week.

Epilepsy: Doses of 200 mg/day should be avoided, as seizure risk may increase.

▷ **Dosing Instructions:** May be taken with or following meals. Can open the capsule to take it.

Usual Duration of Use: Use on a regular schedule for up to 2 weeks is usually needed to see this drug's effectiveness in relieving symptoms of parkinsonism. Long-term use (months to years) requires periodic check of response and dose changes. See your doctor on a regular basis.

Following exposure to influenza type A, peak protection requires continual daily dosage for at least 10 days. During influenza epidemics, this drug may be given for 6 to 8 weeks.

▷ **This Drug Should Not Be Taken If**

• you have had an allergic reaction to it previously.

▷ **Inform Your Physician Before Taking This Drug If** ·

• you have any type of seizure disorder.
• you have a history of a serious emotional or mental disorder.
• you have a history of heart disease, especially previous heart failure.
• you have impaired liver or kidney function.
• you have a history of lowering of blood pressure when you stand (orthostatic hypotension).
• you have a history of peptic ulcer disease.
• you have eczema or recurring eczemalike skin rashes.
• you are taking any drugs for emotional or mental disorders.

- you take other prescription or nonprescription medications that were not discussed when amantadine was prescribed for you.
- you have a history of low white blood cell counts.
- you are unsure of how much amantadine to take or how often to take it.

Possible Side Effects (natural, expected, and unavoidable drug actions)

Light-headedness, dizziness, weakness, feeling of impending faint in upright position (see Orthostatic Hypotension in Glossary). Dry mouth, constipation. Reddish-blue network pattern or patchy discoloration of the skin of the legs and feet (livedo reticularis); this is transient and unimportant.

▷ **Possible Adverse Effects** (unusual, unexpected, and infrequent reactions)

If any of the following develop, consult your physician promptly for guidance.

Mild Adverse Effects

Allergic reaction: skin rash.

Headache, nervousness, irritability, inability to concentrate, insomnia, nightmares—rare to infrequent.

Unsteadiness, visual disturbances, slurred speech—infrequent.

Swelling (fluid retention) of the arms, feet, or ankles—case report.

Difficulty breathing—possible.

Urine retention—rare.

Loss of appetite, nausea, vomiting—infrequent.

Serious Adverse Effects

Allergic reaction: severe eczemalike skin rashes.

Idiosyncratic reactions: confusion, depression, hallucinations—rare.

Increased seizure activity in presence of epilepsy—increased risk.

Development of congestive heart failure—rare.

Aggravation of prostatism (see Glossary)—possible.

Elevated liver function tests—rare.

Abnormally low white blood cell counts: fever, sore throat, infections—rare.

Catatonia or seizures (if abruptly stopped).

▷ **Possible Effects on Sexual Function:**   None reported.

Adverse Effects That May Mimic Natural Diseases or Disorders

Mood changes, confusion, or hallucinations may suggest a psychotic disorder.

Swelling of the legs and feet may suggest (but not necessarily be indicative of) heart, liver, or kidney disorder.

Natural Diseases or Disorders That May Be Activated by This Drug

Latent epilepsy, incipient congestive heart failure.

Possible Effects on Laboratory Tests

Liver function tests: increased liver enzymes (AST/GOT, alkaline phosphatase).

Kidney function tests: Transient increase in blood urea nitrogen (BUN).

CAUTION

1. NARROW margin of safety. Do not exceed a total dose of 400 mg every 24 hours. Watch closely for adverse effects with doses over 200 mg every 24 hours.
2. Initial benefit may only last 3 to 6 months in treatment of parkinsonism. If this occurs, ask your doctor if the dose should be adjusted or the drug changed.

3. May increase susceptibility to German measles. Avoid exposure to anyone with active German measles.

4. Watch for early signs of congestive heart failure: shortness of breath on exertion or during the night while sleeping, mild cough, swelling of the feet and ankles. Report these developments promptly to your doctor.

Precautions for Use

By Infants and Children: Safety and effectiveness for use by those under 1 not established.

By Those Over 60 Years of Age: Confusion, delirium, hallucinations, and disorderly conduct may develop. Prostatism may be aggravated by this drug.

▷ **Advisability of Use During Pregnancy**

Pregnancy Category: C. See Pregnancy Risk Categories at the back of this book.
Animal studies: Birth defects reported in rat studies; no defects reported in rabbit studies.
Human studies: Adequate studies of pregnant women are not available. Avoid this drug during the first 3 months if possible. Ask your doctor for help.

Advisability of Use If Breast-Feeding

Presence of this drug in breast milk: Yes.
Nursing infant may develop skin rash, vomiting, or retention of urine. Avoid drug or refrain from nursing.

Habit-Forming Potential: This drug has a potential for abuse because of its ability to cause euphoria, hallucinations, and feelings of detachment.

Effects of Overdosage: Hyperactivity, disorientation, confusion, visual hallucinations, aggressive behavior, severe toxic psychosis, seizures, heart rhythm disturbances, drop in blood pressure.

Possible Effects of Long-Term Use: Livedo reticularis (see "Possible Side Effects" above). Congestive heart failure in predisposed individuals.

Suggested Periodic Examinations While Taking This Drug (at physician's discretion)

White blood cell counts, liver and kidney function tests.
Evaluation of heart function.

▷ **While Taking This Drug, Observe the Following**

Foods: No restrictions.
Beverages: No restrictions. May be taken with milk.
▷ *Alcohol:* This combination may impair mental function and lower blood pressure excessively.
Tobacco Smoking: No interactions expected, but I advise everyone to quit smoking.
Marijuana Smoking: No interactions expected.
▷ *Other Drugs*

Amantadine may *increase* the effects of
• atropinelike drugs that are used to treat parkinsonism, especially benztropine (Cogentin), orphenadrine (Disipal), and trihexyphenidyl (Artane). Amantadine can increase their therapeutic effectiveness, but if the doses are too large, these drugs (taken concurrently with amantadine) may cause mental confusion, delirium, hallucinations, and nightmares.
• levodopa (Dopar, Larodopa, Sinemet, etc.), and enhance its therapeutic effectiveness. Combination may cause acute mental disturbances.
The following drugs may *increase* the effects of amantadine:

- amphetamine and amphetaminelike stimulant drugs may cause excessive stimulation and adverse behavioral effects.
- hydrochlorothiazide with triamterene may increase the blood level of amantadine and cause toxicity.

Amantadine taken *concurrently* with
- cotrimoxazole may increase risk of CNS stimulation or arrhythmias.
- hydrochlorothiazide (Dyazide, Esidrix, others) may increase risk of amantadine toxicity.
- sulfamethoxazole may increase risk of CNS stimulation or arrhythmia.
- trimethoprim may increase risk of CNS stimulation or arrhythmias.

▷ *Driving, Hazardous Activities:* This drug may cause drowsiness, dizziness, blurred vision, or confusion. If these drug effects occur, avoid all hazardous activities.

Aviation Note: The use of this drug *may be a disqualification* for piloting. Consult a designated Aviation Medical Examiner.

Exposure to Sun: No restrictions.

Exposure to Heat: No restrictions.

Exposure to Cold: Use caution. Excessive chilling may enhance the development of livedo reticularis (see "Possible Side Effects" above).

Discontinuation: When used to treat parkinsonism, this drug should not be stopped abruptly. Sudden discontinuation may cause an acute parkinsonian crisis. When used to treat influenza A infections, this drug should be continued for 48 hours after the disappearance of all symptoms.

AMILORIDE (a MIL oh ride)

Introduced: 1967　　**Class:** Diuretic　　**Prescription:** USA: Yes　　**Controlled Drug:**　USA: No; Canada: No　　**Available as Generic:**　Yes

Brand Names: ✦Apo-Amilzide, Midamor, ✦Moduret [CD], Moduretic [CD], ✦Nu-Amilzide [CD]

BENEFITS versus RISKS	
Possible Benefits	*Possible Risks*
EFFECTIVE DIURETIC WITH DECREASED POTASSIUM LOSS	ABNORMALLY HIGH BLOOD POTASSIUM with excessive use
	Rare bone marrow depression
	Rare heart arrhythmias
	Rare kidney failure
	Rare liver toxicity

▷ **Principal Uses**

As a Single Drug Product: Uses currently included in FDA-approved labeling: (1) Eliminates excessive fluid (edema) seen in congestive heart failure; (2) treats high blood pressure, especially good in those prone to low potassium; (3) treatment of thiazide-caused low blood potassium.

As a Combination Drug Product [CD]: Combined with other thiazide diuretics to prevent excess potassium loss.

Other (unlabeled) generally accepted uses: (1) May be able to help dissolve kidney stones in patients unable to tolerate surgery; (2) can help correct increased urination that occurs in patients taking lithium.

How This Drug Works: This drug promotes loss of sodium and water from the body and potassium retention by altering kidney enzymes that control urine formation.

Available Dosage Forms and Strengths
    Tablets — 5 mg

▷ **Usual Adult Dosage Range:**   One 5-mg dose a day, preferably in the morning. May increase up to 15 mg daily as needed and tolerated. Should not exceed 20 mg every 24 hours. **Note: Actual dosage and administration schedule must be determined for each patient individually.**

Conditions Requiring Dosing Adjustments
    Liver Function: Use with extreme caution in patients with severe liver disease.
    Kidney Function: Should NOT be used in patients who can't make urine or who have acute kidney failure or creatinine clearance less than 50 ml/min.

▷ **Dosing Instructions:**   Best taken when you wake up, with food. Tablet may be crushed for administration.

Usual Duration of Use: As needed to lose abnormal fluid or normalize normal blood pressure. Intermittent or alternate-day use is recommended to minimize imbalance of sodium and potassium. See your doctor on a regular basis.

▷ **This Drug Should Not Be Taken If**
    • you have had an allergic reaction to any form of it previously.
    • your blood potassium level is above the normal range.
    • you have nerve damage caused by diabetes (diabetic nephropathy).
    • your kidneys are not producing urine.

▷ **Inform Your Physician Before Taking This Drug If**
    • you are allergic to this drug or one similar to it.
    • you have diabetes or glaucoma.
    • you have a history of kidney disease or impaired kidney function.
    • you take any other diuretic, blood pressure drug, any form of digitalis, or lithium.
    • you are unsure of how much amiloride to take or how often to take it.

Possible Side Effects (natural, expected, and unavoidable drug actions)
    Abnormally high blood potassium level (10% of users), abnormally low blood sodium level, dehydration, decreased blood magnesium, constipation.
    Dizziness on standing (orthostatic hypotension)—possible.

▷ **Possible Adverse Effects** (unusual, unexpected, and infrequent reactions)
    If any of the following develop, consult your physician promptly for guidance.
    Mild Adverse Effects
    Allergic Reactions: skin rash, itching—rare.
    Headache—infrequent.
    Dizziness, weakness, fatigue, numbness, and tingling—case reports (related to electrolyte problems).
    Dry mouth, nausea, vomiting, stomach pains, diarrhea—infrequent.
    Decreased ability to taste salt—possible.
    Loss of scalp hair—rare.

Serious Adverse Effects
Idiosyncratic reactions: joint and muscle pains.
Liver or kidney toxicity—rare.
Abnormally low sodium level—case reports.
Increased internal eye pressure (of concern in glaucoma)—rare.
Mental depression, visual disturbances, ringing in ears, tremors—infrequent.
Aplastic anemia (see Glossary): unusual fatigue or weakness, fever, sore throat, abnormal bleeding or bruising—case reports and questionable cause.
Palpitations and arrhythmias—rare.

▷ **Possible Effects on Sexual Function:** More than 1%: decreased libido and impotence (5 to 10 mg per day).

Adverse Effects That May Mimic Natural Diseases or Disorders
Nervousness, confusion, or depression may mimic spontaneous mental disorder.

Natural Diseases or Disorders That May Be Activated by This Drug
Preexisting peptic ulcer, latent glaucoma.

Possible Effects on Laboratory Tests
Blood cholesterol level: decreased.
Blood creatinine level: increased with long-term use.
Blood potassium level: increased.
Blood uric acid level: increased with long-term use, especially if taken with thiazide diuretics.
Blood sodium level: decreased.

CAUTION
1. Do **NOT** take potassium supplements or eat more high potassium foods.
2. More frequent potassium levels are needed if you take digitalis compounds.
3. Do not stop this drug abruptly unless your doctor says you must.

Precautions for Use
By Infants and Children: Oral dosing with 0.625 mg per kg of body mass daily has been used to promote water loss (diuresis) in young patients weighing from 6 to 20 kg.
By Those Over 60 Years of Age: Declines in kidney function may make it likely that you will retain potassium. Limit use of this drug to periods of 2 to 3 weeks if possible. The dose MUST be reduced. This drug can cause excessive water loss, increased tendency of the blood to clot, and increased risk of clots (thrombosis, heart attack, stroke).

▷ **Advisability of Use During Pregnancy**
Pregnancy Category: B. See Pregnancy Risk Categories at the back of this book.
Animal studies: No birth defects reported.
Human studies: Adequate studies of pregnant women are not available.
Use only if clearly needed.

Advisability of Use If Breast-Feeding
Presence of this drug in breast milk: Unknown, but probably present.
This drug may suppress milk production.

Avoid drug if possible. If use is necessary, watch nursing infant closely and stop drug or nursing if adverse effects develop.

Habit-Forming Potential: None.

Effects of Overdosage: Thirst, drowsiness, fatigue, weakness, nausea, vomiting, confusion, numbness and tingling of face and extremities, irregular heart rhythm, shortness of breath.

Suggested Periodic Examinations While Taking This Drug (at physician's discretion)

Complete blood counts; blood levels of sodium, potassium, magnesium, and chloride; kidney function tests; and check of water balance (state of hydration).

▷ **While Taking This Drug, Observe the Following**

Foods: Avoid excessive salt restriction and high potassium foods.

Beverages: No restrictions. May be taken with milk.

▷   *Alcohol:* Use caution. Alcohol can exaggerate the blood-pressure-lowering effect of this drug and cause orthostatic hypotension (see Glossary).

Tobacco Smoking: No interactions expected, but I advise everyone to quit smoking.

▷   *Other Drugs*

Amiloride may *increase* the effects of
• other blood-pressure-lowering drugs. Dosage decreases may be needed.

Amiloride may *decrease* the effects of
• digoxin (Lanoxin, etc.), and reduce its effect in treating heart failure.

Amiloride *taken concurrently* with
• ACE inhibitors (see Drug Classes) such as benazepril may result in abnormally high blood potassium.
• lithium (Lithobid) may cause lithium accumulation to toxic levels.
• metformin (Glucophage) may increase glucophage levels and increase risk of lactic acidosis or excessively lowered blood sugar (hypoglycemia).
• NSAIDs (see Drug Classes) may decrease the lowering of blood pressure.
• potassium supplements may result in extremely elevated blood potassium levels.
• spironolactone (Aldactone, Aldactazide) or triamterene (Dyrenium, Dyazide) may cause dangerous blood potassium levels. Avoid these combinations.

▷   *Driving, Hazardous Activities:* May cause drowsiness, dizziness, and orthostatic hypotension. If these drug effects occur, avoid hazardous activities.

Aviation Note: The use of this drug *may be a disqualification* for piloting. Consult a designated Aviation Medical Examiner.

Exposure to Sun: No restrictions.

Exposure to Heat: Caution is advised. Excessive sweating can cause water, sodium, and potassium imbalance. Hot environments can cause lowering of blood pressure.

Occurrence of Unrelated Illness: Call your doctor if you contract an illness causing vomiting or diarrhea.

Discontinuation: With high dosage or prolonged use, withdraw this drug gradually. Sudden withdrawal can cause excessive loss of potassium from the body.

AMINOPHYLLINE (am in OFF i lin)

Other Name: Theophylline ethylenediamine
Introduced: 1910   **Class:** Antiasthmatic, bronchodilator, xanthines
Prescription: USA: Yes   **Controlled Drug:** USA: No; Canada: No   **Available as Generic:** Yes
Brand Names: Aminophyllin, Mudrane [CD], Mudrane GG [CD], ✦Palaron, Phyllocontin, Somophyllin, ✦Somophyllin-12, Truphylline

BENEFITS versus RISKS	
Possible Benefits	*Possible Risks*
EFFECTIVE PREVENTION AND RELIEF OF ACUTE BRONCHIAL ASTHMA	NARROW TREATMENT RANGE FREQUENT STOMACH DISTRESS Gastrointestinal bleeding
MODERATELY EFFECTIVE CONTROL OF CHRONIC, RECURRENT BRONCHIAL ASTHMA	Central nervous system toxicity, seizures Heart rhythm disturbances
Moderately effective symptomatic relief in chronic bronchitis and emphysema	

Author's Note: This medicine is active (79%) as theophylline. See the theophylline profile for further details.

AMITRIPTYLINE (a mee TRIP ti leen)

Introduced: 1961   **Class:** Antidepressant   **Prescription:** USA: Yes
Controlled Drug: USA: No; Canada: No   **Available as Generic:** Yes
Brand Names: Amitril, ✦Apo-Amitriptyline, Elavil, ✦Elavil Plus [CD], Emitrip, Endep, Enovil, Etrafon [CD], ✦Etrafon-A [CD], Etrafon-Forte [CD], ✦Levate, PMS-Levazine [CD], SK-Amitriptyline, ✦Triavil [CD]

BENEFITS versus RISKS	
Possible Benefits	*Possible Risks*
EFFECTIVE RELIEF OF ENDOGENOUS DEPRESSION	ADVERSE BEHAVIORAL EFFECTS: Confusion, disorientation, hallucinations
Additive (adjunctive) therapy in some pain syndromes	CONVERSION OF DEPRESSION TO MANIA in manic-depressive disorders
	Irregular heart rhythms—possible Blood cell abnormalities—rare

▷ **Principal Uses**

As a Single Drug Product: Uses currently included in FDA-approved labeling: (1) Relieves symptoms seen in spontaneous (endogenous) depression—should be used only when a diagnosis of a true, primary depression of significant degree has been made; (2) has a role in relieving depression that is resistant (refractory) to single agent therapy.

Other (unlabeled) generally accepted uses: (1) Additive (adjuvant) therapy in chronic pain and other pain syndromes; (2) helps ease agitation; (3) may have a role in diabetic neuropathic pain; (4) is an alternative in intractable hiccups; (5) used in combination with other medicines to ease the pain of postherpetic neuralgia; (6) may be of some benefit in easing the pain of chronic vulvar burning (vulvodynia); (7) used in fish (ciguatera) poisoning.

As a Combination Drug Product [CD]: Combined with chlordiazepoxide to relieve anxiety that may accompany depression. Also available in combination with perphenazine, a strong phenothiazine tranquilizer, to relieve severe agitation that may accompany depression.

How This Drug Works: Relieves depression by slowly restoring normal levels of norepinephrine and serotonin, chemicals that transmit nerve impulses.

Available Dosage Forms and Strengths
Injection — 10 mg/ml
Oral suspension — 10 mg/5 ml
Tablets — 10 mg, 25 mg, 50 mg, 75 mg, 100 mg, 150 mg

▷ **Usual Adult Dosage Range:** Intramuscular injection is given as 80 to 120 mg per day divided into four doses. A switch to the oral form is made as rapidly as possible. Oral dosing starts with 25 mg two to four times daily. Dose may be increased cautiously as needed and tolerated by 10 to 25 mg daily at intervals of 1 week. Usual maintenance dose is 50 to 100 mg daily. Total dose should not exceed 150 mg daily. When the best dose is found, it may be taken at bedtime as one dose. Some clinicians start with 50 mg at bedtime. **Note: Actual dosage and administration schedule must be determined for each patient individually.**

Conditions Requiring Dosing Adjustments
Liver Function: Specific guidelines are not available; however, low doses and a check of blood levels is prudent.
Kidney Function: Lower doses and blood level checks are needed with kidney failure (18% of drug is removed this way).

▷ **Dosing Instructions:** May be taken without regard to meals. Tablet may be crushed to take it.

Usual Duration of Use: Some benefit may occur in 1 to 2 weeks, but adequate response may require continual use for 4 to 6 weeks or longer. Long-term use should not exceed 6 months without follow-up evaluation.

▷ **This Drug Should Not Be Taken If**
- you are allergic to any of the brand names listed above.
- you are taking or have taken within the past 14 days any monoamine oxidase (MAO) type A inhibitor drug (see Drug Classes).
- you have heart-induced chest pain (angina pectoris).
- you have a rapid heart rate that occurs spontaneously (paroxysmal tachycardia).
- you have heart (cardiovascular) disease or abnormal heart rhythms.
- you are recovering from a recent heart attack.
- you have narrow-angle glaucoma.
- you are pregnant.
- you have congestive heart failure.

▷ **Inform Your Physician Before Taking This Drug If**
- you are allergic to any tricyclic antidepressant (see Drug Classes).
- you have a history of: diabetes, epilepsy (or other seizure disorder), glaucoma, heart disease, prostate gland enlargement, or overactive thyroid function.
- you plan to have surgery under general anesthesia in the near future.
- you take other prescription or nonprescription medications that were not discussed when amitriptyline was prescribed for you.
- you are unsure of how much amitriptyline to take or how often to take it.
- you have a history of schizophrenia—this drug may worsen any paranoia.
- you have a history of prostate problems.
- you have a liver or kidney disorder.
- you have a blood cell disorder.
- you have a history of intestinal block (ileus).
- you have a history of sexual dysfunction.

Possible Side Effects (natural, expected, and unavoidable drug actions)
Drowsiness, blurred vision, dry mouth, constipation, impaired urination.

▷ **Possible Adverse Effects** (unusual, unexpected, and infrequent reactions)
If any of the following develop, consult your physician promptly for guidance.

Mild Adverse Effects
Allergic reactions: skin rash, hives, swelling of face or tongue, drug fever (see Glossary).
Headache, dizziness, weakness, fainting, unsteady gait, tremors—infrequent.
Peculiar taste, irritation of tongue or mouth, nausea, indigestion—rare to infrequent.
Fluctuation of blood sugar levels—possible.
Increased dental cavities (caries)—increased risk.
Restlessness and nightmares—rare.
Change in the ability to perceive tones—case report.

Serious Adverse Effects
Allergic reactions: hepatitis, with or without jaundice (see Glossary).
Idiosyncratic reactions: neuroleptic malignant syndrome (see Glossary).
Confusion or hallucinations—may be more likely in older patients and with higher doses.
Bowel obstruction (ileus)—rare.
SIADH (see Glossary)—rare.
Excessively low blood pressure (hypotension)—possible.
Seizures—rare.
Severe eye or other movement problems—case reports.
Heart palpitation and irregular rhythm—rare and more likely with increasing doses or overdose.
Bone marrow depression (see Glossary): fatigue, weakness, fever, sore throat, abnormal bleeding or bruising—rare.
Peripheral neuritis (see Glossary): numbness, tingling, pain, loss of arm or leg strength—possible.
Parkinson-like disorders (see Glossary): usually mild and infrequent—more likely to occur in the elderly.

Liver toxicity—rare.

Worsening of paranoid psychosis in schizophrenic patients—possible.

▷ **Possible Effects on Sexual Function:** Decreased libido—rare; increased libido (possible antidepressant effect), inhibited female orgasm, inhibited ejaculation—case reports; male and female breast enlargement, milk production, swelling of testicles, impotence—case reports. These effects usually disappear within 2 to 10 days after discontinuation of the drug.

Adverse Effects That May Mimic Natural Diseases or Disorders
Liver toxicity may suggest viral hepatitis.

Natural Diseases or Disorders That May Be Activated by This Drug
Latent diabetes, epilepsy, glaucoma, impaired urination due to prostate.

Possible Effects on Laboratory Tests
Complete blood counts: decreased white cells and platelets; increased eosinophils.

Liver function tests: increased ALT/GPT, AST/GOT, alkaline phosphatase, increased bilirubin.

Blood glucose levels: increased or decreased (fluctuations).

CAUTION
1. Dosage must be individualized. Report for follow-up evaluation and laboratory tests.
2. It is best to withhold this drug if electroconvulsive therapy (ECT, "shock" treatment) is to be used.

Precautions for Use
By Infants and Children: Safety and effectiveness for those under 12 years old not established.

By Those Over 60 Years of Age: During the first 2 weeks of treatment watch for confusion, agitation, forgetfulness, disorientation, delusions, and hallucinations. Decreased dose or discontinuation may be needed. Unsteadiness may predispose to falling and injury. May worsen impaired urination associated with prostate gland enlargement (prostatism).

▷ **Advisability of Use During Pregnancy**
Pregnancy Category: D. See Pregnancy Risk Categories at the back of this book.

Animal studies: Skull deformities reported in rabbits.

Human studies: No defects reported in 21 exposures, one case report of a leg deformity in a woman also taking prochlorperazine. Adequate studies of pregnant women are not available.

Avoid use of drug during first 3 months. Use during last 6 months only if clearly needed.

Advisability of Use If Breast-Feeding
Presence of this drug in breast milk: Yes, in small amounts.

Watch nursing infant closely and stop drug or nursing if adverse effects start.

Habit-Forming Potential: If prolonged therapy has been given, stopping this medicine suddenly can lead to headache, nausea, and weakness (malaise). Rare reports of hypomania or mania have been made 2 to 7 days after stopping therapy with tricyclic antidepressants.

Effects of Overdosage: Confusion, hallucinations, marked drowsiness, heart palpitations, dilated pupils, tremors, stupor, deep sleep, coma, convulsions.

Suggested Periodic Examinations While Taking This Drug (at physician's discretion)
>   Complete blood cell counts, liver function tests, serial blood pressure readings, and electrocardiograms.
▷ **While Taking This Drug, Observe the Following**
>   *Foods:* Excessive vitamin C can result in an unexpected increase in decreased therapeutic benefit of amitriptyline. May also increase appetite and cause excessive weight gain.
>   *Beverages:* No restrictions. May be taken with milk.
▷   *Alcohol:* Avoid completely. Can markedly increase the intoxicating effects of alcohol and brain function depression.
>   *Tobacco Smoking:* May hasten the elimination of this drug. Higher doses may be necessary. I advise you to quit smoking.
▷   *Other Drugs*
>   Amitriptyline may ***increase*** the effects of
>   • albuterol or other direct sympathomimetic drugs (amphetamines, epinephrine).
>   • antihistamines (such as diphenhydramine—Benadryl, others) can increase the risk of urinary retention, chronic glaucoma, and bowel obstruction (ileus). This is especially problematic in the elderly.
>   • atropinelike drugs (see Drug Classes).
>   • cimetidine (Tagamet).
>   • disulfiram (Antabuse) can worsen the disulfiram effect if alcohol is consumed.
>   • phenytoin (Dilantin).
>   Amitriptyline may ***decrease*** the effects of
>   • clonidine (Catapres).
>   • guanethidine (Ismelin).
>   • guanfacine (Hytrin).
>   • methyldopa; can result in reduced amitriptyline and/or methyldopa benefits.
>   Amitriptyline ***taken concurrently*** with
>   • amphetamines can result in abnormally increased responses to amitriptyline.
>   • anticoagulants such as warfarin (Coumadin) may cause an increased risk of bleeding.
>   • carbamazepine (Tegretol) may decrease the blood level of amitriptyline.
>   • epinephrine may cause an increased risk of rapid heart rate and high blood pressure.
>   • estrogens (see Drug Classes) may result in abnormal body movements.
>   • ethanol (alcohol) may result in additive toxicity to the central nervous system.
>   • fluoxetine (Prozac) can result in very high levels of amitriptyline.
>   • fluvoxamine (Luvox) can result in very high levels of amitriptyline.
>   • meperidine (Demerol) may worsen chances of breathing (respiratory) depression.
>   • monoamine oxidase (MAO) type A inhibitor drugs may cause high fever, delirium, and convulsions (see Drug Classes).
>   • quinidine (Quinaglute, etc.) can result in increased antidepressant blood levels.

- ritonavir (Norvir) and perhaps other protease inhibitors (see Drug Classes) can lead to amitriptyline toxicity.
- thyroid preparations may impair heart rhythm and function. Ask your doctor for help with adjustment of thyroid dose.
- tramadol (Ultram) may increase risk of seizures. This combination is not advised.

▷ *Driving, Hazardous Activities:* This drug may impair mental alertness, judgment, physical coordination, and reaction time. Avoid hazardous activities.

Aviation Note: The use of this drug *is a disqualification* for piloting. Consult a designated Aviation Medical Examiner.

Exposure to Sun: This drug may cause photosensitivity (see Glossary).

Exposure to Heat: This drug can inhibit sweating and impair the body's adaptation to hot environments, increasing the risk of heatstroke. Avoid saunas.

Exposure to Cold: The elderly should avoid conditions conducive to hypothermia (see Glossary).

Discontinuation: It is best to stop this drug gradually. Abrupt withdrawal after long-term use can cause headache, malaise, and nausea.

AMLODIPINE (am LOH di peen)

Introduced: 1986   **Class:** Anti-anginal, antihypertensive, calcium channel blocker   **Prescription:** USA: Yes   **Controlled Drug:** USA: No; Canada: No   **Available as Generic:** No

Brand Names: Lotrel [CD], Norvasc

Controversies in Medicine: Medicines in this class have been subject to much conflicting data. There have also been several FDA hearings held on the calcium channel blocker class. **This medicine became the first calcium channel blocker to be FDA approved as safe for use in treating hypertension or angina in patients who also have congestive heart failure.** More recent data found the long-acting forms of calcium channel blockers to be safe and effective.

BENEFITS versus RISKS	
Possible Benefits	*Possible Risks*
EFFECTIVE PREVENTION OF BOTH MAJOR TYPES OF ANGINA	DOSE-RELATED CHANGES IN HEART RHYTHM
EFFECTIVE TREATMENT OF HYPERTENSION	Peripheral edema (fluid retention in feet and ankles)
	Dose-related palpitations

▷ **Principal Uses**

As a Single Drug Product: Uses currently included in FDA-approved labeling: Treatment of (1) angina pectoris due to coronary artery spasm (Prinzmetal's variant angina) that happens spontaneously and is not associated with exertion; (2) classical angina-of-effort (due to atherosclerotic disease of the coronary arteries) in people who have not responded to or can't tolerate nitrates or beta-blocker drugs; (3) mild to moderate hypertension; (4) hypertension or angina in patients who also have congestive heart failure.

Other (unlabeled) generally accepted uses: (1) Research indicates that calcium channel blockers may keep early atherosclerotic lesions from progressing; established or older lesions may not be affected to a smaller extent. Medicines in this class may also help after heart transplants; (2) can help stop premature labor; (3) may help prevent migraine headaches.

How This Drug Works: By blocking the normal passage of calcium through cell walls, this drug inhibits the contraction of coronary arteries and peripheral arterioles. As a result of these combined effects, this drug

- prevents spontaneous spasm of the coronary arteries (Prinzmetal's type of angina).
- decreases rate and contraction force of the heart during exertion, reducing frequency of effort-induced angina.
- reduces contraction of peripheral arterial walls, resulting in lower blood pressure. This decreases the work of the heart during exertion and helps prevent angina.

Available Dosage Forms and Strengths

Lotrel tablets — 2.5/10 mg, 5/10 mg and 5/20 mg
Tablets — 2.5 mg, 5 mg, 10 mg

▷ **Recommended Dosage Ranges** (Actual dosage and administration schedule must be determined for each patient individually.)
Infants and Children: Dosage not established.
12 to 60 Years of Age: High blood pressure: 2.5 to 10 mg daily, in a single dose.
Chronic angina: 5 to 10 mg daily; 10 mg may improve exercise ability in stable angina patients.
Congestive heart failure: 5 mg once daily for 2 weeks with increase to 10 mg as needed and tolerated.
Over 65 Years of Age: Lower doses (2.5 mg for high blood pressure and 5 mg for angina) are prudent and effective.

Conditions Requiring Dosing Adjustments
Liver Function: Patients with damaged livers should be started on a daily 2.5-mg dose for high blood pressure and 5 mg for angina, and have the medicine slowly increased as needed or tolerated.
Kidney Function: No adjustment in dosing is needed.
Low Protein or Starvation: This drug is transported in the body by a protein called albumin. If protein is low, as in liver failure or starvation, an increased effect may be seen with "normal" doses. Therapy should be started with low doses and increased only if needed or tolerated.

▷ **Dosing Instructions:**   May be taken with or following food to reduce stomach irritation. The tablet may be crushed for administration.

Usual Duration of Use: Use on a regular schedule for 2 to 4 weeks is usually needed to see this drug's effectiveness in reducing the frequency and severity of angina and in controlling hypertension. For long-term use (months to years), determine the smallest effective dose. Periodic evaluation by your doctor is needed.

Possible Advantages of This Drug
Slow onset and prolonged effect, allowing effective once-a-day treatment for both angina and hypertension.
No adverse effects on heart function.

▷ **This Drug Should Not Be Taken If**
- you have had an allergic reaction to it previously.
- you have active liver disease.
- you have low blood pressure—systolic pressure below 90 mm Hg.
- you have atrioventricular block or sick sinus syndrome (talk to your doctor).
- you have a severe problem (dysfunction) in your left ventricle.
- you have a seriously contracted or narrowed (stenosed) aorta.

▷ **Inform Your Physician Before Taking This Drug If**
- you have had an unfavorable response to any calcium blocker drug.
- you are currently taking any form of digitalis or a beta-blocker drug (see Drug Classes).
- you are taking any drugs that lower blood pressure.
- you have had congestive heart failure, heart attack, or stroke.
- you are subject to disturbances of heart rhythm.
- you have a history of drug-induced liver damage.
- you develop a rash while taking this medicine.
- you are unsure of how much amlodipine to take or how often to take it.
- you have circulation problems in your hands.
- you have muscular dystrophy.

Possible Side Effects (natural, expected, and unavoidable drug actions)
Swelling of feet and ankles, flushing (4.5% in women and 1.5 % in men) and sensation of warmth.
Impaired sense of smell.

▷ **Possible Adverse Effects** (unusual, unexpected, and infrequent reactions)
If any of the following develop, consult your physician promptly for guidance.
Mild Adverse Effects
Allergic reactions: skin rash (call your doctor, as persistent rashes may become serious).
Headache (up to 12%), dizziness (dose related)—infrequent; fatigue—infrequent.
Nausea, constipation—infrequent.
Dose-related palpitations—rare at low dose, infrequent at 10-mg doses.
Overgrowth of the gums (gingival hyperplasia)—up to 10% with drugs in the same class.
Increased urge to urinate at night—rare.
Visual changes (eye pain, double vision)—rare.
Ringing in the ears (tinnitus)—rare.
Cough, muscle pain—rare.
Dose-related flushing (4.5% in women and 1.5% in men)—infrequent.
Elevated liver enzymes (may be a hypersensitivity—usually resolves)—rare.
Serious Adverse Effects
Allergic reactions: none reported.
Idiosyncratic reactions: Parkinson-like symptoms—case report.
Dose-dependent edema (up to 6.2 % in those over 65)—infrequent.
Exfoliative dermatitis or erythema multiforme—rare.
Agranulocytosis; reported with other medicines in this class—case reports.
Rebound angina—if drug is abruptly stopped.
Difficulty breathing (dyspnea)—infrequent.

▷ **Possible Effects on Sexual Function:**   Sexual dysfunction has been reported in both men and women as frequently as 1–2%.

Swelling and tenderness of male breast tissue (gynecomastia)—case report.

Adverse Effects That May Mimic Natural Diseases or Disorders

An allergic rash and swelling of the legs may resemble erysipelas.

Possible Effects on Laboratory Tests

Liver function tests: transient increases in liver enzymes.

CAUTION

1. Tell all health care providers involved in your care that you are taking this drug. Note the use of this drug on your card of personal identification.
2. You may use nitroglycerin and other nitrate drugs as needed to relieve acute episodes of angina pain. If you notice that your angina attacks are becoming more frequent or intense, call your doctor promptly.

Precautions for Use

By Infants and Children: Safety and effectiveness for use by those under 12 not established.

By Those Over 60 Years of Age: May be more susceptible to the development of weakness, dizziness, fainting, and falling. Take necessary precautions to prevent injury. Starting doses should be lower in this age bracket.

▷ **Advisability of Use During Pregnancy**

Pregnancy Category: C. See Pregnancy Risk Categories at the back of this book.

Animal studies: No information available.

Human studies: Adequate studies of pregnant women are not available.

Avoid this drug during the first 3 months. Use during the last 6 months only if clearly needed. Ask your physician for guidance.

Advisability of Use If Breast-Feeding

Presence of this drug in breast milk: Unknown.

Avoid drug or refrain from nursing.

Habit-Forming Potential: None.

Effects of Overdosage: Weakness, light-headedness, fainting, fast pulse, low blood pressure, slow heartbeat, sinus arrest, heart attack, shortness of breath, flushed and warm skin, seizures, metabolic acidosis, low potassium and calcium.

Possible Effects of Long-Term Use: Possible overgrowth of the gums.

Suggested Periodic Examinations While Taking This Drug (at physician's discretion)

Evaluations of heart function, including electrocardiograms; measurements of blood pressure in supine, sitting, and standing positions.

▷ **While Taking This Drug, Observe the Following**

Foods: One medicine in this class is increased by grapefruit or grapefruit juice. Avoid eating grapefruit for an hour after taking this medicine. Avoid excessive salt intake.

Beverages: One medicine in this class is increased by grapefruit juice. Do not take this medicine with grapefruit juice. Avoid grapefruit juice for an hour after you take this medicine. May be taken with milk.

▷ *Alcohol:* Use caution. Alcohol may exaggerate the drop in blood pressure.

Tobacco Smoking: Nicotine may reduce the effectiveness of this drug. I advise everyone to quit smoking.

Marijuana Smoking: Possible reduced effectiveness of this drug; mild to moderate increase in angina; possible changes in electrocardiogram, confusing interpretation.

▷ *Other Drugs*

Amlodipine *taken concurrently* with

- adenosine (Adenocard) may cause extended problems with slow heart rate.
- azole antifungals (such as fluconazole [Diflucan] or itraconazole [Sporanox]), and imidazoles (see Drug Classes) such as ketoconazole (Nizoral) may lead to toxic amlodipine blood levels.
- beta-blocker drugs or digitalis preparations (see Drug Classes) may cause heart rate and rhythm problems.
- cyclosporine (Sandimmune) causes increased cyclosporine blood levels and increased risk of toxicity.
- rifampin (Rifater, others) may result in decreased therapeutic benefit of amlodipine.
- ritonavir (Norvir) and probably other protease inhibitors (see Drug Classes) may lead to amlodipine toxicity.

The following drug may *increase* the effects of amlodipine

- cimetidine (Tagamet).

▷ *Driving, Hazardous Activities:* This drug may cause dizziness. Restrict activities as necessary.

Aviation Note: Coronary artery disease *is a disqualification* for piloting. Consult a designated Aviation Medical Examiner.

Exposure to Sun: No restrictions.

Exposure to Heat: Caution is advised. Hot environments can exaggerate the blood-pressure-lowering effects of this drug. Observe for light-headedness or weakness.

Heavy Exercise or Exertion: This drug may improve your ability to be more active without resulting angina pain. Use caution.

Discontinuation: Do not stop this drug abruptly. Ask your doctor about gradual withdrawal. Observe for the possible development of rebound angina.

AMOXAPINE (a MOX a peen)

Introduced: 1970 **Class:** Antidepressant **Prescription:** USA: Yes
Controlled Drug: USA: No; Canada: No **Available as Generic:** Yes
Brand Name: Asendin

BENEFITS versus RISKS	
Possible Benefits	*Possible Risks*
EFFECTIVE RELIEF OF PRIMARY DEPRESSIONS: Endogenous, neurotic, reactive	ADVERSE BEHAVIORAL EFFECTS: Confusion, delusions, disorientation, hallucinations CONVERSION OF DEPRESSION TO MANIA in manic-depressive disorders Rare blood cell abnormalities Rare movement disorders Rare seizures Rare liver toxicity

Author's Note: Since use of this medicine has declined in favor of newer medicines, the information in this profile has been shortened.

AMOXICILLIN (a mox i SIL in)

AMOXICILLIN/CLAVULANATE (a mox i SIL in/KLAV yu lan ayt)

AMPICILLIN (am pi SIL in)

See the new penicillins profile for further information on these medicines.

ANTI-ALZHEIMER'S DRUGS

Donepezil (DON ep a zill)   **Tacrine** (TA kreen)

Introduced: 1993, 1996   **Class:** Acetylcholinesterase inhibitor, anti-Alzheimer's drug   **Prescription:** USA: Yes   **Controlled Drug:** USA: No; Canada: No   **Available as Generic:** USA: No
Brand Names: Donepezil: Aricept; Tacrine: Cognex

BENEFITS versus RISKS	
Possible Benefits	*Possible Risks*
IMPROVEMENT OF MEMORY IN MILD TO MODERATE ALZHEIMER'S DISEASE IMPROVEMENT OF SYMPTOMS IN MILD TO MODERATE ALZHEIMER'S DISEASE	LIVER TOXICITY (tacrine) Nausea Dizziness

▷ **Principal Uses**

As a Single Drug Product: Uses currently included in FDA-approved labeling: Treatment of symptoms of mild to moderate Alzheimer's disease (both medicines).

Author's Note: Recent guidelines from the American Psychiatric Association (APA) recommend use of vitamin E alone or in combination with donepezil as first-line therapy for delaying symptoms of patients with mild to moderate Alzheimer's.

Other (unlabeled) generally accepted uses: (1) Significant increases in protective white blood cells (CD4 lymphocytes) occurred when tacrine was used to treat AIDS dementia; (2) some early data indicated a benefit in movement disorders (tardive dyskinesia) for tacrine.

How These Drugs Work: Alzheimer's disease is thought to be caused by a loss of nerve cells that make a nerve transmitter (acetylcholine). Donepezil and tacrine act to increase levels of a neurotransmitter (acetylcholine) in the brain.

Available Dosage Forms and Strengths
Donepezil:
Tablets — 5 mg, 10 mg
Tacrine:
Capsules — 10 mg, 20 mg, 30 mg, 40 mg

▷ **Recommended Dosage Ranges** (Actual dosage and administration schedule must be determined for each patient individually.)

Infants and Children: No data are available on use of these drugs in infants and children.

18 to 60 Years of Age: Donepezil: Dosing is started with 5 mg once daily at bedtime. Patients are continued on this dose for 4 to 6 weeks. The dose may be increased to 10 mg after 4 to 6 weeks as needed and tolerated. The 10-mg dose has been associated with increased risk of side effects.

Tacrine: Adult starting dose is 10 mg taken four times a day. The dose can be increased at 6-week intervals if needed. Maximum daily dose is 160 mg.

Over 60 Years of Age: Same as 12 to 60 years of age.

Conditions Requiring Dosing Adjustments
Liver Function: Donepezil doses should be decreased in patients with liver compromise and their blood levels checked. Tacrine should be used with great caution or not at all in liver compromise.

Kidney Function: Dose decreases in kidney compromise are not presently indicated.

▷ **Dosing Instructions:** The donepezil tablet may be crushed and is not effected by food. The tacrine capsule may be opened and is best taken 1 hour before meals. Food decreases the amount of tacrine that gets into your body by 30 to 40%.

Usual Duration of Use: Use on a regular schedule for 3 to 4 weeks is usually needed to see improvement from donepezil or tacrine. Dose increases are made at 4- to 6-week intervals. Long-term use (months to years) requires periodic physician evaluation of response and dosage adjustment.

Possible Advantages of These Drugs
Improvement of memory and other symptoms of mild to moderate Alzheimer's with fewer side effects than other available agents. Donepezil appears to offer a more favorable side effect profile than tacrine, and it avoids liver damage.

Currently a "Drug of Choice"
Donepezil—because of its more favorable side-effect profile—is preferred for treatment of symptoms of mild to moderate Alzheimer's disease.

These Drugs Should Not Be Taken If
DONEPEZIL:
- you have had an allergic reaction to any dosage form of it previously.

TACRINE:
- you have had an allergic reaction to any dosage form of it previously.
- you have had tacrine-caused hepatoxicity and blood bilirubin levels greater than 3 mg/dl.
- you have bronchial asthma.
- you have a slow heartbeat (bradycardia), an abnormal electrical conduction system in your heart (AV conduction defect), or excessively low blood pressure.

- you have an overly active thyroid (hyperthyroidism).
- you have peptic ulcer disease.
- you have an intestinal or urinary tract obstruction.

▷ **Inform Your Physician Before Taking These Drugs If**
- you have a history of seizure disorder.
- you have had liver disease.
- you have a history of peptic ulcer disease.
- you have a history of a slow heartbeat.
- you take an NSAID (see Drug Classes).
- you take muscle relaxants.
- you have glaucoma (angle closure).

Possible Side Effects (natural, expected, and unavoidable drug actions)
Symptoms of cholinergic excess (abdominal upset, agitation).

▷ **Possible Adverse Effects** (unusual, unexpected, and infrequent reactions)
If any of the following develop, consult your physician promptly for guidance.
Mild Adverse Effects
Allergic reactions: skin rash.
Increased sweating—rare.
Increased urination—infrequent.
Muscle aches—infrequent.
Lowered blood pressure—possible.
Nausea or vomiting, belching and diarrhea, decreased appetite—infrequent to frequent.
Dizziness, confusion, and insomnia—infrequent.
Serious Adverse Effects
Allergic reactions: anaphylactoid reactions.
Dose-related increase in liver function tests (starts 6 to 8 weeks after therapy begins)—frequent for tacrine.
Hallucinations—case report for tacrine.
Purpura—infrequent for tacrine.
Severe decrease in white blood cells—one tacrine case report.
Slow heart rate (bradycardia) or abnormal rhythm—possible to rare.
Seizures—case reports for tacrine.

▷ **Possible Effects on Sexual Function:**   Very rare effect of causing lactation for tacrine.

Possible Delayed Adverse Effects: Liver toxicity (tacrine only), rash, low white blood cell count (tacrine only).

Adverse Effects That May Mimic Natural Diseases or Disorders
Liver toxicity of tacrine may mimic acute hepatitis.

Natural Diseases or Disorders That May Be Activated by These Drugs
May worsen bronchial asthma and precipitate seizures. May exacerbate peptic ulcer disease.

Possible Effects on Laboratory Tests
Tacrine: Liver function tests: increased SGOT, SGPT, and CPK. Complete blood count: decreased white blood cells.
Donepezil: None.

CAUTION
1. These drugs should **NOT** be stopped abruptly as sudden decline in think-ing ability may happen (acute deterioration of cognitive abilities).
2. Changes in color of stools (light or very black—tacrine) should be promptly reported to your doctor.
3. These drugs do **NOT** alter the course of Alzheimer's disease. Over time, benefits may be lost.
4. The dose of tacrine **must** be decreased by 40 mg per day if the liver func-tion levels (transaminases) rise to three to five times the upper normal valuc.
5. Females achieve 50% higher tacrine blood levels than men. Dose-related side effects may occur sooner (with lower doses) in women than in men. Beneficial doses may be lower for women than men.

Precautions for Use
By Infants and Children: Safety and effectiveness for those under 18 years of age not established.
By Those Over 60 Years of Age: No specific changes are presently indicated.

▷ **Advisability of Use During Pregnancy**
Pregnancy Category: C. See Pregnancy Risk Categories at the back of this book.
Animal studies: Data not available.
Human studies: Adequate studies of pregnant women are not available.
Consult your doctor.

Advisability of Use If Breast-Feeding
Presence of these drugs in breast milk: Unknown.
Monitor nursing infant closely and discontinue drug or nursing if adverse effects develop.

Habit-Forming Potential: None.

Effects of Overdosage: May precipitate a cholinergic crisis—severe nausea and vomiting, slow heartbeat, low blood pressure, extreme muscle weakness, collapse, and convulsions.

Suggested Periodic Examinations While Taking These Drugs (at physician's discretion)
Assessment of mental status: periodically to check benefit of therapy and po-tential loss of effectiveness as the underlying disease progresses. For ta-crine, liver function tests should be checked every 2 weeks for the first 16 weeks of therapy, then monthly for 2 months and then every 3 months thereafter if the same dose is maintained. If the dose is increased, liver function tests should be checked weekly for 7 weeks and then the above schedule should be followed. Tacrine patients also need complete blood counts periodically or if symptoms of low blood count occur.

While Taking These Drugs, Observe the Following
Foods: Tacrine is best **NOT** taken with food. Donepezil is not affected by food.
Beverages: No restrictions.
▷ *Alcohol:* Occasional small amounts of alcohol are acceptable. Frequent use of alcohol may worsen memory impairment and adversely effect liver en-zymes.
Tobacco Smoking: No interactions expected, but I advise everyone to quit smok-ing.
Marijuana Smoking: Additive dizziness may occur.

▷ *Other Drugs*
These medicines may ***increase*** the effects of
- bethanechol (Duvoid, others).
- theophylline (Theo-Dur, others) by doubling the drug level (reported for tacrine).
- succinylcholine (Anectine, others).

These medicines may ***decrease*** the effects of
- anticholinergic medications (see Drug Classes).

The following drug may ***increase*** the effects of these medicines:
- cimetidine (Tagamet).

These medicines ***taken concurrently*** with
- dexamethasone, phenobarbital, or phenytoin (Dilantin) may decrease the therapeutic benefits.
- ketoconazole and perhaps ritonavir (Norvir) or other protease inhibitors (see Drug Classes) may lead to increased risk of donepezil or tacrine toxicity.

▷ *Driving, Hazardous Activities:* These drugs may cause confusion or dizziness. Restrict activities as necessary.

Aviation Note: The use of these drugs ***may be a disqualification*** for piloting. Consult a designated Aviation Medical Examiner.

Exposure to Sun: No restrictions.

Exposure to Heat: Increased sweating may occur rarely with tacrine. The combination of increased sweating and hot environments may lead to more rapid dehydration.

Discontinuation: These drugs should **NOT** be abruptly stopped. Some adverse effects are dose related, and may abate if the dose is decreased. Slow withdrawal of the drug is indicated if it is not tolerated.

ANTI-LEUKOTRIENES

Zafirlukast (zah FUR lew kast) **Zileuton** (ZEYE loo ton)

Introduced: 1996, 1997   **Class:** Anti-leukotriene, antiasthmatic   **Prescription:** USA: Yes   **Controlled Drug:** USA: No; Canada: No   **Available as Generic:** No

Brand Names: Zafirlukast: Accolate; Zileuton: Zyflo

BENEFITS versus RISKS	
Possible Benefits	*Possible Risks*
EFFECTIVE PREVENTION AND CHRONIC TREATMENT OF BRONCHIAL ASTHMA	Headache
	Nausea
	Liver enzyme increase
Zafirlukast may have a role in treating bronchospasm caused by exercise	

▷ **Principal Uses**
As a Single Drug Product: Uses currently included in FDA-approved labeling: Used to prevent recurrence of asthmatic episodes and to chronically treat asthmatic episodes.

Author's Note: These medicines are indicated as Step Two medicines (alternatives to low-dose inhaled steroids, cromolyn, or nedocromil in mild persistent asthma) in the National Institutes of Health's (NIH, NHLBI) "Guidelines for Diagnosis and Management of Asthma."

Other (unlabeled) generally accepted uses: (1) Zafirlukast may have a role in preventing spasm of the bronchi caused by exercise; (2) zileuton may have a role in preventing allergic rhinitis or aspirin-sensitive asthma; (3) zileuton may also help symptoms of ulcerative colitis.

How These Drugs Work: Zafirlukast works by blocking (leukotriene receptor antagonist) the action of chemicals called leukotrienes (formerly known as slow-reacting substances of anaphylaxis). Zileuton works by blocking the formation (leukotriene pathway inhibitor) of leukotrienes by inhibiting a chemical called 5-lipoxygenase inhibitor. By inhibiting the action or formation of leukotrienes, both medicines help keep the airways open.

Available Dosage Forms and Strengths

Zafirlukast:

Accolate tablet — 20 mg

Zileuton:

    Tablets — 600 mg

▷ **Recommended Dosage Ranges** (Actual dosage and administration schedule must be determined for each patient individually.)

Children 12 or Older: Zafirlukast and zileuton: Same as adult dose.

12 to 60 Years of Age: Zafirlukast: 20 mg twice daily.

Zileuton: 600 mg four times a day.

Over 60 Years of Age: Zafirlukast: Removal (clearance) is changed such that the maximum blood level is twice that of younger patients. It appears prudent to lower the dose, but specific guidelines have not been developed. The current package insert notes that using the typical dose in these patients did not result in adverse effects in clinical trials.

Zileuton: Same as those for 12 to 60 years old. **Note: These medicines may be continued during an acute worsening (exacerbation) of asthma, but are not to be used to treat an sudden (acute) asthma attack.**

Conditions Requiring Dosing Adjustments

Liver Function: Zafirlukast remains in the body up to 60% longer in patients with alcoholic cirrhosis. Specific guidelines are not available, but lower doses and blood levels appear prudent. Zileuton should not be given if active liver disease is present.

Kidney Function: Dosage changes are not needed for either medicine in patients with compromised kidneys.

▷ **Dosing Instructions:** Zafirlukast should be taken on an empty stomach, 1 hour before or 2 hours after a meal. Zileuton may be given with or without food. NEITHER medicine is to be used to stop a sudden (acute) attack.

Usual Duration of Use: Zafirlukast appears to have a significant effect on bronchoconstriction 30 minutes after the medicine is taken, and lasts 12 hours after a typical dose. Zileuton reaches a significant effect 5 to 8 hours after the medication is taken, and the effect continued for up to 7 days in single-dose clinical studies. Ongoing use requires periodic follow-up with your doctor.

These Drugs Should Not Be Taken If
- you have had an allergic reaction to them, or to any other form of these drugs.
- you have active liver disease or increased liver enzymes (transaminases) greater than three times the upper normal limit (zileuton).

▷ **Inform Your Physician Before Taking This Drug If**
- you have a liver disease (zafirlukast).
- you are having a sudden (acute) asthma attack.
- you have impaired kidney function.

Possible Side Effects (natural, expected, and unavoidable drug actions)
Not defined at present.

▷ **Possible Adverse Effects** (unusual, unexpected, and infrequent reactions)
If any of the following develop, consult your physician promptly for guidance.
Mild Adverse Effects
Allergic reactions: skin rash, hives.
Headache, fatigue, weakness—infrequent.
Dizziness—rare for zafirlukast, infrequent for zileuton.
Nausea or abdominal pain—infrequent.
Muscle pain—rare for zafirlukast, infrequent for zileuton.
Serious Adverse Effects
Allergic reactions: not reported as yet.
Idiosyncratic reactions; none reported as yet.
Liver toxicity (increased enzyme tests)—rare for zafirlukast, infrequent for for zileuton.

▷ **Possible Effects on Sexual Function:**   None reported.

Natural Diseases or Disorders That May Be Activated by This Drug
Since both medicines may increase liver enzymes, hidden (subclinical) liver problems may be activated.

Possible Effects on Laboratory Tests
Liver function tests (SGPT, SGOT, LDH): may be increased.

CAUTION
1. Other medicines which you take for asthma should be discussed with your doctor to see if he or she wants you to continue taking them.
2. Since both medicines can (1.5 % and 2% of the time) affect the liver, it is critical that you have blood drawn for laboratory testing of liver function as your doctor orders the tests.

Precautions for Use
By Children: Make certain that these medicines are taken in the amount and for the number of times they are ordered.
By Those Over 65 Years of Age: Zafirlukast goes to higher peak blood levels and remains in the body longer in those over 65. It appears that smaller starting doses are indicated. Zileuton is not changed by age.

▷ **Advisability of Use During Pregnancy**
Pregnancy Category: zafirlukast: B; zileuton: C. See Pregnancy Risk Categories at the back of this book.
Animal studies: Zafirlukast: no teratogenicity up to 160 times the maximum

recommended dose given to mice. Zileuton: Adverse effects were seen in rats given 18 times the typical human dose.

Human studies: Adequate studies of pregnant women are not available. Ask your doctor for guidance.

Advisability of Use If Breast-Feeding
Presence of this drug in breast milk: Zafirlukast: Yes. Zileuton: Unknown. Avoid drug or refrain from nursing.

Habit-Forming Potential: None.

Effects of Overdosage: No overdose experience in humans for zafirlukast. Zileuton overdose experience is limited. One patient received between 6.6 and 9.0 g of zileuton, which caused vomiting, and recovered without ill effects.

Possible Effects of Long-Term Use: Not defined.

Suggested Periodic Examinations While Taking This Drug (at physician's discretion)
Periodic liver function tests.

▷ **While Taking This Drug, Observe the Following**
Foods: Zafirlukast should be taken on an empty stomach; no restrictions for zileuton.
Beverages: No restrictions.
▷ *Alcohol:* May worsen drowsiness.
Tobacco Smoking: I advise everyone to quit smoking.
Marijuana Smoking: May cause additive drowsiness.
▷ *Other Drugs*
These medicines *taken concurrently* with
- aspirin (various brands) may cause zafirlukast toxicity.
- beta-blocker drugs (see Drug Classes) may cause beta-blocker toxicity if combined with zileuton.
- erythromycin (E-Mycin, Erythrocin, etc.) may decrease zafirlukast's benefits.
- terfenadine (Seldane) may decrease zafirlukast blood levels and its therapeutic benefits. Zileuton may decrease terfenadine (and perhaps other similarly structured minimally sedating antihistamine levels) and lead to toxicity. DO NOT combine.
- theophylline (Theo-Dur, others) may decrease zafirlukast blood levels and its therapeutic benefits. Zileuton may result in doubling of theophylline levels and require reduced theophylline doses.
- warfarin (Coumadin) may lead to increased risk of bleeding. More frequent INRs are needed.
▷ *Driving, Hazardous Activities:* These drugs may cause dizziness. Restrict activities as necessary.
Aviation Note: The use of this drug *may be a disqualification* for piloting. Consult a designated Aviation Medical Examiner.
Exposure to Sun: No restrictions.
Discontinuation: Do not stop this medicine without first talking with your doctor.

ASPIRIN* (AS pir in)

Other Names: ASA, acetylsalicylic acid

Introduced: 1899   **Class:** Analgesics, mild; antiplatelet, antipyretic, NSAIDs, salicylates **Prescription:** USA: No   **Controlled Drug:** USA: No; Canada: No   **Available as Generic:** Yes

Brand Names: Added Strength Analgesic Pain Reliever, Alka-Seltzer Effervescent Pain Reliever & Antacid [CD], Alka Seltzer Night Time [CD], Alka-Seltzer Plus [CD], Alka-Seltzer Plus Cold [CD], Anacin [CD], Anacin Maximum Strength [CD], ✦Anacin w/Codeine [CD], ✦Ancasal, APC [CD], APC with Codeine [CD], Arthritis Pain Formula [CD], Arthritis Strength Bufferin, A.S.A. Enseals, ✦Asasantine [CD], Ascriptin [CD], Ascriptin A/D [CD], Aspergum, ✦Aspirin*, Asprimox, ✦Astrin, Axotal [CD], Azdone [CD], Bayer Aspirin, Bayer Children's Chewable Aspirin, Bayer Enteric Aspirin, Bayer Plus, Buffaprin, Bufferin [CD], Bufferin Arthritis Strength [CD], Bufferin Extra Strength [CD], Bufferin w/Codeine [CD], Cama Arthritis Pain Reliever [CD], Carisoprodol Compound [CD], Cope [CD], Coricidin [CD], ✦Coryphen, ✦Coryphen-Codeine [CD], ✦C2 Buffered [CD], Darvon Compound [CD], Direct Formulary Aspirin, ✦Dristan [CD], Easprin, Ecotrin, 8-Hour Bayer, Empirin, Empirin w/Codeine No. 2, 4 [CD], ✦Entrophen, Excedrin [CD], Excedrin Extra Strength Geltabs [CD], Fiorinal [CD], ✦Fiorinal-C 1/4, -C 1/2 [CD], Fiorinal w/Codeine [CD], Genprin, Halprin, Hepto [CD], Lortab ASA [CD], Low Dose Adult Chewable Aspirin, Marnal [CD], Maximum Bayer Aspirin, Measurin, Midol Caplets [CD], Momentum [CD], Norgesic [CD], Norgesic Forte [CD], Norwich Aspirin, ✦Novasen, Orphenadrine [CD], PAP with Codeine [CD], Percodan [CD], Percodan-Demi [CD], ✦Phenaphen [CD], ✦Phenaphen No. 2, 3, 4 [CD], Propoxyphene Compound [CD], ✦Riphen-10, Robaxisal [CD], ✦Robaxisal-C [CD], Roxiprin [CD], SK-65 Compound [CD], Soma Compound [CD], St. Joseph Children's Aspirin, ✦Supasa, Synalgos [CD], Synalgos-DC [CD], Talwin Compound [CD], Talwin Compound-50 [CD], ✦Tecnal tablet [CD], ✦Triaphen-10, ✦217 [CD], ✦217 Strong [CD], ✦292 [CD], ✦692 [CD], Vanquish [CD], Verin, Wesprin, Zorprin

---

BENEFITS versus RISKS

Possible Benefits	Possible Risks
EFFECTIVE RELIEF OF MILD TO MODERATE PAIN AND INFLAMMATION	Stomach irritation, bleeding, and/or ulceration
REDUCTION OF FEVER	Decreased numbers of white blood cells and platelets
PREVENTION OF BLOOD CLOTS	Hemolytic anemia—rare
PREVENTION OF HEART ATTACK	Liver toxicity—rare
PREVENTION OF STROKE	Bronchospasm in asthmatics—possible
PREVENTION OF COLON CANCER MAY ACT TO LIMIT THE SIZE AND SEVERITY OF A HEART ATTACK ONCE IT HAS STARTED	

---

*In the United States *aspirin* is an official generic designation. In Canada *Aspirin* is the Registered Trade Mark of the Bayer Company Division of Sterling Drug Limited.

▷ **Principal Uses**

As a Single Drug Product: Uses currently included in FDA-approved labeling: (1) Relieves mild to moderate pain, and provides symptomatic relief in conditions causing inflammation or high fever. Treats musculoskeletal disorders, especially acute and chronic arthritis, as well as painful menstruation (dysmenorrhea). Used selectively to (2) reduce the risk of first heart attack; (3) reduce the risk of recurrent heart attack; (4) prevent platelet embolism to the brain (in men); (5) reduce the risk of clots (thromboembolism) in heart attack patients and in people with artificial heart valves and after hip surgery (scc Blood Platelets in Glossary); (6) help prevent recurrence of stroke in people who have suffered a stroke; (7) help prevent stroke in patients who have had a transient ischemic attack (TIA); (8) help prevent migraine headaches.

Other (unlabeled) generally accepted uses: (1) Can help prevent toxemia of pregnancy when used in low doses; (2) a very recent, well-designed, large-sample-size study shows that long-term use may decrease the risk of colon polyps or colon cancer in females. The data are large enough to be expected to apply to men as well; (3) another very recent study shows that aspirin may limit the size and severity of a heart attack when it is taken immediately after symptoms are recognized and is continued for at least 30 days after the heart attack; (4) can help reduce flushing caused by niacin.

As a Combination Drug Product [CD]: Frequently combined with other mild or strong analgesic drugs to enhance pain relief. Also combined with antihistamines and decongestants in many cold preparations to relieve headache and general discomfort.

How This Drug Works: Reduces prostaglandins, chemicals involved in the production of inflammation and pain. By modifying the temperature-regulating center in the brain, dilating blood vessels, and increasing sweating, aspirin reduces fever. By preventing the production of thromboxane in blood platelets, aspirin inhibits formation of blood clots.

Available Dosage Forms and Strengths

Capsules, enteric coated —	500 mg
Capsules, enteric-coated granules —	325 mg
Gum tablets —	227.5 mg
Suppositories —	60 mg, 120 mg, 125 mg, 130 mg, 195 mg, 200 mg, 300 mg, 325 mg, 600 mg, 650 mg, 1.2 g
Tablets —	65 mg, 81 mg, 325 mg, 500 mg
Tablets, chewable —	81 mg
Tablets, enteric coated —	81 mg, 165 mg, 325 mg, 500 mg, 650 mg, 975 mg
Tablets, prolonged action —	650 mg, 800 mg

▷ **Usual Adult Dosage Range:**   For pain or fever—325 to 650 mg every 4 hours as needed. For arthritis (and related conditions)—3600 to 5400 mg daily in divided doses. For the prevention of blood clots—80 to 150 mg daily or every other day. Low-dose, long-term daily aspirin may also decrease risk of colon cancer. Some patients are given aspirin every other day to help prevent heart attacks. **Note: For long-term use, actual dosage and administration schedule must be determined for each patient individually.**

Conditions Requiring Dosing Adjustments
Liver Function: This medication should be avoided in severe liver disease.
Kidney Function: It should be avoided or used with caution in patients with kidney problems, and not at all in severe (creatinine clearance less than 10 ml/min) kidney failure.
Glucose-6-Phosphate Dehydrogenase (G6PD) Deficiency: May cause destruction of red blood cells in patients with G6PD deficiency.

▷ **Dosing Instructions:**   Take with food, milk, or a full glass of water to reduce stomach upset. Regular tablets may be crushed and capsules opened for administration. Enteric-coated tablets, prolonged-action tablets, A.S.A. En-seals, Cama tablets, and Ecotrin tablets should not be crushed.

Usual Duration of Use: Short-term use is recommended—3 to 5 days. Daily use should not exceed 10 days without physician supervision. Use on a regular schedule for 1 week is usually needed to determine this drug's effectiveness in relieving the symptoms of chronic arthritis. Response must be evaluated and dose adjusted in long-term use. Long-term use for prevention of heart attack, colon cancer, or stroke certainly requires ongoing physician super-vision, even though aspirin is not a prescription drug. Consult your doctor on a regular basis.

▷ **This Drug Should Not Be Taken If**
- you have had an allergic reaction to any form of aspirin.
- you have any type of bleeding disorder (such as hemophilia).
- you have active peptic ulcer disease.
- you are in the last 3 months of pregnancy.
- it smells like vinegar. This indicates decomposition of aspirin.

▷ **Inform Your Physician Before Taking This Drug If**
- you are taking any anticoagulant drug.
- you are taking oral antidiabetic drugs.
- you have a history of peptic ulcer disease or gout.
- you have lupus erythematosus.
- you are pregnant or planning pregnancy.
- you have asthma, carditis, or nasal polyps.
- you plan to have surgery of any kind in the near future.
- you take other prescription or nonprescription medications that were not discussed when aspirin was prescribed for you.
- you are unsure of how much aspirin to take or how often to take it.
- you have a history of liver or kidney problems.
- you have a deficiency of glucose-6-phosphate dehydrogenase (G6PD).
- you have a history of angina (may be worsened by this drug).

Possible Side Effects (natural, expected, and unavoidable drug actions)
Mild drowsiness in sensitive patients.

▷ **Possible Adverse Effects** (unusual, unexpected, and infrequent reactions)
If any of the following develop, consult your physician promptly for guidance.
Mild Adverse Effects
Allergic reactions: skin rash, hives, nasal discharge (resembling hay fever), nasal polyps.
Stomach irritation, heartburn, nausea, vomiting, constipation—infrequent to frequent.
Lowering of the blood sugar—rare.

Serious Adverse Effects

Allergic reactions: acute anaphylactic reaction (see Glossary), allergic destruction of blood platelets (see Glossary) and bruising—rare.

Idiosyncratic reactions: hemolytic anemia (see Glossary)—rare.

Stevens-Johnson syndrome—possible.

Erosion of stomach lining, with silent bleeding—may be dose and frequency related.

Activation of peptic ulcer, with or without hemorrhage—frequent with long-term nonenteric coated use.

Bone marrow depression (see Glossary): fatigue, weakness, fever, sore throat, abnormal bleeding or bruising—possible.

Hepatitis with jaundice (see Glossary): yellow skin and eyes, dark-colored urine, light-colored stool—possible.

Hearing toxicity (ototoxicity)—more common with higher doses and long-term use.

Kidney damage, if used in large doses or for a prolonged period of time—possible.

Bronchospasm when used in patients with nasal polyps, asthma—possible.

May worsen angina attacks and increase their frequency—possible.

Reye syndrome if used during viral illness—DO NOT USE.

▷ **Possible Effects on Sexual Function:**   None reported.

Adverse Effects That May Mimic Natural Diseases or Disorders

Liver damage may suggest viral hepatitis or reveal (unmask) low level (subclinical) liver disease.

Possible Effects on Laboratory Tests

Complete blood counts: decreased red cells, hemoglobin, white cells, and platelets.

Bleeding time: prolonged.

INR (prothrombin time): increased by large doses; decreased by small doses.

Blood glucose level: decreased in diabetics.

Blood uric acid level: increased by small doses; decreased by large doses.

Liver function tests: increased ALT/GPT, AST/GOT, alkaline phosphatase.

Kidney function tests: increased blood creatinine and urea nitrogen levels with long-term use; increased protein and kidney cells in urine.

Thyroid function tests: increased T_3 uptake, free T_3 and free T_4; decreased TSH, T_3, T_4, and free thyroxine index (FTI).

Urine sugar tests: false positive with Clinitest or Benedict's solution.

Fecal occult blood test: positive with large doses of aspirin.

CAUTION

1. Remember that aspirin is a drug. Although it is one of our most useful drugs, we have an unrealistic sense of its safety and its potential for adverse effects.

2. Make it a point to learn the contents of all drugs you take—those prescribed by your physician and over-the-counter (OTC) medicines.

3. Do NOT take more than 3 tablets (975 mg) at one time; allow at least 4 hours between doses; and do not take more than 10 tablets (3250 mg) in 24 hours without physician supervision.

4. Remember that aspirin can
   • cause new illnesses.
   • complicate existing illnesses.

- complicate pregnancy.
- complicate surgery.
- interact unfavorably with other drugs.

5. When your physician asks, "Are you taking any drugs?" the answer is **yes** if you are taking aspirin. This also applies to *any* nonprescription drug you may be taking (see Over-the-Counter Drugs in Glossary).

Precautions for Use

By Infants and Children: Reye syndrome (brain and liver damage in children, often fatal) can follow flu or chickenpox in children and teenagers. Some reports suggest that the use of aspirin by children with flu or chickenpox can increase the risk of developing this complication. Consult your physician before giving aspirin to a child or teenager with chickenpox, flu, or similar infection.

Usual dosage schedule for children:

Up to 2 years of age—consult physician.
2 to 4 years of age—160 mg/4 hours, up to 5 doses/24 hours.
4 to 6 years of age—240 mg/4 hours, up to 5 doses/24 hours.
6 to 9 years of age—320 mg/4 hours, up to 5 doses/24 hours.
9 to 11 years of age—400 mg/4 hours, up to 5 doses/24 hours.
11 to 12 years of age—480 mg/4 hours, up to 5 doses/24 hours.

Do not exceed 5 days of continual use without consulting your physician.
Give all doses with food, milk, or a full glass of water.

By Those Over 60 Years of Age: Watch for signs of excessive dosage: nervous irritability, confusion, ringing in the ears, deafness, loss of appetite, nausea, and stomach upset. Aspirin can cause serious bleeding from the stomach. This can occur as "silent" bleeding of small amounts over a long time, resulting in anemia. Sudden hemorrhage can occur, even without a history of stomach ulcer. Watch for gray- to black-colored stools, an indication of stomach bleeding.

▷ **Advisability of Use During Pregnancy**

Pregnancy Category: C. See Pregnancy Risk Categories at the back of this book. Animal studies: Significant birth defects due to this drug have been reported. Human studies: Information from studies of pregnant women indicates no increased risk of birth defects in 32,164 pregnancies exposed to aspirin. However, studies show that the regular use of aspirin during pregnancy is often detrimental to the health of the mother and the welfare of the fetus. Anemia, hemorrhage before and after delivery, and an increased incidence of stillbirths and newborn deaths have been reported. It is advisable to limit aspirin use during pregnancy to small doses and for brief periods of time. There are data which support use of aspirin in low doses to prevent toxemia of pregnancy in some women with a history of this problem. Ask your doctor for help. Avoid aspirin altogether during the last 3 months.

Advisability of Use If Breast-Feeding

Presence of this drug in breast milk: Yes.
Avoid drug or refrain from nursing.

Habit-Forming Potential: Extended high dose use may cause a psychological dependence (see Glossary).

Effects of Overdosage: Stomach distress, nausea, vomiting, ringing in the ears, dizziness, impaired hearing, blood chemistry imbalance, sweating, stupor, fever, deep and rapid breathing, muscular twitching, delirium, shock, hallucinations, convulsions.

Possible Effects of Long-Term Use
A form of psychological dependence (see Glossary).
Anemia due to chronic blood loss from erosion of stomach lining.
The development of stomach ulcer.
The development of "aspirin allergy"—nasal discharge, nasal polyps, asthma.
Kidney damage.
Prolonged bleeding time, critical in the event of injury or surgery.

Suggested Periodic Examinations While Taking This Drug (at physician's discretion)
Complete blood cell counts.
Kidney function tests and urine analyses.
Liver function tests.

▷ **While Taking This Drug, Observe the Following**
Foods: May decrease the total amount of aspirin per dose which is absorbed.
Nutritional Support: Do not take large doses of vitamin C while taking aspirin regularly.
Beverages: No restrictions. May be taken with milk.
▷ *Alcohol:* Concurrent use of alcohol and aspirin may significantly increase the risk of stomach damage and may prolong bleeding time.
Tobacco Smoking: No interactions expected, but I advise everyone to quit smoking.
▷ *Other Drugs*
Aspirin may ***increase*** the effects of
- adrenocortical steroids (see Drug Classes) may lead to additive stomach irritation and bleeding.
- insulin (various brands) and require dosage adjustment.
- oral anticoagulants (see Drug Classes), and cause abnormal bleeding.
- oral antidiabetic drugs, and cause hypoglycemia (see Drug Classes). Dosage adjustments are often necessary.
- heparin, and cause abnormal bleeding.
- methotrexate, and increase its toxic effects.
- valproic acid (Depakene).

Aspirin may ***decrease*** the effects of
- beta-adrenergic-blocking drugs (see Drug Classes).
- captopril (Capoten).
- furosemide (Lasix).
- other NSAIDs (see Drug Classes).
- probenecid (Benemid), and reduce its effectiveness in the treatment of gout—with aspirin doses of less than 2 g every 24 hours.
- spironolactone (Aldactazide, Aldactone, others), and reduce its diuretic effect.
- sulfinpyrazone (Anturane), and reduce its effectiveness in the treatment of gout—with aspirin doses of less than 2 g every 24 hours.

Aspirin ***taken concurrently*** with
- diltiazem (Cardizem) may result in increased risk of bleeding.
- high blood pressure (antihypertensive) medicines may blunt their thera-

peutic benefit, especially those that are diuretics such as furosemide (Lasix), spironolactone, or thiazides (see Drug Classes).

- intrauterine devices (IUDs) may result in decreased IUD effectiveness.
- lithium (Lithobid) may increase lithium blood levels.
- methotrexate (Mexate) may cause toxicity.
- valproic acid (Depakote) may cause toxic blood levels.
- varicella vaccine (Varivax) may result in Reye syndrome. **Avoid aspirin and other salicylates for 6 weeks following Varivax inoculation.**
- verapamil (Calan, others) may cause increased bleeding risk.
- zafirlukast (Accolate) may increase zafirlukast blood levels and increase adverse effects.

The following drugs may *increase* the effects of aspirin:

- acetazolamide (Diamox).
- cimetidine (Tagamet).
- para-aminobenzoic acid (Pabalate).

The following drugs may *decrease* the effects of aspirin:

- antacids, with regular continual use.
- cortisonelike drugs (see Drug Classes).
- urinary alkalinizers (sodium bicarbonate, sodium citrate).

▷ *Driving, Hazardous Activities:* No restrictions or precautions.

Aviation Note: It is advisable to watch for mild drowsiness and restrict activities accordingly.

Exposure to Sun: Use caution; may cause photosensitivity.

Discontinuation: Aspirin should be stopped at least 1 week before surgery of any kind.

ASTEMIZOLE (a STEM i zohl)

See the new minimally sedating antihistamines profile for further information.

ATENOLOL (a TEN oh lohl)

Introduced: 1973   **Class:** Anti-anginal, antihypertensive, beta-adrenergic blocker   **Prescription:** USA: Yes   **Controlled Drug:** USA: No; Canada: No   **Available as Generic:** Yes

Brand Names: ✦Apo-Atenolol, ✦Novo-Atenolol, ✦Nu-Atenolol, Tenoretic [CD], Tenormin

BENEFITS versus RISKS	
Possible Benefits	*Possible Risks*
EFFECTIVE ANTI-ANGINAL DRUG in the management of effort-induced angina	CONGESTIVE HEART FAILURE in advanced heart disease
EFFECTIVE, WELL-TOLERATED ANTIHYPERTENSIVE in mild to moderate high blood pressure	Worsening of angina in coronary heart disease (abrupt withdrawal)
	Masking of low blood sugar (hypoglycemia) in drug-treated diabetes
	Provocation of bronchial asthma (with high doses)

▷ **Principal Uses**

As a Single Drug Product: Uses currently included in FDA-approved labeling: (1) Treats classical, effort-induced angina pectoris; (2) used for mild to moderately severe high blood pressure. May be used alone or in combination with other antihypertensive drugs, such as diuretics; (3) used following heart attacks to prolong life, **helps decrease risk of a second heart attack**, decrease the size of the heart attack, and reduce risk of abnormal heartbeats.

Other (unlabeled) generally accepted uses: (1) Can help people with stage fright; (2) may have a role in preventing migraine headaches; (3) can have an adjunctive role in alcohol withdrawal.

As a Combination Drug Product [CD]: Used in combination with a thiazide diuretic to combine the benefits of a beta-blocker with the excess-fluid-losing properties of a thiazide. This attacks high blood pressure using two different mechanisms.

How This Drug Works: By blocking certain actions of the sympathetic nervous system, this drug reduces the rate and contraction force of the heart, reducing the oxygen requirement for the heart as it works and reduces blood vessel wall contraction, resulting in their relaxation and expansion and consequent lowering of blood pressure.

Available Dosage Forms and Strengths

Tablets — 25 mg, 50 mg, 100 mg

▷ **Usual Adult Dosage Range:**   Hypertension: Initially 50 mg once daily. Dose may be increased gradually at intervals of 7 to 10 days as needed and tolerated up to 100 mg every 24 hours. The usual maintenance dose is 50 to 100 mg every 24 hours. The total dose should not exceed 100 mg every 24 hours.

Angina: Starting dose is 50 mg once daily. Dose may be increased gradually at intervals of 7 to 10 days as needed and tolerated up to 100 mg every 24 hours. The usual maintenance dose is 50 to 100 mg every 24 hours. Some patients have required 200 mg daily.

After a heart attack (post MI): Within 12 hours after the attack, 5 mg of this drug is given intravenously. This is followed by a second 5-mg intravenous dose 10 minutes later. Twelve hours after the second intravenous dose, 50 mg is given orally, followed by a second 50 mg 12 hours later. Oral dosing is continued at 100 mg orally for the next 10 days. **Note: Actual dosage and administration schedule must be determined for each patient individually.**

Conditions Requiring Dosing Adjustments

Liver Function: No decreases needed as the liver has a small role in eliminating atenolol.

Kidney Function: The dose must be decreased with 25 mg a day as a maximum dose in some people.

▷ **Dosing Instructions:**   May be taken without regard to eating. Tablet may be crushed to take it. **DO NOT** stop this drug abruptly.

Usual Duration of Use: Use on a regular schedule for 3 to 7 days is usually needed to see this drug's effectiveness in lowering blood pressure. Long-term use of this drug will be decided by how much your blood pressure decreases over time in response to an overall treatment program (weight reduction, salt restriction, smoking cessation, etc.). It may take 3 months for peak chest pain benefits. See your doctor on a regular basis.

Possible Advantages of This Drug: Least likely of all beta-blocker drugs to cause central nervous system adverse effects: confusion, hallucinations, nervousness, nightmares.

▷ **This Drug Should Not Be Taken If**
- you have had an allergic reaction to it previously.
- you are in heart failure (overt).
- you have an abnormally slow heart rate or a serious form of heart block.
- you are taking, or have taken within the past 14 days, any monoamine oxidase (MAO) type A inhibitor drug (see Drug Classes).
- you are in cardiogenic shock.

▷ **Inform Your Physician Before Taking This Drug If**
- you have had an adverse reaction to any beta-blocker drug (see Drug Classes).
- you have a history of serious heart disease, with or without episodes of heart failure.
- you have a history of hay fever (allergic rhinitis), asthma, chronic bronchitis, chronic obstructive pulmonary disease (COPD), or emphysema.
- you have been taking clonidine.
- you have a history of overactive thyroid function (hyperthyroidism).
- you have a history of low blood sugar (hypoglycemia)—this drug may hide some of the symptoms occurring with hypoglycemia.
- you have impaired liver or kidney function.
- you have diabetes or myasthenia gravis.
- you currently take any form of digitalis, quinidine, or reserpine, or any calcium blocker drug (see Drug Classes).
- you plan to have surgery under general anesthesia in the near future.
- you take other prescription or nonprescription medications that were not discussed when atenolol was prescribed for you.
- you are unsure of how much atenolol to take or how often to take it.

Possible Side Effects (natural, expected, and unavoidable drug actions)
Lethargy, fatigability, cold extremities, slow heart rate, light-headedness in upright position (see Orthostatic Hypotension in Glossary)—all reported during treatment.

▷ **Possible Adverse Effects** (unusual, unexpected, and infrequent reactions)
If any of the following develop, consult your physician promptly for guidance.
Mild Adverse Effects
Allergic reactions: skin rash, itching.
Headache, dizziness, drowsiness, abnormal dreams—infrequent.
Indigestion, nausea, diarrhea—infrequent.
Joint and muscle discomfort, fluid retention (edema)—possible.
Serious Adverse Effects
Mental depression—frequent.
Chest pain, shortness of breath, can lead to congestive heart failure—rare.
Induction of bronchial asthma (in asthmatic patients)—possible.
Angina or rebound hypertension—if abruptly stopped.
Difficulty walking (intermittent claudication)—controversial.
Psychosis—case reports.
Systemic lupus erythematosus—case reports.

▷ **Possible Effects on Sexual Function:**   Decreased libido and impaired potency (50 to 100 mg per day). This drug is less likely to cause reduced erectile capacity than most drugs of its class. Impotence—rare.

Possible Effects on Laboratory Tests

Blood cholesterol levels: no effect with doses of 50 mg/day; increased with doses of 100 mg/day.

Blood HDL cholesterol levels: no effect with doses of 50 mg/day; decreased with doses of 100 mg/day.

Blood LDL cholesterol levels: no effect with doses of 50 mg/day; increased with doses of 100 mg/day.

Blood VLDL cholesterol levels: no effect with doses of 50 mg/day; increased with doses of 100 mg/day.

Blood triglyceride levels: no effect with doses of 50 mg/day; increased with doses of 100 mg/day.

CAUTION

1. *DO NOT stop this drug suddenly* without the knowledge and guidance of your physician. Always carry a note that says you take this drug.
2. Consult your physician or pharmacist before using nasal decongestants. These can cause sudden increases in blood pressure when combined with beta-blocker drugs.
3. Report the development of any tendency to emotional depression.

Precautions for Use

By Infants and Children: Safety and effectiveness by those under 12 years of age not established. However, if this drug is used, watch for development of low blood sugar (hypoglycemia), especially if meals are skipped.

By Those Over 60 Years of Age: Proceed *cautiously* with all antihypertensive drugs. High blood pressure should be reduced slowly, avoiding excessively low blood pressure. Small doses and frequent blood pressure checks are needed. Sudden and excessive decrease in blood pressure can predispose to stroke or heart attack. Maximum daily dosage is 100 mg. Watch for dizziness, unsteadiness, tendency to fall, confusion, hallucinations, depression, or urinary frequency.

▷ **Advisability of Use During Pregnancy**

Pregnancy Category: D. See Pregnancy Risk Categories at the back of this book.

Animal studies: Increased resorptions of embryo and fetus reported in rats, but no birth defects.

Human studies: Adequate studies of pregnant women are not available, but the drug has caused fetal harm.

This drug has been used during the last three months of pregnancy; however, fetal growth may be slowed and the child may be born with low blood pressure and temperature. Ask your doctor for guidance.

Advisability of Use If Breast-Feeding

Presence of this drug in breast milk: Yes.

Avoid drug if possible. If drug is necessary, observe nursing infant for slow heart rate and indications of low blood sugar.

Habit-Forming Potential: None.

Effects of Overdosage: Weakness, slow pulse, low blood pressure, fainting, cold and sweaty skin, congestive heart failure, possible coma, and convulsions.

Possible Effects of Long-Term Use: Reduced heart reserve and eventual heart failure in some people with advanced heart disease.

Suggested Periodic Examinations While Taking This Drug (at physician's discretion)
Measurements of blood pressure, evaluation of heart function.

▷ **While Taking This Drug, Observe the Following**
Foods: Can decrease total atenolol absorption by 20%. It is also best to avoid excessive salt intake.

Beverages: No restrictions. May be taken with milk.

▷ *Alcohol:* Use caution. Alcohol may exaggerate this drug's ability to lower blood pressure and may increase its mild sedative effect.

Tobacco Smoking: Nicotine may reduce this drug's effectiveness in treating high blood pressure. High doses may worsen bronchial tightening caused by regular smoking. I advise everyone to quit smoking.

▷ *Other Drugs*
Atenolol may ***increase*** the effects of
- other antihypertensive drugs and cause excessive lowering of blood pressure. Dosage adjustments may be necessary.
- reserpine (Ser-Ap-Es, etc.) and cause sedation, depression, slowing of heart rate, and lowering of blood pressure.

Atenolol ***taken concurrently*** with
- amiodarone (Cordarone) may result in cardiac arrest.
- ampicillin or bacampicillin may result in lower blood levels of atenolol.
- calcium (various) may result in large decreases in atenolol blood levels.
- clonidine (Catapres) requires close monitoring for rebound high blood pressure if clonidine is stopped while atenolol is still being taken.
- insulin requires close monitoring to avoid undetected hypoglycemia (see Glossary).
- oral antidiabetic drugs (see Drug Classes) may result in prolonged low blood sugar.
- phenothiazines (see Drug Classes) may increase the effects of both agents and result in phenothiazine toxicity or excessively low blood pressure.
- quinidine (Quinaglute) may cause additive lowering of the blood pressure.
- verapamil can result in undesirable slowing of the heart rate and excessively low blood pressure.

The following drugs may ***decrease*** the effects of atenolol:
- antacids can decrease atenolol absorption.
- fluvoxamine (Luvox).
- indomethacin (Indocin), and possibly other "aspirin substitutes," or NSAIDs, may impair atenolol's antihypertensive effect.

▷ *Driving, Hazardous Activities:* Use caution until the full extent of drowsiness, lethargy, and blood pressure change has been determined.

Aviation Note: The use of this drug ***is a disqualification*** for piloting. Consult a designated Aviation Medical Examiner.

Exposure to Sun: No restrictions.

Exposure to Heat: Caution is advised. Hot environments can lower blood pressure and exaggerate the effects of this drug.

Exposure to Cold: Caution is advised. Can enhance the circulatory deficiency that may occur with this drug. The elderly should be careful to prevent hypothermia (see Glossary).

Heavy Exercise or Exertion: Avoid exertion that causes light-headedness, excessive fatigue, or muscle cramping. This drug may worsen the blood pressure response to isometric exercise.

Occurrence of Unrelated Illness: Fever can lower blood pressure and require a decreased dose. Nausea or vomiting may interrupt the dosing schedule. Ask your physician for help.

Discontinuation: Avoid stopping this drug suddenly. If possible, gradual reduction of dose over a period of 2 to 3 weeks is recommended. Ask your physician for help.

ATORVASTATIN (a TOR va stat in)

Introduced: 1996 **Class:** Cholesterol-lowering agent, HMG-CoA reductase inhibitor **Prescription:** USA: Yes **Controlled Drug:** USA: No; Canada: No **Available as Generic:** No

Brand Name: Lipitor

BENEFITS versus RISKS	
Possible Benefits	*Possible Risks*
EFFECTIVE REDUCTION OF TOTAL BLOOD CHOLESTEROL AND LDL CHOLESTEROL	Drug-induced hepatitis (without jaundice)—rare
DECREASED TRIGLYCERIDES	Drug-induced myositis (muscle inflammation)—rare

▷ **Principal Uses**

As a Single Drug Product: Uses currently included in FDA-approved labeling: (1) Treats high total blood cholesterol levels (in people with Types IIa and IIb hypercholesterolemia) due to increased fractions of low-density lipoprotein (LDL) cholesterol. It is used in conjunction with a cholesterol-lowering diet. It should not be used until an adequate trial of nondrug methods for lowering cholesterol has proved to be ineffective; (2) also helps familial hypercholesterolemia; (3) the only "statin" that also lowers triglycerides.

Other (unlabeled) generally accepted uses: None at present.

How This Drug Works: This drug blocks the liver enzyme that starts production of cholesterol. It works to lower blood levels of low-density lipoproteins (LDL), the fraction of total cholesterol thought to increase the risk of coronary heart disease. Since the amount of cholesterol is reduced in the liver, the VLDL fraction may also be decreased.

Available Dosage Forms and Strengths

Tablets — 10 mg, 20 mg, 40 mg

Recommended Dosage Ranges: (Actual dosage and administration schedule must be determined for each patient individually.)

Infants and Children: Data are not available.

18 to 65 Years of Age: Dosing is stared with 10 mg once daily. This can be increased as needed and tolerated to a maximum of 80 mg daily. Lipid levels are best rechecked within 2 to 4 weeks of starting or changing the dose of this medicine.

Over 65 Years of Age: Some research has shown that usual doses of this medicine may result in higher blood levels of atorvastatin than seen in younger patients. It appears prudent from this data that the lowest dose (10 mg) be used in treatment and LDL-C levels be obtained to guide any dose increases. Dose increases must be made by the prescriber after weighing the benefits to risks, mindful that any given dose may result in a higher than expected blood level of atorvastatin.

Conditions Requiring Dosing Adjustments

Liver Function: Caution should be used in patients with liver compromise. Research has shown specifically that in those with liver damage caused by alcohol, elimination of this medicine has been prolonged. The 10-mg dose appears prudent in those patients. Like other HMG-CoA medicines, atorvastatin should not be given during active liver disease.

Kidney Function: Dosing changes are not recommended by the manufacturer.

Dosing Instructions: The tablet may be crushed and while the amount that gets into the body is decreased if atorvastatin is taken with food, LDL-C levels are still lowered. Since cholesterol is made at the fastest rate between midnight and 5 A.M., many clinicians advise patients to take such medicines at bedtime.

Usual Duration of Use: Use on a regular schedule for 2 to 4 weeks usually determines the effectiveness of this drug in reducing blood levels of total and LDL-C cholesterol. Long-term use (months to years) requires periodic physician evaluation.

Possible Advantages of This Drug

Recent studies indicate that drugs of this class (HMG-CoA reductase inhibitors) are more effective and better tolerated than other drugs currently available for reducing total and LDL-C cholesterol. Since this medicine is so new, head-to-head trials with other HMG-CoA medicines have not been done.

This Drug Should Not Be Taken If

- you have had an allergic reaction to it previously.
- you have active liver disease or increased liver function tests that are unexplained.
- you are pregnant or are breast-feeding your infant.

Inform Your Physician Before Taking This Drug If

- you have previously taken any other drugs in this class: lovastatin (Mevacor), simvastatin (Zocor).
- you have a history of liver disease or impaired liver function.
- you have kidney disease.
- you are not using any method of birth control, or you are planning pregnancy.
- you regularly consume substantial amounts of alcohol.
- you develop any kind of unexplained muscle weakness, pain, or tenderness.
- you have any type of chronic muscular disorder.
- you plan to have major surgery in the near future.

Possible Side Effects (natural, expected, and unavoidable drug actions)
None with usual doses.

Possible Adverse Effects (unusual, unexpected, and infrequent reactions)
If any of the following develop, consult your physician promptly for guidance.

Mild Adverse Effects
Allergic reactions: skin rash—infrequent.
Headache—infrequent to frequent, rare drowsiness.
Flu-like syndrome—infrequent.
Diarrhea, constipation, or gas (flatulence)—infrequent.
Muscle pain (myalgia)—infrequent with 20-mg dose.

Serious Adverse Effects
Allergic reactions: not reported as yet.
Marked and persistent abnormal liver function tests (without jaundice)—rare.
Acute myositis (muscle pain and tenderness)—rare to infrequent with 10- to 80-mg doses.
Rhabdomyolysis with sudden kidney failure—rarely reported with other HMG-CoA medicines.
One case report of euphoria, confusion, and short-term memory problems.

Possible Effects on Sexual Function: Decreased libido or impotence (2%).

Possible Delayed Adverse Effects: Rare muscle changes.

Natural Diseases or Disorders That May Be Activated by This Drug
Latent liver disease.

Possible Effects on Laboratory Tests
Blood total cholesterol, LDL cholesterol, and triglyceride levels: decreased.

CAUTION
1. If pregnancy occurs while taking this drug, discontinue it immediately and consult your physician.
2. Report promptly any development of muscle pain or tenderness, especially if accompanied by fever or malaise.
3. Report promptly the development of altered or impaired vision so that appropriate evaluation can be made (visual changes have been reported with some other HMG-CoA medicines).
4. If CPK levels become markedly elevated, this medicine should be stopped.

Precautions for Use
By Infants and Children: Safety and effectiveness for those under 18 years of age not established.
By Those Over 60 Years of Age: Blood levels for those over 65 may be higher than those reached by the same dose in younger people. Tell your doctor about any changes that appear to be one of the listed side effects right away.

Advisability of Use During Pregnancy
Pregnancy Category: X. See Pregnancy Risk Categories at the back of this book.
Animal studies: Rat studies reveal decreased pup survival and maturity with high-dose studies.
Human studies: Adequate studies of pregnant women are not available.
This drug should be avoided during entire pregnancy.

Advisability of Use If Breast-Feeding
Presence of this drug in breast milk: Yes, in rats; expected in humans.
Avoid drug or refrain from nursing.

Habit-Forming Potential: None.

Effects of Overdosage: Increased indigestion, stomach distress, nausea, diarrhea with other HMG-CoA medicines.

Possible Effects of Long-Term Use: Abnormal liver function tests.

Suggested Periodic Examinations While Taking This Drug (at physician's discretion)

Blood cholesterol studies: total cholesterol, HDL, and LDL fractions.

Liver function tests before treatment, every 6 weeks during the first 3 months of use, every 8 weeks for the rest of the first year, and at 6-month intervals thereafter have been recommended for other HMG-CoA inhibitors. Ask your physician for guidance.

▷ **While Taking This Drug, Observe the Following**

Foods: Follow a standard low cholesterol diet.

Beverages: No restrictions. May be taken with milk.

Alcohol: Excessive alcohol not recommended.

Tobacco Smoking: No interactions expected, but I advise everyone to quit smoking.

Other Drugs

Atorvastatin may **increase** the effects of

• clofibrate (Atromid-S) and other fibric acid derivatives; has been associated with increased risk of muscle damage (rhabdomyolysis).

Atorvastatin **taken concurrently** with

• antacids may decrease the amount of atorvastatin that gets into your body, yet lowering of LDL-C appears to remain the same.

• azole antifungals (such as itraconazole or Sporanox) may increase the risk for myopathy.

• birth control pills (oral contraceptives) may decrease the levels of the contraceptives (certain kinds) and could blunt effectiveness and result in pregnancy.

• colestipol (Colestid) results in lowered atorvastatin blood levels, but better lowering of LDL-C.

• cyclosporine (Sandimmune) may increase the risk for myopathy.

• digoxin (Lanoxin, others) can decrease digoxin levels (and possibly therapeutic effects).

• erythromycin (and perhaps other macrolide antibiotics) may increase the risk for myopathy.

• niacin (various) may increase the risk for myopathy.

• warfarin (Coumadin) does not appear at present to have a clinically significant effect.

Driving, Hazardous Activities: This drug may cause drowsiness. Restrict activities as necessary.

Aviation Note: The use of this drug **may be a disqualification** for piloting. Consult a designated Aviation Medical Examiner.

Exposure to Sun: No restrictions.

Occurrence of Unrelated Illness: Call your doctor if another physician (such as a specialist) diagnoses a sudden liver problem.

Discontinuation: Do not stop this drug without your doctor's knowledge and help. There may be a significant increase in blood cholesterol levels if this medicine is stopped.

AURANOFIN (aw RAY noh fin)

Introduced: 1976   **Class:** Antiarthritic   **Prescription:** USA: Yes
Controlled Drug: USA: No; Canada: No   **Available as Generic:** Yes
Brand Name: Ridaura

BENEFITS versus RISKS	
Possible Benefits	*Possible Risks*
REDUCTION OF JOINT PAIN, TENDERNESS, AND SWELLING in active, severe RHEUMATOID ARTHRITIS	SIGNIFICANTLY REDUCED LEVELS OF RED AND WHITE BLOOD CELLS AND BLOOD PLATELETS—rare
Medication effective when taken by mouth	LIVER DAMAGE WITH JAUNDICE—rare
	Diarrhea
	Ulcerative colitis—rare
	Skin rash
	Mouth sores
	Kidney toxicity (protein in the urine)
	Lung damage—rare

▷ **Principal Uses**

As a Single Drug Product: Uses currently included in FDA-approved labeling: Used *only* for severe rheumatoid arthritis in adults who have had an inadequate response to aspirin, aspirin substitutes, or other antiarthritic drugs and treatment programs. Usually added to a well-established program of antiarthritic drugs of the aspirin-substitute (NSAID) class.

Other (unlabeled) generally accepted uses: (1) May have a role in helping decrease the need for steroid use in people with asthma; (2) can ease the symptoms of nodular vasculitis.

How This Drug Works: Unknown. It suppresses but does not cure arthritis and associated synovitis. It has an effect on specific cells (macrophages) and stops them from engulfing cell debris and also inhibits lysosomes.

Available Dosage Forms and Strengths

Capsules — 3 mg

▷ **Usual Adult Dosage Range:**   6 mg daily, taken either as one dose every 24 hours or as two doses of 3 mg each every 12 hours. If 6 months of regular continual use does not produce an adequate response, the dose may be increased to 9 mg daily, taken as three doses of 3 mg each. If response remains inadequate after 3 months of 9 mg daily, this drug should be stopped. **Note: Actual dosage and administration schedule must be determined for each patient individually.**

Conditions Requiring Dosing Adjustments

Liver Function: The liver is not involved in auranofin elimination. No dose decreases needed.

Kidney Function: Blood levels are recommended, and decreased doses may be needed.

▷ **Dosing Instructions:**   Take with or following food to reduce stomach irritation. Take the capsule whole with milk or a full glass of water.

Usual Duration of Use: Use on a regular schedule for 3 to 4 months is usually needed to see this drug's effectiveness in reducing joint pain, tenderness, and swelling associated with rheumatoid arthritis. Long-term use will depend on how much benefit or the pattern of adverse effects experienced. Consult your physician on a regular basis.

Author's Note: The information in this profile has been shortened to make room for medicines which are more widely used.

AZATHIOPRINE (ay za THI oh preen)

Introduced: 1965   **Class:** Antiarthritic, immunosuppressive   **Prescription:** USA: Yes   **Controlled Drug:** USA: No; Canada: No   **Available as Generic:** Yes

Brand Name: Imuran

BENEFITS versus RISKS	
Possible Benefits	*Possible Risks*
REDUCTION OF JOINT PAIN, TENDERNESS, AND SWELLING in active, severe RHEUMATOID ARTHRITIS	UNACCEPTABLE ADVERSE EFFECTS IN 15% OF USERS
PREVENTION OF REJECTION IN ORGAN TRANSPLANTATION	REDUCED LEVELS OF WHITE BLOOD CELLS
	REDUCED LEVELS OF RED BLOOD CELLS AND PLATELETS
	LIVER DAMAGE WITH JAUNDICE—rare
	POSSIBLE INCREASED RISK OF MALIGNANCY—rare

▷ **Principal Uses**

As a Single Drug Product: Uses currently included in FDA-approved labeling: (1) Used to prevent rejection of transplanted organs (mainly kidney transplants); (2) also used in active, severe rheumatoid arthritis (in adults) that has failed conventional treatment.

Other (unlabeled) generally accepted uses: (1) Used to treat lupus erythematosus, ulcerative colitis, chronic active hepatitis, and other "autoimmune" disorders; (2) decreases rejection rates as part of combination therapy in preventing heart transplant failures.

How This Drug Works: It is thought that by impairing purine metabolism, DNA, and RNA, and inhibiting cell multiplication, this drug decreases the immune reaction that is responsible for rheumatoid arthritis, lupus erythematosus, etc.

Available Dosage Forms and Strengths

Injection — 100 mg per 20-ml vial

Tablets — 50 mg

▷ **Usual Adult Dosage Range:**   As immunosuppressant—3 to 5 mg per kg of body mass daily, 1 to 3 days before transplantation surgery; for postoperative maintenance—1 to 2 mg per kg of body mass daily. In rheumatoid arthritis—1 mg per kg of body mass daily for 6 to 8 weeks; increase dose by 0.5

mg per kg of body mass every 4 weeks as needed and tolerated. Maximal daily dose is 2.5 mg per kg of body mass. Total dose may be taken once daily or divided into two equal doses taken 12 hours apart. **Note: Actual dosage and administration schedule must be determined for each patient individually.**

Conditions Requiring Dosing Adjustments
Liver Function: No specific dosing guidelines are available; however, the drug may need to be stopped if jaundice occurs. Liver function must be closely watched.

Kidney Function: The dose must be decreased by up to 50% in kidney failure.

▷ **Dosing Instructions:** Take with or following food to reduce stomach upset. Tablet may be crushed.

Usual Duration of Use: Use on a regular schedule for 12 weeks is usually needed to determine this drug's effectiveness in helping rheumatoid arthritis. Successful use for up more than a decade has been reported. See your physician regularly.

▷ **This Drug Should Not Be Taken If**
- you have had an allergic reaction to it previously.
- you are pregnant, and this drug is prescribed to treat rheumatoid arthritis.
- you have an active blood cell or bone marrow disorder.
- you are taking, or have recently taken, any form of chlorambucil (Leukeran), cyclophosphamide (Cytoxan), or melphalan (Alkeran).

▷ **Inform Your Physician Before Taking This Drug If**
- you have any kind of active infection.
- you have any form of cancer.
- you have gout or are taking allopurinol (Zyloprim).
- you have a history of blood cell or bone marrow disorders.
- you have impaired liver or kidney function.
- you are taking a drug in the ACE inhibitor (see Drug Classes) class. Combination use of azathioprine with these medicines has severely lowered white blood cell counts.
- you are taking any form of gold, penicillamine, or an antimalarial drug for arthritis.
- you plan pregnancy in the near future.
- you take other prescription or nonprescription medications that were not discussed when azathioprine was prescribed for you.
- you are unsure of how much azathioprine to take or how often to take it.

Possible Side Effects (natural, expected, and unavoidable drug actions)
Development of infection.

▷ **Possible Adverse Effects** (unusual, unexpected, and infrequent reactions)
If any of the following develop, consult your physician promptly for guidance.
Mild Adverse Effects
Allergic reaction: skin rash—rare.
Loss of appetite, nausea, vomiting, diarrhea—infrequent.
Sores on lips and in mouth—possible.
Muscle aches—infrequent.

Serious Adverse Effects
Allergic reactions: drug fever (see Glossary), joint and muscle pain—rare.
Pancreatitis: severe stomach pain with nausea and vomiting—rare.
Bone marrow depression (see Glossary): fatigue, weakness, fever, sore throat, abnormal bleeding or bruising—dose dependent.
Liver damage: yellow eyes and skin, dark-colored urine, light-colored stools (see Hepatitis and Jaundice in Glossary)—rare.
Drug-induced pneumonia: cough, shortness of breath—possible.
Development of cancer: skin cancer, reticulum-cell sarcoma, lymphoma, leukemia—possible.

▷ **Possible Effects on Sexual Function:**   Reversal of male infertility due to sperm antibodies; this drug suppresses autoantibodies and permits the normal accumulation of sperm. May also decrease sperm counts.

Possible Delayed Adverse Effects: Bone marrow depression may occur many weeks after stopping this drug.

Adverse Effects That May Mimic Natural Diseases or Disorders
Liver damage may suggest viral hepatitis.

Possible Effects on Laboratory Tests
Complete blood cell counts: decreased red cells, hemoglobin, white cells, and platelets.
Blood amylase and lipase levels: increased—possible pancreatitis.
Blood uric acid levels: increased with rapid tissue destruction; decreased in patients with gout.
Liver function tests: increased liver enzymes (ALT/GPT, AST/GOT, and alkaline phosphatase); increased bilirubin.
Sperm counts: decreased.

CAUTION
1. Promptly report any indications of a developing infection—fever, chills, lip or mouth sores, etc.
2. Inform your physician promptly if you become pregnant.
3. Periodic blood counts are mandatory for the safe use of this drug.

Precautions for Use
By Infants and Children: Safety and effectiveness in those under 12 years of age not established.
By Those Over 60 Years of Age: The smallest effective dose should be used, as this reduces the risk of toxic reactions.

▷ **Advisability of Use During Pregnancy**
Pregnancy Category: D. See Pregnancy Risk Categories at the back of this book.
Animal studies: Birth defects reported in rodent studies.
Human studies: This drug exhibits teratogenic effects and also poses a risk of suppression of the immune system of the newborn. Adequate studies of pregnant women are not available. **Avoid completely** during entire pregnancy if possible.

Advisability of Use If Breast-Feeding
Presence of this drug in breast milk: Yes.
Avoid drug or refrain from nursing.

Habit-Forming Potential: None.

Effects of Overdosage: Immediate—nausea, vomiting, diarrhea. Delayed—lowered white blood cell and platelet counts, liver and kidney toxicity.

Possible Effects of Long-Term Use: Susceptibility to infection, bone marrow depression, development of malignancies.

Suggested Periodic Examinations While Taking This Drug (at physician's discretion)
Complete blood cell counts, liver function tests.

▷ **While Taking This Drug, Observe the Following**
Foods: No restrictions.
Beverages: No restrictions. May be taken with milk.
▷ *Alcohol:* No interactions expected.
Tobacco Smoking: No interactions expected, but I advise everyone to quit smoking.
▷ *Other Drugs*
Azathioprine may *decrease* the effects of
- certain muscle relaxants (gallamine, pancuronium, tubocurarine), and make it necessary to increase their dosage.
- oral anticoagulants (warfarin, etc.), and requires increased doses.
The following drugs may *increase* the effects of azathioprine
- allopurinol (Zyloprim); may increase its activity and toxicity and make it necessary to reduce its dosage.
Azathioprine *taken concurrently* with
- ACE inhibitors (see Drug Classes) such as captopril or enalapril may cause severe white blood cell count lowering or anemia.
- cotrimoxazole (Bactrim, others) can cause severe lowering of white blood cell counts.
- prednisolone will result in lower prednisolone blood levels and risk of decreased therapeutic benefit.
- warfarin (Coumadin) may result in decreased anticoagulant effectiveness.
▷ *Driving, Hazardous Activities:* No restrictions.
Aviation Note: The use of this drug *may be a disqualification* for piloting. Consult a designated Aviation Medical Examiner.
Exposure to Sun: No restrictions.
Discontinuation: A gradual reduction in dosage is preferable. Consult your physician for a withdrawal schedule.

AZITHROMYCIN (a zith roh MY sin)

See the new macrolide antibiotics profile for further information.

BACAMPICILLIN (bak am pi SIL in)

See the new penicillins profile for further information.

BECLOMETHASONE (be kloh METH a sohn)

Introduced: 1976   **Class:** Antiasthmatic, cortisonelike drugs   **Prescription:** USA: Yes   **Controlled Drug:** USA: No; Canada: No   **Available as Generic:** No

Brand Names: ✦Beclodisk, ✦Becloforte, Beclovent, ✦Beclovent Rotacaps, ✦Beclovent Rotahaler, Beconase AQ Nasal Spray, Beconase Nasal Inhaler, ✦Propaderm, ✦Propaderm-C, Vancenase AQ Nasal Spray, Vancenase Nasal Inhaler, Vanceril

```
┌──────────────────────────────────────────────────────────────┐
│                    BENEFITS versus RISKS                       │
│     Possible Benefits              Possible Risks              │
│ EFFECTIVE RELIEF OF ALLERGIC   FUNGUS INFECTIONS OF THE        │
│   RHINITIS                       MOUTH AND THROAT              │
│ EFFECTIVE CONTROL OF SEVERE,   Localized areas of "allergic"   │
│   CHRONIC ASTHMA                 pneumonia                     │
│                                Changes in lining of the nose (nasal │
│                                  mucosa)                       │
│                                Increased cataract risk         │
└──────────────────────────────────────────────────────────────┘
```

▷ **Principal Uses**

As a Single Drug Product: Uses currently included in FDA-approved labeling: (1) Treats bronchial asthma in people who do not respond to bronchodilators and who need cortisonelike drugs for asthma control. This inhalation dosage form is much more advantageous than cortisone taken by mouth (swallowed) or by injection in that it works directly on the respiratory tract and does not require absorption and systemic distribution. This prevents the more serious adverse effects of long-term systemic cortisone use; (2) prevention of nasal polyps once they have been surgically removed; (3) treats seasonal and perennial rhinitis in children and adults (AQ nasal forms).

Other (unlabeled) generally accepted uses: (1) Has a role in lung disease (bronchopulmonary dysplasia) in helping decrease the required daily dose of prednisone; (2) could be of use in inflammatory bowel disease while avoiding pituitary gland problems.

How This Drug Works: By increasing the amount of cyclic AMP, this drug may increase epinephrine, which opens the bronchial tubes and fights asthma. The drug can also reduce local inflammation in the lining of the respiratory tract.

Available Dosage Forms and Strengths

Inhalant — 17 g (50 mcg)
Nasal inhaler — 16.8 g (200 doses of 42 mcg each)
Nasal spray — 0.042%
Oral inhaler — 16.8 g (200 doses of 42 mcg each, 50 mcg in Canada)
Rotacaps (Canada) — 100- and 200-mcg capsules
Topical lotion (Canada) — 0.025%

▷ **Usual Adult Dosage Range:**

Infants and Children: Data are not available for infants. Children 6–12 years old may receive: Nasal inhaler—one inhalation (42 mcg) in each nostril three times a day. Oral inhalation—maximum is 10 inhalations (420 mcg).

18 to 65 Years of Age: Nasal inhaler—one inhalation (42 mcg) two to four times daily. Oral inhaler—two inhalations (84 mcg) three or four times daily. For severe asthma—12 to 16 inhalations daily. The maximal daily dose should not exceed 20 inhalations.

By Those Over 65 Years of Age: Doses similar to those used in younger patients have been effective and safe. In some cases, oral-steroid-dependent patients have been able to slowly taper, then stop oral steroids while taking beclomethasone.

Note: Actual dosage and administration schedule must be determined for each patient individually.

Conditions Requiring Dosing Adjustments

Liver Function: Use with caution in patients with liver compromise.

Kidney Function: No adjustments in dosing expected to be needed.

▷ **Dosing Instructions:** May be used without regard to eating. Rinse the mouth and throat (gargle) with water thoroughly after each inhalation.

Usual Duration of Use: Use on a regular schedule for 1 to 4 weeks is usually needed to see this drug's effectiveness in relieving severe, chronic allergic rhinitis and in controlling severe, chronic asthma. Long-term use must be physician supervised. See your doctor on a regular basis.

▷ **This Drug Should Not Be Taken If**
- you have had an allergic reaction to any of the brand names listed above.
- you are experiencing severe acute asthma or status asthmaticus that requires more intense treatment for prompt relief.
- your asthma can be controlled by other antiasthmatic drugs that are not related to cortisone.
- your asthma requires cortisonelike drugs infrequently for control.
- you have a form of nonallergic bronchitis with asthmatic features.

▷ **Inform Your Physician Before Taking This Drug If**
- you are now taking or have recently taken any cortisone-related drug (including ACTH by injection) for any reason (see Drug Classes).
- you have a history of tuberculosis of the lungs.
- you have chronic bronchitis or bronchiectasis.
- you think you have an active infection of any kind, especially a respiratory infection.
- you have recently been exposed to chickenpox or other viral illnesses.
- you are prone to nosebleeds (epistaxis) (nasal forms).
- you are unsure of how much or how often to take beclomethasone.

Possible Side Effects (natural, expected, and unavoidable drug actions)

Fungus infections (thrush) of the mouth and throat.

▷ **Possible Adverse Effects** (unusual, unexpected, and infrequent reactions)

If any of the following develop, consult your physician promptly for guidance.

Mild Adverse Effects

Allergic reaction: skin rash—rare.

Dryness of mouth, hoarseness, sore throat, cough—possible.
Nosebleeds (epistaxis)—infrequent.
Serious Adverse Effects
Allergic reaction: localized areas of "allergic" pneumonitis (lung inflammation).
Bronchospasm, asthmatic wheezing—rare.
Shrinking of the nasal tissues (nasal atrophy)—possible.
Yeast infections (up to 41%)—frequent.
Increased risk of cataracts with chronic use.
Osteoporosis (any corticosteroid can cause this)—possible.

▷ **Possible Effects on Sexual Function:**   None reported.

Natural Diseases or Disorders That May Be Activated by This Drug
Cortisone-related drugs having systemic effects impair immunity and lead to reactivation of "healed" or dormant tuberculosis. People with a history of tuberculosis must be watched closely while using this drug.

Possible Effects on Laboratory Tests
Blood cortisol levels: decreased.

CAUTION
1. This drug should not be relied upon for immediate relief of acute asthma.
2. If you were using cortisone-related drugs for your asthma *before* starting this inhaler, it may be necessary to resume the former cortisone-related drug if you experience injury or infection of any kind, or if you require surgery. Tell your doctor of your prior use of cortisone-related drugs taken either by mouth or by injection.
3. If severe asthma returns while using this drug, notify your doctor immediately so that supportive treatment with cortisone-related drugs by mouth or injection can be provided as needed.
4. Carry a personal identification card with a notation (if applicable) that you have used cortisone-related drugs within the past year. During periods of stress it may be necessary to resume cortisone treatment.
5. Wait 5 to 10 minutes after using a bronchodilator inhaler like epinephrine, isoetharine, or isoproterenol (which should be used first) before inhalation of this drug. This will permit greater penetration of beclomethasone into the bronchial tubes. The delay between inhalations will also reduce the possibility of adverse propellant effects.
6. This drug does NOT replace systemic steroids, but may allow dosage decreases in some patients.

Precautions for Use
By Infants and Children: Safety and effectiveness for use of the nasal inhaler by those under 6 years of age have not been established. Safety and effectiveness for use of the oral inhaler by those under 6 years of age have not been established. The maximal daily dose in children 6 to 12 years of age should not exceed 10 inhalations.
By Those Over 60 Years of Age: People with bronchiectasis should be watched closely for the development of lung infections.

▷ **Advisability of Use During Pregnancy**
Pregnancy Category: C. See Pregnancy Risk Categories at the back of this book.
Animal studies: Mouse, rat, and rabbit studies reveal significant birth defects due to this drug.

Human studies: Adequate studies of pregnant women are not available. Avoid drug during the first 3 months. Use infrequently and only as clearly needed during the last 6 months.

Advisability of Use If Breast-Feeding
Presence of this drug in breast milk: Probably yes.
Avoid drug or refrain from nursing.

Habit-Forming Potential: With recommended dosage, a state of functional dependence (see Glossary) is not likely to develop. There have been a small number of cases reported where the aerosol was abused for the fluorocarbon propellants.

Effects of Overdosage: Indications of cortisone excess (due to systemic absorption)—fluid retention, flushing of the face, stomach irritation, nervousness.

Suggested Periodic Examinations While Taking This Drug (at physician's discretion)
Inspection of nose, mouth, and throat for evidence of fungus infection. Inspection of the nose tissues for nasal atrophy. Assessment of adrenal function status in people who have used cortisone-related drugs over an extended period of time prior to using this drug. Lung X ray of people with a prior history of tuberculosis. Measures of bone mineral density (long-term use can lead to osteoporosis).

▷ **While Taking This Drug, Observe the Following**
Foods: No specific restrictions beyond those advised by your physician.
Beverages: No specific restrictions.
▷ *Alcohol:* No interactions expected.
Tobacco Smoking: No interactions expected. However, smoking can reduce the effectiveness of this drug. I advise everyone to quit smoking.
▷ *Other Drugs*
The following drugs may ***increase*** the effects of beclomethasone:
- flunisolide (Nasalide).
- inhalant bronchodilators—epinephrine, isoetharine, isoproterenol.
- oral bronchodilators—aminophylline, ephedrine, terbutaline, theophylline, etc.
▷ *Driving, Hazardous Activities:* No restrictions.
Aviation Note: The use of this drug and the disorder for which this drug is prescribed ***may be disqualifications*** for piloting. Consult a designated Aviation Medical Examiner.
Exposure to Sun: No restrictions.
Occurrence of Unrelated Illness: Acute infections, serious injuries, and surgical procedures can create an urgent need for additional supportive cortisone-related drugs given by mouth and/or injection. Notify your physician immediately in the event of new illness or injury of any kind.
Discontinuation: If the regular use of this drug has made it possible to reduce or discontinue maintenance doses of cortisonelike drugs by mouth, ***do not*** stop this drug abruptly. If you must stop this drug, call your doctor. It may be necessary to resume cortisone preparations and to institute other measures for satisfactory management.
Special Storage Instructions: Store at room temperature. Avoid exposure to temperatures above 120 degrees F (49 degrees C). Do not store or use this inhaler near heat or open flame. Protect from light.

BENAZEPRIL (ben AY ze pril)

Introduced: 1985   **Class:** Antihypertensive, ACE inhibitor   **Prescription:** USA: Yes   **Controlled Drug:** USA: No; Canada: No   **Available as Generic:** No

Brand Names: Lotensin, Lotensin HCT [CD], Lotrel [CD]

BENEFITS versus RISKS	
Possible Benefits	*Possible Risks*
EFFECTIVE CONTROL OF MILD TO MODERATE HIGH BLOOD PRESSURE	Headache, dizziness, fatigue, low blood pressure—rare
	Allergic swelling of face, tongue, throat, vocal cords—rare
	Decreased hemoglobin—rare

▷ **Principal Uses**

As a Single Drug Product: Uses currently included in FDA-approved labeling: Treatment of mild to moderate high blood pressure, alone or in combination with a thiazide diuretic.

Other (unlabeled) generally accepted uses: (1) Helps relieve symptoms of congestive heart failure; (2) of benefit when added to usual therapies after a heart attack (MI).

As a Combination Drug Product [CD]: Used to treat high blood pressure which has not responded to single agent treatment. The combination products have hydrochlorothiazide, a diuretic. or amlodipine, a calcium channel blocker.

How This Drug Works: By blocking certain enzyme systems (angiotensin-converting enzyme, ACE) that affect arteries, benazepril helps relax arterial walls throughout the body and lowers the blood pressure. This, in turn, reduces the workload of the heart and improves its performance. The combination products use a diuretic (eases fluid load) or a calcium channel blocker.

Available Dosage Forms and Strengths

Lotensin tablets — 5 mg, 10 mg, 20 mg, 40 mg

▷ **Recommended Dosage Ranges** (Actual dosage and administration schedule must be determined for each patient individually.)

Infants and Children: Dosage not established.

12 to 60 Years of Age: Initially 10 mg once daily for those not taking a diuretic; 5 mg once daily for those taking a diuretic. Usual maintenance dose is 20 to 40 mg daily, taken in a single dose. If once-a-day dosing does not give stable control of blood pressure over a 24-hour period, divide the dose equally into morning and evening doses. The total daily dosage should not exceed 80 mg.

Over 60 Years of Age: Same as 12 to 60 years of age, if kidney function is normal. If kidney function is significantly impaired, reduce dose by 50%. The total daily dose should not exceed 40 mg in those with impaired kidneys.

Conditions Requiring Dosing Adjustments

Liver Function: Dosage adjustment in cirrhosis is not currently considered necessary.

Kidney Function: Some of this medicine is removed by the kidneys. For people with creatinine clearances of less than 30 ml/min., or serum creatinine concentrations of greater than 3 mg/dl, the initial dose should be 5 mg once daily.

▷ **Dosing Instructions:** Take on an empty stomach or with food, at same time each day. The tablet may be crushed for administration.

Usual Duration of Use: Use on a regular schedule for 2 to 3 weeks is usually needed to see this drug's peak effect in controlling high blood pressure. Therapy may be long term. See your physician on a regular basis.

Possible Advantages of This Drug
Usually controls blood pressure effectively with one daily dose.
Relatively low incidence of adverse effects.
No adverse influence on asthma, cholesterol blood levels, or diabetes.
Sudden withdrawal does not result in a rapid increase in blood pressure.

▷ **This Drug Should Not Be Taken If**
- you have had an allergic reaction to this or any ACE inhibitor before (see Drug Classes).
- you are pregnant.
- you currently have a blood cell or bone marrow disorder.
- you have an abnormally high level of blood potassium.
- you are being dialyzed with PAN high flux dialyzers (may result in serious allergic reactions).

▷ **Inform Your Physician Before Taking This Drug If**
- you are planning pregnancy.
- you have a history of kidney disease or impaired kidney function.
- you have scleroderma or systemic lupus erythematosus or other autoimmune disease.
- you have cerebral artery disease.
- you have any form of heart disease.
- you are breast-feeding your infant.
- you are taking: other antihypertensives, diuretics, nitrates, or potassium supplements.
- you plan to have surgery under general anesthesia in the near future.
- you are unsure of how much benazepril to take or how often to take it.
- you have renal artery stenosis (ask your doctor).
- you have liver disease.
- your face or tongue becomes swollen after you start taking this drug.
- you are taking an immunosuppressant drug or have a low white blood cell count.
- you think you are dehydrated.

Possible Side Effects (natural, expected, and unavoidable drug actions)
Dizziness, orthostatic hypotension (see Glossary)—rare; fainting—rare; increased blood potassium level—rare.

▷ **Possible Adverse Effects** (unusual, unexpected, and infrequent reactions)
If any of the following develop, consult your physician promptly for guidance.
Mild Adverse Effects
Allergic reactions: skin rash, itching—rare.
Headache, fatigue, drowsiness , numbness and tingling, weakness—rare.

Cough—rare.

Indigestion, nausea, vomiting, constipation—rare.

Back pain—rare.

Serious Adverse Effects

Allergic reactions: swelling (angioedema) of face, tongue, and/or vocal chords; can be life threatening—rare.

Pancreatitis (reported with other ACE inhibitors)—case reports.

Impairment of kidney function—rare.

Decreased white blood cell counts or hemoglobin—rare.

Asthmalike symptoms—rare.

Angina and palpitations—case reports.

First-dose low blood pressure (reported with other ACE inhibitors)—case reports.

Elevated blood potassium—rare.

Psoriasis—rare.

▷ **Possible Effects on Sexual Function:**   Decreased libido, impotence—less than 1%. Enlargement and tenderness of male breast tissue (gynecomastia)—case reports with other ACE inhibitors.

Possible Effects on Laboratory Tests

Blood potassium level: increased.

Kidney function tests: blood urea nitrogen (BUN) and creatinine increased.

Blood glucose: rare increases.

Uric acid: rare increases.

Amylase and lipase: increased if pancreatitis (rare) develops.

Blood cholesterol: decreased (7.6–13.1%).

CAUTION

1. Ask your doctor if you should stop other antihypertensive drugs (especially diuretics) for 1 week before starting this drug.

2. **Inform your physician immediately if you become pregnant.** This drug should not be taken beyond the first 3 months of pregnancy.

3. **Report promptly** any signs of infection (fever, sore throat), and any weight gain, puffiness, swollen feet or ankles.

4. Do not use a salt substitute without your physician's knowledge and approval. (Many salt substitutes contain potassium.)

5. It is advisable to obtain blood cell counts and urine analyses **before** starting this drug.

Precautions for Use

By Infants and Children: Safety and effectiveness for use by those in this age group not established.

By Those Over 60 Years of Age: Small starting doses are advisable. Sudden or excessive lowering of blood pressure can cause stroke or heart attack in people with impaired brain circulation or coronary artery heart disease.

▷ **Advisability of Use During Pregnancy**

Pregnancy Category: C during the first 3 months of pregnancy; D during the second or third trimester. See Pregnancy Risk Categories at the back of this book.

Animal studies: No birth defects found in mouse, rat, or rabbit studies.

Human studies: The use of ACE inhibitor drugs during the last 6 months of pregnancy is known to possibly cause very serious injury and possible death to the fetus; skull and limb malformations, lung defects, and kidney failure have been reported in over 50 cases worldwide.

Avoid this drug completely during the last 6 months. During the first 3 months of pregnancy, use this drug only if clearly needed. Ask your physician for guidance.

Advisability of Use If Breast-Feeding
Presence of this drug in breast milk: Yes, in small amounts.
Ask your doctor for guidance.

Habit-Forming Potential: None.

Effects of Overdosage: Excessive drop in blood pressure, light-headedness, dizziness, fainting.

Possible Effects of Long-Term Use: Gradual increase in blood potassium level.

Suggested Periodic Examinations While Taking This Drug (at physician's discretion)
Before starting drug: Complete blood cell counts; urine analysis with measurement of protein content; blood potassium level.
During use of drug: Blood cell counts; measurements of blood potassium.

▷ **While Taking This Drug, Observe the Following**
Foods: Consult physician regarding salt intake. Ask about the benefits of weight loss if you are above your ideal body weight.
*Nutritional Support: **Do not** take potassium supplements unless directed by your physician.
Beverages: No restrictions. May be taken with milk.
▷ *Alcohol:* Use caution. Alcohol may enhance the blood-pressure-lowering effect of this drug.
Tobacco Smoking: No interactions expected, but I advise everyone to quit smoking.
▷ *Other Drugs*
Benazepril *taken concurrently* with
- aspirin may decrease the benefit of benazepril on heart function.
- bumetanide (Bumex) or furosemide (Lasix) may cause severe lowering of blood pressure if the patient suddenly stands.
- chlorpromazine (Thorazine) may cause excessive lowering of blood pressure.
- cyclosporine (Sandimmune) may cause increased kidney toxicity.
- interferon alpha or beta may result in blood cell (low platelets or granulocytopenia) problems.
- ketorolac (Toradol) or other NSAIDs can increase the risk of kidney (renal) toxicity.
- lithium (Lithobid, others) may triple blood levels of lithium and result in lithium toxicity.
- phenothiazines (see Drug Classes) may cause sudden lowering of the blood pressure to undesirable levels.
- potassium preparations (K-Lyte, Slow-K, etc.) may cause increased blood levels of potassium with risk of serious heart rhythm disturbances.
- potassium-sparing diuretics—amiloride (Moduretic), spironolactone (Aldactazide), triamterene (Dyazide)—may cause increased blood levels of potassium with risk of serious heart rhythm disturbances.

- thiazide diuretics (see Drug Classes) may cause excessive lowering of blood pressure.

▷ *Driving, Hazardous Activities:* Be aware of possible drops in blood pressure with resultant dizziness or faintness.

Aviation Note: The use of this drug *may be a disqualification* for piloting. Consult a designated Aviation Medical Examiner.

Exposure to Sun: Caution is advised. A similar drug of this class can cause photosensitivity.

Exposure to Heat: Caution is advised. Excessive perspiring with resultant loss of body water may drop blood pressure.

Occurrence of Unrelated Illness: Promptly report vomiting or diarrhea. Fluid and chemical imbalances must be corrected as soon as possible.

Discontinuation: Talk to your doctor about withdrawal of this drug for any reason.

BENZTROPINE (BENZ troh peen)

Introduced: 1954   **Class:** Anti-parkinsonism, atropinelike drugs   **Prescription:** USA: Yes   **Controlled Drug:** USA: No; Canada: No   **Available as Generic:** USA: Yes; Canada: Yes

Brand Names: ✦Apo-Benztropine, ✦Bensylate, Cogentin, ✦PMS Benztropine

BENEFITS versus RISKS	
Possible Benefits	*Possible Risks*
PARTIAL RELIEF OF SYMPTOMS OF PARKINSON'S DISEASE RELIEF OF DRUG-INDUCED EXTRAPYRAMIDAL REACTIONS	Atropinelike side effects: blurred vision, dry mouth, constipation, impaired urination Toxic psychosis—rare Tardive dyskinesia—rare

▷ **Principal Uses**

As a Single Drug Product: Uses currently included in FDA-approved labeling: (1) Used in combination with other therapy in of all types of parkinsonism to relieve the characteristic rigidity, tremor, and sluggish movement. If relief is inadequate, it may be supplemented with more potent drugs such as levodopa and bromocriptine; (2) also used to control parkinsonian reactions that can result from some antipsychotic drugs, such as phenothiazines and related medicines; (3) used to help parkinsonian symptoms that can occur after encephalitis.

Other (unlabeled) generally accepted uses: (1) Combined with psychotherapy, this drug can help excessively sweaty palms; (2) can help drooling in developmentally disabled patients; (3) can relieve painful erections (priapism).

How This Drug Works: It decreases the symptoms of parkinsonism by restoring a more normal balance of chemicals responsible for nerve impulses in the brain (basal ganglia).

Available Dosage Forms and Strengths

Injection — 1 mg/ml

Tablets — 0.5 mg, 1 mg, 2 mg

▷ **Usual Adult Dosage Range:**   For Parkinson's disease: 0.5 to 2 mg daily, taken in a single dose at bedtime. For drug-induced parkinsonian reactions: 1 to 4 mg daily, either in a single dose or in two to three divided doses. The total daily dose should not exceed 6 mg. For Parkinson's symptoms that occur after encephalitis: starting doses of 2 mg/day are used. The dose can then be increased as needed or tolerated to 4 to 6 mg per day. **Note: Actual dosage and administration schedule must be determined for each patient individually.**

Conditions Requiring Dosing Adjustments
Liver Function: Use with caution in patients with impaired liver function.
Kidney Function: **Caution:** Decreased kidney function may lead to an increased blood level and an increased risk of adverse effects.

▷ **Dosing Instructions:**   May be taken with or following food to reduce stomach irritation. Tablet may be crushed.

Usual Duration of Use: Use on a regular schedule for 2 to 4 weeks is usually necessary to see this drug's peak benefit in relieving symptoms of parkinsonism and to determine the best dosage schedule. Long-term use (months to years) requires physician supervision. See your doctor regularly.

▷ **This Drug Should Not Be Taken If**
- you have had an allergic reaction to any dosage form of it previously.
- it is prescribed for a child under 3 years of age.
- you have tardive dyskinesia.
- you have narrow angle glaucoma.

▷ **Inform Your Physician Before Taking This Drug If**
- you have had an unfavorable reaction to atropine or atropinelike drugs.
- you have glaucoma or myasthenia gravis.
- you have heart disease or high blood pressure.
- you have a history of liver or kidney disease.
- you have difficulty emptying the urinary bladder, especially if due to an enlarged prostate gland.
- you are taking, or have taken within the past 2 weeks, any monoamine oxidase (MAO) type A inhibitor drug (see Drug Classes).
- you take other prescription or nonprescription medications that were not discussed when benztropine was prescribed for you.
- you are unsure of how much benztropine to take or how often to take it.
- you will be exposed to extreme heat for extended periods, such as some iron smelters or traveling to tropical climates.
- you have a history of bowel obstructions.

Possible Side Effects (natural, expected, and unavoidable drug actions)
Nervousness, blurring of vision, dryness of mouth, constipation, impaired urination. (These often subside as drug use continues.)

▷ **Possible Adverse Effects** (unusual, unexpected, and infrequent reactions)
If any of the following develop, consult your physician promptly for guidance.
Mild Adverse Effects
Allergic reaction: skin rashes—rare.
Headache, dizziness, drowsiness, muscle cramps—possible.
Indigestion, nausea, vomiting—reported.

Fast heart rate (tachycardia)—infrequent.

Memory problems—possible.

Serious Adverse Effects

Idiosyncratic reactions: abnormal behavior, confusion, delusions, hallucinations, agitation—case reports.

Tardive dyskinesia—case reports.

Dystonia—rare.

Bowel obstruction—case reports.

Abnormal elevations of temperature (hyperthermia)—case reports.

▷ **Possible Effects on Sexual Function**

Reversal of male impotence due to the use of fluphenazine (a phenothiazine antipsychotic drug).

Male infertility (0.5 to 6 mg per day).

May help treat priapism.

Natural Diseases or Disorders That May Be Activated by This Drug

Latent glaucoma, latent myasthenia gravis.

Possible Effects on Laboratory Tests

Prolactin: may be increased (especially if taken with haloperidol).

CAUTION

1. Many over-the-counter (OTC) medications for allergies, colds, and coughs contain drugs that should NOT be combined with benztropine. Ask your physician or pharmacist for help.
2. This drug may aggravate tardive dyskinesia (see Glossary). Ask your physician for guidance.

Precautions for Use

By Infants and Children: Safety and effectiveness for those under 3 years of age not established. Children are especially susceptible to the atropinelike effects.

By Those Over 60 Years of Age: Small starting doses are advisable. Increased susceptibility to impaired thinking, confusion, nightmares, hallucinations, increased internal eye pressure (glaucoma), and impaired urination associated with prostate gland enlargement (prostatism).

▷ **Advisability of Use During Pregnancy**

Pregnancy Category: C. See Pregnancy Risk Categories at the back of this book.

Animal studies: No data available.

Human studies: Adequate studies of pregnant women are not available.

Avoid use if possible, especially close to delivery. This drug can impair the infant's intestinal tract following birth.

Advisability of Use If Breast-Feeding

Presence of this drug in breast milk: Unknown.

Ask your doctor for guidance.

Habit-Forming Potential: Occasional reports of anti-parkinsonian drug abuse have been made. Sudden withdrawal of benztropine may lead to craving, restlessness, nervousness, and depression. Propranolol (20–80 mg three times daily) or diazepam (Valium) have been used to ease these symptoms.

Effects of Overdosage: Weakness; drowsiness; stupor; impaired vision; rapid pulse; excitement; confusion; hallucinations; dry, hot skin; skin rash; dilated pupils.

Possible Effects of Long-Term Use: Increased internal eye pressure—possible glaucoma, especially in the elderly.

Suggested Periodic Examinations While Taking This Drug (at physician's discretion)
Measurement of internal eye pressure at regular intervals.

▷ **While Taking This Drug, Observe the Following**
Foods: No restrictions.
Beverages: No restrictions.
▷ *Alcohol:* Use caution. Alcohol may increase the sedative effects of this drug.
Tobacco Smoking: No interactions expected, but I advise everyone to quit smoking.
Marijuana Smoking: May increase heart rate to unacceptable levels. Avoid completely if this increased heart rate will be a problem for you.
▷ *Other Drugs*
Benztropine may *decrease* the effects of
• cisapride (Propulsid).
• haloperidol (Haldol).
• phenothiazines (Thorazine, etc.).
The following drugs may *increase* the effects of benztropine:
• antihistamines may add to the dryness of mouth and throat.
• monoamine oxidase (MAO) type A inhibitor drugs may intensify all effects of this drug (see Drug Classes).
• tricyclic antidepressants (Elavil, etc.) may add to eye effects and further increase internal eye pressure (dangerous in glaucoma).
Benztropine *taken concurrently* with
• amantadine (Symmetrel) may cause increased confusion and possible hallucinations.
• clozapine (Clozaril) can cause increased risk of elevated temperatures, neurological adverse effects, and bowel obstruction (ileus).
▷ *Driving, Hazardous Activities:* Drowsiness and dizziness may occur in sensitive individuals. Avoid hazardous activities until full effects and tolerance have been determined.
Aviation Note: The use of this drug *is a disqualification* for piloting. Consult a designated Aviation Medical Examiner.
Exposure to Sun: No restrictions.
Exposure to Heat: Use caution. This drug may reduce sweating, cause an increase in body temperature, and increase risk of heatstroke.
Heavy Exercise or Exertion: Use caution. Avoid in hot environments.
Discontinuation: Do not stop this drug abruptly. Ask your doctor how to reduce the dose gradually.

BETAXOLOL (be TAX oh lohl)

Introduced: 1983   **Class:** Antihypertensive, beta-adrenergic blocker
Prescription: USA: Yes   **Controlled Drug:** USA: No; Canada: No   **Available as Generic:** No
Brand Names: Betoptic, Betoptic-Pilo [CD], Betoptic-S, Kerlone

> **BENEFITS versus RISKS**
>
> | *Possible Benefits* | *Possible Risks* |
> |---|---|
> | EFFECTIVE, WELL-TOLERATED ANTIHYPERTENSIVE in mild to moderate high blood pressure | CONGESTIVE HEART FAILURE in advanced heart disease |
> | EFFECTIVE TREATMENT OF CHRONIC, OPEN-ANGLE GLAUCOMA | Worsening of angina in coronary heart disease (abrupt withdrawal) |
> | PROLONGATION OF LIFE AFTER A HEART ATTACK | Masking of low blood sugar (hypoglycemia) in drug-treated diabetes |
> | Treatment of ocular hypertension | Provocation of bronchial asthma (with high doses) |
> | | Rare anemia and low blood platelets |

▷ **Principal Uses**

As a Single Drug Product: Uses currently included in FDA-approved labeling: Used to treat: (1) mild to moderate high blood pressure; (2) chronic open-angle glaucoma (eyedrops). May be used alone or combined with other antihypertensive drugs, such as diuretics; (3) ocular hypertension; (4) Betoptic-Pilo: approved for use in reducing elevated intraocular pressure in patients with primary open-angle glaucoma who have failed Betoptic-S therapy.

Other (unlabeled) generally accepted uses: (1) The oral form may help decrease death (mortality) by reducing damage from a heart attack and making abnormal heartbeats less likely; (2) helps decrease the occurrence and severity of chest pain (angina); (3) can be of help in easing aggressive behavior in selected psychiatric patients; (4) may help panic attacks; (5) can treat selected cases of stuttering.

How This Drug Works: By blocking certain actions of the sympathetic nervous system, this drug reduces the rate and contraction force of the heart, lowering blood ejection pressure and reducing the oxygen needed by the heart to work; relaxes contracted blood vessel walls, resulting in expansion and consequent lowering of blood pressure; reduces the internal pressure of the eye.

Available Dosage Forms and Strengths

Eyedrops — 2.8 mg/ml
— 5.6 mg/ml
Tablets — 10 mg, 20 mg

▷ **Usual Adult Dosage Range:**   Hypertension: Initially 10 mg once daily. Dose may be increased gradually at intervals of 7 to 14 days as needed and tolerated up to 20 mg every 24 hours. The usual maintenance dose is 10 to 15 mg daily. Some patients have tolerated 40 mg daily well, but have not shown increased benefits in reduced blood pressure. The total dose should not exceed 20 mg daily.

For use in glaucoma: One or two drops of the 2.8 mg/ml solution or one drop of the 5.6 mg/ml.

Betoptic-Pilo: Reducing elevated intraocular pressure in patients with primary open-angle glaucoma who have failed Betoptic-S therapy: Follow label instructions. **Note: Actual dosage and administration schedule must be determined for each patient individually.**

Conditions Requiring Dosing Adjustments
  Liver Function: Use with caution; this drug is metabolized in the liver. Dose decreases are not, however, routinely needed.
  Kidney Function: Up to 12% of a dose is removed by the kidney. Starting dose is 5 mg in this case, and the dose is only increased as needed and tolerated by 5 mg every 2 weeks for a maximum of 20 mg daily.

▷ **Dosing Instructions:**   May be taken without regard to eating. The tablet may be crushed. Do not stop this drug abruptly.

Usual Duration of Use: Use on a regular schedule for 10 to 14 days is usually needed to see this drug's effectiveness in lowering blood pressure. Long-term use will be determined by the success in lowering your blood pressure over time and your response to an overall treatment program of weight reduction, salt restriction, smoking cessation, etc. See your doctor regularly.

Possible Advantages of This Drug: Usually effective and well tolerated with a single dose daily, which is easier to remember to take.

▷ **This Drug Should Not Be Taken If**
  • you have had an allergic reaction to it previously.
  • you have heart (overt) failure.
  • you have an abnormally slow heart rate or a serious heart block.
  • you are taking, or have taken within the past 14 days, any monoamine oxidase (MAO) type A inhibitor drug (see Drug Classes).

▷ **Inform Your Physician Before Taking This Drug If**
  • you have had an adverse reaction to any beta-blocker drug (see Drug Classes).
  • you have a history of serious heart disease or episodes of heart failure.
  • you have a history of hay fever (allergic rhinitis), asthma, chronic bronchitis, or emphysema. Some drugs in this class are contraindicated in asthmatics.
  • you have a history of overactive thyroid function (hyperthyroidism).
  • you have a history of low blood sugar (hypoglycemia).
  • you have impaired liver or kidney function.
  • you have narrowing of the vessels in your legs or arms (peripheral vascular disease). Discuss this with your doctor.
  • you have diabetes or myasthenia gravis.
  • you take digitalis, quinidine, or reserpine, or any calcium blocker drug (see Drug Classes).
  • you plan to have surgery under general anesthesia in the near future.
  • you take other prescription or nonprescription medications that were not discussed when betaxolol was prescribed for you.
  • you are unsure of how much betaxolol to take or how often to take it.

Possible Side Effects (natural, expected, and unavoidable drug actions)
  Lethargy, fatigue (up to 10%), cold extremities—rare; slow heart rate, lightheadedness in upright position (see Orthostatic Hypotension in Glossary).

▷ **Possible Adverse Effects** (unusual, unexpected, and infrequent reactions)
  If any of the following develop, consult your physician promptly for guidance.

Mild Adverse Effects
Allergic reactions: skin rash, itching—rare.
Hair loss—rare.
Headache (up to 15%)—frequent.
Dizziness, fatigue—infrequent.
Insomnia or abnormal dreams—infrequent.
Indigestion, nausea, diarrhea—infrequent.
Joint and muscle discomfort—infrequent.
Fluid retention (edema)—rare.
Difficulty breathing—infrequent.

Serious Adverse Effects
Mental depression or anxiety—rare.
Increased blood sugar (hyperglycemia) in noninsulin-dependent diabetics—possible.
Chest pain, shortness of breath, congestive heart failure—rare.
Induction of bronchial asthma (in asthmatic individuals)—possible.
Low blood platelets and anemia—rare.
Congestive heart failure—rare.
Angina (if drug abruptly stopped).
Intermittent problems walking (intermittent claudication)—possible.
Heart attack (myocardial infarction)—rare.

▷ **Possible Effects on Sexual Function:** Decreased libido, impotence—rare.
Altered menstrual patterns (reported rarely with other medicines in this class)—possible.

Adverse Effects That May Mimic Natural Diseases or Disorders
Reduced blood flow to extremities may mimic Raynaud's disease (see Glossary).

Possible Effects on Laboratory Tests
Glaucoma-screening test (measurement of internal eye pressure): pressure is decreased (false low or normal value).
Antinuclear antibodies (ANA) test: positive in 5.3% of users.
Blood potassium: slightly increased.
Blood platelet counts and hemoglobin: decreased—rare.
Blood glucose: increased in noninsulin-dependent diabetics.

CAUTION
1. ***Do not stop this drug suddenly*** without the knowledge of your doctor. Always carry a note with you that says you are taking this drug.
2. Ask your physician or pharmacist before using nasal decongestants. These can cause sudden increases in blood pressure when combined with beta-blocker drugs.
3. Report the development of any tendency to emotional depression.

Precautions for Use
By Infants and Children: Safety and effectiveness for those under 12 years of age not established.
*By Those Over 60 Years of Age: **Caution**:* High blood pressure should be slowly reduced, avoiding risks associated with excessively low blood pressure. Treatment should be started with 5 mg daily and blood pressure checked often. Sudden, rapid, and excessive reduction of blood pressure can cause stroke or heart attack. Total daily dosage should not exceed 10 to 15 mg.

Watch for dizziness, unsteadiness, tendency to fall, confusion, hallucinations, depression, or urinary frequency. This age group is more prone to develop excessively slow heart rates and hypothermia.

▷ **Advisability of Use During Pregnancy**

Pregnancy Category: C. See Pregnancy Risk Categories at the back of this book.

Animal studies: Rat studies reveal increased resorptions of embryo and fetus, retarded growth and development of newborn, and mild skeletal defects.

Human studies: Adequate studies of pregnant women are not available.

Avoid use of drug during the first 3 months if possible. Avoid use during labor and delivery because of the possible effects on the newborn infant.

Advisability of Use If Breast-Feeding

Presence of this drug in breast milk: Yes.

Avoid drug if possible. If drug is necessary, observe nursing infant for slow heart rate and indications of low blood sugar.

Habit-Forming Potential: None.

Effects of Overdosage: Weakness, slow pulse, low blood pressure, fainting, cold and sweaty skin, congestive heart failure, possible coma, and convulsions.

Possible Effects of Long-Term Use: Reduced heart reserve and eventual heart failure in susceptible individuals with advanced heart disease.

Suggested Periodic Examinations While Taking This Drug (at physician's discretion)

Measurements of blood pressure, evaluation of heart function.

▷ **While Taking This Drug, Observe the Following**

Foods: No restrictions. Avoid excessive salt intake.

Beverages: No restrictions. May be taken with milk.

▷ *Alcohol:* Use with caution. Alcohol may exaggerate this drug's ability to lower blood pressure and may increase its mild sedative effect.

Tobacco Smoking: Nicotine may reduce this drug's effectiveness in treating high blood pressure. In addition, high drug doses worsen the constriction of bronchial tubes caused by regular smoking. I advise everyone to quit smoking.

▷ *Other Drugs*

Betaxolol may ***increase*** the effects of

- other antihypertensive drugs and cause excessive lowering of blood pressure. Dosage decreases may be necessary.
- reserpine (Ser-Ap-Es, etc.) and cause sedation, depression, slowing of heart rate, and lowering of blood pressure (light-headedness, fainting).
- verapamil and cause additive risk of congestive heart failure and slow heart rate (bradycardia).

Betaxolol ***taken concurrently*** with

- amiodarone (Cordarone) may result in extremely slow heart rate and arrest.
- calcium channel blockers (see Drug Classes) may cause severe lowering of blood pressure.
- clonidine (Catapres) requires close monitoring for rebound high blood pressure if clonidine is stopped while betaxolol is still being taken.
- fluoroquinolone (see Drug Classes) antibiotics may cause an increase in betaxolol blood levels and lead to toxicity.

- fluvoxamine (Luvox) may cause excessive slowing of the heart and very low blood pressure.
- insulin requires close supervision to avoid hypoglycemia (see Glossary).
- oral antidiabetic drugs (see Drug Classes) may prolong recovery from low blood sugars.
- phenothiazines (see Drug Classes) may result in additive blood-pressure-lowering effects.
- ritonavir (Norvir) and perhaps other protease inhibitors (see Drug Classes) may decrease betaxolol benefits.
- venlafaxine (Effexor) may cause excessive slowing of the heart and very low blood pressure.

The following drugs may *decrease* the effects of betaxolol:
- indomethacin (Indocin), and possibly other "aspirin substitutes" or NSAIDs, may impair betaxolol's antihypertensive effect.

▷ *Driving, Hazardous Activities:* Use caution until the full extent of drowsiness, lethargy, and blood pressure change has been determined.

Aviation Note: The use of this drug *is a disqualification* for piloting. Consult a designated Aviation Medical Examiner.

Exposure to Sun: No restrictions.

Exposure to Heat: Caution is advised. Hot environments can lower blood pressure and exaggerate the effects of this drug.

Exposure to Cold: Caution is advised. Cold environments can enhance the circulatory deficiency in the extremities that may occur with this drug. The elderly should be careful to prevent hypothermia (see Glossary).

Heavy Exercise or Exertion: It is advisable to avoid exertion that produces light-headedness, excessive fatigue, or muscle cramping. The use of this drug may intensify the hypertensive response to isometric exercise.

Occurrence of Unrelated Illness: Fever can lower blood pressure and require adjustment of dosage. Nausea or vomiting may interrupt the dosing schedule. Ask your physician for help.

Discontinuation: Avoid sudden discontinuation of this drug in all situations. If possible, gradual reduction of dose over a period of 2 to 3 weeks is recommended. Ask your physician for specific guidance.

BITOLTEROL (bi TOHL ter ohl)

Introduced: 1985   **Class:** Antiasthmatic, bronchodilator   **Prescription:** Yes   **Controlled Drug:** No   **Available as Generic:** No
Brand Name: Tornalate

BENEFITS versus RISKS	
Possible Benefits	*Possible Risks*
EFFECTIVE PREVENTION AND RELIEF OF ASTHMA	Fine hand tremor
	Nervousness
	Throat irritation
	Irregular heart rhythm (with excessive use)

▷ **Principal Uses**

As a Single Drug Product: Uses currently included in FDA-approved labeling: (1) To relieve acute bronchial asthma and to reduce the frequency and severity of chronic, recurrent asthmatic attacks; (2) used to help those asthmatics dependent on steroids.

Other (unlabeled) generally accepted uses: (1) May be more useful than other agents in helping open the bronchi in patients with chronic obstructive pulmonary disease (COPD); (2) may have a role in preventing exercise-induced asthma.

How This Drug Works: By increasing cyclic AMP, this drug relaxes bronchial muscles and relieves asthmatic wheezing.

Available Dosage Forms and Strengths

Aerosol inhaler — 15 ml (300 inhalations of 0.37 mg each)

▷ **Usual Adult Dosage Range:**   For acute bronchospasm—two inhalations at intervals of 1 to 3 minutes, followed by a third inhalation in 3 to 4 minutes if needed. For prevention of bronchospasm—two inhalations every 8 hours. Maximum inhalation dose is two inhalations every 4 hours.

For children over 12: same as adult bronchospasm dose. **Note: Actual dosage and administration schedule must be determined for each patient individually.**

Conditions Requiring Dosing Adjustments

Liver Function: Use with caution in severe liver compromise.

Kidney Function: Significant kidney removal; however, specific dosage guidelines are unavailable.

▷ **Dosing Instructions:**   May be used without regard to eating. Follow the written directions for use carefully. **Do not overuse**.

Usual Duration of Use: Do not use beyond the time needed to stop episodes of acute asthma. Ask your physician for help regarding use in preventing asthma attacks.

▷ **This Drug Should Not Be Taken If**

- you have had an allergic reaction to it previously.
- you currently have an irregular heart rhythm.
- you are taking, or have taken within the past 2 weeks, any monoamine oxidase (MAO) type A inhibitor drug (see Drug Classes).

▷ **Inform Your Physician Before Taking This Drug If**

- you have any type of heart or circulatory disorder, especially high blood pressure or coronary heart disease.
- you have diabetes, epilepsy, or an overactive thyroid gland.
- you are taking any form of digitalis or any stimulant drug.
- you are unsure of how much bitolterol to take or how often to take it.
- you are pregnant and are nearing the time of delivery of your baby (may complicate labor and delivery).

Possible Side Effects (natural, expected, and unavoidable drug actions)

Dryness or irritation of mouth or throat.

▷ **Possible Adverse Effects** (unusual, unexpected, and infrequent reactions)

If any of the following develop, consult your physician promptly for guidance.

Mild Adverse Effects
Headache, dizziness, nervousness, insomnia—infrequent.
Fine tremor of hands—frequent.
Nausea, indigestion—infrequent.
Coughing—infrequent.
Fast heart rate (tachycardia)—rare.

Serious Adverse Effects
Excessive use can cause irregular heart rate or rhythm or increased blood pressure.
Paradoxical bronchospasm—rare.

▷ **Possible Effects on Sexual Function:**   None reported.

Natural Diseases or Disorders That May Be Activated by This Drug
Latent coronary artery disease, diabetes, or high blood pressure.

Possible Effects on Laboratory Tests
None reported.

CAUTION
1. Combination use of this drug by inhalation with beclomethasone aerosol (Beclovent, Vanceril) may increase the risk of toxicity due to fluorocarbon propellants. Use bitolterol aerosol 20 to 30 minutes *before* beclomethasone aerosol. This will reduce toxicity risk and enhances penetration of beclomethasone.
2. Excessive or prolonged use of this drug by inhalation can reduce effectiveness and cause serious heart rhythm disturbances.

Precautions for Use
By Infants and Children: Safety and effectiveness for children under 12 years of age not established.
By Those Over 60 Years of Age: Avoid excessive and continual use. If acute asthma is not relieved promptly, other drugs will be needed. Watch for development of nervousness, palpitations, irregular heart rhythm, and muscle tremors.

▷ **Advisability of Use During Pregnancy**
Pregnancy Category: C. See Pregnancy Risk Categories at the back of this book.
Animal studies: Cleft palate reported in mice.
Human studies: Adequate studies of pregnant women are not available.
Avoid use during first 3 months if possible.

Advisability of Use If Breast-Feeding
Presence of this drug in breast milk: Unknown.
Avoid drug or refrain from nursing.

Habit-Forming Potential: None.

Effects of Overdosage: Nervousness, palpitation, rapid heart rate, sweating, headache, tremor, vomiting, abnormal heart rhythms, chest pain.

Possible Effects of Long-Term Use: Loss of effectiveness.

Suggested Periodic Examinations While Taking This Drug (at physician's discretion)
Blood pressure measurements, evaluation of heart status.

▷ **While Taking This Drug, Observe the Following**
Foods: No restrictions.
Beverages: Avoid excessive caffeine—coffee, tea, cola, chocolate.

▷ *Alcohol:* No interactions expected.

Tobacco Smoking: No interactions expected, but the smoke itself can irritate airways. I advise everyone to quit smoking.

▷ *Other Drugs*

Bitolterol *taken concurrently* with

• monoamine oxidase (MAO) type A inhibitor drugs (see Drug Classes) may cause large increases in blood pressure and undesirable heart stimulation.

▷ *Driving, Hazardous Activities:* Use caution if excessive nervousness or dizziness occurs.

Aviation Note: The use of this drug *is a disqualification* for piloting. Consult a designated Aviation Medical Examiner.

Exposure to Sun: No restrictions.

Heavy Exercise or Exertion: Use caution. Excessive exercise can induce asthma in some people.

BROMOCRIPTINE (broh moh KRIP teen)

Introduced: 1975 **Class:** Anti-parkinsonism, ergot derivative **Prescription:** USA: Yes **Controlled Drug:** USA: No; Canada: No **Available as Generic:** No

Brand Names: Parlodel, Normatine

BENEFITS versus RISKS	
Possible Benefits	*Possible Risks*
PARTIAL RELIEF OF SYMPTOMS OF PARKINSON'S DISEASE CORRECTION OF INFERTILITY AND ABSENT MENSTRUATION in women with high prolactin levels	ABNORMAL INVOLUNTARY MOVEMENTS AND ALTERED BEHAVIOR in users taking high doses Raynaud's phenomenon (see Glossary) in users taking high doses Low blood pressure

▷ **Principal Uses**

As a Single Drug Product: Uses currently included in FDA-approved labeling: (1) Can be used to treat early-stage symptoms of Parkinson's disease. Often it is used in conjunction with levodopa when levodopa starts to lose its effectiveness, or the patient cannot tolerate the adverse effects of levodopa and dosage adjustment or withdrawal is necessary; (2) treats disorders due to excessive production of prolactin by the pituitary gland: absence of menstruation, infertility, and inappropriate production of milk; (3) helps as an adjunct to surgery in acromegaly; (4) eases breast engorgement and galactorrhea in stress-induced hyperprolactinemia; (5) can help in functional infertility in females; (6) reduces the size of pituitary tumors.

Other (unlabeled) generally accepted uses: (1) Can help in patients who have had a stroke and have problems in speaking; (2) may have a small role in helping cocaine withdrawal; (3) may help return growth to normal in children experiencing abnormal skeletal growth.

Author's Note: Bromocriptine is no longer FDA approved for the treatment of physiological lactation. This indication was withdrawn be-

cause the risks of the use of the drug outweigh the benefits for this indication.

How This Drug Works: By stimulating receptor sites (dopamine) in the brain (corpus striatum), this drug helps increase dopamine and relieve rigidity, tremor, and sluggish movement characteristic of Parkinson's disease. By inhibiting the production of the hormone prolactin by the anterior pituitary gland, this drug reduces the amount of prolactin in the blood and blocks breast milk production; reduces abnormally high levels of prolactin in the blood, restoring it to normal levels that permit menstrual regularity and fertility.

Available Dosage Forms and Strengths

    Capsules — 5 mg
    Tablets — 2.5 mg
    Elixir — 4 mg/5 ml

▷ **Usual Adult Dosage Range:** For Parkinson's disease—initially 1.25 mg twice daily. Patients should be checked every 14 days to assess benefits of bromocriptine. The dose may be increased as needed and tolerated by no more than 2.5 mg daily every 14 to 28 days. The usual dosage range is 10 to 40 mg daily. Do not exceed 100 mg daily. The lowest possible dose should be used. For absent menstruation and infertility—initially 2.5 mg one to three times daily with meals. Total dose can be increased by 2.5 mg every 3 to 7 days. Effective response may be seen at 2.5 to 15 mg per day. **Note: Actual dosage and administration schedule must be determined for each patient individually.**

Conditions Requiring Dosing Adjustments

Liver Function: The dose should be decreased or the dosing interval lengthened; however, specific guidelines are not available.

Kidney Function: Use with caution in severe renal failure only.

▷ **Dosing Instructions:** Take with food or milk to reduce stomach irritation. Capsule may be opened and tablet may be crushed for administration.

Usual Duration of Use: Use on a regular schedule for 3 to 4 months is usually needed to determine this drug's effectiveness in controlling the symptoms of Parkinson's disease. Treatment for 4 to 12 weeks restores fertility and normal menstruation in most women; however, treatment may be necessary for 6 to 12 months. Long-term use (up to 3 years or more) must be under physician supervision and guidance. See your doctor regularly.

▷ **This Drug Should Not Be Taken If**
  • you have had an allergic reaction to it previously.
  • you have had a serious adverse effect from any ergot preparation.
  • you have severe coronary artery disease or peripheral vascular disease.
  • you are pregnant.
  • you are nursing your infant (will disrupt milk formation).

▷ **Inform Your Physician Before Taking This Drug If**
  • you have constitutionally low blood pressure.
  • you are taking any antihypertensive drugs or phenothiazines (see Drug Classes).
  • you have coronary artery disease, especially with a history of heart attack (myocardial infarction).

- you have a history of heart rhythm abnormalities.
- you have impaired liver function.
- you have a seizure disorder (epilepsy).
- you take other prescription or nonprescription medications that were not discussed when bromocriptine was prescribed for you.
- you have an ulcer.
- you have a history of mental illness.
- you take other medicines that can lower blood pressure.
- you are unsure of how much bromocriptine to take or how often to take it.

Possible Side Effects (natural, expected, and unavoidable drug actions)
Fatigue, lethargy, light-headedness in upright position (see Orthostatic Hypotension in Glossary). Lowering of blood pressure (hypotension)—frequent. Swelling of feet and ankles (edema).

▷ **Possible Adverse Effects** (unusual, unexpected, and infrequent reactions)
If any of the following develop, consult your physician promptly for guidance.
Mild Adverse Effects
Allergic reaction: skin rash.
Headache, dizziness—frequent.
Fainting (syncope)—rare.
Nightmares—possible.
Nasal congestion, dry mouth—reported.
Loss of appetite, nausea—frequent.
Indications of "ergotism": numbness and tingling of fingers, cold hands and feet, muscle cramps of legs and feet—frequent.
Serious Adverse Effects
Abnormal involuntary movements—possible.
Hallucinations, psychosis—case reports.
Seizures—case reports.
Stroke—case reports.
Loss of urinary bladder control, inability to empty bladder—possible.
Retroperitoneal fibrosis—case reports.
May worsen existing ulcers.
Excessive lowering of blood pressure—possible.
Worsening of mania in manic patients—possible.
Abnormal heart rhythms—possible.
Vasospasms and potential for heart attack—very rare.
Lung changes (pulmonary fibrosis) with long-term use—rare.

▷ **Possible Effects on Sexual Function:** Impotence—rare. However, this drug can correct impotence and reduced libido when the problem is due to high blood levels of prolactin (a pituitary hormone).

Adverse Effects That May Mimic Natural Diseases or Disorders
Effects on mental function and behavior may resemble psychotic disorders.

Natural Diseases or Disorders That May Be Activated by This Drug
Coronary artery disease with anginal syndrome, Raynaud's phenomenon.

Possible Effects on Laboratory Tests
Blood alkaline phosphatase level: increased.
White blood cell count and platelets: lowered (single case report).

CAUTION

1. During treatment of parkinsonism, avoid excessive and hurried activity as improvement occurs; this will reduce the risk of falls and injury.
2. The neurological and psychiatric disturbances due to this drug may last for 2 to 6 weeks after stopping it.
3. During treatment to reduce the blood level of prolactin and restore normal menstruation and fertility, it is mandatory that you use a barrier method of contraception to prevent pregnancy. Oral contraceptives should not be used while taking bromocriptine.
4. If pregnancy occurs, notify your physician **immediately**.

Precautions for Use

By Infants and Children: Safety and effectiveness for those under 15 years of age not established.

By Those Over 60 Years of Age: Your initial test dose should be 1.25 mg. Watch closely for light-headedness or faintness on attempting to stand after this first dose. You may be more susceptible to the development of impaired thinking, confusion, agitation, nightmares, hallucinations, nausea, or vomiting. Close monitoring and careful dosage adjustments are mandatory.

▷ **Advisability of Use During Pregnancy**

Pregnancy Category: B. See Pregnancy Risk Categories at the back of this book. Animal studies: Rabbit studies reveal an increase in cleft lip.

Human studies: Serious birth defects have been reported in infants whose mothers took this drug during early pregnancy. Because the incidence of these defects does not exceed that reported for the general population, a cause-and-effect relationship is uncertain. Information from adequate studies of pregnant women is not available.

Ask your doctor for advice on stopping therapy.

Advisability of Use If Breast-Feeding

This drug prevents the production of milk and makes nursing impossible.

Habit-Forming Potential: Use to treat cocaine craving may result in a chemical dependence on bromocriptine.

Effects of Overdosage: Weakness, low blood pressure, nausea, vomiting, diarrhea, confusion, agitation, hallucinations, loss of consciousness.

Possible Effects of Long-Term Use: Changes in lung tissue, thickening of the pleura and pleural effusion (fluid formation within the chest cage). These changes appear reversible after stopping the drug. Fibrosis (scar tissue formation) in the back wall of the abdominal cavity and contractures of the extremities have been reported.

Suggested Periodic Examinations While Taking This Drug (at physician's discretion)

Blood pressure measurements; CAT scan of the pituitary gland for enlargement due to tumor; pregnancy test; blood tests for anemia; evaluation of heart, lung, and liver functions.

▷ **While Taking This Drug, Observe the Following**

Foods: No restrictions.

Beverages: No restrictions. May be taken with milk.

▷ *Alcohol:* Caution—alcohol can exaggerate the blood-pressure-lowering effects and sedative effects of this drug and also worsen nausea and abdominal side effects.

Tobacco Smoking: Smoking may worsen symptoms of ergotism. I advise everyone to quit smoking.

▷   *Other Drugs*

Bromocriptine *taken concurrently* with

- antihypertensive drugs (and other drugs that can lower blood pressure) requires careful monitoring for excessive drops in pressure. Dosage adjustments may be necessary.
- cyclosporine (Sandimmune) may lead to cyclosporine toxicity.
- erythromycin or other macrolide antibiotics (see Drug Classes) may result
in increased bromocriptine levels and toxicity.
- phenylpropanolamine can result in bromocriptine toxicity.

The following drugs may *decrease* the effects of bromocriptine:

- phenothiazines (see Drug Classes). It is probably best to avoid the concurrent use of these drugs until the results of further studies are available.

▷   *Driving, Hazardous Activities:* Be alert to the possible occurrence of orthostatic
hypotension, dizziness, drowsiness, or impaired coordination.

Aviation Note: Parkinsonism *is a disqualification* for piloting. The use of this
drug otherwise *may be a disqualification* for piloting. Consult a designated Aviation Medical Examiner.

Exposure to Sun: No restrictions.

Discontinuation: Once this medicine is stopped, pituitary tumor regrowth and
symptoms of hyperprolactinemia may occur again.

BUMETANIDE (byu MET a nide)

Introduced: 1983   **Class:** Diuretic   **Prescription:** USA: Yes; Canada:
No   **Controlled Drug:** USA: No   **Available as Generic:** Yes
Brand Name: Bumex

BENEFITS versus RISKS	
Possible Benefits	*Possible Risks*
POTENT, EFFECTIVE DIURETIC BY MOUTH OR INJECTION	ABNORMALLY LOW BLOOD POTASSIUM with excessive use Decreased magnesium with chronic therapy Blood disorders—rare

▷ **Principal Uses**

As a Single Drug Product: Uses currently included in FDA-approved labeling: (1)
Relieves retained fluid associated with congestive heart failure, liver disease, or kidney disease; (2) helps edema in patients who don't respond or
can't tolerate furosemide.

Other (unlabeled) generally accepted uses: (1) Used as an adjunct to other
therapy in high blood pressure (hypertension); (2) can help older people
decrease the number of times they must get up at night to urinate (nocturia); (3) eases the amount of fluid that can build up in the lungs (pulmonary
edema).

How This Drug Works: Increases removal of salt and water from the body
(through increased urine production), and reduces sodium and the volume
of fluid in the blood.

Available Dosage Forms and Strengths
    Injection — 0.25 mg/ml (2-ml ampules)
    Tablets — 0.5 mg, 1 mg, 2 mg

▷ **Usual Adult Dosage Range:**   0.5 to 2 mg daily, usually taken in the morning as a single dose. If needed, an additional second or third dose may be taken later in the day at 4- to 5-hour intervals. The total daily dose should not exceed 10 mg. Alternate-day dosage (taken every other day) may be adequate for some individuals. **Note: Actual dosage and administration schedule must be determined for each patient individually.**

Conditions Requiring Dosing Adjustments
    Liver Function: Rapid body fluid removal can cause a coma in liver failure patients. Use of medicines in this class is only done under close medical supervision as in a hospital or outpatient care center.
    Kidney Function: **NOT** recommended for use in progressive renal failure.

▷ **Dosing Instructions:**   May be crushed when taken and given with or following food to reduce stomach irritation.

Usual Duration of Use: Two to three days of use on a regular schedule is often needed to see peak effect in relieving fluid buildup (edema). Once peak benefit is realized, intermittent use reduces risk of sodium, potassium, magnesium, and water imbalance. Long-term use requires physician supervision.

Possible Advantages of This Drug
    Diuretic effect is usually complete in 4 hours; diuretic effect of furosemide usually lasts from 6 to 8 hours.

▷ **This Drug Should Not Be Taken If**
- you have had an allergic reaction to either dosage form previously.
- coma caused by liver failure is present.
- your kidneys are unable to produce urine.
- you have developed a marked increase in creatinine or blood urea nitrogen (BUN) while taking this drug.
- severe electrolyte or fluid imbalance.

▷ **Inform Your Physician Before Taking This Drug If**
- you are allergic to any form of "sulfa" drug.
- you are pregnant or planning pregnancy.
- you have a blood disorder.
- you have impaired liver or kidney function.
- you have diabetes, a diabetic tendency, or a history of gout.
- you have impaired hearing, or develop hearing loss during therapy.
- you are taking: cortisone, digitalis, oral antidiabetic drugs, insulin, probenecid (Benemid), indomethacin (Indocin), lithium, or drugs for high blood pressure.
- you plan to have surgery under general anesthesia in the near future.
- you are unsure of how much to take or how often to take bumetanide.

Possible Side Effects (natural, expected, and unavoidable drug actions)
    Light-headedness on arising from sitting or lying position (see Orthostatic Hypotension in Glossary).
    Increase in level of blood sugar, affecting control of diabetes.
    Increase in level of blood uric acid, affecting control of gout.

Decreased blood potassium and sodium with muscle weakness and cramping.
Decreased blood magnesium.

▷ **Possible Adverse Effects** (unusual, unexpected, and infrequent reactions)
**If any of the following develop, consult your physician promptly for
guidance.**
Mild Adverse Effects
Allergic reactions: skin rashes, hives, itching.
Headache, dizziness, vertigo, fatigue, weakness, sweating, earache—rare.
Nausea, vomiting, stomach pain, diarrhea—infrequent.
Breast nipple tenderness, joint and muscle pains or cramps—rare.
Serious Adverse Effects
Serious skin rash (Stevens-Johnson syndrome)—case reports.
Development of liver coma (in preexisting liver disease)—possible.
Abnormally low magnesium, potassium, and sodium (electrolytes): possible
with long-term or high-dose use—rare to frequent.
Low white blood cells and platelets (leukopenia and thrombocytopenia)—
rare.
Kidney failure—rare.
Pancreatitis—case reports.
Elevated blood glucose—infrequent.
Lung fibrosis—case reports.
Hearing toxicity (ototoxicity)—rare.

▷ **Possible Effects on Sexual Function:**   Difficulty maintaining an erection; premature ejaculation (0.5 to 2 mg daily)—rare.
Male breast enlargement and tenderness (gynecomastia)—case reports.

Natural Diseases or Disorders That May Be Activated by This Drug
Latent diabetes, gout.

Possible Effects on Laboratory Tests
White blood cell counts: increased—usual; decreased—rare.
Blood platelets: decreased.
Blood sugar (glucose): increased.
Blood lithium or uric acid levels: increased.
Blood potassium, magnesium, or chloride: decreased.

CAUTION
1. High doses can cause excessive excretion of water, sodium, and potassium, with loss of appetite, nausea, weakness, confusion, and profound
   drop in blood pressure (circulatory collapse).
2. May cause digitalis toxicity by depleting potassium. If you are taking a
   digitalis preparation (digitoxin, digoxin), ensure an adequate intake of
   high potassium foods.
3. People with cirrhosis of the liver must never increase their dose unless
   told to do so by their doctor. Excess dosing can cause liver coma.
4. People who take lithium may experience lithium toxicity.

Precautions for Use
By Infants and Children: Safety and effectiveness for those under 18 years of age
not established.
By Those Over 60 Years of Age: Small starting doses are advisable. You may be

more susceptible to the development of impaired thinking, orthostatic hypotension, potassium loss, and elevation of blood sugar. Overdosage and prolonged use can cause excessive loss of body water, thickening of the blood, and an increased risk of blood clots, stroke, heart attack, or thrombophlebitis.

▷ **Advisability of Use During Pregnancy**
　　Pregnancy Category: C. See Pregnancy Risk Categories at the back of this book.
　　　Animal studies: Ten times the maximum therapeutic human dose caused bone defects in rabbits.
　　　Human studies: Adequate studies of pregnant women are not available.
　　　Only used in pregnancy if a very serious complication of pregnancy occurs for which this drug is significantly beneficial.

Advisability of Use If Breast-Feeding
　　Presence of this drug in breast milk: Unknown.
　　Avoid drug or refrain from nursing.

Habit-Forming Potential: None.

Effects of Overdosage: Weakness, lethargy, dizziness, confusion, nausea, vomiting, muscle cramps, thirst, electrolyte disturbances, drowsiness progressing to deep sleep or coma, weak and rapid pulse.

Possible Effects of Long-Term Use: Impaired balance of water, salt, and potassium in blood and body tissues. Dehydration with resultant increase in blood viscosity and potential for abnormal clotting. Increased blood sugar in some patients.

Suggested Periodic Examinations While Taking This Drug (at physician's discretion)
　　Complete blood counts; blood levels of sodium, potassium, magnesium, chloride, sugar, uric acid; liver and kidney function tests.

▷ **While Taking This Drug, Observe the Following**
　　Foods: Salt restriction and a high potassium diet may be needed. Ask your doctor. See Section Six for Table 13, "High Potassium Foods."
　　Beverages: No restrictions unless directed by your doctor. May be taken with milk.
▷　*Alcohol:* Alcohol can exaggerate the blood-pressure-lowering effect of this drug and cause orthostatic hypotension (see Glossary).
　　Tobacco Smoking: No interactions expected, but I advise everyone to quit smoking.
▷　*Other Drugs*
　　Bumetanide may *increase* the effects of
　　• antihypertensive drugs. Careful decreases in dose are needed to prevent excessive lowering of the blood pressure.
　　Bumetanide *taken concurrently* with
　　• ACE inhibitors (see Drug Classes) may result in severe lowering of blood pressure on standing (postural or orthostatic hypotension).
　　• aminoglycoside antibiotics (amikacin, gentamicin, kanamycin, neomycin, streptomycin, tobramycin, viomycin) increases the risk of hearing loss.
　　• cephalosporins (see Drug Classes) may increase risk of kidney toxicity.
　　• cortisone-related drugs may cause excessive potassium loss.

- digitalis-related drugs requires very careful monitoring and dose adjustments to prevent serious disturbances of heart rhythm.
- lithium (Lithobid, others) may increase the risk of lithium toxicity.

The following drugs may **decrease** the effects of bumetanide:

- indomethacin (Indocin) or other NSAIDs (see Drug Classes) may reduce its diuretic effect.

▷ *Driving, Hazardous Activities:* **Caution**: Varying degrees of dizziness, weakness, or orthostatic hypotension (see Glossary) may occur.

Aviation Note: The use of this drug *may be a disqualification* for piloting. Consult a designated Aviation Medical Examiner.

Exposure to Sun: No restrictions.

Occurrence of Unrelated Illness: Report vomiting or diarrhea promptly to your doctor.

Discontinuation: It may be advisable to stop this drug 5 to 7 days before major surgery. Consult your physician, surgeon, or anesthesiologist for help.

BUPROPION (byu PROH pee on)

Other Name: Amfebutamone

Introduced: 1986 **Class:** Antidepressant **Prescription:** USA: Yes
Controlled Drug: USA: No; Canada: No **Available as Generic:** USA: No
Brand Names: Wellbutrin, Zyban

BENEFITS versus RISKS	
Possible Benefits	*Possible Risks*
ZYBAN HAS BEEN APPROVED FOR USE IN SMOKING CESSATION	DRUG-INDUCED SEIZURES—rare
EFFECTIVE TREATMENT OF MAJOR DEPRESSIVE DISORDERS	Excessive mental stimulation: excitement, anxiety, confusion, hallucinations, insomnia
Offers a different class than tricyclic, MAO, or SSRI antidepressants	Conversion of depression to mania in manic-depressive disorders

▷ **Principal Uses**

As a Single Drug Product: Uses currently included in FDA-approved labeling: (1) Helps smokers quit smoking (Zyban); (2) treatment of major depressive disorders.

Other (unlabeled) generally accepted uses: (1) Chronic fatigue syndrome symptoms may be relieved by this medicine; (2) can significantly reduce cocaine craving when combined with psychotherapy; (3) is the agent of choice in patients who have had significant weight gain while taking tricyclic antidepressants; (4) has been helpful in a limited number of cases of low back pain that did not respond to other agents.

How This Drug Works: Bupropion increases the levels of two nerve transmitters (norepinephrine and dopamine). Animal studies demonstrate that this drug is primarily a brain stimulant.

Available Dosage Forms and Strengths

Tablets — 75 mg, 100 mg
Tablets, sustained release — 100 mg, 150 mg

▷ **Recommended Dosage Ranges** (Actual dosage and administration schedule must be determined for each patient individually.)

Infants and Children: Dosage not established for those under 18 years of age.

18 to 60 Years of Age: Depression: Initially (first 3 days) 100 mg in the morning, 100 mg in the evening; total daily dose of 200 mg. On the fourth day, if needed and tolerated, increase dose to 100 mg in the morning, at noon, and in the evening; total daily dose of 300 mg. This schedule of 100 mg, three times daily, 6 hours apart, is now continued for 3 to 4 weeks. If tolerated and improvement continues, the dose may be slowly increased if needed up to a maximum of 450 mg daily. Increases should not exceed 100 mg per day within a period of 3 days. No single dose should exceed 150 mg. If a daily dose of 450 mg is reached, take 150 mg in the morning, then 100 mg every 4 hours for three more doses.

The lowest dose that maintains remission of depression should be used. This drug should be stopped if significant improvement is not seen after an adequate trial of 450 mg daily. Doses higher than 450 mg daily appear to only increase the risk of seizures.

Smoking cessation: 150 mg once a day for 3 days, then 150 mg twice daily for up to 90 days.

Over 60 Years of Age: Same as 18 to 60 years of age.

Conditions Requiring Dosing Adjustments

Liver Function: Lower dosages and caution in monitoring should be used.

Kidney Function: The dose **must** be decreased in patients with compromised kidneys or who develop kidney compromise while taking this medicine.

▷ **Dosing Instructions:** May be taken with food to reduce stomach upset. Best to swallow the tablet whole, not chewing or crushing it; this drug has a bitter taste and a local numbing effect on the lining of the mouth. Sustained-release forms should never be crushed or altered.

Usual Duration of Use: Use on a regular schedule for 3 to 4 weeks is usually needed to realize this drug's effectiveness in decreasing the symptoms of depression. Long-term use (months to years) requires periodic evaluation of response and dosage adjustment. For use as an aid in quitting smoking: use for up to 90 days. See your doctor regularly.

Possible Advantages of This Drug

Causes less atropinelike side effects: Blurred vision, dry mouth, constipation, impaired urination.

Does not cause sedation or orthostatic hypotension (see Glossary).

▷ **This Drug Should Not Be Taken If**
- you have had an allergic reaction to it previously.
- you have a history of anorexia nervosa or bulimia (may be associated with increased seizure risk).
- you have a seizure disorder of any kind.
- you are taking, or have taken within the past 14 days, any monoamine oxidase (MAO) type A inhibitor drug (see Drug Classes).

▷ **Inform Your Physician Before Taking This Drug If**
- you have had any adverse effects from antidepressant drugs.
- you are pregnant or planning pregnancy.
- you are breast-feeding your infant.
- you have a history of mental illness, head injury, or brain tumor.

- you have a history of alcoholism or drug abuse.
- you have any kind of heart disease, especially a recent heart attack.
- you have impaired liver or kidney function.
- you take other prescription or nonprescription medications that were not discussed when bupropion was prescribed for you.
- you are unsure of how much to take or how often to take bupropion.

Possible Side Effects (natural, expected, and unavoidable drug actions)
Nervousness, anxiety, confusion, insomnia.
Weight loss of more than 5 pounds—frequent.

▷ **Possible Adverse Effects** (unusual, unexpected, and infrequent reactions)
If any of the following develop, consult your physician promptly for guidance.
Mild Adverse Effects
Allergic reactions: skin rash, itching—rare.
Headache, dizziness, tremor, agitation (9.7 % more than placebo), or blurred vision (4.3 % more than placebo)—infrequent.
Indigestion, nausea and vomiting, constipation—infrequent.
Dry mouth—frequent.
Excessive sweating (diaphoresis)—frequent.
Serious Adverse Effects
Drug-induced seizures—rare, more common with high doses.
Change of depression to mania in manic-depressive disorders—possible.
Psychosis in patients with psychotic predisposition—possible.
Decreased (by 10–15%) white blood cell counts—possible.
Liver toxicity—case reports.
Ringing in the ears (tinnitus)—possible.

▷ **Possible Effects on Sexual Function:**   A recent University of Alabama at Birmingham study found 77% of patients to experience increased sexual desire. Impotence—infrequent; however, another study reported a decrease in sexual dysfunction when patients were switched from fluoxetine (Prozac) to bupropion; altered menstruation up to 3.6% more than placebo in clinical trials—infrequent.

Possible Delayed Adverse Effects: None reported.

Natural Diseases or Disorders That May Be Activated by This Drug
Latent epilepsy, latent psychosis, manic phase of bipolar affective disorder.

Possible Effects on Laboratory Tests
White blood cell count: decreased.

CAUTION
1. Take exactly the amount prescribed; rapid dose increases can cause seizures. Watch closely for excessive stimulation.
2. Ask your physician or pharmacist before taking any other prescription or over-the-counter drug while taking this drug.
3. Do not take any monoamine oxidase (MAO) type A inhibitor drug while taking this drug (see Drug Classes). If you have taken a MAO inhibitor, then stopped it, wait 2 weeks before starting bupropion.

Precautions for Use
By Infants and Children: Safety and effectiveness for those under 18 years of age not established.

By Those Over 60 Years of Age: Age-related liver or kidney function decline may require dose decreases.

▷ **Advisability of Use During Pregnancy**
Pregnancy Category: B. See Pregnancy Risk Categories at the back of this book.
Animal studies: Rat and rabbit studies reveal no significant birth defects.
Human studies: Adequate studies of pregnant women are not available.
Use this drug only if clearly needed. Ask your physician for guidance.

Advisability of Use if Breast-Feeding
Presence of this drug in breast milk: Yes.
Avoid drug or refrain from nursing.

Habit-Forming Potential: Remote with use of recommended doses. Slight potential for abuse by those who abuse stimulant drugs.

Effects of Overdosage: Headache, agitation, confusion, hallucinations, seizures, loss of consciousness.

Possible Effects of Long-Term Use: Not reported.

Suggested Periodic Examinations While Taking This Drug (at physician's discretion)
Liver and/or kidney function tests as appropriate.

▷ **While Taking This Drug, Observe the Following**
Foods: No restrictions.
Beverages: No restrictions. May be taken with milk.
▷ *Alcohol:* Avoid completely. Alcohol may predispose to the development of seizures.
Tobacco Smoking: No interactions expected, but I advise everyone to quit smoking.
Marijuana Smoking: Avoid completely; it may induce psychotic behavior.
▷ *Other Drugs*
The following drugs *taken concurrently* with bupropion may increase the risk of major seizures:
• antidepressants (tricyclic).
• clozapine (Clozaril).
• fluoxetine (Prozac).
• haloperidol (Haldol).
• lithium (Lithobid, others).
• loxapine (Loxitane).
• maprotiline (Ludiomil).
• molindone (Moban).
• phenothiazines (see Drug Classes).
• thioxanthenes (see Xanthine Drug Class).
• trazodone (Desyrel).
Bupropion *taken concurrently* with
• carbamazepine (Tegretol) may result in lowered carbamazepine levels.
• levodopa results in increased nausea, restlessness, and tremor.
• MAO inhibitors (see Drug Classes) can lead to sudden toxicity. Do not combine.
• phenobarbital may result in decreased levels.
• phenytoin (Dilantin) may result in decreased phenytoin levels.

- ritonavir (Norvir) and probably other protease inhibitors may lead to increased blood levels of bupropion and toxicity—do not combine.
▷ *Driving, Hazardous Activities:* This drug may cause dizziness, drowsiness, or seizures. Restrict activities as necessary.
Aviation Note: The use of this drug *is a disqualification* for piloting. Consult a designated Aviation Medical Examiner.
Exposure to Sun: No restrictions.
Discontinuation: Do not stop this drug abruptly. Ask your physician for help.

BUSPIRONE (byu SPI rohn)

Introduced: 1979   **Class:** Antianxiety drug   **Prescription:** USA: Yes
Controlled Drug: USA: No; Canada: No   **Available as Generic:** No
Brand Name: Buspar

BENEFITS versus RISKS	
Possible Benefits	*Possible Risks*
EFFECTIVE RELIEF OF MILD TO MODERATE ANXIETY	Mild dizziness, faintness, or headache—uncommon
DECREASED RISK OF SEDATION OR DEPENDENCE THAN OTHER AGENTS	Tachycardia—rare Restlessness, depression, tremor, or rigidity (with high doses)—rare

▷ **Principal Uses**
As a Single Drug Product: Uses currently included in FDA-approved labeling: (1) Relieves mild to moderate anxiety and nervous tension. Particularly useful in the elderly, alcoholics, and addiction-prone people because of its lack of significant sedative effects or abuse potential; (2) beneficial in decreasing self-injurious behaviors or aggression in developmentally disabled adults.
Other (unlabeled) generally accepted uses: (1) May have a benefit in reducing alcohol craving in alcoholics; (2) can help aggression or hyperactivity in autistics; (3) may decrease symptoms in obsessive-compulsive disorder; (4) can be of help in sexual dysfunction in people with generalized anxiety disorder; (4) may help decrease the urge to smoke in those addicted to nicotine.
How This Drug Works: This drug is thought to be a "midbrain modulator" that causes changes in brain chemicals (dopamine, norepinephrine, and serotonin), resulting in a calming effect. It is also a partial agonist at serotonin reuptake sites.
Available Dosage Forms and Strengths
Tablets — 5 mg, 10 mg
▷ **Usual Adult Dosage Range:**   Initially 5 mg three times daily; if needed, increase dose by 5 mg/day every 2 to 3 days, with individual doses every 6 to 8 hours. The total daily dose should not exceed 60 mg. **Note: Actual dosage and administration schedule must be determined for each patient individually.**
Conditions Requiring Dosing Adjustments
Liver Function: Use with caution in severe liver failure. Doses must be decreased.

Kidney Function: Use with caution in severe kidney problems. Dose should be decreased to 25–50% of normal dose.

▷ **Dosing Instructions:**   The tablet may be crushed and taken without regard to food.

Usual Duration of Use: Use on a regular schedule for up to 7 days may be needed to see this drug's full benefit in relieving anxiety and nervous tension. Avoid uninterrupted use. Use intermittently and only as needed.

Possible Advantages of This Drug
Relieves anxiety or tension without severe sedation or impaired thinking.
Does not cause withdrawal when it is stopped.
Actually appears to improve driving-related skills in one study.

▷ **This Drug Should Not Be Taken If**
- you have had an allergic reaction to this or similar medicines previously.
- you take, or have taken in the last 2 weeks, one of the MAO inhibitor drugs (see Drug Classes). May increase blood pressure.

▷ **Inform Your Physician Before Taking This Drug If**
- you take other drugs that affect the brain or nervous system: tranquilizers, sedatives, hypnotics, analgesics, narcotics, antidepressants, antipsychotic drugs, anticonvulsants, or anti-parkinsonism drugs.
- you have impaired liver or kidney function.
- you take fluoxetine (Prozac) for depression.

Possible Side Effects (natural, expected, and unavoidable drug actions)
Mild drowsiness (less than with benzodiazepines) (up to 16%)—frequent; lethargy is possible.

▷ **Possible Adverse Effects** (unusual, unexpected, and infrequent reactions)
If any of the following develop, consult your physician promptly for guidance.
Mild Adverse Effects
Headache, faintness, excitement—infrequent.
Dizziness—infrequent to frequent.
Tingling and touch sensation changes (paresthesias)—rare.
Insomnia and dream disturbances, depression—possible.
Increased blood pressure—case reports.
Nausea—infrequent.
Serious Adverse Effects
Tachycardia—infrequent.
With high doses: dysphoria, restlessness, rigidity, tremors—possible.
Movement disorders—case reports.

▷ **Possible Effects on Sexual Function:**   Increased or decreased libido, difficult or absent orgasm, inhibited ejaculation, impotence, breast milk production, altered timing or pattern of menstruation (10 to 40 mg daily)—all case reports.
May increase prolactin; however no reports of male breast tenderness or enlargement have been reported.

Possible Effects on Laboratory Tests
Growth hormone: Conflicting increases or lack of effect on growth hormone levels. Blood prolactin levels: dose-related increase.

CAUTION
> This drug is reported to have very mild sedative effects and no abuse potential; however, it should be used with caution and only when clearly needed. Most use has been short term. Some unexpected side effects or adverse effects may still be reported. Actual dysphoria has been reported with higher doses and may preclude its recreational use.

Precautions for Use
> *By Infants and Children:* Safety and effectiveness by those under 18 years of age not established.
> *By Those Over 60 Years of Age:* Expected to be tolerated much better than benzodiazepines and barbiturates. Watch for increased dizziness or weakness and avoid falls.

▷ **Advisability of Use During Pregnancy**
> *Pregnancy Category:* B. See Pregnancy Risk Categories at the back of this book.
> Animal studies: No birth defects found in rat and rabbit studies.
> Human studies: Adequate studies of pregnant women are not available.
> Use this drug during pregnancy only when clearly needed. It is advisable to avoid this drug during the first 3 months of pregnancy.

Advisability of Use If Breast-Feeding
> Presence of this drug in breast milk: Excreted in rat milk; probably also in humans.
> Avoid drug or refrain from nursing.

Habit-Forming Potential: Does not appear to cause addiction; however, more studies are needed. Higher doses result in a dysphoric reaction, which may keep it from becoming a drug involved in recreational use.

Effects of Overdosage: Drowsiness, fatigue, nausea, dysphoria, tingling sensations (paresthesias), and a rare chance of seizures.

Possible Effects of Long-Term Use: None reported.

Suggested Periodic Examinations While Taking This Drug (at physician's discretion)
> Periodic check of heart rate.

▷ **While Taking This Drug, Observe the Following**
> *Foods:* No restrictions; taking with food may result in a clinically insignificant increase in absorption of this drug.
> *Beverages:* No restrictions.
▷ *Alcohol:* Milder problems than diazepam (Valium); however, avoid the combination.
> *Tobacco Smoking:* No interactions expected, but I advise everyone to quit smoking.
> *Marijuana Smoking:* Additive increase in drowsiness.
▷ *Other Drugs:*
> Buspirone *taken concurrently* with
> - fluoxetine (Prozac) may increase underlying anxiety or mental disorder such as obsessive-compulsive disorder. Do not combine.
> - fluvoxamine (Luvox) may result in serious slowing of the heart (bradycardia). Doses must be decreased.
> - MAO inhibitors (see Drug Classes) such as phenelzine (Parnate) may result in large blood pressure increases. Do not combine.

- narcotics such as oxycodone (Percodan) may result in additive sedation and potential decreases in breathing (respiratory depression).
- venlafaxine (Effexor) may lead to decreased buspirone benefits or venlafaxine toxicity.

▷ *Driving, Hazardous Activities:* This drug may cause dizziness, faintness, or fatigue. Restrict activities as necessary.

Aviation Note: The use of this drug *may be a disqualification* for piloting. Consult a designated Aviation Medical Examiner.

Exposure to Sun: No restrictions.

CALCITONIN (kal si TOH nin)

Other Names: Salcatonin, thyrocalcitonin

Introduced: 1977, nasal spray form 1995   **Class:** Anti-osteoporotic, hormones   **Prescription:** USA: Yes   **Controlled Drug:** USA: No; Canada: No   **Available as Generic:** USA: No; Canada: No

Brand Names: Calcimar, Cibacalcin, Miacalcin Injection, Miacalcin Nasal Spray

---

BENEFITS versus RISKS

Possible Benefits	*Possible Risks*
PARTIAL RELIEF OF SYMPTOMS OF PAGET'S DISEASE OF BONE	Nausea (with or without vomiting)
NASAL FORM CAN INCREASE BONE MASS	Allergic reactions
Effective adjunctive treatment of postmenopausal osteoporosis	
Effective adjunctive treatment of abnormally high blood calcium levels (associated with malignant disease)	

▷ **Principal Uses**

As a Single Drug Product: Uses currently included in FDA-approved labeling: (1) Treatment of symptomatic Paget's disease of bone (excessive bone growth of skull, spine, and long bones); (2) combination treatment of postmenopausal osteoporosis, taken with calcium and vitamin D (also has an effect on the pain of osteoporosis); (3) nasal form approved for treatment of postmenopausal osteoporosis in women with low bone mass who had menopause 5 years previously; (4) adjunctive treatment of high blood calcium levels seen in bone cancer; (5) relieves symptoms of neurologic compression in Paget's disease.

Other (unlabeled) generally accepted uses: (1) Combination treatment of osteoporosis due to medicinal drugs, hormonal disorders, or immobilization, taken with calcium and vitamin D; (2) may help aneurysmal bone cysts when directly injected into the cyst; (3) preliminary study indicates that this drug may be of benefit in preventing migraine headaches and reduce or eliminate the need for prophylactic medicines; (4) useful adjunct in cancer pain; (5) very beneficial in treating pain that occurs when an arm or leg has been amputated (phantom limb); (6) data gathered from several studies show this drug may also decrease risk of bone fractures in those with osteoporosis in the spine (no hip data).

How This Drug Works: This hormone slows abnormally accelerated "bone turnover" that occurs in Paget's disease. Excessive replacement of bone loss is gradually reduced and a more normal balance is restored. In cancer of the bone, this drug slows bone destruction and decreases the transfer of calcium from bone to bloodstream. In osteoporosis, this drug acts primarily on bone by blocking resorption (inhibiting osteoclasts) and allowing bone-building cells to act. There are also effects on the intestine (calcium absorption) and the kidney (decreased calcium elimination) that are not fully defined.

Available Dosage Forms and Strengths

Calcitonin-human
    Injection — 500 mcg (0.5 mg)
Calcitonin-salmon
    Injection — 200 IU per ml
Nasal spray — 200 IU per spray

▷ **Recommended Dosage Ranges** (Actual dosage and administration schedule must be determined for each patient individually.)
Skin Testing: Skin testing is accomplished by diluting 10 IU to 1 ml with 0.9% sodium chloride. 0.1 ml of this dilution is injected into the inner forearm (about 1 IU). A positive reaction occurs if more than mild skin reddening or a weal is seen within 15 minutes. The drug should NOT be used if this positive reaction is seen.
Infants and Children: Dosage not established.
12 to 60 Years of Age: Calcitonin-human: For Paget's disease—Initially 500 mcg (0.5 mg) daily, injected subcutaneously; after adequate response, dose may be decreased to 250 mcg (0.25 mg) daily, or 500 mcg (0.5 mg) two or three times per week. Severe cases may require 1 mg/day.
Calcitonin-salmon: For Paget's disease—50 to 100 IU daily or every other day, injected subcutaneously or intramuscularly; after adequate response, dose may be decreased to 50 IU daily, every other day, or three times per week.
For postmenopausal osteoporosis—100 IU daily, every other day, or three times per week, injected under the skin. If adverse effects are marked, reduce dose to 50 IU daily; then increase dose gradually over a period of 2 weeks.
Nasal spray: 200 IU (one spray) daily. Nostrils should be alternated daily to help avoid nasal irritation. Calcium and vitamin D replacement is strongly recommended—such replacement can help keep you from drawing on your "bone bank" (your bones) to maintain adequate calcium. For high blood calcium levels—Initially 4 IU per kg of body mass every 12 hours, injected subcutaneously or intramuscularly; as needed and tolerated, increase dose to 8 IU per kg of body mass every 12 hours; if necessary, the dose may be increased to a maximum of 8 IU per kg of body mass every 6 hours.

For adjunctive pain treatment: 100 to 200 IU daily, given intramuscularly or subcutaneously. Some clinicians have started using the nasal spray form (200 IU daily) for adjunctive pain therapy.

Over 60 Years of Age: Same as 12 to 60 years of age.

Conditions Requiring Dosing Adjustments

Liver Function: No changes indicated.

Kidney Function: Should be used with caution in blocked kidneys, as the attempt to lose water via the kidney (diuresis) will put added pressure on an overloaded system.

▷ **Dosing Instructions:**   **The nasal spray** form should be activated (as in package instructions), then the head placed upright, the spray tip placed firmly into the chosen nostril (remember to use a different nostril every day), and the pump depressed toward the bottle. Call your doctor if your nose becomes ulcerated. **Subcutaneous** (under the skin) injection is preferred for self-administration of the injectable form. Your doctor will teach you about proper injection technique. The daily dose may be given at bedtime with the stomach empty if you become nauseated.

Usual Duration of Use: Peak effect in treating Paget's disease is usually seen after 1–3 months of use on a regular schedule. If effective, the usual treatment is 6 months; and if response continues, the dose may be reduced during the next 6 months. Peak response may require treatment for up to 24 months. Long-term use (months to years) requires periodic physician evaluation. Bone mineral density testing is strongly recommended. Osteoporosis benefits should be followed by bone mineral density testing to decide the ongoing success of therapy or the need to change to another medicine.

Possible Advantages of This Drug

Calcitonin-human is less likely to induce allergic reactions than calcitonin-salmon, permitting treatment for longer periods of time.

▷ **This Drug Should Not Be Taken If**
- you have had an allergic reaction to it previously.
- you recently fractured a bone that has not healed completely.

▷ **Inform Your Physician Before Taking This Drug If**
- you are allergic by nature (history of eczema, hives, hay fever, asthma).
- you have known allergies to foreign proteins.
- you are unsure of how much to take or how often to take it.
- you develop sores in the nose following repeated intranasal use.
- you will be unable to have follow-up laboratory testing of blood calcium.

Possible Side Effects (natural, expected, and unavoidable drug actions)

Salty or metallic taste in mouth—possible.

▷ **Possible Adverse Effects** (unusual, unexpected, and infrequent reactions)

If any of the following develop, consult your physician promptly for guidance.

Mild Adverse Effects

Allergic reactions: skin rash, hives, itching—rare.

Headache, dizziness, weakness—rare.

Loss of appetite, nausea, vomiting, stomach pain, diarrhea—infrequent.

Increased frequency of urination or urination at night (nocturia)—case reports.

Abnormal fluid accumulation (pedal edema)—rare.

Flushing of the face—may be frequent with human calcitonin injection.

Irritation of the nose (with nasal spray use)—infrequent.

Serious Adverse Effects

Allergic reactions: flushing, redness, anaphylaxis—rare.

Sugar (glucose) intolerance—possible.

Excessive lowering of calcium and rigidity (tetany) of muscles due to lack of calcium—possible.

Severe ulceration of the nose (with nasal spray use)—rare.

▷ **Possible Effects on Sexual Function:**   None reported.

Possible Effects on Laboratory Tests

Blood alkaline phosphatase levels: decreased.

Blood calcium levels: decreased.

Urine hydroxyproline values: decreased.

Blood glucose: lack of diabetic control, glucose intolerance.

Bone mineral density: increased.

CAUTION

1. It is best that your doctor perform a skin test before beginning treatment with calcitonin-salmon.
2. Eat a well-balanced diet with adequate calcium and vitamin D.
3. Tell your doctor if bone pain persists while taking this drug.
4. Talk to your doctor about decreasing risk factors for osteoporosis and also ask how much exercise is appropriate for you.

Precautions for Use

By Infants and Children: No specific information.

By Those Over 60 Years of Age: Watch fluid balance closely if this drug is given to lower blood calcium.

▷ **Advisability of Use During Pregnancy**

Pregnancy Category: C. See Pregnancy Risk Categories at the back of this book.

Animal studies: No drug-induced birth defects reported.

Human studies: Adequate studies of pregnant women are not available.

Use this drug only if clearly needed. Ask your physician for help.

Advisability of Use if Breast-Feeding

Presence of this drug in breast milk: Yes.

Calcitonin taken in with breast milk is typically destroyed by infant stomach acids before it has any effect. Ask your doctor for guidance.

Habit-Forming Potential: None.

Effects of Overdosage: Nausea, vomiting.

Possible Effects of Long-Term Use: Antibodies may cause resistance and loss of effect with pork or salmon calcitonin. This occurs in up to 70% of people after 2 to 18 months of treatment. Antibodies to human calcitonin are rare but have been reported.

Suggested Periodic Examinations While Taking This Drug (at physician's discretion)

Measurements of blood calcium, phosphate, and alkaline phosphatase levels.

Measurement of urine hydroxyproline content.

Measurement of bone mineral density (BMD) by DEXA densitometry scanning.

▷ **While Taking This Drug, Observe the Following**
Foods: No restrictions.
Nutritional Support: Ensure adequate intake of calcium and vitamin D.
Beverages: No restrictions.
▷ *Alcohol:* No interactions expected, but alcohol (in higher doses) acts as a bone-forming cell (osteoblast) poison and is a risk factor for osteoporosis.
Tobacco Smoking: No interactions expected, but smoking is a risk factor for osteoporosis. I advise everyone to quit smoking.
▷ *Other Drugs*
Calcitonin **taken concurrently** with
• ketoprofen may inhibit the calcium and uric acid distribution in the urine by calcitonin of pig origin. Changes with other calcitonins are not defined.
• plicamycin will cause additive loss of calcium.
▷ *Driving, Hazardous Activities:* No restrictions.
Aviation Note: The use of this drug **may be a disqualification** for piloting. Consult a designated Aviation Medical Examiner.
Exposure to Sun: No restrictions.
Heavy Exercise or Exertion: As defined by your doctor. Remember, weight-bearing exercise (if not contraindicated for you) actually helps fight osteoporosis by stimulating receptors (mechanoreceptors) to release factors that help structure healthy (normal architecture) bone.
Discontinuation: Your doctor should decide when to stop this drug.
Special Storage Instructions: Calcitonin-human—Store at a temperature below 77 degrees F (25 degrees C). Do not refrigerate. Protect from light.
Calcitonin-salmon—Store in refrigerator, between 36 and 46 degrees F (2 and 8 degrees C). Do not freeze.
Calcitonin-salmon nasal spray—Store unopened in the refrigerator. Once it has been opened, the bottle can be kept at room temperature for 2 weeks.

CAPTOPRIL (KAP toh pril)

Introduced: 1979   **Class:** Antihypertensive, ACE inhibitor   **Prescription:** USA: Yes   **Controlled Drug:** USA: No; Canada: No   **Available as Generic:** Yes, recently approved.

Brand Names: ✤Apo-Capto, Capoten, Capozide [CD], ✤Novo-Captopril, ✤Nu-Capto, ✤Syn-Captopril

BENEFITS versus RISKS	
Possible Benefits	*Possible Risks*
EFFECTIVE CONTROL OF MILD TO SEVERE HIGH BLOOD PRESSURE	Impaired white blood cell production—rare
USEFUL ADJUNCTIVE TREATMENT FOR CONGESTIVE HEART FAILURE	Bone marrow depression—rare Kidney damage—rare Liver damage—rare
MAY DECREASE RISK OF KIDNEY PROBLEMS IN DIABETICS TAKING INSULIN	
MAY REDUCE RISK OF DEATH AFTER A HEART ATTACK	

▷ **Principal Uses**

As a *Single Drug Product:* Uses currently included in FDA-approved labeling: (1) Treats all degrees of high blood pressure; (2) may help prevent death after heart attacks; (3) used in advanced heart failure; (4) used in type one insulin-dependent diabetics who have kidney problems and damage to the retina of the eye; (5) helps people live longer (improves survival) in cases of congestive heart failure.

Other (unlabeled) generally accepted uses: (1) Helps relieve symptoms of cystinuria; (2) may have some role in easing rheumatoid arthritis symptoms; (3) can help Raynaud's phenomenon symptoms.

As a *Combination Drug Product* [CD]: In combination with hydrochlorothiazide, this medicine offers the benefits of an ACE inhibitor and a diuretic.

How This Drug Works: It is thought that by blocking an enzyme system, this drug relaxes arterial walls and lowers the blood pressure. This, in turn, decreases the heart's workload and improves its performance. Use after heart attack appears to result from captopril blunting of response to catecholamines, free-radical scavenging, as well as increased prostacyclin or bradykinin. Use in combination with a diuretic helps ease fluid load.

Available Dosage Forms and Strengths

Tablets — 12.5 mg, 25 mg, 50 mg, 100 mg

▷ **Usual Adult Dosage Range:** Congestive heart failure (CHF): Doses of 25 mg three times daily are suggested. Lower doses (6.25 to 12.5 mg) three times daily may reduce the risk of excessive lowering of blood pressure. For high blood pressure: 25 mg two or three times daily for 1–2 weeks. If necessary, dose may be increased to 50 mg three times daily. If blood pressure response is still not acceptable, addition of a diuretic or change to the combination form may be needed. Total daily dose should not exceed 450 mg.

After a heart attack: A test dose of 6.25 mg is given to see if excessive lowering of the blood pressure occurs. If the test is tolerated, 12.5 mg is given three times a day. This dose is then increased toward a goal of 50 mg three times a day.

Diabetic kidney problems (nephropathy) and eye problems (retinopathy): Success has been achieved with 50 mg twice daily in two large studies. The manufacturer suggests a starting dose of 25 mg three times a day. Children (1.5 to 18 years old) with severe high blood pressure caused by the kidneys (renal hypertension) have been successfully treated using 1.3 mg per kg of body mass per day, progressing to 2.2 mg per kg of body mass per day. **Note: Actual dosage and administration schedule must be determined for each patient individually.**

Conditions Requiring Dosing Adjustments

Liver Function: Must be used with extreme caution, and started at a lower dose in liver failure.

Kidney Function: Increased blood level and risk of adverse effects (low blood counts and protein in the urine) if used in kidney failure. **Must** decrease dose according to decreases in creatinine clearance. The lowest effective dose must be used.

▷ **Dosing Instructions:** Take on empty stomach, 1 hour before meals, at same time each day. Tablet may be crushed.

Usual Duration of Use: Several weeks of use on a regular schedule is usually needed to see high blood pressure control. Use may be continued for life.

▷ **This Drug Should Not Be Taken If**
- you have had an allergic reaction to it previously.
- you are pregnant (last 6 months).
- you currently have a blood cell or bone marrow disorder.
- you undergo dialysis with polyacrylonitrile (PAN) high-flux dialyzers.
- you have an abnormally high level of blood potassium.

▷ **Inform Your Physician Before Taking This Drug If**
- you are allergic to ACE inhibitors (see Drug Classes).
- you are planning pregnancy or to breast-feed your child.
- you have a history of kidney disease or impaired kidney function.
- you have scleroderma or systemic lupus erythematosus.
- you have any form of heart or liver disease.
- you have diabetes.
- you develop swelling of the tongue, face, or throat while taking this drug.
- you have an elevated potassium level.
- you have a blood cell disorder.
- you take other antihypertensives, diuretics, nitrates, allopurinol (Zyloprim), Indocin, or potassium supplements.
- you plan to have surgery under general anesthesia in the near future.
- you have renal artery stenosis (ask your doctor).
- you are taking medicines that suppress the immune system.
- you are unsure of how much to take or how often to take captopril.

Possible Side Effects (natural, expected, and unavoidable drug actions)
Dizziness, light-headedness, fainting (excessive drop in blood pressure).

▷ **Possible Adverse Effects** (unusual, unexpected, and infrequent reactions)
If any of the following develop, consult your physician promptly for guidance.
Mild Adverse Effects
Allergic reactions: skin rash—infrequent.
Swelling of face, hands, or feet; fever—rare.
Lost or altered (metallic or salty) taste, mouth or tongue sores—case reports.
Nightmares, joint pain—rare.
Cough—infrequent.
Increased temperature (hyperthermia)—case reports.
Rapid heart rate on standing—case reports.
Serious Adverse Effects
Bone marrow depression (neutropenia, anemia, or aplastic anemia): weakness, fever, sore throat, bleeding or bruising—rare (infrequent in those with kidney failure and collagen vascular disease).
Hemolytic or aplastic anemia—case reports.
Kidney damage: water retention (edema)—case reports.
Elevated blood potassium (hyperkalemia)—case reports.
Rare accumulation of fluid around the heart (pericarditis)—case reports.
Hallucinations—rare.
Stevens-Johnson syndrome, lupus erythematosus, or other serious skin conditions—rare.

Pancreatitis—case reports.

Liver damage (with or without jaundice)—rare.

▷ **Possible Effects on Sexual Function:** Decreased male libido (20% to 30%) with recommended dosage. Impotence. Swelling and tenderness of male breast tissue (gynecomastia)—rare.

Possible Effects on Laboratory Tests

Complete blood counts: decreased red cells, hemoglobin, white cells, and platelets; increased eosinophils.

Blood antinuclear antibodies (ANA): increased.

Blood cholesterol and triglycerides: no effects.

Blood sodium level: decreased.

Blood urea nitrogen level (BUN): increased.

Liver function tests: increased liver enzymes (alkaline phosphatase, AST/ GOT, LDH), increased bilirubin.

Urine ketone tests: false positive results with Keto-Diastix and Chemstrip-6.

Blood sugar (glucose): decreased—case reports.

Venereal Disease Research Laboratory (VDRL): rare false positive results.

CAUTION

1. If possible, it is advisable to stop all other antihypertensive drugs (especially diuretics) for 1 week before starting captopril.
2. **Tell your doctor immediately if you become pregnant.** This drug should not be taken beyond the first 3 months of pregnancy.
3. **Report promptly** any signs of infection (fever, sore throat), and any indications of water retention (weight gain, swollen feet or ankles).
4. Many salt substitutes contain potassium; ask your doctor before using.
5. Blood counts and urine analyses are needed **before** taking captopril.

Precautions for Use

By Infants and Children: One study used a starting dose of 0.01 to 0.25 mg per kg of body mass every 12 hours in infants; 0.05 to 0.5 mg per kg of body mass three times daily has been used in older children.

By Those Over 60 Years of Age: Small starting doses are advisable. Sudden and excessive lowering of blood pressure can cause stroke or heart attack.

▷ **Advisability of Use During Pregnancy**

Pregnancy Category: C during the first 3 months; **D during the last 6 months** (last two trimesters). See Pregnancy Risk Categories at the back of this book.

Animal studies: No birth defects found in rat, rabbit, or hamster studies. However, this drug was found to be toxic to the embryo and newborn.

Human studies: The use of ACE inhibitor drugs during the last 6 months of pregnancy is known to possibly cause very serious injury and possible death to the fetus; skull and limb malformations, lung defects, and kidney failure have been reported in over 50 cases worldwide.

Avoid this drug completely during the last 6 months. During the first 3 months of pregnancy, use this drug only if clearly needed. Ask your physician for guidance.

Advisability of Use If Breast-Feeding

Presence of this drug in breast milk: Yes, in small amounts.

Monitor nursing infant closely and discontinue drug or nursing if adverse effects develop.

Habit-Forming Potential: None.

Effects of Overdosage: Excessive drop in blood pressure—light-headedness, dizziness, fainting.

Possible Effects of Long-Term Use: Gradual increase in blood potassium level.

Suggested Periodic Examinations While Taking This Drug (at physician's discretion)

Complete blood cell count, urine analysis and blood potassium level before drug is started. Once started: Blood counts every 2 weeks during the first 3 months, then periodically for duration of use. Urine protein every month for the first 9 months of treatment, then periodically for duration of use. Periodic measurements of blood potassium.

▷ **While Taking This Drug, Observe the Following**

Foods: Consult your physician regarding salt intake.

Nutritional Support: **Do not** take potassium supplements unless directed by your physician. Case reports of zinc deficiency have been made.

Beverages: No restrictions. May be taken with milk.

▷ *Alcohol:* Alcohol can further lower blood pressure. Use with caution.

Tobacco Smoking: No interactions expected, but I advise everyone to quit smoking.

▷ *Other Drugs*

Captopril *taken concurrently* with

- allopurinol (Zyloprim) may increase risk of serious skin reactions.
- azathioprine (Imuran) may result in severe anemia.
- cyclosporine (Sandimmune) may result in kidney failure that takes a while to appear (delayed acute renal dysfunction).
- lithium (Lithobid, others) may result in three times the expected lithium levels and **toxicity**.
- loop diuretics (such as Lasix or Bumex; see Drug Classes) may result in excessively low blood pressure on standing (postural hypotension).
- phenothiazines (see Drug Classes) may result in postural hypotension.
- potassium preparations (K-Lyte, Slow-K, etc.) will increase blood potassium with risk of serious heart rhythm disturbances.
- potassium-sparing diuretics—amiloride (Moduretic), spironolactone (Aldactazide), triamterene (Dyazide)—may increase blood levels of potassium with risk of serious heart rhythm disturbances.

The following drugs may *decrease* the effects of captopril

- antacids—by decreasing captopril absorption. Separate doses by 2 hours.
- ibuprofen (Motrin), indomethacin (Indocin), or other NSAIDs (see Drug Classes).
- naloxone (Narcan).
- salicylates (aspirin, etc.).

▷ *Driving, Hazardous Activities:* Usually no restrictions. Be aware of possible drops in blood pressure with resultant dizziness or faintness.

Aviation Note: The use of this drug *may be a disqualification* for piloting. Consult a designated Aviation Medical Examiner.

Exposure to Sun: Caution is advised. This drug can cause photosensitivity.

Exposure to Heat: Caution is advised. Excessive perspiring may drop blood pressure.

Occurrence of Unrelated Illness: Report promptly any disorder that causes nausea, vomiting, or diarrhea. Fluid and chemical imbalances must be corrected as soon as possible.

CARBAMAZEPINE (kar ba MAZ e peen)

Introduced: 1962   **Class:** Anticonvulsant, antineuralgic, pain syndrome modifier   **Prescription:** USA: Yes   **Controlled Drug:** USA: No; Canada: No   **Available as Generic:** Yes

Brand Names: ✦Apo-Carbamazepine, Epitol, ✦Mazepine, ✦Novo-Carbamaz, ✦PMS Carbamazepine, Tegretol, Tegretol Chewable Tablet, Tegretol-XR

BENEFITS versus RISKS	
Possible Benefits	*Possible Risks*
RELIEF OF PAIN IN TRIGEMINAL NEURALGIA	BONE MARROW DEPRESSION (reduced formation of all blood cells)—RARE
EFFECTIVE CONTROL OF CERTAIN TYPES OF EPILEPTIC SEIZURES	Liver damage with jaundice—rare
Relief of pain in some rare forms of nerve pain (neuralgia)	

▷ **Principal Uses**

As a Single Drug Product: Uses currently included in FDA-approved labeling: (1) For relief of pain in true trigeminal neuralgia (tic douloureux) and glossopharyngeal neuralgia; (2) for control of several types of epilepsy, namely grand mal, tonic-clonic, psychomotor or temporal lobe, complex partial and mixed seizure patterns. Precise diagnosis and careful management are mandatory for its proper use.

Other (unlabeled) generally accepted uses: Beneficial in (1) bipolar affective disorders; (2) schizoaffective disorders; (3) resistant schizophrenia; (4) post-traumatic stress disorder; (5) tabes dorsalis; (6) diabetic neuropathy; (7) hemifacial spasm; (8) cocaine withdrawal; (9) helping aggression in some Alzheimer's patients; (10) helping hiccups and belching associated with flutter of the diaphragm; (11) treating nerve problems resulting from thiamine deficiency; (12) possibly having a role in treating pain that occurs when an arm or leg is amputated (phantom limb pain); (13) possibly being of great benefit in a form of perceived repetitive ear noise called clicking tinnitus.

How This Drug Works: By reducing impulses at certain nerve terminals, this drug relieves or reduces pain (of trigeminal neuralgia) and also reduces the excitability of nerve fibers in the brain, decreasing the likelihood of seizures or reducing their frequency and severity.

Available Dosage Forms and Strengths

Oral suspension — 100 mg/5 ml

Tablets — 200 mg (400 mg in Canada)

Tablets, chewable — 100 mg, 200 mg

Tablets, extended release — 10 mg, 200 mg, 400 mg

▷ **Usual Adult Dosage Range:** Initially 200 mg every 12 hours (regular or extended-release tablets). Dose may be increased at weekly intervals by 200 mg daily as needed and tolerated. The dose is given twice daily for the extended-release tablets or three times daily for the regular tablets. Total daily dosage should not exceed 1200 mg.

Infants and Children: Children under age 6 are given 10 to 20 mg per kg of body mass. This dose is divided into three equal doses and is given three times daily. This dose is then increased as needed or tolerated based on clinical response and blood levels. Children 6–12 are given 100 mg twice daily or 50 mg of the suspension four times daily. The dose can then be increased by 100 mg a day after a week, as needed and tolerated. Maximum is 1000 mg or lower. **Note: Actual dosage and administration schedule must be determined for each patient individually. Dosing must be guided by blood levels.**

Conditions Requiring Dosing Adjustments

Liver Function: Use with extreme caution, in lower doses and with close supervision in liver compromise patients. This medicine may have to be stopped in active liver disease.

Kidney Function: Capable of being toxic to the kidneys. Use with extreme caution and in decreased dose in patients with kidneys that already do not work well.

Heart Attack: Changes in blood distribution (perfusion) and protein binding may result in much higher than expected blood levels. Blood levels should be obtained more frequently to guide dose decreases and avoid toxicity.

▷ **Dosing Instructions:** Take at same time each day, with or following food to reduce stomach irritation. Regular-release tablet may be crushed for administration. Extended-release tablet should not be altered.

Usual Duration of Use: Use on a regular schedule for 3 months may be needed to see this drug's effect in relieving the pain of trigeminal neuralgia. Longer periods, with dosage adjustment, may be required for control of epileptic seizures. Careful evaluation of individual tolerance and response should be made every 3 months during long-term treatment.

Currently a "Drug of Choice"

For patients with grand mal or partial seizures.

▷ **This Drug Should Not Be Taken If**
- you have had an allergic reaction to it previously.
- you have active liver disease.
- you currently have a blood cell or bone marrow disorder.
- you currently take, or have taken within the past 14 days, a monoamine oxidase (MAO) type A inhibitor (see Drug Classes).

▷ **Inform Your Physician Before Taking This Drug If**
- you have had an allergic reaction to any tricyclic antidepressant drug (see Drug Classes).
- you have taken this drug in the past.
- you have had any blood or bone marrow disorder, especially drug induced.
- you have a history of liver or kidney disease.
- you have had serious mental depression or other mental disorder.
- you have had thrombophlebitis.
- you have high blood pressure, heart disease, or glaucoma.
- you take more than two alcoholic drinks a day.
- you take other prescription or nonprescription medications that were not discussed when carbamazepine was prescribed for you.

- you are unsure of how much to take or how often to take carbamazepine.
- you are pregnant or are breast-feeding your baby.

Possible Side Effects (natural, expected, and unavoidable drug actions)
Dry mouth and throat, constipation, impaired urination.

▷ **Possible Adverse Effects** (unusual, unexpected, and infrequent reactions)
If any of the following develop, consult your physician promptly for guidance.

Mild Adverse Effects

Allergic reactions: skin rash, hives, itching, drug fever—rare to infrequent.

Dizziness, drowsiness, unsteadiness—may be frequent when therapy is started.

Fatigue, blurred vision, confusion—infrequent.

Exaggerated hearing, ringing in ears—case reports.

Loss of appetite, nausea, vomiting, indigestion, diarrhea—may be frequent when starting therapy.

Decreased sense of taste —possible.

Aching of muscles and joints, leg cramps—case reports.

Serious Adverse Effects

Allergic reactions: severe dermatitis with peeling of skin, irritation of mouth and tongue, swelling of lymph glands—case reports.

Idiosyncratic reactions: lung inflammation (pneumonitis): cough, shortness of breath. Agranulocytosis may also be idiosyncratic—case reports.

Lowering of white blood cells (leukopenia): may be up to 10%—infrequent.

Low thyroid hormones—rare.

Bone marrow depression (see Glossary) (agranulocytosis, hemolytic or aplastic anemia) or thrombocytopenia: fatigue, weakness, fever, sore throat, abnormal bleeding or bruising—case reports.

Pseudolymphoma or systemic lupus erythematosus—case reports.

Abnormal heartbeats (bradyarrhythmias)—case reports.

Liver damage with jaundice (see Glossary): yellow eyes or skin, dark-colored urine, light-colored stools—case reports.

Kidney damage or porphyria—case reports.

Mental depression or agitation/psychosis or paradoxical increase in seizures—case reports.

Abnormally elevated urine output (SIADH)—case reports.

Neuroleptic malignant syndrome or aseptic meningitis—case reports.

Abnormal movement and muscle contractions—case reports.

Pancreatitis—case reports.

Retinopathy, visual hallucinations, peripheral neuritis (see Glossary)—case reports.

Vitamin D deficiency (especially if other risk factors are present). This may lead to osteoporosis.

▷ **Possible Effects on Sexual Function**

Decreased libido and/or impotence—case reports. Possible male infertility. This drug is used to control hypersexuality (exaggerated sexual behavior) that can result from injury to the temporal lobe of the brain.

Adverse Effects That May Mimic Natural Diseases or Disorders

Liver reactions may suggest viral hepatitis. Lung reactions may suggest interstitial pneumonitis.

Natural Diseases or Disorders That May Be Activated by This Drug
Latent psychosis, systemic lupus erythematosus.

Possible Effects on Laboratory Tests
Complete blood cell: decreased red cells, hemoglobin, white cells, and platelets; increased eosinophils, increased white cells.
Blood calcium level: decreased.
INR (prothrombin time): decreased.
Thyroid hormones: falsely decreased blood levels.
Blood urea nitrogen level (BUN): increased.
Liver function tests: increased liver enzymes (ALT/GPT, AST/GOT, and alkaline phosphatase), increased bilirubin.
Urine pregnancy tests: false negative or inconclusive results with Prepurex, Predictor, Gonavislide, Pregnosticon.

CAUTION
1. This drug should be used only after less toxic drugs have failed.
2. *Before* the first dose is taken, blood cell counts, liver function tests, and kidney function tests should be obtained.
3. Careful periodic testing for blood cell or bone marrow toxicity is *mandatory.*
4. *This drug should not be used* to prevent recurrence of trigeminal neuralgia when it is in remission.
5. *Do not stop this drug suddenly* if it is being used to control seizures.
6. If exposed to humidity, the tablet form hardens; this results in poor absorption from the gastrointestinal tract and erratic control of seizures. Store this drug in a cool, dry place; avoid bathrooms or other humid areas. Try a locking cabinet in the kitchen.

Precautions for Use
By Infants and Children: Careful testing of blood production and liver and kidney function must be performed regularly. This drug can reduce the effectiveness of other anticonvulsant drugs. Blood levels of all anticonvulsant drugs should be checked if this drug is added to the treatment program.
By Those Over 60 Years of Age: Can cause confusion and agitation. Watch for aggravation of glaucoma, coronary artery disease (angina), or prostatism (see Glossary).

▷ **Advisability of Use During Pregnancy**
Pregnancy Category: C. See Pregnancy Risk Categories at the back of this book.
Animal studies: Rat studies reveal significant birth defects.
Human studies: Adequate studies of pregnant women are not available.
Avoid completely during the first 3 months. Use during the last 6 months only if clearly needed.

Advisability of Use If Breast-Feeding
Presence of this drug in breast milk: Yes.
Avoid drug or refrain from nursing.

Habit-Forming Potential: None.

Effects of Overdosage: Dizziness, drowsiness, disorientation, tremor, involuntary movements, nausea, vomiting, flushed skin, dilated pupils, stupor progressing to coma.

Possible Effects of Long-Term Use: Water retention (edema), impaired liver function, possible jaundice.

Suggested Periodic Examinations While Taking This Drug (at physician's discretion)
Complete blood counts weekly during the first 3 months of treatment, and then monthly until the drug is stopped. Liver and kidney function tests. Complete eye examinations.

▷ **While Taking This Drug, Observe the Following**
Foods: No restrictions. There may be a minor increase in absorption if taken with food.
Beverages: No restrictions. May be taken with milk.
▷ *Alcohol:* Avoid alcohol use, unless your doctor approves alcohol use.
Tobacco Smoking: No interactions expected, but I advise everyone to quit smoking.
▷ *Other Drugs*
Carbamazepine may *increase* the effects of
- sedatives, tranquilizers, hypnotics, and narcotics, and enhance their sedative effects.

Carbamazepine may *decrease* the effects of
- adrenocortical steroids (see Drug Classes).
- antidepressants (see Drug Classes).
- birth control pills (oral contraceptives) and result in pregnancy.
- cyclosporine (Sandimmune).
- doxycycline (Doxy-II, Vibramycin, etc.).
- felodipine (Plendil).
- haloperidol (Haldol) or other phenothiazines.
- isradipine (DynaCirc).
- itraconazole (Sporanox).
- tetracyclines (see Drug Classes).
- valproic acid (Depakene, etc.).
- warfarin (Coumadin). Increased frequency of INR testing is indicated.

Carbamazepine *taken concurrently* with
- clozapine (Clozaril) may result in serious bone marrow suppression.
- felbamate (Felbatol) may result in decreased carbamazepine levels and seizures.
- lithium (Lithobid, others) may cause serious neurological problems: confusion, drowsiness, weakness, unsteadiness, tremors, and twitching.
- monoamine oxidase (MAO) type A inhibitor drugs (see Drug Classes) may cause severe toxic reactions.
- phenytoin (Dilantin, etc.) may cause unpredictable fluctuations of blood levels of both drugs and impair seizure control.
- terfenadine (Seldane), and perhaps other nonsedating antihistamines, may result in carbamazepine toxicity.
- theophylline (Theo-Dur, etc.) may reduce the effects of both drugs.

The following drugs may *increase* the effects of carbamazepine:
- cimetidine (Tagamet).
- danazol (Danocrine).
- diltiazem (Cardizem)—and perhaps other calcium channel blockers.
- flu shots (influenza vaccine).

- fluoxetine (Prozac); may lead to toxicity.
- fluvoxamine (Luvox); may result in toxicity.
- isoniazid (INH).
- macrolide antibiotics—erythromycins, clarithromycin, or troleandomycin.
- nicotinamide (nicotinic acid amide).
- propoxyphene (Darvon, Darvocet, etc.).
- rifampin; may result in toxicity.
- ritonavir (Norvir) and perhaps other protease inhibitors (see Drug Classes).
- verapamil (Calan, Isoptin).

▷ *Driving, Hazardous Activities:* Can cause dizziness, drowsiness, or blurred vision. Adjust activities.

Aviation Note: The use of this drug *is a disqualification* for piloting. Consult a designated Aviation Medical Examiner.

Exposure to Sun: This drug can cause photosensitivity (see Glossary). Use caution until sensitivity to sun is known.

Heavy Exercise or Exertion: Use caution if you have coronary artery disease. Can intensify angina and reduce tolerance for physical activity.

Occurrence of Unrelated Illness: Because of potential for serious adverse effects, you MUST tell each physician and dentist you see that you take carbamazepine.

Discontinuation: If treating trigeminal neuralgia, every 3 months attempts to reduce the maintenance dose or to stop this drug are needed. If used to control epilepsy, this drug *must not be stopped abruptly.*

Special Storage Instructions: Store the tablet form of this drug in a cool, dry place. Protect it from exposure to humid conditions **(do NOT store in a bathroom medicine cabinet),** as the tablets may lose potency.

CARTEOLOL (KAR tee oh lohl)

Introduced: 1983   **Class:** Antihypertensive, beta-adrenergic blocker
Prescription: USA: Yes   **Controlled Drug:** USA: No; Canada: No   **Available as Generic:** No

Brand Names: Cartrol, Ocupress, Optipress

BENEFITS versus RISKS	
Possible Benefits	*Possible Risks*
EFFECTIVE, WELL-TOLERATED ANTIHYPERTENSIVE	Congestive heart failure
EFFECTIVE GLAUCOMA TREATMENT	Worsening of angina in coronary heart disease (abrupt withdrawal)
Prevention of angina	Masking of low blood sugar (hypoglycemia) in drug-treated diabetics
	Provocation of asthma in asthmatics

▷ **Principal Uses**

As a Single Drug Product: Uses currently included in FDA-approved labeling: (1) Treatment of mild to moderate high blood pressure. May be used alone or in combination with other drugs, such as diuretics; (2) helps lower eye (intraocular) pressure in people with glaucoma.

Other (unlabeled) generally accepted uses: (1) Effective in helping increase the amount of exercise that can be performed before angina occurs; (2) can have a role in helping decrease aggressive behavior; (3) decreases the occurrence of abnormal heart rhythms; (3) other beta-blockers have shown benefits in treating patients after heart attacks; however, studies using carteolol have not been performed; (4) may help lessen panic attacks.

How This Drug Works: By blocking certain actions of the sympathetic nervous system, this drug
- reduces the rate and contraction force of the heart, lowering the ejection pressure of blood leaving the heart.
- reduces the extent of blood vessel wall contraction, resulting in relaxation and expansion and lowering of blood pressure.
- reduces elevated eye pressure (intraocular) and relieves glaucoma symptoms.

Available Dosage Forms and Strengths
Tablets — 2.5 mg, 5 mg
Ophthalmic solution — 5 ml, 10 ml (1%)

▷ **Usual Adult Dosage Range:**   For high blood pressure (hypertension): Initially 2.5 mg once daily. The dose may be increased gradually by 2.5 mg/day at intervals of 2 weeks, as needed and tolerated, up to 10 mg/day. For maintenance, 2.5 to 7.5 mg once daily is usually adequate. The total daily dose should not exceed 10 mg.

For glaucoma: One drop in the affected eye or eyes two times a day. **Note: Actual dosage and administration schedule must be determined for each patient individually.**

Conditions Requiring Dosing Adjustments
Liver Function: Decreased doses needed in severe liver failure.
Kidney Function: The kidney is the main route of elimination for this drug. Dosing interval **MUST** be decreased in kidney failure. In severe compromise, the drug is given every 48 to 72 hours.

▷ **Dosing Instructions:**   Tablet may be crushed and taken without regard to eating. Do not stop this drug abruptly.

Usual Duration of Use: Use on a regular schedule for up to 3 weeks may be needed to see this drug's effectiveness in lowering blood pressure. Long-term use of this drug (months to years) will be determined by the benefit in lowering your blood pressure over time and your response to a treatment program of weight reduction, salt restriction, smoking cessation, etc. See your doctor on a regular basis.

Possible Advantages of This Drug
Adequate control of blood pressure with a single daily dose. Causes less slowing of the heart rate than most other beta-blocker drugs.

▷ **This Drug Should Not Be Taken If**
- you have bronchial asthma.
- you have had an allergic reaction to it previously.
- you have congestive heart failure.
- you have an abnormally slow heart rate or a serious heart block.
- you have a dissecting aortic aneurysm (ask your doctor).

▷ **Inform Your Physician Before Taking This Drug If**
- you have had an adverse reaction to any beta-blocker (see Drug Classes).
- you have serious heart disease or episodes of heart failure.

- you have had hay fever (allergic rhinitis), asthma, chronic bronchitis, or emphysema.
- you have a history of overactive thyroid function (hyperthyroidism).
- you have a history of low blood sugar (hypoglycemia), diabetes, or myasthenia gravis.
- you have impaired liver or kidney function.
- you have a circulation problem (Raynaud's phenomenon, claudication pains in legs).
- you take any form of digitalis, quinidine, or reserpine, or any calcium blocker drug (see Drug Classes).
- you plan to have surgery under general anesthesia in the near future.

Possible Side Effects (natural, expected, and unavoidable drug actions)
Lethargy and fatigability, cold extremities, slow heart rate, light-headedness in upright position (see Orthostatic Hypotension in Glossary).

▷ **Possible Adverse Effects** (unusual, unexpected, and infrequent reactions)
If any of the following develop, consult your physician promptly for guidance.
Mild Adverse Effects
Allergic reactions: skin rash—rare.
Headache, dizziness, nervousness, drowsiness—infrequent.
Indigestion, nausea, vomiting, constipation, diarrhea—infrequent.
Slight increase in blood potassium—possible.
Cough, wheezing, or sinusitis—rare.
Joint and muscle discomfort, numbness of fingers or toes—rare.
Episodic difficulty walking (intermittent claudication with peripheral vascular disease)—possible.
Tearing and irritation (with use in the eye)—infrequent to frequent.
Serious Adverse Effects
Mental depression—possible, but less likely than some other beta-blockers.
Chest pain, irregular heartbeat, shortness of breath; can cause congestive heart failure—possible.
Induction of bronchial asthma (in asthmatic patients)—possible.
Aggravation of myasthenia gravis—possible.
May hide symptoms of low blood sugar.

▷ **Possible Effects on Sexual Function:** Decreased libido, impotence—case reports.

Adverse Effects That May Mimic Natural Diseases or Disorders
Decreased extremity blood flow may mimic Raynaud's phenomenon (see Glossary).

Natural Diseases or Disorders That May Be Activated by This Drug
Raynaud's disease, intermittent claudication, myasthenia gravis.

Possible Effects on Laboratory Tests
Blood creatine kinase level: increased.
Blood potassium: slight increase.

CAUTION
1. ***Do not stop this drug suddenly*** without the knowledge of your doctor. Carry a note that says you are taking this drug.
2. Ask your physician or pharmacist before using nasal decongestants.

These can cause sudden increases in blood pressure when combined with beta-blocker drugs.

3. Report any new tendency to emotional depression.

Precautions for Use

By Infants and Children: Safety and effectiveness by those under 12 years of age not established. However, if this drug is used, watch for the development of low blood sugar (hypoglycemia), especially if meals are skipped.

By Those Over 60 Years of Age: **Caution**: Unacceptably high blood pressure should be reduced without creating excessively low blood pressure. Treatment should begin with small doses, and blood pressure should be checked often. Sudden and excessive reduction of blood pressure can lead to stroke or heart attack. Watch for dizziness, tendency to fall, confusion, hallucinations, depression, or urinary frequency.

▷ **Advisability of Use During Pregnancy**

Pregnancy Category: C. See Pregnancy Risk Categories at the back of this book. Animal studies: No birth defects due to this drug found in rat or rabbit studies.

Human studies: Adequate studies of pregnant women are not available. Use this drug only if clearly needed. Ask your physician for guidance.

Advisability of Use If Breast-Feeding

Presence of this drug in breast milk: Unknown in humans; yes in animals. Avoid drug or refrain from nursing.

Habit-Forming Potential: None.

Effects of Overdosage: Weakness, slow pulse, low blood pressure, fainting, cold and sweaty skin, congestive heart failure, possible coma, and convulsions.

Possible Effects of Long-Term Use: Reduced heart reserve and eventual heart failure in susceptible individuals with advanced heart disease.

Suggested Periodic Examinations While Taking This Drug (at physician's discretion)

Measurements of blood pressure, evaluation of heart function.

▷ **While Taking This Drug, Observe the Following**

Foods: No restrictions. Avoid excessive salt intake.

Beverages: No restrictions. May be taken with milk.

▷ *Alcohol:* Use caution. Alcohol may exaggerate this drug's ability to lower the blood pressure and may increase its mild sedative effect.

Tobacco Smoking: Nicotine may reduce this drug's effectiveness in treating high blood pressure. In addition, high doses may worsen constriction of the bronchial tubes caused by regular smoking. I advise everyone to quit smoking.

▷ *Other Drugs*

Carteolol may *increase* the effects of

• other antihypertensive drugs, and cause excessive lowering of the blood pressure. Dosage adjustments may be necessary.

• reserpine (Ser-Ap-Es, etc.), and cause sedation, depression, slowing of the heart rate, and low blood pressure. This combination is best avoided.

• theophyllines (aminophylline, dyphylline, oxtriphylline, etc.).

- verapamil (Calan, Isoptin), and cause excessive depression of heart function; monitor this combination closely.

Carteolol *taken concurrently* with

- amiodarone (Cordarone) may cause severe slowing of the heart and sinus arrest. Do not combine these agents.
- clonidine (Catapres) requires close monitoring for rebound high blood pressure if clonidine is stopped while carteolol is still being taken. Severe rebound hypertension may occur.
- digoxin (Lanoxin) may lead to abnormal heart conduction. Caution is prudent.
- diltiazem (Cardizem) (like verapamil) may be very helpful in patients with normal heart function, but may result in AV conduction problems.
- epinephrine (Adrenalin, etc.) may cause sudden rise in blood pressure followed by slowing of the heart rate. Avoid this combination.
- ergot preparations (ergotamine, methysergide, etc.) may enhance serious ergot-induced constriction of peripheral circulation.
- fluoxetine (Prozac) may result in dangerous slowing of the heart or dangerously low blood pressure.
- fluvoxamine (Luvox) may result in dangerous slowing of the heart or dangerously low blood pressure.
- insulin requires close monitoring to avoid hypoglycemia (see Glossary).
- nifedipine (dihydroperidine) may result in excessive lowering of the blood pressure.
- oral antidiabetic drugs (see Drug Classes) may cause prolonged recovery from hypoglycemia should it occur.
- phenothiazines (see Drug Classes) can cause increased effects of both drugs.
- rifabutin (Mycobutin) may reduce carteolol's effectiveness.
- venlafaxine (Effexor) may lead to toxicity from either drug.

The following drugs may *decrease* the effects of carteolol:

- indomethacin (Indocin), and possibly other "aspirin substitutes" or NSAIDs, may impair carteolol's antihypertensive effect.

▷ *Driving, Hazardous Activities:* Use caution until the full extent of fatigue, dizziness, and blood pressure change have been determined.

Aviation Note: The use of this drug *is a disqualification* for piloting. Consult a designated Aviation Medical Examiner.

Exposure to Sun: No restrictions.

Exposure to Heat: Caution is advised. Hot environments can lower the blood pressure and exaggerate the effects of this drug.

Exposure to Cold: Caution is advised. The elderly should take precautions to prevent hypothermia (see Glossary).

Heavy Exercise or Exertion: Avoid exertion that produces light-headedness, excessive fatigue, or muscle cramping. The use of this drug can cause dangerously increased blood pressure with isometric exercise.

Occurrence of Unrelated Illness: Fever can lower the blood pressure and require decreased doses. Illnesses that cause nausea or vomiting may interrupt the regular dosage schedule. Ask your physician for guidance.

Discontinuation: **DO NOT STOP this drug suddenly**. If possible, gradual reduction of dose over a period of 2 to 3 weeks is recommended. Ask your physician for help.

CEPHALOSPORINS (SEF a low spoar ins)

Cefaclor (SEF a klor); **Cefadroxil** (SEF a drox il); **Cefixime** (SE fix eem); **Cefprozil** (SEF proh zil); **Ceftriaxone** (SEF try ax own); **Cefuroxime** (SEF yur ox eem); **Cephalexin** (SEF ah lex in)

Introduced: 1979, 1977, 1986, 1991, 1984, 1974, 1969, respectively   **Class:** Antibiotics, cephalosporins   **Prescription:** USA: Yes   **Controlled Drugs:** USA: No; Canada: No   **Available as Generic:** Cefaclor: yes; cefadroxil: yes; cefixime: no; cefprozil: no; ceftriaxone: no; cefuroxime: yes; cephalexin: yes.

Brand Names: Cefaclor: Ceclor; Cefadroxil: Duricef, Ultracef; Cefixime: Su-prax; Cefprozil: Cefzil; Ceftriaxone: Rocephin; Cefuroxime: Ceftin, Kefu-rox, Zinacef; Cephalexin: ✦Apo-Cephalex, Cefanex, ✦Ceporex, Keflet, Ke-flex, Keftab, ✦Novo-Lexin✦Nu-Cephalex

---

BENEFITS versus RISKS

Possible Benefits	*Possible Risks*
EFFECTIVE TREATMENT OF INFECTIONS due to susceptible microorganisms	ALLERGIC REACTIONS, mild to severe (may also be seen in those allergic to penicillin)
HOME INTRAVENOUS TREATMENT OF SERIOUS INFECTIONS (ceftriaxone)	Drug-induced colitis—rare
	Superinfections (see Glossary)
ONE INJECTION TREATMENT OF SOME CHILDHOOD EAR INFECTIONS	Low white blood cell or platelet counts (cefixime or ceftriaxone)—rare
	Anemia (ceftriaxone)—rare

▷ **Principal Uses**

As a Single Drug Product: Uses currently included in FDA-approved labeling: (1) To treat some infections of the skin and skin structures, the upper and lower respiratory tract (including middle ear infections and "strep" throat), some urinary tract and some postoperative wound infections; (2) treatment of advanced Lyme disease (stage 2 or 3) via home intravenous (home IV) services (ceftriaxone); (3) treatment of serious bone infections (osteomyeli-tis) via home IV; (4) treatment of gonorrhea (cefuroxime).

Other unlabeled, generally accepted uses: (1) May have an alternative role in helping prevent rheumatic fever if the bacteria are resistant to erythromy-cin (cefaclor); (2) may help treat resistant cervical infections (cefixime); part of combination treatment of Whipple's disease (cefixime); (3) treats sexual assault cases and chancroid (ceftriaxone); (4) used in *Shigella* infec-tions; (5) used to change from an intravenous medicine to one taken by mouth in order to shorten hospital stays and preserve results (cefuroxime).

How These Drugs Work: These drugs destroy susceptible infecting bacteria by interfering with their ability to produce new protective cell walls as they multiply and grow.

Available Dosage Forms and Strengths

Cefaclor:
Capsules — 250 mg, 500 mg
Oral suspension — 125 mg, 187 mg, 250 mg, 375 mg/5 ml

Cefadroxil:
>   Capsules — 500 mg, 1000 mg
> Gelatin capsules (Canada) — 500 mg
>   Oral suspension — 125 mg, 250 mg, 500 mg/5 ml
>   Tablets — 1000 mg (1 g)

Cefixime:
>   Oral suspension — 100 mg/5 ml
>   Tablets — 200 mg, 400 mg

Cefprozil:
>   Oral suspension — 125 mg, 250 mg/5 ml
>   Tablets — 250 mg, 500 mg

Ceftriaxone:
>   250 mg of Rocephin — Boxes of 1 or 10 vial(s)
>   500 mg of Rocephin — Boxes of 1 or 10 vial(s)
>   1 g of Rocephin — Boxes of 1 or 10 vial(s) or piggyback bottles of 10
>   2 g of Rocephin — Boxes of 10 vials, or piggyback bottles of 10
>   10 g of Rocephin — Box of one
> 1 g or 2 g ADD-Vantage
>   packaging

Cefuroxime:
>   Tablets — 125 mg, 250 mg, 500 mg
>   Intravenous — 750 mg/10 ml
>   — 750 mg/50 ml
>   — 750 mg/100 ml
>   — 1.5 g/100 ml
>   — 1.5 g/50 ml
>   — 1.5 g/20 ml
>   — 7.5 g/127 ml
>   Oral suspension — 125 mg/5 ml

Cephalexin:
>   Capsules — 250 mg, 500 mg
>   Oral suspension — 125 mg, 250 mg/5 ml
> Pediatric oral suspension — 100 mg/ml
>   Tablets — 250 mg, 500 mg, 1000 mg (1 g)

▷ **Usual Adult Dosage Ranges:**   Cefaclor: 250 to 500 mg every 8 hours. Total daily dose should not exceed 4 g (4000 mg).

Cefadroxil: Skin infections—500 mg every 12 hours, or 1 g daily. "Strep" throat—500 mg every 12 hours for 10 days. Urinary tract infections—500 mg to 1 g every 12 hours, or 1 to 2 g daily. Total daily dosage should not exceed 6 g.

Cefixime: 400 mg daily, taken as a single dose or as 200 mg every 12 hours. For treatment of multidrug-resistant *Salmonella*: 20 mg per kg of body mass per day in divided doses every 12 hours, for at least 12 days. For treatment of uncomplicated gonorrhea: 400 to 800 mg as a single dose.

Cephalexin: 250 to 500 mg every 6 hours. Total daily dose should not exceed 4 g.

Infants and Children: Cefaclor: 20 to 40 mg per kg of body mass per day is given in divided doses every 8 hours. Maximum dose is 1 g (1000 mg) daily.

Cefadroxil: 30 mg per kg of body mass per day, given in divided doses every 12 hours.

Cefixime: For children over 6 months of age: 8 mg per kg of body mass per day, all in one dose or divided into two doses.

Cefprozil: For otitis media (6 months to 12 years of age)—15 mg per kg of body mass every 12 hours, for 10 days.

Ceftriaxone: For neonates and children less than 12 for treatment of serious infections caused by susceptible organisms (other than CNS infections such as meningitis): 50 to 75 mg per kg of body mass per day, given in two equally divided doses 12 hours apart (not to exceed 2 g daily). Some doctors suggest that neonates 1 week old or younger be given 50 mg per kg of body mass per day; that neonates older than 1 week and weighing 2 kg or less also receive 50 mg per kg of body mass per day; and 50–75 mg per kg of body mass per day be given to neonates older than 1 week and weighing more than 2 kg.

For meningitis (caused by susceptible organisms) the dose for neonates and children 12 or younger is 100 mg per kg of body mass daily, divided into two equal doses given every 12 hours. The American Academy of Pediatrics suggests 80–100 mg per kg of body mass be given once daily or in two equally divided doses every 12 hours for children older than 1 month. Because the once-daily regimen is relatively new, I suggest that the 12-hour regimen be used. Serious CNS disease—children can be treated with 75–100 mg per kg of body mass IV daily for 21 days. Cardiac disease—children can be given 75–100 mg per kg of body mass per day IV. Treatment of serious arthritis, cardiac or neurologic complications of early or late (stage 2 or 3) Lyme disease: Arthritis: 75–100 mg per kg of body mass per day IV. One recent article advocated a single dose of ceftriaxone for some childhood ear infections.

For otitis media: 75–100 mg per kg of body mass per day, in four divided doses.

Cefuroxime: For children over 2: Oral: 125 mg twice a day, 250 mg twice daily for treatment of otitis media. Intravenous: Those over 3 months should be given 50 to 100 mg per kg of body mass per day, divided every 6 to 8 hours. Maximum dose is 4 g.

Cephalexin: 25 to 50 mg per kg of body mass per day in two to four divided doses. Maximum dose is 4 g (4000 mg).

12 to 60 Years of Age: Cefprozil: Pharyngitis or tonsillitis—500 mg every 24 hours (once daily), for 10 days. Acute or chronic bronchitis—500 mg every 12 hours, for 10 days. Bacterial pneumonia—250 mg three times a day for 14 days. Skin or skin structure infections—250 to 500 mg every 12 to 24 hours, for 10 days.

The dosing of ceftriaxone for treatment of most infections (caused by susceptible organisms) is: 1–2 g daily or in equally divided doses two times a day depending on the type and severity of the infection. Children older than 12 can be given the adult dose. Some physicians recommend that CNS infections in adults may require 4 g daily. This is the maximum adult dosage recommended by the manufacturer. Uncomplicated gonorrhea caused by penicillinase-producing strains of *Neisseria* gonorrhea (PPNG) or non-penicillinase-producing strains may be treated by a single IM 250-mg dose of ceftriaxone. Disseminated gonococcal infection should be treated by 1 g of ceftriaxone IV or IM once a day for 7 days. Acute sexually transmitted epididymitis in adults may be treated with a single 250-mg IM dose of ceftriaxone followed by 7 days of oral tetracycline or erythromycin. For treatment of acute pelvic inflammatory disease (PID), a single 250-mg IM dose of ceftriaxone should be given and then followed by 100 mg of oral doxycycline two times a day for 10–14 days. Treatment of serious arthritis, cardiac or neurologic complications of early or late (stage 2 or 3) Lyme disease: Arthritis—ceftriaxone at a dose of 2 g IV daily for adults. Serious CNS disease—ceftriaxone at a dose of 2 g IV daily for 21 days in adults. Cardiac disease—ceftriaxone 2 g IV per day for 21 days in adults. Surgical prophylaxis—although ceftriaxone is FDA approved for surgical prophylaxis, we do not recommend its routine use. Other readily available agents are equally as effective, and much less expensive. Ceftriaxone use for surgical prophylaxis also increases the potential for resistance to this drug, and could decrease its usefulness in treating later infections.

Cefuroxime: Oral: 250 to 500 mg every 12 hrs. Total daily dosage should not exceed 4 g.

Intravenous: 750 mg to 1.5 g every 8 hours.

Over 60 Years of Age: Cefprozil: Same as 12 to 60 years of age. Decreased dose in kidney failure.

Ceftriaxone: Same as 12 to 60 years of age.

Note: Actual dosage and administration schedule must be determined for each patient individually for ALL of these medicines.

Conditions Requiring Dosing Adjustments

Liver Function: Cefaclor, cefixime, cefprozil, cefuroxime, or cephalexin: No changes in dosing needed at present.

Cefadroxil: The liver is involved to a minimal degree, and no dosing changes are anticipated in liver compromise.

Ceftriaxone: Patients with both liver and kidney problems should have blood levels checked and a maximum dose of 2 g given.

Kidney Function: Cefaclor is 40–80% eliminated by the kidney. For creatinine clearances (CrCl) of 10–50 ml/min., 50–100% of the usual dose at the normal interval is used. For creatinine clearances of less than 10 ml/min., 50% of the usual dose at the usual time is given.

Cefadroxil: With creatinine clearances of 10–50 ml/min., use the usual doses every 12 to 24 hours. For creatinine clearances less than 10 ml/min., usual doses are given every 24–48 hours.

Cefixime: Dose **must be decreased** in mild to moderate kidney problems. In severe failure, a single dose every 48 hours is often used.

Cefprozil: With severe kidney failure, **half** the dose can be given at the usual time.

Ceftriaxone: Patients with kidney compromise must be carefully followed for adverse effects.

Cefuroxime: 750 mg once daily for most kidney compromise. Dose must be repeated after dialysis, as this medicine is dialyzable.

Cephalexin: For creatinine clearances of 10–50 ml/min., usual dose every 6 hours. For creatinine clearances less than 10 ml/min., usual dose every 8–12 hours.

Phenylketonuria (PKU): Cefprozil only: The suspension has 28 mg of phenylalanine in every 5 ml. This may preclude use of this drug in these patients.

▷ **Dosing Instructions:**   May be taken on an empty stomach or with food if stomach irritation occurs. Capsule (cefaclor, cefadroxil) may be opened and tablet forms crushed for administration. Cefuroxime tablet can give a bitter taste that lingers. Shake suspension forms well before measuring (use a measured dose cup or other calibrated dose measure) dose. Intravenous forms should be brought to room temperature if they were previously refrigerated. Take the full course prescribed.

Usual Duration of Use: Continual use on a regular schedule for 3 to 5 days is usually needed to determine the effectiveness of these drugs in controlling the infection under treatment. Response varies with the nature of the infection. Total treatment time will vary from 1 (for some minor infections) to 6 (as in some bone infections) weeks. Some infections **require 10 consecutive days** of treatment to prevent the development of rheumatic fever. Follow your doctor's instructions about how long to take this medicine. Many clinicians ask that you call them if symptoms worsen or fever persists for 24 to 48 hours after you start to take these medicines.

These Drugs Should Not Be Taken If
- you are allergic to any cephalosporin antibiotic (see Drug Classes).
- you have pseudomembranous colitis.

▷ **Inform Your Physician Before Taking This Drug If**
- you have a history of allergy to any penicillin (see Drug Classes).
- you have a history of regional enteritis or ulcerative colitis.
- you have impaired kidney function.
- you have a history of blood clotting disorders.
- you have a history of low platelets or white blood cell count (cefprozil, cefixime, or ceftriaxone).

Possible Side Effects (natural, expected, and unavoidable drug actions)
Superinfections (see Glossary).

▷ **Possible Adverse Effects** (unusual, unexpected, and infrequent reactions)
If any of the following develop, consult your physician promptly for guidance.
Mild Adverse Effects
Allergic reactions: skin rash, itching, hives.
Nausea and vomiting or mild diarrhea—most common adverse effects.
Sore mouth or tongue—possible.
Mild and reversible decrease in white blood cells (neutrophils) (cefaclor).
Confusion, nervousness, insomnia, dizziness—rare.
Serious Adverse Effects
Allergic reactions: drug fever (see Glossary), anaphylactic reaction (see Glossary), Stevens-Johnson syndrome—rare.
Idiosyncratic reactions: lowered white blood cell counts or platelets (cefixime, ceftriaxone, cefuroxime)—rare; rare and idiosyncratic (cephalexin).
Extended time for blood to clot (reported with chronic use of other second or third generation cephalosporins in debilitated patients)—rare.
Genital itching (may represent a fungus superinfection)—possible.
Serum sickness (itching, joint pain, and irritated swellings)—rare.
Increased blood urea nitrogen (BUN) or serum creatinine—rare.
Gall bladder concretions (ceftriaxone)—rare.
Severe diarrhea, possibly indicating a drug-induced form of colitis—rare.

Increases in liver enzymes (cefadroxil) and jaundice (cholestatic—cefaclor)—
rare.

▷ **Possible Effects on Sexual Function:**   None reported.

Adverse Effects That May Mimic Natural Diseases or Disorders
Skin rash and fever may resemble measles.

Possible Effects on Laboratory Tests
Blood platelet counts: decreased—rare (see above).
INR: may be increased (cefixime, ceftriaxone)—rare.
PTT: extended (cefprozil)—rare.
Liver enzymes: increased (cefaclor, cefuroxime, cefprozil, ceftriaxone)—rare.
BUN and creatinine: increased (cefaclor, cefprozil, cefuroxime, ceftriax-
one)—rare.
White blood cell counts: decreased (cefprozil, cefixime, cefuroxime, ceftriax-
one, cephalexin)—rare.

CAUTION
Some drugs in this class can cause a false positive test result for urine sugar
when using Clinitest tablets, Benedict's solution, or Fehling's solution, but
not with Tes-Tape.

Precautions for Use
By Infants and Children: Not recommended for use in infants less than 1 month
old (cefaclor), or 1 year old (cephalexin). The maximal dose in children
should not exceed 1 g every 24 hours (cefaclor). Dosing of other medicines
in this class is based on weight. Follow the dosing instructions exactly.
Safety and effectiveness for those under 6 months not established (cefixime, cefprozil).
By Those Over 60 Years of Age: Dosage must be carefully individualized and
based upon evaluation of kidney function. Natural changes in the skin may
predispose to severe and prolonged itching reactions in the genital and anal
regions. Such reactions should be reported promptly. The natural decline
in kidney function often requires a decrease in dose and achieves the same
effect as a larger dose (all but ceftriaxone).

▷ **Advisability of Use During Pregnancy**
Pregnancy Category: B. See Pregnancy Risk Categories at the back of this book.
Animal studies: No birth defects reported.
Human studies: Information from adequate studies of pregnant women is not
available.
Generally considered to be safe. Ask your physician for guidance.

Advisability of Use If Breast-Feeding
Presence of this drug in breast milk: Yes, in small amounts (cefaclor, cefadroxil, ceftriaxone, cefuroxime, and cephalexin); unknown (cefixime, cefprozil).
Ask your doctor for advice.

Habit-Forming Potential: None.

Effects of Overdosage: Nausea, vomiting, stomach cramps, and/or diarrhea.

Possible Effects of Long-Term Use: Superinfections (see Glossary).

Suggested Periodic Examinations While Taking This Drug (at physician's discretion)
Complete blood cell counts.

Liver enzymes.

INR or PTT (for some of these medicines).

BUN and creatinine with long-term therapy.

▷ **While Taking This Drug, Observe the Following**

Foods: Delays the absorption of this drug and may result in decreased antibiotic effect (cefaclor). No restrictions (cefadroxil, cefprozil, cefixime, ceftriaxone, cefuroxime, or cephalexin).

Beverages: No restrictions. May be taken with milk.

▷ *Alcohol:* Ceftriaxone: May cause severe nausea and vomiting. Others: No interactions expected, but large amounts of alcohol may blunt the immune system.

Tobacco Smoking: No interactions expected, but I advise everyone to quit smoking.

▷ *Other Drugs*

These medicines *taken concurrently* with

- any aminoglycoside antibiotic (see Drug Classes) may result in increased kidney (renal) toxicity.
- anticoagulants (blood thinners) such as heparin or warfarin (Coumadin) may have anticoagulant effects increased by some medicines in this class.
- birth control pills (oral contraceptives) may result in **decreased effectiveness** in preventing conception and pregnancy.
- cholestyramine may decrease cephalexin (and perhaps other drugs in this class) absorption and blunt the beneficial effects in fighting infection.
- loop diuretics such as ethacrynic acid may result in increased risk of kidney toxicity.
- probenecid (Benemid) will slow the elimination of these drugs, resulting in higher blood levels and prolonged effect.

▷ *Driving, Hazardous Activities:* Usually no restrictions.

Aviation Note: The use of these drugs *may be a disqualification* for piloting. Consult a designated Aviation Medical Examiner.

Exposure to Sun: No restrictions.

Special Storage Instructions: Oral suspension should be kept at room temperature (cefixime). Oral suspensions should be refrigerated (cefaclor, cefadroxil, cefprozil, cephalexin, ceftriaxone IV form). Cefuroxime may be stored at room temperature or in the refrigerator.

Observe the Following Expiration Times: Do not take the oral suspension of this drug if it is older than 14 days (cefaclor, cefadroxil, cefprozil, cephalexin) or 10 days (cefuroxime).

CHLORAMBUCIL (klor AM byu sil)

Introduced: 1974   **Class:** Anticancer, immunosuppressant   **Prescription:** USA: Yes   **Controlled Drug:** USA: No; Canada: No   **Available as Generic:** USA: No; Canada: No

Brand Name: Leukeran

BENEFITS versus RISKS

Possible Benefits	*Possible Risks*
EFFECTIVE PALLIATIVE TREATMENT FOR CHRONIC LYMPHOCYTIC LEUKEMIA	BONE MARROW DEPRESSION (see Glossary)
EFFECTIVE PALLIATIVE TREATMENT FOR HODGKIN'S DISEASE AND OTHER LYMPHOMAS	INCREASED SUSCEPTIBILITY TO INFECTIONS
	CENTRAL NERVOUS SYSTEM TOXICITY
Immunosuppression of nephrotic syndrome	Male and female sterility
	Drug-induced liver or lung damage
Immunosuppression of rheumatoid arthritis	Development of secondary cancers

---

▷ **Principal Uses**

As a Single Drug Product: Uses currently included in FDA-approved labeling: Treats (1) chronic lymphocytic leukemia; (2) Hodgkin's lymphoma and other malignant lymphomas.

Other (unlabeled) generally accepted uses: (1) Hairy cell leukemia; (2) multiple myeloma; (3) Letterer-Siwe disease; (4) nephrotic syndrome; (5) ovarian cancer; (6) may have a role in treating rheumatoid arthritis; (7) can have a short-term role in treating systemic lupus erythematosus.

How This Drug Works: This drug blocks genetic activity (impairs DNA and RNA), and inhibits production of essential proteins. This kills cancerous cells.

Available Dosage Forms and Strengths

Tablets — 2 mg

▷ **Usual Adult Dosage Range:** For leukemia and lymphoma: Initially (induction phase of 3–6 weeks) 0.1 to 0.2 mg per kg of body mass daily, or 3 to 6 mg per square meter of body surface daily (usually 4 to 10 mg daily) as a single dose or in divided doses. Maintenance dose: 2–4 mg per day or a maximum of 0.1 mg per kg of body mass daily.

For immunosuppression: 0.1 to 0.2 mg per kg of body mass daily, in a single dose, for 8 to 12 weeks.

Note: Actual dosage and administration schedule must be determined for each patient individually.

Conditions Requiring Dosing Adjustments

Liver Function: Can cause liver damage. Use with extreme caution in liver compromise. Extensively metabolized.

Kidney Function: Can cause bladder inflammation; caution is advised in cases of compromised urine outflow.

▷ **Dosing Instructions:** Tablet may be crushed; however, food may decrease absorption by up to 20%. Avoid this combination. See your doctor if vomiting prevents you from taking chlorambucil.

Usual Duration of Use: Use on a regular schedule for 3 to 4 weeks is usually required to see this drug's effectiveness in controlling leukemia or lymphoma; several months are needed to assess immunosuppression. Long-term use requires periodic evaluation of response and dose changes.

▷ **This Drug Should Not Be Taken If**
  • you have had an allergic reaction to it previously.
  • you have a significant degree of bone marrow depression.
  • you currently have an uncontrolled infection.

▷ **Inform Your Physician Before Taking This Drug If**
  • you are allergic to melphalan (Alkeran).
  • you are pregnant, planning pregnancy, or breast-feeding.
  • you have a history of bone marrow depression or a blood cell disorder.
  • you have a history of gout or urate kidney stones.
  • you have a seizure disorder of any kind.
  • you have a history of porphyria.
  • you have impaired liver or kidney function.
  • you have had cancer chemotherapy or radiation therapy previously.
  • you are taking drugs that can impair your immunity.
  • you had or recently have been exposed to chickenpox or herpes zoster.

Possible Side Effects (natural, expected, and unavoidable drug actions)
  Decreased white blood cell and platelet counts.
  Decreased immunity; susceptibility to infections.
  Increased blood levels of uric acid, formation of kidney stones.

▷ **Possible Adverse Effects** (unusual, unexpected, and infrequent reactions)
  If any of the following develop, consult your physician promptly for guidance.
  Mild Adverse Effects
  Allergic reactions: skin rash, itching, drug fever (see Glossary)—rare.
  Mouth and lip sores, nausea, vomiting—infrequent.
  Serious Adverse Effects
  Allergic reactions: drug-induced hepatitis with jaundice—case reports.
  Cataract formation with high-dose usage—case reports.
  Central nervous system toxicity: agitation, confusion, hallucinations, seizures, tremors, paralysis—case reports.
  Peripheral neuritis (see Glossary)—possible.
  Lung damage: cough, shortness of breath—case reports.
  Bone marrow damage, aplastic anemia (see Glossary)—possible (dose related and can be dose limiting).
  Leukemia (may depend on dose and length of treatment)—possible.
  Liver damage (hepatotoxicity and jaundice)—case reports.
  Severe skin damage (toxic epidermal necrolysis)—case reports.

▷ **Possible Effects on Sexual Function:**   Can inhibit reproduction: stops sperm production (male sterility); altered menstrual patterns, blocks ovulation and menstruation (female sterility)—possible.

Possible Delayed Adverse Effects
  Severe bone marrow depression can happen after the drug has been stopped.
  Secondary cancers (especially leukemia) have been reported.
  Lung damage (pulmonary fibrosis).

Adverse Effects That May Mimic Natural Diseases or Disorders
  Drug-induced seizures may suggest epilepsy.
  Drug-induced jaundice may suggest viral hepatitis.

Natural Diseases or Disorders That May Be Activated by This Drug
Gout, urate kidney stones, porphyria, latent epilepsy.

Possible Effects on Laboratory Tests
Complete blood counts: decreased red cells, hemoglobin, white cells, and platelets.
Blood uric acid level: increased.
Liver function tests: increased liver enzymes (ALT/GPT, AST/GOT), increased bilirubin, increased icterus index.
Sperm counts: decreased or absent.

CAUTION
1. Long-term use of this drug in noncancerous conditions requires extreme caution. Risks include permanent sterility, lung damage, and the development of secondary cancers. It should only be used where less toxic medicines have failed.
2. It is advisable to have any needed dental work done prior to using this drug. The bone marrow depression could lead to gum infection, excessive bleeding, and delayed healing.
3. If gout develops, allopurinol is the drug of choice for chlorambucil-caused gout symptoms.
4. This drug impairs the body's ability to produce protective antibodies. Both killed virus vaccines and live virus vaccines will not work. There is an increased risk that live virus vaccines may actually cause infection. Three months to 1 year is needed for the immune system to recover after stopping this and similar drugs. Family members or people in close contact with chlorambucil patients should not receive the oral poliovirus vaccine. This eliminates risk of accidental exposure.
5. Immediately report: Onset of infection, unusual bruising or bleeding, excessive fatigue, tremors or muscle twitching, difficulty walking, loss of appetite with nausea or vomiting.
6. It is advisable to avoid pregnancy while taking this drug. A nonhormonal method of contraception is recommended. Call your doctor promptly if you think pregnancy has occurred.

Precautions for Use
By Infants and Children: Dosage schedules and treatment monitoring should be supervised by a qualified pediatrician. Children with nephrotic syndrome can be more prone to drug-induced seizures.
By Those Over 60 Years of Age: Watch closely for central nervous system toxicity.

▷ **Advisability of Use During Pregnancy**
Pregnancy Category: D. See Pregnancy Risk Categories at the back of this book.
Animal studies: Rat studies reveal drug-associated defects of the nervous system, palate, skeleton, and urogenital system.
Human studies: Adequate studies of pregnant women are not available. There are two known cases of an infant born with an absent kidney and ureter following exposure to this drug during early pregnancy.
If possible, this drug should be avoided during pregnancy, especially the first 3 months.

A nonhormonal contraceptive is generally advisable during treatment with this and similar drugs.

Advisability of Use If Breast-Feeding
Presence of this drug in breast milk: Unknown.
Avoid drug or refrain from nursing.

Habit-Forming Potential: None.

Effects of Overdosage: Fatigue, weakness, fever, sore throat, bruising, agitation, unstable gait, bone marrow depression, seizures.

Possible Effects of Long-Term Use: Permanent sterility; secondary cancers (leukemia); lung damage (pulmonary fibrosis).

Suggested Periodic Examinations While Taking This Drug (at physician's discretion)
Before drug treatment and *periodically* during drug use: Complete blood counts, uric acid levels, liver function tests, sperm counts.

▷ **While Taking This Drug, Observe the Following**
Foods: No restrictions.
Beverages: No restrictions. May be taken with milk. It is advisable to drink 2 to 3 quarts of liquids daily to reduce the risk of kidney stone formation.
▷ *Alcohol:* Use with caution. Avoid if platelet counts are low and there is a risk of stomach bleeding.
Tobacco Smoking: No interactions expected, but I advise everyone to quit smoking.
Marijuana Smoking: Best avoided. This could increase the risk of central nervous system toxicity. Some fungal infections (toxoplasmosis) may be contracted from marijuana in patients with immune system suppression.
Other Drugs
Chlorambucil *taken concurrently* with
- amphotericin B (Abelcet) may increase risk of bronchial spasm, low blood pressure, and kidney (nephrotoxicity) toxicity.
- antidepressant or antipsychotic (neuroleptic) drugs requires careful monitoring; these drugs lower the seizure threshold and increase the risk of chlorambucil-induced seizures.
- aspirin may increase the risk of bruising or bleeding; the platelet-reduction effects of chlorambucil and the antiplatelet action of aspirin are additive; avoid aspirin while taking chlorambucil.
- other immunosuppressant drugs can increase the risk of infection and the development of secondary cancers.
▷ *Driving, Hazardous Activities:* This drug may cause nervous agitation, confusion, hallucinations, or seizures. Restrict activities as necessary.
Aviation Note: The use of this drug *may be a disqualification* for piloting. Consult a designated Aviation Medical Examiner.
Exposure to Sun: No restrictions.
Discontinuation: Whether this drug is used as an anticancer drug or immunosuppressant, many factors will determine when and how this drug should be stopped. In order to get the greatest benefit, follow your doctor's advice.

CHLORAMPHENICOL (klor am FEN i kohl)

Introduced: 1947   **Class:** Antibiotic   **Prescription:** USA: Yes   **Controlled Drug:** USA: No; Canada: No   **Available as Generic:** USA: Yes; Canada: No

Brand Names: Ak-Chlor, Chloracol, Chlorofair, Chloromycetin, Chloroptic, Chloroptic SOP, Econochlor, ✦Elase-Chloromycetin, I-Chlor, ✦Isopto Fenicol, ✦Minims, ✦Nova-Phenicol, ✦Novochlorocap, ✦Ocu-Chlor, Ophthochlor, ✦Ophtho-Chloram, Ophthocort, ✦PMS-Chloramphenicol, ✦Sopamycetin, ✦Sopamycetin/HC

BENEFITS versus RISKS

Possible Benefits	*Possible Risks*
VERY EFFECTIVE TREATMENT OF INFECTIONS due to susceptible microorganisms	BONE MARROW DEPRESSION APLASTIC ANEMIA (see Glossary) Peripheral neuritis (see Glossary) Liver damage, jaundice

---

Author's Note: Risks are largely as defined for systemic use, not ophthalmic.

▷ **Principal Uses**

As a Single Drug Product: Uses currently included in FDA-approved labeling: (1) Very effective in a broad spectrum of serious infections. However, because of serious toxicity (fatal aplastic anemia), it is now reserved for life-threatening (such as meningitis) infections caused by resistant organisms, and for infections in people who cannot tolerate other appropriate anti-infective drugs; (2) used in eye (intraocular) infections.

Other (unlabeled) generally accepted uses: (1) May have a role in prevention of plague; (2) can help when applied topically to pressure sores; (3) can be used topically to treat acne.

How This Drug Works: This drug prevents the growth and multiplication of susceptible microorganisms by interfering with their formation of essential proteins.

Available Dosage Forms and Strengths

Previously available capsules and oral suspensions are no longer made.

Cream — 1%
Eye/ear solutions — 0.5%
Eye ointment — 1%
Injection — 100 mg/ml
Ophthalmic/otic suspension — 2 mg/ml

▷ **Usual Adult Dosage Range:** Ophthalmic: Chloramphenicol plus hydrocortisone suspension or solution is given as two drops to the affected eye every 3 hours day and night for 48 hours. After this, the time between doses is usually lengthened and therapy continued until 48 hours after the eye appears normal. Intravenous: Total daily dose is 50 to 100 mg per kg of body mass divided into four doses, 6 hours apart. **Note: Actual dosage and administration schedule must be determined for each patient individually.**

Conditions Requiring Dosing Adjustments

Liver Function: Must be adjusted in liver failure based on blood levels.

Kidney Function: Adjustments in dose or dosing interval are suggested based on blood levels.

▷ **Dosing Instructions:** Shake ophthalmic or otic suspension well before dosing.

Usual Duration of Use: Use of the ophthalmic or otic preparations every 3 hours for 48 hours is needed to assess the benefit in fighting the infection. Use of the intravenous form on a regular schedule for 3 to 5 days is needed to see this drug's effectiveness in controlling the infection. Limit use to the time required to treat the infection. Repeated intravenous courses should be avoided if possible.

Author's Note: Since use of this medicine has declined, the profile has been shortened in order to make room for more widely used medicines.

CHLOROQUINE (KLOR oh kwin)

Introduced: 1964   **Class:** Amebecide, antimalarial   **Prescription:** USA: Yes   **Controlled Drug:** USA: No; Canada: No   **Available as Generic:** USA: Yes; Canada: No

Brand Names: Aralen, Kronofed-A-JR

Warning: The brand names Aralen and Arlidin are similar and can be mistaken for each other; this can lead to serious medication errors. These names represent very different drugs. Verify that you are taking the correct drug.

BENEFITS versus RISKS

Possible Benefits	*Possible Risks*
EFFECTIVE PREVENTION AND TREATMENT OF CERTAIN FORMS OF MALARIA	INFREQUENT BUT SERIOUS DAMAGE OF CORNEAL AND RETINAL EYE TISSUES
EFFECTIVE COMBINATION TREATMENT OF SOME FORMS OF AMEBIC INFECTION	RARE BUT SERIOUS BONE MARROW DEPRESSION; aplastic anemia, deficient white blood cells and platelets
Possibly effective in palindromic rheumatism	Heart muscle damage—rare
Possibly effective in short-term treatment of systemic lupus erythematosus	Ear damage; hearing loss, ringing in ears—rare
Can be of help in refractory rheumatoid arthritis	Eye damage—rare

---

▷ **Principal Uses**

As a Single Drug Product: Uses currently included in FDA-approved labeling: (1) Treatment of acute attacks of certain types of malarial infection; (2) treatment for certain forms of amebic infection.

Other (unlabeled) generally accepted uses: (1) Reduces disease activity in refractory rheumatoid and juvenile arthritis; (2) suppress disease activity in certain types of lupus erythematosus (patients are switched to hydroxychloroquine as soon as possible); (3) treatment of sarcoidosis, polymorphous light eruption, and porphyria; (4) may give dramatic results in palindromic rheumatism; (5) second-line agent for people traveling in areas where there is risk of malaria.

How This Drug Works: In treating malaria and amebiasis, this drug impairs the function of DNA in the protozoa that cause these diseases. As an antiarthritic and anti-lupus drug, it acts as a mild immunosuppressant. It accumulates in white blood cells and blocks many enzymes involved in tissue destruction.

Available Dosage Forms and Strengths

Injection — 50 mg/ml
Tablets — 250 mg, 500 mg

▷ **Usual Adult Dosage Range:**   For malaria suppression: 500 mg once every 7 days.

For malaria treatment: Initially 1 g, followed by 500 mg in 6 to 8 hours; then 500 mg once a day on the second and third days.

For amebiasis (other than intestinal): Initially 250 mg four times daily for 2 days; then 250 mg two times daily for 2 to 3 weeks.

For rheumatoid arthritis: Up to 4 mg per kg of lean body weight daily.

For lupus erythematosus: Up to 4 mg per kg of lean body weight daily.

Note: Actual dosage and administration schedule must be determined for each patient individually.

Conditions Requiring Dosing Adjustments

Liver Function: Blood levels are needed, and the dose should be adjusted appropriately. Half of the medicine is removed by the liver.

Kidney Function: In severe kidney failure 50% of the normal dose should be used. If therapy is extended, 50 to 100 mg of chloroquine base should be given daily.

▷ **Dosing Instructions:**   Tablet may be crushed and taken with food or milk to reduce stomach irritation. Take full course of treatment as prescribed. For malaria prevention, begin medication 2 weeks before entering malarious area; continue medication while in the area and for 4 weeks after leaving the area. When treating arthritis or lupus, take medication on a regular schedule daily; use for 6 months may be needed to see peak effect.

Usual Duration of Use: Use on a regular schedule for 2 weeks before exposure, during period of exposure, and 4 weeks after exposure is needed to realize effectiveness in preventing malaria. Use on a regular schedule for up to 6 months may be required to evaluate benefits in treating rheumatoid arthritis and lupus erythematosus. The drug is changed to hydroxychloroquine because it is less toxic. Long-term use (months to years) requires periodic physician evaluation of response and dose adjustments.

Possible Advantages of This Drug

May be more effective than hydroxychloroquine in some cases of lupus erythematosus.

▷ **This Drug Should Not Be Taken If**

- you have an allergy to chloroquine or hydroxychloroquine.
- you have an active bone marrow or blood cell disorder.
- you have significant pathology of the heart muscle (cardiomyopathy).
- you have existing visual field or retinal changes.

▷ **Inform Your Physician Before Taking This Drug If**
- you are pregnant or planning pregnancy.
- you have bone marrow depression or a blood cell disorder.
- you have a deficiency of glucose-6-phosphate dehydrogenase (G6PD).
- you have any eye disorder, especially disease of the cornea or retina, or visual field changes.
- you have a history of mental illness.
- you have impaired hearing or ringing in the ears.
- you have a seizure disorder, movement disorders, or a history of peripheral neuritis.
- you have low blood pressure or a heart rhythm disorder.
- you have a history of peptic ulcer disease, Crohn's disease, or ulcerative colitis.
- you have impaired liver or kidney function or porphyria.
- you have any form of psoriasis.
- you are taking antacids, cimetidine, or penicillamine.

Possible Side Effects (natural, expected, and unavoidable drug actions)
Light-headedness (low blood pressure); blue-black discoloration of skin, fingernails, or mouth lining with long-term use.

▷ **Possible Adverse Effects** (unusual, unexpected, and infrequent reactions)
If any of the following develop, consult your physician promptly for guidance.

Mild Adverse Effects
Allergic reactions: skin rash, itching (more common in African-Americans)—possible.
Loss of hair color, loss of hair—case reports.
Headache, blurring of near vision (reading), ringing in ears—case reports.
Loss of appetite, nausea, vomiting, stomach cramps, diarrhea—possible.

Serious Adverse Effects
Allergic reactions: severe skin rash (erythema multiforme)—case reports.
Idiosyncratic reactions: hemolytic anemia in those with glucose-6-phosphate dehydrogenase (G6PD) deficiency in red blood cells.
Aplastic anemia (see Glossary): abnormally low red cells (fatigue and weakness), low white blood cell counts (fever, sore throat, infections), abnormally low platelets (abnormal bruising or bleeding)—case reports.
Emotional or psychotic mental changes; seizures—case reports.
Movement disorders (ataxia, dyskinesias)—case reports.
Muscle damage (myopathy)—case reports.
Loss of hearing, ringing in the ears—case reports.
Low blood sugar (hypoglycemia)—case reports.
Eye damage (cornea and retina), with significant impairment of vision—possible.
Heart rhythm abnormalities—case reports.

▷ **Possible Effects on Sexual Function:**   None reported.

Possible Delayed Adverse Effects: Retinal damage (reports of development 7 years after stopping) is more likely to occur following high-dose and/or long-term use.

Adverse Effects That May Mimic Natural Diseases or Disorders

Central nervous system toxicity mimics unrelated neuropsychiatric disorder. Seizures may suggest the onset of epilepsy.

Natural Diseases or Disorders That May Be Activated by This Drug

Porphyria, psoriasis.

Possible Effects on Laboratory Tests

Complete blood counts: decreased red cells, hemoglobin, white cells, and platelets.

Liver function tests: increased liver enzymes (AST/GOT) and bilirubin.

Urine tests for drug abuse: *initial* test result may be falsely **positive**; *confirmatory* test will be **negative**. (Test results depend upon amount of drug taken and testing method used.)

Blood sugar (glucose): decreased.

Electrocardiogram: conduction abnormalities, prolonged QRS interval, T wave changes, heart block.

CAUTION

1. Will not prevent relapses in certain types of malaria. Ask your doctor for advice.
2. Not effective in treating acute amebic dysentery (intestinal infection) or asymptomatic carriers.
3. High-dose and/or long-term use of this drug may cause irreversible retinal damage; such use may also cause hearing loss due to nerve damage. Promptly report any vision or hearing changes.

Precautions for Use

By Infants and Children: This age group is very sensitive to the effects of this drug. Dosages should be chosen and therapy monitored by a qualified pediatrician.

By Those Over 60 Years of Age: Reduced tolerance for high-dose and/or long-term use. Watch for behavioral changes, low blood pressure, heart rhythm disturbances, muscle weakness, and changes in vision or hearing.

▷ Advisability of Use During Pregnancy

Pregnancy Category: C. See Pregnancy Risk Categories at the back of this book.

Animal studies: 47% of rat fetuses revealed undeveloped or partially developed eyes.

Human studies: Adequate studies of pregnant women are not available. A 1964 report includes drug-induced congenital deafness, retinal damage, gait instability, and asymmetric body growth. A 1991 study of use in systemic lupus erythematosus concluded that the benefit outweighed the fetal risk. Avoid use during pregnancy except for the suppression or treatment of malaria or amebic infection of the liver. Seek your doctor's advice.

Advisability of Use If Breast-Feeding

Presence of this drug in breast milk: Yes.

Avoid drug or refrain from nursing.

Habit-Forming Potential: None.

Effects of Overdosage: Drowsiness, headache, blurred vision, excitability, low blood pressure, seizures, coma.

Possible Effects of Long-Term Use: Irreversible eye damage (cornea and retina), hearing loss, myocarditis, muscle weakness, aplastic anemia.

Suggested Periodic Examinations While Taking This Drug (at physician's discretion)

    Complete blood counts; liver and kidney function tests. Serial blood pressure readings and electrocardiograms. Neurological examinations for significant muscle weakness.

    Complete eye examinations before starting high-dose or long-term treatment, then every 3 to 6 months during drug use. Hearing tests as indicated.

▷ **While Taking This Drug, Observe the Following**

    Foods: No restrictions.

    Beverages: No restrictions. May be taken with milk.

▷   *Alcohol:* Use sparingly to minimize stomach irritation.

    Tobacco Smoking: No interactions expected, but I advise everyone to quit smoking.

▷   *Other Drugs*

    Chloroquine may *increase* the effects of
- cyclosporine (Sandimmune) and increase risk of kidney toxicity.
- penicillamine (Cuprimine, Depen), and increase its toxic potential.

    Chloroquine may *decrease* the effects of
- ampicillin (Amcil) or bacampicillin (Spectrobid).
- methotrexate (Mexate, others).
- rabies vaccine.

    The following drug may *increase* the effects of chloroquine:
- cimetidine (Tagamet).

    The following drugs may *decrease* the effects of chloroquine:
- magnesium salts and antacids.

▷   *Driving, Hazardous Activities:* This drug may cause light-headedness, blurred vision, or impaired hearing. Restrict activities as necessary.

    Aviation Note: The use of this drug *may be a disqualification* for piloting. Consult a designated Aviation Medical Examiner.

    Exposure to Sun: This drug may cause photosensitivity (see Glossary).

    Discontinuation: This drug should be stopped and prompt evaluation made if any changes in vision or hearing, seizures, unusual muscle weakness, infection (fever, sore throat, etc.), or abnormal bruising or bleeding occurs.

CHLOROTHIAZIDE (klor oh THI a zide)

See the thiazide diuretics profile for further information.

CHLORPROMAZINE (klor PROH ma zeen)

Introduced: 1952   **Class:** Antipsychotic, strong tranquilizer, phenothiazines   **Prescription:** USA: Yes   **Controlled Drug:** USA: No; Canada: No   **Available as Generic:** Yes

Brand Names: ✦Chlorpromanyl, ✦Largactil, ✦Novochlorpromazine, Ormazine, Thora-Dex, Thorazine, Thorazine SR

```
┌─────────────────────────────────────────────────────────────┐
│                    BENEFITS versus RISKS                      │
│      Possible Benefits              Possible Risks            │
│ EFFECTIVE CONTROL OF ACUTE    Toxic effects on the brain with │
│   MENTAL DISORDERS              long-term use—rare but possible│
│ Beneficial effects on thinking, mood,  Liver damage with jaundice—rare │
│   and behavior                Rare blood disorders: hemolytic │
│ Moderately effective control of nausea  anemia, abnormally low white │
│   and vomiting                  blood count                   │
│                               Eye toxicity                    │
└─────────────────────────────────────────────────────────────┘
```

▷ **Principal Uses**

As a Single Drug Product: Uses currently included in FDA-approved labeling: (1) Treats acute and chronic psychotic disorders such as agitated depression, schizophrenia, and mania; (2) can be used for presurgical anxiety; (3) helps reduce symptoms in porphyrias and tetanus; (4) is used to stop prolonged hiccups; (5) lessens or stops vomiting caused by toxic chemotherapy or a potent drug used to treat fungal infections (amphotericin B).

Other (unlabeled) generally accepted uses: (1) Can be of help in complicated drug withdrawal cases; (2) lessens the symptoms of Tourette's syndrome; (3) may be of help in combination therapy of tuberculosis; (4) can be used intravenously after some heart surgeries.

How This Drug Works: By inhibiting the action of dopamine, this drug acts to correct an imbalance of nerve impulses found in some mental disorders.

Available Dosage Forms and Strengths

Capsules, prolonged action — 30 mg, 75 mg, 150 mg, 200 mg, 300 mg

Concentrate — 30 mg/ml and 100 mg/ml

Oral drops — 40 mg/ml

Injection — 25 mg/ml

Suppositories — 25 mg, 100 mg

Syrup — 10 mg/5 ml

Tablets — 10 mg, 25 mg, 50 mg, 100 mg, 200 mg

▷ **Usual Adult Dosage Range:**   Initially 10 to 25 mg three or four times daily. Dose may be increased by 20 to 50 mg at 3- to 4-day intervals as needed and tolerated. Usual dosage range is 300 to 800 mg daily. Extreme range is 25 to 2000 mg daily. Total daily dosage should not exceed 2000 mg. **Note: Actual dosage and administration schedule must be determined for each patient individually.**

Conditions Requiring Dosing Adjustments

Liver Function: Use with caution and in decreased dose in patients with compromised livers. Can also be a cause of a specific kind of (cholestatic) jaundice.

Kidney Function: Blood levels are recommended if used in severe kidney compromise.

▷ **Dosing Instructions:**   Tablets may be crushed and taken with or after meals to reduce stomach irritation. Prolonged-action capsules may be opened, but not crushed or chewed.

Usual Duration of Use: Use on a regular schedule for several weeks is usually needed to see this drug's effectiveness in controlling psychotic disorders. If benefits are not seen in 6 weeks, it should be stopped. Long-term use (months to years) requires periodic physician evaluation.

▷ **This Drug Should Not Be Taken If**
- you are allergic to any form of this drug.
- you have active liver disease.
- you have taken a large amount of alcohol or narcotics.
- you have cancer of the breast.
- you have a current blood cell or bone marrow disorder.

▷ **Inform Your Physician Before Taking This Drug If**
- you are allergic or very sensitive to any phenothiazine drug (see Drug Classes).
- you have impaired liver or kidney function.
- you have any type of seizure disorder.
- you have diabetes, glaucoma, or heart disease.
- you have a history of lupus erythematosus.
- you have experienced neuroleptic malignant syndrome previously.
- you work in extreme heat or are typically exposed to organophosphorous insecticides.
- you are taking any drug with sedative effects.
- you plan to have surgery with anesthesia (general or spinal) soon.

Possible Side Effects (natural, expected, and unavoidable drug actions)
Drowsiness (usually during the first 2 weeks), orthostatic hypotension (see Glossary), blurred vision, dry mouth, nasal congestion, constipation, impaired urination.
Pink or purple coloration of urine, of no clinical significance.

▷ **Possible Adverse Effects** (unusual, unexpected, and infrequent reactions)
If any of the following develop, consult your physician promptly for guidance.
Mild Adverse Effects
Allergic reactions: skin rash, hives, low-grade fever—case reports.
Lowering of body temperature, especially in the elderly—possible.
Increased appetite and weight gain.
Weakness, agitation, insomnia, impaired day and night vision.
Chronic constipation, fecal impaction—possible.
Serious Adverse Effects
Allergic reactions: hepatitis with jaundice (see Glossary), usually between second and fourth week; high fever; asthma; anaphylactic reaction (see Glossary): case reports—rare.
Idiosyncratic reactions: neuroleptic malignant syndrome (see Glossary)—rare.
Depression, disorientation, seizures—possible.
Eye (ocular) toxicity—case reports.
Disturbances of heart rhythm—case reports.
Hemolytic or aplastic anemia (see Glossary)—case reports.
Low blood platelets or low white blood cells: fever, sore throat, infections—case reports.
Parkinson-like disorders (see Glossary): muscle spasms of face, jaw, neck, back, extremities—rare to frequent.
Prolonged drop in blood pressure with weakness, perspiration, and fainting

or drop in blood pressure on standing (orthostatic hypotension)—infrequent.

▷ **Possible Effects on Sexual Function**

Decreased libido and impotence (1200 mg/day); inhibited ejaculation (400 mg/day); priapism (see Glossary) (250 mg/day); male infertility (30 to 800 mg/day); enlargement of male breasts (gynecomastia)—case reports; enlargement of female breasts with milk production, cessation of menstruation (30 to 800 mg/day).

Adverse Effects That May Mimic Natural Diseases or Disorders

Nervous system reactions may suggest Parkinson's disease. Liver reactions may suggest viral hepatitis. Reactions resembling systemic lupus erythematosus can occur.

Natural Diseases or Disorders That May Be Activated by This Drug

Latent epilepsy, glaucoma, diabetes mellitus (25%), prostatism (see Glossary).

Possible Effects on Laboratory Tests

Complete blood counts: decreased red cells, hemoglobin, white cells, and platelets; increased eosinophils (often warns of jaundice).

Antinuclear antibodies (ANA): positive in 63% of long-term users.

Blood cholesterol level: increased (with liver damage).

Blood glucose level: increased with long-term use.

Glucose tolerance test (GTT): decreased; 40% abnormal with chronic use.

Partial thromboplastin time (PTT): increased.

Blood uric acid level: decreased.

Liver function tests: increased liver enzymes (ALT/GPT, AST/GOT, and alkaline phosphatase); increased bilirubin.

Urine pregnancy tests: false positive results with frog, rabbit, and immunological tests.

CAUTION

1. Many over-the-counter medications (see Glossary) for allergies, colds, and coughs should not be combined with this drug. Ask your physician or pharmacist for help.
2. Antacids that contain aluminum and/or magnesium can lower absorption of this drug and reduce its effect.
3. Obtain prompt evaluation of any change or disturbance of vision.
4. This drug can cause false positive pregnancy test results.

Precautions for Use

By Infants and Children: This drug has been used in neonates. Younger children may require more frequent dosing. Do not use in children of any age with symptoms suggestive of Reye syndrome (see Glossary). Watch carefully for blood cell changes.

By Those Over 60 Years of Age: You may be more susceptible to the development of drowsiness, lethargy, constipation, lowering of body temperature (hypothermia), and orthostatic hypotension (see Glossary). Can worsen existing prostatism (see Glossary). Parkinson-like reactions and/or tardive dyskinesia (see discussion of these terms in Glossary) are more likely. Symptoms must be recognized early, since they may become irreversible.

▷ **Advisability of Use During Pregnancy**

Pregnancy Category: C. See Pregnancy Risk Categories at the back of this book.

Animal studies: No birth defects reported in rodent studies. However, rodent studies suggest possible permanent neurological damage to the fetus.

Human studies: No increase in birth defects reported in 284 exposures. Adequate studies of pregnant women are not available. Limit use to small and infrequent doses only when clearly needed. Avoid drug during the last month of pregnancy.

Advisability of Use If Breast-Feeding

Presence of this drug in breast milk: Yes, in small amounts.

Ask your doctor for advice.

Habit-Forming Potential: None.

Effects of Overdosage: Marked drowsiness, weakness, tremor, agitation, unsteadiness, deep sleep, coma, convulsions.

Possible Effects of Long-Term Use: Tardive dyskinesia in 10% to 20% (see Glossary); eye changes—cataracts and pigmentation of retina; gray to violet pigmentation of skin in exposed areas, more common in women; severe ulcerative colitis.

Suggested Periodic Examinations While Taking This Drug (at physician's discretion)

Complete blood counts, especially between 4 to 10 weeks of treatment.

Liver function tests, electrocardiograms.

Complete eye examinations—eye structures and vision.

Careful tongue inspection for fine, involuntary, wavelike movements that could be the beginning of tardive dyskinesia.

▷ **While Taking This Drug, Observe the Following**

Foods: No restrictions.

Nutritional Support: A riboflavin (vitamin B_2) supplement should be taken with long-term use. Vitamin C may blunt therapeutic benefits.

Beverages: Caffeine may lessen calming effect of drug. May be taken with milk.

▷ *Alcohol:* Avoid completely. Increases phenothiazine sedative action and accentuates their depressant effects on brain function and blood pressure. Phenothiazines can increase the intoxicating effects of alcohol.

Tobacco Smoking: Possible reduction of drowsiness from drug, but I advise everyone to quit smoking.

Marijuana Smoking: Moderate increase in drowsiness; worsened orthostatic hypotension; increased risk of precipitating latent psychoses.

▷ *Other Drugs*

Chlorpromazine may ***increase*** the effects of

• all atropinelike drugs, and cause nervous system toxicity.

• all sedatives or narcotics, especially meperidine (Demerol).

• zolpidem (Ambien).

Chlorpromazine may ***decrease*** the effects of

• guanethidine (Ismelin, Esimil), and reduce its effectiveness in lowering blood pressure.

• oral antidiabetic drugs (see Drug Classes).

Chlorpromazine ***taken concurrently*** with

• ACE inhibitors (see Drug Classes) causes excessive lowering of blood pressure.

- amphetamine will cause decreased effects of both drugs.
- beta-blockers (see Drug Classes) can intensify the effects of both drugs.
- birth control pills (oral contraceptives) may lead to increased chlorpromazine levels.
- lithium (Lithobid, others) may result in a decrease in lithium or chlorpromazine effectiveness.
- propranolol (Inderal) may cause increased effects of both drugs; watch drug effects closely—doses may have to be decreased.
- ritonavir (Norvir) and perhaps other protease inhibitors (see Drug Classes) may lead to chlorpromazine toxicity.
- valproic acid (Depakene) can result in elevated valproic acid blood levels and toxicity.

The following drugs may *decrease* the effects of chlorpromazine:
- antacids containing aluminum and/or magnesium.
- benztropine (Cogentin).
- trihexyphenidyl (Artane).

▷ *Driving, Hazardous Activities:* This drug can impair mental alertness, judgment, and physical coordination. Avoid hazardous activities.

Aviation Note: The use of this drug *is a disqualification* for piloting. Consult a designated Aviation Medical Examiner.

Exposure to Sun: Use caution. Some phenothiazines cause photosensitivity (see Glossary).

Exposure to Heat: Use caution and avoid excessive heat. This drug can impair body temperature regulation and increase the risk of heatstroke.

Exposure to Cold: Use caution and dress warmly. Increased risk of hypothermia in the elderly.

Discontinuation: After long-term use, do not stop this drug suddenly. Gradually withdraw over 2 to 3 weeks. Do not stop this drug without your physician's knowledge and approval. Schizophrenia relapse rate after discontinuation is 50% to 60%.

CHLORPROPAMIDE (klor PROH pa mide)

Introduced: 1958   **Class:** Antidiabetic, sulfonylureas   **Prescription:** USA: Yes   **Controlled Drug:** USA: No; Canada: No   **Available as Generic:** Yes

Brand Names: ✦Apo-Chlorpropamide, ✦Chloronase, Diabinese, Glucamide

BENEFITS versus RISKS	
Possible Benefits	*Possible Risks*
Helps in regulating blood sugar in noninsulin-dependent diabetes (adjunctive to appropriate diet and weight control)	HYPOGLYCEMIA, severe and prolonged
	Allergic skin reactions (some severe)
	Water retention
Tight blood sugar control may avoid or delay blood vessel, heart, nerve, and vision damage possible with uncontrolled increased in blood sugar	Liver damage or blood cell and bone marrow disorders—rare

▷ **Principal Uses**
   As a Single Drug Product: Uses currently included in FDA-approved labeling:
   Helps control mild to moderate type II diabetes mellitus (adult, maturity-
   onset) that does not require insulin, but is not adequately controlled by diet
   alone.
   Other (unlabeled) generally accepted uses: (1) May be of help in easing abnormal urine output (SIADH); (2) can be used as a test to define some genetic
   characteristics of diabetes (CPAF test); (3) can be of benefit for some people
   who have an excessive reaction to sugar (reactive hypoglycemia).

How This Drug Works: This drug (1) stimulates the secretion of insulin if the
   pancreas is capable of responding to stimulation, and (2) enhances the utilization of insulin by appropriate tissues.

Available Dosage Forms and Strengths
   Tablets — 100 mg, 250 mg

▷ **Usual Adult Dosage Range:**   Initially 250 mg daily with breakfast. After 5 to 7
   days, dose may be increased to 500 mg daily if needed and tolerated. Total
   daily dosage should not exceed 750 mg. **Note: Actual dosage and administration schedule must be determined for each patient individually.**

Conditions Requiring Dosing Adjustments
   Liver Function: The dose **must** be decreased in patients with liver compromise.
   Kidney Function: One researcher advocated a 50% decrease in dose in mild to
   moderate kidney failure and that this medicine should be avoided (and a
   different oral hypoglycemic used) in patients with moderate to severe kidney failure.

▷ **Dosing Instructions:**   Tablet may be crushed when taken. Taking with food
   reduces stomach irritation.

Usual Duration of Use: Use on a regular schedule for 1 to 2 weeks is usually
   needed to see peak effect in controlling diabetes. Failure to respond to maximum doses in 1 month is a primary failure. Up to 15% of those who respond initially may develop secondary failure of the drug within a year.
   Periodic measurement of blood sugar is needed. See your physician on a
   regular basis.

▷ **This Drug Should Not Be Taken If**
   • you have had an allergic reaction to it previously.
   • you have severe impairment of liver or kidney function.
   • you are pregnant.
   • you make ketone bodies (ketosis). Ask your doctor.
   • you are a brittle, juvenile, or unstable diabetic.

▷ **Inform Your Physician Before Taking This Drug If**
   • you are allergic to other sulfonylurea drugs or "sulfa" drugs.
   • your diabetes has been unstable or "brittle" in the past.
   • you have a history of blood disorders.
   • you do not know how to recognize or treat hypoglycemia (see Glossary).
   • you have a history of congestive heart failure, kidney disease, peptic ulcer
     disease, cirrhosis of the liver, hypothyroidism, or porphyria.
   • you have glucose-6-dehydrogenase (G6PD) deficiency (ask your doctor).

Possible Side Effects (natural, expected, and unavoidable drug actions)

If drug dose is excessive or food intake is delayed or inadequate, low blood sugar (hypoglycemia) will occur as a drug effect.

▷ **Possible Adverse Effects** (unusual, unexpected, and infrequent reactions)

If any of the following develop, consult your physician promptly for guidance.

Mild Adverse Effects

Allergic reactions: skin rash, hives, itching, drug fever—rare to infrequent.

Headache, ringing in ears, weakness, numbness and tingling—rare.

Indigestion, nausea, vomiting, diarrhea (may be severe)—rare to infrequent.

Water retention (edema), weight gain—case reports.

Serious Adverse Effects

Allergic reactions: hepatitis with jaundice (see Glossary)—rare; severe skin reactions—case reports.

Idiosyncratic reaction: hemolytic anemia (see Glossary)—case reports.

Disulfiramlike reaction (see Glossary) with concurrent use of alcohol—possible.

SIADH (ask your doctor)—rare, but more likely in women over 60 years old taking more than 500 mg daily.

Lowered thyroid function (hypothyroidism)—case reports.

Bone marrow depression (see Glossary)—fatigue, weakness, fever, sore throat, abnormal bleeding or bruising—case reports, rare.

Abnormal heartbeats—case report with a 2500-mg dose.

Persistent diarrhea (pseudomembranous colitis)—case reports.

Severe skin reactions (Stevens-Johnson syndrome)—rare.

▷ **Possible Effects on Sexual Function:**   None reported.

Adverse Effects That May Mimic Natural Diseases or Disorders

Liver reactions may suggest viral hepatitis.

Natural Diseases or Disorders That May Be Activated by This Drug

Acute intermittent porphyria, congestive heart failure (in predisposed individuals), peptic ulcer disease.

Possible Effects on Laboratory Tests

Complete blood cell counts: decreased red cells, hemoglobin, white cells, and platelets; increased eosinophils (allergic reaction).

Blood sodium: increased or decreased.

INR (prothrombin time): increased (with liver damage).

Blood thyroxine (T_4) level: decreased.

Liver function tests: increased liver enzymes (ALT/GPT, AST/GOT, and alkaline phosphatase), increased bilirubin.

CAUTION

1. This drug must be only one part of a total diabetes management program. It is not a substitute for a prescribed diet and regular exercise.
2. Over time (usually several months), this drug may lose its effectiveness in controlling blood sugar levels. Periodic follow-up examinations are necessary.
3. This drug has a long duration of action (up to 60 hours). It can produce severe and prolonged hypoglycemia, especially in the elderly.

Precautions for Use

By Infants and Children: This drug does not work in type I (juvenile, growth-onset) insulin-dependent diabetes.

By Those Over 60 Years of Age: Should be avoided in this age group. Because its effect lasts such a long time, it can accumulate and cause marked and prolonged hypoglycemia. Repeated hypoglycemia in the elderly can cause brain damage.

▷ **Advisability of Use During Pregnancy**

Pregnancy Category: C by manufacturer; D by some researchers. See Pregnancy Risk Categories at the back of this book.

Animal studies: Specific studies have not been conducted in animals.

Human studies: Adequate studies of pregnant women are not available.

Ask your doctor for guidance. Insulin is clearly the drug of choice during pregnancy to control glucose levels.

Advisability of Use If Breast-Feeding

Presence of this drug in breast milk: Yes.

Avoid drug or refrain from nursing.

Habit-Forming Potential: None.

Effects of Overdosage: Symptoms of mild to severe hypoglycemia: headache, light-headedness, faintness, nervousness, confusion, tremor, sweating, heart palpitation, weakness, hunger, nausea, vomiting, stupor progressing to coma.

Possible Effects of Long-Term Use: Reduced function of the thyroid gland (hypothyroidism). Reports of increased frequency and severity of heart and blood vessel diseases associated with long-term use of this class of drugs was based on a study of tolbutamide, but may apply to any drug in this class. A direct cause-and-effect relationship (see Glossary) is tenuous. Ask your physician for guidance.

Suggested Periodic Examinations While Taking This Drug (at physician's discretion)

Complete blood cell counts, liver function tests, thyroid function tests, periodic evaluation of heart and circulatory system, hemoglobin A1-C.

▷ **While Taking This Drug, Observe the Following**

Foods: Follow the diabetic diet prescribed by your physician.

Beverages: As directed in the diabetic diet. May be taken with milk.

▷ *Alcohol:* Avoid this combination. Alcohol can exaggerate this drug's hypoglycemic effect. This drug can also cause a disulfiramlike reaction (see Glossary): facial flushing, sweating, palpitation.

Tobacco Smoking: No interactions expected, but I advise everyone to quit smoking.

▷ *Other Drugs*

The following drugs may ***increase*** the effects of chlorpropamide:

- ammonium chloride.
- aspirin, aspirin-containing combination drugs (see aspirin profile), and other salicylates.
- beta-blockers (see Drug Classes) and cause slowed recovery from any low blood sugars that may occur.
- calcium channel blockers (see Drug Classes).

- chloramphenicol (Chloromycetin).
- clofibrate (Atromid-S).
- dicumarol.
- fenfluramine (Pondimin).
- monoamine oxidase (MAO) type A inhibitor drugs (see Drug Classes).
- NSAIDs (see Drug Classes).
- some "sulfa" drugs: sulfamethoxazole (Gantanol), sulfisoxazole (Gantrisin), Septra, Bactrim.

The following drugs may *decrease* the effects of chlorpropamide:
- diazoxide (Proglycem).
- estrogens.
- phenothiazines (see Drug Classes).
- phenytoin (Dilantin).
- rifampin (Rifadin, Rimactane).
- sodium bicarbonate.
- steroids or cortisonelike medicines (see Drug Classes).
- thiazide diuretics (see Drug Classes).

Chlorpropamide **taken concurrently** with
- acarbose (Precose) may further lower blood sugar. This may be a therapeutic benefit or a cause for caution.

▷ *Driving, Hazardous Activities:* Dosing, eating schedule, and physical activities must be carefully regulated to prevent hypoglycemia. Know the early symptoms of hypoglycemia so you can avoid hazardous activities and take corrective measures.

Aviation Note: Diabetes *is a disqualification* for piloting. Consult a designated Aviation Medical Examiner.

Exposure to Sun: Use caution. Drugs of this class can cause photosensitivity (see Glossary).

Occurrence of Unrelated Illness: Acute infections, illnesses causing vomiting or diarrhea, serious injuries, and surgical procedures can change diabetic control and may require insulin use. Consult your physician promptly.

Discontinuation: Only about 12% of patients remain well controlled by this drug for more than 6 to 7 years. It is advisable to evaluate the continued benefit of this drug every 6 months.

CHLORTHALIDONE (klor THAL i dohn)

See the thiazide diuretics profile for further information.

CHOLESTYRAMINE (koh LES tir a meen)

Introduced: 1959   **Class:** Anticholesterol   **Prescription:** USA: Yes
Controlled Drug: USA: No; Canada: No   **Available as Generic:** USA: No; Canada: No
Brand Names: Questran, Questran Light
   Author's Note: Questran and Questran Light have been proposed to the FDA to be changed from prescription to nonprescription status. To date, approval has not been granted.

```
┌─────────────────────────────────────────────────────────────────┐
│                     BENEFITS versus RISKS                          │
│        Possible Benefits                  Possible Risks           │
│  EFFECTIVE REDUCTION OF TOTAL    Constipation (may be severe)      │
│    CHOLESTEROL AND               Reduced absorption of fat, fat-soluble │
│    LOW-DENSITY CHOLESTEROL         vitamins (A, D, E, and K), and folic │
│    IN TYPE IIa CHOLESTEROL         acid                            │
│    DISORDERS                     Reduced formation of prothrombin  │
│  Reduction of total cholesterol and   with possible bleeding      │
│    reduction of LDL cholesterol                                    │
│  EFFECTIVE RELIEF OF ITCHING                                       │
│    associated with biliary obstruction                            │
│  Effective binding of medicines in                                 │
│    some drug overdoses                                             │
└─────────────────────────────────────────────────────────────────┘
```

▷ **Principal Uses**

As a Single Drug Product: Uses currently included in FDA-approved labeling: Used to (1) treat a new condition called arteriohepatic dysplasia, which results in liver and heart problems; (2) reduces abnormally high blood levels of total cholesterol and low-density (LDL) cholesterol in Type IIa cholesterol disorders; (3) relieves itching due to the deposit of bile acids in the skin associated with partial biliary obstruction; (4) reduces risk of heart disease in type II hyperlipoproteinemia; (5) reduces progression of disease in coronary arteries in people with type II hyperlipoproteinemia.

Other (unlabeled) generally accepted uses: (1) May be of help in biliary fistulas and skin irritations seen in colostomy; (2) can help lower thyroid hormone levels if too much thyroid hormone has been given in error; (3) may help treat cholesterol ester storage disease (CESD); (4) helps relapses of resistant diarrhea (pseudomembranous colitis); (5) may help regression of atherosclerosis (increase coronary lumen size).

How This Drug Works: It combines with bile acids and bile salts in the intestinal tract, and forms insoluble complexes that are excreted in the feces. This process stimulates conversion of cholesterol to bile acids to replace the loss, and reduces cholesterol levels. By reducing the blood levels of bile acids, this drug reduces bile acids deposited in the skin and relieves itching.

Available Dosage Forms and Strengths
    Cans — 378 g
    Packets — 4 g, 9 g

▷ **Usual Adult Dosage Range:** Diarrhea (pseudomembranous colitis): 2–4 g two or three times daily.

Hypercholesterolemia: 9 g of powder (equivalent to 4 g of cholestyramine) one to six times daily. Dose may be increased slowly as needed and tolerated. The total daily dosage should not exceed 72 g of powder (32 g of cholestyramine). **Note: Actual dosage and administration schedule must be determined for each patient individually.**

Conditions Requiring Dosing Adjustments

Liver Function: Cholestyramine is eliminated via the feces—no liver involvement.

Kidney Function: This medication is **not** absorbed, and the kidney is not involved.

▷ **Dosing Instructions:**   Always take just before or with a meal; this drug is ineffective when taken without food. Mix the powder thoroughly in 4 to 6 ounces of water, fruit juice, milk, thin soup, or a soft food like applesauce; do not use carbonated beverages. **Do not take it in its dry form.**

Usual Duration of Use: Use on a regular schedule for up to 3 weeks may be needed to see this drug's benefit in lowering excessively high cholesterol. Duration of use should not exceed 3 months if an adequate response does not occur. Long-term use (months to years) requires periodic evaluation of response.

▷ **This Drug Should Not Be Taken If**
- you have had an allergic reaction to it previously.
- you have complete obstruction of the bile duct (biliary obstruction).
- you have type III, IV, or V hyperlipoproteinemia, as this drug does not work in these conditions. Ask your doctor.

▷ **Inform Your Physician Before Taking This Drug If**
- you are prone to constipation.
- you have peptic ulcer disease.
- you have a bleeding disorder of any kind.
- you have impaired kidney function.
- you have phenylketonuria (PKU), as Questran Light has aspartame.
- you have a bleeding disorder.

Possible Side Effects (natural, expected, and unavoidable drug actions)
Constipation; interference with normal fat digestion and absorption; reduced absorption of vitamins A, D, E, and K and folic acid. Possible tooth discoloration with prolonged contact with teeth. (Do not swish this product in the mouth.)

▷ **Possible Adverse Effects** (unusual, unexpected, and infrequent reactions)
If any of the following develop, consult your physician promptly for guidance.
Mild Adverse Effects
Allergic reactions: skin rash, hives, tongue irritation, anal itching—rare.
Loss of appetite, heartburn, abdominal discomfort, excessive gas, nausea, vomiting, diarrhea—possible.
Constipation—frequent.
Serious Adverse Effects
Allergic reaction: asthmalike wheezing.
Vitamin K deficiency and increased bleeding tendency—case reports.
Impaired absorption of calcium; predisposition to osteoporosis—possible.
Gallbladder colic—case reports.
Disruption of acid–base balance (acidosis, hyperchloremic)—case reports.

▷ **Possible Effects on Sexual Function:**   Increased libido (questionable).

Natural Diseases or Disorders That May Be Activated by This Drug
Peptic ulcer disease; steatorrhea (excessive fat in stools) with large doses.

Possible Effects on Laboratory Tests
Blood cholesterol and triglyceride levels: decreased (therapeutic effect).
Blood hemoglobin and iron levels: decreased (drug impairs absorption of iron).
INR (prothrombin time): increased (drug impairs absorption of vitamin K).

Liver function tests: increased liver enzymes (ALT/GPT, AST/GOT) in a few cases; not thought to be liver damage.

Urine calcium: increased (drug impairs absorption of calcium from intestine).

CAUTION

1. The powder should never be taken in its dry form; always mix it thoroughly with a suitable liquid before swallowing.
2. Use stool softeners and laxatives as needed if constipation develops.
3. This drug may bind other drugs and impair their absorption. It is advisable to take *all other drugs* 1 to 2 hours before or 4 to 6 hours after taking this drug.

Precautions for Use

By Infants and Children: Safety and effectiveness for those under 6 years of age not established. Watch carefully for development of acidosis and vitamin A or folic acid deficiency. (Ask your doctor for help.)

By Those Over 60 Years of Age: Increased risk of developing severe constipation. Impaired kidney function may predispose to the development of acidosis.

▷ **Advisability of Use During Pregnancy**

Pregnancy Category: C. See Pregnancy Risk Categories at the back of this book.

Animal studies: No information available.

Human studies: Adequate studies of pregnant women are not available.

Use this drug only if clearly needed. Ensure adequate intake of vitamins and minerals. Ask your physician for guidance.

Advisability of Use If Breast-Feeding

Presence of this drug in breast milk: No.

However, since it causes problems in absorbing fat-soluble vitamins, caution is advised.

Habit-Forming Potential: None.

Effects of Overdosage: Progressive constipation.

Possible Effects of Long-Term Use

Deficiencies of vitamins A, D, E, and K and folic acid.

Calcium deficiency, osteoporosis. Bone mineral density testing is recommended.

Acidosis due to excessive retention of chloride.

Suggested Periodic Examinations While Taking This Drug (at physician's discretion)

Measurements of blood levels of total cholesterol, low-density (LDL) cholesterol, and high-density (HDL) cholesterol.

Hemoglobin and red blood cell studies for possible anemia.

▷ **While Taking This Drug, Observe the Following**

Foods: Avoid foods that tend to constipate (cheeses, etc.).

Nutritional Support: Ask your doctor about the need for supplements of vitamins A, D, E, and K, folic acid, and calcium.

Beverages: Avoid carbonated beverages. Ensure adequate liquid intake (up to 2 quarts daily). This drug may be taken with milk.

▷   *Alcohol:* No interactions expected.

Tobacco Smoking: No interactions expected, but I advise everyone to quit smoking.

▷   *Other Drugs*
   Cholestyramine may ***decrease*** the effects of
   • acetaminophen; take 2 hours before cholestyramine.
   • digitoxin and digoxin; take 2 hours before cholestyramine.
   • fluvastatin (Lescol).
   • furosemide (Lasix).
   • iron preparations; separate from cholestyramine doses by 4 hours.
   • methotrexate (Mexate); take 3 hours before cholestyramine.
   • metronidazole (Flagyl).
   • NSAIDs (some acidic ones, such as piroxicam and sulindac) (see Drug Classes).
   • oral antidiabetic drugs (see Drug Classes).
   • penicillin G (Pentids).
   • phenobarbital; take 2 hours before cholestyramine.
   • thiazide diuretics (see Drug Classes); take 2 hours before cholestyramine.
   • thyroxin; take 5 hours before cholestyramine.
   • warfarin; take 6 hours after cholestyramine.
   Cholestyramine ***taken concurrently*** with
   • amiodarone (Cordarone) can result in lowered amiodarone blood levels and decreased effectiveness.
▷   *Driving, Hazardous Activities:* No restrictions.
   Aviation Note: The use of this drug ***is usually not a disqualification*** for piloting. Consult a designated Aviation Medical Examiner.
   Exposure to Sun: No restrictions.
   Discontinuation: The dose of any potentially toxic drug taken concurrently must be reduced appropriately when this drug is discontinued.

CIMETIDINE (si MET i deen)

See the histamine (H$_2$) blocking drugs profile for further information.

CIPROFLOXACIN (sip roh FLOX a sin)

See the fluoroquinolone antibiotics profile for more information.

CISAPRIDE (SIS a pryde)

Introduced: 1993   **Class:** Gastrointestinal drug   **Prescription:** USA: Yes   **Controlled Drug:** USA: No; Canada: No   **Available as Generic:** USA: No; Canada: No

Brand Names: ✚Prepulsid, Propulsid

BENEFITS versus RISKS	
Possible Benefits	*Possible Risks*
EFFECTIVE TREATMENT OF NOCTURNAL HEARTBURN	Diarrhea, cramping
FEW CENTRAL NERVOUS SIDE EFFECTS	Joint pain
May have a role in helping diabetic gastroparesis	

▷ **Principal Uses**

As a Single Drug Product: Uses currently included in FDA-approved labeling: (1) Used to relieve symptoms of reflux esophagitis; (2) helps decrease nocturnal heartburn caused by gastroesophageal reflux disease; (3) eases heartburn that happens at night (nocturnal heartburn).

Other (unlabeled) generally accepted uses: (1) May have a role in helping improve delayed stomach emptying that may lead to anorexia nervosa; (2) can help children with chronic constipation; (3) helps relieve slow emptying of the stomach (diabetic gastroparesis) often seen in diabetes; (4) relieves slowed stomach emptying caused by morphine; (5) decreases pain and flatulence in irritable bowel syndrome; (6) helps the gallbladder work better in patients with myotonic muscular dystrophy; (7) can be of help in promoting defecation in patients with spinal cord injury.

How This Drug Works: Increases the movement of the esophagus (by activating a specific muscarinic receptor) and increases contractions in the stomach and helps it to empty.

Available Dosage Forms and Strengths

Tablets — 10 mg, 20 mg

Oral suspension — 1 mg/ml

▷ **Recommended Dosage Ranges** (Actual dosage and administration schedule must be determined for each patient individually.)

Infants and Children: Safety and efficacy not established in children or infants.

12 to 60 Years of Age: For relief of nocturnal heartburn: 10 to 20 mg four times a day given 15 minutes before meals and at bedtime.

For reflux esophagitis: 10 mg four times a day combined with cimetidine (1 g a day).

For diabetic gastroparesis: 10 mg four times a day given 15 minutes before meals and at bedtime.

Over 60 Years of Age: Same as 12 to 60 years of age.

Conditions Requiring Dosing Adjustments

Liver Function: Patients with liver failure should be given 50% of the usual dose. The dose may then be increased (titrated upward) as needed and tolerated.

Kidney Function: Dose changes are not needed in kidney failure, but metabolites may accumulate.

▷ **Dosing Instructions:**   This medicine should be taken 15 minutes before meals and at bedtime for best effect.

Usual Duration of Use: Use on a regular schedule for 8 to 12 weeks may be needed to see the peak benefit in treating chronic functional constipation. Up to 12 weeks may be needed to realize the full therapeutic effect when used in therapy of reflux esophagitis. Long-term use (months to years) requires periodic physician evaluation of response and dosage adjustment.

Possible Advantages of This Drug
Significant decrease in central nervous side effects compared to metoclopramide.

Currently a "Drug of Choice"
For patients who are unable to tolerate metoclopramide and require it for a condition that cisapride effectively treats.

▷ **This Drug Should Not Be Taken If**
- you have had an allergic reaction to any dosage form of it previously.
- you have gastrointestinal obstruction, hemorrhage, or perforation.
- you are taking fluconazole, miconazole, itraconazole, ketoconazole, or macrolide antibiotics such as clarithromycin, erythromycin, or troleandomycin.

▷ **Inform Your Physician Before Taking This Drug If**
- you currently take a benzodiazepine drug (see Drug Classes).
- you have an abnormally fast heartbeat.
- you take other prescription or nonprescription medicines that were not discussed with your doctor when cisapride was prescribed.

Possible Side Effects (natural, expected, and unavoidable drug actions)
Sleepiness and fatigue—rare.

▷ **Possible Adverse Effects** (unusual, unexpected, and infrequent reactions)
If any of the following develop, consult your physician promptly for guidance.
Mild Adverse Effects
Allergic reactions: skin rash and itching—case reports.
Depression, somnolence or fatigue—rare
Joint pain—rare.
Abnormal vision—rare.
Headache, dizziness, and sleep disturbances—infrequent.
Rhinitis, sinusitis, or coughing—rare.
Diarrhea, abdominal pain, joint pain—infrequent.
Urinary incontinence—rare.
Serious Adverse Effects
Allergic reactions: anaphylactic reaction (see Glossary)—case reports.
Rare increases in heart rate, palpitations, or abnormal heartbeat—case reports and intensified by drug interactions.

▷ **Possible Effects on Sexual Function:**   None reported.

Possible Delayed Adverse Effects: None defined.

Possible Effects on Laboratory Tests
Liver function tests: increased liver enzymes (SGOT, SGPT, and CPK).

CAUTION
1. May cause increased heart rate. Notify your physician if this occurs.
2. Report promptly any increased tendency to depression.

Precautions for Use
By Infants and Children: Safety and effectiveness for children not established.
By Those Over 60 Years of Age: Specific changes not required.

▷ **Advisability of Use During Pregnancy**

Pregnancy Category: C. See Pregnancy Risk Categories at the back of this book.
Animal studies: Has caused prolongation of breeding interval in female rats.
Embryotoxic and fetotoxic in high-dose studies in rats.
Human studies: Adequate studies of pregnant women are not available.
A benefit-to-risk decision in pregnancy. Ask your doctor for help.

Advisability of Use If Breast-Feeding

Presence of this drug in breast milk: Yes.
Monitor nursing infant closely and discontinue drug or nursing if adverse effects develop.

Habit-Forming Potential: None.

Effects of Overdosage: Nausea, vomiting, flatulence, increased urination, and diarrhea.

Possible Effects of Long-Term Use: None defined.

Suggested Periodic Examinations While Taking This Drug (at physician's discretion)

Complete blood counts: Periodically.

▷ **While Taking This Drug, Observe the Following**

Foods: No restrictions, but food may actually increase the blood level obtained.
Beverages: No restrictions.
▷ *Alcohol:* Sedative effects of alcohol will be increased.
Tobacco Smoking: No interactions expected, but I advise everyone to quit smoking.
Marijuana Smoking: May cause additive drowsiness.
▷ *Other Drugs*

Cisapride may *decrease* the effects of

- warfarin (Coumadin) and decrease benefits. More frequent INR (prothrombin times) are indicated, and dosing should be adjusted if needed.

Cisapride *taken concurrently* with

- benzodiazepines (see Drug Classes) may result in increased blood levels and increased effects.
- cimetidine (Tagamet) or ranitidine (Zantac) results in increased cisapride levels and potential cisapride toxicity. Cisapride dose may need to be decreased.
- diazepam (Valium) can lead to up to a 17% increase in the peak drug level.
- fluvoxamine (Luvox) may lead to heart (cardiac) toxicity. Do not combine.
- indinavir (Crixivan), and perhaps other protease inhibitors (see Drug Classes), can lead to cisapride toxicity. DO NOT mix these two medicines.
- itraconazole (Sporanox), ketoconazole (Nizoral), fluconazole (Diflucan), or miconazole (Monistat IV) can lead to cisapride toxicity and abnormal heart effects.
- macrolide antibiotics such as clarithromycin (Biaxin), erythromycin (E-Mycin, others), or troleandomycin can lead to cisapride toxicity. Do not combine.
- nefazodone (Serzone) increases risk of heart (cardiac) toxicity. Do not combine.
- warfarin (Coumadin) may lead to excessive lowering of prothrombin and increased risk of bleeding. More frequent INR testing is needed with warfarin dosing adjusted to lab results.

▷ *Driving, Hazardous Activities:* This drug may cause some drowsiness. Restrict
activities as necessary.
Aviation Note: The use of this drug ***may be a disqualification*** for piloting. Consult a designated Aviation Medical Examiner.
Exposure to Sun: No restrictions.
Discontinuation: If this medication is stopped and you have been taking an anticoagulant, INR (prothrombin time) testing will be needed.

CLARITHROMYCIN (klar ith roh MY sin)

See the new macrolide antibiotics profile for more information.

CLINDAMYCIN (klin da MY sin)

Introduced: 1973   **Class:** Antibiotic   **Prescription:** USA: Yes   **Controlled Drug:** USA: No; Canada: No   **Available as Generic:** USA: Yes; Canada: No

Brand Names: Cleocin, Cleocin Pediatric, Cleocin T, Cleocin Vaginal Cream,
❧Dalacin C❧Dalacin T

BENEFITS versus RISKS	
Possible Benefits	*Possible Risks*
EFFECTIVE TREATMENT FOR SERIOUS INFECTIONS OF THE LOWER RESPIRATORY TRACT, ABDOMINAL CAVITY, GENITAL TRACT IN WOMEN, BLOODSTREAM (SEPTICEMIA), SKIN AND RELATED TISSUES caused by susceptible organisms Combination treatment of *Pneumocystis carinii* pneumonia Effective for the local treatment of acne	SEVERE DRUG-INDUCED COLITIS (fatalities reported) Liver injury with jaundice—rare Reduction in white blood cell and platelet counts—rare

▷ **Principal Uses**
As a Single Drug Product: Uses currently included in FDA-approved labeling: (1)
Treats serious and unusual infections of the lungs and bronchial tubes, organs and tissues within the abdominal cavity, the genital tract and pelvic
organs in women, the skin and soft tissue structures, and generalized infections involving the bloodstream; (2) used in topical form to treat acne.
Other (unlabeled) generally accepted uses: (1) Treatment of resistant gum
disease and malaria; (2) prevention of infection of the heart; (3) combination treatment of *Pneumocystis carinii* pneumonia (PCP), an infection associated with AIDS; (4) may have a role in combination therapy of toxoplasmosis infections of the brain in AIDS patients.

How This Drug Works: By blocking the formation of critical growth and reproductive proteins, this drug (in low concentrations) stops multiplication of bacteria and (in high concentrations) kills bacteria.

Available Dosage Forms and Strengths

Capsules — 75 mg, 150 mg, 300 mg
Injection — 150 mg/ml
Oral solution — 75 mg/5 ml
Topical gel — 10 mg/ml
Topical lotion — 1%
Topical solution — 10 mg/ml
Vaginal cream — 2%

▷ **Usual Adult Dosage Range:** For infections of average severity: 150 to 300 mg every 6 hours; for more severe infections: 300 to 450 mg every 6 hours. The total daily dosage should not exceed 1800 mg. In treating acne: The topical formulation is applied to the affected area twice daily. In *Pneumocystis carinii* pneumonia in AIDS patients: Intravenous or oral therapy: 900 to 2700 mg daily given in divided doses every 6 hours in combination with primaquine (15 to 30 mg of base daily). **Note: Actual dosage and administration schedule must be determined for each patient individually.**

Conditions Requiring Dosing Adjustments

Liver Function: The dose must be decreased with liver compromise, and blood levels checked.

Kidney Function: Serum levels should be checked in patients with renal compromise, and the dose adjusted appropriately.

▷ **Dosing Instructions:** Take the capsule with a full glass of water or with food to prevent irritation. The capsule may be opened and the contents mixed with food for administration. Shake the oral solution well before measuring the dose. Do not refrigerate the oral solution; chilling can cause it to thicken, making it difficult to take. The topical lotion should be shaken well before it is applied.

Usual Duration of Use: Use on a regular schedule for 3 to 5 days is usually needed to see this drug's effect in controlling infections.

Possible Advantages of This Drug: Bacterial sensitivity testing may show this drug to be more effective than other antibiotics in treating some severe infections.

▷ **This Drug Should Not Be Taken If**
- you are allergic to either clindamycin or lincomycin.
- it is prescribed for a mild or trivial infection.
- you have a history of Crohn's disease or ulcerative colitis.

▷ **Inform Your Physician Before Taking This Drug If**
- you have a history of allergy to any drug.
- you have a history of drug-induced colitis.
- you are allergic by nature: hay fever, asthma, hives, eczema.
- you have a history of previous yeast infections.
- you have a blood disorder.
- you have myasthenia gravis.
- you have impaired liver or kidney function.
- you plan to have surgery under general anesthesia in the near future.

Possible Side Effects (natural, expected, and unavoidable drug actions)
Superinfections (see Glossary).
Ringing in the ears (tinnitus).

▷ **Possible Adverse Effects** (unusual, unexpected, and infrequent reactions)
If any of the following develop, consult your physician promptly for guidance.
Mild Adverse Effects
Allergic reactions: skin rashes, hives—rare.
Nausea, vomiting, mild diarrhea, stomach pain—rare to infrequent.
Multiple joint pains—rare.
Serious Adverse Effects
Allergic reactions: severe skin reactions: erythema multiforme (Stevens-Johnson syndrome)—case reports.
Toxic liver reaction with jaundice (see Glossary)—case reports.
Severe colitis with persistent diarrhea; stools may contain blood and/or mucus—rare.
Reduction of white blood cell and platelet counts—case reports.
Neuromuscular blockade (dose related)—rare.

▷ **Possible Effects on Sexual Function:**   None reported.

Possible Delayed Adverse Effects: Severe colitis with diarrhea (pseudomembranous colitis) may start several weeks after stopping this drug.

Adverse Effects That May Mimic Natural Diseases or Disorders
Liver reactions may suggest viral hepatitis.
Multiple joint pains may suggest the onset of arthritis.

Natural Diseases or Disorders That May Be Activated by This Drug
Crohn's disease, ulcerative colitis, myasthenia gravis.

Possible Effects on Laboratory Tests
Complete blood counts: decreased white cells and platelets; increased eosinophils (allergic reaction).
Liver function tests: uncommon, mild, and transient increases in liver enzymes (ALT/GPT, AST/GOT, alkaline phosphatase).

CAUTION
1. Persistent diarrhea can develop in some patients. If diarrhea persists longer than 24 hours, stop the drug and call your doctor.
2. If surgery under general anesthesia is planned, the anesthetic must be carefully chosen to prevent clindamycin-induced excessive muscle relaxation (neuromuscular blockade) and breathing problems.

Precautions for Use
By Infants and Children: Safety and effectiveness for those under 1 month of age not established. Use with caution.
By Those Over 60 Years of Age: Diarrhea will be more common in this age group. Watch for development of yeast infection of the skin in the genital and anal regions, a form of superinfection (see Glossary). Report such developments promptly to your physician.

▷ **Advisability of Use During Pregnancy**
Pregnancy Category: B. See Pregnancy Risk Categories at the back of this book.
Animal studies: No birth defects due to this drug found in mouse or rat studies.

Human studies: Adequate studies of pregnant women are not available. Use this drug only if clearly needed. Ask your physician for guidance.

Advisability of Use If Breast-Feeding
Presence of this drug in breast milk: Yes.
Avoid drug or refrain from nursing.

Habit-Forming Potential: None.

Effects of Overdosage: Nausea, vomiting, cramping, diarrhea.

Possible Effects of Long-Term Use
Superinfections, especially from yeast organisms.
Severe colitis with persistent diarrhea.

Suggested Periodic Examinations While Taking This Drug (at physician's discretion)
Complete blood cell counts, liver function tests.

▷ **While Taking This Drug, Observe the Following**
Foods: No restrictions.
Beverages: No restrictions. May be taken with milk.
▷ *Alcohol:* No interactions expected.
Tobacco Smoking: No interactions expected.
▷ *Other Drugs*
Clindamycin *taken concurrently* with
- antidiarrheal drugs (diphenoxylate, loperamide, paregoric) may result in worsening of the underlying colitis. Avoid the combination.
- antimyasthenic drugs (ambenonium, neostigmine, pyridostigmine) may reduce their benefits in relieving muscle weakness of myasthenia gravis.
- carisoprodol (Soma) may result in increased and perhaps undesirable muscle relaxation.
- cholestyramine (Questran) may blunt therapeutic benefits of clindamycin.
- dantrolene or other skeletal muscle relaxants may result in enhanced or protracted and potentially dangerous muscle relaxation.
- saquinavir (Invirase) and perhaps other protease inhibitors (see Drug Classes) may lead to toxic clindamycin blood levels.

The following drugs may *decrease* the effects of clindamycin:
- chloramphenicol (Chloromycetin).
- macrolide antibiotics such as erythromycin (E.E.S., E-Mycin, etc.), clarithromycin, or azithromycin.

▷ *Driving, Hazardous Activities:* This drug may cause nausea and diarrhea. Restrict activities as necessary.
Aviation Note: The use of this drug *may be a disqualification* for piloting. Consult a designated Aviation Medical Examiner.
Exposure to Sun: Use caution until sensitivity is determined.
Discontinuation: If tolerated, take the full course prescribed. When used to treat infections that may predispose to rheumatic fever or nephritis, take continually in full dosage for no less than 10 days.
Special Storage Instructions: Oral solution should be kept at room temperature; do not refrigerate.
Observe the Following Expiration Times: Do not take the oral solution if it is older than 14 days.

CLOMIPRAMINE (kloh MI pra meen)

Introduced: 1970   **Class:** Antidepressant   **Prescription:** USA: Yes
Controlled Drug: USA: No; Canada: No   **Available as Generic:** USA: No;
Canada: No
Brand Name: Anafranil

BENEFITS versus RISKS	
Possible Benefits	*Possible Risks*
EFFECTIVE TREATMENT OF SEVERE OBSESSIVE-COMPULSIVE NEUROSIS Effective relief of symptoms of some types of endogenous depression	DRUG-INDUCED SEIZURES—rare ADVERSE BEHAVIORAL EFFECTS Conversion of depression to mania in manic-depressive (bipolar) disorders Aggravation of schizophrenia Liver toxicity—rare Bone marrow depression and blood cell disorders—rare

▷ **Principal Uses**

As a Single Drug Product: Uses currently included in FDA-approved labeling: Relieves manifestations of severe, disabling obsessive-compulsive disorder. Other (unlabeled) generally accepted uses: (1) Relieves symptoms of panic attacks; (2) helps some phobias; (3) may help repetitive symptoms in autistics; (4) could have a role in diabetic neuropathy; (5) can help premature ejaculation; (6) may relieve severity of hair-pulling syndromes, severe nail biting and arm burning in obsessive-compulsive patients; (7) can help relieve symptoms in severe premenstrual syndrome.

How This Drug Works: By increasing brain levels of some nerve transmitters, principally serotonin, this drug reduces the frequency and intensity of obsessive and compulsive behavior patterns.

Available Dosage Forms and Strengths

Capsules — 10 mg (Canada only), 25 mg, 50 mg, 75 mg

▷ **Usual Adult Dosage Range:** Initially 25 mg daily, taken in the evening. Dose may be increased as needed and tolerated by 25 mg daily at intervals of 3 to 4 days until a dose of 100 mg daily is reached in 2 weeks. This larger dose should be divided and taken after meals. The usual maintenance dose is 50 mg to 150 mg daily. The total daily dosage should not exceed 250 mg. (When determined, the optimal daily requirement may be given at bedtime as a single dose.) **Note: Actual dosage and administration schedule must be determined for each patient individually.**

Conditions Requiring Dosing Adjustments

Liver Function: The dose should be decreased in patients with liver compromise.
Kidney Function: Changes in dose are not usually needed.

▷ **Dosing Instructions:** May be taken without regard to meals. If needed, the capsule may be opened and may be taken with or following food to reduce stomach upset.

Usual Duration of Use: Use on a regular schedule for 3 to 4 weeks is usually needed to see this drug's benefit in controlling obsessive-compulsive behavior; peak response may require 3 or more months of use. Long-term use (months to years) requires periodic evaluation.

▷ **This Drug Should Not Be Taken If**
- you have had an allergic reaction to it previously.
- you are taking, or have taken within the past 14 days, any monoamine oxidase (MAO) type A inhibitor drug (see Drug Classes).
- you have active bone marrow depression or a current blood cell disorder.
- you have had a recent heart attack (myocardial infarction).
- you have narrow-angle glaucoma.

▷ **Inform Your Physician Before Taking This Drug If**
- you have had an adverse reaction to an antidepressant drug, especially one of the tricyclic class.
- you have a history of bone marrow or blood cell disorder.
- you have any type of seizure disorder.
- you have increased internal eye pressure.
- you have any type of heart disease, especially coronary artery disease or a heart rhythm disorder.
- you are subject to bronchial asthma.
- you have impaired liver or kidney function.
- you have any type of thyroid disorder or are taking thyroid medication.
- you have a history of suicide attempts.
- you have an adrenaline-producing tumor.
- you have prostatism (see Glossary).
- you have a history of alcoholism.
- you plan to have surgery under general anesthesia in the near future.

Possible Side Effects (natural, expected, and unavoidable drug actions)
Drowsiness, increased sweating, light-headedness, blurred vision, dry mouth, constipation, impaired urination.

▷ **Possible Adverse Effects** (unusual, unexpected, and infrequent reactions)
If any of the following develop, consult your physician promptly for guidance.
Mild Adverse Effects
Allergic reactions: skin rash, itching, drug fever (see Glossary)—case reports.
Headache, dizziness, nervousness, impaired memory, weakness, tremors, insomnia, muscle cramps, flushing—infrequent.
Sweating—infrequent.
Increased appetite, weight gain—infrequent.
Altered taste, indigestion, nausea, vomiting, diarrhea—infrequent.
Serious Adverse Effects
Allergic reactions: drug-induced hepatitis, with or without jaundice—case reports.
Idiosyncratic reactions: neuroleptic malignant syndrome (see Glossary)—case reports.
Adverse behavioral effects: confusion, delirium, delusions, hallucinations, paranoia—case reports.
Seizures; reduced control of epilepsy—rare.

Aggravation of paranoid psychoses and schizophrenia—case reports.

Heart rhythm disturbances—rare.

Bone marrow depression (see Glossary): fatigue, weakness, fever, sore throat, infections, abnormal bleeding or bruising—case reports.

SIADH and severe lowering of blood sodium—case reports.

Liver toxicity—infrequent.

Serotonin syndrome—case reports.

▷ **Possible Effects on Sexual Function:** Altered libido, impaired (delayed) ejaculation, impotence, inhibited male orgasm, inhibited female orgasm, abnormal sperm formation, female breast enlargement with milk production, absence of menstruation—case reports.

Adverse Effects That May Mimic Natural Diseases or Disorders

Liver toxicity may suggest viral hepatitis.

Natural Diseases or Disorders That May Be Activated by This Drug

Latent epilepsy, glaucoma, prostatism, schizophrenia.

Possible Effects on Laboratory Tests

Complete blood cell counts: decreased red cells, hemoglobin, white cells, and platelets.

Liver function tests: increased liver enzymes (ALT/GPT, AST/GOT)—liver damage.

Thyroid function tests: decreased TT3 and FT3.

Blood sodium: severely lowered in cases of drug-induced SIADH.

CAUTION

1. Watch for toxicity: confusion, agitation, rapid heart rate, heart irregularity. Blood levels will clarify the situation.
2. Use with caution in schizophrenia. Watch closely for deterioration of thinking or behavior.
3. Use with caution in epilepsy. Watch for any change in the frequency or severity of seizures.
4. Complete blood counts should be obtained in patients who develop sore throat or fever while taking this medicine.

Precautions for Use

By Infants and Children: Safety and effectiveness for those under 10 years of age not established. Dose and management should be supervised by a properly trained pediatrician. Total daily dosage should not exceed 200 mg or 3 mg per kg of body mass, whichever number is smaller.

By Those Over 60 Years of Age: Start treatment with 10 mg at bedtime. Dose may be increased gradually as needed and tolerated to 75 mg daily in divided doses. During the first 2 weeks of treatment, watch for behavioral reactions: restlessness, agitation, forgetfulness, disorientation, delusions, or hallucinations. Also observe for unsteadiness and instability that may predispose to falling. This drug may aggravate prostatism.

▷ **Advisability of Use During Pregnancy**

Pregnancy Category: C. See Pregnancy Risk Categories at the back of this book.

Animal studies: No drug-induced birth defects reported in mouse or rat studies.

Human studies: Adequate studies of pregnant women are not available.

Use only if clearly needed. Avoid use during the last 3 months, if possible, to prevent withdrawal symptoms in the newborn infant: irritability, tremors, seizures.

Advisability of Use If Breast-Feeding
Presence of this drug in breast milk: Yes.
Avoid drug or refrain from nursing.

Habit-Forming Potential: Psychological or physical dependence is rare and unexpected. This drug is not liable to abuse.

Effects of Overdosage: Confusion, delirium, hallucinations, drowsiness, tremors, unsteadiness, heart irregularity, seizures, stupor, sweating, fever.

Possible Effects of Long-Term Use: Neuroleptic malignant syndrome (see Glossary): Fever, fast or irregular heartbeat, fast breathing, sweating, weakness, muscle stiffness, seizures, loss of bladder control.

Suggested Periodic Examinations While Taking This Drug (at physician's discretion)
Monitoring of blood drug levels as appropriate.
Complete blood cell counts; liver and kidney function tests.
Serial blood pressure readings and electrocardiograms.
Measurement of internal eye pressure.

▷ **While Taking This Drug, Observe the Following**
Foods: No specific restrictions. May need to limit food intake to avoid excessive weight gain.
Beverages: No restrictions. May be taken with milk.
▷ *Alcohol:* Avoid completely. This drug can markedly increase the intoxicating effects of alcohol; the combination can depress brain function significantly.
Tobacco Smoking: May delay the elimination of this drug and require dosage adjustment. I advise everyone to quit smoking.
Marijuana Smoking: Increased drowsiness and mouth dryness; and reduced effectiveness.
▷ *Other Drugs*
Clomipramine may *increase* the effects of
• all drugs with atropinelike effects (see Drug Classes).
• all drugs with sedative effects; observe for excessive sedation.
Clomipramine may *decrease* the effects of
• clonidine (Catapres).
• guanadrel (Hylorel).
• guanethidine (Ismelin, Esimil).
Clomipramine *taken concurrently* with
• anticonvulsants such as carbamazepine (Tegretol) (see Drug Classes) requires careful monitoring for changes in seizure patterns and the need to adjust anticonvulsant dosage.
• monoamine oxidase (MAO) type A inhibitor drugs (see Drug Classes) may cause high fever, seizures, and excessive rise in blood pressure; avoid combining these drugs and provide periods of 14 days between administration of either.
• stimulant drugs (amphetamine, cocaine, epinephrine, phenylpropanolamine, etc.) may cause severe high blood pressure and/or high fever.
• thyroid preparations may increase the risk of heart rhythm disorders.

- warfarin (Coumadin) may cause an increased warfarin effect and bleeding. More frequent INR (prothrombin time) testing is needed.

The following drugs may *increase* the effects of clomipramine:
- ACE inhibitors (see Drug Classes).
- birth control pills (oral contraceptives).
- cimetidine (Tagamet).
- estrogens.
- fluoxetine (Prozac).
- fluvoxamine (Luvox).
- haloperidol (Haldol).
- methylphenidate (Ritalin).
- phenothiazines (see Drug Classes).
- quinidine.
- ranitidine (Zantac).
- ritonavir (Norvir) and perhaps other protease inhibitors (see Drug Classes).
- sertraline (Zoloft).
- verapamil (Calan, others).

The following drugs may *decrease* the effects of clomipramine:
- barbiturates (see Drug Classes).
- carbamazepine (Tegretol).
- chloral hydrate (Noctec, Somnos, etc.).
- lithium (Lithobid, Lithotab, etc.).
- reserpine (Serpasil, Ser-Ap-Es, etc.).

▷ *Driving, Hazardous Activities:* This drug may cause seizures and impair alertness, judgment, physical coordination, and reaction time. Restrict activities as necessary.

Aviation Note: The use of this drug *is a disqualification* for piloting. Consult a designated Aviation Medical Examiner.

Exposure to Sun: No restrictions.

Exposure to Heat: Use caution. This drug may impair the body's adaptation to hot environments, increasing the risk of heatstroke. Avoid saunas.

Exposure to Environmental Chemicals: This drug may mask the symptoms of poisoning due to handling certain insecticides (organophosphorous types). Read their labels carefully.

Discontinuation: It is best to slowly reduce the dose over a period of 3 to 4 weeks. Abrupt withdrawal after prolonged use may cause nausea, vomiting, diarrhea, headache, dizziness, malaise, disturbed sleep, and irritability. Obsessive-compulsive behavior may worsen when this drug is stopped. It may be necessary to adjust the dosages of other drugs taken concurrently when this drug is discontinued.

CLONAZEPAM (kloh NA ze pam)

Introduced: 1977   **Class:** Anticonvulsant, benzodiazepines   **Prescription:** USA: Yes   **Controlled Drug:** USA: C-IV*; Canada: No   **Available as Generic:** Yes

*See Schedules of Controlled Drugs at the back of this book.

Brand Names: Klonopin, ✦Rivotril

Warning: The brand name Klonopin and the generic name clonidine are similar and can be mistaken for each other; this can lead to serious medication errors. These names represent very different drugs. Verify that you are taking the correct drug.

BENEFITS versus RISKS	
Possible Benefits	*Possible Risks*
EFFECTIVE CONTROL OF SOME TYPES OF PETIT MAL, AKINETIC, AND MYOCLONIC SEIZURES	Paradoxical reactions: excitement, agitation, hallucinations
Possibly effective in the management of panic disorders	Minor impairment of mental functions
Can help restless leg syndrome	Blood cell disorders: anemia, abnormally low white blood cell and platelet counts—rare
	Increased salivation (of concern for those with chronic lung disease)

▷ **Principal Uses**

> *As a Single Drug Product:* Uses currently included in FDA-approved labeling: (1) Treats several types of epilepsy: petit mal variations, akinetic, myoclonic, and absence seizure patterns; (2) used in panic disorder.
>
> Other (unlabeled) generally accepted uses: (1) Eases symptoms of Tourette's syndrome; (2) relieves trigeminal neuralgia; (3) helps resistant depression; (4) can ease drug-induced mania; (5) may be of help in restless leg syndrome (Ekbom syndrome); (6) may help essential tremor symptoms.

How This Drug Works: This drug produces an anticonvulsant effect by increasing the action of a nerve transmitter (gamma-aminobutyric acid), which then blocks seizures.

Available Dosage Forms and Strengths

> Tablets — 0.125 mg, 0.25 mg, 0.5 mg, 1 mg, 2 mg

▷ **Usual Adult Dosage Range:**   Initially 0.5 mg three times daily. The dose may be increased by 0.5 mg to 1.0 mg every 3 days, as needed and tolerated, until seizures are controlled. Total daily dose should not exceed 20 mg. **Note: Actual dosage and administration schedule must be determined for each patient individually.**

Conditions Requiring Dosing Adjustments

> *Liver Function:* The dose **must** be decreased in liver compromise.
> *Kidney Function:* Watch for signs and symptoms of accumulation (see "Effects of Overdosage" below).

▷ **Dosing Instructions:**   May be taken on empty stomach or with food or milk. The tablet may be crushed for administration. Do not stop this drug abruptly if taken for control of seizures, or if taken for more than 4 weeks to control panic attacks.

Usual Duration of Use: Use on a regular schedule for 2 to 3 weeks may be needed to see this drug's benefit in reducing the frequency and severity of seizures. Peak control will require careful dosage adjustments over a period of several months. Long-term use (months to years) requires ongoing supervision and periodic evaluation by your physician.

▷ **This Drug Should Not Be Taken If**
- you have had an allergic reaction to it previously.
- you have acute narrow-angle glaucoma.
- you have active liver disease.

▷ **Inform Your Physician Before Taking This Drug If**
- you are allergic to any benzodiazepine (see Drug Classes).
- you have a history of alcoholism or drug abuse.
- you are pregnant or planning pregnancy.
- you have palpitations, as this drug may worsen palpitations.
- you have impaired liver or kidney function.
- you have a history of serious depression or mental disorder.
- you have any of the following: asthma, emphysema, chronic bronchitis, myasthenia gravis.
- you have acute intermittent porphyria.

Possible Side Effects (natural, expected, and unavoidable drug actions)
Drowsiness—frequent (may diminish with time); increased salivation.

▷ **Possible Adverse Effects** (unusual, unexpected, and infrequent reactions)
If any of the following develop, consult your physician promptly for guidance.
Mild Adverse Effects
Allergic reactions: skin rash, hives, itching.
Ataxia—frequent.
Weight gain—frequent.
Headache, dizziness, blurred vision, double vision, slurred speech, impaired memory, confusion, depression—possible.
Muscle weakness, uncontrolled body movements—possible.
Palpitations or hair loss—rare.
Nausea, vomiting, constipation, diarrhea, impaired urination, incontinence—case reports in older patients.
Serious Adverse Effects
Idiosyncratic reactions: paradoxical responses of excitement, hyperactivity, agitation, anger, hostility—case reports.
Hallucinations, seizures—case reports.
Blood disorders: abnormally low red blood cell, white blood cell, and platelet counts—case reports.
Porphyria—case reports.
Increased secretions and breathing problems, especially in those with chronic lung disease—case reports.

▷ **Possible Effects on Sexual Function:** Increased libido, enlargement of male breasts. May cause abnormally early (precocious) secondary sex characteristics in children—case reports.

Possible Effects on Laboratory Tests
Complete blood cell counts: decreased red cells, hemoglobin, white cells, and platelets.
Urine screening tests for drug abuse: may be *positive*. (Test results depend upon amount of drug taken and testing method used.)
Liver function tests: increased.

CAUTION
1. This drug should not be stopped abruptly if used to control seizures.
2. Some over-the-counter drug products that contain antihistamines (allergy and cold preparations, sleep aids) can cause excessive sedation if combined with clonazepam.
3. Adverse behavioral reactions are more common in people with brain damage, mental retardation, or psychiatric disorders.
4. A decreased response to this drug occurs in approximately 30% of users within 3 months after initiating treatment. Dosage adjustment may be necessary to restore seizure control.

Precautions for Use

By Infants and Children: This drug is used to treat infants and children of all ages. Careful dosage adjustment based on weight and age is mandatory. Abnormal behavioral responses are more common in children.

By Those Over 60 Years of Age: Smaller doses and longer intervals are suggested. Watch for development of lethargy, indifference, fatigue, weakness, unsteadiness, disturbing dreams, nightmares, and paradoxical reactions of excitement, agitation, anger, hostility, and rage.

▷ **Advisability of Use During Pregnancy**

Pregnancy Category: C. See Pregnancy Risk Categories at the back of this book. Animal studies: This drug causes cleft palates, open eyelids, fused rib structures, and limb defects in rabbits.

Human studies: Adequate studies of pregnant women are not available.

It is advisable to avoid this drug during the first 3 months if possible. Frequent use in late pregnancy may cause the "floppy infant" syndrome in the newborn: weakness, lethargy, unresponsiveness, depressed breathing, low body temperature.

Advisability of Use If Breast-Feeding

Presence of this drug in breast milk: Yes.
Avoid drug or refrain from nursing.

Habit-Forming Potential: This drug can produce psychological and/or physical dependence (see Glossary) if used in large doses for an extended period of time.

Effects of Overdosage: Marked drowsiness, weakness, confusion, slurred speech, staggering gait, tremor, stupor progressing to deep sleep or coma.

Possible Effects of Long-Term Use: Benefits versus risks must be considered carefully during the extended use of this drug in children. Possible adverse effects on physical or mental development may not be apparent for many years.

Suggested Periodic Examinations While Taking This Drug (at physician's discretion)

During long-term use: Complete blood cell counts; liver function tests.

▷ **While Taking This Drug, Observe the Following**

Foods: No restrictions.
Beverages: No restrictions. May be taken with milk.
▷   *Alcohol:* Use with extreme caution. Alcohol may increase the depressant effects of this drug on the brain. It is advisable to avoid alcohol completely—

throughout the day and night—if it is necessary to drive or to engage in any hazardous activity.

Tobacco Smoking: No interactions expected, but I advise everyone to quit smoking.

Marijuana Smoking: Increased sedation and significant impairment of intellectual and physical performance.

▷ *Other Drugs*

Clonazepam *taken concurrently* with

- amiodarone (Cordarone) may decrease elimination of clonazepam and also worsen toxicity by causing low thyroid function.
- carbamazepine (Tegretol) may decrease blood levels and hence benefits of both medications.
- desipramine, imipramine, and other tricyclic antidepressants (see Drug Classes) can decrease the tricyclic antidepressant blood level and lessen its therapeutic benefit.
- MAO inhibitors (see Drug Classes) may result in very low blood pressure and worsening of sedation and respiratory depression.
- phenytoin (Dilantin) may result in decreased phenytoin levels.
- ritonavir (Norvir), and perhaps other protease inhibitors (see Drug Classes), may lead to clonazepam toxicity.
- valproic acid (Depakene, etc.) may cause continuous absence seizures.

The following drugs may *increase* the effects of clonazepam:

- cimetidine (Tagamet).
- disulfiram (Antabuse).
- macrolide antibiotics such as azithromycin, clarithromycin, or erythromycin (see Drug Classes).
- omeprazole (Prilosec).
- oral contraceptives (birth control pills).

The following drugs may *decrease* the effects of clonazepam:

- theophylline (aminophylline, Theo-Dur, etc.).

▷ *Driving, Hazardous Activities:* This drug can impair mental alertness, judgment, physical coordination, and reaction time. Avoid hazardous activities accordingly.

Aviation Note: The use of this drug *is a disqualification* for piloting. Consult a designated Aviation Medical Examiner.

Exposure to Sun: No restrictions.

Discontinuation: Do not stop clonazepam suddenly if it is being used to control any type of seizure, or if it has been taken for more than 4 weeks to treat other conditions. Dosage should be tapered gradually to prevent a withdrawal syndrome that could include depression, confusion, hallucinations, tremor, seizures, muscle cramping, sweating, and vomiting.

CLONIDINE (KLOH ni deen)

Introduced: 1969   **Class:** Antihypertensive   **Prescription:** USA: Yes
Controlled Drug: USA: No; Canada: No   **Available as Generic:** USA: Yes; Canada: No

Brand Names: ✦Apo-Clonidine, Catapres, Catapres-TTS, Combipres [CD], ✦Dixarit, ✦Nu-Clonidine

BENEFITS versus RISKS	
Possible Benefits	*Possible Risks*
EFFECTIVE ANTIHYPERTENSIVE in mild to moderate high blood pressure	ACUTE WITHDRAWAL SYNDROME (rebound hypertension) with abrupt discontinuation
Effective control of menopausal hot flashes (in selected cases)	Raynaud's phenomenon (cold fingers or toes)
Effective help in narcotic withdrawal	

▷ **Principal Uses**

As a Single Drug Product: Uses currently included in FDA-approved labeling: Used in combination with other medicines that are usually drugs of first choice in starting treatment of mild to moderate high blood pressure. Generally not used to start therapy. It may also be added later, replacing drugs that cause marked orthostatic hypotension (see Glossary).

Other (unlabeled) generally accepted uses: (1) Helps prevent migraine headache; (2) may help improve outcomes in patients with head injuries; (3) can aid menopausal hot flashes and treat severe menstrual cramps; (4) helps to lessen symptoms of alcohol or narcotic drug withdrawal; (5) has a role in some cases of abnormal heart rhythms (atrial fibrillation); (6) some data suggest a role for intravenous use after a heart attack to limit the size of the heart damage (infarct); (7) may have a benefit in attention deficit disorder (ADD).

As a Combination Drug Product [CD]: Available in combination with chlorthalidone. The different ways in which these drugs work complement each other, making the combination a more effective antihypertensive.

How This Drug Works: By decreasing the activity of part of the brain (vasomotor center), this drug limits the ability of the sympathetic nervous system to constrict blood vessels and increase blood pressure.

Available Dosage Forms and Strengths

Patches — 2.5 mg, 5.0 mg, 7.5 mg

Tablets — 0.1 mg, 0.2 mg, 0.3 mg

▷ **Usual Adult Dosage Range:**   Tablets—initially 0.1 mg twice daily. Increased by 0.1 to 0.2 mg daily as needed and tolerated. Usual range is 0.2 to 0.6 mg daily, taken in two doses. Total daily dosage should not exceed 2.4 mg, and some researchers have recommended a maximum of 1.2 mg daily. Medicated patches are applied once a week. Hypertension in children has been treated with 5 to 10 mcg per kg of body mass per day, divided into two or three doses. Some children (4–17 years old) with ADD have been given 0.05 mg per kg of body mass at bedtime to help reduce sleep problems.

Note: Actual dosage and administration schedule must be determined for each patient individually.

Conditions Requiring Dosing Adjustments

Liver Function: This drug is changed into six active forms. The dose **must** be decreased in liver compromise.

Kidney Function: Presently, dosing changes are not thought to be needed in mild to severe kidney failure. Some kidney patients may require higher maintenance doses to get the best blood pressure.

▷ **Dosing Instructions:** Tablets may be taken without regard to eating. The tablet may be crushed for administration.

Usual Duration of Use: Use on a regular schedule for 2 to 3 weeks is usually needed to see this drug's benefit in lowering high blood pressure. Long-term use (months to years) requires physician supervision and guidance.

▷ **This Drug Should Not Be Taken If**
- you have had an allergic reaction to it previously.
- you have a problem in your heart that impacts the timing of the heartbeat or transmission of electrical impulses through the heart.

▷ **Inform Your Physician Before Taking This Drug If**
- you have a circulatory disorder of the brain.
- you have angina or coronary artery disease.
- you have or have had serious emotional depression.
- you have a very slow heart rate.
- you have Buerger's disease or Raynaud's phenomenon.
- you are taking a tricyclic antidepressant (see Drug Classes).
- you are taking any sedative or hypnotic drugs or an antidepressant.
- you plan to have surgery under general anesthesia in the near future.

Possible Side Effects (natural, expected, and unavoidable drug actions)
Drowsiness, dry nose and mouth, constipation—common; decreased heart rate, mild orthostatic hypotension (see Glossary).

▷ **Possible Adverse Effects** (unusual, unexpected, and infrequent reactions)
If any of the following develop, consult your physician promptly for guidance.
Mild Adverse Effects
Allergic reactions: skin rash, hives, localized swellings, itching—rare to infrequent.
Drowsiness—infrequent to frequent.
Headache, dizziness, fatigue, anxiety, sleep disorders (nightmares or vivid dreaming), dry and burning eyes—possible.
Painful parotid (salivary) gland, nausea, vomiting—case reports.
Dry mouth—frequent.
Urination at night—rare.
Increased liver function tests—case reports.
Serious Adverse Effects
Idiosyncratic reaction: Raynaud's phenomenon (see Glossary)—case reports.
Aggravation of congestive heart failure, heart rhythm disorders—case reports.
Depression, hallucinations, or psychosis—case reports.

▷ **Possible Effects on Sexual Function:** Decreased libido in 10% (0.2 to 0.8 mg/day); impotence in 8 to 24% (0.5 to 3.6 mg/day); impaired ejaculation—rare; enlargement of male breasts (gynecomastia) (0.2 to 0.8 mg/day)—rare. Precocious puberty in females.

Possible Effects on Laboratory Tests
Blood cholesterol or triglyceride levels: no consistent or significant effects.
Blood sodium level: increased.
Liver function: Rare increases of enzymes (ALT/GPT, AST/GOT, alkaline phosphatase).

CAUTION
1. ***Do not stop this drug suddenly.*** Sudden withdrawal can cause a severe and possibly fatal reaction.
2. Hot weather or fever can reduce blood pressure significantly. Dose adjustments may be necessary.
3. Report the development of any tendency to emotional depression.

Precautions for Use
By Infants and Children: Initial doses of 5–10 mcg per kg of body mass per day, divided into two or three doses, have been used. A larger evening dose and smaller morning dose can help minimize sedation during school hours when used for ADD.

By Those Over 60 Years of Age: ***Proceed cautiously*** with this drug. High blood pressure should be reduced slowly without the risks associated with excessively low blood pressure. Low initial doses and frequent blood pressure checks are needed. Watch for development of light-headedness, dizziness, unsteadiness, fainting, and falling. Sedation and dry mouth occur in 50% of elderly users. Promptly report any changes in mood or behavior: depression, delusions, hallucinations.

▷ ### Advisability of Use During Pregnancy
Pregnancy Category: C. See Pregnancy Risk Categories at the back of this book.
Animal studies: No birth defects reported. However, this drug is toxic to the embryo in low dosage.
Human studies: Adequate studies of pregnant women are not available.
The manufacturer recommends that this drug be avoided by women who are or who may become pregnant. Ask your physician for guidance.

Advisability of Use If Breast-Feeding
Presence of this drug in breast milk: Yes.
This drug may impair milk production. Monitor nursing infant closely and discontinue drug or nursing if adverse effects begin.

Habit-Forming Potential:
A small number of reports regarding abuse of this drug have surfaced. It may cause extreme grogginess and lethargy when combined with diazepam (Valium).

Effects of Overdosage:
Marked drowsiness, weakness, dry mouth, slow pulse, low blood pressure, vomiting, stupor progressing to coma.

Possible Effects of Long-Term Use:
Development of tolerance (see Glossary) with loss of drug effect; weight gain due to salt and water retention; temporary sexual impotence.

Suggested Periodic Examinations While Taking This Drug (at physician's discretion)
Blood pressure measurements, monitoring of body weight.

▷ ### While Taking This Drug, Observe the Following
Foods: Avoid excessive salt. Ask your physician for help with degree of salt restriction.
Beverages: No restrictions. May be taken with milk.
▷ *Alcohol:* Use with extreme caution. Combined effects can cause marked drowsiness and exaggerated reduction of blood pressure.
Tobacco Smoking: No expected interactions, but I advise everyone to quit smoking.

▷ *Other Drugs*
Clonidine may *decrease* the effects of
- levodopa (Larodopa, Sinemet, etc.), causing an increase in parkinsonism symptoms.

Clonidine *taken concurrently* with
- beta-adrenergic-blocking drugs (Inderal, Lopressor, etc.) may increase the risk of rebound hypertension if clonidine is stopped first. It is best to stop the beta-blocker first, and then withdraw clonidine gradually.
- naloxone (Narcan, Talwin NX) may blunt the therapeutic effect of clonidine and result in a hypertensive response.
- niacin may decrease the facial flushing side effect of niacin.
- nonsteroidal anti-inflammatory drugs NSAIDs (see Drug Classes) may blunt blood-pressure-lowering benefits of clonidine.
- verapamil (Calan, others) may lead to problems in conduction of the heart.

The following drugs may *decrease* the effects of clonidine:
- tricyclic antidepressants (Elavil, Sinequan, etc.; see Drug Classes); may reduce its effectiveness in lowering blood pressure.

▷ *Driving, Hazardous Activities:* Use caution. This drug can cause drowsiness and can impair mental alertness, judgment, and coordination.
Aviation Note: Hypertension (high blood pressure) *is a disqualification* for piloting. Consult a designated Aviation Medical Examiner.
Exposure to Sun: No restrictions.
Exposure to Heat: Use caution. Hot environments may reduce blood pressure; be alert to the possibility of orthostatic hypotension (see Glossary).
Exposure to Cold: Use caution. May cause painful blanching and numbness of the hands and feet on exposure to cold air or water (Raynaud's phenomenon).
Heavy Exercise or Exertion: Use caution. Isometric exercises—the "overload" technique for strengthening individual muscles—can raise blood pressure significantly. This drug may intensify the hypertensive response to isometric exercise. Ask your physician for guidance.
Occurrence of Unrelated Illness: Fever may lower blood pressure. Repeated vomiting may prevent the regular use of this drug and cause an acute withdrawal reaction. Consult your physician.
*Discontinuation: **Do not stop this drug suddenly.*** A severe withdrawal reaction can occur within 12 to 48 hours after the last dose. It is best to gradually decrease the dose over 3 to 4 days, and check blood pressure often.

CLOTRIMAZOLE (kloh TRIM a zohl)

Introduced: 1976   **Class:** Antifungal   **Prescription:** USA: Yes, though some are nonprescription   **Controlled Drug:** USA: No; Canada: No   **Available as Generic:** USA: Yes; Canada: No

Brand Names: ✤Canesten, Clotrimaderm, Clotrimazole, Femcare, Gyne-Lotrimin (1% cream and insert are nonprescription), ✤Lotriderm, Lotrimin, Lotrimin AF (nonprescription), Lotrisone, Mycelex (1% vaginal cream is nonprescription), Mycelex-7, Mycelex-G, ✤Myclo, ✤Neo-Zol

Warning: The brand names Mycelex and Myoflex are similar and can be mistaken for each other; this can lead to serious medication errors. These names represent very different drugs. Verify that you are using the correct drug.

BENEFITS versus RISKS	
Possible Benefits	*Possible Risks*
EFFECTIVE TREATMENT AND PREVENTION OF *CANDIDA* (YEAST) INFECTIONS OF THE MOUTH AND THROAT (THRUSH)	Skin and mucous membrane irritation due to sensitization (drug-induced allergy)
EFFECTIVE TREATMENT OF *CANDIDA* (YEAST) INFECTIONS OF THE SKIN	Nausea, vomiting, stomach cramping, diarrhea (when swallowed)
EFFECTIVE TREATMENT OF *CANDIDA* (YEAST) INFECTIONS OF THE VULVA AND VAGINA	
EFFECTIVE TREATMENT OF TINEA (RINGWORM) INFECTIONS OF THE SKIN	

▷ **Principal Uses**

As a Single Drug Product: Uses currently included in FDA-approved labeling: (1) Treatment of *Candida* (yeast) infections of the skin, mouth, throat, vulva, and vagina; (2) treatment of tinea and related infections: ringworm of the body, groin (jock itch), and feet (athlete's foot), due to susceptible fungal organisms.

Other (unlabeled) generally accepted uses: Prevention of *Candida* (yeast) infections of the mouth and throat in the management of AIDS.

How This Drug Works: By damaging cell walls and blocking essential enzymes, this drug inhibits fungal cell growth and reproduction (with low drug concentrations) and kills fungus (with high drug concentrations).

Available Dosage Forms and Strengths

Cream — 1% (10 mg/g)
Lotion — 1% (10 mg/g)
Topical solution — 1% (10 mg/ml)
Mouth lozenges — 10 mg
Vaginal cream — 1% (10 mg/g), 2%
Vaginal tablets — 100 mg, 200 mg, 500 mg

▷ **Recommended Dosage Ranges** (Actual dosage and administration schedule must be determined for each patient individually.)

Infants and Children: Use of lozenges not recommended for children under 5 years of age; for 5 years and older—dissolve one lozenge slowly and completely in mouth five times a day for 14 days, longer if necessary.

12 to 60 Years of Age: For *Candida* infections of mouth and throat—dissolve 1 lozenge slowly and completely in mouth five times a day for 14 days; extended treatment will be necessary for people with AIDS.

For *Candida* and tinea infections of skin—apply cream, lotion, or solution to infected areas twice a day, morning and evening.

For *Candida* infections of vulva and vagina—one applicatorful (5 g) of cream intravaginally at bedtime for 7 to 14 consecutive days; or one 100-mg tablet intravaginally at bedtime for 7 days; or two 100-mg tablets intravaginally at bedtime for 3 days; single-dose treatment: one 500-mg tablet intravaginally at bedtime, one time only.

Over 60 Years of Age: Same as 12 to 60 years of age.

Conditions Requiring Dosing Adjustments

Liver Function: This drug is removed via the bile—dose should be decreased if bile duct is blocked.

Kidney Function: Dosing changes are not needed.

▷ **Dosing Instructions:** Dissolve lozenge in mouth completely, swallowing saliva as it accumulates. Do not chew the lozenge or swallow it whole. Take full course prescribed. If symptoms persist after or worsen during a course of nonprescription forms, see your doctor.

Usual Duration of Use: Use on a regular schedule for 1 to 2 weeks is usually needed to see this drug's benefit in controlling yeast or tinea infection. Some single-, 3-, or 7-day courses are appropriate for some of the creams or tablets. Long-term use (as in management of AIDS) requires periodic evaluation of response and dosage adjustment. Treatment failure may also be an indication to change to combination HIV therapy or change agents.

Possible Advantages of This Drug

Reasonably effective with minimal toxicity.

More palatable than nystatin.

▷ **This Drug Should Not Be Taken If**
- you have had an allergic reaction to it previously.

▷ **Inform Your Physician Before Taking This Drug If**
- you are allergic to related antifungal drugs: fluconazole, itraconazole, ketoconazole, miconazole.
- you have liver problems and are taking the oral clotrimazole troche.

Possible Side Effects (natural, expected, and unavoidable drug actions)

None.

▷ **Possible Adverse Effects** (unusual, unexpected, and infrequent reactions)

If any of the following develop, consult your physician promptly for guidance.

Mild Adverse Effects

Allergic reactions: skin rash, hives, itching, burning, swelling, blistering (not present prior to treatment)—possible.

Depression, disorientation, or drowsiness—may be frequent with oral therapy.

Nausea, vomiting, stomach cramping, diarrhea (when swallowed)—frequent.

Serious Adverse Effects

Allergic reactions: sensitization of tissues (where applied locally) that will react allergically with future drug application—possible.

Liver toxicity (with oral form)—infrequent.

▷ **Possible Effects on Sexual Function:** None.

Possible Delayed Adverse Effects: Local tissue sensitization to this drug.

Possible Effects on Laboratory Tests

Liver function tests: increased liver enzyme AST/GOT in 15% of users.

CAUTION
1. Avoid contact of cream, lotion, and solution with the eyes.
2. Do not cover applied cream or lotion with an occlusive dressing.

Precautions for Use
By Infants and Children: Use of lozenges by those under 5 years of age is not recommended.
By Those Over 60 Years of Age: No specific problems reported.

▷ **Advisability of Use During Pregnancy**
Pregnancy Category: B. See Pregnancy Risk Categories at the back of this book.
Animal studies: No drug-induced birth defects were found in mouse, rat, or rabbit studies.
Human studies: Adequate studies of pregnant women are not available.
Use this drug only if clearly needed. Ask your physician for guidance.

Advisability of Use If Breast-Feeding
Presence of this drug in breast milk: Unknown.
Watch infant closely and stop drug or nursing if adverse effects start.

Habit-Forming Potential: None.

Effects of Overdosage: Excessive use of lozenges may cause nausea, vomiting, or diarrhea.

Possible Effects of Long-Term Use: None reported.

Suggested Periodic Examinations While Taking This Drug (at physician's discretion)
Chronic oral use: liver function tests.

▷ **While Taking This Drug, Observe the Following**
Foods: No restrictions.
Beverages: No restrictions.
▷ *Alcohol:* No interactions expected.
Tobacco Smoking: No interactions expected, but I advise everyone to quit smoking.
▷ *Other Drugs:* Clotrimazole (oral dosage forms) *taken concurrently* with
• cyclosporine (Sandimmune) may result in cyclosporine toxicity.
• tacrolimus (Prograf) can result in kidney toxicity and increased potassium and glucose.
▷ *Driving, Hazardous Activities:* No restrictions.
Aviation Note: No restrictions.
Exposure to Sun: No restrictions.
Discontinuation: As directed by your physician.

CLOXACILLIN (klox a SIL in)

See the new penicillin combination profile for more information.

CLOZAPINE (KLOH za peen)

Introduced: 1975   **Class:** Strong tranquilizer (antipsychotic)   **Prescription:** USA: Yes   **Controlled Drug:** USA: No   **Available as Generic:** USA: No

Brand Name: Clozaril

Note: In the United States, this drug is available only by special arrangement through the Clozaril Patient Management System, which was administered by Caremark Homecare Corporation, and is now administered by HMI. The toll-free number is 1–800–648–1975. Ask your doctor for help.

BENEFITS versus RISKS	
Possible Benefits	*Possible Risks*
EFFECTIVE CONTROL OF SEVERE SCHIZOPHRENIA that has failed to respond adequately to other appropriate drugs Improvement in many refractory cases Useful in patients who have tardive dyskinesia	SERIOUS BLOOD CELL DISORDERS: abnormally low white blood cell and platelet counts—rare DRUG-INDUCED SEIZURES (depending upon size of dose)

▷ **Principal Uses**

As a Single Drug Product: Uses currently included in FDA-approved labeling: Used in managing severe schizophrenia that has failed to respond to adequate trials of other standard antipsychotic medications (treatment resistant). Because of its potential for causing serious blood cell disorders and seizures, its use is reserved for the severely ill schizophrenic patient.

Other (unlabeled) generally accepted uses: (1) Severe and refractory bipolar disorder; (2) severe tardive dyskinesia (dystonic subtype)—a syndrome that can happen after some medicines are used to treat psychosis; (3) psychosis occurring after labor with lactation.

How This Drug Works: By blocking the place (receptor) where dopamine works in some parts of the brain, this drug helps correct an imbalance of nerve impulses that causes schizophrenic thought disorders.

Available Dosage Forms and Strengths

Tablets — 25 mg, 100 mg

▷ **Usual Adult Dosage Range:** Initially 12.5 mg two times a day; the dose is gradually increased by 25 mg to 50 mg daily, as tolerated, to reach a dose of 300 mg to 450 mg daily (divided into three doses) by the end of 2 weeks. Later increases should be limited to 100 mg one or two times a week. Average dosage requirements are 600 mg daily. Total daily dosage should not exceed 900 mg. **Note: Actual dosage and administration schedule must be determined for each patient individually.**

Conditions Requiring Dosing Adjustments

Liver Function: Eliminated in the liver; however, no specific dosing guidelines are available.

Kidney Function: Patients with kidney failure should be watched closely for adverse effects.

▷ **Dosing Instructions:** May be taken without regard to meals or with food if necessary to reduce stomach irritation. The tablet may be crushed.

Usual Duration of Use: This drug's benefits may be seen after 2 to 4 weeks of regular use. Peak effect may require 3 months; some patients have required 12 months. If no significant benefit is seen within 6 to 8 weeks, the drug should be stopped. Long-term use requires periodic evaluation of response, dosage adjustment, and laboratory testing.

Possible Advantages of This Drug

Rarely causes significant sexual dysfunction.
Low incidence of Parkinson-like reactions (see Glossary).
Only case reports of tardive dyskinesia (see Glossary).

Currently a "Drug of Choice"

For treatment of severe schizophrenia in patients who have not responded to other standard antipsychotic drugs.

▷ This Drug Should Not Be Taken If

- you have had an allergic reaction to it previously.
- you have experienced severe bone marrow depression (impaired white blood cell production) with previous use of this drug.
- you presently have any type of bone marrow or blood cell disorder.
- you are currently taking any other drug that can cause bone marrow depression (see Glossary).

▷ Inform Your Physician Before Taking This Drug If

- you have a history of any type of seizure disorder.
- you have a history of narrow-angle glaucoma.
- you have any type of heart or circulatory disorder, especially heart rhythm abnormalities or hypertension.
- your body is very depleted (cachectic).
- you have impaired liver or kidney function.
- you have prostatism (see Glossary).

Possible Side Effects (natural, expected, and unavoidable drug actions)

Drowsiness, sedation—frequent.
Weight gain—frequent.
Dizziness, light-headedness—infrequent to frequent.
Orthostatic hypotension (see Glossary)—possible.
Blurred vision, salivation, dry mouth, impaired urination, constipation—possible.

▷ Possible Adverse Effects (unusual, unexpected, and infrequent reactions)

If any of the following develop, consult your physician promptly for guidance.

Mild Adverse Effects

Allergic reactions: skin rash; drug fever (see Glossary), which usually occurs within the first 3 weeks of treatment and is self-limiting—rare.
Headache, tremor, fainting, sleep disorders, restlessness, confusion, depression—rare.
Increased salivation—frequent.
Rapid heartbeat, hypertension, chest pain—rare to infrequent.
Nausea, indigestion, vomiting, diarrhea—rare.

Serious Adverse Effects

Allergic reactions: asthmatic-type respiratory reaction—case reports.
Bone marrow depression: specific impairment of white blood cell production with potential for serious infection—rare.
Drug-induced seizures, dose related—rare.
Tardive dyskinesia—case reports.

Abnormally low blood pressure on standing (orthostatic hypotension)—possible.

Anticholinergic syndrome—rare.

Neuroleptic malignant syndrome—case reports.

▷ **Possible Effects on Sexual Function:** Decreased libido and impotence (infrequent and dose related—over 150 mg), abnormal ejaculation or priapism (see Glossary)—rare.

Adverse Effects That May Mimic Natural Diseases or Disorders

Drug-induced fever may suggest systemic infection. Because of the risk of bone marrow depression and secondary infection, any occurrence of fever must be carefully evaluated.

Drug-induced seizures may suggest the possibility of epilepsy.

Natural Diseases or Disorders That May Be Activated by This Drug

Latent glaucoma, prostatism.

Possible Effects on Laboratory Tests

White blood cell counts: decreased.

CAUTION

1. Baseline white blood cell counts must be checked before clozapine treatment is started; follow-up counts must be made every week during the entire course of treatment and for 4 weeks after discontinuation of clozapine.
2. Promptly report any signs of infection: fever, sore throat, flu-like symptoms, skin infections, painful urination, etc.
3. Report promptly light-headedness or dizziness on rising from a sitting or lying position; this could be orthostatic hypotension (see Glossary).
4. Call your doctor before taking any other medication. This includes all prescription and over-the-counter drugs.

Precautions for Use

By Infants and Children: An open label trial of 11 patients from 12 to 17 years old used 12.5 to 25 mg per day as a starting dose, and increased every 4 days by one or two times the starting dose. This dosing strategy was used to treat refractory childhood onset schizophrenia. Mean trial dose was 370 mg per day.

By Those Over 60 Years of Age: Increased risk of orthostatic hypotension, confusion, blood problems, and prostatism. Report related symptoms promptly.

▷ **Advisability of Use During Pregnancy**

Pregnancy Category: B. See Pregnancy Risk Categories at the back of this book.

Animal studies: No birth defects due to this drug reported.

Human studies: Adequate studies of pregnant women are not available.

Use this drug only if clearly needed.

Advisability of Use If Breast-Feeding

Presence of this drug in breast milk: Unknown.

Avoid drug or refrain from nursing.

Habit-Forming Potential: None, but a withdrawal syndrome has been reported after suddenly stopping long-term therapy.

Effects of Overdosage: Marked drowsiness, delirium, hallucinations, rapid and irregular heartbeat, irregular breathing, fainting.

Possible Effects of Long-Term Use: Tardive dyskinesia—case report.

Suggested Periodic Examinations While Taking This Drug (at physician's discretion)

White blood and differential counts prior to starting therapy, every week during therapy, and for 4 weeks after stopping therapy.

Serial blood pressure measurements and electrocardiograms.

▷ **While Taking This Drug, Observe the Following**

Foods: No restrictions.

Beverages: No restrictions. May be taken with milk.

▷   *Alcohol:* Avoid completely. Alcohol increases sedation and accentuates its brain function and blood pressure depression. This drug can increase the intoxicating effects of alcohol.

Tobacco Smoking: May accelerate the elimination of this drug and require increased dosage. I advise everyone to quit smoking.

Marijuana Smoking: Moderate increase in drowsiness; accentuation of orthostatic hypotension; increased risk of aggravating psychosis.

▷   *Other Drugs*

Clozapine may ***increase*** the effects of

- antihypertensive drugs; observe for excessive lowering of blood pressure.
- drugs with atropinelike actions (see Drug Classes).
- drugs with sedative actions; observe for excessive sedation.

Clozapine ***taken concurrently*** with

- cimetidine (Tagamet) can result in a toxic level of clozapine.
- erythromycin (E-Mycin, others) can result in increased clozapine concentrations and potential toxicity. This has been seen in a single case report, but caution is advised.
- fluoxetine (Prozac) can result in clozapine toxicity.
- fluvoxamine (Luvox) can result in clozapine toxicity.
- lithium (Lithobid, Lithotab, etc.) may increase the risk of confusional states, seizures, and neuroleptic malignant syndrome (see Glossary).
- monoamine oxidase inhibitors (MAO inhibitors; see Drug Class) may cause abnormally low blood pressure and exaggerated central nervous system response.
- other bone marrow depressant drugs, such as carbamazepine (Tegretol), may increase the risk of impaired white blood cell production.
- paroxetine (Paxil) may lead to toxicity from either medicine.
- phenytoin (Dilantin) can cause a decreased clozapine level and result in breakthrough schizophrenia.
- risperidone (Risperdal).
- ritonavir (Norvir), and perhaps other protease inhibitors (see Drug Classes), may lead to increased risk of blood adverse effects or other adverse effects. DO NOT COMBINE.
- sertraline (Zoloft) can result in clozapine toxicity.
- venlafaxine (Effexor) may lead to clozapine toxicity.

▷   *Driving, Hazardous Activities:* This drug may cause drowsiness, dizziness, blurred vision, confusion, and seizures. Restrict activities as necessary.

Aviation Note: The use of this drug ***is a disqualification*** for piloting. Consult a designated Aviation Medical Examiner.

Exposure to Sun: No restrictions.

Exposure to Heat: Use caution. This drug can cause fever and can impair the body's adaptation to heat.

Occurrence of Unrelated Illness: Infections must be vigorously treated. White blood cell response to infection must be followed closely.

Discontinuation: If possible, this drug should be discontinued gradually over a period of 1 to 2 weeks. If abrupt withdrawal is necessary, observe carefully for recurrence of psychotic symptoms.

CODEINE (KOH deen)

Introduced: 1886   **Class:** Analgesic, narcotic, opioid   **Prescription:** USA: Yes   **Controlled Drug:** USA: C-II*; Canada: No   **Available as Generic:** Yes

Brand Names: A.B.C. Compound with Codeine [CD], AC & C [CD], Accopain, Actagen-C [CD], Actifed w/Codeine [CD], Afed-C [CD], Alamine-C [CD], Alamine Expectorant [CD], Ambenyl Expectorant [CD], Ambenyl Syrup [CD], Anacin 3 with Codeine #2–4, Anacin w/Codeine [CD], APC with Codeine [CD], Atasol-8, -15, -30 [CD], Ban-Tuiss C [CD], Benylin Syrup w/Codeine [CD], Bromanyl Cough Syrup [CD], Bromotuss, Bromphen DC [CD], Bufferin w/Codeine [CD], Butalbital Compound [CD], Chemdal Expectorant [CD], Chem-Tuss NE [CD], Chlor-Trimeton Expectorant [CD], Coactifed [CD], Codehist DH, Codehist Elixir, ✦Coricidin with Codeine [CD], ✦Coryphen-Codeine [CD], ✦C2 Buffered, ✦C2 with Codeine, Deproist [CD], Dimetane Cough Syrup-DC [CD], Dimetane Expectorant-C [CD], Dimetapp-C [CD], Dimetapp w/Codeine [CD], Empirin w/Codeine No. 2, 4 [CD], ✦Empracet-30, -60 [CD], Empracet w/Codeine No. 3, 4 [CD]✦Emtec-30 [CD], ✦Exdol-8, -15, -30 [CD], ✦Extra Strength Acetaminophen, ✦Fiorinal-C 1/4, -C 1/2 [CD], Fiorinal w/Codeine No. 1, 2, 3 [CD], Gecil [CD], Glydeine, Isoclor Expectorant [CD], ✦Lenoltec w/Codeine No. 1, 2, 3, 4 [CD], ✦Mersyndol, Naldecon-CX [CD], Normatane [CD], Novadyne DH [CD], ✦Novahistex C [CD], ✦Novo-Gesic, Nucochem [CD], Nucofed [CD], ✦Omni-Tuss [CD], Oridol-C [CD], Panadol with Codeine [CD], ✦Paveral, Pediacof [CD], Penntuss [CD], ✦Phenaphen No. 2, 3, 4 [CD], Phenaphen w/Codeine No. 2, 3, 4 [CD], Phenergan w/Codeine [CD], Poly-Histine [CD], Promethazine CS [CD], Pyra-Phed [CD], ✦Robaxacet-8, Robaxisal-C [CD], ✦Rounox w/Codeine [CD], SK-Apap [CD], Tamine Expectorant DC [CD], ✦Tecnal C [CD], Terpin Hydrate and Codeine [CD], Triafed with Codeine [CD], Triaminic Expectorant w/Codeine [CD], ✦Triatec-8, 30 [CD], ✦Tussaminic C Forte [CD], ✦Tussaminic C Ped [CD], ✦Tussi-Organidin [CD], ✦Tylenol w/Codeine [CD], Tylenol w/Codeine No. 1, 2, 3, 4 [CD], Tylenol w/Codeine Elixir [CD], ✦222 [CD], ✦282 [CD], ✦292 [CD], ✦318 A.C. & C. [CD], ✦VC Expectorant with Codeine, ✦Veganin [CD]

*See Schedules of Controlled Drugs at the back of this book.

BENEFITS versus RISKS	
Possible Benefits	**Possible Risks**
EFFECTIVE RELIEF OF MODERATE TO SEVERE PAIN	Potential for habit formation (dependence)
VERY EFFECTIVE CONTROL OF COUGH	Mild allergic reactions—infrequent Nausea, constipation

▷ **Principal Uses**

As a *Single Drug Product:* Uses currently included in FDA-approved labeling: (1) relieves moderate to severe pain; (2) controls cough. Its widest use is as an ingredient in analgesic preparations and cough remedies.

Other (unlabeled) generally accepted uses: May have a limited role in controlling diarrhea.

As a *Combination Drug Product* [CD]: Codeine is combined with other analgesics (aspirin and acetaminophen) on the World Health Organization pain ladder to increase overall pain control. It is also added to cough mixtures containing antihistamines, decongestants, and expectorants.

How This Drug Works: By depressing some brain functions, this drug decreases pain perception, calms emotional responses to pain, and reduces cough reflex sensitivity.

Available Dosage Forms and Strengths

Injection — 30 mg/ml, 60 mg/ml

Tablets — 15 mg, 30 mg, 60 mg

Tablets, soluble — 15 mg, 30 mg, 60 mg

▷ **Usual Adult Dosage Range:** As analgesic—15 to 60 mg every 4 hours. Current pain theory says that the drug should be scheduled, not taken in response to pain as in the past. For cough—10 to 20 mg every 4 to 6 hours as needed. Total daily dosage should not exceed 200 mg for pain or 120 mg for cough. **Note: Actual dosage and administration schedule must be determined for each patient individually.**

Conditions Requiring Dosing Adjustments

Liver Function: The dose must be decreased in liver compromise.

Kidney Function: In moderate to severe kidney failure, the dose is decreased by up to 50%.

▷ **Dosing Instructions:** Tablet may be crushed, then taken with or following food to reduce stomach irritation or nausea.

Usual Duration of Use: As required to control pain or cough. Continual use should not exceed 5 to 7 days without reassessment of need.

▷ **This Drug Should Not Be Taken If**
- you have had an allergic reaction to any dosage form of it previously.
- you are having an acute attack of asthma.
- your breathing is depressed (respiratory depression).

▷ **Inform Your Physician Before Taking This Drug If**
- you have a history of drug abuse or alcoholism.
- you have impaired liver or kidney function.
- you have gallbladder disease, a seizure disorder, or an underactive thyroid gland.
- you have chronic obstructive pulmonary disease (COPD).

- you have low blood calcium (increased sensitivity to this medicine).
- you have a history of porphyria.
- you tend to be constipated.
- you are taking any other drugs that have a sedative effect.
- you plan to have surgery under general anesthesia in the near future.

Possible Side Effects (natural, expected, and unavoidable drug actions)
Drowsiness, light-headedness, dry mouth, urinary retention—possible.
Constipation—frequent and dose related.

▷ **Possible Adverse Effects** (unusual, unexpected, and infrequent reactions)
If any of the following develop, consult your physician promptly for guidance.
Mild Adverse Effects
Allergic reactions: skin rash, hives, itching—case reports.
Dizziness, impaired concentration, sensation of drunkenness, confusion, depression, blurred or double vision—infrequent.
Nausea, vomiting—frequent and may be dose related.
Serious Adverse Effects
Allergic reactions: anaphylaxis, severe skin reactions—case reports.
Idiosyncratic reactions: delirium, hallucinations, excitement, increased sensitivity to pain after the analgesic effect has worn off.
Seizures—rare.
Impaired breathing—dose related.
Porphyria—case reports.
Liver toxicity—case reports.

▷ **Possible Effects on Sexual Function:** Opiates have a variety of effects on sexual response. These may range from blunting of sexual response to increased response if anxiety has been a factor inhibiting response—case reports.

Adverse Effects That May Mimic Natural Diseases or Disorders
Paradoxical behavioral disturbances may suggest psychotic disorder.

Possible Effects on Laboratory Tests
Blood platelet counts: decreased.
Blood amylase and lipase levels: increased (natural side effect).
Urine screening tests for drug abuse: may be **positive**. (Test results depend upon amount of drug taken and testing method used.)

CAUTION
1. If you have asthma, chronic bronchitis, or emphysema, excessive use of this drug may cause respiratory difficulty, thickening of bronchial secretions, and decrease of needed cough reflex.
2. Combining this drug with atropinelike drugs can increase the risk of urinary retention and reduced intestinal function.
3. Do not take this drug following acute head injury.

Precautions for Use
By Infants and Children: Do not use this drug in children under 2 years of age because of their vulnerability to life-threatening respiratory depression. Children 2 to 6 years old: 1 mg per kg of body mass per day, divided into four equal doses. Maximum dose is 30 mg per day. Children 6–12 years of age can receive 5 to 10 mg per dose every 4 to 6 hours, to a maximum of 60 mg every 24 hours.

By Those Over 60 Years of Age: Small starting doses and short-term use is indicated. Expect increased risk of drowsiness, dizziness, unsteadiness, falling, urinary retention, and constipation (often leading to fecal impaction).

▷ **Advisability of Use During Pregnancy**

Pregnancy Category: C; D if used in high doses or for prolonged periods near the time the baby is about to be born. See Pregnancy Risk Categories at the back of this book.

Animal studies: Skull defects reported in hamster studies.

Human studies: Adequate studies of pregnant women are not available. Some studies suggest an increase in significant birth defects when this drug is taken during the first 6 months of pregnancy. Codeine taken during the last few weeks before delivery can cause withdrawal symptoms in the newborn. Use this drug only if clearly needed and in small, infrequent doses.

Advisability of Use If Breast-Feeding

Presence of this drug in breast milk: Yes, in small amounts.

Avoid drug or refrain from nursing.

Habit-Forming Potential: Psychological and/or physical dependence can develop with use of large doses for an extended period of time. However, true dependence is infrequent and unlikely with prudent use.

Effects of Overdosage: Drowsiness, restlessness, agitation, nausea, vomiting, dry mouth, vertigo, weakness, lethargy, stupor, coma, seizures.

Possible Effects of Long-Term Use: Psychological and physical dependence, chronic constipation.

Suggested Periodic Examinations While Taking This Drug (at physician's discretion)

None.

▷ **While Taking This Drug, Observe the Following**

Foods: No restrictions.

Beverages: No restrictions. May be taken with milk.

▷   *Alcohol:* Use extreme caution. Codeine intensifies the intoxicating effects of alcohol, and alcohol intensifies the depressant effects of codeine on brain function, breathing, and circulation. DO NOT COMBINE.

Tobacco Smoking: No interactions expected, but tobacco smoking may cause a decrease in pain tolerance and require an increased or more frequent dose of codeine. I advise everyone to quit smoking.

Marijuana Smoking: Increased drowsiness and pain relief; mental and physical performance will be impaired.

▷   *Other Drugs*

Codeine may *increase* the effects of

- atropinelike drugs, and increase the risk of constipation and urinary retention.
- monoamine oxidase (MAO) inhibitors and also increase central nervous symptoms and depression.
- other drugs with sedative effects.
- tramadol (Ultram).

Codeine *taken concurrently* with

- quinidine may decrease codeine pain control.
- rifabutin (Mycobutin) may decrease codeine's effectiveness.

▷ *Driving, Hazardous Activities:* This drug can impair mental alertness, judgment, reaction time, and physical coordination. Avoid hazardous activities accordingly.

Aviation Note: The use of this drug *is a disqualification* for piloting. Consult a designated Aviation Medical Examiner.

Exposure to Sun: No restrictions.

Discontinuation: It is best to limit this drug to short-term use. If extended use occurs, discontinuation should be gradual to minimize possible effects of withdrawal (usually mild with codeine).

COLCHICINE (KOL chi seen)

Introduced: 1763   **Class:** Anti-gout   **Prescription:** USA: Yes   **Controlled Drug:** USA: No; Canada: No   **Available as Generic:** Yes

Brand Names: Colbenemid [CD], Col-Probenecid [CD], Cosalide, Proben-C [CD]

BENEFITS versus RISKS	
Possible Benefits	*Possible Risks*
EFFECTIVE RELIEF OF ACUTE GOUT SYMPTOMS	Loss of hair
Prevention of recurrent gout attacks	Rare bone marrow depression (see Glossary)
Prevention of attacks of Mediterranean fever	Rare peripheral neuritis (see Glossary)
	Rare liver damage

▷ **Principal Uses**

As a Single Drug Product: Uses currently included in FDA-approved labeling: (1) Reduces the pain, swelling, and inflammation associated with acute attacks of gout (however, many rheumatologists prefer NSAIDs [see Drug Classes] as drugs of first choice in acute gout); (2) it is also used in smaller doses to prevent recurrent gout attacks.

Other (unlabeled) generally accepted uses: (1) Prevention and control of attacks of familial Mediterranean fever; (2) may have a role in easing symptoms of Behçet's disease; (3) limited use in cirrhosis of the liver; (4) damaged disk syndrome may be helped in some patients; (5) may have a role in recurrent pericarditis; (6) can be of help in pseudogout; (7) appears to be of benefit in some lung disease (idiopathic pulmonary fibrosis); (8) has a role in treatment of some cases of refractory immune thrombocytopenic purpura.

As a Combination Drug Product [CD]: Colchicine combined with probenecid enhances its ability to prevent recurrent attacks of gout. Colchicine is most effective in relieving acute gout; it has some effect in preventing recurrent and chronic discomfort. Probenecid increases removal of uric acid by the kidneys and reduces risk of acute gout. This dual action is more effective than either drug used alone in the long-term management of gout.

How This Drug Works: By decreasing joint tissue acid, this drug decreases painful deposit of uric acid crystals and acute inflammation and pain. (Colchicine does not lower uric acid in the blood or increase urine removal.)

Available Dosage Forms and Strengths
Injection — 1 mg/2 ml
Tablets — 0.5 mg, 0.6 mg (also 1 mg in Canada)

▷ **Usual Adult Dosage Range:**   For acute attack—0.5 to 1.2 mg initially, followed by 0.5 to 0.65 mg every 1 to 2 hours until pain is relieved or nausea, vomiting, or diarrhea occurs. Maximum total dose is 8 mg. For prevention of recurrent attacks—0.5 to 0.65 mg, one to three times per day. Pericarditis: 1 mg daily to start, followed by 0.5 mg daily has been effective in treating recurrent heart inflammation (pericarditis). **Note: Actual dosage and administration schedule must be determined for each patient individually.**

Conditions Requiring Dosing Adjustments
Liver Function: Caution must be used, and the dose decreased, if there is a bile obstruction. This drug should NOT be used in people with both liver and kidney compromise.
Kidney Function: For severe kidney failure, 50% of the usual dose should be given. Ongoing prophylactic use should NOT occur in moderate (creatinine clearance less than 50 ml/min) kidney problems. Those with creatinine clearances less than 10 ml/min should NOT be given this medicine.

▷ **Dosing Instructions:**   The tablet may be crushed, then either taken on an empty stomach or with food to reduce nausea or stomach irritation. Start treatment at the first sign of an acute attack. Take the exact dose prescribed.

Usual Duration of Use: For acute attack—stop the drug when pain is relieved or when nausea, vomiting, or diarrhea occurs; do not start this drug for 3 days without asking your doctor. For prevention—use the smallest dose that works; consult your doctor about dosage schedule and duration.

▷ **This Drug Should Not Be Taken If**
• you have had an allergic reaction to it previously.
• you have an active stomach or duodenal ulcer.
• you have active ulcerative colitis.
• you have a severe kidney or liver disorder.
• you have a serious heart disorder.
• you have a history of blood cell disorders.

▷ **Inform Your Physician Before Taking This Drug If**
• you have a history of peptic ulcer disease or ulcerative colitis.
• you develop diarrhea and vomiting while taking this drug.
• you have any type of heart disease.
• you have impaired liver or kidney function.
• you plan to have surgery in the near future.

Possible Side Effects (natural, expected, and unavoidable drug actions)
Nausea, vomiting, abdominal cramping, diarrhea—frequent, especially with maximum doses.

▷ **Possible Adverse Effects** (unusual, unexpected, and infrequent reactions)
If any of the following develop, consult your physician promptly for guidance.
Mild Adverse Effects
Allergic reactions: skin rash, hives, fever—rare.
Hair loss—reported after overdoses.

Serious Adverse Effects
Allergic Reaction: Anaphylactic reaction (see Glossary)—case reports.
Bone marrow depression (see Glossary): fatigue, weakness, fever, sore throat, abnormal bleeding or bruising—case reports.
Peripheral neuritis (see Glossary): numbness, tingling, pain, weakness in hands and/or feet, or myopathy with nerve symptoms (facial palsy and weakness, especially with long-term use in patients with declines in kidney function)—case reports.
Rhabdomyolysis—case reports.
Porphyria—case reports.
Drooping of the eyes (ptosis)—case reports.
Inflammation of colon with bloody diarrhea—case reports.
Thrombophlebitis with intravenous use—case reports.

▷ **Possible Effects on Sexual Function:**   Reversible absence of sperm (azoospermia).

Possible Delayed Adverse Effects: Impaired production of sperm, possibly resulting in birth defects of a child conceived while the father was taking this drug.

Natural Diseases or Disorders That May Be Activated by This Drug
Peptic ulcer disease, ulcerative colitis.

Possible Effects on Laboratory Tests
Complete blood cell counts: decreased red cells, hemoglobin, white cells, and platelets; increased white cells (follows initial decrease).
Prothrombin time: decreased (with concurrent use of warfarin).
Blood vitamin B_{12} level: decreased.
Liver function tests: increased liver enzymes (ALT/GPT, AST/GOT, and alkaline phosphatase), increased bilirubin.
Fecal occult blood test: positive.
Sperm counts: decreased (may be marked).

CAUTION
1. If this drug causes vomiting and/or diarrhea before relief of joint pain, discontinue it and inform your physician.
2. Try to limit each course of treatment for acute gout to 4 to 8 mg. Do not exceed 3 mg every 24 hours or a total of 10 mg per course.
3. Omit drug for 3 days between courses to avoid toxicity.
4. Carry this drug with you while traveling if you are subject to attacks of acute gout.
5. The stress of surgery can cause an acute attack of gout. Ask your doctor how much colchicine should be taken before and after surgery to prevent gout.

Precautions for Use
By Infants and Children: Use for preventing (prophylaxis) familial Mediterranean fever in children 6 to 13 years of age was given as 0.5 mg per day and increased by 0.5 mg per day, to symptom control or a maximum of 2 mg per day. For other uses in children, dosage has not been established. Ask your physician for guidance.
By Those Over 60 Years of Age: Because the dosage needed to relieve acute gout often causes vomiting and/or diarrhea, extreme caution is advised if you

have heart or circulatory disorders, reduced liver or kidney function, or general debility.

▷ **Advisability of Use During Pregnancy**
Pregnancy Category: C by one manufacturer, and D by another. See Pregnancy Risk Categories at the back of this book.
Animal studies: This drug causes significant birth defects in hamsters and rabbits.
Human studies: Adequate studies of pregnant women are not available. However, it is reported that colchicine can cause harm to the fetus.
Avoid during entire pregnancy if possible. Ask your physician for guidance.

Advisability of Use If Breast-Feeding
Presence of this drug in breast milk: Yes.
Ask your doctor for help.

Habit-Forming Potential: None.

Effects of Overdosage: Nausea, vomiting, abdominal cramping, diarrhea (may be bloody), burning sensation in throat and skin, weak and rapid pulse, progressive paralysis, inability to breathe.

Possible Effects of Long-Term Use: Hair loss, aplastic anemia (see Glossary), peripheral neuritis (see Glossary).

Suggested Periodic Examinations While Taking This Drug (at physician's discretion)
Complete blood cell counts, uric acid blood levels to monitor status of gout, sperm analysis for quantity and condition, liver function tests.

▷ **While Taking This Drug, Observe the Following**
Foods: Follow your physician's advice regarding the need for a low purine diet.
Beverages: Drink at least 3 quarts of liquids every 24 hours. This drug may be taken with milk. Some "herbal teas" (promoted as being beneficial for arthritis) contain phenylbutazone and other potentially toxic ingredients. Avoid herbal teas if you are not certain of their source, content, and medicinal effects.
▷ *Alcohol:* No interactions expected. Combination may increase the risk of gastrointestinal irritation or bleeding and raise uric acid blood levels.
Tobacco Smoking: No interactions expected, but I advise everyone to quit smoking.
▷ *Other Drugs*
Colchicine *taken concurrently* with
• allopurinol (Zyloprim), probenecid (Benemid), or sulfinpyrazone (Anturane) can prevent attacks of acute gout that often occur when treatment with these drugs is first started.
• cyanocobalamin will decrease absorption of the vitamin B_{12}. Higher doses of oral cyanocobalamin may be required by patients on colchicine.
• cyclosporine (Sandimmune) may increase cyclosporine levels and result in toxicity.
• erythromycins (E.E.S., azithromycin, clarithromycin) can result in toxic colchicine blood levels.
• insulin may inhibit the response (biphasic) of the body to sugar.
▷ *Driving, Hazardous Activities:* Usually no restrictions when taken continually in

small (preventive) doses. May cause nausea, vomiting, and/or diarrhea when taken in larger (treatment) doses.

Aviation Note: The use of this drug **may be a disqualification** for piloting. Consult a designated Aviation Medical Examiner.

Exposure to Sun: No restrictions.

Exposure to Cold: This drug can lower body temperature. Use caution to prevent excessive lowering (hypothermia), especially in those over 60 years of age.

Occurrence of Unrelated Illness: Acute attacks of gout may result from injury or illness. Call your doctor for dosing adjustment if injury or new illness occurs.

COLESTIPOL (koh LES ti pohl)

Introduced: 1974   **Class:** Anticholesterol   **Prescription:** USA: Yes
Controlled Drug: USA: No; Canada: No   **Available as Generic:** USA: No;
Canada: No
Brand Name: Colestid

BENEFITS versus RISKS	
Possible Benefits	*Possible Risks*
EFFECTIVE REDUCTION OF TOTAL CHOLESTEROL AND LOW-DENSITY CHOLESTEROL IN TYPE IIa CHOLESTEROL DISORDERS EFFECTIVE RELIEF OF ITCHING associated with biliary obstruction	Constipation (may be severe) Reduced absorption of fat, fat-soluble vitamins (A, D, E, and K), and folic acid Reduced formation of prothrombin with resultant bleeding

▷ **Principal Uses**

As a Single Drug Product: Uses currently included in FDA-approved labeling: (1) Used in combination with diet changes to decrease blood cholesterol and low-density (LDL) cholesterol in Type IIa cholesterol disorders; (2) eases itching due to the deposit of bile acids in the skin associated with partial biliary obstruction; (3) helps remove buildup on interior of blood vessels (atherosclerosis).

Other (unlabeled) generally accepted uses: (1) Data from one study showed that colestipol in combination with lovastatin actually caused regression of plaque buildup (atherosclerosis) inside blood vessels; (2) some data show that colestipol is useful in pseudomembranous colitis.

How This Drug Works: This drug combines with bile acids and salts and is excreted in the feces. This removal of bile acids stimulates conversion of cholesterol to bile acids to replace the loss; this in turn reduces the blood levels of cholesterol. By reducing the blood levels of bile acids, this drug hastens clearance of bile acids in the skin and relieves itching.

Available Dosage Forms and Strengths

Bottles — 250 g, 500 g
Packets — 5 g
Flavored Colestid Granules for oral suspension — 5 g per dose

▷ **Usual Adult Dosage Range:** Initially 5 g of powder is mixed in an approved liquid (such as orange juice, apple juice, water, or grape juice) and taken three times daily. Dose may be increased slowly as needed and tolerated to 30 g daily in two to four divided doses. **Note: Actual dosage and administration schedule must be determined for each patient individually.**

Conditions Requiring Dosing Adjustments

Liver Function: This medication is eliminated via the feces, and the liver is not involved.

Kidney Function: No changes are needed in renal compromise, as the drug is not absorbed.

▷ **Dosing Instructions:** Always take just before or with a meal; this drug is ineffective when taken without food. Mix the powder thoroughly in 4 to 6 ounces of water, fruit juice, tomato juice, milk, thin soup, or a soft food like applesauce. **Do not take it in its dry form.**

Usual Duration of Use: Use on a regular schedule for up to a month may be needed to see peak benefits in lowering cholesterol. The drug should be stopped if an acceptable response is not seen after 3 months. Long-term use (months to years) requires periodic physician evaluation of response and dosage adjustment.

▷ **This Drug Should Not Be Taken If**
- you have had an allergic reaction to it previously.
- you have complete biliary obstruction.

▷ **Inform Your Physician Before Taking This Drug If**
- you are prone to constipation.
- you have low thyroid function (hypothyroidism).
- you have peptic ulcer disease.
- you have a bleeding disorder of any kind.
- you have impaired kidney function.

Possible Side Effects (natural, expected, and unavoidable drug actions)

Constipation; interference with normal fat digestion and absorption; reduced absorption of vitamins A, D, E, and K and folic acid. Binds to vitamin B_{12}—intrinsic factor complex.

▷ **Possible Adverse Effects** (unusual, unexpected, and infrequent reactions)

If any of the following develop, consult your physician promptly for guidance.

Mild Adverse Effects

Allergic reactions: skin rash—rare; hives, tongue irritation, anal itching—case reports.

Headache, dizziness, weakness, muscle and joint pains—possible.

Constipation—most frequent.

Loss of appetite, indigestion, heartburn, abdominal discomfort, excessive gas, nausea, vomiting, diarrhea—case reports.

Serious Adverse Effects

Vitamin K deficiency and increased bleeding tendency—possible.

Impaired absorption of calcium; predisposition to osteoporosis—possible.

Hypothyroidism—possible.

Disruption of normal acid–base balance of the body (metabolic acidosis)—possible with long-term use.

▷ **Possible Effects on Sexual Function:**   None reported.

Natural Diseases or Disorders That May Be Activated by This Drug

Peptic ulcer disease; steatorrhea (excessive fat in stools) with large doses.

Possible Effects on Laboratory Tests

Blood cholesterol and triglyceride levels: decreased (therapeutic effect).

Blood thyroxine (T_4) level: decreased when colestipol and niacin are taken concurrently (in presence of normal thyroid function).

CAUTION

1. Never take the powder in its dry form; always mix it thoroughly with a suitable liquid before swallowing.
2. Watch carefully for constipation; use stool softeners and laxatives as needed.
3. This drug may bind other drugs taken concurrently and impair their absorption. It is advisable to take **all other drugs** 1 to 2 hours before or 4 to 6 hours after taking this drug.

Precautions for Use

By Infants and Children: Safety and effectiveness for those under 12 years of age not established. Watch carefully for the possible development of acidosis and vitamin A or folic acid deficiency. (Ask your physician for guidance.)

By Those Over 60 Years of Age: Increased risk of severe constipation. Impaired kidney function may predispose to the development of acidosis.

▷ **Advisability of Use During Pregnancy**

Pregnancy Category: C. See Pregnancy Risk Categories at the back of this book.

Animal studies: No information available.

Human studies: Adequate studies of pregnant women are not available.

Use this drug only if clearly needed. Ensure adequate intake of vitamins and minerals to satisfy needs of mother and fetus.

Advisability of Use If Breast-Feeding

Presence of this drug in breast milk: None.

Breast-feeding is permitted.

Habit-Forming Potential: None.

Effects of Overdosage: Progressive constipation, skin changes (skin drying).

Possible Effects of Long-Term Use: Deficiencies of vitamins A, D, E, and K and folic acid. Calcium deficiency, osteoporosis. Acidosis due to excessive retention of chloride. Binding of the B-12 intrinsic factor complex may lead to blood cell problems.

Suggested Periodic Examinations While Taking This Drug (at physician's discretion)

Measurements of blood levels of total cholesterol, low-density (LDL) cholesterol, and high-density (HDL) cholesterol. Hemoglobin and red blood cell studies for possible anemia. Thyroid function tests.

▷ **While Taking This Drug, Observe the Following**

Foods: Avoid foods that tend to constipate (cheeses, etc.).

Nutritional Support: Ask your doctor if you need supplements of vitamins A, D, E, and K, folic acid, and calcium.

Beverages: Ensure adequate liquid intake (up to 2 quarts daily). This drug may be taken with milk.

▷ *Alcohol:* No interactions expected.

Tobacco Smoking: No interactions expected, but I advise everyone to quit smoking.

▷ *Other Drugs*

Colestipol may *decrease* the effects of
- acetaminophen (Tylenol); take 2 hours before colestipol.
- aspirin; take 2 hours before colestipol.
- digitoxin and digoxin (Lanoxin); take 2 hours before colestipol.
- folic acid; take 2 hours before colestipol.
- furosemide (Lasix); take 4 hours before colestipol.
- hydrocortisone; take 2 hours before colestipol.
- iron preparations; take 2 to 3 hours before colestipol.
- penicillin G; take 2 hours before colestipol.
- phenobarbital; take 2 hours before colestipol.
- tetracycline (Achromycin); take 2 hours before colestipol.
- thiazide diuretics (see Drug Classes); take 2 hours before colestipol.
- thyroxine (see Thyroid Hormones Drug Class); take 5 hours before colestipol.
- vitamin B_{12}.

▷ *Driving, Hazardous Activities:* No restrictions.

Aviation Note: The use of this drug *is usually not a disqualification* for piloting. Consult a designated Aviation Medical Examiner.

Exposure to Sun: No restrictions.

Discontinuation: The dose of any toxic drug combined with colestipol must be reduced when this drug is stopped. Once colestipol is stopped, cholesterol levels usually return to pretreatment levels in 1 month.

CROMOLYN (KROH moh lin)

Other Names: Cromolyn sodium, sodium cromoglycate

Introduced: 1968 **Class:** Antiasthmatic drug, preventive **Prescription:** USA: Yes **Controlled Drug:** USA: No; Canada: No **Available as Generic:** USA: No; Canada: No

Brand Names: Crolom, Gastrocrom, Intal, ✦Intal Spincaps, ✦Intal Syncroner, ✦Nalcrom, Nasalcrom, Opticrom, ✦Rynacrom

BENEFITS versus RISKS	
Possible Benefits	*Possible Risks*
LONG-TERM PREVENTION OF RECURRENT ASTHMA ATTACKS	Anaphylactic reaction (see Glossary)
Prevention of acute asthma due to allergens or exercise	Spasm of bronchial tubes, increased wheezing
Prevention and treatment of allergic rhinitis	Allergic pneumonitis (allergic reaction in lung tissue)
Prevention of bronchospasm	
Relief of allergic conjunctivitis	
Treatment of giant papillary conjunctivitis	

▷ **Principal Uses**

As a Single Drug Product: Uses currently included in FDA-approved labeling: (1) Prevents allergic reactions in the nose (allergic rhinitis, hay fever) and the bronchial tubes (bronchial asthma). Does not help asthma once an attack starts; (2) it is also used to treat allergic rhinitis; (3) helps conjunctivitis (allergic); (4) helps prevent exercise- or environmentally-induced asthma; (5) treatment of mastocytosis and management of several allergy-related skin disorders.

Other (unlabeled) generally accepted uses: (1) Helps modify the reactions in food allergies; (2) may have a small part in the therapy of Bell's palsy.

How This Drug Works: It blocks the release of histamine (and other chemicals) that worsen allergic reactions. This drug prevents the sequence of events that lead to swelling and itching and to constriction of bronchial tubes (asthma).

Available Dosage Forms and Strengths

Capsules, oral — 100 mg
Eyedrops — 2% and 4%
Inhalation aerosol — 0.8 mg per metered spray
Inhalation capsules (powder) — 20 mg
Inhalation solution — 20 mg per ampule
Nasal insufflation (powder) — 10 mg per cartridge
Nasal solution — 40 mg/ml

▷ **Usual Adult Dosage Range**

Eyedrops: one to two drops four to six times daily at regular intervals.

Inhalation aerosol: 1.6 mg (two inhalations) four times daily at regular intervals for prevention of asthma, or a single dose 10 to 15 minutes before exposure to prevent allergen-induced or exercise-induced asthma.

Inhalation powder: 20 mg (one capsule) four times daily at regular intervals for long-term prevention of asthma; 20 mg (one capsule) as a single dose 10 to 15 minutes before exposure to prevent acute allergen-induced or exercise-induced asthma. Total daily maximum dosage is 160 mg (eight capsules).

Inhalation solution: Same as inhalation powder.

Nasal insufflation: Initially 10 mg in each nostril every 4 to 6 hours as needed; reduce to every 8 to 12 hours for maintenance.

Nasal solution: 2.6 mg to 5.2 mg in each nostril three to six times daily as needed.**Note: Actual dosage and administration schedule must be determined for each patient individually.**

Conditions Requiring Dosing Adjustments

Liver Function: If the bile duct is damaged by liver disease, the dose must be decreased.

Kidney Function: The dose should be decreased in kidney failure.

▷ **Dosing Instructions:**   Follow instructions provided with all of the dosage forms, especially the inhalers. Do not swallow the capsules; the powder is intended for inhalation. (If the capsule is accidentally swallowed, the drug will cause no beneficial or adverse effects). Contents of capsules for mouth (oral) use can be poured into 4 ounces (one half glass) of hot water and then stirred until completely dissolved.

Usual Duration of Use: Use on a regular schedule for 6 weeks or more is often needed to see benefit in preventing asthma attacks or allergic rhinitis. Long-term use (months to years) requires periodic physician evaluation.

Possible Advantages of This Drug
May be quite effective in the young asthmatic.
Usually well tolerated. Serious adverse effects are very rare.

▷ **This Drug Should Not Be Taken If**
- you have had an allergic reaction to any dosage form of it previously.

▷ **Inform Your Physician Before Taking This Drug If**
- you are allergic to milk, milk products, or lactose. (The inhalation powder contains lactose.)
- you have impaired liver or kidney function.
- you have soft contact lenses (these should not be worn while using the eye-drops).
- you have angina or a heart rhythm disorder. (The inhalation aerosol contains propellants that could be hazardous.)

Possible Side Effects (natural, expected, and unavoidable drug actions)
Unpleasant taste with use of inhalation aerosol.
Mild throat irritation, hoarseness, cough. (These can be minimized by a few swallows of water after each inhalation of powder.)

▷ **Possible Adverse Effects** (unusual, unexpected, and infrequent reactions)
If any of the following develop, consult your physician promptly for guidance.
Mild Adverse Effects
Allergic reactions: skin rash, hives, itching—possible.
Headache, dizziness, drowsiness—rare.
Nausea, vomiting, urinary urgency and pain (dysuria), joint pain—infrequent.
Muscle pain (myositis)—rare.
Stinging or burning of the eyes with ophthalmic use—possible.
Cough and bronchial irritation—rare.
Nosebleed or itching with nasal solution use—rare.
Serious Adverse Effects
Allergic reactions: rare anaphylactic reaction (see Glossary). Allergic pneumonitis (allergic reaction in lung tissue)—case reports.
Propellants in the metered dose inhaler may cause problems in patients with disease of the heart arteries or a history of abnormal heart rhythms—possible.
Inflammation of the arteries—case reports.

▷ **Possible Effects on Sexual Function:**   None reported.

Possible Effects on Laboratory Tests
None reported.

CAUTION
1. This drug only helps **prevent** bronchial asthma—used **before** the start of acute bronchial constriction (asthmatic wheezing).
2. *Do not* use this drug during an acute attack of asthma; it could worsen and prolong asthmatic wheezing.
3. This drug does *not* block the benefits of drugs that relieve acute asthma

attacks after they start. Cromolyn is used *before and between* acute attacks to help keep them from starting; bronchodilators are used *during* acute attacks.

4. If you are using a bronchodilator drug by inhalation, it is best to take it about 5 minutes before inhaling cromolyn.

5. If this drug has allowed you to decrease or eliminate steroids, and you are unable to tolerate it, ask your doctor about the need to start steroids once again.

Precautions for Use

By Infants and Children: Safety and effectiveness for those under 5 years of age not established for the metered dose inhaler. Inhalation capsules: For children 2 years and older: 20 mg (contents of one capsule) inhaled four times a day. Young children may find a nebulized solution easier than the powder.

By Those Over 60 Years of Age: This drug does not work in the management of chronic bronchitis or emphysema.

▷ **Advisability of Use During Pregnancy**

Pregnancy Category: B. See Pregnancy Risk Categories at the back of this book.
Animal studies: Mouse, rat, and rabbit studies revealed no birth defects due to this drug.
Human studies: Adequate studies of pregnant women are not available.
Use this drug only if clearly needed.

Advisability of Use If Breast-Feeding

Presence of this drug in breast milk: Unknown.
Avoid drug or refrain from nursing.

Habit-Forming Potential: None.

Effects of Overdosage: No significant effects reported.

Possible Effects of Long-Term Use: Allergic reaction of lung tissue (allergic pneumonitis)—very rare.

Suggested Periodic Examinations While Taking This Drug (at physician's discretion)

Sputum analysis and X ray if symptoms suggest allergic pneumonitis.

▷ **While Taking This Drug, Observe the Following**

Foods: Follow physician-prescribed diet. Avoid all foods to which you are allergic.

Beverages: Avoid all beverages to which you may be allergic.

▷   *Alcohol:* No interactions expected.

Tobacco Smoking: No interactions with the medicine, but smoking can irritate your airways. I advise everyone to quit smoking.

▷   *Other Drugs:* Cromolyn may allow reduced dosage of cortisonelike drugs in the management of chronic asthma. Ask your doctor about dosage adjustment.

▷   *Driving, Hazardous Activities:* This drug may cause dizziness. Restrict activities as necessary.

Aviation Note: The use of this drug *may be a disqualification* for piloting. Consult a designated Aviation Medical Examiner.

Exposure to Sun: No restrictions.

Heavy Exercise or Exertion: This drug may prevent exercise-induced asthma if taken 10 to 15 minutes before exertion. It is most effective in young people.

Discontinuation: If cromolyn has made it possible to reduce or stop maintenance doses of cortisonelike drugs, and you find it necessary to discontinue
cromolyn, watch closely for a sudden return of asthma. You may have to
start a cortisonelike drug as well as other measures to control asthma.

Special Storage Instructions: Keep the powder cartridges in a dry, tightly closed
container. Store in a cool place, but not in the refrigerator. Do not handle
the cartridges or the inhaler when hands are wet.

CYCLOPHOSPHAMIDE (si kloh FOSS fa mide)

Introduced: 1959   **Class:** Anticancer, immunosuppressive   **Prescription:** USA: Yes   **Controlled Drug:** USA: No; Canada: No   **Available as
Generic:** No

Brand Names: Cytoxan, Neosar, ✚Procytox

BENEFITS versus RISKS	
Possible Benefits	*Possible Risks*
CURE OR CONTROL OF CERTAIN TYPES OF CANCER	REDUCED WHITE BLOOD CELL COUNT
PREVENTION OF REJECTION IN ORGAN TRANSPLANTATION	SECONDARY INFECTION
	URINARY BLADDER BLEEDING
Possibly beneficial in the treatment of rheumatoid arthritis and lupus erythematosus	HEART, LUNG, LIVER, OR KIDNEY DAMAGE
	Loss of hair
Possibly beneficial in selected cases of nephrotic syndrome in children	

▷ **Principal Uses**

As a Single Drug Product: Uses currently included in FDA-approved labeling: (1)
Treatment of various forms of cancer, notably malignant lymphomas, multiple myeloma, sarcomas, retinoblastomas, leukemias, and cancers of the
breast and ovary; (2) because this drug exerts a suppressant effect on the
immune system, it is also used to prevent rejection in organ transplantation
and treat certain autoimmune disorders; (3) also used to treat some resistant forms of nephrotic syndrome.

Other (unlabeled) generally accepted uses: (1) Used to prepare patients for
autologous bone marrow transplants; (2) part of several combination chemotherapy regimens; (3) helps overall survival in combination therapy of
lung or fallopian tube cancer; (4) can be part of combination therapy for
Ewing's sarcoma; (5) may be of help in patients with lupus erythematosus
who have interstitial lung disease or nephritis; (6) secondary role in prostate cancer; (7) has a role in treating serious anemia (aplastic anemia) with
high-dose treatment. This was recently evaluated as an alternative to bone
marrow transplantation.

How This Drug Works: Because of its ability to kill cancer cells during all
phases of their development and reproduction, this drug suppresses the
primary growth and secondary spread (metastasis) of certain types of cancer.

Available Dosage Forms and Strengths

Injection — vials of 100 mg, 200 mg, 500 mg, 1 g, and 2 g

Tablets — 25 mg, 50 mg

▷ **Usual Adult Dosage Range:**   Oral form: 60 to 120 mg per square meter of body surface area daily or 400 mg per square meter of body surface area on days 1 to 5, every 3 to 4 weeks. As therapy continues, the dose is adjusted according to how the tumor responds or unacceptable low white blood cell counts develop. Intravenous: 1000 to 1500 mg per square meter every 3 to 4 weeks, adjusted the same as the oral form. **Note: Actual dosage and administration schedule must be determined for each patient individually.**

Conditions Requiring Dosing Adjustments

Liver Function: Dose changes are not required in liver compromise.

Kidney Function: In moderate to severe kidney problems, the dose is decreased by 25–50%.

▷ **Dosing Instructions:**   Tablets may be crushed, and are best taken on an empty stomach. However, if nausea or indigestion occurs, this drug may be taken with or following food. Total liquid intake should be no less than 3 quarts every 24 hours to reduce the risk of bladder irritation.

Usual Duration of Use: Use on a regular schedule is required to achieve and maintain a significant remission of the cancer. Duration of use depends on the response of the cancer and patient tolerance of the drug.

▷ **This Drug Should Not Be Taken If**

• you have had an allergic reaction to any dosage form of it previously.
• you have an active infection of any kind.
• you have bloody urine for any reason.
• you have kidney (renal) failure with creatinine clearance less than 30 ml/min (talk with your doctor).
• you are pregnant.

▷ **Inform Your Physician Before Taking This Drug If**

• you have impaired liver or kidney function.
• you have a blood cell or bone marrow disorder.
• you have had previous chemotherapy or X-ray therapy for any type of cancer.
• you take, or have taken within the past year, any cortisonelike drug (adrenal corticosteroids).
• you have diabetes.
• you plan to have surgery under general anesthesia in the near future.

Possible Side Effects (natural, expected, and unavoidable drug actions)

Bone marrow depression (see Glossary)—low production of white blood cells and, to a lesser degree, red blood cells and blood platelets (see Glossary). Possible effects include fever, chills, sore throat, fatigue, weakness, abnormal bleeding or bruising.

Leukemia has been reported following cyclophosphamide therapy.

Impairment of natural resistance (immunity) to infection.

Weakening of the heart muscle (cardiomyopathy).

Excessive urination (SIADH).

Cystitis or hemorrhagic cystitis.

Ninefold increase in bladder cancer risk.

▷ **Possible Adverse Effects** (unusual, unexpected, and infrequent reactions)
   If any of the following develop, consult your physician promptly for guidance.
   Mild Adverse Effects
   Allergic reaction: skin rash—rare.
   Headache, dizziness, blurred vision—possible.
   Loss of scalp hair (50% of users), darkening of skin and fingernails, transverse ridging of nails.
   Nausea, vomiting (dose related)—frequent.
   Ulceration of mouth, diarrhea (may be bloody)—possible.
   Serious Adverse Effects
   Idiosyncratic reaction: hemolytic anemia—case reports.
   Liver damage with jaundice: yellow eyes and skin, dark-colored urine, light-colored stools—rare.
   Kidney damage: impaired kidney function, reduced urine volume, bloody urine—case reports.
   Severe inflammation of bladder: painful urination, bloody urine—infrequent to frequent.
   Drug-induced damage of heart and lung (interstitial pneumonitis) tissue—case reports.
   Pancreatitis—case reports.

▷ **Possible Effects on Sexual Function**
   Suppression of ovarian function—irregular menstrual pattern or cessation of menstruation (18 to 57%, depending upon dose and duration of use).
   Testicular suppression—reduced or no sperm production (100% of users).

Possible Delayed Adverse Effects
   Development of other types of cancer (secondary malignancies). Development of severe cystitis with bleeding from the bladder wall. (May occur many months after the last dose.)

Possible Effects on Laboratory Tests
   Complete blood cell counts: decreased red cells, hemoglobin, white cells, and platelets.
   INR (prothrombin time): increased.
   Liver function tests: increased liver enzymes (ALT/GPT, AST/GOT, and alkaline phosphatase), increased bilirubin.

CAUTION
   1. This drug may interfere with the normal healing of wounds.
   2. This drug can cause significant changes in genetic material in both men and women (sperm and eggs or ova). Patients taking this drug **must** understand the potential for serious defects in children that are conceived during or following the course of medication.
   3. This drug can suppress natural resistance (immunity) to infection, resulting in life-threatening illness.
   4. Avoid live virus vaccines while taking this drug (talk with your doctor about this).

Precautions for Use
   By Infants and Children: This drug should not be given if the child is dehydrated. Adequate fluid intake to ensure a copious urine volume for 4 hours following each dose is needed. Prevent exposure of child to anyone

with active chickenpox or shingles. This drug may cause ovarian or testicular sterility.

By Those Over 60 Years of Age: Increased risk of serious bladder problems (chemical cystitis). Patients **MUST** drink large amounts of water in order to keep the bladder flushed. This may increase the risk of urinary retention in men with prostatism (see Glossary).

▷ **Advisability of Use During Pregnancy**

Pregnancy Category: D. See Pregnancy Risk Categories at the back of this book.

Animal studies: Significant birth defects reported in mice, rat, and rabbit studies.

Human studies: Information from studies of pregnant women indicates that this drug can cause serious birth defects or fetal death.

Avoid completely during the first 3 months. Use of this drug during the last 6 months must be carefully individualized.

Advisability of Use If Breast-Feeding

Presence of this drug in breast milk: Yes.

Avoid drug or refrain from nursing.

Habit-Forming Potential: None.

Effects of Overdosage: Nausea, vomiting, diarrhea, bloody urine, water retention, weight gain, severe bone marrow depression, severe infections.

Possible Effects of Long-Term Use: Development of fibrous tissue in lungs; secondary malignancies.

Suggested Periodic Examinations While Taking This Drug (at physician's discretion)

Complete blood cell counts, every 2 to 4 days during initial treatment; then every 3 to 4 weeks during maintenance treatment.

Liver and kidney function tests.

Thyroid function tests (if symptoms warrant).

▷ **While Taking This Drug, Observe the Following**

Foods: No restrictions.

Beverages: No restrictions. May be taken with milk.

▷ *Alcohol:* No interactions expected.

Tobacco Smoking: No interactions expected, but I advise everyone to quit smoking.

▷ *Other Drugs*

Cyclophosphamide *taken concurrently* with

- allopurinol (Zyloprim) may increase the extent of bone marrow depression.
- amphotericin (Abelcet and others) may increase risk of kidney toxicity.
- chloramphenicol can decrease cyclophosphamide effectiveness.
- ciprofloxacin (Cipro) can result in lowered ciprofloxacin levels and the need for a larger than usual dose.
- digoxin may decrease digoxin absorption and impair digoxin's effectiveness.
- flu (influenza) vaccine, and perhaps other vaccines, may decrease the vaccine's ability to confer immunity.
- hydrochlorothiazide and other thiazide diuretics (see Drug Classes) may worsen the lowering of white blood cells (myelosuppression) caused by cyclophosphamide.
- indomethacin (Indocin) can cause fluid retention.

- pentostatin may cause fatal heart damage.
- succinylcholine can result in succinylcholine toxicity.

▷ *Driving, Hazardous Activities:* Use caution if dizziness occurs.

Aviation Note: The use of this drug **may be a disqualification** for piloting. Consult a designated Aviation Medical Examiner.

Exposure to Sun: No restrictions.

Occurrence of Unrelated Illness: Any signs of infection—fever, chills, sore throat, cough, or flu-like symptoms—must be promptly reported. This drug may have to be stopped until the infection is controlled. Consult your physician.

CYCLOSPORINE (SI kloh spor een)

Other Names: Ciclosporin, cyclosporin A

Introduced: 1983   **Class:** Immunosuppressant   **Prescription:** USA: Yes   **Controlled Drug:** USA: No; Canada: No   **Available as Generic:** USA: No; Canada: No

Brand Names: Neoral, Sandimmune

BENEFITS versus RISKS	
Possible Benefits	*Possible Risks*
EFFECTIVE PREVENTION AND TREATMENT OF REJECTION IN ORGAN TRANSPLANTATION	MARKED KIDNEY TOXICITY DEVELOPMENT OF HYPERTENSION
Limited effectiveness in the treatment of Crohn's disease, myasthenia gravis, or severe psoriasis and other inflammatory (autoimmune) conditions	Liver toxicity Low white blood cell count Development of lymphoma Excessive hair growth Overgrowth of gums
Neoral form has been approved for rheumatoid arthritis	

▷ **Principal Uses**

As a Single Drug Product: Uses included in FDA-approved labeling: (1) Helps prevent (in conjunction with cortisonelike drugs) organ rejection in kidney, liver, and heart transplantation; (2) helps treat rejection crisis; (3) the Neoral microemulsion form has recently been approved for use in severe active rheumatoid arthritis that has not responded to methotrexate therapy.

Other (unlabeled) generally accepted uses: (1) Used in transplantation of the bone marrow; (2) used investigationally in a variety of diseases involving the immune system such as: Sjögren's, Crohn's, and Grave's diseases; psoriasis; myasthenia gravis; bullous pemphigoid; pulmonary fibrosis associated with rheumatoid arthritis; rheumatoid arthritis; Sweet's syndrome; insulin-dependent diabetes; and aplastic anemia; (3) may have a role in helping severe, steroid-dependent asthma; (4) can have a role in treating severe skin reactions (toxic epidermal necrolysis) to phenytoin (Dilantin).

How This Drug Works: By inhibiting some lymphocytes (white blood cells) and their growth factors, this drug suppresses the rejection of transplanted organs.

Available Dosage Forms and Strengths
  Capsules, soft gelatin — 25 mg, 100 mg
  Injection, intravenous — 50 mg/ml
  Oral solution (Note: The microemulsion, Neoral, is NOT the same as
  Sandimmune.)   — 100 mg/ml

▷ **Usual Adult Dosage Range:**   Initially 15 mg per kg of body mass per day, taken
    4 to 12 hours prior to transplantation surgery. This dose is continued fol-
    lowing surgery for 1 to 2 weeks; then the dose is gradually reduced by 5%
    per week to a maintenance dose of 5 to 10 mg per kg of body mass per day.
    A new dosing strategy NOT using weight (using only the lowest blood level
    or trough) has been developed. Rectal dosing for ulcerative colitis has been
    given in a range of 250 to 350 mg per day. The microemulsion formulation
    offers more consistent pharmacokinetics. If Neoral is used, it should be
    given at the same time each day in two equally divided doses. If a conver-
    sion is made from oral Sandimmune to Neoral, the Neoral dose is usually
    started at the same daily dose as the Sandimmune. Cyclosporine trough
    levels should be measured twice a week when patients are converted to
    Neoral who were taking more than 10 mg per kg of body mass per day of
    Sandimmune.
  Interstitial cystitis: 2.5–5 mg per kg of body mass daily, adjusted to blood
    levels (80–200 mcg/L) has been used for up to 6 months. **Note: Actual do-
    sage and administration schedule must be determined for each pa-
    tient individually.**

Conditions Requiring Dosing Adjustments
  Liver Function: The dose must be adjusted (based on blood levels) in liver com-
    promise. Much of the drug is eliminated in the bile.
  Kidney Function: This drug is capable of causing marked kidney toxicity. Cau-
    tion is critical. Dosing usually does not change, but more frequent blood
    levels are indicated.
  Diabetes: People who are diabetic and subsequently have kidney or pancreatic
    transplants will need larger than usual doses.
  Hypercholesterolemia: If the blood cholesterol is 50% above normal, the dose
    must be decreased by 50% in order to avoid toxicity.
  Obesity: Because of the way the drug is distributed in the body, the dosing of this
    medication **must** be based on ideal (a calculation which helps eliminate the
    weight which is fat) body weight.
  Cystic Fibrosis: It is very difficult to appropriately dose this medication in pa-
    tients who have this disease. Some patients will require as much as two
    times the usual dose. The dose should be adjusted to drug levels.
  Multiple Organ Transplants: Patients with multiple transplants (such as pan-
    creas and kidney) often need an increased dose of cyclosporine in order to
    achieve the desired effect. The dose should be determined based on blood
    levels.

▷ **Dosing Instructions:**   Preferably taken with or immediately following food to
    reduce stomach irritation. The capsule should be swallowed whole; do not
    open, crush, or chew. The oral solution should be mixed with milk, choco-
    late milk, or orange juice (at room temperature) in a glass or ceramic cup;
    do not use a wax-lined or plastic container. Stir well and drink immedi-

ately. It is advisable to take this drug at the same time each day to maintain steady blood levels.

Usual Duration of Use: Use on a regular schedule for several weeks is usually needed to see this drug's effectiveness in preventing organ rejection or stopping rejection that is already underway. Long-term use (months to years) requires periodic evaluation of response, blood tests, and dosage adjustment.

▷ **This Drug Should Not Be Taken If**
- you have had an allergic reaction to it previously.
- you are taking any immunosuppressant drug other than cortisonelike preparations.
- you have an active lymphoma of any type.
- you have an active, uncontrolled infection, especially chickenpox or shingles.

▷ **Inform Your Physician Before Taking This Drug If**
- you are pregnant or breast-feeding.
- you have a history of liver or kidney disease, or impaired liver or kidney function.
- you have a history of hypertension or gout.
- you have a chronic gastrointestinal disorder.
- you are taking a potassium supplement or drugs that can raise the blood level of potassium.
- you have a seizure disorder.
- you have a history of a blood cell disorder.
- you are taking other medicines that may be toxic to the kidney.

Possible Side Effects (natural, expected, and unavoidable drug actions)
Predisposition to infections.

▷ **Possible Adverse Effects** (unusual, unexpected, and infrequent reactions)
If any of the following develop, consult your physician promptly for guidance.

Mild Adverse Effects
Allergic Reactions: Skin rash, itching—case reports.
Excessive hair growth—frequent in transplant patients; acne—rare.
Headache, confusion—infrequent.
Tremors (dose dependent)—frequent.
Mouth sores—rare; gum overgrowth—frequent in some reports; nausea/vomiting, diarrhea—infrequent.
Changes in facial features (dysmorphosis)—possible with longer-term therapy.

Serious Adverse Effects
Allergic Reactions: Anaphylactic reaction (see Glossary) to intravenous solution—case reports.
Kidney injury (25% kidney transplant, 37% liver, and 38% heart)—frequent.
Hypertension, mild to severe (up to half)—frequent.
Seizures—rare to frequent (kidney—1.8%, bone marrow—5.5%, and up to 25% of liver transplant patients).
Cortical blindness—case reports.
Liver injury—infrequent.

Pancreatitis—rare.

Low white blood cell count (leukopenia)—infrequent.

Low blood platelets—rare.

High blood potassium levels, blood glucose, uric acid levels (and gout), increased blood cholesterol, or low blood magnesium—all possible.

Lymphoma, possibly drug induced—rare to infrequent.

Relapse of lupus erythematosus—case reports.

Increased risk of skin cancers (risk increased by sun or UV light exposure).

▷ **Possible Effects on Sexual Function**

Enlargement and tenderness of male breast (1 to 4%)—rare to infrequent.

Adverse Effects That May Mimic Natural Diseases or Disorders

Liver toxicity may suggest viral hepatitis.

Natural Diseases or Disorders That May Be Activated by This Drug

Latent infections, hypertension, gout.

Possible Effects on Laboratory Tests

Complete blood cell counts: decreased red cells, hemoglobin, and white cells.

Blood potassium level or uric acid level: increased.

Blood platelets, white cells, magnesium: decreased.

Liver function tests: increased liver enzymes (ALT/GPT, AST/GOT, and alkaline phosphatase), increased bilirubin.

Kidney function tests: blood creatinine and urea nitrogen levels (BUN) increased; urine casts present.

CAUTION

1. Report promptly any indications of infection of any kind.
2. Promptly report swollen glands, sores or lumps in the skin, abnormal bleeding or bruising.
3. Inform your physician promptly if you become pregnant.
4. Periodic laboratory tests are mandatory.
5. It is best to avoid immunizations and contact with people who have recently taken oral poliovirus vaccine.

Precautions for Use

By Infants and Children: This drug has been used successfully and safely in children of all ages. Dosing is made on the adult schedule in some cases, while others require increased dosing.

By Those Over 60 Years of Age: The dose must be adjusted to any decline in kidney function.

▷ **Advisability of Use During Pregnancy**

Pregnancy Category: C. See Pregnancy Risk Categories at the back of this book.

Animal studies: Rat and rabbit studies reveal that this drug is toxic to the embryo and fetus. No drug-induced birth defects were found.

Human studies: Adequate studies of pregnant women are not available.

Avoid this drug during entire pregnancy unless it is clearly needed.

Advisability of Use If Breast-Feeding

Presence of this drug in breast milk: Yes.

Avoid drug or refrain from nursing.

Habit-Forming Potential: None.

Effects of Overdosage: Headache, painful sensations in hands and feet, flushing of the face, gum soreness and bleeding, high blood pressure, atrial fibrillation, respiratory distress syndrome, seizures, coma, hallucinations, neurotoxicity, electrolyte disturbances, liver toxicity.

Possible Effects of Long-Term Use: Irreversible kidney damage, severe hypertension, abnormal growth of gums.

Suggested Periodic Examinations While Taking This Drug (at physician's discretion)

Measurement of cyclosporine blood levels. Complete blood cell counts.

Liver and kidney function tests. Measurement of magnesium, potassium, and uric acid blood levels.

Serial blood pressure measurements.

▷ **While Taking This Drug, Observe the Following**

Foods: Avoid excessive intake of high potassium foods. See Table 13, Section Six. Food may also increase the peak blood level of cyclosporine.

Beverages: Grapefruit juice increases blood levels. Milk may increase blood levels.

▷ *Alcohol:* Large amounts of alcohol may increase blood levels of cyclosporine.

Tobacco Smoking: This interaction has not been well studied, but I advise everyone to quit smoking.

▷ *Other Drugs*

Cyclosporine *taken concurrently* with

- ACE inhibitors (see Drug Classes) may increase the risk of kidney problems.
- aminoglycoside antibiotics (see Drug Classes) may increase kidney toxicity.
- amphotericin B (Abelcet, others) can cause serious kidney toxicity.
- aspirin substitutes (nonsteroidal anti-inflammatory drugs or NSAIDs) may increase kidney toxicity.
- azathioprine (Imuran) may increase immunosuppression.
- calcium channel blockers (see Drug Classes) may result in cyclosporine toxicity.
- ciprofloxacin (and other fluoroquinolones—see Drug Classes) may increase risk of kidney toxicity.
- cotrimoxazole (Bactrim, others) may result in decreased cyclosporine effectiveness as well as kidney toxicity.
- cyclophosphamide (Cytoxan) may increase immunosuppression.
- digoxin (Lanoxin) may result in serious digoxin toxicity.
- furosemide (Lasix) may result in increased risk of gout.
- ganciclovir (Cytovene) may result in increased kidney toxicity.
- histamine (H_2) inhibitors (see Drug Classes) and ketoconazole may experience decreased cyclosporine blood levels.
- imipenem/cilastatin (Primaxin) may result in neurotoxicity.
- lovastatin (Mevacor) and other HMG-CoA reductase inhibitors may increase risk of muscle toxicity (myopathy) or kidney failure.
- methylprednisolone (Medrol) may cause seizures.
- metronidazole (Flagyl) may result in increased cyclosporine levels and toxicity.
- nifedipine (Adalat) may worsen abnormal gum growth (gingival hyperplasia) and also cause nifedipine toxicity (low blood pressure and abnormal heartbeats).
- pravastatin (Pravachol) can cause myopathy.

- simvastatin (Zocor) may cause myopathy.
- sulfamethoxazole and/or trimethoprim (Septra) may increase kidney toxicity.
- tacrolimus (Prograf) can cause kidney toxicity.
- thiazide diuretics (see Drug Classes) may increase adverse effects on the blood (myelosuppression).
- vaccines may blunt the benefit of the vaccine.
- verapamil (Calan) may increase immunosuppression.

The following drugs may ***increase*** the effects of cyclosporine

- acetazolamide.
- allopurinol (Zyloprim).
- amiodarone (Cordarone).
- ceftriaxone (Rocephin).
- clarithromycin (Biaxin).
- colchicine (ColBENEMID).
- danazol or other anabolic steroids.
- diltiazem (Cardizem).
- econazole (Spectazole).
- erythromycin (E.E.S., others).
- fluconazole (Diflucan).
- itraconazole (Sporanox).
- ketoconazole (Nizoral).
- methyltestosterone.
- metoclopramide (Reglan).
- miconazole (Lotrimin, Micatin).
- oral contraceptives (birth control pills).
- terconazole (Terazol).

The following drugs may ***decrease*** the effects of cyclosporine

- carbamazepine (Tegretol).
- isoniazid (INH).
- nafcillin.
- octreotide (Sandostatin).
- phenobarbital.
- phenytoin (Dilantin).
- quinine.
- rifabutin (Mycobutin).
- rifampin (Rifadin).
- sulfadimidine, sulfadiazine, and/or trimethoprim.
- ticlopidine (Ticlid).

▷ *Driving, Hazardous Activities:* This drug may cause confusion or seizures. Restrict activities as necessary.

Aviation Note: The use of this drug ***may be a disqualification*** for piloting. Consult a designated Aviation Medical Examiner.

Exposure to Sun: Exposure to sunlight or other ultraviolet (UV) radiation may increase the risk of skin cancer.

Discontinuation: Do not stop this drug without your physician's guidance.

Special Storage Instructions: Keep the gelatin capsules in the blister packets until ready for use. Store below 77 degrees F (25 degrees C).

Keep the oral solution in a tightly closed container. Store below 86 degrees F (30 degrees C). Do not refrigerate.

Observe the Following Expiration Times: The oral solution must be used within 2 months after opening.

DESIPRAMINE (des IP ra meen)

Introduced: 1964 **Class:** Antidepressant **Prescription:** USA: Yes
Controlled Drug: USA: No; Canada: No **Available as Generic:** USA: Yes; Canada: Yes

Brand Names: Norpramin, Pertofrane

```
┌─────────────────────────────────────────────────────────────────┐
│                   BENEFITS versus RISKS                           │
```

Possible Benefits	*Possible Risks*
EFFECTIVE RELIEF OF ENDOGENOUS DEPRESSION	ADVERSE BEHAVIORAL EFFECTS: confusion, disorientation, delusions, hallucinations
Possibly beneficial in other depressive disorders	CONVERSION OF DEPRESSION TO MANIA in manic-depressive (bipolar) disorders
	Aggravation of paranoia and schizophrenia
	Drug-induced heart rhythm disorders
	Abnormally low white blood cell and platelet counts

▷ **Principal Uses**

As a Single Drug Product: Uses currently included in FDA-approved labeling: Relieves severe depression. This drug is more likely to work in primary (endogenous) depression than in secondary, reactive (exogenous) depression. Other (unlabeled) generally accepted uses: (1) Chronic pain syndromes, including diabetic neuropathy; (2) treatment of attention deficit disorder in children over 6 years of age and in adolescents; (3) decreases the symptoms of panic disorder; (4) helps treat resistant malaria; (5) may help reduce binge eating in bulimia.

How This Drug Works: By increasing brain concentrations of some nerve impulse transmitters (norepinephrine and serotonin), this drug relieves the symptoms associated with depression.

Available Dosage Forms and Strengths

Capsules — 25 mg, 50 mg
Tablets — 10 mg, 25 mg, 50 mg, 75 mg, 100 mg, 150 mg

▷ **Usual Adult Dosage Range:** Initially 25 mg two to four times daily. Dose may be increased cautiously as needed and tolerated by 25 mg daily at intervals of 1 week. The usual maintenance dose is 100 mg to 200 mg daily. The total daily dosage should not exceed 300 mg. (When determined, the optimal daily requirement may be given at bedtime as a single dose.) **Note: Actual dosage and administration schedule must be determined for each patient individually.**

Conditions Requiring Dosing Adjustments

Liver Function: The dose should be decreased in patients with compromised livers.

Kidney Function: Can cause urine retention—use with caution in kidney compromise with urine outflow problems.

▷ **Dosing Instructions:** May be taken without regard to meals. The capsule may be opened and the tablet may be crushed for administration.

Usual Duration of Use: Use on a regular schedule for 3 to 4 weeks is usually needed to see this drug's effectiveness in relieving depression; peak response may require 3 months of use. Delusional patients may require 7 weeks to benefit. Long-term use (months to years) requires periodic evaluation of response and dosage adjustment.

▷ **This Drug Should Not Be Taken If**
- you have had an allergic reaction to it previously.
- you are taking, or have taken within the past 14 days, any monoamine oxidase (MAO) type A inhibitor drug (see Drug Classes).
- you have had a recent heart attack (myocardial infarction).
- you have narrow-angle glaucoma.

▷ **Inform Your Physician Before Taking This Drug If**
- you have had an adverse reaction to any other antidepressant drug.
- you have any type of seizure disorder.
- you have increased internal eye pressure.
- you have any type of heart disease, especially a heart rhythm disorder.
- you have any type of thyroid disorder or are taking thyroid medication.
- you have thought about or attempted suicide.
- you have diabetes or sugar intolerance.
- you take levodopa (increased risk of heart rhythm problems with high desipramine doses).
- you have prostatism (see Glossary).
- you plan to have surgery under general anesthesia in the near future.

Possible Side Effects (natural, expected, and unavoidable drug actions)

Mild drowsiness, light-headedness (low blood pressure), blurred vision, dry mouth, constipation, impaired urination.

▷ **Possible Adverse Effects** (unusual, unexpected, and infrequent reactions)

If any of the following develop, consult your physician promptly for guidance.

Mild Adverse Effects

Allergic Reactions: Skin rash, hives, swelling of face or tongue, drug fever (see Glossary)—case reports.

Headache, dizziness, weakness, unsteadiness, tremors, fainting—infrequent.

Irritation of tongue or mouth, altered taste, difficulty talking—rare; indigestion, nausea—infrequent.

Fluctuations of blood sugar—possible.

Serious Adverse Effects

Allergic Reactions: Drug-induced hepatitis, with or without jaundice; anaphylactic reaction (see Glossary)—case reports.

Adverse behavioral effects: delusions, hallucinations—case reports.

Seizures; reduced control of epilepsy—case reports.

Aggravation of paranoid psychoses and schizophrenia—possible.

Heart rhythm disturbances, myocarditis—case reports.

Parkinson-like disorders, peripheral neuritis (see both terms in Glossary)—rare to infrequent.

Abnormally low white blood cell and platelet counts: fever, sore throat, infections, abnormal bleeding or bruising—case reports.

Neuroleptic malignant syndrome—case reports.

▷ **Possible Effects on Sexual Function:** Decreased libido, increased libido (antidepressant effect), impotence, painful male orgasm, male breast enlargement (gynecomastia), female breast enlargement with milk production, swelling of testicles, decreased sperm viability—case reports.

Adverse Effects That May Mimic Natural Diseases or Disorders

Liver toxicity may suggest viral hepatitis.

Natural Diseases or Disorders That May Be Activated by This Drug

Latent diabetes, epilepsy, glaucoma, prostatism.

Possible Effects on Laboratory Tests

Complete blood cell counts: decreased red cells, hemoglobin, white cells, and platelets; increased eosinophils (allergic reaction).

Blood glucose levels: unexplained fluctuations.

Liver function tests: increased liver enzymes (ALT/GPT, AST/GOT, and alkaline phosphatase), increased bilirubin—all rare.

Thyroid function tests: decreased TSH and mean free thyroxin.

CAUTION

1. Should only be used when a true, primary, endogenous depression (not reactive) has been diagnosed.
2. Watch for indications of toxicity: confusion, agitation, rapid heart rate, heart irregularity. Blood levels will be needed.
3. It is advisable to withhold this drug if electroconvulsive therapy (ECT) is to be used to treat the depression.

Precautions for Use

By Infants and Children: Safety and effectiveness for those under 6 years of age not established. This drug is being used to treat children who have attention deficit disorder, with or without hyperactivity. Dosage and management must be supervised by a properly trained pediatrician.

By Those Over 60 Years of Age: Initiate treatment with 25 mg one or two times daily to evaluate tolerance. During the first 2 weeks of treatment, watch for confusion, restlessness, agitation, forgetfulness, disorientation, delusions, or hallucinations. Also observe for unsteadiness and instability that may predispose to falling. This drug may aggravate prostatism.

▷ **Advisability of Use During Pregnancy**

Pregnancy Category: C. See Pregnancy Risk Categories at the back of this book.

Animal studies: Birth defects reported in rat and rabbit studies.

Human studies: Adequate studies of pregnant women are not available.

Use only if clearly needed. Avoid during the first 3 months if possible.

Advisability of Use If Breast-Feeding

Presence of this drug in breast milk: Yes, in small amounts.

Monitor nursing infant closely and discontinue drug or nursing if adverse effects develop.

Habit-Forming Potential: Psychological or physical dependence is rare and unexpected. Some patients may seek to abuse this medicine for its ability to create anticholinergic delirium.

Effects of Overdosage: Confusion, hallucinations, drowsiness, tremors, heart irregularity, seizures, stupor, hypothermia (see Glossary).

Possible Effects of Long-Term Use: None reported.

Suggested Periodic Examinations While Taking This Drug (at physician's discretion)

Complete blood cell counts, liver function tests.
Serial blood pressure readings and electrocardiograms.

▷ **While Taking This Drug, Observe the Following**

Foods: No specific restrictions. Limiting food intake may avoid excess weight gain.

Nutritional Support: High doses of vitamin C may blunt the therapeutic effects of desipramine.

Beverages: No restrictions. May be taken with milk.

▷ *Alcohol:* **Avoid completely.** This drug can markedly increase the intoxicating effects of alcohol; the combination can depress brain function.

Tobacco Smoking: May accelerate the elimination of this drug and require increased dosage. I advise everyone to quit smoking.

Marijuana Smoking

Occasional (once or twice weekly): transient increase in drowsiness and mouth dryness as well as possible unacceptable increases in heart rate.

Daily: persistent drowsiness and mouth dryness; possible reduced effectiveness of this drug.

▷ *Other Drugs*

Desipramine may *increase* the effects of
• all drugs with atropinelike effects (see Drug Classes).
• all drugs with sedative effects; watch for excessive sedation.

Desipramine may *decrease* the effects of
• clonidine (Catapres).
• guanethidine (Ismelin, Esimil).
• guanfacine (Tenex).
• levodopa by decreasing absorption of the levodopa.

Desipramine *taken concurrently* with
• albuterol (Ventolin) may increase the effect of albuterol on the blood vessels.
• anticonvulsants requires careful monitoring for changes in seizure patterns and need to adjust anticonvulsant dosage (carbamazepine–Tegretol or phenytoin–Dilantin are examples).
• ethchlorvynol (Placidyl) may cause delirium; avoid concurrent use.
• large doses (greater than 2 g/day) of vitamin C may lead to increased removal of desipramine and the need to increase the dose.
• monoamine oxidase (MAO) type A inhibitor drugs (see Drug Classes) may cause high fever, seizures, and excessive rise in blood pressure; avoid concurrent use of these drugs and provide periods of 14 days between administration of either.
• quinidine may cause desipramine toxicity.
• stimulant drugs (amphetamine, cocaine, epinephrine, phenylpropanolamine, etc.) may cause severe high blood pressure and/or high fever.

- thyroid preparations may increase the risk of heart rhythm disorders.
- tramadol (Ultram) may increase seizure risk.
- warfarin may cause an increased risk of bleeding. Increased testing of INR is indicated.

The following drugs may *increase* the effects of desipramine

- cimetidine (Tagamet).
- fluoxetine (Prozac).
- fluvoxamine (Luvox).
- methylphenidate (Ritalin).
- phenothiazines (see Drug Classes).
- ritonavir (Norvir) and perhaps other protease inhibitors (see Drug Classes).

The following drugs may *decrease* the effects of desipramine

- barbiturates (see Drug Classes).
- chloral hydrate (Noctec, Somnos, etc.).
- clonazepam (Klonopin).
- estrogen (see profile for brand names).
- lithium (Lithobid, Lithotab, etc.).
- oral contraceptives (birth control pills; see profile for brand names).
- reserpine (Serpasil, Ser-Ap-Es, etc.).

▷ *Driving, Hazardous Activities:* This drug may impair mental alertness, judgment, physical coordination, and reaction time. Restrict activities as necessary.

Aviation Note: The use of this drug *is a disqualification* for piloting. Consult a designated Aviation Medical Examiner.

Exposure to Sun: Use caution. This drug may cause photosensitivity (see Glossary) and changes in iris and skin pigment color with sun exposure.

Exposure to Heat: Use caution. This drug can inhibit sweating and impair adaptation to hot environments, increasing the risk of heatstroke. Avoid saunas.

Exposure to Cold: The elderly should use caution and avoid conditions conducive to hypothermia (see Glossary).

Exposure to Environmental Chemicals: This drug may mask the symptoms of poisoning due to handling certain insecticides (organophosphorous types). Read labels carefully.

Discontinuation: It is advisable to stop this drug gradually. Abrupt withdrawal after prolonged use may cause headache, malaise, and nausea. When this drug is stopped, it may be necessary to adjust the dosages of other drugs taken concurrently.

DEXAMETHASONE (dex a METH a sohn)

Introduced: 1958   **Class:** Cortisonelike drugs   **Prescription:** USA: Yes
Controlled Drug: USA: No; Canada: No   **Available as Generic:** USA: Yes;
Canada: Yes

Brand Names: Acroseb-Dex, ✚Ak-Dex, Ak-Trol [CD], Baldex, Dalalone, Dalalone DP, Dalalone LA, Decaderm, Decadron, Decadron Nasal Spray, Decadron-LA, Decadron Phosphate Ophthalmic, Decadron Phosphate Respihaler, Decadron Phosphate Turbinaire, Decadron w/Xylocaine [CD], Decaject, Decaject LA, Decaspray, Deenar [CD], ✚Deronil, Dex-4, Dexacen-4, Dexacen LA-8, Dexacidin[CD], Dexacort, Dexameth, Dexasone,

Dexasone-LA, Dexo-LA, Dexon, Dexone, Dexone-E, Dexone-LA, Hexadrol, Maxidex, Mymethasone, ✦Neodecadron Eye-Ear, Neodexair, Neomycin-Dex, Ocu-Trol [CD], ✦Oradexon, ✦PMS-Dexamethasone, ✦SK-Dexamethasone, ✦Sofracort, Solurex, Solurex-LA, ✦Spersadex, Tobradex, Turbinaire

BENEFITS versus RISKS	
Possible Benefits	*Possible Risks*
EFFECTIVE RELIEF OF SYMPTOMS IN A WIDE VARIETY OF INFLAMMATORY AND ALLERGIC DISORDERS EFFECTIVE IMMUNOSUPPRESSION in selected benign and malignant disorders	Long-term systemic use (exceeding 2 weeks) is associated with many possible adverse effects: ALTERED MOOD AND PERSONALITY, CATARACTS, GLAUCOMA, HYPERTENSION, ARRHYTHMIAS, PEPTIC ULCERS, PANCREATITIS, OSTEOPOROSIS, ASEPTIC BONE NECROSIS, INCREASED SUSCEPTIBILITY TO INFECTIONS

▷ **Principal Uses**

As a Single Drug Product: Uses currently included in FDA-approved labeling: (1) Used in the management of serious skin disorders, asthma, allergic rhinitis, lymphoma, brain edema, shock, systemic lupus erythematosus, and all types of major rheumatic disorders including bursitis, systemic lupus erythematosus, tendonitis, and most forms of arthritis; (2) ulcerative disease of the colon; (3) topical cream is used to treat eczema, psoriasis, dermatitis, and lichen planus; (4) used in conjunction with antibiotics in meningitis; (5) helps ease swelling in otitis media.

Other (unlabeled) generally accepted uses: (1) Adrenal insufficiency; (2) acute airway obstruction; (3) mountain sickness; (4) vomiting caused by chemotherapy; (5) cardiopulmonary bypass; (6) refractory depression; (7) relief of symptoms of cancer that has spread to the brain (metastasis); (8) used in combination regimens to control multiple myeloma; (9) may have a role in extreme cases of *Pneumocystis carinii* pneumonia; (10) can help suppress male hormones (androgens) in women with acne, hirsutism, or hair loss (androgenic alopecia) caused by androgens.

How This Drug Works: Inhibits defensive functions of certain white blood cells. It reduces the production of lymphocytes and some antibodies and acts as an immunosuppressant.

Available Dosage Forms and Strengths

Aerosol — 0.01% and 0.04%
Aerosol inhaler — 84 mcg per spray
Cream — 0.1%
Elixir — 0.5 mg/5 ml
Eye ointment — 0.05%
Eye solution — 0.1%
Gel — 0.1%
Injection — 4 mg/ml, 8 mg/ml, 10 mg/ml, 16 mg/ml, 20 mg/ml, 24 mg/ml
Oral solution — 0.5 mg/0.5 ml, 0.5 mg/5 ml

Solution — 0.1%
Spray, topical — 10 mg/25 g
Suspension — 0.1%
Tablets — 0.25 mg, 0.5 mg, 0.75 mg, 1 mg, 1.5 mg, 2 mg, 4 mg, 6 mg

▷ **Usual Adult Dosage Range:**   Oral: 0.75 to 9 mg daily divided into two to four doses.

Topical (0.1% cream): apply thin film of medicine on the affected area three or four times a day.

Oral dose for children: 0.03 to 0.15 mg per kg of body mass per day, divided into equal doses given every 6 to 12 hours. Or 1–5 mg per square meter divided into equal doses and given every 6 to 12 hours. **Note: Actual dosage and administration schedule must be determined for each patient individually.**

Conditions Requiring Dosing Adjustments

Liver Function: This drug is eliminated via the liver; however, no specific guidelines for dosing adjustments are available.

Kidney Function: Use with caution as it can cause alkalosis (a change toward a more basic condition in the body's chemistry).

Obesity: Dosing on a mg-per-kg-of-body-mass-per-day basis is recommended. It is best to measure free urinary cortisol as well.

▷ **Dosing Instructions:**   Tablet may be crushed and taken with or following food to prevent stomach irritation, preferably in the morning.

Usual Duration of Use: For acute disorders: 4 to 10 days. For chronic disorders: according to individual requirements. Length of therapy should not exceed the time needed to obtain adequate symptomatic relief in acute self-limiting conditions, or the time required to stabilize a chronic condition and permit gradual withdrawal. Because of its long duration of action, this drug is not appropriate for alternate-day administration.

▷ **This Drug Should Not Be Taken If**
- you have had an allergic reaction to any dosage form of it previously.
- you have active peptic ulcer disease.
- you have an active herpes simplex infection of the eye.
- you have a systemic fungal infection (talk with your doctor).
- your sputum consistently grows *Candida albicans* (a yeast that may grow very quickly if steroids suppress your immune system).
- you have a psychoneurosis or psychosis.
- you have active tuberculosis.

▷ **Inform Your Physician Before Taking This Drug If**
- you have had an unfavorable reaction to any cortisonelike drug.
- you have a history of peptic ulcer disease, thrombophlebitis, or tuberculosis.
- you have: diabetes, glaucoma, high blood pressure, deficient thyroid function, or myasthenia gravis.
- you start to have restricted motion, increased pain, fever, or joint swelling; these may be early signs of a septic arthritis.
- you have osteoporosis.
- you plan to have surgery of any kind in the near future.

Possible Side Effects (natural, expected, and unavoidable drug actions)

Increased appetite, weight gain, retention of salt and water, excretion of potassium, increased susceptibility to infection (yeast infections can be frequent in cancer patients treated with a corticosteroid).

Increased white blood cell count (release from the bone marrow versus a sign of infection).

▷ **Possible Adverse Effects** (unusual, unexpected, and infrequent reactions)

If any of the following develop, consult your physician promptly for guidance.

Mild Adverse Effects

Allergic Reaction: Skin rash—case reports

Headache, dizziness, insomnia—possible.

Mild euphoria or depression—most common possible central nervous system (CNS) effects.

High blood pressure (may be lessened by alternate-day therapy): more likely in older patients and those who already have high blood pressure—possible.

Acid indigestion, abdominal distention—possible.

Muscle cramping and weakness—case reports.

Easy bruising (ecchymosis) or acnelike lesions—case reports.

Vaginal itching—may be frequent with intravenous dosing.

Serious Adverse Effects

Allergic Reaction: Anaphylaxis—case reports.

Mental and emotional disturbances of serious magnitude—infrequent.

Reactivation of latent tuberculosis—possible. *Pneumocystis carinii* pneumonia—possible with immunosuppression and chronic use.

Development of peptic ulcer—rare, but risk increases with higher doses and preexisting ulcers.

Inflammation of the pancreas—rare.

Thrombophlebitis (inflammation of a vein with the formation of blood clot): pain or tenderness in thigh or leg, or swelling of the foot, ankle, or leg—possible with intravenous use.

Abnormal lipids (cholesterol, triglycerides, LDLs)—possible.

Abnormal heart rhythm—case reports.

Cushing's syndrome—possible with chronic use and high doses (supraphysiologic).

Suppression of the adrenal gland—possible with chronic use and more common with larger doses.

High blood sugar—risk increases with use in diabetics and with higher doses.

Excessively low blood potassium—case reports.

Abnormally slow heartbeat in infants—case reports.

Increased pressure in the eye or cataracts or glaucoma—rare to frequent.

Precipitation of porphyria—case reports.

Excessive thyroid function (questionable causality)—case reports.

Muscle changes (myopathy)—infrequent, but more likely with higher doses and some steroids.

Bone death (aseptic necrosis or avascular necrosis)—infrequent, but more likely with high initial doses.

Osteoporosis—more likely with long-term and higher-dose use.

▷ **Possible Effects on Sexual Function:**   Altered timing and pattern of menstruation—case reports.

Adverse Effects That May Mimic Natural Diseases or Disorders
Pattern of symptoms and signs resembling Cushing's syndrome.

Natural Diseases or Disorders That May Be Activated by This Drug
Latent diabetes, glaucoma, peptic ulcer disease, tuberculosis.

Possible Effects on Laboratory Tests
Blood amylase level: increased (possible pancreatitis).
Blood glucose level: increased.
Digoxin testing: may falsely increase digoxin results.
Glucose tolerance test (GTT): increased.
Blood potassium level: decreased.
Thyroid function tests: decreased.
Cholesterol: increased in some studies while decreased in others.

CAUTION
1. It is best to carry a card noting that you are taking this drug, if your course of treatment is to exceed 1 week.
2. Do not stop this drug abruptly if it is used for long-term treatment.
3. If vaccination against measles, rabies, smallpox, or yellow fever is required, stop this drug 72 hours before vaccination and do not resume it for at least 14 days after vaccination.
4. Children may be more sensitive to topical application since there is a larger skin surface area to body weight (ratio).

Precautions for Use
By Infants and Children: Avoid prolonged use if possible. During long-term use, watch for suppression of normal growth and the possibility of increased intracranial pressure. Following long-term use, the child may be at risk for adrenal gland deficiency during stress for as long as 18 months after cessation.
By Those Over 60 Years of Age: Avoid prolonged use of this drug. Continual use (even in small doses) can increase the severity of diabetes, enhance fluid retention, raise blood pressure, weaken resistance to infection, induce stomach ulcer, and accelerate the development of cataracts and osteoporosis.

▷ **Advisability of Use During Pregnancy**
Pregnancy Category: C. See Pregnancy Risk Categories at the back of this book.
Animal studies: Birth defects reported in mice, rats, and rabbits.
Human studies: Adequate studies of pregnant women are not available.
Avoid completely during the first 3 months. Limit use during the last 6 months as much as possible. If used, examine infant for possible deficiency of adrenal gland function.

Advisability of Use If Breast-Feeding
Presence of this drug in breast milk: Yes.
Avoid drug or refrain from nursing.

Habit-Forming Potential: Use to suppress symptoms over an extended period of time may produce a state of functional dependence (see Glossary). In treating asthma and rheumatoid arthritis, it is best to keep the dose as small as possible and to attempt drug withdrawal after periods of reasonable improvement. Such procedures may reduce the degree of "steroid rebound"—the return of symptoms as the drug is withdrawn.

Effects of Overdosage: Fatigue, muscle weakness, stomach irritation, acid indigestion, excessive sweating, facial flushing, fluid retention, swelling of extremities, increased blood pressure.

Possible Effects of Long-Term Use: Increased blood sugar (possible diabetes), increased fat deposits on the trunk of the body ("buffalo hump"), rounding of the face ("moon face"), thinning and fragility of skin, loss of texture and strength of bones (osteoporosis, aseptic necrosis), cataracts, glaucoma, retarded growth and development in children.

Suggested Periodic Examinations While Taking This Drug (at physician's discretion)

Measurements of blood pressure, blood sugar, and potassium levels.

Complete eye examinations at regular intervals. Chest X ray if history of tuberculosis.

Determination of the rate of development of the growing child to detect retardation of normal growth.

Bone mineral density testing to assess risk of osteoporosis.

▷ **While Taking This Drug, Observe the Following**

Foods: No interactions expected. Ask your physician about salt restriction or need for potassium-rich foods. During long-term use of this drug, it is advisable to eat a high protein diet.

Nutritional Support: During long-term use, take a vitamin D supplement and increase calcium. During wound repair, take a zinc supplement.

Beverages: No restrictions. Drink all forms of milk liberally.

▷ *Alcohol:* No interactions expected. Caution if you are prone to peptic ulcer disease.

Tobacco Smoking: Nicotine increases the blood levels of naturally produced cortisone and related hormones. Heavy smoking may add to the expected actions of this drug and requires close observation for excessive effects. I advise everyone to quit smoking.

Marijuana Smoking: May cause additional impairment of immunity, and also is a risk factor for toxoplasmosis.

▷ *Other Drugs*

Dexamethasone may ***decrease*** the effects of

• isoniazid (INH, Niconyl, etc.).
• salicylates (aspirin, sodium salicylate, etc.).
• vaccines (such as flu vaccine), by blunting the immune response to them.

Dexamethasone ***taken concurrently*** with

• birth control pills (oral contraceptives) may increase dexamethasone's therapeutic effects.
• carbamazepine (Tegretol) will reduce the effectiveness of dexamethasone.
• loop diuretics such as furosemide (Lasix) or bumetanide (Bumex) can result in additive potassium loss.
• oral anticoagulants may either increase or decrease their effectiveness; ask your doctor about prothrombin time testing and dosage adjustment.
• oral antidiabetic drugs (see Drug Classes) will decrease their effectiveness.
• ritonavir (Norvir), and perhaps other protease inhibitors (see Drug

Classes), may decrease ritonavir blood levels and increase dexamethasone blood levels.
- thiazide diuretics (see Drug Classes) will decrease their blood-pressure-lowering ability.

The following drugs may **decrease** the effects of dexamethasone
- antacids: may reduce its absorption.
- barbiturates (Amytal, Butisol, phenobarbital, etc.).
- phenobarbital.
- phenytoin (Dilantin, etc.).
- primidone (Mysoline).
- rifabutin (Mycobutin).
- rifampin (Rifadin, Rimactane, etc.).

▷ *Driving, Hazardous Activities:* Usually no restrictions. Be alert to the rare occurrence of dizziness.

Aviation Note: The use of this drug **may be a disqualification** for piloting. Consult a designated Aviation Medical Examiner.

Exposure to Sun: No restrictions.

Occurrence of Unrelated Illness: This drug may decrease natural resistance to infection. Call your doctor if you develop an infection of any kind. It may also reduce your body's ability to respond to the stress of acute illness, injury, or surgery. Keep your physician fully informed of any significant health changes.

Discontinuation: Do not stop this drug abruptly after chronic use. Ask your doctor for help regarding gradual withdrawal. For a period of 2 years after discontinuing this drug, it is essential in the event of illness, injury, or surgery that you inform attending medical personnel that you have used this drug in the past.

DEXFENFLURAMINE (DEX fen flur a MEEN)

Introduced: 1996   **Class:** Serotonin reuptake inhibitor, weight loss agent
Prescription: USA: Yes   **Controlled Drug:** USA: Yes, C-IV; Canada: Yes
Available as Generic: USA: No

Brand Name: Redux

Warning: Because of new data showing a large increase in the number of patients in one study who suffered heart valve damage, this medicine has been recalled. At present, it appears that benefits do not outweigh the risks for any use.

BENEFITS versus RISKS

Possible Benefits	*Possible Risks*
EFFECTIVE WEIGHT LOSS FOR 6 MONTHS (longer-term use carries an increased risk of pulmonary hypertension)	HEART VALVE OR LUNG DAMAGE

▷ **Principal Uses**
As a Single Drug Product: Uses currently included in FDA-approved labeling: (1)

Used in the management of obesity, including weight loss and helping to maintain weight loss in people on a reduced calorie diet; (2) recommended for use by obese people with an initial body mass index (BMI, a calculation that takes the patient's weight in kg divided by their height in meters squared) greater than 30 kg per square meter or 27 kg per square meter in the presence of other risk factors (such as diabetes, hyperlipidemia, or hypertension).

Other (unlabeled) generally accepted uses: None.

How This Drug Works: This medicine helps treat obesity by decreasing the desire to eat by increasing serotonin (a nerve transmitter) in brain synapses. It accomplishes this effect by both stimulating release of serotonin from synaptosomes and also inhibiting serotonin reuptake. Clinical trial data showed that dexfenfluramine resulted in decreased appetite and possible slowing of stomach (gastric) emptying. Patients also ate fewer carbohydrates and had decreased craving between meals for high carbohydrate snack foods.

Available Dosage Forms and Strengths

Capsules — 15 mg

▷ **Recommended Dosage Ranges** (Actual dosage and administration schedule must be determined for each patient individually.)

One capsule (15 mg) twice a day, with meals. Doses greater than 30 mg daily are not recommended.

Conditions Requiring Dosing Adjustments

Liver Function: This drug is metabolized in the liver; however, no specific guidelines for dosing adjustments are available.

Kidney Function: Fenfluramine and norfenfluramine (a liver metabolite) combined—up to 30% removed by the kidneys; however, no specific guidelines for dosing adjustments are available.

Obesity: No significant differences between final medicine levels (steady-state drug concentrations) in nonobese or obese people.

▷ **Dosing Instructions:** Capsule may be taken with or following food, twice daily.

Usual Duration of Use: Initial studies done in 1995 were 3-month placebo-controlled, and were usually used in conjunction with a low calorie diet or counseling. Longer-term use should be discussed with your doctor. Safety and effectiveness for longer than 1 year have not been determined. Clinical trial data also showed that patients benefited from lower cholesterol and blood pressure while realizing weight loss as well. Patients who do not lose 4 pounds during the initial 4 weeks of therapy should be reevaluated to make certain they are taking their medicine correctly. If dexfenfluramine has been taken correctly, and a 4-pound weight loss has not occurred during the initial 4 weeks of therapy, consideration should be given to stopping dexfenfluramine. Ongoing use requires periodic physician followup.

▷ **This Drug Should Not Be Taken If**
- you have had an allergic reaction to any dosage form of it previously.
- you have pulmonary hypertension.
- you have glaucoma.
- you take or have taken a monoamine oxidase (MAO) inhibitor (see Drug Classes) within the last 14 days.

▷ **Inform Your Physician Before Taking This Drug If**
  - you have cardiovascular disease or have had an unfavorable reaction to any serotonin reuptake inhibitor.
  - you have a history of abnormal heart rhythms.
  - you have a history of kidney or liver compromise.
  - you have a history of psychiatric disorders or drug abuse.
  - you have a history of porphyria.
  - you have taken other weight loss medicines (anorexigens) in the last year.
  - you develop unexplained difficulty in breathing, fainting, chest pain, or swelling of the ankles. These may be early symptoms of pulmonary hypertension.

Possible Side Effects (natural, expected, and unavoidable drug actions)
  None reported as yet.

▷ **Possible Adverse Effects** (unusual, unexpected, and infrequent reactions)
  If any of the following develop, consult your physician promptly for guidance.
  Mild Adverse Effects
  Allergic Reaction: Skin rash.
  Tiredness or drowsiness, headache, dizziness, or sleep disturbances—infrequent.
  Lowering or increase in blood pressure—case reports.
  Chest pain or palpitations—rare.
  Muscle or joint pain—infrequent.
  Dry mouth, nausea, vomiting, or constipation—infrequent.
  Increased urination (polyuria)—infrequent.
  Serious Adverse Effects
  Dysphoria or suicidal tendency—case reports.
  Depression, serious enough for 5% of the patients in clinical trials to discontinue its use—infrequent.
  Vision changes—infrequent.
  Low blood platelets, anemia, or blood clotting disorders—rare.
  Liver toxicity—rare.
  Cases of primary pulmonary hypertension—rare.
  Serotonin syndrome—rare.

▷ **Possible Effects on Sexual Function:**   Menstrual disorders (less than 2% in clinical trials). Infrequent impotence occurred in clinical trials.

Possible Effects on Laboratory Tests
  Serum cholesterol: decreased.
  Drug testing: may cause false positive tests for amphetamines.

CAUTION
  1. It is best to carry a card noting that you are taking this drug, if your course of treatment is to exceed 1 week.
  2. May increase insulin sensitivity in obese patients. If insulin is taken at the same time as this medicine, the dose may be able to be decreased.
  3. This medicine may cause false positive urine drug tests for amphetamines.
  4. Other conditions (organic causes) leading to obesity (such as low activity of the thyroid gland—hypothyroidism) should be ruled out prior to starting this medicine.

5. Safety and efficacy of use of dexfenfluramine with other weight loss agents have NOT been established. Combination therapy is NOT recommended.
6. This medicine was approved with the provision that a study be undertaken to assess dexfenfluramine effects on the brain. Studies of monkeys and baboons showed that high doses destroyed brain cells that make serotonin.

Precautions for Use

By Infants and Children: Safety and effectiveness have not been established in those less than 18 years old.

By Those Over 60 Years of Age: The drug levels this medicine achieves and the places in the body where this medicine goes are no different for those over 60 than those under 60. Caution should be used (as with all medicines active in the central nervous system) in treating elderly patients with dexfenfluramine.

▷ Advisability of Use During Pregnancy

Pregnancy Category: C. See Pregnancy Risk Categories at the back of this book.

Animal studies: Decreased weight gain, reduced numbers of placental implantations, and fewer live young (as well as delayed bone formation or ossification) was reported in rats. These rats were given 2.5–5 times the human dose of dexfenfluramine.

Human studies: Adequate studies of pregnant women are not available.

NOT recommended for pregnant women.

Advisability of Use If Breast-Feeding

Presence of this drug in breast milk: Yes in rats; unknown in humans.

Avoid drug or refrain from nursing.

Habit-Forming Potential:

The possibility of physical dependence is low. Further study is needed to confirm an accurate probability of dependence risk. There was no evidence of addictive or drug-seeking behavior in premarketing studies.

Effects of Overdosage:

During postmarketing reports sent in over 10 years in Europe, 66 cases of overdoses show: agitation, drowsiness, mydriasis, shivering, nausea, and vomiting.

Possible Effects of Long-Term Use:

Weight loss (the desired effect). Some reports of higher occurrence (although still rare) of pulmonary hypertension with long-term use have been made.

Suggested Periodic Examinations While Taking This Drug (at physician's discretion)

Periodic weigh-ins.

▷ While Taking This Drug, Observe the Following

Foods: No interactions expected; follow prescribed diet.

Nutritional Support: Dietary counseling and physician- or dietitian-directed diets are suggested.

Beverages: No restrictions except as described in your dietary guidelines.

▷ *Alcohol:* Since dexfenfluramine may cause drowsiness and also has significant central nervous system (CNS) effects, caution is advised. Discuss this with your doctor before drinking alcohol.

Tobacco Smoking: No interactions are described in the current literature. I advise everyone to quit smoking.

Marijuana Smoking: May cause additive drowsiness.

▷ *Other Drugs*

Dexfenfluramine *taken concurrently* with

- anti-migraine agents (such as sumatriptan or Imitrex) and dihydroergotamine may rarely result in a serotonin syndrome. DO NOT combine.
- central nervous system active medicines (see Drug Classes of benzodiazepines, opioids, phenothiazines, and others) may have additive effects. Caution is advised.
- insulin (various brands) may increase the sensitivity of the body to insulin (in obese patients) and enable a decreased insulin dose to give a larger than expected effect. More frequent fingerstick glucose testing is recommended, with ongoing insulin doses adjusted to blood sugar levels.
- monoamine oxidase (MAO) inhibitors (see Drug Classes) may result in serious, even fatal reactions. Fourteen days should pass after stopping a MAO inhibitor and starting dexfenfluramine. Three weeks should pass after stopping dexfenfluramine and starting a MAO inhibitor.
- some oral antidiabetic drugs (see Drug Classes) may increase their effectiveness.

▷ *Driving, Hazardous Activities:* Use caution. In one large study which lasted a year, this medicine caused tiredness in more than a quarter of patients, but drowsiness in only 5% of those who took this medicine.

Aviation Note: The use of this drug *may be a disqualification* for piloting. Consult a designated Aviation Medical Examiner.

Exposure to Sun: No restrictions at present.

Occurrence of Unrelated Illness: Since weight loss may modify the need for medicines used to control blood pressure and lipids, and dexfenfluramine itself may increase sensitivity to insulin, the medicines used in these conditions may need to be adjusted.

Discontinuation: Ask your doctor for help if you are considering stopping this medicine.

DIAZEPAM (di AZ e pam)

Introduced: 1963   **Class:** Antianxiety drug, mild tranquilizer, benzodiazepines   **Prescription:** USA: Yes   **Controlled Drug:** USA: C-IV*; Canada: No   **Available as Generic:** Yes

Brand Names: ✦Apo-Diazepam, Diastat, ✦Diazemuls, Diazepam Intensol Oral Solution, ✦Meval, ✦Novodipam, ✦Rival, Valcaps, Valium, Valrelease, Vazepam, ✦Vivol, Zetran

*See Schedules of Controlled Drugs at the back of this book.

BENEFITS versus RISKS

Possible Benefits	*Possible Risks*
RELIEF OF ANXIETY AND NERVOUS TENSION	Habit-forming potential with prolonged use
Wide margin of safety with therapeutic doses	Minor impairment of mental functions
	Respiratory depression
	Jaundice—very rare
	Blood cell disorders—case reports

▷ **Principal Uses**

As a Single Drug Product: Uses included in FDA-approved labeling: (1) Provides short-term relief of mild to moderate anxiety; (2) relieves the symptoms of acute alcohol withdrawal: agitation, tremors, hallucinations, incipient delirium tremens; (3) eases skeletal muscle spasm; (4) provides short-term control of certain types of seizures (epilepsy, fever induced, and status epilepticus); (5) short-term relief of insomnia; (6) adjunctive use in endoscopic procedures; (7) decreases anxiety prior to electrical defibrillation of the heart (cardioversion); (8) eases severe muscle spasms.

Other (unlabeled) generally accepted uses: (1) Helps prevent LSD flashbacks; (2) short-term treatment of sleepwalking; (3) treatment of persistent hiccups; (4) adjunctive treatment of catatonia.

How This Drug Works: By enhancing the nerve transmitter gamma-aminobutyric acid (GABA), this drug helps block higher brain centers and causes calming.

Available Dosage Forms and Strengths

Capsules, prolonged action (sustained release) — 15 mg
Concentrate — 5 mg/ml
Injection — 5 mg/ml
Oral solution — 5 mg/ml, 5 mg/5 ml
Tablets — 2 mg, 5 mg, 10 mg

▷ **Usual Adult Dosage Range:** For anxiety: 2 to 10 mg, two to four times daily. Dose may be increased cautiously as needed and tolerated. After 1 week of continual use, the total daily dose may be taken at bedtime. Total daily dose should not exceed 60 mg. The sustained-release form can be given once daily if the total daily dose is determined to be 15 mg given as 5 mg three times daily. **Note: Actual dosage and administration schedule must be determined for each patient individually.**

Conditions Requiring Dosing Adjustments

Liver Function: The dose **must** be decreased by 50% in patients with liver compromise.

Kidney Function: Caution—if 15 mg or more is given daily, diazepam metabolites may accumulate.

Obesity: Obese patients may take longer than nonobese patients to accumulate this medicine. The time that it takes to remove diazepam (elimination half-life) is prolonged in obese people. This means that obese people may take a much longer time to get the peak effect of diazepam and will also take a longer time to remove the drug from their bodies.

▷ **Dosing Instructions:** The tablet may be crushed and taken on empty stomach or with food or milk. The prolonged-action capsule should not be opened. Do not stop this drug abruptly if taken for more than 4 weeks.

Usual Duration of Use: Use on a regular schedule for 3 to 5 days is usually needed to see this drug's effectiveness in relieving moderate anxiety. Limit continual use to 1 to 3 weeks. Avoid uninterrupted and prolonged use.

▷ **This Drug Should Not Be Taken If**
- you have had an allergic reaction to any dosage form of it previously.
- you have acute narrow-angle glaucoma.
- it is prescribed for a child under 6 months of age.

▷ **Inform Your Physician Before Taking This Drug If**
- you are allergic to any benzodiazepine (see Drug Classes).
- you have a history of alcoholism or drug abuse.
- you are pregnant or planning pregnancy.
- you have impaired liver or kidney function.
- you have a history of serious depression or a mental disorder.
- you have asthma, emphysema, epilepsy, or myasthenia gravis.

Possible Side Effects (natural, expected, and unavoidable drug actions)
Drowsiness—frequent; lethargy, unsteadiness—rare; "hangover" effects on the day following bedtime use.

▷ **Possible Adverse Effects** (unusual, unexpected, and infrequent reactions)
If any of the following develop, consult your physician promptly for guidance.

Mild Adverse Effects
Allergic Reactions: Rashes, hives—rare.
Dizziness, fainting, blurred or double vision, slurred speech, sweating, nausea—possible.
Ringing in the ears—case reports.
Impaired motor skills (dose related to some extent)—frequency varies.

Serious Adverse Effects
Allergic Reactions: Liver damage with jaundice (see Glossary), kidney damage, abnormally low blood platelet count, anaphylaxis—case reports.
Respiratory depression—dose related.
Bone marrow depression: low white blood cells, fever, sore throat—case reports.
Severe lowering of blood pressure, slow heart rate, and cardiac arrest has been reported after rapid intravenous dosing—case reports.
Hip fracture—expected to be an indirect effect of the medicine arising from unsteadiness.
Amnesia—dose related.
Obsessive-compulsive disorder following extended use and abrupt withdrawal—possible.
Paradoxical responses of excitement, agitation, anger, rage—case reports.

▷ **Possible Effects on Sexual Function**
Altered timing and pattern of menstruation.
Small doses (2 to 5 mg/day) may help the anxiety seen in many cases of impotence in men and inhibited sexual responsiveness in women.
Larger doses (10 mg/day or more) can decrease libido, impair potency in men, and inhibit orgasm in women.

Swelling and tenderness of male breast tissue (gynecomastia). Abnormally prolonged erections (priapism)—case reports.

Adverse Effects That May Mimic Natural Diseases or Disorders
Liver reaction with jaundice may suggest viral hepatitis.

Possible Effects on Laboratory Tests
White blood cell counts: decreased.

Blood thyroxine (T_4) level: decreased.

Liver function tests: increased liver enzymes (ALT/GPT, AST/GOT, and alkaline phosphatase), increased bilirubin—all rare.

Urine sugar tests: no drug effect with Tes-Tape; low test results with Clinistix and Diastix.

Urine screening tests for drug abuse: may be **positive**. (Test results depend upon amount of drug taken and testing method used.)

CAUTION
1. This drug should not be stopped abruptly if it has been taken continually for more than 4 weeks.
2. Some nonprescription (over-the-counter or OTC) drug products that contain antihistamines (allergy and cold preparations, sleep aids) can cause excessive sedation if combined with diazepam.

Precautions for Use
By Infants and Children: This drug should not be used in hyperactive or psychotic children. Watch for excessive sedation and incoordination. Usual dose in children for muscle relaxation or sedation is 0.1 to 0.8 mg per kg of body mass per day, divided into equal doses and given every 8 hours or as often as every 6 hours. The drug has been used intravenously to help seizures in neonates.

By Those Over 60 Years of Age: Small doses are indicated. Observe for lethargy, indifference, fatigue, weakness, unsteadiness, disturbing dreams, nightmares, and paradoxical reactions of excitement, agitation, anger, hostility, and rage.

▷ Advisability of Use During Pregnancy
Pregnancy Category: D. See Pregnancy Risk Categories at the back of this book.

Animal studies: Cleft palate reported in mice; skeletal defects in rats.

Human studies: Available information is conflicting and inconclusive. Some findings of increased serious birth defects. Other studies have found no significant increase in birth defects.

Frequent use in late pregnancy can cause the "floppy infant" syndrome in the newborn: weakness, lethargy, unresponsiveness, depressed breathing, low body temperature.

Avoid use during entire pregnancy.

Advisability of Use If Breast-Feeding
Presence of this drug in breast milk: Yes.

Avoid drug or refrain from nursing.

Habit-Forming Potential: This drug can produce psychological and/or physical dependence (see Glossary), especially if used in large doses for an extended period of time.

Effects of Overdosage: Marked drowsiness, weakness, feeling of drunkenness, staggering gait, tremor, stupor progressing to deep sleep or coma.

Possible Effects of Long-Term Use: Psychological and/or physical dependence, rare blood cell disorders.

Suggested Periodic Examinations While Taking This Drug (at physician's discretion)
Complete blood cell counts during long-term use.

▷ **While Taking This Drug, Observe the Following**
Foods: No restrictions.
Beverages: Avoid excessive intake of caffeine-containing beverages: coffee, tea, cola. May be taken with milk.

▷ *Alcohol:* **Avoid this combination**. Alcohol increases the absorption of this drug and adds to its depressant effects on the brain. It is advisable to avoid alcohol completely—throughout the day and night—if it is necessary to drive or to engage in any hazardous activity.
Tobacco Smoking: Heavy smoking may reduce the calming action of this drug. I advise everyone to quit smoking.
Marijuana Smoking: Increased sedation and impairment of intellectual and physical performance.

▷ *Other Drugs*
Diazepam may *increase* the effects of
• digoxin (Lanoxin), and cause digoxin toxicity.
• phenytoin (Dilantin), and cause phenytoin toxicity.
Diazepam may *decrease* the effects of
• levodopa (Sinemet, etc.), and reduce its effectiveness in treating Parkinson's disease.
Diazepam *taken concurrently* with
• fluoxetine (Prozac) may lead to diazepam toxicity.
• fluvoxamine (Luvox) can result in serious accumulation of diazepam and toxicity.
• macrolide antibiotics (see Drug Classes) may lead to toxicity.
• MAO inhibitors (see Drug Classes) may exaggerate breathing depression.
• narcotics or other centrally active medicines may cause additive respiratory depression or decreased levels of consciousness.
The following drugs may *increase* the effects of diazepam
• birth control pills (oral contraceptives).
• cimetidine (Tagamet).
• disulfiram (Antabuse).
• isoniazid (INH, Rifamate, etc.).
• itraconazole (Sporanox), ketoconazole (Nizoral).
• omeprazole (Prilosec).
• ritonavir (Norvir), and perhaps other protease inhibitors (see Drug Classes).
• sertraline (Zoloft).
• valproic acid (Depakene).
The following drugs may *decrease* the effects of diazepam
• ranitidine (Zantac).
• rifampin (Rimactane, etc.).

- rifabutin (Mycobutin).
- theophylline (aminophylline, Theo-Dur, etc.).

▷ *Driving, Hazardous Activities:* This drug can impair mental alertness, judgment, physical coordination, and reaction time. Avoid hazardous activities accordingly.

Aviation Note: The use of this drug *is a disqualification* for piloting. Consult a designated Aviation Medical Examiner.

Exposure to Sun: No restrictions.

Exposure to Heat: Because of reduced urine volume, this drug may accumulate in the body and produce effects of overdosage.

Discontinuation: Avoid sudden discontinuation if this drug has been taken for over 4 weeks without interruption. Dosage should be tapered gradually to prevent a withdrawal syndrome that could include depression, confusion, hallucinations, tremor, seizures, muscle cramping, sweating, and vomiting.

DICLOFENAC (di KLOH fen ak)

See the acetic acid (nonsteroidal anti-inflammatory drugs) profile for further information.

DIDANOSINE (di DAN oh seen)

Other Names: Dideoxyinosine, DDI

Introduced: 1991   **Class:** Antiviral   **Prescription:** USA: Yes   **Controlled Drug:** USA: No; Canada: No   **Available as Generic:** USA: No; Canada: No

Brand Name: Videx

BENEFITS versus RISKS	
Possible Benefits	*Possible Risks*
DELAYED PROGRESSION OF DISEASE IN HIV-INFECTED INDIVIDUALS WITH AIDS OR AIDS-RELATED COMPLEX	DRUG-INDUCED PANCREATITIS DRUG-INDUCED PERIPHERAL NEURITIS
USE IN COMBINATION THERAPY OF AIDS	Drug-induced seizures Liver damage—rare

▷ **Principal Uses**

As a Single Drug Product: Uses currently included in FDA-approved labeling: (1) Treats human immunodeficiency virus (HIV) infections in adults and children (6 months of age or older). This drug is **not** a cure for AIDS, and it does **not** reduce the risk of transmission of HIV infection to others through sexual contact or contamination of blood.

Author's Note: The *Panel on Clinical Practices for Treatment of HIV Infection Report* says that the preferred regimen is two nucleoside analogs and one potent protease inhibitor. Single-agent therapy (with the exception of AZT use in preventing HIV transmission from mother to fetus) was rejected by the panel.

Other (unlabeled) generally accepted uses: (1) Used in combination with other antiretroviral medicines (such as protease inhibitors or hydroxyurea [Hydrea]) to treat AIDS.

How This Drug Works: By interfering with essential HIV enzyme systems, this drug prevents growth and reproduction of HIV particles in infected cells, limiting the severity and extent of HIV infection.

Available Dosage Forms and Strengths

  Powder for oral solution — 2 g or 4 g per bottle
  Powder for oral solution — packets of 100 mg, 167 mg, 250 mg, 375 mg
  Tablets, chewable/dispersible — 25 mg, 50 mg, 100 mg, 150 mg

Author's Note: The company is actively investigating other formulations for this medicine.

▷ **Recommended Dosage Ranges** (Actual dosage and administration schedule must be determined for each patient individually.)

Infants and Children: For those 6 months of age or older, dosage is based on dosage form and body surface area:

  Pediatric oral solution (reconstituted and admixed with buffers)—125 mg (12.5 ml) every 12 hours for body surface area of 1.1–1.4 m^2, 94 mg (9.5 ml) every 12 hours for body surface area of 0.8–1 m^2, 62 mg (6 ml) every 12 hours for body surface area of 0.5–0.7 m^2, 31 mg (3 ml) every 12 hours for body surface area of 0.4 m^2 or less.

  Chewable/dispersible tablets—100 mg every 12 hours for body surface area of 1.1–1.4 m^2, 75 mg every 12 hours for body surface area of 0.8–1 m^2, 50 mg every 12 hours for body surface area of 0.5–0.7 m^2, 25 mg every 12 hours for body surface area of 0.4 m^2 or less. In children 1 year of age or older, each dose should be two tablets to ensure that adequate buffering is provided to prevent destruction (degradation) of the drug in stomach acid. In children younger than 1 year of age, one tablet will provide adequate buffering.

12 to 60 Years of Age: Dosing as follows:

  Adult oral solution (buffered)—250 mg every 12 hours for those weighing more than 60 kg, 167 every 12 hours for those weighing less than 60 kg.

  Chewable/dispersible tablets—200 mg every 12 hours for body weight of 60 kg or more, 125 mg every 12 hours for body weight of less than 60 kg.

Over 60 Years of Age: Same as 12 to 60 group. Dose reduced in impaired liver or kidney function.

Conditions Requiring Dosing Adjustments

Liver Function: Up to 60% of a given dose is changed by the liver to other compounds. There is an increased risk of liver toxicity if used in people with compromised livers. Dose must be decreased if used in liver failure.

Kidney Function: Dose **must** be decreased in mild to moderate kidney failure. There is also an increased risk of magnesium toxicity and drug-induced pancreatitis in patients with kidney problems.

▷ **Dosing Instructions:** Best taken on an empty stomach, 2 hours before or 2 hours after eating.

  The pediatric oral solution is first reconstituted with water and then combined with equal quantities of antacid (such as Mylanta or Maalox). This mixture must be shaken thoroughly before measuring each dose.

The adult oral solution is made by stirring one packet into 120 ml (4 ounces) of water until the powder is dissolved; this may take up to 3 minutes. The powder should not be mixed with fruit juice or other acidic liquid. The entire 4-ounce solution should be swallowed immediately.

The chewable/dispersible buffered tablets should be thoroughly chewed, crushed, or dispersed in water before swallowing. To disperse the tablet(s), stir the prescribed number in at least 30 ml (1 ounce) of water until a uniform suspension is obtained. Swallow the entire preparation immediately.

Author's Note: Current HIV therapy involves combination use of agents from different drug classes to attack the AIDS virus from different points and delay resistance. Many clinicians are using viral load or burden (see Glossary) as an indicator for success of treatment or to show a need for changes in therapy.

Usual Duration of Use: Use on a regular schedule for several months is usually needed to see this drug's effectiveness in slowing AIDS progression. Long-term use (months to years) requires periodic physician evaluation.

Possible Advantages of This Drug
Does not cause serious bone marrow depression (production of blood cells). Less frequent liver toxicity.

▷ **This Drug Should Not Be Taken If**
- you have had an allergic reaction to it previously.
- you have active liver disease.
- you have had pancreatitis recently.

▷ **Inform Your Physician Before Taking This Drug If**
- you have had allergic reactions to any drugs in the past.
- you are taking any other drugs currently.
- you have a history of pancreatitis or peripheral neuritis.
- you have a history of gout or high blood uric acid level.
- you have a history of alcoholism.
- you have a history of diarrhea.
- you have a history of phenylketonuria (PKU).
- you have a history of low blood platelets or blood disorder.
- you have a history of low blood potassium.
- you have a history of heart failure.
- you have a seizure disorder.
- you have impaired liver or kidney function.

Possible Side Effects (natural, expected, and unavoidable drug actions)
Mild decreases in red blood cell, white blood cell, and platelet counts in adults. Mild increases in blood uric acid levels. Increased magnesium levels in patients with kidney problems.

▷ **Possible Adverse Effects** (unusual, unexpected, and infrequent reactions)
If any of the following develop, consult your physician promptly for guidance.

Mild Adverse Effects
Allergic Reactions: Skin rash and itching—occasional in adults and common in pediatric patients.
Headache, dizziness, insomnia, nervousness, confusion—infrequent.
Visual disturbances—rare.

Nausea, vomiting—may be frequent in pediatrics; stomach pain and diarrhea (25% of adults and frequent in pediatric patients), dry mouth and altered taste, yeast infection of mouth—rare to infrequent.

Lowered blood pressure—rare to infrequent.

Loss of color in the retina (retinal depigmentation)—case reports.

Asthma, cough—infrequent.

Loss of hair, muscle and joint pains—rare to infrequent.

Serious Adverse Effects

Drug-induced pancreatitis, usually seen in the first 6 months—infrequent.

Drug-induced peripheral neuritis (see Glossary), usually occurring after 2 to 6 months of treatment. This effect also appears to be dose related—infrequent to frequent.

Electrolyte imbalance (low potassium, magnesium, or calcium)—variable.

Abnormal heart rhythm—infrequent.

High blood sugar—possible.

Excessive lowering of blood pressure and passing out (syncope)—case reports.

Serious skin rash (Stevens-Johnson syndrome)—case reports.

Seizures (may be due to electrolyte problems)—rare.

Lowered white blood cell counts, lowered granulocyte (a specific white blood cell) counts, and lowered blood platelets (69%) in pediatric patients—infrequent to frequent.

Optic neuritis and blindness—case reports.

Liver damage—rare to infrequent.

Kidney damage—rare.

▷ **Possible Effects on Sexual Function:**   None reported.

Adverse Effects That May Mimic Natural Diseases or Disorders

Drug-induced liver reaction—rare at less than 0.2%—may suggest viral hepatitis.

Possible Effects on Laboratory Tests

Complete blood cell counts: decreased red cells and white cells (3–5%); decreased platelets (1%).

Blood amylase level: increased (7–18%).

Blood uric acid level: increased—infrequent.

Blood electrolytes: low calcium, potassium, and magnesium.

Liver function tests: increased liver enzymes (ALT/GPT, AST/GOT, and alkaline phosphatase), increased bilirubin (1–9% of adults and higher in pediatric patients).

CAUTION

1. This drug **does not cure HIV infection** or reduce the risk of transmitting infection to others.
2. Report development of stomach pain with nausea and vomiting; this could indicate pancreatitis.
3. Report the development of pain, numbness, tingling or burning in the hands or feet; this could be peripheral neuritis. It may be necessary to stop this drug.
4. If your kidneys are damaged or your creatinine elevated, ask your doctor if accumulating magnesium will be a problem for you.

Precautions for Use

By Infants and Children: Safety and effectiveness for those under 6 months of age not established. Children are also at risk for developing pancreatitis and peripheral neuritis. It is recommended that detailed eye examinations be performed every 6 months and at any time that visual disturbance occurs.

By Those Over 60 Years of Age: Reduced kidney function may require dosage reduction.

▷ **Advisability of Use During Pregnancy**

Pregnancy Category: B. See Pregnancy Risk Categories at the back of this book.
Animal studies: Rat and rabbit studies show no birth defects.
Human studies: Adequate studies of pregnant women not available.
Consult your physician for specific guidance.

Advisability of Use If Breast-Feeding

Presence of this drug in breast milk: Unknown.
Avoid drug or refrain from nursing.
Note: HIV has been found in human breast milk. Breast-feeding may result in transmission of HIV infection to the nursing infant.

Habit-Forming Potential: None.

Effects of Overdosage: Nausea, vomiting, stomach pain, diarrhea, pain in hands and feet, irritability, confusion.

Possible Effects of Long-Term Use: Peripheral neuritis (see Glossary).

Suggested Periodic Examinations While Taking This Drug (at physician's discretion)

Complete blood cell counts before starting treatment and weekly thereafter until tolerance is established.
Electrolytes.
Blood amylase levels, fractionated for salivary gland and pancreatic origin.
Liver and kidney function tests.
Viral load or viral burden in order to assess success of treatment.
CD4 counts.

▷ **While Taking This Drug, Observe the Following**

Foods: High fat foods can decrease didanosine absorption and lower therapeutic benefit.

Beverages: No restrictions.

▷ *Alcohol:* No interactions expected.

Tobacco Smoking: No interactions expected, but I advise everyone to quit smoking.

▷ *Other Drugs*

Didanosine may *increase* the effects of
• zidovudine (Retrovir), and enhance its antiviral effect against HIV.
Didanosine may *decrease* the effects of
• ciprofloxacin (Cipro), if taken at the same time; take ciprofloxacin at least 2 hours before taking didanosine.
• dapsone and render it ineffective; avoid concurrent use.
• indinavir (Crixivan) and blunt therapeutic benefits; separate dosing by 2 hours.
• itraconazole (Sporanox). Separate dosing by at least 2 hours.

- ketoconazole (Nizoral), if taken at the same time; take ketoconazole at least 2 hours before taking didanosine.
- tetracyclines (see Drug Classes), if taken at the same time; take tetracyclines at least 2 hours before taking didanosine.

Didanosine *taken concurrently* with

- antacids will decrease didanosine absorption and lower its therapeutic benefit.
- histamine (H_2) blocking drugs (see Drug Classes)—cimetidine, etc.—may increase didanosine toxicity.
- pentamidine or sulfamethoxazole may increase the risk of drug-induced pancreatitis; watch for significant symptoms.
- triazolam (Halcion) may cause confusion.
- zalcitabine (Hivid) will cause increased neurotoxicity.

▷ *Driving, Hazardous Activities:* This drug may cause dizziness and impaired vision. Restrict activities as necessary.

Aviation Note: The use of this drug *is a disqualification* for piloting. Consult a designated Aviation Medical Examiner.

Exposure to Sun: No restrictions.

Discontinuation: Do not stop this drug without your physician's knowledge and guidance.

DIFLUNISAL (di FLU ni sal)

See the acetic acids (nonsteroidal anti-inflammatory drugs) profile for further information.

DIGITOXIN (di ji TOX in)

See the digoxin profile for further information.

DIGOXIN (di JOX in)

Introduced: 1934   **Class:** Digitalis preparations   **Prescription:** USA: Yes   **Controlled Drug:** USA: No; Canada: No   **Available as Generic:** Yes
Brand Names: Lanoxicaps, Lanoxin, ✦Novodigoxin, SK-Digoxin

BENEFITS versus RISKS	
Possible Benefits	*Possible Risks*
EFFECTIVE HEART STIMULANT IN CONGESTIVE HEART FAILURE	NARROW TREATMENT RANGE
EFFECTIVE PREVENTION AND TREATMENT OF CERTAIN HEART RHYTHM DISORDERS	Frequent and sometimes serious disturbances of heart rhythm

▷ **Principal Uses**

As a Single Drug Product: Uses in current FDA-approved labeling: (1) Treatment of congestive heart failure; (2) restoration and maintenance of normal heart rate and rhythm in cases of atrial fibrillation (second-line agent behind verapamil, diltiazem, or a beta-blocker), atrial flutter, PAT, and atrial/supraventricular tachycardia.

Other (unlabeled) generally accepted uses: (1) postoperative arrhythmias; (2) helps to increase left ventricular function in patients with pacemakers; (3) may have a role in treating Wolff-Parkinson-White syndrome.

How This Drug Works: Increases force of heart muscle contraction by increasing calcium. Slows the pacemaker and delays electrical transmission through the heart and helps restore normal rate and rhythm.

Available Dosage Forms and Strengths
　　Elixir, pediatric — 0.05 mg/ml
　　　　Capsules — 0.05 mg, 0.1 mg, 0.2 mg
　　　　Injection — 0.1 mg/ml, 0.25 mg/ml
　　　　　Tablets — 0.0625 mg (Canada), 0.125 mg, 0.25 mg, 0.5 mg

Author's Note: Dosing and timing of doses is critical for this medication because the difference between toxic blood levels and therapeutic blood levels is small. Be CERTAIN you understand how and when to take this medicine.

▷ **Usual Adult Dosage Range:**   Loading dose: 10 mcg per kilogram of lean body mass; 10–15 mcg per kg of body mass may be needed if digoxin is being used to control abnormal heart rhythms (such as atrial fibrillation). This loading dose can be given orally or intravenously, and once calculated is often given as 50% in the first dose with the remainder divided into smaller doses and given at 6- to 8-hour intervals until the desired response is achieved. The usual maintenance dose (the ongoing dose used after loading is achieved) is 0.125 to 0.5 mg per day. In neonatal and pediatric patients, a similar loading and maintenance dose strategy is used, but the amount on a mg-per-kg-of-body-mass basis is very different than that for adults. **Note: Actual dosage and administration schedule must be determined for each patient individually.**

Conditions Requiring Dosing Adjustments
　Liver Function: Use with caution; blood levels should be obtained more frequently.
　Kidney Function: Dose **must** be adjusted in kidney compromise. Smaller doses and some cases of dosing every other day may be needed.

▷ **Dosing Instructions:**   Tablet may be crushed, and is best taken at the same time each day on an empty stomach. Can be taken with or following food if desired; milk and dairy products may delay absorption but do not reduce the amount of drug absorbed. The capsule should be swallowed whole.

Usual Duration of Use: Use on a regular schedule for 7 to 10 days is needed to see this drug's effectiveness in relieving heart failure or controlling heart rhythm disorders. Long-term use requires physician supervision and periodic assessment of continued need.

▷ **This Drug Should Not Be Taken If**
　• you have had an allergic reaction to any dosage form of it previously.
　• you are in ventricular fibrillation (a life-threatening heart rhythm).

▷ **Inform Your Physician Before Taking This Drug If**
　• you have had an unfavorable reaction to a digitalis preparation.
　• you have taken any digitalis preparation within the past 2 weeks.

- you now take (or have recently taken) any diuretic (urine-producing) drug.
- you have a history of severe lung disease.
- you have abnormal heart rhythms or certain problems with the aorta.
- you have sustained damage to the heart muscle (myocardium).
- you have a history of low blood potassium or magnesium.
- you have impaired liver or kidney function.
- you have a history of thyroid function disorder.

Possible Side Effects (natural, expected, and unavoidable drug actions)
Slow heart rate.
Enlargement or sensitivity of the male breast—rare.

▷ **Possible Adverse Effects** (unusual, unexpected, and infrequent reactions)
If any of the following develop, consult your physician promptly for guidance.
Mild Adverse Effects
Allergic Reactions: Skin rash, hives.
Headache, drowsiness, lethargy, confusion, changes in vision: "halo" effect, blurring, spots, double vision, yellow-green vision—infrequent.
Changes in vaginal tissue (vaginal cornification)—case reports.
Nightmares—case reports.
Loss of appetite, nausea, vomiting, diarrhea (early signs of adult toxicity)—frequent.
Serious Adverse Effects
Idiosyncratic Reactions: Hallucinations, facial neuralgias, peripheral neuralgias, blindness—case reports.
Low blood platelets—case reports and probably an immune reaction.
Psychosis and hallucinations—associated with toxic levels.
Seizures—rare.
Serious skin rash (Stevens-Johnson syndrome)—rare.
Disorientation, most common in the elderly.
Heart rhythm disturbances—possible and dose related.

▷ **Possible Effects on Sexual Function**
Decreased libido and impotence in 35% of male users. Enlargement and tenderness of male breasts (gynecomastia)—case reports.
Both effects are attributed to digoxin's estrogenlike action.

Adverse Effects That May Mimic Natural Diseases or Disorders
Drug-induced mental changes may be mistaken for senile dementia or psychosis.

Possible Effects on Laboratory Tests
White blood cell counts: decreased.
Blood testosterone level: decreased 30% in men with long-term use.

CAUTION
1. Adhere strictly to prescribed dosage schedules. Do not raise or lower the dose without first consulting your doctor.
2. If you take calcium supplements, ask your physician for help. Avoid large doses.
3. It is best to carry a card that says you are taking this drug.
4. Avoid taking over-the-counter antacids and cold, cough, and allergy remedies without consulting your physician.

Precautions for Use

By Infants and Children: Observe carefully for indications of toxicity: slow heart rate (below 60 beats/min), irregular heart rhythms.

By Those Over 60 Years of Age: You may have reduced drug tolerance; smaller doses are advisable. Watch for early toxicity: headache, dizziness, fatigue, weakness, lethargy, depression, confusion, nervousness, agitation, delusions, difficulty with reading. Promptly call your doctor if these happen.

▷ **Advisability of Use During Pregnancy**

Pregnancy Category: C. See Pregnancy Risk Categories at the back of this book. Animal studies: No birth defects reported.

Human studies: Adequate studies of pregnant women not available. However, no birth defects from the therapeutic use of this drug have been reported.

Use this drug only if clearly needed. Overdosage can be harmful to the fetus.

Advisability of Use If Breast-Feeding

Presence of this drug in breast milk: Yes.

Monitor nursing infant closely and discontinue drug or nursing if adverse effects develop.

Habit-Forming Potential: None.

Effects of Overdosage: Loss of appetite, excessive saliva, nausea, vomiting, diarrhea, serious disturbances of heart rate and rhythm, intestinal bleeding, drowsiness, headache, confusion, delirium, hallucinations, convulsions.

Possible Effects of Long-Term Use: None reported.

Suggested Periodic Examinations While Taking This Drug (at physician's discretion)

Measurements of blood levels of digoxin, calcium, magnesium, and potassium; electrocardiograms.

Time to sample blood for digoxin level: 6–8 hours after last dose, or just before next dose.

Recommended therapeutic range: 0.5–2.0 ng/ml.

▷ **While Taking This Drug, Observe the Following**

Foods: Talk to your doctor about the advisability of eating high potassium foods. The peak concentration and absorption rate will be decreased if digoxin is taken with food.

Beverages: Avoid excessive amounts of caffeine-containing beverages: coffee, tea, cola. May be taken with milk.

▷   *Alcohol:* No interactions expected.

Tobacco Smoking: Nicotine can cause heart muscle irritability and predispose to serious rhythm disturbances. It is best to abstain from all forms of tobacco.

Marijuana Smoking: Possible accentuation of heart failure; reduced digoxin effect; possible changes in electrocardiogram, confusing interpretation.

▷   *Other Drugs*

Digoxin ***taken concurrently*** with

• acarbose (Precose) may result in decreased digoxin blood levels and loss of digoxin's benefits.

• calcium (intravenously) may cause a fatal interaction.

• digoxin immune Fab (Digibind) will result in decreased blood levels. This is used to therapeutic advantage in digoxin toxicity.

- diuretics (other than spironolactone and triamterene) can cause serious heart rhythm disturbances due to excessive loss of potassium.
- propranolol or other beta-blocking medicines (see Drug Classes) may cause very slow heart rate.
- quinidine may result in decreased digoxin effectiveness and increased digoxin toxicity; careful dosage adjustments are necessary.
- succinylcholine may lead to abnormal heart rhythms.

The following drugs may *increase* the effects of digoxin

- alprazolam (Xanax).
- amiloride (Midamor).
- amiodarone (Cordarone).
- amphotericin B (Abelcet, Fungizone).
- benzodiazepines (Librium, Valium, etc.; see Drug Classes).
- captopril (Capoten, Capozide).
- cyclosporine (Sandimmune).
- diltiazem (Cardizem) and other calcium channel blockers (see Drug Classes).
- disopyramide (Norpace).
- erythromycin (E.E.S., Erythrocin, etc.). May also occur with clarithromycin and azithromycin.
- ethacrynic acid.
- flecainide (Tambocor).
- hydroxychloroquine.
- ibuprofen (Advil, Medipren, Motrin, Nuprin, etc.).
- indomethacin (Indocin) and other NSAIDs.
- itraconazole (Sporanox).
- methimazole (Tapazole).
- nifedipine (Adalat, Procardia).
- phenytoin (Dilantin).
- propafenone (Rythmol).
- propylthiouracil (Propacil).
- quinine.
- tetracyclines (see Drug Classes).
- tolbutamide (Orinase).
- trazodone (Desyrel).
- verapamil (Calan, Verelan, others).

The following drugs may *decrease* the effects of digoxin

- aluminum-containing antacids (Amphojel, Maalox, etc.).
- bleomycin (Blenoxane).
- carmustine (BiCNU).
- cholestyramine (Questran).
- colestipol (Colestid).
- cyclophosphamide (Cytoxan).
- cytarabine (Cytosar).
- doxorubicin (Adriamycin).
- fluvoxamine (Luvox).
- kaolin/pectin (Donnagel, others).
- methotrexate (Mexate).
- metoclopramide (Reglan).
- neomycin.

- penicillamine (Cuprimine, Depen).
- procarbazine (Matulane).
- rifampin or rifabutin.
- sucralfate (Carafate).
- sulfa antibiotics or sulfasalazine.
- thyroid hormones.
- vincristine (Oncovin).

▷ *Driving, Hazardous Activities:* Usually no restrictions. However, this drug may cause drowsiness, vision changes, and nausea. Restrict activities as necessary.

Aviation Note: Heart function disorders **are a disqualification** for piloting. Consult a designated Aviation Medical Examiner.

Exposure to Sun: No restrictions.

Occurrence of Unrelated Illness: Vomiting or diarrhea can seriously alter this drug's effectiveness. Notify your physician promptly.

Discontinuation: This drug may be continued indefinitely. Do not stop it without consulting your physician.

DILTIAZEM (dil TI a zem)

Introduced: 1977   **Class:** Anti-anginal, antihypertensive, calcium channel blocker   **Prescription:** USA: Yes   **Controlled Drug:** USA: No; Canada: No   **Available as Generic:** Yes

Brand Names: ✦Apo-Diltiaz, Cardizem, Cardizem CD, Cardizem SR, Dilacor XR, Diltiazem, ✦Novo-Diltiazem, ✦Nu-Diltiaz, ✦Syn-Diltiazem, Tiazac

Controversies in Medicine: Medicines in this class have been subject to much conflicting data. There have also been several FDA hearings held on the calcium channel blocker class. **Amlodipine became the first calcium channel blocker to be FDA approved as safe for use in treating hypertension or angina in patients who also have congestive heart failure.** More recent data found the long-acting forms of calcium channel blockers to be safe and effective.

BENEFITS versus RISKS	
Possible Benefits	*Possible Risks*
EFFECTIVE PREVENTION OF BOTH MAJOR TYPES OF ANGINA	Depression, confusion
	Low blood pressure
EFFECTIVE CONTROL OF MILD TO MODERATE HYPERTENSION	Heart rhythm disturbance
	Fluid retention
HELPS CONTROL ATRIAL FIBRILLATION	Liver damage—case reports
	Muscle damage—case reports

▷ **Principal Uses**

As a Single Drug Product: Uses currently included in FDA-approved labeling: Treats (1) angina pectoris due to coronary artery spasm (Prinzmetal's variant angina) that occurs spontaneously or is associated with exertion; (2) classical angina-of-effort (due to atherosclerotic disease); (3) mild to moderate hypertension.

Other (unlabeled) generally accepted uses: (1) unstable angina; (2) congestive heart failure; (3) migraine prophylaxis; (4) prevention of abnormal protein excretion in the urine; (5) treatment of abnormal heart rhythms such as atrial fibrillation; (6) treatment of buildup of abnormal plaques on the inside of blood vessels (atherosclerosis); (7) may help prevent abnormal growth of the left side of the heart (left ventricular hypertrophy) in patients who have suffered a heart attack; (8) can be of benefit in patients with esophageal disorders; (9) may have a role in helping ease the symptoms of an overactive thyroid gland (hyperthyroidism); (10) can ease symptoms of Raynaud's phenomena; (11) can have a role in preserving function in kidney and heart transplant patients; (12) may protect against heart attacks or variant or unstable angina that can occur after (postoperatively) coronary artery bypass grafting.

How This Drug Works: By blocking normal calcium movement through certain cell walls (needed for nerve and muscle tissue), this drug slows electrical activity in the conduction system of the heart and inhibits the contraction of coronary arteries and peripheral arterioles. As a result of these combined effects, this drug

- prevents spontaneous coronary artery spasm (Prinzmetal's angina).
- reduces the rate and contraction force of the heart during exertion, lowers the oxygen needs of heart muscle, and reduces the occurrence of effort-induced angina (classical angina pectoris).
- reduces contraction of peripheral arterial walls, resulting in relaxation and consequent lowering of blood pressure. This further reduces heart workload during exertion and helps prevent angina.

Available Dosage Forms and Strengths

Tablets (immediate release) — 30 mg, 60 mg, 90 mg, 120 mg

Capsules (extended release) — 120 mg, 180 mg, 240 mg, 300 mg, 360 mg (Tiazac only)

Capsules (sustained release) — 60 mg, 90 mg, 120 mg

▷ **Usual Adult Dosage Range:**   Initially 30 mg, three or four times daily. Dose may be increased gradually at 1- to 2-day intervals as needed and tolerated. Sustained-release forms are dosed 120 or 180 mg daily. Total daily dosage should not exceed 360 mg. **Note: Actual dosage and administration schedule must be determined for each patient individually.**

Conditions Requiring Dosing Adjustments

Liver Function: Maximum daily dose in patients with liver compromise should be 90 mg. Rarely causes hepatoxicity, and a benefit-to-risk decision must be made.

Kidney Function: May be one of the best to use in kidney compromise since it has such a large percentage of liver metabolism and fecal excretion. Caution must still be used, however, as the drug can be a rare cause of kidney compromise.

▷ **Dosing Instructions:**   Immediate-release form may be crushed and is best taken before meals and at bedtime. Extended-release forms should NEVER be crushed or altered. Tiazac form may be taken with or without food.

Usual Duration of Use: Use on a regular schedule for 2 to 4 weeks is required to see this drug's effectiveness in decreasing frequency and severity of angina and in lowering elevated blood pressure. The smallest effective dose should be used in long-term therapy (months to years).

Possible Advantages of This Drug
   Often effective as single-drug therapy.
   Does not reduce blood supply to kidneys.
   Does not raise blood cholesterol levels.
   Does not induce asthma in susceptible individuals.

▷ **This Drug Should Not Be Taken If**
- you have had an allergic reaction to it previously.
- you have "sick sinus" syndrome (and do not have an artificial pacemaker).
- you have second- or third-degree heart block.
- you have low blood pressure—systolic pressure below 90.
- you have heart failure (talk with your doctor).
- you have advanced stenosis of the aorta.

▷ **Inform Your Physician Before Taking This Drug If**
- you had an unfavorable response to any calcium blocker drug.
- you currently take any form of digitalis or a beta-blocker (see Drug Classes).
- you have a history of congestive heart failure.
- you have atrial fibrillation (talk with your doctor).
- you have impaired liver or kidney function.
- you have a history of drug-induced liver damage.

Possible Side Effects (natural, expected, and unavoidable drug actions)
Fatigue—rare; light-headedness, heart rate and rhythm changes in some people—rare.

▷ **Possible Adverse Effects** (unusual, unexpected, and infrequent reactions)
If any of the following develop, consult your physician promptly for guidance.
Mild Adverse Effects
Allergic Reactions: Skin rash, hives, itching—rare.
Headache—may be self-limiting but frequent; drowsiness, dizziness—occasional and dose related; nervousness, sleep problems, depression, confusion, hallucinations—case reports.
Desire to be in constant motion (acathisia)—case reports.
Overgrowth of the gums (gingival hyperplasia)—may be frequent.
Impaired sense of smell—possible.
Increased urination—rare.
Flushing, palpitations, fainting, slow heart rate, low blood pressure—rare.
Nausea, indigestion, heartburn, vomiting, diarrhea, constipation—rare to infrequent.
Serious Adverse Effects
Serious disturbances of heart rate and/or rhythm, fluid retention (edema), congestive heart failure—rare.
Drug-induced myopathy or liver damage—rare.
Lowering of a specific kind of white blood cell (granulocytes)—case reports with other calcium channel blockers.
Lowering of blood platelets—case reports.

▷ **Possible Effects on Sexual Function:** Impotence is reported in less than 1% of users. Swelling or tenderness of the male breast tissue (gynecomastia)—case reports. One reported case of heavy vaginal bleeding.

Possible Effects on Laboratory Tests

Blood total cholesterol and triglyceride levels: no effects.

Blood HDL cholesterol level: increased.

Blood LDL and VLDL cholesterol levels: no effects.

CAUTION

1. Tell all physicians and dentists or other people who provide health care that you take this drug. Note the use of this drug on your card of personal identification.
2. You may use nitroglycerin and other nitrate drugs as needed to relieve acute angina pain. However, if your angina attacks become more frequent or intense, call your doctor promptly.

Precautions for Use

By Infants and Children: Safety and effectiveness for those under 12 years of age not established.

By Those Over 60 Years of Age: May be more likely to have weakness, dizziness, fainting, and falling. Take necessary precautions to prevent injury. Report promptly any changes in your pattern of thirst and urination.

▷ **Advisability of Use During Pregnancy**

Pregnancy Category: C. See Pregnancy Risk Categories at the back of this book.

Animal studies: Embryo and fetal deaths and skeletal birth defects reported in mice, rats, and rabbits.

Human studies: Adequate studies of pregnant women not available.

Avoid this drug during the first 3 months.

Use during the last 6 months only if clearly needed. Ask your physician for help.

Advisability of Use If Breast-Feeding

Presence of this drug in breast milk: Yes.

Avoid drug or refrain from nursing.

Habit-Forming Potential: None.

Effects of Overdosage: Weakness, light-headedness, fainting, slow pulse, low blood pressure, shortness of breath, congestive heart failure.

Possible Effects of Long-Term Use: None reported.

Suggested Periodic Examinations While Taking This Drug (at physician's discretion)

Evaluations of heart function, including electrocardiograms; liver and kidney function tests, with long-term use.

▷ **While Taking This Drug, Observe the Following**

Foods: May increase absorption and cause a 30% increase in blood levels. Avoid excessive salt intake.

Beverages: No restrictions. May be taken with milk.

▷ *Alcohol:* Use with caution. Alcohol may exaggerate the drop in blood pressure.

Tobacco Smoking: Nicotine may reduce the effectiveness of this drug. Follow your physician's advice regarding smoking.

Marijuana Smoking: Possible reduced effectiveness of this drug; mild to moderate increase in angina; possible changes in electrocardiogram, confusing interpretation.

▷ *Other Drugs*

Diltiazem *taken concurrently* with

- aspirin can result in prolonged bleeding time or hemorrhage.
- beta-blocker drugs or digitalis preparations (see Drug Classes) may affect heart rate and rhythm. Careful physician monitoring is necessary if these drugs are combined.
- carbamazepine (Tegretol) may result in toxicity and seizures.
- cyclosporine (Sandimmune) may result in cyclosporine toxicity and kidney failure.
- digoxin (Lanoxin) can result in digoxin toxicity.
- lithium (Lithobid, others) can result in psychosis and neurotoxicity.
- oral antidiabetic drugs (see Drug Classes) such as glipizide (Glucotrol) may result in greater than expected lowering of blood sugar and hypoglycemia.
- phenytoin (Dilantin) decreases phenytoin metabolism and causes phenytoin toxicity.
- rifabutin (Mycobutin) may decrease diltiazem blood levels.
- rifampin (Rifadin) may result in decreased diltiazem effectiveness.
- ritonavir (Norvir) and perhaps other protease inhibitors (see Drug Profiles) may lead to diltiazem toxicity.
- tacrolimus (Prograf) may result in tacrolimus accumulation and tacrolimus toxicity.

The following drugs may *increase* the effects of diltiazem

- cimetidine (Tagamet).
- fluoxetine (Prozac).
- fluvoxamine (Luvox).
- ranitidine (Zantac).

▷ *Driving, Hazardous Activities:* Usually no restrictions. This drug may cause drowsiness or dizziness. Limit activities as necessary.

Aviation Note: Coronary artery disease *is a disqualification* for piloting. Consult a designated Aviation Medical Examiner.

Exposure to Sun: This drug may cause photosensitivity (see Glossary).

Exposure to Heat: Caution is advised. Hot environments can exaggerate the blood-pressure-lowering effects of this drug. Observe for light-headedness or weakness.

Heavy Exercise or Exertion: This drug may improve ability to be more active without angina pain. Use caution and avoid excessive exercise that could impair heart function in the absence of warning pain.

Discontinuation: Do not stop this drug abruptly. Ask your doctor about gradual withdrawal.

DIPHENHYDRAMINE (di fen HI dra meen)

Introduced: 1946   **Class:** Hypnotic, antihistamines   **Prescription:** USA: Varies   **Controlled Drug:** USA: No*; Canada: No   **Available as Generic:** Yes

Brand Names: Acetaminophen-PM, AID to Sleep, Allerdryl, Allergy Capsules, Allergy Formula, Allermax, ✦Ambenyl Expectorant [CD], Ambenyl Syrup [CD], Anacin P.M. Aspirin-free, Banophen, Bayer Select, Beldin Syrup,

*Ambenyl Syrup is C-V. See Schedules of Controlled Drugs at the back of this book.

Bena-D, Benahist, Benadryl, Benadryl 25, Benylin, ✤Benylin Decongestant [CD], ✤Benylin Pediatric Syrup, ✤Benylin Syrup w/Codeine [CD], ✤Caladryl [CD], Caldyphen Lotion, Children's Complete Allergy, Complete Allergy Medication, Compoz, Dermarest, Di-Delamine, Dihydrex, Diphendryl, Diphenhist, Dormarex 2, ✤Ergodryl [CD], Excedrin P.M. [CD], Extra Strength Tylenol PM, Gecil, Genahist, Gen-D-Phen, Hydramine, ✤Insomnal, Kolex, ✤Mandrax [CD], Maximum Strength Nytol, Medi-Phedryl, Midol-PM, Nervine Nightime Sleep, Nidryl Elixir, Nighttime Cold Medicine [CD], Nite-Time, Noradryl [CD], Noradryl 25, Nytol, Pain Relief PM [CD], Pathadryl, ✤PMS-Diphenhydramine, Sinutab Maximum Strength, SK-Diphenhydramine, Sleep, Sleep-Eze 3, ✤Sleep-Eze D, Sominex, Sominex 2, Thcraflu Cold Medicine (Nighttime Strength) Twilite, Tylenol PM Extra Strength, Unisom Sleepgels, Valdrene, Valu-Dryl Allergy Medicine [CD], Wal-Ben, Wal-Dryl, Wehydryl

---

BENEFITS versus RISKS

Possible Benefits	*Possible Risks*
EFFECTIVE RELIEF OF ALLERGIC RHINITIS AND ALLERGIC SKIN DISORDERS	Marked sedation
	Atropinelike effects
	Accentuation of prostatism (see Glossary)
EFFECTIVE, NONADDICTIVE SEDATIVE AND HYPNOTIC	
Treatment of anaphylaxis	
Prevention and relief of motion sickness	
Partial relief of symptoms of Parkinson's disease	

▷ **Principal Uses**

As a Single Drug Product: Uses currently included in FDA-approved labeling: (1) Prevention or treatment of motion sickness (control of dizziness, nausea, and vomiting); (2) treatment of drug-induced parkinsonian reactions, especially in children or the elderly; (3) treatment of conditions caused by histamine release (such as allergic drug reactions); (4) used as a short-term sleep aid; (5) helps hives (urticaria) that have an unknown cause (idiopathic).

Other (unlabeled) generally accepted uses: (1) cough suppression; (2) eases the symptoms of the common cold; (3) can have a role in easing the discomfort of mucositis caused by radiation therapy.

As a Combination Drug Product [CD]: This drug may have a mild suppressant effect on coughing. It is combined with expectorants and codeine or dextromethorphan in some cough products.

How This Drug Works: This drug blocks the action of histamine after it has been released. Its natural side effects are used to advantage: sedative action is used to induce drowsiness and sleep; its atropinelike action is used in motion sickness and Parkinson-related disorders.

Available Dosage Forms and Strengths

Capsules — 25 mg (nonprescription), 50 mg (prescription)

Cream — 1%

Elixir — 12.5 mg/5 ml (14% alcohol)

Spray — 1%

Syrup — 12.5 mg, 13.3 mg/5 ml
Tablets — 25 mg (nonprescription), 50 mg (prescription)

▷ **Usual Adult Dosage Range:**   Antihistamine, to prevent motion sickness or in Parkinsonism: 25 to 50 mg every 6 to 8 hours. Cough control (antitussive): 25 to 50 mg every 4 to 6 hours. Total daily dosage should not exceed 300 mg. When used as a sleep aid (hypnotic), 50 mg at bedtime is often used. **Note: Actual dosage and administration schedule must be determined for each patient individually.**

Conditions Requiring Dosing Adjustments

Liver Function: Caution—single doses are not expected to be a problem; however, the use of multiple doses in patients with liver compromise has not been studied.

Kidney Function: In mild kidney failure (creatinine clearance more than 50 ml/min) the usual dose is given every 6 hours, every 6–12 hours in mild–moderate failure, and every 12–18 hours in severe kidney failure.

▷ **Dosing Instructions:**   Tablet may be crushed and capsule may be opened, and is best taken with or following food.

Usual Duration of Use: Use on a regular schedule for 2 to 3 days is needed to see effectiveness in relieving the symptoms of allergic rhinitis and dermatosis. If not effective after 5 days, this drug should be stopped. As a bedtime sedative (hypnotic), use only as needed. Avoid long-term use without interruption.

▷ **This Drug Should Not Be Taken If**
- you have had an allergic reaction to any dosage form of it previously.
- you are taking, or have taken during the past 2 weeks, any monoamine oxidase (MAO) type A inhibitor drug (see Drug Classes).
- you have chickenpox.

▷ **Inform Your Physician Before Taking This Drug If**
- you have had an unfavorable response to any antihistamine drug.
- you have narrow-angle glaucoma.
- you have peptic ulcer disease, with any degree of pyloric obstruction.
- you have prostatism (see Glossary).
- you are subject to bronchial asthma or seizures (epilepsy).
- you have difficulty urinating.
- you have glucose-6-phosphate dehydrogenase (G6PD) deficiency.

Possible Side Effects (natural, expected, and unavoidable drug actions)

Drowsiness (diphenhydramine is the most sedating antihistamine); weakness; dryness of nose, mouth, and throat; constipation.

▷ **Possible Adverse Effects** (unusual, unexpected, and infrequent reactions)

If any of the following develop, consult your physician promptly for guidance.

Mild Adverse Effects

Allergic Reactions: Skin rash, hives—rare.

Headache, dizziness, inability to concentrate, blurred or double vision, difficult urination—infrequent.

Reduced tolerance for contact lenses—possible.

Nausea, vomiting, diarrhea—possible.

Serious Adverse Effects

Allergic Reaction: Anaphylactic reaction (see Glossary)—case reports.

Idiosyncratic Reactions: Insomnia, excitement, confusion—case reports.

Hemolytic anemia (see Glossary) or porphyria—case reports.

Reduced white blood cell count: fever, sore throat, infections, or blood platelet destruction (abnormal bleeding or bruising; see Glossary)—case reports.

Movement disorders (dyskinesias)—case reports.

▷ **Possible Effects on Sexual Function:**   Shortened menstrual cycle (early arrival of expected menstrual onset).

Natural Diseases or Disorders That May Be Activated by This Drug

Latent epilepsy, glaucoma, prostatism.

Possible Effects on Laboratory Tests

Red blood cell counts and hemoglobin: decreased.

Urine screening tests for drug abuse: *initial* test result may be falsely **positive**; *confirmatory* test result will be **negative**. (Test results depend upon amount of drug taken and testing method used.)

CAUTION

1. Stop this drug 5 days before diagnostic skin testing procedures in order to prevent false negative test results.

2. Do not use if you have active bronchial asthma, bronchitis, or pneumonia.

Precautions for Use

By Infants and Children: This drug should not be used in premature or full-term newborn infants. Doses for children should be small, as the young child is especially sensitive to the effects of antihistamines on the brain and nervous system. For use to decrease coughing (antitussive) in children 6 to 12 years old: 12.5 mg every 4 to 6 hours. The maximum daily dose here is 75 mg/day. Avoid the use of this drug in the child with chickenpox or a flu-like infection—may adversely affect Reye syndrome if it develops.

By Those Over 60 Years of Age: Increased risk of drowsiness, dizziness, and unsteadiness, and impairment of thinking, judgment, and memory. Can increase the degree of impaired urination associated with prostate enlargement (prostatism). Sedative effects may be misinterpreted as senility or emotional depression.

▷ **Advisability of Use During Pregnancy**

Pregnancy Category: B by the manufacturer. See Pregnancy Risk Categories at the back of this book.

Animal studies: No birth defects reported in rats or rabbits.

Human studies: Information from studies of pregnant women indicates no significant increase in birth defects in 2,948 exposures to this drug. A withdrawal syndrome of tremor and diarrhea has been reported in a 5-day-old infant whose mother used this drug (150 mg daily) during pregnancy.

Avoid drug during the last 3 months. Use sparingly during the first 6 months, only if clearly needed.

Advisability of Use If Breast-Feeding

Presence of this drug in breast milk: Yes.

Avoid drug or refrain from nursing.

Habit-Forming Potential: Combination use of pentazocine and diphenhydramine has become an abused intravenous drug combination. There have been rare reports of a withdrawal syndrome after use of high diphenhydramine doses.

Effects of Overdosage: Marked drowsiness, confusion, incoordination, unsteadiness, muscle tremors, stupor, coma, seizures, fever, flushed face, dilated pupils, weak pulse, shallow breathing.

Possible Effects of Long-Term Use: The development of tolerance (see Glossary) and reduced effectiveness of drug.

Suggested Periodic Examinations While Taking This Drug (at physician's discretion)
Complete blood cell counts.

▷ **While Taking This Drug, Observe the Following**
Foods: No restrictions.
Beverages: No restrictions. May be taken with milk.
▷ *Alcohol:* Use extreme caution. The combination of alcohol and antihistamines can cause rapid and marked sedation.
Tobacco Smoking: No interactions expected, but I advise everyone to quit smoking.
Marijuana Smoking: Increased drowsiness and mouth dryness; accentuation of impaired thinking.
▷ *Other Drugs*
Diphenhydramine may *increase* the effects of
• all drugs with a sedative effect such as benzodiazepines, tricyclic antidepressants, and narcotics (see Drug Classes), and cause oversedation.
• amitriptyline (Elavil) and cause increased urinary retention.
• atropine and atropinelike drugs (see Drug Classes).
• tramadol (Ultram), leading to increased sedation risk.
The following drugs may *increase* the effects of diphenhydramine
• monoamine oxidase (MAO) type A inhibitor drugs (see Drug Classes): can delay elimination, exaggerating and prolonging its action.
Diphenhydramine *taken concurrently* with
• phenothiazines (see Drug Classes) may result in increased difficulty urinating, intestinal obstruction, or glaucoma, especially in those over 70 years old.
• temazepam (Restoril) in pregnancy may increase risk of death of the fetus.
• tricyclic antidepressants (see Drug Classes) may cause increased risk of urinary retention.
▷ *Driving, Hazardous Activities:* This drug may impair mental alertness, judgment, physical coordination, and reaction time. Restrict activities as necessary.
Aviation Note: The use of this drug *is a disqualification* for piloting. Consult a designated Aviation Medical Examiner.
Exposure to Sun: Caution—this drug may cause photosensitivity (see Glossary).
Exposure to Environmental Chemicals: The insecticides Aldrin, Dieldrin, and Chlordane may decrease the effectiveness of this drug. Sevin may increase the sedative effects of this drug.

DISOPYRAMIDE (di so PEER a mide)

Introduced: 1969   **Class:** Antiarrhythmic   **Prescription:** USA: Yes
Controlled Drug: USA: No; Canada: No   **Available as Generic:** USA: Yes;
Canada: No

Brand Names: Napamide, Norpace, Norpace CR, Pisopyramide, ✦Rythmodan,
✦Rythmodan-LA

BENEFITS versus RISKS	
Possible Benefits	*Possible Risks*
EFFECTIVE TREATMENT OF SELECTED HEART RHYTHM DISORDERS	NARROW TREATMENT RANGE LOW BLOOD PRESSURE LOW BLOOD SUGAR (INFREQUENT) AGRANULOCYTOSIS—RARE Peripheral neuropathy Liver toxicity Heart conduction and rhythm abnormalities Frequent atropinelike side effects

▷ **Principal Uses**

As a Single Drug Product: Uses currently included in FDA-approved labeling:
This drug is used to treat abnormal rhythms in the ventricles of the heart
(ventricular arrhythmias). It is classified as a Type 1 antiarrhythmic agent,
similar to procainamide and quinidine in its actions.

Other (unlabeled) generally accepted uses: (1) It is used to abolish and prevent the recurrence of premature beats arising in the atria (upper chambers) and the ventricles (lower chambers) of the heart; (2) also useful in the
treatment and prevention of abnormally rapid heart rates (tachycardia)
that originate in the atria or the ventricles; (3) eases arrhythmias and abnormal pressures in the heart arising from cardiomyopathy or subaortic
stenosis.

How This Drug Works: By slowing the activity of the pacemaker and delaying
the transmission of electrical impulses through the conduction system and
muscle of the heart, this drug assists in restoring normal heart rate and
rhythm.

Available Dosage Forms and Strengths

Capsules — 100 mg, 150 mg
Capsules, prolonged action — 100 mg, 150 mg, 250 mg LA (in Canada)
Tablet, controlled release — 150 mg, 250 mg (Canada)

▷ **Usual Adult Dosage Range:**   For most adults, 600 mg per day is given. For the
immediate-release form: 150 mg every 6 hours. For the controlled-release
form: 300 mg every 12 hours. Should not exceed 1600 mg every 24 hours—
reserved for refractory cases. A loading dose has been used if there is a
critical need for quick control: for patients weighing more than 50 kg, 300
mg of the immediate-release form is used. For patients weighing less than
50 kg, 200 mg of the immediate-release form is used. **Note: Actual dosage**

and administration schedule must be determined for each patient individually.

Conditions Requiring Dosing Adjustments

Liver Function: The dose should be decreased in patients with liver compromise by 25 to 50%.

Kidney Function: The dose **must** be adjusted in kidney compromise. In moderate to severe kidney failure, the immediate-release form usual dose is only given every 12 to 24 hours. This drug may cause urine retention and should be used with caution in patients with urinary outflow problems.

▷ **Dosing Instructions:** The regular capsules may be opened to take them, and are best taken on an empty stomach, 1 hour before or 2 hours after eating. However, it may be taken with or following food to reduce stomach irritation. The prolonged-action capsules should not be opened, chewed, or crushed.

Usual Duration of Use: Use on a regular schedule for 2 to 4 days is needed to see this drug's effectiveness in correcting or preventing rhythm disorders. Long-term use requires physician supervision and periodic evaluation.

▷ **This Drug Should Not Be Taken If**
- you have had an allergic reaction to it previously.
- you have second- or third-degree heart block.
- you have sick sinus syndrome (talk with your doctor).

▷ **Inform Your Physician Before Taking This Drug If**
- you have had unfavorable reactions to other antiarrhythmic drugs.
- you have heart disease of any kind, especially "heart block."
- you have a history of atrial fibrillation.
- you have a history of low blood potassium.
- you have a history of low blood pressure.
- you have a history of low white blood cells.
- you have impaired liver or kidney function.
- you have glaucoma, a family history of glaucoma, or myasthenia gravis.
- you have an enlarged prostate gland.
- you are prone to low blood sugars.
- you take digitalis or any diuretic drug that can cause loss of body potassium (ask your doctor).

Possible Side Effects (natural, expected, and unavoidable drug actions)

Drop in blood pressure in susceptible individuals. Dry mouth, constipation, blurred vision, impaired urination—may be frequent.

▷ **Possible Adverse Effects** (unusual, unexpected, and infrequent reactions)

If any of the following develop, consult your physician promptly for guidance.

Mild Adverse Effects

Allergic Reactions: Skin rash, itching—case reports.

Headache, nervousness, fatigue, muscular weakness, mild aches—infrequent.

Loss of appetite, indigestion, nausea, vomiting, diarrhea—infrequent to frequent.

Serious Adverse Effects

Idiosyncratic Reaction: Acute psychotic behavior—rare.

Severe drop in blood pressure, fainting—possible.

Progressive heart weakness, predisposing to congestive heart failure.

Inability to empty urinary bladder, prostatism (see Glossary).

Abnormal heart rhythms—case reports, usually happens within the first month of treatment.

Low blood sugar (glucose)—infrequent.

Jaundice (see Glossary) or liver toxicity—case reports.

Porphyria—rare.

Abnormally low white blood cell count—case report.

▷ **Possible Effects on Sexual Function:**   Rare impotence (300 mg/day); enlargement and tenderness of male breasts—case reports.

Adverse Effects That May Mimic Natural Diseases or Disorders

Reversible jaundice may suggest viral hepatitis.

Natural Diseases or Disorders That May Be Activated by This Drug

Glaucoma, myasthenia gravis.

Possible Effects on Laboratory Tests

White blood cell counts: decreased.

Liver function tests: increased liver enzymes (ALT/GPT, AST/GOT, and alkaline phosphatase), increased bilirubin.

CAUTION

1. Thorough heart exam (including electrocardiograms) is critical prior to using this drug.
2. Periodic heart exams are needed to follow drug responses. Some people may have heart rhythm or function declines. Close monitoring of heart rate, rhythm, and overall performance is essential.
3. Dosage must be individualized. Do not change your dosage without the knowledge and supervision of your physician.
4. Talk with your doctor about the signs and symptoms of low blood sugar.
5. Do not take any other antiarrhythmic drug while taking this drug unless directed to do so by your doctor.

Precautions for Use

By Infants and Children: In pediatric patients, disopyramide is given on a mg-per-kg-of-body-mass basis. The dose is then divided into equal doses and given at times determined by the patient response. For example, some patients from 1 to 4 years old will receive 10 to 20 mg per kg of body mass per day, divided into equal doses and given every 6 hours. Initial use of this drug requires hospitalization and supervision by a qualified pediatrician.

By Those Over 60 Years of Age: Reduced kidney function may require dose reductions. This drug can aggravate existing prostatism (see Glossary) and promote constipation. Observe carefully for light-headedness, dizziness, unsteadiness, and tendency to fall.

▷ **Advisability of Use During Pregnancy**

Pregnancy Category: C. See Pregnancy Risk Categories at the back of this book.

Animal studies: No birth defects reported in rats and rabbits.

Human studies: Adequate studies of pregnant women are not available. It has been reported that this drug can cause contractions of the pregnant uterus.

Use this drug only if clearly needed. Ask your physician for guidance.

Advisability of Use If Breast-Feeding

Presence of this drug in breast milk: Yes.

Avoid drug or refrain from nursing.

Habit-Forming Potential: None.

Effects of Overdosage: Dryness of eyes, nose, mouth, and throat; impaired urination; constipation; marked drop in blood pressure; abnormal heart rhythms; congestive heart failure.

Possible Effects of Long-Term Use: None reported.

Suggested Periodic Examinations While Taking This Drug (at physician's discretion)
Electrocardiograms, complete blood counts, potassium blood levels.

▷ **While Taking This Drug, Observe the Following**
Foods: No restrictions. Ask your physician regarding need for salt restriction and advisability of eating potassium-rich foods.
Beverages: No restrictions. May be taken with milk.
▷ *Alcohol:* Use caution. Alcohol can increase the blood-pressure-lowering effects and the blood-sugar-lowering effects of this drug.
Tobacco Smoking: Nicotine can cause irritability of the heart and reduce the effectiveness of this drug. I advise everyone to quit smoking.
▷ *Other Drugs*
Disopyramide may *increase* the effects of
• antihypertensive drugs, and cause excessive lowering of blood pressure.
• atropinelike drugs (see Drug Classes).
• warfarin (Coumadin, etc.); check INR (prothrombin times) more often, adjust dosing.
Disopyramide may *decrease* the effects of
• ambenonium (Mytelase).
• neostigmine (Prostigmin).
• pyridostigmine (Mestinon).
Benefits of these three drugs in treating myasthenia gravis may be reduced.
Disopyramide *taken concurrently* with
• amiodarone (Cordarone) may result in an abnormal heart effect (torsade de pointes).
• beta-blockers (see Drug Classes) may result in abnormally low heart rates.
• digoxin (Lanoxin) can cause digoxin toxicity.
• erythromycins (E.E.S., others) can cause increased disopyramide blood concentrations and abnormal heart effects. Caution is advised in combining with azithromycin, clarithromycin, or dirithromycin because they are structurally similar.
• insulin or oral antidiabetic drugs (see Drug Classes) agents may result in abnormally low blood sugars.
• phenobarbital may result in loss of disopyramide's effectiveness.
• phenytoin (Dilantin)can result in decreased disopyramide effectiveness and accumulation of a metabolite of phenytoin, which causes a severe increase in anticholinergic effects.
• potassium supplements may result in elevated potassium levels, which can lead to disopyramide toxicity.
• quinidine can cause increases in disopyramide blood levels and decreases in quinidine levels.
• ritonavir (Norvir) and perhaps other protease inhibitors (see Drug Classes) may increase disopyramide blood levels and lead to toxicity.

- verapamil (Calan, others) can precipitate or worsen congestive heart failure.
- warfarin (Coumadin) may cause increased risk of bleeding. INR should be checked more frequently if these medicines are combined.

The following drugs may *decrease* the effects of disopyramide

- all diuretics that promote potassium loss.
- rifabutin (Mycobutin).
- rifampin (Rimactane, Rifadin).

▷ *Driving, Hazardous Activities:* May cause dizziness or blurred vision. Limit activities as needed.

Aviation Note: The use of this drug *may be a disqualification* for piloting. Consult a designated Aviation Medical Examiner.

Exposure to Sun: Use caution. This drug causes photosensitization (see Glossary).

Exposure to Heat: Use caution. The use of this drug in hot environments may increase the risk of heatstroke.

Occurrence of Unrelated Illness: Vomiting, diarrhea, or dehydration can affect this drug's action adversely. Report such developments promptly.

Discontinuation: This drug should not be stopped abruptly following long-term use. Ask your doctor for help regarding gradual dose reduction.

DISULFIRAM (di SULF i ram)

Introduced: 1948   **Class:** Antialcoholism   **Prescription:** USA: Yes
Controlled Drug: USA: No; Canada: No   **Available as Generic:** USA: Yes; Canada: No
Brand Name: Antabuse

BENEFITS versus RISKS	
Possible Benefits	*Possible Risks*
EFFECTIVE ADJUNCT IN THE TREATMENT OF CHRONIC ALCOHOLISM	DANGEROUS REACTIONS WITH ALCOHOL INGESTION
	Acute psychotic reactions
	Drug-induced liver damage
	Drug-induced optic and/or peripheral neuritis
	Low blood platelets

▷ **Principal Uses**

As a Single Drug Product: Uses currently included in FDA-approved labeling: Deters abusive drinking of alcoholic beverages. It does not abolish the craving or impulse to drink.

Other (unlabeled) generally accepted uses: (1) Limited use in helping skin problems (dermatitis) caused by nickel exposure; (2) some data showing increase in infection-fighting cells (CD4) in AIDS.

How This Drug Works: After alcohol is taken, this drug blocks normal liver enzyme activity after the conversion of alcohol to acetaldehyde. This causes excessive accumulation of acetaldehyde, and produces the disulfiram (Antabuse) reaction (see Glossary).

Available Dosage Forms and Strengths
   Tablets — 250 mg, 500 mg

▷ **Usual Adult Dosage Range:**   Once all signs of alcoholic intoxication are gone and no less than 12 hours after the last alcohol-containing drink, treatment is started with 500 mg/day for 1 to 2 weeks. This is followed by a maintenance dose of 250 mg/day. The range of the maintenance dose is 125 mg to 500 mg daily and is individually determined. Total daily dosage should not exceed 500 mg. **Note: Actual dosage and administration schedule must be determined for each patient individually.**

Conditions Requiring Dosing Adjustments
   Liver Function: This drug is a benefit-to-risk decision in mild liver compromise. Disulfiram is clearly contraindicated in portal hypertension and active hepatitis.
   Kidney Function: Dosing adjustments are not indicated.
   Diabetes: People with diabetes who take disulfiram can be at increased risk for diabetic blood vessel (micro- and macrovascular) problems. The risk is worsened by potential adverse drug effects such as increased cholesterol levels and peripheral neuropathy.
   Lung Disease: Accumulation of a metabolite may occur in severe lung problems. Drug levels or dose reduction will be needed.

▷ **Dosing Instructions:**   The tablet may be crushed and taken with or following food to decrease stomach irritation.

Usual Duration of Use: Use on a regular schedule for several months is needed to see this drug's effectiveness in deterring alcohol use. If tolerated well, use of this drug should continue until permanent self-control and sobriety is seen.

▷ **This Drug Should Not Be Taken If**
   • you have had a severe allergic reaction to disulfiram. (Note: The interaction of disulfiram and alcohol is *not* an allergic reaction.)
   • you have taken any form of alcohol within the past 12 hours.
   • you are pregnant.
   • you have a history of psychosis.
   • you are taking paraldehyde.
   • you have significant exposure to ethylene dibromide where you live or work. Disulfiram inhibits the removal of this chemical and enhances the ability of ethylene dibromide to cause cancer.
   • you are taking (or have taken recently) metronidazole (Flagyl).
   • you have coronary heart disease or a serious heart rhythm disorder.

▷ **Inform Your Physician Before Taking This Drug If**
   • you have used disulfiram in the past.
   • you do not intend to avoid alcohol completely while taking this drug.
   • you do not understand what will happen if you drink alcohol while taking this drug.
   • you are planning pregnancy in the near future.
   • you have a history of diabetes, epilepsy, or kidney or liver disease.
   • you take oral anticoagulants, digitalis, isoniazid, paraldehyde, or phenytoin (Dilantin).
   • you have a history of low thyroid function (hypothyroidism).

- you have a history of lung disease.
- you plan to have surgery under general anesthesia while taking this drug.

Possible Side Effects (natural, expected, and unavoidable drug actions)
Drowsiness, lethargy during early use.
Offensive breath and body odor.

▷ **Possible Adverse Effects** (unusual, unexpected, and infrequent reactions)
If any of the following develop, consult your physician promptly for guidance.

Mild Adverse Effects
Allergic Reactions: Skin rash, hives—case reports.
Headache, dizziness, restlessness, tremor—infrequent.
Metallic or garliclike taste, indigestion (usually subsides in 2 weeks).
Decreased or increased blood pressure—possible.

Serious Adverse Effects
Allergic Reactions: Severe skin rashes, drug-induced hepatitis—rare.
Idiosyncratic Reaction: Acute toxic effect on brain, including abnormal movements and psychotic behavior—case reports.
Optic or peripheral neuritis (see Glossary)—case reports.
Seizures—case reports.
Decreased thyroid gland function—possible.
May increase risk for blood vessel problems in people with diabetes or cause low blood platelets—case reports.
Carpal tunnel syndrome, peripheral neuropathy—case reports.

▷ **Possible Effects on Sexual Function:**   Decreased libido and/or impaired erection in users taking recommended doses of 125 to 500 mg daily—case reports.

Adverse Effects That May Mimic Natural Diseases or Disorders
Liver reaction may suggest viral hepatitis.
Brain toxicity may suggest spontaneous psychosis.

Possible Effects on Laboratory Tests
Blood cholesterol level: increased.
INR (prothrombin time): increased (taken concurrently with warfarin).
Liver function tests: liver enzymes increased (ALT/GPT, AST/GOT, and alkaline phosphatase), increased bilirubin.

CAUTION
1. No one should take this drug while in a state of alcoholic intoxication.
2. The patient must be fully informed about the purpose and actions of this drug *before* treatment is started.
3. Long-term use requires exam for reduced thyroid function.
4. Carry a personal identification card noting you are taking this drug.

Precautions for Use
By Infants and Children: Safety and effectiveness for those under 12 years of age not established.
By Those Over 60 Years of Age: Watch for excessive sedation when the drug is started. *Do not* perform an "alcohol trial" to see the effects of this drug.

▷ **Advisability of Use During Pregnancy**
Pregnancy Category: C. See Pregnancy Risk Categories at the back of this book.
Animal studies: No defects reported in rats and hamsters.

Human studies: Two reports indicate that four of eight fetuses exposed had serious birth defects. Adequate studies of pregnant women are not available.

Avoid this drug completely if possible.

Advisability of Use If Breast-Feeding
Presence of this drug in breast milk: Unknown.
Talk with your doctor, as this is a question of benefit of the drug versus the risk of adverse effects to the fetus.

Habit-Forming Potential: None.

Effects of Overdosage: Marked lethargy, impaired memory, altered behavior, confusion, unsteadiness, weakness, stomach pain, nausea, vomiting, diarrhea.

Possible Effects of Long-Term Use: Decreased function of thyroid gland.

Suggested Periodic Examinations While Taking This Drug (at physician's discretion)
Visual acuity, liver function tests, thyroid function tests.

▷ **While Taking This Drug, Observe the Following**
Foods: Avoid all foods prepared with alcohol, including sauces, marinades, vinegars, desserts, etc. Ask when dining out about use of alcohol in cooking food.
Beverages: Avoid all punches, fruit drinks, etc., that may contain alcohol. This drug may be taken with milk.

▷   *Alcohol: **Avoid completely in all forms*** while taking this drug and for 14 days following the last dose. Combination of disulfiram and alcohol—even in small amounts—produces the disulfiram (Antabuse) reaction. This starts 5 to 10 minutes after ingesting alcohol and consists of: intense flushing, severe headache, shortness of breath, chest pains, nausea, repeated vomiting, sweating, and weakness. If large amounts of alcohol are taken, the reaction may progress to blurred vision, vertigo, confusion, marked drop in blood pressure, and loss of consciousness. Severe reactions may lead to convulsions and death. The reaction may last from 30 minutes to several hours, depending upon the amount of alcohol and disulfiram in the body.
Tobacco Smoking: No interactions expected, but I advise everyone to quit smoking.
Marijuana Smoking: Possible increase in drowsiness or lethargy.

▷   *Other Drugs*
Disulfiram may ***increase*** the effects of
  • chlordiazepoxide (Librium) and diazepam (Valium), and cause oversedation. Other benzodiazepines such as alprazolam, clonazepam, clorazepate, flurazepam, halazepam, prazepam, or triazolam may also be subject to this interaction.
  • oral anticoagulants (warfarin, etc.), and increase the risk of bleeding; dosage adjustments may be necessary.
  • paraldehyde, and cause excessive depression of brain function.
  • phenytoin (Dilantin), and cause toxicity; dosage must be decreased.
Disulfiram may ***decrease*** the effects of
  • perphenazine (Trilafon, etc.).

Disulfiram *taken concurrently* with
- bacampicillin (Spectrobid) can theoretically cause a disulfiram reaction, but no cases have been reported.
- cisplatin (Platinol) can increase risk of toxicity of cisplatin.
- cyclosporine (Sandimmune) may result in a disulfiram reaction, as there is alcohol in the intravenous and oral forms of cyclosporine.
- isoniazid (INH, etc.) may cause acute mental problems and incoordination.
- metronidazole (Flagyl) may cause acute mental and behavioral disturbances, making it necessary to stop treatment.
- omeprazole (Prilosec) may result in increased disulfiram levels and toxicity.
- over-the-counter (OTC) cough syrups, tonics, etc., containing alcohol may cause a disulfiram (Antabuse) reaction; avoid concurrent use (see Over-the-Drugs in Glossary).
- paraldehyde may result in a disulfiram reaction.
- theophylline (Theo-Dur, others) can lead to theophylline toxicity because the metabolism of theophylline is decreased.
- warfarin will result in an increased risk of bleeding. Increased INR testing is recommended.

The following drugs may *increase* the effects of disulfiram
- amitriptyline (Elavil), and perhaps other tricyclic antidepressants may enhance the disulfiram + alcohol interaction; avoid concurrent use of these drugs.

▷ *Driving, Hazardous Activities:* This drug may cause drowsiness or dizziness. Limit activities as necessary.

Aviation Note: Alcoholism *is a disqualification* for piloting. Consult a designated Aviation Medical Examiner.

Exposure to Sun: No restrictions.

Exposure to Environmental Chemicals: Thiram, a pesticide, and carbon disulfide, a pesticide and industrial solvent, can have additive toxic effects. Watch for toxic effects on the brain and nervous system.

Discontinuation: Drug treatment is only part of your total program. Do not stop it without the knowledge and guidance of your physician. If it must be stopped abruptly, there are no symptoms. However, no alcohol should be ingested for 14 days following discontinuation.

DORNASE ALPHA (DOOR nase AL fa)

Introduced: 1994   **Class:** Anti-cystic-fibrosis agent   **Prescription:** USA: Yes   **Controlled Drug:** USA: No; Canada: No   **Available as Generic:** USA: No; Canada: No

Brand Name: Pulmozyme

BENEFITS versus RISKS	
Possible Benefits	*Possible Risks*
DECREASED MUCOUS VISCOSITY	Hoarseness
IMPROVED LUNG FUNCTION	Antibodies to DNA
DECREASED OCCURRENCE OF	Facial swelling (edema)
RESPIRATORY INFECTIONS	
DECREASED NUMBER OF	
HOSPITALIZATIONS	

▷ **Principal Uses**

As a Single Drug Product: Uses currently included in FDA-approved labeling: Management of cystic fibrosis in conjunction with standard therapies.

Other (unlabeled) generally accepted uses: May have a role in treating chronic bronchitis.

How This Drug Works: The sputum of people with cystic fibrosis contains large amounts of DNA and is much thicker than normal. Dornase breaks the DNA down, making the sputum easier to remove. Other undiscovered mechanisms may also account for its benefits.

Available Dosage Forms and Strengths

Solution — 2.5 ml ampules of 1.0 mg/ml dornase alpha (2.5 mg)

▷ **Recommended Dosage Ranges** (Actual dosage and administration schedule must be determined for each patient individually.)

Infants and Children: Safety and efficacy for those under 5 not established.

5 to 60 Years of Age: One 2.5-mg dose administered by one of the tested nebulizers each day. Some selected patients may benefit from twice-daily dosing (older patients).

Over 60 Years of Age: Same as 12 to 60 years of age.

Conditions Requiring Dosing Adjustments

Liver Function: Not defined.

Kidney Function: Not defined.

▷ **Dosing Instructions:**   The solution must be kept in the refrigerator and protected from strong light. The drug should not be used if it is cloudy or discolored. Do **not** mix dornase with other medications. Clinical trials have only been conducted with the Hudson T Up-Draft 2, Marquest Acorn ll, and Pulmo-Aide compressor. The reusable PARI LC Jet nebulizer and PARI PRONEB compressor were also tested. Do **not** use with other equipment.

Usual Duration of Use: Use on a regular schedule for 8 days usually determines effectiveness in cystic fibrosis. Long-term use (up to 12 months has been studied) requires periodic physician evaluation of response and dosage adjustment.

Possible Advantages of This Drug

Reduction in number of infections, use of antibiotics and hospitalizations with minimal side effects.

▷ **This Drug Should Not Be Taken If**
- you have had an allergic reaction to any dosage form of it previously.
- you have an allergy to Chinese hamster ovary cells.

▷ **Inform Your Physician Before Taking This Drug If**
- you had a rash after the last dose was taken.

- you are uncertain how to use the nebulizer or compressor.
- you are uncertain of how much dornase to take or how often to take it.

Possible Side Effects (natural, expected, and unavoidable drug actions)
Hoarseness—may be frequent.

▷ **Possible Adverse Effects** (unusual, unexpected, and infrequent reactions)
If any of the following develop, consult your physician promptly for guidance.
Mild Adverse Effects
Allergic Reactions: Rash—infrequent.
Mild pharyngitis or laryngitis—infrequent.
Conjunctivitis—infrequent.
Chest pain—has been reported. Facial swelling—rare.
Serious Adverse Effects
Allergic Reactions: None defined at present.
Antibodies to DNA (2–4%).

▷ **Possible Effects on Sexual Function:**   None reported.

Possible Delayed Adverse Effects: None reported.

Possible Effects on Laboratory Tests
Antibodies to DNA.

CAUTION
1. This drug should only be used with one of the studied nebulizers and compressors.
2. Do not use the drug if it is cloudy or discolored.

Precautions for Use
By Infants and Children: Safety and effectiveness for those under 5 years of age not established.
By Those Over 60 Years of Age: No changes or precautions.

▷ **Advisability of Use During Pregnancy**
Pregnancy Category: B. See Pregnancy Risk Categories at the back of this book.
Animal studies: Studies in rats and rabbits at up to 600 times the usual human dose have not revealed any harm to the fetus.
Human studies: Adequate studies of pregnant women are not available.
Ask your doctor for guidance.

Advisability of Use If Breast-Feeding
Presence of this drug in breast milk: Unknown.
Avoid drug or refrain from nursing.

Habit-Forming Potential: None.

Effects of Overdosage: Single doses of up to 180 times the usual human dose in rats and monkeys have been well tolerated.

Possible Effects of Long-Term Use: Not defined.

Suggested Periodic Examinations While Taking This Drug (at physician's discretion)
Periodic pulmonary function tests.

▷ **While Taking This Drug, Observe the Following**
Foods: No restrictions.
Nutritional Support: Continued enzyme and nutritional support is still needed.
Beverages: No specific restrictions.

▷   *Alcohol:* Follow your doctor's advice relative to alcohol use.
    Tobacco Smoking: No specific drug interactions, but I advise everyone to quit smoking.
▷   *Other Drugs:* Clinical studies have revealed that dornase is compatible with medications typically used in management of cystic fibrosis. Specific adverse drug interactions are not documented at present.
▷   *Driving, Hazardous Activities:* Specific limitations because of drug effects are not defined at present.
    Aviation Note: The use of this drug *may be a disqualification* for piloting. Consult a designated Aviation Medical Examiner.
    Exposure to Sun: No restrictions.
    Discontinuation: This drug's benefits stop soon after its regular use is stopped. It must be continued indefinitely to continue to benefit.
    Special Storage Instructions: This drug should be stored at 36–46 degrees F and should be protected from light. Unused ampules should be stored in their protective pouch in the refrigerator.

DOXAZOSIN (dox AY zoh sin)

Introduced: 1986   **Class:** Antihypertensive   **Prescription:** USA: Yes
Controlled Drug: USA: No   **Available as Generic:** No
Brand Name: Cardura

BENEFITS versus RISKS	
Possible Benefits	*Possible Risks*
EFFECTIVE TREATMENT OF MILD TO MODERATE HYPERTENSION when used alone or in combination with other antihypertensive drugs	"First-dose" drop in blood pressure, but without fainting
	Dizziness
	Fluid retention
TREATMENT OF BENIGN PROSTATIC HYPERPLASIA	Rapid heart rate

▷ **Principal Uses**

    As a Single Drug Product: Uses currently included in FDA-approved labeling: (1) Once-daily treatment of mild to moderate hypertension; (2) used in treatment of benign prostatic hypertrophy/hyperplasia.
        Other (unlabeled) generally accepted uses: (1) Used in conjunction with other drugs to treat congestive heart failure; (2) used to treat pheochromocytoma.

How This Drug Works: By blocking certain actions of the sympathetic nervous system, this drug causes direct relaxation of blood vessel walls and lower blood pressure. Decreases the peak pressure of the detrusor muscle, prevents alpha-1 receptor stimulation and, as such occurs, prevents smooth muscle contractions in the prostatic urethra and bladder neck and helps urine outflow.

Available Dosage Forms and Strengths
    Tablets — 1 mg, 2 mg, 4 mg, 8 mg

▷ **Usual Adult Dosage Range:**   Starts with a "test dose" of 1 mg to check patient's response within the first 2 to 6 hours. If tolerated, dose is increased cautiously (as needed and tolerated) every 2 weeks and taken as a single dose at bedtime. Doses in excess of 4 mg may increase the occurrence of light-headedness or dizziness, and should be avoided. Total daily dosage should not exceed 16 mg. For benign prostatic hyperplasia (BPH), a similar test dose is used; usual effective doses are from 4 to 8 mg. **Note: Actual dosage and administration schedule must be determined for each patient individually.**

Conditions Requiring Dosing Adjustments
Liver Function: Extreme caution and lower doses **must** be used if the drug is used in patients with liver compromise.
Kidney Function: Doses of 1–16 mg have been used. In one study of kidney compromise, 1 mg decreased the blood pressure for 3 days.

▷ **Dosing Instructions:**   The tablet may be crushed and is best taken at bedtime to avoid orthostatic hypotension (see Glossary). May be taken without regard to food.

Usual Duration of Use: Use on a regular schedule for 6 to 8 weeks is needed to see this drug's benefit in controlling hypertension. Long-term use (months to years) requires physician supervision and evaluation.

Possible Advantages of This Drug
May be used to initiate treatment.
Effective with once-a-day dosage.
Causes depression or impotence infrequently.
Lowers blood cholesterol and sugar levels.
Does not lose effectiveness with long-term use.

▷ **This Drug Should Not Be Taken If**
• you have had an allergic reaction to this drug or to prazosin (Minipres) or terazosin (Hytrin).
• you have active liver disease.

▷ **Inform Your Physician Before Taking This Drug If**
• you have had orthostatic hypotension (see Glossary) when using other antihypertensive drugs.
• you have a history of mental depression.
• you have impaired circulation to the brain, or a history of stroke.
• you have coronary artery disease.
• you are taking other medicine to help lower your blood pressure.
• you have had a stroke and have high blood pressure.
• you have a history of low white blood cells.
• you have active liver disease or impaired liver function.
• you have impaired kidney function.
• you have angina (active coronary artery disease) and you are not taking a beta-blocking drug. (Consult your physician.)
• you plan to have surgery under general anesthesia in the near future.

Possible Side Effects (natural, expected, and unavoidable drug actions)
Orthostatic hypotension—infrequent; drowsiness, salt and water retention, dry mouth—rare; nasal congestion, constipation—rare.

▷ **Possible Adverse Effects** (unusual, unexpected, and infrequent reactions)
   If any of the following develop, consult your physician promptly for guidance.
   Mild Adverse Effects
   Allergic Reaction: Skin rash or itching—rare.
   Headache, dizziness, fatigue, nervousness, numbness and tingling, blurred vision—rare to infrequent.
   Palpitation, rapid heart rate, or shortness of breath—rare.
   Nausea, diarrhea, indigestion—rare to infrequent.
   Increased urination—rare.
   Serious Adverse Effects
   Mental depression—rare.
   Arrhythmias—case reports.
   Decreased blood sugar (glucose)—case reports.
   Low white blood cell counts (has not caused symptoms in patients who had follow-up visits).

▷ **Possible Effects on Sexual Function:**   Impotence—rare.

Natural Diseases or Disorders That May Be Activated by This Drug
   Latent coronary artery insufficiency.

Possible Effects on Laboratory Tests
   White blood cell counts: rare occurrence of mild decrease while taking drug.
   Blood lipid tests: decreased total cholesterol, LDL cholesterol, and cholesterol/HDL ratio; decreased triglycerides; increased HDL.
   Blood sugar level: variable decreases.

CAUTION
   1. Watch for "first-dose" response of precipitous drop in blood pressure, with or without fainting; this usually happens in the first 6 hours. Starting dose is 1 mg taken at bedtime for the first week; remain supine after taking these trial doses.
   2. Impaired liver function will increase drug level and require smaller than usual doses.
   3. Ask your doctor or pharmacist before you take over-the-counter remedies for allergic rhinitis or head colds; these preparations contain drugs that may interact with doxazosin.

Precautions for Use
   By Infants and Children: Safety and effectiveness for those under 12 years of age not established.
   By Those Over 60 Years of Age: Therapy is started with no more than 1 mg/day for the first week. Subsequent increases in dose must be very gradual. Orthostatic hypotension can cause unexpected falls and injury; sit or lie down promptly if you feel light-headed or dizzy. Report dizziness or chest pain promptly.

▷ **Advisability of Use During Pregnancy**
   Pregnancy Category: B. See Pregnancy Risk Categories at the back of this book.
   Animal studies: No birth defects found in rat or rabbit studies.
   Human studies: Adequate studies of pregnant women are not available.
   Use this drug only if clearly needed. Ask your physician for guidance.

Advisability of Use If Breast-Feeding
   Presence of this drug in breast milk: Unknown.
   Watch nursing infant closely and discontinue drug or nursing if adverse effects develop.

Habit-Forming Potential: None.

Effects of Overdosage: Orthostatic hypotension, headache, generalized flushing, rapid heart rate, extreme weakness, irregular heart rhythm, circulatory collapse.

Possible Effects of Long-Term Use: None reported.

Suggested Periodic Examinations While Taking This Drug (at physician's discretion)
   Measurements of blood pressure in lying, sitting, and standing positions.
   Measurements of body weight to check for fluid retention.

▷ **While Taking This Drug, Observe the Following**
   Foods: No restrictions. Avoid excessive salt intake.
   Beverages: No restrictions. May be taken with milk.
▷ *Alcohol:* Use with extreme caution. Alcohol can exaggerate the blood-pressure-lowering actions of this drug and cause excessive reduction.
   Tobacco Smoking: Nicotine can contribute to this drug's ability to intensify coronary insufficiency. All forms of tobacco should be avoided.
▷ *Other Drugs*
   The following drugs may *increase* the effects of doxazosin
   • beta-adrenergic-blocking drugs (see Drug Classes); severity and duration of the "first-dose" response may be increased.
   The following drugs may *decrease* the effects of doxazosin
   • estrogens.
   • indomethacin (Indocin) and other NSAIDs.
▷ *Driving, Hazardous Activities:* This drug may cause dizziness or drowsiness. Restrict activities as necessary.
   Aviation Note: The use of this drug *is a disqualification* for piloting. Consult a designated Aviation Medical Examiner.
   Exposure to Sun: No restrictions.
   Exposure to Cold: Use caution. Cold environments may increase coronary insufficiency (angina) and hypothermia (see Glossary).
   Heavy Exercise or Exertion: Excessive exertion can augment this drug's ability to induce angina.
   Discontinuation: If you are taking this drug for congestive heart failure, do not stop it abruptly. Ask your physician for guidance.

DOXEPIN (DOX e pin)

Introduced: 1969   **Class:** Antidepressant   **Prescription:** USA: Yes
Controlled Drug: USA: No; Canada: No   **Available as Generic:** USA: Yes; Canada: No

Brand Names: Adapin, Sinequan, ♣Triadapin, Zonalon

BENEFITS versus RISKS

Possible Benefits	*Possible Risks*
EFFECTIVE RELIEF OF ENDOGENOUS DEPRESSION	ADVERSE BEHAVIORAL EFFECTS: Confusion, disorientation, hallucinations, delusions
EFFECTIVE RELIEF OF ANXIETY AND NERVOUS TENSION	CONVERSION OF DEPRESSION TO MANIA in manic-depressive (bipolar) disorders
EFFECTIVE RELIEF OF SOME KINDS OF ITCHING (TOPICAL FORM)	Aggravation of schizophrenia and paranoia
Possibly beneficial in other depressive disorders	Rare blood cell disorders
	Rare liver toxicity
	Low blood pressure on standing

▷ **Principal Uses**

As a Single Drug Product: Uses currently included in FDA-approved labeling: (1) Relieves the symptoms associated with spontaneous (endogenous) depression, refractory depression, neurotic depression, mixed depression anxiety, and depression and anxiety in alcoholism; (2) helps treat sleep disturbances; (3) treats depression and anxiety associated with alcoholism.

Other (unlabeled) generally accepted uses: (1) Helps decrease the frequency of urination at night in patients with excessive activity of the detrusor muscle; (2) has a role in pain management in cancer patients; (3) can ease the extent of lowered blood glucose (postprandial hypoglycemia) that occurs after meals in some patients; (4) may help in the management of posttraumatic stress disorder; (5) helps people troubled by itching and swelling of unknown cause (idiopathic urticaria); (6) may help ease the craving that occurs when people try to stop smoking.

How This Drug Works: Relieves depression by slowly restoring to normal levels chemicals (norepinephrine and serotonin) that transmit nerve impulses.

Available Dosage Forms and Strengths

Capsules — 10 mg, 25 mg, 50 mg, 75 mg, 100 mg, 150 mg
Oral concentrate — 10 mg/ml
Topical cream — 50 mg/g

▷ **Usual Adult Dosage Range:**   Initially 25 mg three to four times daily. Dose may be increased cautiously as needed and tolerated by 10 to 25 mg daily at intervals of 1 week. Usual maintenance dose is 75 to 150 mg daily. Usually there is no greater benefit achieved by using more than 300 mg/day. There have been rare uses of 500 mg/day. When the optimal requirement is determined, it may be taken at bedtime as one dose.

Topical cream: The cream is applied four times daily for up to 8 days. **Note: Actual dosage and administration schedule must be determined for each patient individually.**

Conditions Requiring Dosing Adjustments

Liver Function: Doxepin has rarely caused hepatitis. This drug should be used with caution and in reduced doses in patients with liver compromise.

Kidney Function: Use with caution in patients with compromised kidneys and urine outflow problems.

▷ **Dosing Instructions:** May be taken without regard to meals. Capsule may be opened for administration. The cream may be applied four times a day for up to 8 days. DO NOT cover the area where the cream was applied with an occlusive (water-tight) dressing, as this may lead to excessive drug absorption.

Usual Duration of Use: Some benefit may be apparent within to 2 weeks, but adequate response may require continual use for 3 weeks or longer. Long-term use should not exceed 6 months without evaluation regarding the need for continuation of the drug. Consult your physician on a regular basis.

▷ **This Drug Should Not Be Taken If**
- you have had an allergic reaction to it previously.
- you are taking or have taken within the past 14 days any monoamine oxidase (MAO) type A inhibitor drug (see Drug Classes).
- you are recovering from a recent heart attack.
- you have significant urine retention.
- you have narrow-angle glaucoma.

▷ **Inform Your Physician Before Taking This Drug If**
- you are allergic or sensitive to any other tricyclic antidepressant (see Drug Classes).
- you have a history of any of the following: diabetes, epilepsy, glaucoma, heart disease, liver compromise, prostate gland enlargement, or overactive thyroid function.
- you are pregnant or are breast-feeding.
- you plan to have surgery under general anesthesia in the near future.

Possible Side Effects (natural, expected, and unavoidable drug actions)
Drowsiness—frequent and may be dose related.
Blurred vision, dry mouth, constipation, impaired urination, low blood pressure on standing—infrequent to frequent.

▷ **Possible Adverse Effects** (unusual, unexpected, and infrequent reactions)
If any of the following develop, consult your physician promptly for guidance.
Mild Adverse Effects
Allergic Reactions: Skin rash, hives, swelling of face or tongue, drug fever (see Glossary)—possible.
Ringing in the ears—rare.
Stinging or burning of the skin with application of doxepin cream—possible.
Headache, dizziness, drowsiness, weakness, fainting, unsteady gait, tremors—case reports.
Increased appetite, craving for sweets, weight gain—case reports.
Peculiar taste, irritation of tongue or mouth, nausea, indigestion—case reports.
Fluctuation of blood sugar levels—case reports.
Serious Adverse Effects
Allergic Reactions: Hepatitis, with or without jaundice (see Glossary).
Confusion, hallucinations, agitation, restlessness, delusions—rare with systemic use.
Bone marrow depression (see Glossary): fatigue, weakness, fever, sore throat, abnormal bleeding or bruising—case reports.

Peripheral neuritis (see Glossary): numbness, tingling, pain, loss of strength in arms and legs—case reports.

Elevations in temperature or seizures—case reports.

Kidney or liver damage—case reports.

Parkinson-like disorders (see Glossary)—usually mild and infrequent; more likely to occur in the elderly.

Abnormal heart rhythm or rate—case reports.

▷ **Possible Effects on Sexual Function:** Female breast enlargement with milk production.

Swelling of testicles. Enlargement and tenderness of male breast tissue (gynecomastia). Ejaculation disorder. Painful and persistent erection (priapism)—case reports.

Adverse Effects That May Mimic Natural Diseases or Disorders

Liver toxicity may suggest viral hepatitis.

Natural Diseases or Disorders That May Be Activated by This Drug

Latent diabetes, epilepsy, glaucoma, impaired urination due to prostate gland enlargement (prostatism; see Glossary).

Possible Effects on Laboratory Tests

White blood cell and platelet counts: may be decreased.

Liver function tests: increased.

Blood sugar (glucose): may be increased.

CAUTION

1. Dosage must be adjusted for each person individually. Report for follow-up evaluation and laboratory tests as directed by your physician.
2. It is advisable to withhold this drug if electroconvulsive therapy (ECT, "shock" treatment) is to be used to treat your depression.

Precautions for Use

By Infants and Children: Safety and effectiveness for those under 12 years of age not established.

By Those Over 60 Years of Age: During the first 2 weeks of treatment, watch for development of confusion, agitation, forgetfulness, disorientation, delusions, and hallucinations. Reduction of dosage or discontinuation may be necessary. Unsteadiness may predispose to falling and injury. This drug can increase the degree of impaired urination associated with prostate gland enlargement (prostatism).

▷ **Advisability of Use During Pregnancy**

Pregnancy Category: C. See Pregnancy Risk Categories at the back of this book.

Animal studies: No birth defects reported in rats, rabbits, dogs, or monkeys.

Human studies: Adequate studies of pregnant women are not available.

Use this drug only if clearly needed. If possible, avoid use during the first 3 months and the last month. Ask your physician for guidance.

Advisability of Use If Breast-Feeding

Presence of this drug in breast milk: Yes.

Monitor nursing infant very closely and discontinue drug or nursing if adverse effects develop.

Habit-Forming Potential: None.

Effects of Overdosage: Confusion, hallucinations, marked drowsiness, heart palpitations, dilated pupils, tremors, stupor, deep sleep, coma, convulsions.

Suggested Periodic Examinations While Taking This Drug (at physician's discretion)

Complete blood cell counts, liver function tests, serial blood pressure readings, and electrocardiograms.

▷ **While Taking This Drug, Observe the Following**

Foods: No restrictions. This drug may increase the appetite and cause excessive weight gain.

Beverages: No restrictions. May be taken with milk.

▷   *Alcohol:* Avoid completely. This drug can markedly increase the intoxicating effects of alcohol and accentuate its depressant action on brain function.

Tobacco Smoking: May hasten the elimination of this drug; higher doses may be necessary. I advise everyone to quit smoking.

Marijuana Smoking: Possible increase in heart rate.

▷   *Other Drugs*

Doxepin may *increase* the effects of

• albuterol (Ventolin) on blood vessels.
• atropinelike drugs (see Drug Classes).
• dicumarol, and increase the risk of bleeding; dosage adjustments may be necessary.
• other drugs with central nervous system effects (narcotics, benzodiazepines, etc.; see Drug Classes).
• phenytoin (Dilantin).
• thyroid hormones.

Doxepin may *decrease* the effects of

• clonidine (Catapres).
• guanethidine (Ismelin).

Doxepin *taken concurrently* with

• carbamazepine (Tegretol) may decrease the effectiveness of doxepin.
• cimetidine (Tagamet) may result in doxepin toxicity (urine retention, dry mouth).
• cholestyramine (Questran) may blunt doxepin levels and benefits.
• diphenhydramine (Benadryl) or other drugs with anticholinergic actions may result in increased risk of urine retention or bowel obstruction.
• epinephrine will result in an exaggerated increase in blood pressure.
• estrogens may change the action of doxepin.
• fluoxetine (Prozac) can result in doxepin toxicity.
• meperidine (Demerol) may result in an increased risk of respiratory depression.
• methylphenidate (Ritalin) can result in doxepin toxicity.
• monoamine oxidase (MAO) type A inhibitor drugs (see Drug Classes) may cause high fever, delirium, and convulsions.
• paroxetine (Paxil) can cause increased doxepin levels and toxicity.
• propoxyphene (Darvon) can result in doxepin toxicity.
• pseudoephedrine will result in abnormal increases in blood pressure and should not be combined in therapy.
• quinidine (Quinaglute) can result in doxepin toxicity.
• sertraline (Zoloft) can result in increased doxepin levels.
• verapamil (Calan, Verelan, others) may result in increased doxepin levels.

- vitamin C (ascorbic acid) may result in decreased doxepin benefits.
- warfarin will result in prolonged action of the anticoagulant. More frequent INR testing is needed.

▷ *Driving, Hazardous Activities:* This drug may impair mental alertness, judgment, physical coordination, and reaction time. Avoid hazardous activities.

Aviation Note: The use of this drug *is a disqualification* for piloting. Consult a designated Aviation Medical Examiner.

Exposure to Sun: Use caution until sensitivity has been determined. This drug may cause photosensitivity (see Glossary).

Exposure to Heat: This drug can inhibit sweating and impair the body's adaptation to hot environments, increasing the risk of heatstroke. Avoid saunas.

Exposure to Cold: The elderly should use caution and avoid conditions conducive to hypothermia (see Glossary).

Discontinuation: It is advisable to discontinue this drug gradually. Abrupt withdrawal after long-term use can cause headache, malaise, and nausea.

DOXYCYCLINE (dox ee SI kleen)

Introduced: 1967   **Class:** Antibiotic, tetracyclines   **Prescription:** USA: Yes   **Controlled Drug:** USA: No; Canada: No   **Available as Generic:** USA: Yes; Canada: No

Brand Names: Apo-Doxy, Apo-Doxy-Tabs, ✦Doryx, Doryx, Doxy 100, 200, Doxy Caps, Doxychel, ✦Doxycin, Doxy-Lemmon, Novopharm, Vibramycin, Vibra-Tabs, ✦Vibra-Tabs C-Pak

BENEFITS versus RISKS	
Possible Benefits	*Possible Risks*
EFFECTIVE TREATMENT OF INFECTIONS due to susceptible microorganisms	ALLERGIC REACTIONS, mild to severe
	Liver reaction with jaundice
	Kidney toxicity
	Fungal superinfections
	Drug-induced colitis
	Blood cell disorders

▷ **Principal Uses**

As a Single Drug Product: Uses currently included in FDA-approved labeling: (1) Treats a broad range of infections caused by susceptible bacteria and protozoa; (2) treats and prevents "traveler's diarrhea"; (3) treats syphilis in people who are penicillin-allergic; (4) helps prevent malaria in travelers; (5) helpful in acne.

Other (unlabeled) generally accepted uses: (1) treatment of early Lyme disease; (2) treatment of sexual assault victims; (3) treatment of prostatitis; (4) can help in some cases of PMS; (5) may be of benefit in some cases of male infertility of unexplained origin.

How This Drug Works: Prevents growth and multiplication of susceptible bacteria by interfering with formation of essential proteins and causing leaky cell walls.

Available Dosage Forms and Strengths

Capsules — 50 mg, 100 mg
Capsules, coated pellets — 100 mg
Capsule, delayed release — 100 mg
Injection — 100 mg per vial, 200 mg per vial
Oral suspension — 25 mg/5 ml
Syrup — 50 mg/5 ml
Tablets — 50 mg, 100 mg

▷ **Usual Adult Dosage Range:** 100 mg every 12 hours the first day, then 100 mg once daily. Some severe infections may require ongoing therapy of 100 mg every 12 hours. Total daily dosage should not exceed 300 mg. **Note: Actual dosage and administration schedule must be determined for each patient individually.**

Conditions Requiring Dosing Adjustments

Liver Function: Patients with both liver and kidney compromise should have the dose decreased. This drug can cause liver problems, and a benefit-to-risk decision should be made for patients with liver compromise.

Kidney Function: Patients with moderate to severe kidney failure should be given the usual dose, but only every 12 to 24 hours.

Malnutrition: Lower than expected levels may occur in patients with malnutrition. If clinical progress is not as expected, the dose may need to be increased.

▷ **Dosing Instructions:** The tablet may be crushed and the capsule opened; best taken on an empty stomach, 1 hour before or 2 hours after eating. If stomach irritation occurs, it may be taken with food or milk. (Unlike other tetracyclines, the doxycycline absorption is not significantly changed by food or milk.) Take at same time each day, with a full glass of water or milk. Take the full course prescribed.

Usual Duration of Use: The time needed to control the infection and be free of fever and symptoms for 48 hours. This varies with the nature of the infection.

▷ **This Drug Should Not Be Taken If**
- you are allergic to any tetracycline drug (see Drug Classes).
- you are pregnant or breast-feeding.
- you have severe liver disease.

▷ **Inform Your Physician Before Taking This Drug If**
- you are taking a penicillin antibiotic (see Drug Classes).
- you have a history of any of the following: liver or kidney disease, lupus erythematosus.
- it is prescribed for a child under 8 years old.
- you are taking any anticoagulant drug.
- you plan to have surgery under general anesthesia in the near future.

Possible Side Effects (natural, expected, and unavoidable drug actions)
Superinfections (see Glossary), often due to yeast organisms. These can occur in the mouth, intestinal tract, rectum, and/or vagina, resulting in rectal and vaginal itching.

▷ **Possible Adverse Effects** (unusual, unexpected, and infrequent reactions)
If any of the following develop, consult your physician promptly for guidance.

Mild Adverse Effects
> Allergic Reactions: Skin rash, hives, itching of hands and feet, swelling of face or extremities—rare.
>
> Loss of appetite, nausea, vomiting, diarrhea—infrequent.
>
> Loss of smell (anosmia) or distortion of smell (dysosmia)—rare.
>
> Irritation of mouth or tongue, "black tongue," sore throat, abdominal cramping or pain—possible.
>
> Increased eosinophils—possible.

Serious Adverse Effects
> Allergic Reactions: Anaphylactic reaction (see Glossary), asthma, fever, swollen joints, abnormal bleeding or bruising, jaundice (see Glossary)—case reports.
>
> Permanent discoloration and/or malformation of teeth when taken by children under 8 years of age, including unborn child and infant.
>
> Ulceration of the esophagus—infrequent.
>
> Liver or kidney toxicity—rare.
>
> Systemic lupus erythematosus—case reports.
>
> Blood cell disorders (hemolytic anemia, thrombocytopenia, neutropenia, or eosinophilia)—case reports.
>
> Serious skin reactions (erythema multiforme or Stevens-Johnson syndrome)—case reports.

▷ **Possible Effects on Sexual Function:**   None reported.

Natural Diseases or Disorders That May Be Activated by This Drug
> Systemic lupus erythematosus.

Possible Effects on Laboratory Tests
> Complete blood cell counts: decreased red cells, hemoglobin, white cells, and platelets; increased eosinophils (allergic reaction).
>
> Prothrombin time: increased.
>
> Kidney function tests: increased blood creatinine and urea nitrogen (BUN) levels; increased urine protein (kidney damage).

CAUTION
1. Antacids and preparations containing aluminum, bismuth, iron, magnesium, or zinc can prevent adequate drug absorption.
2. Troublesome and persistent diarrhea can occur. If diarrhea persists for more than 24 hours, stop this drug and call your doctor.

Precautions for Use
> *By Infants and Children:* If possible, tetracyclines should not be given to those under 8 years old because of the risk of permanent tooth discoloration and deformity. Rarely, infants may develop increased intracranial pressure within the first 4 days of receiving this drug. Tetracyclines may inhibit normal bone growth and development.
>
> *By Those Over 60 Years of Age:* Natural skin changes may predispose to severe and prolonged itching reactions in the genital and anal regions.

▷ **Advisability of Use During Pregnancy**
> *Pregnancy Category:* D. See Pregnancy Risk Categories at the back of this book.
> Animal studies: Tetracycline causes limb defects in rats, rabbits, and chickens.
> Human studies: Information from studies of pregnant women indicates that

drugs of this class can cause impaired development and discoloration of teeth and other developmental defects.

It is advisable to avoid this drug completely during entire pregnancy.

Advisability of Use If Breast-Feeding
Presence of this drug in breast milk: Yes.
Avoid drug or refrain from nursing.

Habit-Forming Potential: None.

Effects of Overdosage: Nausea, vomiting, diarrhea, acute liver damage—rare.

Possible Effects of Long-Term Use: Superinfections (see Glossary), prolongation of prothrombin time.

Suggested Periodic Examinations While Taking This Drug (at physician's discretion)
Complete blood cell counts, liver and kidney function tests.
During extended use, sputum and stool examinations may detect early superinfection due to yeast organisms.

▷ **While Taking This Drug, Observe the Following**
Foods: Avoid meats and iron-fortified cereals and supplements for 2 hours before and after taking this drug. Avoid combination with dairy products or calcium supplements.
Beverages: No restrictions. May be taken with milk or carbonated beverages.
▷ *Alcohol:* Shortened half-life and decreased antibiotic benefit. Best avoided if you have active liver disease.
Tobacco Smoking: No interactions expected, but I advise everyone to quit smoking.
▷ *Other Drugs*
Doxycycline may *increase* the effects of
- oral anticoagulants such as warfarin (Coumadin). More frequent INR tests are advised.
- digoxin (Lanoxin), and cause digitalis toxicity.
- lithium (Eskalith, Lithane, etc.), and increase the risk of lithium toxicity.
Doxycycline may *decrease* the effects of
- birth control pills (oral contraceptives), and **impair their effectiveness, resulting in pregnancy.**
- penicillins, and impair their effectiveness in treating infections.
The following drugs may *decrease* the effects of doxycycline
- antacids (aluminum and magnesium preparations, sodium bicarbonate, etc.); may reduce drug absorption.
- barbiturates (see Drug Classes).
- bismuth preparations (Pepto-Bismol, etc.).
- calcium supplements (various).
- carbamazepine (Tegretol).
- cimetidine (Tagamet).
- iron and mineral preparations (such as zinc salts); may reduce drug absorption.
- phenobarbital.
- phenytoin (Dilantin).
- rifampin (Rifadin, others).
- zinc salts.

▷ *Driving, Hazardous Activities:* Usually no restrictions. Watch for nausea or diarrhea.

Aviation Note: The use of this drug *may be a disqualification* for piloting. Consult a designated Aviation Medical Examiner.

Exposure to Sun: Use caution—tetracyclines can cause photosensitivity (see Glossary).

ENALAPRIL (e NAL a pril)

Introduced: 1981 **Class:** Antihypertensive, ACE inhibitor **Prescription:** USA: Yes **Controlled Drug:** USA: No **Available as Generic:** Yes

Brand Names: ✦Vaseretic (also available in U.S.) [CD], Vasotec

BENEFITS versus RISKS	
Possible Benefits	*Possible Risks*
EFFECTIVE CONTROL OF MILD TO SEVERE HIGH BLOOD PRESSURE	Headache, dizziness, fatigue, and low blood pressure
THIS AND OTHER DRUGS OF THE SAME CLASS MAY BE DRUGS OF FIRST CHOICE FOR PATIENTS WITH HIGH BLOOD PRESSURE WHO EXERCISE	Bone marrow depression
	Allergic swelling of face, tongue, or vocal cords
	Increased blood potassium
Possibly beneficial as adjunctive treatment in selected cases of congestive heart failure	

▷ **Principal Uses**

As a Single Drug Product

Uses currently included in FDA-approved labeling: (1)Treats high blood pressure; (2) adjunctive treatment of symptomatic congestive heart failure; (3) pheochromocytoma (a rare tumor that increases blood pressure); (4) kidney crisis in scleroderma.

Other (unlabeled) generally accepted uses: (1) Angina therapy; (2) captopril-induced protein in the urine; (3) kidney failure in diabetics.

How This Drug Works: By blocking certain enzyme systems (angiotensin-converting enzymes—ACE) that influence arterial function, this drug contributes to relaxation of arterial walls and lowers blood pressure. This reduces the workload of the heart and improves its performance.

Available Dosage Forms and Strengths

Injection — 1.25 mg/ml

Tablets — 2.5 mg, 5 mg, 10 mg, 20 mg

▷ **Usual Adult Dosage Range:** For high blood pressure (if not also taking a diuretic): Initially 5 mg once daily. Usual maintenance dose is 10 to 40 mg daily in a single dose or divided into two equal doses. Total daily dose should not exceed 40 mg if kidney function is impaired.

For heart failure: 2.5 to 10 mg once or twice daily. Usually combined with other medications. Maximum is 40 mg daily. **Note: Actual dosage and** administration schedule must be determined for each patient individually.

Conditions Requiring Dosing Adjustments

Liver Function: In patients with liver compromise, the dose may need to be **increased** because less of the drug is activated.

Kidney Function: Patients with mild to moderate kidney failure can be given 5 mg/day. In severe kidney failure, maximum dose is 2.5 mg/day.

Diabetes: Patients with diabetes with decreased creatinine clearance and protein in the urine (proteinuria) should be given decreased doses.

▷ **Dosing Instructions:**   Tablet may be crushed and taken on an empty stomach or with food, at same time each day.

Usual Duration of Use: Use on a regular schedule for several weeks is needed to see this drug's effectiveness in controlling high blood pressure. Treatment of high blood pressure usually requires the long-term therapy.

▷ **This Drug Should Not Be Taken If**
- you have had an allergic reaction to it previously.
- you have angioedema from other ACE inhibitors (swelling of the tongue, face, or glottis).
- you are pregnant (last 6 months).
- you have active liver disease.

▷ **Inform Your Physician Before Taking This Drug If**
- you have had an allergic reaction (or other adverse effect) from any ACE inhibitor (see Drug Classes).
- you are planning pregnancy.
- you have severe liver disease.
- you take immunosuppressant medicines.
- you currently have a blood cell or bone marrow disorder or an autoimmune disorder.
- you have a history of kidney disease or impaired kidney function.
- you have scleroderma or systemic lupus erythematosus.
- you have an abnormally high level of blood potassium.
- you have any form of heart disease or diabetes.
- you have renal artery stenosis (talk with your doctor).
- you are taking other antihypertensives, diuretics, nitrates, or potassium supplements.
- you have swelling of the face or tongue. Call your doctor immediately if this occurs.
- you plan to have surgery under general anesthesia in the near future.

Possible Side Effects (natural, expected, and unavoidable drug actions)

Dizziness, light-headedness, fainting (excessive drop in blood pressure). Impaired sense of smell.

▷ **Possible Adverse Effects** (unusual, unexpected, and infrequent reactions)

If any of the following develop, consult your physician promptly for guidance.

Mild Adverse Effects

Allergic Reactions: Skin rash, itching.

Headache, fatigue, dizziness, drowsiness—infrequent.

Insomnia, nervousness, numbness and tingling—rare.

Rapid heart rate, palpitation—rare.

Indigestion, taste disorders, stomach pain, nausea, vomiting, diarrhea—rare.

Vulvovaginal itching—case reports.

Excessive sweating, muscle cramps—rare.

Cough—infrequent.

Ringing in the ears—case reports.

Serious Adverse Effects

Allergic Reactions: Swelling (angioedema) of face, tongue, and/or vocal cords; can be life-threatening—case reports.

Bone marrow depression: fatigue, weakness, fever, sore throat, abnormal bleeding or bruising—very rare.

Problems with blood clotting (reduced platelet aggregation)—possible.

Excessively low blood pressure—possible.

Pancreatitis—case reports.

Kidney or liver toxicity—rare.

Rare peripheral neuropathy.

Depression or hallucinations—case reports.

Elevated blood potassium—rare.

Serious skin reactions (Stevens-Johnson, etc.)—case reports to rare.

▷ **Possible Effects on Sexual Function:**   Impotence—case reports. Swelling and tenderness of male breast tissue (gynecomastia)—rare.

Itching of the vulva and vagina—case reports.

Possible Effects on Laboratory Tests

Blood eosinophil counts: increased (allergic reaction).

Blood creatinine or potassium level: increased.

Blood uric acid level: decreased.

CAUTION

1. Consult your physician regarding the advisability of discontinuing other antihypertensive drugs (especially diuretics) for 1 week before starting this drug.

2. **Tell your doctor immediately if you become pregnant.** This drug should not be taken beyond the first 3 months of pregnancy.

3. **Report promptly** any signs of infection (fever, sore throat), or water retention (weight gain, puffiness, swollen feet or ankles).

4. Do not use a salt substitute without your physician's knowledge and approval. (Many salt substitutes contain potassium.)

5. Blood counts and urine analyses are needed **before** starting this drug.

Precautions for Use

By Infants and Children: Safety and effectiveness for those in this age group are not established.

By Those Over 60 Years of Age: Small starting doses are advisable. Sudden or excessive lowering of blood pressure can predispose to stroke or heart attack.

▷ **Advisability of Use During Pregnancy**

Pregnancy Category: D during the final 6 months (second and third trimesters). C during the first 3 months. See Pregnancy Risk Categories at the back of this book.

Animal studies: No birth defects found in rat or rabbit studies.

Human studies: Use of ACE inhibitor drugs during the final 6 months of pregnancy is known to possibly cause very serious injury and death to the fetus; skull and limb malformations, lung defects, and kidney failure have been reported in over 50 cases worldwide.

Avoid this drug completely during the final 6 months of pregnancy. During the first 3 months, ask your physician for help.

Advisability of Use If Breast-Feeding
Presence of this drug in breast milk: Yes.
Watch nursing infant closely and discontinue drug or nursing if adverse effects develop.

Habit-Forming Potential: None.

Effects of Overdosage: Excessive drop in blood pressure—light-headedness, dizziness, fainting.

Possible Effects of Long-Term Use: Gradual increase in blood potassium level.

Suggested Periodic Examinations While Taking This Drug (at physician's discretion)
Before starting drug: Complete blood cell counts; urine analysis with measurement of protein content; blood potassium level.
During use of drug: Blood cell counts; measurements of blood potassium.

▷ **While Taking This Drug, Observe the Following**
Foods: Consult your physician regarding salt intake.
Nutritional Support: **Do not** take potassium supplements unless directed by your physician.
Beverages: No restrictions. May be taken with milk.
▷ *Alcohol:* Use caution until combined effect has been determined. Alcohol may enhance the blood-pressure-lowering effect of this drug.
Tobacco Smoking: No interactions expected, but I advise everyone to quit smoking.
▷ *Other Drugs*
Enalapril *taken concurrently* with
• allopurinol (Zyloprim) can result in serious skin reactions.
• aspirin or other NSAIDs (see Drug Classes) can lessen therapeutic benefit of enalapril.
• azathioprine (Imuran) can cause severe impairment of blood formation (myelosuppression).
• cyclosporine (Sandimmune) can cause acute kidney failure.
• ethacrynic acid (Edecrin) can cause excessive lowering of blood pressure.
• interferon alfa (and perhaps beta) can lead to severe blood (hematological) problems.
• lithium (Lithobid, others) can lead to lithium toxicity.
• loop diuretics (see Drug Classes) can cause severe lowering of blood pressure upon standing up from a sitting position.
• oral hypoglycemic agents (glyburide—Glynase, others) may result in decreased insulin resistance and the need to decrease the dose of the oral hypoglycemic agent.
• phenothiazines (see Drug Classes) can cause additive lowering of blood pressure.
• potassium preparations (K-Lyte, Slow-K, etc.) may cause increased blood levels of potassium with risk of serious heart rhythm disturbances.

- potassium-sparing diuretics—amiloride (Moduretic), spironolactone (Aldactazide), triamterene (Dyazide)—may cause increased potassium with risk of serious heart rhythm disturbances.
- rifampin (Rifadin) or rifabutin (Mycobutin) may cause decreased therapeutic benefit from enalapril.
- thiazide diuretics (hydrochlorothiazide, others) may result (especially in older people) in increased levels of enalaprilat (the active medicine) and increased reduction in blood pressure. Doses may need to be decreased if this combination is used.

▷ *Driving, Hazardous Activities:* Usually no restrictions. Be aware of possible drops in blood pressure with resultant dizziness or faintness.

Aviation Note: The use of this drug *may be a disqualification* for piloting. Consult a designated Aviation Medical Examiner.

Exposure to Sun: Caution is advised. A similar drug from this class can cause photosensitivity.

Exposure to Heat: Caution is advised. Avoid excessive perspiring with resultant loss of body water and drop in blood pressure.

Occurrence of Unrelated Illness: Promptly report any nausea, vomiting, or diarrhea. Fluid and chemical imbalances must be corrected as soon as possible.

EPINEPHRINE (ep i NEF rin)

Other Name: Adrenaline

Introduced: 1900   **Class:** Antiasthmatic, anti-glaucoma, decongestant
Prescription: USA: Varies   **Controlled Drug:** USA: No; Canada: No
Available as Generic: USA: Yes; Canada: No

Brand Names: Adrenalin, Adreno-Mist, Ana-Kit, Asthmahaler, Asthmanephrine, Bronkaid Mist, ✦Bronkaid Mistometer, ✦Citanest Forte, Duranest [CD], ✦Dysne-Inhal, Epifrin, E-Pilo Preparations [CD], Epinal Ophthalmic, EpiPen, Epitrate, Marcaine, Medihaler-Epi Preparations, Micronephrine, Norocaine, Octocaine, P1E1, P2E1, P3E1, P4E1, P6E1, Primatene Mist, Propine Ophthalmic, Sensoricaine, Sus-Phrine, Thalfed [CD], Therex [CD], ✦Ultracaine, Vaponefrin, Xylocaine

BENEFITS versus RISKS	
Possible Benefits	*Possible Risks*
EFFECTIVE RELIEF OF SEVERE ALLERGIC (ANAPHYLACTIC) REACTIONS	Significant increase in blood pressure (in sensitive people)
TEMPORARY RELIEF OF ACUTE BRONCHIAL ASTHMA	Idiosyncratic reaction: Pulmonary edema (fluid formation in lungs)
Reduction of internal eye pressure (treatment of glaucoma)	Heart rhythm disorders (in sensitive individuals)
Relief of allergic congestion of the nose and sinuses	

▷ **Principal Uses**

As a Single Drug Product: Uses currently included in FDA-approved labeling: (1) Inhalation to relieve acute attacks of bronchial asthma; (2) as a decongestant for symptomatic relief of allergic nasal congestion and as eyedrops in the management of glaucoma; (3) used in treatment of anaphylactic shock; (4) used in emergency situations to treat abnormal heart rhythms and in cardiopulmonary resuscitation; (5) used as an aid to increase the beneficial effects of topical anesthetics.

Other (unlabeled) generally accepted uses: (1) Septic shock; (2) wheezing in infants; (3) croup; (4) can have a role in easing painful erections (priapism).

How This Drug Works: By stimulating some nerve terminals (sympathetic), this drug acts to
- contract blood vessel walls and raise the blood pressure.
- inhibit release of histamine into skin and internal organs.
- dilate constricted bronchial tubes, increasing the size of the airways and improving the ability to breathe.
- decrease fluid formation in the eye, increase its outflow from the eye, and reduce internal eye pressure.
- decrease the amount of blood in the nose, shrinking swelling (decongestion) and expanding the nasal airway.

Available Dosage Forms and Strengths

> Aerosol — 0.2, 0.27, and 0.3 mg per spray
> Eyedrops — 0.1%, 0.25%, 0.5%, 1%, 2%
> Injection — 0.01, 0.1, 1, and 5 mg/ml
> Nose drops — 0.1%
> Solution for nebulizer — 1%, 1.25%, 2.25%

▷ **Usual Adult Dosage Range:** Aerosols: One inhalation, repeated in 1 to 2 minutes if needed; wait 4 hours before next inhalation. Eyedrops: One drop every 12 hours. Dosage may vary with product; follow printed instructions and label directions. **Note: Actual dosage and administration schedule must be determined for each patient individually.**

Conditions Requiring Dosing Adjustments
Liver Function: Dosage reduction is not needed in liver compromise.
Kidney Function: Dosage adjustment is not defined in kidney compromise.

▷ **Dosing Instructions:** Aerosols and inhalation solutions: After first inhalation, wait 1 to 2 minutes to determine if a second inhalation is necessary.
If relief does not occur within 20 minutes of use, and difficult breathing persists, stop this drug and seek medical attention **promptly. Avoid prolonged and excessive use**. Eyedrops: During instillation of drops and for 2 minutes following, press finger against the tear sac (inner corner of eye) to prevent rapid absorption of drug into body circulation.

Usual Duration of Use: According to individual needs. Long-term use requires physician supervision.

▷ **This Drug Should Not Be Taken If**
- you have had an allergic reaction to any dosage form of it previously.
- you have narrow-angle glaucoma.
- you are in shock.
- you have organic brain damage.
- you are in labor—it may delay the second stage of labor.
- you are to undergo general anesthesia with cyclopropane or halogenated hydrocarbons.

- your heart is dilated and you have a coronary deficiency.
- you have experienced a recent stroke or heart attack.

▷ **Inform Your Physician Before Taking This Drug If**
- you have any degree of high blood pressure.
- you have any form of heart disease, especially coronary heart disease (with or without angina), or a heart rhythm disorder.
- you have diabetes or overactive thyroid function (hyperthyroidism).
- you have a history of stroke.
- you have a chronic lung disease
- you take monoamine oxidase (MAO) type A inhibitors, phenothiazines (see Drug Classes), digitalis preparations, or quinidine.

Possible Side Effects (natural, expected, and unavoidable drug actions)
In some people—restlessness, anxiety, headache, tremor, palpitation, cold hands and feet, dryness of mouth and throat (with use of aerosol).

▷ **Possible Adverse Effects** (unusual, unexpected, and infrequent reactions)
If any of the following develop, consult your physician promptly for guidance.
Mild Adverse Effects
Allergic Reactions: Skin rash; eyedrops may cause redness, swelling, and itching of the eyelids.
Weakness, dizziness, pallor.
Serious Adverse Effects
Idiosyncratic Reaction: Sudden development of excessive fluid in the lungs (pulmonary edema).
In predisposed individuals—excessive rise in blood pressure with risk of stroke (cerebral hemorrhage).
Rapid heart rate and arrhythmias—case reports.
Seizures or porphyria—rare.
Pulmonary edema—case reports.
Pigmentation of the eye—case reports.
Kidney toxicity—rare.

▷ **Possible Effects on Sexual Function:** May be of help in painful and abnormally prolonged erections (priapism).

Possible Effects on Laboratory Tests
Complete blood counts: red cells and white cells increased; eosinophils decreased.
Blood glucose level: increased.
Urine sugar tests: false low or negative results with Clinistix; true positive with Benedict's or Fehling's solution.
Acidosis.
Blood platelets: temporarily increased.

CAUTION
1. Medication failure can result from frequent repeat use at short intervals. If this develops, avoid use for 12 hours, and a normal response should return.
2. Excessive use of aerosol preparations in asthmatics has been associated with sudden death.

3. This drug can cause significant irritability of the nerve pathways (conduction system) and muscles of the heart, predisposing to serious heart rhythm disorders. Consult your doctor if you have a heart disorder.
4. This drug can increase blood sugar level. If you have diabetes, test for sugar often to detect significant changes.
5. If you become unresponsive to this drug and you substitute isoproterenol (Isuprel), allow an interval of 4 hours between drugs.
6. Promptly throw this drug away if a pinkish-red to brown coloration or cloudiness (precipitation) occurs.

Precautions for Use

By Infants and Children: Use cautiously in small doses until tolerance is determined. Watch for any indications of weakness, light-headedness, or inclination to faint.

By Those Over 60 Years of Age: Small doses are indicated. Observe for nervousness, headache, tremor, rapid heart rate. If you have hardening of the arteries (arteriosclerosis), heart disease, high blood pressure, Parkinson's disease, or prostatism (see Glossary), this drug may aggravate your disorder. Ask your doctor for help.

▷ **Advisability of Use During Pregnancy**

Pregnancy Category: C. See Pregnancy Risk Categories at the back of this book.
Animal studies: Birth defects reported in rats.
Human studies: Adequate studies of pregnant women are not available.
This drug can cause significant reduction of oxygen supply to the fetus. Use it only if clearly needed and in small, infrequent doses. Avoid during the first 3 months and during labor and delivery.

Advisability of Use If Breast-Feeding

Presence of this drug in breast milk: Yes.
Avoid drug or refrain from nursing.

Habit-Forming Potential: Tolerance to this drug (see Glossary) can develop with frequent use, but dependence does not occur.

Effects of Overdosage: Nervousness, throbbing headache, dizziness, tremor, palpitation, disturbance of heart rhythm, difficult breathing, abdominal pain, vomiting of blood.

Possible Effects of Long-Term Use: "Epinephrine fastness": loss of ability to respond to this drug's bronchodilator effect. With long-term treatment of glaucoma: pigment deposits on eyeballs and eyelids, possible damage to retina, impaired vision, blockage of tear ducts.

Suggested Periodic Examinations While Taking This Drug (at physician's discretion)

Blood pressure measurements; blood or urine sugar measurements in diabetics; vision testing and measurement of internal eye pressure in glaucoma.

▷ **While Taking This Drug, Observe the Following**

Foods: No restrictions, except those that cause you to have asthma.
Beverages: No restrictions.
▷ *Alcohol:* Alcoholic beverages can increase the urinary excretion of this drug.
Tobacco Smoking: No interactions expected, but I advise everyone to quit smoking.

▷   *Other Drugs*
     Epinephrine *taken concurrently* with
     • some beta-blockers (carteolol, nadolol, propranolol) may cause increased
       blood pressure and decreased heart rate.
     • chlorpromazine (Thorazine) or other phenothiazines (see Drug Classes)
       may cause decreased blood pressure and increased heart rate.
     • furazolidone (Furoxone) may cause increased blood pressure.
     • guanethidine (Esimil, Ismelin) may cause increased blood pressure.
     • halothane may cause abnormal heartbeats.
     • pilocarpine (Ocusert) may cause increased myopia.
     • tricyclic antidepressants (amitriptyline, etc.) may cause increased blood
       pressure and heart rhythm disturbances.

▷   *Driving, Hazardous Activities:* This drug may cause dizziness or nervousness.
     Limit activities as necessary.
     Aviation Note: The use of this drug *may be a disqualification* for piloting. Con-
     sult a designated Aviation Medical Examiner.
     Exposure to Sun: No restrictions.
     Heavy Exercise or Exertion: No interactions expected. However, exercise can
     induce asthma in sensitive individuals.
     Occurrence of Unrelated Illness: Use caution in presence of severe burns. This
     drug can increase drainage from burned tissue and cause significant loss of
     tissue fluids and blood proteins.
     Discontinuation: If this drug fails to provide relief after an adequate trial, stop
     using it and call your doctor. It is dangerous to increase the dosage or fre-
     quency.
     Special Storage Instructions: Protect drug from exposure to air, light, and heat.
     Keep in a cool place, preferably in the refrigerator.

ERGOTAMINE (er GOT a meen)

Introduced: 1926   **Class:** Anti-migraine, ergot derivative   **Prescription:**
USA: Yes   **Controlled Drug:**   USA: No; Canada: No   **Available as Generic:**
No

Brand Names: ✦Bellergal [CD], Bellergal-S [CD], ✦Bellergal Spacetabs [CD],
     Cafergot [CD], Cafergot P-B [CD], Cafetrate [CD], Ercaf [CD], ✦Ergodryl
     [CD], Ergomar, Ergostat, Genergen, ✦Gravergol [CD], ✦Gynergen, Medi-
     haler Ergotamine, ✦Megral [CD], Oxoids, Spastrin [CD], Wigraine [CD],
     ✦Wigraine [CD]

BENEFITS versus RISKS	
Possible Benefits	*Possible Risks*
PREVENTION AND RELIEF OF VASCULAR HEADACHES: migraine, migrainelike, and histamine headaches	GANGRENE OF THE FINGERS, TOES, OR INTESTINE AGGRAVATION OF CORONARY ARTERY DISEASE (ANGINA) INCREASED RISK OF ABORTION (if used during pregnancy)

▷ **Principal Uses**
     As a Single Drug Product: Uses currently included in FDA-approved labeling:
     This drug is used to treat vascular headaches, especially migraine and

"cluster" headaches. It is often effective in stopping the headache if taken within the first hour following the onset of pain. It may be used on a short-term basis in an attempt to prevent or abort "cluster" headaches during the period of their occurrence. The inhalation form provides rapid onset of action.

Other (unlabeled) generally accepted uses: Helps to ease the symptoms of narcolepsy.

As a Combination Drug Product [CD]: This drug is combined with caffeine to take advantage of caffeine's ability to enhance its absorption. This makes a smaller dose of ergotamine effective, and reduces the risk of adverse effects with repeated use. This drug is also combined with belladonna (atropine) and one of the barbiturates to provide preparations that help premenstrual tension and the menopausal syndrome—nervousness, nausea, hot flushes, and sweating.

How This Drug Works: By constricting the walls of blood vessels in the head, this drug prevents or relieves the excessive expansion (dilation) that causes the pain of migrainelike headaches.

Available Dosage Forms and Strengths

Aerosol — 9 mg/ml (0.36 mg/inhalation)
Nasal inhaler (Canada) — 9 mg/ml (360 mcg/dose)
Suppositories — 2 mg (in combination with 100 mg of caffeine)
Tablets, sublingual — 2 mg

▷ **Usual Adult Dosage Range:** Inhalation: One spray (0.36 mg) at the onset of headache; repeat one spray after 30 to 60 minutes as needed for relief, up to a maximum of 6 sprays every 24 hours. Do not exceed 15 sprays per week. Sublingual tablets: Dissolve 2 mg under tongue at the onset of headache; repeat 2 mg in 30 to 60 minutes as needed, up to a maximum of 6 mg per attack. Do not exceed 6 mg every 24 hours or 10 mg/week. **Note: Actual dosage and administration schedule must be determined for each patient individually.**

Conditions Requiring Dosing Adjustments

Liver Function: Should be used with caution by patients with liver compromise.
Kidney Function: This drug is a rare cause of acute renal failure, and should be used with caution by patients with compromised kidneys.

▷ **Dosing Instructions:** Follow written instructions and doses **carefully**. The regular tablets (combination drug) may be crushed for administration; the sustained-release tablets should be taken whole (not crushed). Sublingual tablets should be dissolved under the tongue, not swallowed.

Usual Duration of Use: Use on a regular schedule for several episodes of headache is often needed to see this drug's effectiveness in aborting or relieving the pain of vascular headache. Do not exceed recommended dosage schedules. If headaches are not controlled after several trials of maximal doses, ask your doctor about other treatments.

▷ **This Drug Should Not Be Taken If**
- you have had an allergic reaction to any dosage form.
- you are pregnant.
- you have a severe infection.
- you have any of the following conditions:
    angina pectoris (coronary artery disease)

Buerger's disease
hardening of the arteries (arteriosclerosis)
high blood pressure (severe hypertension)
ischemic heart disease
peptic ulcer
kidney disease or impaired kidney function
liver disease or impaired liver function
Raynaud's phenomenon
thrombophlebitis
severe itching

▷ **Inform Your Physician Before Taking This Drug If**
- you are allergic or overly sensitive to *any* ergot preparation.
- you are planning to have a face-lift (rhytidectomy). This drug may cause serious skin flap problems.

Possible Side Effects (natural, expected, and unavoidable drug actions)
Usually infrequent and mild with recommended doses.
Some people may have cold hands and feet, with mild numbness and tingling.

▷ **Possible Adverse Effects** (unusual, unexpected, and infrequent reactions)
If any of the following develop, consult your physician promptly for guidance.
Mild Adverse Effects
Allergic Reactions: Localized swellings (angioedema), itching—case reports.
Headache, drowsiness, dizziness, confusion—possible.
Chest pain, abdominal pain, numbness and tingling of fingers and toes, muscle pains in arms or legs—infrequent.
Nausea, vomiting, diarrhea—possible.
Serious Adverse Effects
Gangrene of the extremities: coldness; numbness; pain; dark discoloration; eventual loss of fingers, toes, or feet—possible.
Gangrene of the intestine: severe abdominal pain and swelling; emergency surgery required—case reports.
Retroperitoneal fibrosis—case reports.
Fibrous changes in the lung (pleuropulmonary fibrosis)—case reports.
Pain syndromes (reflex sympathetic dystrophy)—possible.
Insufficient blood flow to the heart (myocardial ischemia) or arrhythmias—case reports.
Fibrous changes in the heart (myocardial fibrosis) or porphyria—case reports.
Lesions of the rectum or anus (anorectal lesions)—case reports.
Kidney failure—case reports.

▷ **Possible Effects on Sexual Function:**   None reported.

Natural Diseases or Disorders That May Be Activated by This Drug
Angina pectoris (coronary artery insufficiency), Buerger's disease, Raynaud's phenomenon.

Possible Effects on Laboratory Tests
None reported.

CAUTION
1. Excessive use of this drug can provoke migraine headache and increase the frequency of its occurrence.
2. Do not exceed a total dose of 6 mg daily or 10 mg/week of the oral form.
3. Individual drug sensitivity varies greatly. Some may have early toxic effects while taking recommended doses. Promptly report numbness in fingers or toes, muscle cramping, chest pain.

Precautions for Use
By Infants and Children: Safety and effectiveness for those under 12 years of age are not established.
By Those Over 60 Years of Age: Natural circulation changes may make you more susceptible to adverse effects of this drug. See the preceding list of disorders that are contraindications for the use of this drug.

▷ **Advisability of Use During Pregnancy**
Pregnancy Category: X. See Pregnancy Risk Categories at the back of this book.
Animal studies: Fetal deaths reported due to this drug.
Human studies: Information from studies of pregnant women indicates that this drug can cause abortion.
This drug should be avoided during the entire pregnancy.

Advisability of Use If Breast-Feeding
Presence of this drug in breast milk: Yes.
Avoid drug or refrain from nursing.

Habit-Forming Potential: None.

Effects of Overdosage: Manifestations of "ergotism": coldness of skin, severe muscle pains, tingling and burning pain in hands and feet, loss of blood supply to extremities resulting in tissue death (gangrene) in fingers and toes. Acute ergot poisoning: nausea, vomiting, diarrhea, cold skin, numbness of extremities, confusion, seizures, coma.

Possible Effects of Long-Term Use: A form of functional dependence (see Glossary) may develop, resulting in withdrawal headaches when the drug is discontinued.

Suggested Periodic Examinations While Taking This Drug (at physician's discretion)
Evaluation of circulation (blood flow) to the extremities.

▷ **While Taking This Drug, Observe the Following**
Foods: No interactions expected. Avoid all foods to which you are allergic; some migraine headaches are due to food allergies.
Beverages: No restrictions.
▷   *Alcohol:* Best avoided; alcohol can intensify vascular headache.
Tobacco Smoking: Best avoided; nicotine can further reduce the restricted blood flow produced by this drug.
Marijuana Smoking: Best avoided; additive effects can increase the coldness of hands and feet.
▷   *Other Drugs*
Ergotamine may *decrease* the effects of
- nitroglycerin, and reduce its effectiveness in preventing or relieving angina pain.

The following drugs may *increase* the effects of ergotamine
- beta-blockers (see Drug Classes).
- dopamine (Intropin).
- erythromycins: clarithromycin (Biaxin), dirithromycin (Dynabac), or E-Mycin, ERYC, etc. Azithromycin (Zithromax) has not been reported to cause this effect.
- sumatriptan (Imitrex) can also result in extended vasospastic reactions.
- troleandomycin (TAO).

▷ *Driving, Hazardous Activities:* This drug may cause drowsiness or dizziness. Restrict activities as necessary.

Aviation Note: Vascular headache *is a disqualification* for piloting. Consult a designated Aviation Medical Examiner.

Exposure to Sun: No restrictions.

Exposure to Cold: Avoid as much as possible. Cold further reduces restricted blood flow to the extremities.

Discontinuation: Following long-term use, it may be necessary to withdraw this drug gradually to prevent withdrawal headache. Ask your physician for guidance.

ERYTHROMYCIN (er ith roh MY sin)

See the new macrolide antibiotics profile for more information.

ESTROGENS (ES troh jenz)

Other Names: Chlorotrianisene, conjugated estrogens, esterified estrogens, estradiol, estriol, estrone, estropipate, quinestrol

Introduced: 1933   **Class:** Female sex hormones   **Prescription:** USA: Yes   **Controlled Drug:** USA: No; Canada: No   **Available as Generic:** USA: Yes; Canada: No

Brand Names: ✦C.E.S., ✦Climestrone, ✦Congest, Delestrogen, DV, Estinyl, Estrace, Estraderm, Estraguard, Estratab, Estrovis, Feminone, ✦Femogen, ✦Femogex, Gynetone, Gynogen LA, Menest, Menotab, Menotab-M, Menrium [CD], Milprem [CD], ✦Minestrin, ✦Neo-Pause, ✦Oestrilin, Ogen, PMB [CD], PMS-Estradiol, Premarin, Premphase, Prempro (a single-tablet form with conjugated estrogens and medroxyprogesterone has been FDA approved), Progynon Pellet, TACE, Valergen-10, Vivelle (transdermal), White Premarin
   Author's Note: A generic form (from Duramed) of Premarin is being contended by the FDA regarding bioequivalence.

BENEFITS versus RISKS

Possible Benefits	*Possible Risks*
RELIEF OF MENOPAUSAL HOT FLASHES AND NIGHT SWEATS	INCREASED RISK OF CANCER OF THE UTERUS with 3 years of continual use
PREVENTION OR RELIEF OF ATROPHIC VAGINITIS, ATROPHY OF THE VULVA AND URETHRA	INCREASED RISK OF BREAST CANCER (EVEN IF COMBINED WITH A PROGESTERONE)
PREVENTION OF POSTMENOPAUSAL OSTEOPOROSIS	Increased frequency of gallstones
	Accelerated growth of preexisting fibroid tumors of the uterus
EARLY DATA APPEARS TO SHOW A BENEFIT IN PREVENTING ALZHEIMER'S	Fluid retention
Prevention of thinning of the skin	Postmenopausal bleeding
Mental tonic effect	Deep vein thrombophlebitis and thromboembolism (less likely with
Prevention of postmenopausal cardiovascular disease	conjugated estrogens, more likely with synthetic unconjugated hormones)
	Increased blood pressure
	Decreased sugar tolerance

▷ **Principal Uses**

As a Single Drug Product: This widely used hormone is very effective when administered in proper dosage and carefully supervised. Its primary use is "replacement" therapy in: (1) ovarian failure or removal; (2) the menopausal syndrome; (3) postmenopausal atrophy of genital tissues; (4) postmenopausal osteoporosis; (5) also used in selected cases of breast cancer and prostate cancer.

As a Combination Drug Product [CD]: Estrogen is available in combination with chlordiazepoxide (Librium) and with meprobamate (Equanil, Miltown). These mild tranquilizers are added to provide a calming effect that makes the combination more effective in treating selected cases of the menopausal syndrome. See the Profile for oral contraceptives for a discussion of the combination of estrogens and progestins.

How This Drug Works: When used to correct hormonal deficiency states, estrogens restore normal cellular activity by increasing nuclear material and protein synthesis. The frequency and intensity of menopausal symptoms are reduced when normal tissue levels of estrogen are restored.

Available Dosage Forms and Strengths

Capsules — 12 mg, 25 mg, 72 mg (TACE)

Tablets — 0.02 mg, 0.05 mg, 0.1 mg, 0.3 mg, 0.5 mg, 0.625 mg, — 0.9 mg, 1.25 mg, 2.5 mg

Transdermal patch — 0.025 mg (2 mg), 0.05 mg (4 mg), 0.1 mg (8 mg) — 2 mg (only in Canada)

Vaginal cream — 0.1, 0.625, and 1.5 mg/g

▷ **Usual Adult Dosage Range:** For conjugated and esterified estrogens: 0.3 to 1.25 mg daily for 21 days. Omit for 7 days. Repeat cyclically as needed. Progestin is typically added during the final 10 days in order to avoid effects of estrogen alone (unopposed) on the endometrium. For other forms of estrogen:

consult your physician. **Note: Actual dosage and administration schedule must be determined for each patient individually.**

Conditions Requiring Dosing Adjustments

Liver Function: The dose should be decreased in mild liver disease. Estrogens should not be used in acute or severe liver compromise. This drug can be lithogenic (capable of causing stones) in the bile.

Kidney Function: No expected dosing changes in kidney compromise.

▷ **Dosing Instructions:**   The tablets may be crushed and taken without regard to food. The capsules should be taken whole.

Usual Duration of Use: Use on a regular schedule for 10 to 20 days is needed to see this drug's effectiveness in menopausal symptoms. Long-term use requires supervision and periodic evaluation by your physician every 6 months.

▷ **This Drug Should Not Be Taken If**
- you have had an allergic reaction to any form of it previously.
- you have a history of thrombophlebitis, embolism, heart attack, or stroke.
- you have seriously impaired liver function or recent onset of liver disease.
- you have abnormal and unexplained vaginal bleeding.
- you have sickle cell disease.
- you have or are suspected to have breast cancer (may be used to treat some kinds of breast cancer).
- your have known or suspected estrogen-dependent cancer (your doctor would determine this).
- you are pregnant.

▷ **Inform Your Physician Before Taking This Drug If**
- you have had an unfavorable reaction to estrogen therapy previously.
- you have a history of cancer of the breast or reproductive organs.
- you have: fibrocystic breast changes, fibroid tumors of the uterus, endometriosis, migrainelike headaches, epilepsy, asthma, heart disease, high blood pressure, gallbladder disease, diabetes, or porphyria.
- you smoke tobacco on a regular basis.
- you have a history of blood-clotting disorders.
- you plan to have surgery in the near future.

Possible Side Effects (natural, expected, and unavoidable drug actions)

Fluid retention, weight gain, "breakthrough" bleeding (spotting in middle of menstrual cycle), altered menstrual pattern, resumption of menstrual flow (bleeding from the uterus) after a period of natural cessation (postmenopausal bleeding), increased susceptibility to yeast infection of the genital tissues.

▷ **Possible Adverse Effects** (unusual, unexpected, and infrequent reactions)

If any of the following develop, consult your physician promptly for guidance.

Mild Adverse Effects

Allergic Reactions: Skin rash, hives, itching—rare.

Headache, nervous tension, irritability, depression, accentuation of migraine headaches—infrequent.

Nausea, vomiting, bloating, diarrhea—infrequent to frequent.

Tannish pigmentation of the face—possible.

Serious Adverse Effects

Allergic Reactions: Anaphylaxis—case reports.

Idiosyncratic Reaction: Cutaneous porphyria—fragility and scarring of the skin.

Can produce or worsen high blood pressure—more likely with higher doses.

Gallbladder disease, benign liver tumors, jaundice, rise in blood sugar—case reports.

Erosion of uterine cervix, enlargement of uterine fibroid tumors—possible.

Thrombophlebitis (inflammation of a vein with formation of blood clot): pain or tenderness in thigh or leg, with or without swelling of foot or leg—low dose has minimal increased risk; higher doses may carry more risk.

Pulmonary embolism (movement of blood clot to lung): sudden shortness of breath, pain in chest, coughing, bloody sputum—case reports.

Benign liver tumors (adenomas)—possible.

Systemic lupus erythematosus or porphyria—rare.

Stroke (blood clot in brain): headaches, blackout, sudden weakness or paralysis of any part of the body, severe dizziness, altered vision, slurred speech, inability to speak—case reports.

Endometrial cancer (how long increased risk continues if the drug is stopped is not clear).

Retinal thrombosis (blood clot in eye vessels): sudden impairment or loss of vision—case reports.

Heart attack (blood clot in coronary artery)—sudden pain in chest, neck, jaw, or arm; weakness; sweating; nausea. Has been associated with women taking higher doses and with men using estrogen to treat prostate cancer; however, this is not clearly decided as yet. Estrogen in lower doses appears to decrease overall risk of heart attack.

Increased risk of breast cancer, even if combined with a progesterone (with long-term use—9 years).

Conjugated estrogens were not associated with increased overall relative risk of breast cancer in one large study.

▷ **Possible Effects on Sexual Function:** Swelling and tenderness of breasts, milk production.

Increased vaginal secretions.

Possible Delayed Adverse Effects: Estrogens taken during pregnancy can predispose the female child to the later development of cancer of the vagina or cervix following puberty.

▷ **Adverse Effects That May Mimic Natural Diseases or Disorders**

Liver reactions may suggest viral hepatitis.

Natural Diseases or Disorders That May Be Activated by This Drug

Latent hypertension, diabetes mellitus, acute intermittent porphyria.

Possible Effects on Laboratory Tests

Red blood cells, hemoglobin, and platelets: decreased.

Blood calcium level: increased.

Blood total cholesterol level: decreased (treatment effect); increased in postmenopausal women.

Blood LDL cholesterol level: decreased in postmenopausal women.

Blood triglyceride level: no drug effect in postmenopausal women.

Blood glucose level: increased.

Glucose tolerance test (GTT): decreased.

Blood thyroid hormone (T_3 and T_4) levels: increased.

Blood uric acid level: decreased.

Liver function tests: increased liver enzymes (ALT/GPT, AST/GOT, and alkaline phosphatase), increased bilirubin.

CAUTION

1. To avoid prolonged (uninterrupted) stimulation of breast and uterine tissues, estrogen should be taken in cycles of 3 weeks on and 1 week off of medication.
2. The estrogen in estrogen vaginal creams is absorbed systemically. It may also be absorbed through the penis during sexual intercourse and can cause enlargement and tenderness of male breast tissue.

Precautions for Use

By Those Over 60 Years of Age: Very limited usefulness after 60. Restricted to women who are at increased risk for osteoporosis. In this age group, it is advisable to attempt relief of hot flushes with nonestrogenic medications. During use, report promptly any indications of impaired circulation: speech disturbances, altered vision, sudden hearing loss, vertigo, sudden weakness or paralysis, angina, leg pains.

▷ **Advisability of Use During Pregnancy**

Pregnancy Category: X. See Pregnancy Risk Categories at the back of this book.

Animal studies: Genital defects reported in mice and guinea pigs; cleft palate reported in rodents.

Human studies: Information from studies of pregnant women indicates that estrogens can masculinize the female fetus. In addition, limb defects and heart malformations have been reported.

It is now known that estrogens taken during pregnancy can predispose the female child to the development of cancer of the vagina or cervix following puberty. *Avoid estrogens completely during entire pregnancy.*

Advisability of Use If Breast-Feeding

Presence of this drug in breast milk: Yes, in minute amounts.

Estrogens in large doses can suppress milk formation.

Breast-feeding is considered to be safe during the use of estrogens.

Malnourished mothers may have unacceptable decreases in protein and nitrogen in their breast milk if this drug is used while breast-feeding.

Habit-Forming Potential: There has been some suggestion of estrogens having potential for psychological dependence and tolerance because of their mood-elevating properties, but clinical reports have not been presented.

Effects of Overdosage: Headache, drowsiness, nausea, vomiting, fluid retention, abnormal vaginal bleeding, breast enlargement and discomfort.

Possible Effects of Long-Term Use: High blood pressure, gallbladder disease with gallstone formation, increased growth of benign fibroid tumors of the uterus. Several reports suggest possible association between the long-term use (3+ years) of estrogens and the development of cancer of the lining of the uterus. Further studies are needed to establish a definite cause-and-effect relationship (see Glossary). Prudence dictates that women with intact uteri should use estrogens only when symptoms justify it and with proper supervision.

Suggested Periodic Examinations While Taking This Drug (at physician's discretion)

Regular (every 6 months) evaluation of the breasts and pelvic organs, including Pap smears.

Liver function tests as indicated.

▷ **While Taking This Drug, Observe the Following**

Foods: Avoid excessive use of salt if fluid retention occurs. Combined use of calcium can be a further step to help avoid osteoporosis.

Beverages: No restrictions. May be taken with milk.

▷ *Alcohol:* No interactions expected.

Tobacco Smoking: Recent studies indicate that heavy smoking (15 or more cigarettes daily) in association with the use of estrogen-containing oral contraceptives significantly increases the risk of heart attack (coronary thrombosis). I advise everyone to stop smoking.

▷ *Other Drugs*

Estrogens *taken concurrently* with

- alendronate (Fosamax) have not been studied.
- antidiabetic drugs may cause unpredictable fluctuations of blood sugar.
- oral antidiabetic drugs (see Drug Classes) or oral blood-sugar-lowering medicines may cause loss of glucose control and high blood sugars.
- thyroid hormones may increase the bound (inactive) drug and require an increase in thyroid dose.
- tricyclic antidepressants (Elavil, Sinequan, etc.) may enhance their adverse effects and reduce their antidepressant effectiveness.
- vitamin C (ascorbic acid, various brands) in higher doses may result in increased estrogen effects. A lower dose of estrogens may be indicated if higher-dose vitamin C will be taken on an ongoing basis.
- warfarin (Coumadin) may cause alterations of prothrombin activity. Increased doses may be needed.

The following drugs may *decrease* the effects of estrogens

- carbamazepine (Tegretol).
- phenobarbital (Belladenal, others).
- phenytoin (Dilantin).
- primidone (Mysoline).
- rifampin (Rifadin, Rimactane).

▷ *Driving, Hazardous Activities:* Usually no restrictions. Consult your physician for assessment of individual risk and for guidance regarding specific restrictions.

Aviation Note: Usually no restrictions. However, watch for the rare occurrence of disturbed vision and restrict activities accordingly. Consult a designated Aviation Medical Examiner.

Exposure to Sun: Use caution—these drugs can cause photosensitivity (see Glossary).

Discontinuation: Best to stop estrogens periodically to see if they are still needed. The dose is reduced gradually to prevent acute withdrawal hot flushes. Avoid continual, uninterrupted use of large doses. Stop altogether when a definite need for replacement therapy has ended. Ask your doctor for help.

ETHAMBUTOL (eth AM byu tohl)

Introduced: 1971   **Class:** Anti-infective, antituberculosis drug   **Prescription:** USA: Yes   **Controlled Drug:** USA: No; Canada: No   **Available as Generic:** USA: No; Canada: No

Brand Names: ✦Etibi, Myambutol

BENEFITS versus RISKS	
Possible Benefits	*Possible Risks*
EFFECTIVE ADJUNCTIVE TREATMENT OF PULMONARY TUBERCULOSIS	RARE OPTIC NEURITIS WITH IMPAIRMENT OR LOSS OF VISION
EFFECTIVE ADJUNCTIVE TREATMENT OF AIDS-RELATED *MYCOBACTERIUM AVIUM-INTRACELLULARE* COMPLEX INFECTIONS	Rare peripheral neuritis (see Glossary) Activation of gout
Possibly effective treatment of tuberculous meningitis	

▷ **Principal Uses**

As a Single Drug Product: Uses currently included in FDA-approved labeling: Treatment of pulmonary tuberculosis, in combination with other antitubercular drugs (currently three other medicines are added to ethambutol).

Other (unlabeled) generally accepted uses: (1) Treatment of tuberculous meningitis; (2) treatment of AIDS-related *Mycobacterium avium-intracellulare* (MAI) *complex* infections, in combination with other anti-mycobacterial drugs.

How This Drug Works: It enters mycobacterial cells that are actively dividing, and keeps them from reproducing by interfering with nuclear material (RNA).

Available Dosage Forms and Strengths

Tablets — 100 mg, 400 mg

▷ **Recommended Dosage Ranges** (Actual dosage and administration schedule must be determined for each patient individually.)

Infants and Children: Dosage not established. Some authorities recommend that children under 6 years of age not be given this drug.

13 to 60 Years of Age: For initial treatment of tuberculosis—15 mg per kg of body mass, once daily. The total daily dose should not exceed 500–1500 mg.

For retreatment of tuberculosis—25 mg per kg of body mass, once daily for 60 days; then 15 mg per kg of body mass. The total daily dose should not exceed 900–2500 mg.

For tuberculous meningitis or AIDS-related MAI infections—15 to 25 mg per kg of body mass, once daily.

Over 60 Years of Age: Same as 13 to 60 years of age.

Conditions Requiring Dosing Adjustments

Liver Function: No dose decreases are anticipated in mild to moderate liver compromise.

Kidney Function: For mild to moderate kidney failure, the usual dose can be given every 24–36 hours. Severe kidney failure only requires a dose every 48 hours.

▷ **Dosing Instructions:** The tablet may be crushed and taken with food to reduce stomach irritation. Take full course prescribed.

Usual Duration of Use: Use on a regular schedule for 4 to 6 weeks is necessary to determine this drug's effectiveness in controlling infections. Long-term use (6 months to 2 or more years) requires periodic physician evaluation.

▷ **This Drug Should Not Be Taken If**
- you have had an allergic reaction to it previously.
- you currently have optic neuritis or peripheral neuritis.
- you currently have active gout.

▷ **Inform Your Physician Before Taking This Drug If**
- you have a history of gout.
- you have a history of optic neuritis or peripheral neuritis.
- you have diabetes or a history of alcoholism; these conditions predispose to eye problems (optic neuritis).
- you have impaired kidney function.
- you have a history of low blood platelets.

Possible Side Effects (natural, expected, and unavoidable drug actions)
Increased blood level of uric acid (50–66% of users).

▷ **Possible Adverse Effects** (unusual, unexpected, and infrequent reactions)
If any of the following develop, consult your physician promptly for guidance.
Mild Adverse Effects
Allergic Reactions: Skin rash, itching, fever.
Headache, confusion, disorientation—case reports to infrequent.
Loss of appetite, nausea, vomiting, stomach pain—possible.
Serious Adverse Effects
Allergic Reactions: Severe skin reactions, painful joints.
Optic neuritis (one or both eyes): eye pain, blurred vision, red–green color blindness—case reports.
Peripheral neuritis (see Glossary): numbness, tingling, burning, pain, and/or weakness in hands or feet.
Low blood platelets or white blood cells—case reports.
Hallucinations—possible.
Porphyria or kidney problems (interstitial nephritis)—rare.
Gouty arthritis—possible.

▷ **Possible Effects on Sexual Function:** None reported.

Possible Delayed Adverse Effects: Optic neuritis may not happen until many months of therapy. Visual loss may continue for up to a year after stopping this drug, and may be permanent.

Natural Diseases or Disorders That May Be Activated by This Drug
Latent gout.

Possible Effects on Laboratory Tests
Complete blood cell counts: decreased white cells and platelets.
Blood uric acid levels: increased.
Liver function tests: increased liver enzymes (ALT/GPT, AST/GOT).

Kidney function tests: increased blood urea nitrogen (BUN) and creatinine (rare kidney damage).

CAUTION
1. Promptly report any vision changes; this could be the start of optic neuritis. Immediate evaluation is mandatory.
2. Report promptly any unusual sensations in the hands or feet; these could indicate the onset of peripheral neuritis.

Precautions for Use

By Infants and Children: Safety and effectiveness for those under 13 years of age not established.

By Those Over 60 Years of Age: Confusion or disorientation more likely. Age-related decrease in kidney function may require decreased doses.

▷ **Advisability of Use During Pregnancy**

Pregnancy Category: B. See Pregnancy Risk Categories at the back of this book.

Animal studies: Mouse and rabbit studies confirm multiple drug-induced birth defects.

Human studies: Adequate studies of pregnant women are not available.

Use this drug only if clearly needed. Ask your physician for guidance.

Advisability of Use If Breast-Feeding

Presence of this drug in breast milk: Yes.

Avoid drug or refrain from nursing.

Habit-Forming Potential: None.

Effects of Overdosage: Nausea, vomiting, stomach discomfort, confusion, possible blurred vision.

Possible Effects of Long-Term Use: Optic neuritis with significant visual impairment.

Suggested Periodic Examinations While Taking This Drug (at physician's discretion)

Complete eye examinations (including visual fields and color vision) should be performed before treatment is started and monthly during therapy.

Blood uric acid levels.

Liver and kidney function tests.

▷ **While Taking This Drug, Observe the Following**

Foods: Follow your physician's advice regarding high-purine foods.

Beverages: Avoid excessive caffeine-containing beverages such as coffee or some sodas.

▷ *Alcohol:* No interactions expected.

Tobacco Smoking: No interactions expected, but I advise everyone to stop smoking.

▷ *Other Drugs*

The following drugs may *decrease* the effects of ethambutol
- antacids containing aluminum salts can slow and reduce absorption.

Ethambutol *taken concurrently* with
- BCG vaccine may blunt the immune response that can be given by the vaccine.

▷ *Driving, Hazardous Activities:* This drug may cause confusion, disorientation, and impaired vision. Restrict activities as necessary.

Aviation Note: The use of this drug *is a disqualification* for piloting. Consult a designated Aviation Medical Examiner.

Exposure to Sun: No restrictions.

Discontinuation: This drug is generally used for long-term treatment—months to years. Ask your doctor about the appropriate time to stop this medicine.

ETHANOL (ETH an all)

Other Names: Prescription: None
   Nonprescription: Moonshine, alcohol, jack, white lightning, wine, beer, whiskey, vodka, others

Introduced: 1980 (prescription); 6,000 years ago (nonprescription—Babylonian beer)   **Class:** Antianxiety drug (nonprescription form)   **Prescription:** USA: Yes (IV)   **Controlled Drug:** USA: No; Canada: Yes (IV)   **Available as Generic:** USA: Yes; Canada: Yes

Brand Names: Prescription: Tuss-Ornade (5%), Vicks Formula 44D, Temaril (5.7%), Nyquil Nightime Cold Medicine, Novahistine DMX Liquid, Eskaphen B, ✦Dilusol (38.7%), Nonprescription: Robert Alison Chardonnay (12% by volume), Bud Dry, Glenlivet, Smirnoff (40% by volume), others

Warning: The clinical use of this medication is limited to intravenous treatment of methanol and antifreeze (ethylene glycol) poisoning, and as a preservative. There are a huge number of products containing alcohol. Ask your pharmacist for help with ingredients if alcohol is forbidden for you. Past use has included treatment of premature labor (tocolytic).

This drug is widely used in its nonprescription form as an antianxiety agent. Recent data appear to show this as a benefit of moderate use—however, there are some data regarding increased cancer risks. Some people may not experience any mental or physical changes even though a breath or blood alcohol test shows they are "legally drunk."

BENEFITS versus RISKS	
Possible Benefits	*Possible Risks*
EFFECTIVE TREATMENT OF POISONING	WITHDRAWAL SYMPTOMS
	SEIZURES
MODERATE use may decrease heart disease/heart attack risk	LIVER DAMAGE (with prolonged use)
	Possible increased cancer risk
	Pancreatitis
	Encephalopathy
	Low white blood cell counts and anemia
	Myopathy

▷ **Principal Uses**

As a Single Drug Product: Uses currently included in FDA-approved labeling: Supplementation of caloric intake intravenously in very specific cases.

   Other (unlabeled) generally accepted uses: (1) Treatment of methanol or antifreeze (ethylene glycol) poisoning; (2) adjunctive treatment of cancer pain; (3) intravenous treatment of DTs (delirium tremens); (4) used to sclerose esophageal varices and stop bleeding; (5) treatment of hepatocellular cancer where severe liver problems preclude surgery; (6) used to sclerose thyroid cysts; (7) used to destroy nerve tissue (neurolytic block) in chronic pain therapy; (8) widely used in nonprescription form as an antianxiety agent; (9) recent data appear to show that use ranging up to moderate (and NO GREATER than 0.7 mg per kg of body mass for 3 days in a row) may actually help prevent coronary heart disease and heart attacks.

As a Combination Drug Product [CD]: Uses currently included in FDA-approved labeling: Widely present in elixirs and other liquid vehicles for drugs as a preservative, and partial drug action enhancer.

How This Drug Works: In antifreeze (ethylene glycol) or methanol poisoning, ethanol prevents the ethylene glycol from being oxidized or prevents methanol from being changed (metabolized) into toxic chemicals, and lets the body remove the antifreeze or methanol harmlessly. When used in its nonprescription form in excess, it depresses nerve function and leads to emotional changes and disturbances of perception, coordination, and intoxication.

Nonprescription use of up to moderate amounts appears to decrease risk of heart and blood vessel disease, but the way in which it does this is not known.

Available Dosage Forms and Strengths
  Intravenous: — 5%, 10%, 95%
  Nonprescription: — Each ounce of 100-proof whiskey has 15 ml of ethanol
         — 6 ounces (12%) wine has 22 ml of ethanol
         — 12 ounces of beer (4.9%) has 18 ml of ethanol

▷ **Recommended Dosage Ranges** (Actual dosage and administration schedule must be determined for each patient individually.)

Infants and Children: Methanol or ethylene glycol poisoning: 40 ml per kg of body mass per day.

18 to 60 Years of Age: Methanol or ethylene glycol poisoning: A loading dose of 0.6 mg per kg of body mass is given, and followed by 109 to 125 mg per kg of body mass per hour to maintain a blood level of 100 mg/dl.

Coronary heart disease or heart attack prevention: It APPEARS THAT use of moderate amounts (up to 0.8 g per kg of body mass per day or no more than 0.7 mg per kg of body mass per day for 3 days in a row) of alcohol may help in preventing risk of this kind of blood vessel disease and myocardial infarctions.

Over 60 Years of Age: Same as 12 to 60 years of age for poisonings. The amount consumed versus the collective mental and physical effects may decrease in older people for the nonprescription products. It will generally take less of a dose to cause an equal or greater change in coordination or mental ability. There is also an increased risk of hypothermia.

Conditions Requiring Dosing Adjustments

Liver Function: Ethanol is extensively metabolized in the liver to acetaldehyde and acetyl Co-A. The drug is also a clear cause of liver toxicity. The dose must be decreased in liver compromise.

Kidney Function: Minimal involvement of the kidney in the elimination of this drug.

▷ **Dosing Instructions:**   If methanol or ethylene glycol poisoning is suspected— the nearest poison control center should be contacted, and oral dosing (use of a strong vodka mixed in orange juice) may be of benefit, depending on your distance from a hospital or freestanding emergency center.

For nonprescription antianxiety use, the specific dose of this drug and the resulting blood level of alcohol depends on many factors; however, the more important ones are the weight of the person, the metabolic activity of the liver, food content in the stomach, the strength of the alcohol in the consumed beverage, the number of "drinks" consumed over a given period of time, and how well hydrated (whether there has been extreme exercise and fluid loss) you are. Again, although a blood or breath alcohol test may be a marker for mental or physical changes, some people may not have physical or mental changes and have a blood or breath alcohol level that is in the state-defined range that constitutes being "legally drunk." Specific levels of blood or breath alcohol do not absolutely predict impairment.

Each 10 ml of ethanol increases the blood ethanol level of an average 150-lb (70-kg) man by 16.6 mg percent (3.6 mmol/L). The legal definition of intoxication is a blood alcohol level of 0.10% or 100 mg/dl. "Under the influence" in Maryland is .07% or 70 mg/dL. Driving impairment **may** occur at blood levels of 0.05% (50 mg/dl) or lower.

Usual Duration of Use: Use on a regular schedule for 48 hours determines effectiveness in methanol overdose. Long-term excessive use as an antianxiety agent is NOT recommended.

▷ **This Drug Should Not Be Taken If**
- you have had an allergic reaction to any dosage form of it previously.
- you have epilepsy.
- you have a history of alcohol addiction.
- you have a urinary tract infection.
- you are pregnant.
- you are in diabetic coma.

▷ **Inform Your Physician Before Taking This Drug If**
- you have liver or kidney compromise.
- you have gout.
- you are prone to low blood sugars.
- you are a diabetic.
- you have congestive heart failure.

Possible Side Effects (natural, expected, and unavoidable drug actions)
Intoxication, perception, coordination, and mood changes.

▷ **Possible Adverse Effects** (unusual, unexpected, and infrequent reactions)
If any of the following develop, consult your physician promptly for guidance.

Mild Adverse Effects
Allergic Reactions: Itching, rash, hives, and flushing.
Headache, "hangover:" nausea, headache, malaise—dose related.
Sedation—dose dependent.
Disorientation, memory loss—dose dependent.
Color blindness or neuropathy (tingling, burning, or numbness)—with chronic use.
Vitamin deficiency or muscle changes (myopathy)—with chronic use.
Stomach irritation—frequent.

Serious Adverse Effects
Allergic Reactions: Anaphylaxis: rash, swelling of tongue, breathing problems, flushing—case reports.

Bronchospasm (asthmatics at increased risk)—case reports.
Respiratory depression—dose related.
Elevated or decreased white blood cell count—possible.
Increased or decreased platelets—case reports.
Heart dysfunction (myopathy) or anemia (megaloblastic)—with chronic use.
High blood pressure—possible to frequent.
Abnormal heart rhythms (atrial and ventricular) or chest pain (angina)—increased risk.
Liver toxicity—cirrhosis with chronic use possible.
Osteoporosis—increased risk with chronic use.
Pancreatitis—increased risk with chronic higher-dose use.
Encephalopathy or cerebrovascular bleeding—increased risk with higher-dose chronic use.
Low blood sugar or ketoacidosis—especially if meals are missed or with chronic use.
Vitamin deficiency (folic acid, vitamins B_1 and B_6) or low magnesium—with chronic use.
Low potassium (especially with acute intoxication in children)—possible.
Gout (precipitated by alcohol use in those with gout)—possible.
Tolerance (with chronic use)—possible.
Withdrawal: nausea, fever, rapid heart rate, hallucinations. May progress to delirium tremens (5%): profound confusion, hallucinations, etc.—possible.

▷ **Possible Effects on Sexual Function:**   Decreased libido, impotence (with excessive chronic use). Difficulty achieving an erection in males and decreased vaginal dilation in females. Chronic alcohol use may lead to tenderness and swelling of male and female breast tissue, testicular atrophy, low sperm counts, decreased menstrual blood flow, and diminished capability for orgasm in females.

Possible Delayed Adverse Effects: Liver toxicity, anemia, low or high platelets, vitamin deficiency.

▷ **Adverse Effects That May Mimic Natural Diseases or Disorders**
Alcoholic cirrhosis may mimic hepatitis.

Natural Diseases or Disorders That May Be Activated by This Drug
Peptic ulcer disease.

Possible Effects on Laboratory Tests
Liver function tests: elevated ALT.
Complete blood count: decreased white blood cells, decreased hemoglobin, increased or decreased platelets.
Amylase: elevated.
Sperm count: decreased with chronic use.
Magnesium: decreased with chronic use.

CAUTION
1. This drug in its nonprescription form may cause fatal increases in blood pressure if combined with cocaine.
2. With high doses (nearly pure "grain" alcohol) or many drinks (frequent dosing) over a short period of time, fatal blood alcohol levels may be reached with the nonprescription form.

Precautions for Use

By Infants and Children: Safety and effectiveness for those under 12 years of age not established. Accidental and unsupervised drinking of the nonprescription form may result in severe consequences in children. Seriously low blood sugar may happen and be delayed up to 6 hours after drinking. Low potassium may also occur with high ethanol levels. Therapy is guided by blood sugar, potassium, and blood alcohol (ethanol) levels. Fatality caused by low blood sugar was reported in a 4-year-old child who drank 12 ounces of a mouthwash that contained 10% ethanol.

By Those Over 60 Years of Age: Poisoning with methanol or ethylene glycol is an emergency situation, and while there may be an increased sensitivity to effects, dosing is adjusted to blood levels. The nonprescription form dosing (number of drinks) tolerated would be expected to decrease with increasing age.

▷ **Advisability of Use During Pregnancy**

Pregnancy Category: D, X if used for long periods. See Pregnancy Risk Categories at the back of this book.

Human studies: Fetal alcohol syndrome—a collection of limb, neurological, and behavioral defects—occurs with excessive alcohol use.

Avoid use of this drug during your **entire** pregnancy.

Advisability of Use If Breast-Feeding

Presence of this drug in breast milk: Yes.

Avoid drug or refrain from nursing.

Habit-Forming Potential: Clearly defined alcoholism exists and occurs.

Effects of Overdosage: Toxic levels result in ataxia, loss of consciousness progressing to coma, anesthesia, respiratory failure, and death. Levels of 150 to 300 mg per dl may result in exaggerated emotional states, confusion, and incoordination. Fatalities most often result with blood concentrations greater than 400 mg/dl. Fatal blood levels vary greatly, however, and death has been reported following levels as low as 260 mg/dl. Once again, some people will not have any mental or physical changes with an alcohol level that is in the "legally drunk" range and even with higher levels.

Possible Effects of Long-Term Use: Liver toxicity, anemia, esophageal varices, low white blood cell counts, compromised heart function, high blood pressure, arrhythmias, depression, peripheral neuropathy, seizures, cerebrovascular accident (with acute high levels), water intoxication, vitamin deficiency, electrolyte disturbances, gastritis or ulcers, pancreatitis, muscle pain, osteoporosis, tolerance, and withdrawal on discontinuation.

Suggested Periodic Examinations While Taking This Drug (at physician's discretion)

Blood alcohol levels and methanol or ethylene glycol levels guide therapy in poisonings.

Chronic alcohol abuse: Complete blood counts, liver function tests, amylase and lipase, electrocardiograms.

▷ **While Taking This Drug, Observe the Following**

Foods: Food may decrease the absorption of ethanol from the stomach.

Nutritional Support: Vitamin support, particularly thiamin (B$_1$), folic acid, and B$_6$ are needed with chronic use. Magnesium replacement is also needed. Vitamin C may help eliminate ethanol.

Tobacco Smoking: No interactions expected, but I advise everyone to quit smoking.

Marijuana Smoking: Additive central nervous system depression.

▷   *Other Drugs*

Ethanol may *increase* the effects of

- central nervous system depressants such as benzodiazepines, barbiturates, opioids, and anesthetic agents.
- chlorpromazine (Thorazine) will result in increased sedation.
- cocaine and result in dangerous increases in blood pressure.
- cyclosporine (Sandimmune) if the ethanol is taken in large doses.
- diphenhydramine (Benadryl, others) will increase sedation.
- warfarin (Coumadin) and require more frequent INR testing and possible dose changes.

Ethanol may *decrease* the effects of

- phenytoin (Dilantin) by reducing blood phenytoin levels.
- propranolol (Inderal) by increasing propranolol elimination.

Ethanol *taken concurrently* with

- acetaminophen (Tylenol) poses an increased risk of liver damage.
- some antihistamines may increase sedation.
- aspirin may result in increased blood loss from the stomach.
- cefamandole (Mandol), cefotetan (Cefotan), metronidazole (Flagyl), and cefoperazone (Cefobid) may result in disulfiramlike reaction (see Glossary).
- cimetidine (Zantac) may decrease the amount of alcohol that it takes to make you drunk (intoxicated).
- disulfiram (Antabuse) will result in severe vomiting and intolerance.
- griseofulvin (Fulvicin) can increase the effects of alcohol.
- insulin may result in potential severe hypoglycemia.
- isoniazid may result in elevated isoniazid levels.
- ketoconazole (Nizoral) may result in disulfiramlike reactions.
- lithium (Lithobid) may result in worsened impairment of coordination and intoxication.
- methotrexate (especially with long-term ethanol use) may increase risk of liver damage.
- metronidazole (Flagyl) may result in a disulfiramlike reaction.
- nitroglycerin (Nitrostat, others) may result in excessive decreases in blood pressure.
- oral hypoglycemic agents poses an increased risk of seriously low glucose levels.
- tricyclic antidepressants may result in increased antidepressant levels and toxicity.
- verapamil (Calan, others) may increase the amount of time ethanol stays in the body and may pose an increased risk of intoxication.

▷   *Driving, Hazardous Activities:* This drug may cause drowsiness, mental impairment, and coordination problems.

Driving skill may be impaired at very low blood levels with the perception that capabilities are **not** reduced. Drinking and driving is **not** recommended. Restrict activities as necessary.

Aviation Note: The use of this drug *is a disqualification* for piloting. Consult a designated Aviation Medical Examiner.

Exposure to Sun: May result in additive dehydration.

Heavy Exercise or Exertion: May worsen the adverse effects of this drug.

Discontinuation: Abrupt discontinuation after chronic use may result in a serious withdrawal syndrome known as DT or delirium tremens.

ETHOSUXIMIDE (eth oh SUX i mide)

Introduced: 1960   **Class:** Anticonvulsant   **Prescription:** USA: Yes
Controlled Drug: USA: No; Canada: No   **Available as Generic:** Yes
Brand Name: Zarontin

BENEFITS versus RISKS	
Possible Benefits	*Possible Risks*
EFFECTIVE CONTROL OF ABSENCE SEIZURES (PETIT MAL EPILEPSY)	RARE APLASTIC ANEMIA (see Aplastic Anemia and Bone Marrow Depression in Glossary)
EFFECTIVE CONTROL OF MYOCLONIC AND AKINETIC EPILEPSY in some individuals	Rare decrease in white blood cells and blood platelets

▷ **Principal Uses**

As a Single Drug Product: Uses currently included in FDA-approved labeling: Used to treat petit mal epilepsy and is a drug of choice in absence seizures. Other (unlabeled) generally accepted uses: None at present.

How This Drug Works: By altering certain nerve impulses, this drug suppresses abnormal electrical activity that causes absence seizures of petit mal epilepsy.

Available Dosage Forms and Strengths

Capsules — 250 mg
   Syrup — 250 mg/5 ml

▷ **Usual Adult Dosage Range:** 20 to 30 mg per kg of body mass every 24 hours. Initially 500 mg daily.

Dosage may be increased cautiously by 250 mg every 4 to 7 days until satisfactory control is achieved. The total daily dosage should not exceed 1500 mg. IMPORTANT: Blood levels increase more quickly dose to dose in females than males.

For children 3 to 6 years old: Usual starting dose is 250 mg per day. The dose is then increased by 250-mg doses every 4 to 7 days as needed. Usually 20–30 mg per kg of body mass every 24 hours is used as a once-daily dose.

Those more than 6 years old with absence seizures: same as adult dose.

Note: Actual dosage and administration schedule must be determined for each patient individually.

Conditions Requiring Dosing Adjustments

Liver Function: Blood levels are recommended if this medication is used in liver compromise.

Kidney Function: In severe kidney failure, 75% of the usual dose should be given at the usual intervals.

▷ **Dosing Instructions:**   Capsule may be opened and taken with food to reduce stomach irritation.

Usual Duration of Use: Use on a regular schedule for 1 to 2 weeks is usually needed to see this drug's effectiveness in reducing the frequency of absence seizures. Long-term use requires physician supervision.

▷ **This Drug Should Not Be Taken If**
  • you are allergic to this or any succinimide anticonvulsant (see Drug Classes).
  • you have active liver disease.
  • you currently have a blood cell or bone marrow disorder.

▷ **Inform Your Physician Before Taking This Drug If**
  • you have a history of liver or kidney disease.
  • you have any type of blood disorder, especially one caused by drugs.
  • you have a history of serious depression or other mental illness.

Possible Side Effects (natural, expected, and unavoidable drug actions)
  Drowsiness, lethargy, fatigue.

▷ **Possible Adverse Effects** (unusual, unexpected, and infrequent reactions)
  If any of the following develop, consult your physician promptly for guidance.
  Mild Adverse Effects
  Allergic Reactions: Skin rash, hives—case reports.
  Headache, unsteadiness, euphoria, impaired vision, numbness and tingling in extremities—infrequent.
  Loss of appetite, nausea, vomiting, hiccups, stomach pain, diarrhea—infrequent to frequent.
  Thickening and overgrowth of gums—possible.
  Serious Adverse Effects
  Allergic Reaction: Swelling of tongue—case reports.
  Aggravation of emotional depression and paranoid mental disorders—case reports.
  Severe bone marrow depression: fatigue, fever, sore throat, abnormal bleeding or bruising—case reports.
  Porphyria, myasthenia gravis, or systemic lupus erythematosus—rare.

▷ **Possible Effects on Sexual Function:**   Increased libido (questionable); non-menstrual vaginal bleeding—case reports.

Natural Diseases or Disorders That May Be Activated by This Drug
  Latent psychosis, systemic lupus erythematosus.

Possible Effects on Laboratory Tests
  Complete blood cell counts: decreased red cells, hemoglobin, white cells, and platelets; increased eosinophils.
  Blood aspartate aminotransferase (AST) level: increased in 33% of users.
  Blood bilirubin level: increased (rare liver damage).
  Blood lupus erythematosus (LE) cells: positive—rare.
  Kidney function tests: increased blood urea nitrogen (BUN) level, increased urine protein content.

CAUTION
  1. May increase the frequency of grand mal seizures in people with mixed seizure disorders.
  2. Periodic blood counts and other tests are mandatory.

Precautions for Use
By Infants and Children: If a single-daily dose causes nausea or vomiting, give in two or three divided doses 8 to 12 hours apart. Large differences in response occur, and require blood levels. Watch for a lupuslike reaction: fever, rash, arthritis.
By Those Over 60 Years of Age: Rarely used in this age group.

▷ **Advisability of Use During Pregnancy**
Pregnancy Category: C. See Pregnancy Risk Categories at the back of this book.
Animal studies: Bone defects reported in rodents.
Human studies: Three instances of birth defects have been reported. Adequate studies of pregnant women are not available.
Avoid during first 3 months. Use only if clearly needed during the final 6 months.

Advisability of Use If Breast-Feeding
Presence of this drug in breast milk: Yes.
Watch nursing infant closely and discontinue drug or nursing if adverse effects develop. If mother requires high doses, refrain from nursing. Ask your doctor for help.

Habit-Forming Potential: None.

Effects of Overdosage: Increased drowsiness, lethargy, weakness, dizziness, unsteadiness, nausea, vomiting, stupor progressing to coma.

Possible Effects of Long-Term Use: Systemic lupus erythematosus.

Suggested Periodic Examinations While Taking This Drug (at physician's discretion)
Complete blood counts every 2 weeks during the first months of use, then monthly thereafter; liver and kidney function tests.

▷ **While Taking This Drug, Observe the Following**
Foods: No restrictions.
Beverages: No restrictions. May be taken with milk.
▷ *Alcohol:* Use caution—this drug may increase the sedative effects of alcohol. Excessive alcohol may precipitate seizures.
Tobacco Smoking: No interactions expected, but I advise everyone to quit smoking.
▷ *Other Drugs*
Ethosuximide may *increase* the effects of
• phenytoin (Dilantin), by slowing its elimination.
Ethosuximide *taken concurrently* with
• carbamazepine (Tegretol) may change ethosuximide blood levels.
• phenobarbital may decrease seizure control success.
• ritonavir (Norvir) and perhaps other protease inhibitors (see Drug Classes) may lead to toxicity.
• valproic acid (Depakene) may unpredictably alter ethosuximide effects.
The following drug may *increase* the effects of ethosuximide
• isoniazid (INH, Niconyl, etc.).
▷ *Driving, Hazardous Activities:* This drug may cause drowsiness, dizziness, unsteadiness, and impaired vision. Restrict activities as necessary.
Aviation Note: Seizure disorders and the use of this drug *are disqualifications* for piloting. Consult a designated Aviation Medical Examiner.

Exposure to Sun: No restrictions.

Discontinuation: Do not stop taking this drug abruptly. Ask your physician for help with gradual dose reduction.

ETIDRONATE (e ti DROH nate)

Introduced: 1976   **Class:** Anti-osteoporotic   **Prescription:** USA: Yes
Controlled Drug: USA: No; Canada: No   **Available as Generic:** USA: No; Canada: No

Brand Name: Didronel

BENEFITS versus RISKS	
Possible Benefits	*Possible Risks*
PARTIAL RELIEF OF SYMPTOMS OF PAGET'S DISEASE OF BONE	Increased bone pain
	Bone fractures
EFFECTIVE PREVENTION AND TREATMENT OF ABNORMAL CALCIFICATION	Kidney failure
	Focal osteomalacia
Effective adjunctive treatment of abnormally high blood calcium levels (associated with malignant disease)	
Treatment of postmenopausal osteoporosis	

▷ **Principal Uses**

As a Single Drug Product: Uses currently included in FDA-approved labeling: (1) Treatment of symptomatic Paget's disease of bone (excessive bone growth of skull, spine, and long bones); (2) prevention and treatment of abnormal bone formation (ossification) following total hip replacement or spinal cord injury; (3) adjunctive treatment of excessively high blood calcium levels due to malignant bone disease.

Other (unlabeled) generally accepted uses: (1) treatment of Paget's disease of bone that is not yet causing symptoms; (2) treatment of abnormal calcium levels that may result from prolonged immobilization; (3) helps hyperparathyroidism; (4) helps pulmonary alveolar microlithiasis (PAM).

How This Drug Works: This drug attaches to the surface of bone and slows the abnormally accelerated processes of "bone turnover" that occur in Paget's disease. In malignant bone disease, this drug slows bone destruction and reduces excessive transfer of calcium from bone to blood.

Available Dosage Forms and Strengths

Injection — 50 mg/ml

Tablets — 200 mg, 400 mg

▷ **Recommended Dosage Ranges** (Actual dosage and administration schedule must be determined for each patient individually.)

Infants and Children: Dosage not established.

12 to 60 Years of Age: For Paget's disease: Initially 5 mg per kg of body mass daily, as a single dose, for up to 6 months. Discontinue for a drug-free period of 6 months. As needed, repeat, alternating 6-month courses of drug treatment and abstention. Doses above 10 mg per kg of body mass per day are only used if there is a critical need to decrease increased work output of the heart or to quickly slow down increased bone turnover.

For ossification associated with hip replacement: 20 mg per kg of body mass daily for 1 month before and 3 months after surgery.

For ossification associated with spinal cord injury: Initially 20 mg per kg of body mass daily for 2 weeks after injury; then decrease dose to 10 mg per kg of body mass daily for an additional 10 weeks.

For high blood calcium associated with malignant bone disease: 20 mg per kg of body mass daily for 30 days; if needed and tolerated, continue for a maximum of 90 days.

The total daily dose should not exceed 20 mg per kg of body mass.

Over 60 Years of Age: Same as 12 to 60 years of age.

Conditions Requiring Dosing Adjustments

Liver Function: This drug is not known to be metabolized in the liver.

Kidney Function: The drug should be used with caution, if at all, in patients with steady-state creatinines (a measure of kidney function) greater than 2.5. Etidronate should never be used in patients with steady-state creatinines greater than 5.0.

▷ **Dosing Instructions:** The tablet may be crushed and taken with water on an empty stomach, 2 hours before or after food; suggested times—on arising, midmorning, or at bedtime. Do not take with milk. If nausea or diarrhea occurs, the daily dose may be divided into two or three portions.

Usual Duration of Use: Use on a regular schedule for 1 to 3 months will determine this drug's effectiveness in relieving the symptoms of Paget's disease. If effective, the standard course of treatment is 6 months. Long-term use (months to years) requires periodic physician evaluation.

Possible Advantages of This Drug

Effective orally, with once-a-day dosage.

Less expensive than calcitonin.

▷ **This Drug Should Not Be Taken If**
- you have had an allergic reaction to it previously.
- you recently fractured a bone that has not healed completely.

▷ **Inform Your Physician Before Taking This Drug If**
- you have a history of heart disease, especially congestive heart failure.
- you have impaired kidney function.
- you are subject to enterocolitis or recurrent diarrhea.

Possible Side Effects (natural, expected, and unavoidable drug actions)

Increased bone pain or tenderness (usually starts 4 to 6 weeks after beginning treatment).

▷ **Possible Adverse Effects** (unusual, unexpected, and infrequent reactions)

If any of the following develop, consult your physician promptly for guidance.

Mild Adverse Effects

Allergic Reactions: Skin rash, hives, itching.

Nausea, diarrhea—dose related, may be frequent with 20 mg per kg of body mass per day.

Taste disorders—frequent.

Serious Adverse Effects

Allergic Reactions: Angioedema (swelling of face, lips, tongue, throat, and/or vocal cords); may be life-threatening—case reports.

Osteomalacia (thinning and weakening of bone) with fractures.

Pseudomembranous colitis—rare.

Ulcers or kidney failure—case reports.

▷ **Possible Effects on Sexual Function:**   None reported.

Natural Diseases or Disorders That May Be Activated by This Drug

Senile osteomalacia.

Possible Effects on Laboratory Tests

Blood alkaline phosphatase levels: decreased.

Blood calcium levels and urine hydroxyproline values: decreased.

Blood phosphate levels: increased.

CAUTION

1. Maintain a well-balanced diet with adequate calcium and vitamin D.
2. Mineral supplements and drugs containing aluminum, calcium, iron, or magnesium can prevent etidronate absorption; separate doses by at least 2 hours.
3. Tell your doctor if nausea or diarrhea persists; dosage adjustment (multiple small doses) can help.
4. Call your physician if bone pain persists or increases.

Precautions for Use

By Infants and Children: Avoid large doses or prolonged use to reduce the risk of inducing rickets.

By Those Over 60 Years of Age: Watch fluid balance carefully if this drug is given intravenously to lower blood calcium levels.

▷ **Advisability of Use During Pregnancy**

Pregnancy Category: C. See Pregnancy Risk Categories at the back of this book.

Animal studies: Rat and rabbit studies revealed no drug-induced birth defects.

Human studies: Adequate studies of pregnant women are not available.

Use this drug only if clearly needed. Ask your doctor for help.

Advisability of Use If Breast-Feeding

Presence of this drug in breast milk: Unknown.

Avoid drug or refrain from nursing.

Habit-Forming Potential: None.

Effects of Overdosage: Nausea, vomiting, diarrhea.

Possible Effects of Long-Term Use: Development of osteomalacia (softening and weakening of bone structure).

Suggested Periodic Examinations While Taking This Drug (at physician's discretion)

Measurements of blood calcium, phosphate, and alkaline phosphatase levels.

Measurement of urine hydroxyproline content.

Kidney function tests.

▷ **While Taking This Drug, Observe the Following**

Foods: Avoid all foods, especially dairy products, for 2 hours before and after taking this drug.

Nutritional Support: Ensure adequate intake of calcium and vitamin D.

Beverages: Take this drug with water. Avoid all forms of milk for 2 hours before and after taking this drug.

▷ *Alcohol:* No interactions expected.

Tobacco Smoking: No interactions expected, but I advise everyone to quit smoking.

▷ *Other Drugs*

The following drugs may **decrease** the effects of etidronate
- all antacids containing aluminum, calcium, or magnesium.
- all iron preparations.

Etidronate **taken concurrently** with
- foscarnet (Foscavir) may lead to additive decreases in calcium.
- plicamycin can lead to additive calcium decreases.

▷ *Driving, Hazardous Activities:* No restrictions.

Aviation Note: The use of this drug **may be a disqualification** for piloting. Consult a designated Aviation Medical Examiner.

Exposure to Sun: No restrictions.

Discontinuation: Take this medicine exactly as prescribed. Your doctor should decide when to stop this drug.

ETODOLAC (E TOE do lak)

See the acetic acids (nonsteroidal anti-inflammatory drugs) profile for further information.

ETRETINATE (e TRET i nayt)

Introduced: 1976   **Class:** Anti-psoriasis   **Prescription:** USA: Yes
Controlled Drug: USA: No; Canada: No   **Available as Generic:** USA: No; Canada: No
Brand Name: Tegison

BENEFITS versus RISKS	
Possible Benefits	*Possible Risks*
EFFECTIVE TREATMENT FOR SEVERE, RESISTANT PSORIASIS	MAJOR DRUG-INDUCED BIRTH DEFECTS
	RARE DRUG-INDUCED HEPATITIS
	Adverse effects on eyes and vision
	Adverse effects on musculoskeletal structures
	Adverse effects on blood cholesterol and triglycerides
	Increased intracranial pressure—very rare
	Extended PTT
	Increased triglycerides

▷ **Principal Uses**

As a Single Drug Product: Uses currently included in FDA-approved labeling: Treatment of severe, generalized forms of psoriasis (and related skin disorders) that have failed to respond to conventional, less hazardous treatments.

Other (unlabeled) generally accepted uses: (1) Treatment of acne; (2) local treatment of warts; (3) treatment of cutaneous neoplasia in kidney transplant patients; (4) eases symptoms of Darier's disease; (5) can help symptoms in a variety of abnormal keratin conditions; (6) eases cutaneous systemic lupus erythematosus; (7) helps Reiter's syndrome in AIDS patients.

How This Drug Works: Regulates cell differentiation in the skin; this results in a more normal pattern of cell growth, with reduction of inflammation and scale formation.

Available Dosage Forms and Strengths

Capsules — 10 mg, 25 mg

▷ **Usual Adult Dosage Range:** Initially 1 mg per kg of body mass per day, in divided doses, until satisfactory response is obtained (usually 8 to 16 weeks). Maintenance: 0.5 to 0.75 mg per kg of body mass per day, beginning after initial response. Total daily dosage should not exceed 1.5 mg per kg of body mass per day. **Note: Actual dosage and administration schedule must be determined for each patient individually.**

Conditions Requiring Dosing Adjustments

Liver Function: This drug is a rare cause of hepatitis. It should be used with caution in liver compromise, and the dose should be decreased.

Kidney Function: The kidneys are not a significant factor in the elimination of this drug. Etretinate is a rare cause of kidney toxicity, and it should be used with caution by patients with compromised kidneys.

▷ **Dosing Instructions:** Take with or immediately following meals, preferably with whole milk. Do not suck or chew the capsule; swallow it whole.

Usual Duration of Use: Use on a regular schedule for 2 to 4 weeks is usually necessary to see this drug's benefit in reversing the skin changes of psoriasis. The full effect of treatment may not be apparent for 2 to 3 months of continual use. Long-term use (months to years) requires periodic physician evaluation. Due to the potential for accumulation and toxicity with long-term use, this drug should be temporarily discontinued after 18 months of treatment; it may be resumed as needed. Consult your physician on a regular basis.

Possible Advantages of This Drug: When used in conjunction with other anti-psoriasis drugs and procedures, this drug can enhance the therapeutic response and reduce the total dosage or length of treatment required.

▷ **This Drug Should Not Be Taken If**
- you have had an allergic reaction to any dosage form of it previously.
- you are pregnant or breast-feeding.
- you currently take vitamin A therapy.
- you plan to donate blood in the near future.

▷ **Inform Your Physician Before Taking This Drug If**
- you are allergic to vitamin A or other vitamin A derivatives: isotretinoin (Accutane), tretinoin (Retin-A).
- you are allergic to parabens (preservatives).
- you have cerebral or coronary artery disease.
- you have high blood cholesterol or triglyceride levels.

- you have diabetes.
- your night vision is of critical use to you.
- you have impaired liver or kidney function.
- you have alcoholism.
- you have a history of Crohn's disease or ulcerative colitis.

Possible Side Effects (natural, expected, and unavoidable drug actions)
Dry nose, nosebleed, dry lips, sore mouth and tongue, bleeding gums. Loss of hair, skin peeling of hands and feet, dry skin, itching, bruising—frequent. Thickening of bone (hyperostosis), calcification of tendons and ligaments, bone and joint pain. Thirst or baldness—frequent.

▷ **Possible Adverse Effects** (unusual, unexpected, and infrequent reactions)
If any of the following develop, consult your physician promptly for guidance.

Mild Adverse Effects
Allergic Reactions: Skin rash, hives, itching.
Headache, dizziness, fatigue, fever, emotional irritability—infrequent to frequent.
Eye irritation, blurred or double vision, sensitivity to bright light, decreased night vision, decreased tolerance for contact lenses, earache, impaired hearing—infrequent to frequent.
Altered taste, loss of appetite, nausea, stomach pain, constipation, diarrhea—rare to infrequent.
Muscle cramps—frequent.

Serious Adverse Effects
Increased intracranial pressure: headache, nausea, vomiting, visual disturbances—rare.
Hepatitis; 4 reported deaths worldwide—case reports (lab values may increase frequently).
Kidney damage (nephrotoxicity) or low blood platelets—case reports.
Eye reactions: corneal erosion, abrasion, staining; cataract; retinal hemorrhage; visual field defects; reduced night vision—infrequent to frequent.
Inflammatory bowel disease (Crohn's disease)—rare.
Altered blood fat levels—frequent: increased triglycerides (45%), increased total cholesterol (16%), decreased HDL cholesterol (37%); any of these changes may increase the risk for the development of atherosclerotic heart disease.
Muscle damage—case reports.
Extended PTT (a measure of blood clotting)—case reports.

▷ **Possible Effects on Sexual Function:**   Altered timing and pattern of menstruation.
Loss of libido. Erectile dysfunctions—case reports.

Possible Delayed Adverse Effects: This drug has been found in the blood 2.9 years after use was stopped. It has not been determined how long pregnancy should be avoided after therapy has been stopped.

▷ **Adverse Effects That May Mimic Natural Diseases or Disorders**
Increased intracranial pressure may suggest brain tumor. Liver reactions may suggest viral hepatitis. Joint pains due to calcification of ligaments and tendons may suggest arthritis.

Natural Diseases or Disorders That May Be Activated by This Drug

Angina may start in the people with coronary artery heart disease. Heart attack (myocardial infarction) has been associated with this drug.

Possible Effects on Laboratory Tests

Red blood cell counts: decreased.

Blood eosinophil counts: increased.

Blood total cholesterol, LDL cholesterol, and triglyceride levels: increased.

Liver function tests: increased liver enzymes (ALT/GPT, AST/GOT, and alkaline phosphatase.

PTT: increased.

CAUTION

1. *This drug should not be taken during pregnancy.* A pregnancy test should be performed within 2 weeks prior to taking this drug. In the absence of pregnancy, the drug should be started on the second or third day of the next normal menstrual period. An effective form of contraception should be used for 1 month before the drug is started, during the entire period of treatment, and for an indefinite period (minimum of 3 years) after the drug is discontinued. If pregnancy does occur, stop this drug immediately and consult your physician.
2. *Do not donate blood to a blood bank if you are taking this drug.* Blood containing this drug could pose a serious risk to the developing fetus of a pregnant patient who receives it. Avoid blood donation for a minimum of 3 years if use of the blood is beyond your control.
3. *Comply fully with your physician's recommendations for periodic examinations before, during, and following treatment with this drug.* These are mandatory for safe and effective use.
4. Avoid concurrent use of vitamin A supplements.
5. Call your doctor promptly if you have significant eye reactions or altered vision.
6. Your psoriasis may appear to worsen during the early period of treatment with this drug. Call your doctor if symptoms become severe or prolonged.
7. If dry mouth or sore and bleeding gums persist, consult your dentist.

Precautions for Use

By Infants and Children: This drug should be used only after all less hazardous treatments have failed. It is best to obtain pretreatment X rays to determine bone age and monitor bone growth and development by yearly X-ray studies. This drug can impair normal bone maturation.

By Those Over 60 Years of Age: Watch for development of anemia, impaired kidney function, and fluctuation of blood potassium levels.

▷ **Advisability of Use During Pregnancy**

Pregnancy Category: X. See Pregnancy Risk Categories at the back of this book.

Animal studies: No information available.

Human studies: Major birth defects occur in association with the use of this drug: malformations of the skull, vertebrae, face, extremities, brain, and spinal cord.

Avoid this drug completely during entire pregnancy. See "CAUTION," above.

Advisability of Use If Breast-Feeding
Presence of this drug in breast milk: Unknown.
Avoid drug or refrain from nursing.

Habit-Forming Potential: None.

Effects of Overdosage: Severe headache, irritability, drowsiness, itching, nausea, vomiting.

Possible Effects of Long-Term Use: Hyperostosis (84%): abnormal thickening of bone (pelvis), calcification of ligaments and tendons (knees and ankles).

Suggested Periodic Examinations While Taking This Drug (at physician's discretion)
Complete blood counts; tests of blood sugar, potassium, sodium, and chloride.
Blood cholesterol profiles, before and during treatment.
Liver and kidney function tests.
Complete eye examinations.
Bone X rays, especially for children.

▷ **While Taking This Drug, Observe the Following**
Foods: No restrictions. High-fat foods increase absorption of this drug.
Beverages: No restrictions. Whole milk increases absorption of this drug.
▷   *Alcohol:* No interactions expected. Use moderately; excessive intake can increase blood triglyceride levels.
Tobacco Smoking: No interactions expected, but I advise everyone to quit smoking.
▷   *Other Drugs*
Etretinate may *increase* the effects of
• vitamin A and its derivatives (isotretinoin and tretinoin) and increase the risk of vitamin A toxicity.
Etretinate *taken concurrently* with
• carbamazepine (Tegretol) may result in decreased etretinate effectiveness.
• methotrexate (Rheumatrex) may increase the risk of liver toxicity.
• tetracyclines may increase the risk of elevated intracranial pressure.
• warfarin (Coumadin) may cause a decreased effectiveness of warfarin.
▷   *Driving, Hazardous Activities:* This drug may cause dizziness and blurred vision. Limit activities as necessary.
Aviation Note: The use of this drug *may be a disqualification* for piloting. Consult a designated Aviation Medical Examiner.
Exposure to Sun: Use caution. This drug can cause photosensitivity (see Glossary).
Discontinuation: If this drug doesn't help after 4 months of continual use, it should be stopped. If response is adequate to justify long-term use, it should be stopped temporarily ("drug holiday") after 18 months of continual treatment. Once the skin has cleared, this drug should be stopped. Most people have some degree of recurrence after 2 months. Subsequent treatment courses of 4 to 9 months can be started as required.

FAMCICLOVIR (fam SEYE klo veer)

Introduced: 1994   **Class:** Antiviral   **Prescription:** USA: Yes   **Controlled Drug:** USA: No   **Available as Generic:** USA: No
Brand Name: Famvir

BENEFITS versus RISKS	
Possible Benefits	*Possible Risks*
EFFECTIVE TREATMENT OF HERPES ZOSTER (SHINGLES)	Diarrhea
	Purpura
TREATS AN INFECTION THAT MAY BE LIFE-THREATENING IN AIDS AND MARROW TRANSPLANT PATIENTS	Paresthesias
TREATS RECURRENT GENITAL HERPES	

▷ **Principal Uses**

As a Single Drug Product: Uses currently included in FDA-approved labeling: (1) Treatment of acute herpes zoster (shingles); (2) recently approved for treatment of recurrent genital herpes.

Other (unlabeled) generally accepted uses: May have a role in treating hepatitis B.

How This Drug Works: This drug is changed in the body to the active penciclovir. Penciclovir inhibits the virus by blocking DNA synthesis and viral reproduction (replication).

Available Dosage Forms and Strengths

Tablets — 250 mg (Germany), 500 mg

▷ **Recommended Dosage Ranges** (Actual dosage and administration schedule must be determined for each patient individually.)

Infants and Children: Safety and efficacy for those under 18 not established.

18 to 60 Years of Age: Shingles (herpes zoster): 500 to 750 mg is given every 8 hours for 7 days. It is important to start this medicine promptly after the diagnosis is made.

Recurrent genital herpes: 125 mg twice a day for 5 days.

Over 60 Years of Age: Same as 12 to 60 years of age, except for those with compromised livers or kidneys.

Conditions Requiring Dosing Adjustments

Liver Function: No dose changes are needed in well-compensated liver impairment.

Kidney Function: In people with mild kidney compromise (creatinine clearance greater than 60 ml/min), 500 mg is given every 8 hours. People with mild to moderate compromise (creatinine clearance 40 to 59 ml/min) receive 500 mg every 12 hours. Patients with moderate to severe kidney compromise (creatinine clearance 20 to 39 ml/min) receive 500 mg every 24 hours.

Usual Duration of Use: Use on a regular schedule for 2 days usually determines effectiveness in treating herpes zoster, and the medicine is typically continued for 7 days. Physician evaluation is needed to determine when this medicine should be stopped.

For recurrent genital herpes: dosing is started at the first sign of recurrence and dosing is continued for 5 days.

▷ **This Drug Should Not Be Taken If**
- you have had an allergic reaction to any dosage form of it previously.

▷ **Inform Your Physician Before Taking This Drug If**
- you are uncertain how much famciclovir to take or how often to take it.
- you have a history of kidney or liver problems.
- your immune system is compromised.

▷ **Possible Adverse Effects** (unusual, unexpected, and infrequent reactions)
If any of the following develop, consult your physician promptly for guidance.

Mild Adverse Effects
Allergic Reactions: Itching.
Fever, headache or fatigue—infrequent.
Nausea or diarrhea—infrequent to frequent.

Serious Adverse Effects
Allergic Reactions: Unknown.
Purpura or paresthesias—case reports.
Rigors—rare.

▷ **Possible Effects on Sexual Function:**   None reported.

Possible Delayed Adverse Effects: Unknown.

Possible Effects on Laboratory Tests
Unknown.

CAUTION
1. The best effect is achieved with this medicine if it is started very soon after the condition is diagnosed. If used for recurrent genital herpes, it is best started as soon as signs of recurrence occur.

Precautions for Use
By Infants and Children: Safety and effectiveness for those under 18 years of age are not established.
By Those Over 60 Years of Age: Specific adjustments or precautions are not defined except for those with compromised livers or kidneys.

▷ **Advisability of Use During Pregnancy**
Pregnancy Category: B. See Pregnancy Risk Categories at the back of this book.
Human studies: Adequate studies of pregnant women are not available.
Ask your doctor for guidance.

Advisability of Use If Breast-Feeding
Presence of this drug in breast milk: Unknown.
Stop nursing or discontinue the drug.

Effects of Overdosage: Unknown.

▷ **While Taking This Drug, Observe the Following**
Foods: No restrictions.
Tobacco Smoking: No interactions expected, but I advise everyone to quit smoking.

▷ *Other Drugs*
No interactions reported.

▷ *Driving, Hazardous Activities:* This drug may cause dizziness or fatigue. Restrict activities as necessary.

Aviation Note: The use of this drug *may be a disqualification* for piloting. Consult a designated Aviation Medical Examiner.

Exposure to Sun: No restrictions.

FAMOTIDINE (fa MOH te deen)

See the histamine (H$_2$) blocking drugs profile for further information.

FELODIPINE (fe LOH di peen)

Introduced: 1986   **Class:** Antihypertensive, calcium channel blocker
Prescription: USA: Yes   **Controlled Drug:** USA: No   **Available as Generic:** No

Brand Name: Plendil

Controversies in Medicine: Medicines in this class have been subject to much conflicting data. There have also been several FDA hearings held on the calcium-channel-blocker class. **This medicine became the first calcium channel blocker to be FDA approved as safe for use in treating hypertension or angina in patients who also have congestive heart failure.** More recent data found the long-acting forms of calcium channel blockers to be safe and effective.

BENEFITS versus RISKS	
Possible Benefits	*Possible Risks*
EFFECTIVE TREATMENT OF MILD TO MODERATE HYPERTENSION	Peripheral edema (fluid retention in feet and ankles)

▷ **Principal Uses**

As a Single Drug Product: Uses currently included in FDA-approved labeling: Treatment of mild to moderate hypertension.

Other (unlabeled) generally accepted uses: (1) Treatment of angina; (2) treatment of arrhythmias; (3) adjunctive treatment of congestive heart failure; (4) useful in inhibiting the progression of atherosclerosis.

How This Drug Works: By blocking the normal passage of calcium through certain cell walls (which is necessary for the function of nerve and muscle tissue), this drug slows the spread of electrical activity and reduces contraction of peripheral arterial walls, lowering the blood pressure.

Available Dosage Forms and Strengths

Tablets, sustained release — 5 mg, 10 mg

▷ **Recommended Dosage Ranges** (Actual dosage and administration schedule must be determined for each patient individually.)

Infants and Children: Dosage not established.

12 to 60 Years of Age: High blood pressure: Initially 5 mg, once daily. Increase dose as needed and tolerated at intervals of 2 weeks. The usual dosage range is 5–10 mg, once daily. The total daily dose should not exceed 10 mg, once daily.

Over 65 Years of Age: Starting dose is 2.5 mg daily. The total daily dose should not exceed 10 mg, once daily.

Conditions Requiring Dosing Adjustments

Liver Function: When felodipine is used in patients with liver compromise, the starting dose should be 2.5 mg daily, with a maximum of 10 mg daily.

Kidney Function: The kidneys are not significantly involved in elimination of felodipine.

▷ **Dosing Instructions:**   May be taken with or following food to reduce stomach irritation. The tablet should be swallowed whole; do not crush or chew.

Usual Duration of Use: Use on a regular schedule for 2 to 4 weeks is needed to determine this drug's effectiveness in controlling hypertension. The smallest effective dose should be used in long-term (months to years) therapy. Supervision and periodic physician visits are essential.

Possible Advantages of This Drug

Gradual onset and prolonged duration of action, permitting effective once-a-day treatment.

▷ **This Drug Should Not Be Taken If**
- you have had an allergic reaction to it or similar medicines previously.
- you have active liver disease.
- you have severe lowering of the blood pressure.
- you have severe problems (dysfunction) in the left side of your heart.
- you have atrioventricular blockade or sick sinus syndrome (talk with your doctor).
- you have uncorrected congestive heart failure.

▷ **Inform Your Physician Before Taking This Drug If**
- you have had an unfavorable response to any calcium-channel-blocker drug.
- you currently take any form of digitalis or a beta-blocker drug (see Drug Classes).
- you are taking any other drugs that lower blood pressure.
- you have a history of congestive heart failure, heart attack, or stroke.
- you are subject to disturbances of heart rhythm (such as atrial fibrillation).
- you develop a skin reaction while taking this medicine.
- you have circulatory impairment to the fingers.
- you have muscular dystrophy or myasthenia gravis.
- you have a history of impaired liver or kidney function.

Possible Side Effects (natural, expected, and unavoidable drug actions)

Swelling of feet and ankles, flushing and sensation of warmth.

▷ **Possible Adverse Effects** (unusual, unexpected, and infrequent reactions)

If any of the following develop, consult your physician promptly for guidance.

Mild Adverse Effects

Allergic Reactions: Skin rash—rare.

Headache—frequent; dizziness, fatigue, or sleep disorders—infrequent.

Indigestion, nausea, stomach pain, constipation, or diarrhea—all rare.

Palpitations or fast heart rate (tachycardia)—infrequent to frequent.

Dose-related flushing—possible.

Impaired sense of smell—possible.

Cough or pharyngitis—infrequent.
Increased urination—possible.
Abnormal growth of the gums (gingival hyperplasia)—rare.
Serious Adverse Effects
Allergic Reactions: None reported.
Idiosyncratic Reactions: None reported.
Aggravation of angina—possible.
Decreased hemoglobin, hematocrit, and red blood cell count (reported with other drugs in the same family—case reports.

▷ **Possible Effects on Sexual Function:**   Impotence (0.5–1.5%)—rare.

▷ **Adverse Effects That May Mimic Natural Diseases or Disorders**
An allergic rash and swelling of the legs may resemble erysipelas.

Possible Effects on Laboratory Tests
Liver function tests: minor and short-term increases.

CAUTION
1. Tell all of your health care providers that you are taking this drug. Carry a note that says you take felodipine.
2. You may use nitroglycerin and other nitrate drugs as needed to relieve acute episodes of angina pain. However, if your angina attacks become more frequent or intense, call your doctor promptly.

Precautions for Use
By Infants and Children: Safety and effectiveness for those under 12 years of age are not established.
By Those Over 60 Years of Age: You may be more susceptible to the development of weakness, dizziness, fainting, and falling. Take necessary precautions to prevent injury.

▷ **Advisability of Use During Pregnancy**
Pregnancy Category: C. See Pregnancy Risk Categories at the back of this book.
Animal studies: No information available.
Human studies: Adequate studies of pregnant women are not available.
Avoid this drug during the first 3 months. Use during the final 6 months only if clearly needed. Ask your physician for guidance.

Advisability of Use If Breast-Feeding
Presence of this drug in breast milk: Unknown.
Avoid drug or refrain from nursing.

Habit-Forming Potential: None.

Effects of Overdosage: Weakness, light-headedness, fainting, fast pulse, low blood pressure, shortness of breath, flushed and warm skin, tremors.

Possible Effects of Long-Term Use: None reported.

Suggested Periodic Examinations While Taking This Drug (at physician's discretion)
Evaluations of heart function, including electrocardiograms and measurements of blood pressure in supine, sitting, and standing positions.

▷ **While Taking This Drug, Observe the Following**
Foods: Avoid eating grapefruit for 1 hour after taking this medicine. Avoid excessive salt intake.
Beverages: Grapefruit juice can cause **a serious increase** in the absorption of

this drug—levels may be increased by over 400%. Do **not** take this drug with grapefruit juice. May be taken with milk or water.

▷ *Alcohol:* Use with caution—alcohol may exaggerate the drop in blood pressure experienced by some individuals.

Tobacco Smoking: Nicotine may reduce the effectiveness of this drug. I advise everyone to quit smoking.

▷ *Other Drugs*

Felodipine *taken concurrently* with

- adenosine may result in an extended slowing of the heart.
- beta-blocker drugs or digitalis preparations (see Drug Classes) may affect heart rate and rhythm adversely. Careful monitoring by your physician is necessary if these drugs are taken concurrently.
- carbamazepine (Tegretol) may result in decreased felodipine effectiveness.
- digoxin (Lanoxin) may increase digoxin levels and result in toxicity.
- itraconazole, fluconazole, or ketoconazole (see Antifungal Drugs in Drug Classes) may lead to felodipine toxicity.
- magnesium (particularly in high doses) may cause low blood pressure (not specifically reported for felodipine, but another drug in the calcium-channel-blocker class does this).
- phenobarbital can cause decreased felodipine benefits.
- phenytoin (Dilantin) may cause decreased phenytoin levels.
- rifampin (Rifadin) may cause decreased felodipine benefits (reported with other calcium channel blockers).
- ritonavir (Norvir) and perhaps other protease inhibitors (see Drug Classes) may lead to toxicity.

The following drugs may *increase* the effects of felodipine

- cimetidine (Tagamet).
- erythromycin—may also occur with other macrolide antibiotics (see Drug Classes), since they are structurally similar.

▷ *Driving, Hazardous Activities:* Usually no restrictions. This drug may cause dizziness. Restrict activities as necessary.

Aviation Note: Hypertension *is a disqualification* for piloting. Consult a designated Aviation Medical Examiner.

Exposure to Sun: No restrictions.

Exposure to Heat: Caution is advised. Hot environments can exaggerate the blood-pressure-lowering effects of this drug. Observe for light-headedness or weakness.

Discontinuation: Do not stop this drug abruptly. Ask your physician about gradual withdrawal. Watch for development of rebound hypertension.

FENAMATES
(Nonsteroidal Anti-Inflammatory Drugs)

Meclofenamate (MEK low fen a mate)   **Mefenamic Acid** (MEF en amik a sid)

Introduced: 1977, 1966   **Class:** Analgesic, mild; NSAIDs   **Prescription:** USA: Yes   **Controlled Drug:** USA: No; Canada: No   **Available as Generic:** Yes

Brand Names: Meclofenamate: Meclodium, Meclomen; Mefenamic Acid: Ponstel, ✦Ponstan

---

BENEFITS versus RISKS

Possible Benefits	*Possible Risks*
EFFECTIVE RELIEF OF MILD TO MODERATE PAIN AND INFLAMMATION	Gastrointestinal pain, ulceration, bleeding
	Kidney damage
	Fluid retention
	Bone marrow depression (mefenamic acid)
	Hemolytic anemia (mefenamic acid)
	Systemic lupus erythematosus (mefenamic acid)
	Pancreatitis (mefenamic acid)

Author's Note: All these risks are rare.

▷ **Principal Uses**

As a Single Drug Product: Uses currently included in FDA-approved labeling: (1) Meclofenamate is used to relieve pain of osteoarthritis and rheumatoid arthritis; (2) mefenamic acid is used to relieve chronic pain, painful menstruation (dysmenorrhea), and postoperative pain.

Other (unlabeled) generally accepted uses: (1) Meclofenamate is used to treat temporal arteritis and the nephrotic syndrome; (2) mefenamic acid is used to treat PMS, osteoarthritis (maximum 1 week), and temporal arteritis.

How These Drugs Work: These drugs reduce tissue levels of prostaglandins (and related substances), chemicals involved in the production of inflammation and pain.

Available Dosage Forms and Strengths

Meclofenamate (Meclomen):

Capsules — 50 mg, 100 mg
Mefenamic acid (Ponstel):
Capsule — 250 mg

▷ **Usual Adult Dosage Range:**   Meclofenamate: (osteoarthritis or rheumatoid arthritis) 200 to 400 mg daily, in three or four divided doses. Total daily dosage should not be more than 400 mg.

Mefenamic acid: 500 mg initially, then 250 mg every 6 hours, taken with food.

Note: Actual dosage and administration schedule must be determined for each patient individually.

Conditions Requiring Dosing Adjustments

Liver Function: Changes in dosing are not presently recommended in liver compromise.

Kidney Function: Meclofenamate is eliminated by the kidneys; however, specific dosing guidelines have not been specified. Mefenamic acid should **not** be used by patients with compromised kidneys.

▷ **Dosing Instructions:**   Take with food or milk to prevent stomach irritation. Take with a full glass of water and remain upright (do not lie down) for 30 minutes. The capsule may be opened for administration.

Usual Duration of Use: Meclofenamate: Use on a regular schedule for 2 to 3 weeks usually determines its effectiveness in arthritis therapy. Long-term use (months to years) requires physician supervision and periodic evaluation.

Mefenamic acid: Peak levels occur in up to 4 hours. Use beyond 7 days is **not recommended**.

▷ **These Drugs Should Not Be Taken If**
- you have had an allergic reaction to them previously.
- you are subject to asthma or nasal polyps caused by aspirin.
- you have active peptic ulcer disease, regional enteritis, ulcerative colitis, or gastrointestinal bleeding.
- you have a bleeding disorder or a blood cell disorder.
- you have severe impairment of kidney function (mefenamic acid).
- you have systemic lupus erythematosus (mefenamic acid).
- you have recently had pancreatitis (mefenamic acid).

▷ **Inform Your Physician Before Taking These Drugs If**
- you are allergic to aspirin or to other aspirin substitutes.
- you have a history of peptic ulcer disease, regional enteritis, or ulcerative colitis.
- you have a history of any type of bleeding disorder.
- you have impaired liver or kidney function.
- you have high blood pressure or a history of heart failure.
- you take acetaminophen, aspirin, or other aspirin substitutes; anticoagulants; oral antidiabetic drugs; or cortisonelike drugs.

Possible Side Effects (natural, expected, and unavoidable drug actions)
Ringing in ears, fluid retention, or drowsiness.

▷ **Possible Adverse Effects** (unusual, unexpected, and infrequent reactions)
If any of the following develop, consult your physician promptly for guidance.
Mild Adverse Effects
Allergic Reactions: Skin rash, hives, itching.
Headache, dizziness, altered or blurred vision, depression—possible.
Mouth sores, indigestion, nausea, vomiting, diarrhea (10–33%, sometimes severe).
Serious Adverse Effects
Allergic Reactions: Severe skin reactions, drug fever (see Glossary)—case reports.
Active peptic ulcer, with or without bleeding—possible.
Kidney damage with painful urination, bloody urine, reduced urine formation—case reports.
Bone marrow depression (see Glossary) (mefenamic acid): fatigue, weakness, fever, sore throat, abnormal bleeding or bruising—case reports.
Mefenamic acid: Also causes rare hemolytic anemia, seizures, porphyria, liver damage, pancreatitis, and systemic lupus erythematosus.

▷ **Possible Effects on Sexual Function:**   None reported.

Possible Delayed Adverse Effects: Mild anemia due to "silent" blood loss from the stomach (less than that caused by aspirin).

Natural Diseases or Disorders That May Be Activated by These Drugs
Peptic ulcer disease, ulcerative colitis.

Possible Effects on Laboratory Tests
Complete blood cell counts: decreased red cells, hemoglobin, white cells, and platelets—all rare. For mefenamic acid, also add SLE test.

CAUTION
1. Dosage should always be limited to the smallest amount that produces reasonable improvement.
2. This drug may mask early indications of infection. Inform your physician if you think you are developing an infection of any kind.
3. Mefenamic acid should be used for a maximum of 7 days.

Precautions for Use
By Infants and Children: Safety and effectiveness for those under 14 years of age have not been established for meclofenamate, and under 18 years of age for mefenamic acid.
By Those Over 60 Years of Age: Small doses are advisable until tolerance is determined. Observe for any indications of liver or kidney toxicity, fluid retention, dizziness, confusion, impaired memory, stomach bleeding, or diarrhea.

▷ **Advisability of Use During Pregnancy**
Pregnancy Category: Meclofenamate: B normally and D in the final 3 months of pregnancy. Mefenamic acid: C. See Pregnancy Risk Categories at the back of this book.
Animal studies: Some minor birth defects reported in rodents for meclofenamate. Increased fetal resorption in rabbits with 2.5 times the human mefenamic acid dose.
Human studies: Adequate studies of pregnant women are not available.
The manufacturer does not recommend the use of meclofenamate during pregnancy.
Use of mefenamic acid in late pregnancy should be avoided. Ask your doctor for help regarding mefenamic acid use in pregnancy.

Advisability of Use If Breast-Feeding
Presence of these drugs in breast milk: Yes.
Avoid drug or refrain from nursing.

Habit-Forming Potential: None.

Effects of Overdosage: Drowsiness, nausea, vomiting, diarrhea, marked agitation, irrational behavior, metabolic acidosis, and seizures.

Possible Effects of Long-Term Use: None identified.

Suggested Periodic Examinations While Taking These Drugs (at physician's discretion)
Complete blood cell counts, kidney function tests, complete eye examinations if vision is altered in any way.

▷ **While Taking These Drugs, Observe the Following:**
   Foods: No restrictions.
   Beverages: No restrictions. May be taken with milk.
▷ *Alcohol:* Use with caution. The irritant action of alcohol on the stomach lining, added to the irritant action of this drug in sensitive individuals, can increase the risk of stomach ulceration and/or bleeding.
   Tobacco Smoking: No interactions expected, but I advise everyone to quit smoking.
▷ *Other Drugs*
   Meclofenamate may *increase* the effects of
   • acetaminophen (Tylenol, etc.), and increase the risk of kidney damage; avoid prolonged use of this combination.
   • anticoagulants (Coumadin, etc.), and increase the risk of bleeding; monitor INR (prothrombin time), adjust dose accordingly.
   Meclofenamate *taken concurrently* with the following drugs may increase the risk of bleeding; avoid these combinations:
   • aspirin (various).
   • dipyridamole (Persantine).
   • sulfinpyrazone (Anturane).
   • valproic acid (Depakene).
   Mefenamic acid *taken concurrently* with
   • anticoagulants (Coumadin, etc.) will displace the drugs from binding sites and increase bleeding risk.
   • aspirin, dipyridamole, or sulfinpyrazone may result in increased bleeding risk.
   • cyclosporine (Sandimmune) may result in increased cyclosporine levels and toxicity.
   • magnesium-containing antacids may result in rapid mefenamic acid toxicity.
   Meclofenamate or mefenamic acid *taken concurrently* with
   • diuretics (see Drug Classes) may result in decreased effectiveness of the diuretic in controlling blood pressure.
   • enoxaparin may result in increased surgical blood loss if patients receiving this combination undergo surgery.
   • lithium (Lithobid, others) will increase blood lithium levels over time and may result in toxicity.
   • methotrexate (Mexate) can result in serious methotrexate toxicity.
▷ *Driving, Hazardous Activities:* This drug may cause dizziness or altered vision. Restrict activities as necessary.
   Aviation Note: The use of these drugs *may be a disqualification* for piloting. Consult a designated Aviation Medical Examiner.
   Exposure to Sun: No restrictions.

FENOPROFEN (fen oh PROH fen)

See the propionic-acids (nonsteroidal anti-inflammatory drugs) profile for further information.

FENTANYL (FEN ta nil)

Introduced: 1991   **Class:** Analgesic, strong   **Prescription:** USA: Yes
Controlled Drug: USA: C-ll*; Canada: Yes   **Available as Generic:** USA: No;
Canada: No

Brand Names: Duragesic, Oralet, ✦Innovar, Sublimaze

┌───┐
| **BENEFITS versus RISKS** |
Possible Benefits	*Possible Risks*
EFFECTIVE PAIN RELIEF	Habit-forming potential with
SKIN PATCH APPLICATION	prolonged use
NEEDED ONLY ONCE EVERY 3	Impairment of mental function
DAYS	Methemoglobinemia
	Respiratory depression
└───┘

▷ **Principal Uses**

As a Single Drug Product: Uses currently included in FDA-approved labeling:
Treatment of chronic pain.

Other (unlabeled) generally accepted uses: None.

How This Drug Works: This drug acts at specific pain receptors (Mu agonist) to
block pain.

Available Dosage Forms and Strengths

Transdermal patch — 2.5 mg, 5 mg, 7.5
mg, 10 mg

Lozenge on a handle (has been likened to a lollipop) — 200 mcg, 300 mcg,
400 mcg

Author's Note: Injectable forms are not presented in this profile.

▷ **Recommended Dosage Ranges** (Actual dosage and administration schedule
must be determined for each patient individually.)

Infants and Children: Safety and efficacy for those under 12 years of age are not
established.

18 to 60 Years of Age: Patch: Not indicated for patients 18 years old who weigh
less than 50 kg (110 lb).

In patients who have not been using opioids such as morphine, the 25 mcg
per hour (2.5-mg) patch should be used. In people who used opioids previously, the amount needed to control pain on a 24-hour basis is calculated,
converted to an equal amount of morphine (morphine equianalgesic dose),
and then converted to fentanyl.

Lozenge (sucker): Used to treat pain/anxiety before surgery; 400 mcg for
those with a body mass of 50 kg or more.

Over 60 Years of Age: These people should receive the 25 mcg per hour (2.5-mg)
patch, unless they were already receiving the equivalent of 135 mg of oral
morphine daily. Intravenous fentanyl clears more slowly in this population
than in younger patients, and careful observation for overdose should be
made.

*See schedules of Controlled Drugs at the back of this book.

Conditions Requiring Dosing Adjustments
Liver Function: The dose **must be decreased** in liver compromise.
Kidney Function: In moderate to severe kidney failure, 75% of the usual dose should be taken.
In severe kidney failure, the dose should be reduced by 50%. Patients in end-stage kidney disease may be more sensitive to this medicine.

▷ **Dosing Instructions:**   Take the patch from its protective pouch, and remove the stiff protective liner from the sticky side of the patch. Do not cut the system. The sticky side of the patch is placed on a nonhairy, dry area (back, chest, flank, or upper arm). Avoid skin which is burned, irritated, or excessively oily. Wash your hands once you have applied the patch. A new patch should be applied to a different area after 3 days. Fold the old patch onto itself and flush it down the toilet. Avoid exposing the patch to heat such as electric blankets or heating pads. The lozenge or sucker should be allowed to slowly dissolve in the mouth. It should not be bitten or chewed.

Usual Duration of Use: Use on a regular schedule for 1 to 3 days usually determines effectiveness in controlling pain. An immediate-release form of morphine or similar drug should be available while this drug reaches its peak effect. Long-term use (months) requires periodic physician evaluation of response and dosage adjustment.

Possible Advantages of This Drug
Effective pain relief with patch placement once every 3 days and no injections.

▷ **This Drug Should Not Be Taken If**
   • you have had an allergic reaction to any dosage form of it previously.
   • you have had an allergic reaction to the adhesive in the patch before.
   • you are less than 12 years old.
   • you weigh less than 50 kg and are less than 18 years old.
   • you have mild or intermittent pain.
   • you have acute or postoperative pain without opportunity for proper dose adjustment.

▷ **Inform Your Physician Before Taking This Drug If**
   • you have liver or kidney compromise.
   • you have chronic lung disease (such as COPD).
   • you have an abnormally slow heartbeat or other heart disease.
   • you develop a high fever.
   • you have not taken narcotic pain medicines before and you are given a dose more than 25 mcg per hour.
   • you take an MAO inhibitor (see Drug Classes).
   • you have a brain tumor.
   • you are anemic.
   • you have a history of alcoholism or drug abuse.
   • you take other prescription or nonprescription medicines that were not discussed with your doctor when transdermal fentanyl was prescribed.

Possible Side Effects (natural, expected, and unavoidable drug actions)
Constipation, dry mouth. Sleepiness (somnolence) or euphoria—infrequent.

▷ **Possible Adverse Effects** (unusual, unexpected, and infrequent reactions)
   If any of the following develop, consult your physician promptly for guidance.

Mild Adverse Effects
  Allergic Reactions: Skin rash and itching.
  Blurred vision or amblyopia—rare to infrequent.
  Nausea or vomiting—infrequent.
  Urinary retention—infrequent.
  Tremor or muscular rigidity—possible.
Serious Adverse Effects
  Allergic Reactions: Exfoliative dermatitis and/or anaphylactic reactions—
    case reports.
  Arrhythmias—rare.
  Paranoid reaction, depersonalization, speech problems (aphasia)—rare, dose
    related.
  Seizures or hallucinations—case reports.
  Methemoglobinemia or porphyrias—rare.
  Paresthesias—rare.
  Respiratory depression. This effect may last longer than the pain-relieving
    effect—dose related.

▷ **Possible Effects on Sexual Function:**   Impotence and blunted orgasm sensa-
    tion in men. Irregular menstrual periods and blunted orgasm sensation in
    women.

Possible Delayed Adverse Effects: Dependence and tolerance.

Possible Effects on Laboratory Tests
  Methemoglobinemia.

CAUTION
  1. Extreme caution should be used if this drug is combined with other opi-
     oids, narcotic drugs, benzodiazepines, or alcohol.
  2. May cause serious constipation in older patients.
  3. Do not expose the patch site to external sources of heat such as heating
     pads or electric blankets, as an increased rate of drug release may occur.

Precautions for Use
  By Infants and Children: Safety and effectiveness for those under 12 years of age
    are not established.
  By Those Over 60 Years of Age: The 2.5-mg patch should **NOT** be used as a start-
    ing dose unless you are already taking more than 135 mg of morphine daily.
    Those with cardiac, respiratory, kidney, or liver compromise should be
    given low doses and carefully monitored.

▷ **Advisability of Use During Pregnancy**
  Pregnancy Category: C, D if used in high doses when the baby is born or for
    prolonged periods. See Pregnancy Risk Categories at the back of this book.
  Animal studies: Some fetal death data with intravenous use in rats.
  Human studies: Adequate studies of pregnant women are not available.
  Ask your doctor for guidance.

Advisability of Use If Breast-Feeding
  Presence of this drug in breast milk: Yes.
  Avoid drug or refrain from nursing.

Habit-Forming Potential: Fentanyl is a Schedule II narcotic and can cause de-
    pendence resembling morphine dependence. Physical and psychological
    dependence and tolerance can occur with repeated use.

Effects of Overdosage: Dizziness, amnesia, and stupor. Respiratory depression and apnea may occur.

Possible Effects of Long-Term Use: Tolerance and physical or psychological dependence.

Suggested Periodic Examinations While Taking This Drug (at physician's discretion)
  Liver function tests.

▷ **While Taking This Drug, Observe the Following**
  Foods: No restrictions.
  Beverages: No restrictions.
▷ *Alcohol:* **DO NOT DRINK ALCOHOL** while you are taking this drug—leads to additive loss of mental status, respiratory depression, and confusion.
  Tobacco Smoking: No interactions expected, but I advise everyone to quit smoking.
  Marijuana Smoking: Additive adverse effects; however, marijuana may block the vomiting effect of fentanyl.
▷ *Other Drugs*
  Fentanyl may *increase* the effects of
  • benzodiazepines such as diazepam (Valium) and alprazolam (Xanax).
  • central nervous system depressants such as opiates, barbiturates, tranquilizers, and tricyclic antidepressants.
  Fentanyl *taken concurrently* with
  • amiodarone (Cordarone) may result in heart (cardiac) toxicity.
  • clonidine (Catapres, others) may result in greater than expected fentanyl effects. The fentanyl dose may need to be decreased if these medicines are to be combined.
  • MAO inhibitors (see Drug Classes) may worsen the lowering of blood pressure and depression of breathing seen with fentanyl.
  • ritonavir (Norvir) and perhaps other protease inhibitors (see Drug Classes) can lead to major fentanyl toxicity.
▷ *Driving, Hazardous Activities:* This drug may cause drowsiness, sedation, and respiratory depression. Restrict activities as necessary.
  Aviation Note: The use of this drug *is a disqualification* for piloting. Consult a designated Aviation Medical Examiner.
  Exposure to Sun: No restrictions.
  Discontinuation: The patch may be removed if it is not tolerated or to be stopped. Once the patch is removed, fentanyl will still continue to be released from the patch site for 17 hours or more. Ideally, if pain medicine is still needed, the chosen alternative should be substituted, and fentanyl transdermal will slowly taper.

FILGRASTIM (fil GRA stem)

Other Names: Recombinant G-CSF

Introduced: 1991   **Class:** Hematopoietic agent   **Prescription:** USA: Yes   **Controlled Drug:** USA: No; Canada: No   **Available as Generic:** USA: No; Canada: No

Brand Name: Neupogen

BENEFITS versus RISKS	
Possible Benefits	*Possible Risks*
PREVENTION OF INFECTIONS DUE TO LOWERED WHITE BLOOD CELL COUNTS: FOLLOWING CHEMOTHERAPY FOLLOWING BONE MARROW TRANSPLANT IN PATIENTS WITH CHRONIC OR CYCLIC NEUTROPENIA INCREASED BLOOD CELLS IN AIDS PATIENTS CORRECTION OF DRUG-INDUCED LOWERING OF WHITE BLOOD CELLS	Bone pain Changes in heart waves

▷ **Principal Uses**

As a Single Drug Product: Uses currently included in FDA-approved labeling: (1) Used to help white blood cell counts recover after chemotherapy and bone marrow transplants; (2) used subcutaneously or intravenously to reduce or prevent low white blood cell counts that occur after cancer chemotherapy; (3) treats patients who have an absence of white blood cells at birth; (4) used to help patients with Kostmann syndrome have improved white blood cell counts; (5) used to help patients who have low white blood cell counts (neutropenia) of unknown cause (idiopathic).

Other (unlabeled) generally accepted uses: (1) Helps patients recover from a particular kind of lack of white blood cells (agranulocytosis) that has been caused by medications (drug induced); (2) used in AIDS (orphan drug status) patients (taking ganciclovir) to help restore white blood cell counts; (3) used to treat patients with severe long-term (chronic) low white blood cell counts; (4) used to treat patients with abnormally low white blood cell and neutrophil counts (myelodysplastic syndrome).

How This Drug Works: This drug is made by recombinant technology and is one of the many acknowledged hematopoietic growth factors. Filgrastim regulates the proliferation and release of early (progenitor) forms of white blood cells. This medicine also can tell the bone marrow to increase the rate at which it makes white blood cells. Filgrastim may also work with other factors to increase the production of blood platelets.

Available Dosage Forms and Strengths

Solution for injection — 300 mcg/ml (supplied as a 300- or 480-mcg vial)

How to Store

The prepared solution should be stored at 36 to 46 degrees F (2 to 8 degrees C). This medicine **should not** be frozen. Some centers draw up a 7-day supply of syringes that are then stored in a refrigerator.

▷ **Recommended Dosage Ranges** (Actual dosage and administration schedule must be determined for each patient individually.)

Infants and Children: The medicine has been studied in this population and doses of 0.6 to 120 mcg per kg of body mass per day for up to 3 years have been well tolerated. These doses have been used in children 3 months to 18 years of age. In chronic low white blood cell counts (chronic neutropenia), doses of 5 to 10 mcg per kg of body mass per day have been used.

18 to 60 Years of Age: Patients receiving therapy that destroys the bone marrow (myeloablative treatment) and then receive a bone marrow transplant: Should wait 24 hours after the chemotherapy was given and 24 hours after bone marrow transplant, then are given 10 mcg per kg of body mass per day as a starting dose. This dose is adjusted depending on the degree of increase of white blood cells (absolute neutrophil count).

Patients receiving medicine that suppresses the bone marrow should wait until 24 hours after or before the chemotherapy is given. In this population, filgrastim therapy is started with 5 mcg per kg of body mass per day. Doses may be increased by 5 mcg per kg of body mass per day for each cycle of chemotherapy, based on the severity of the lowering of white blood cell count (nadir) and how long the lowered white cell (absolute neutrophil) count lasts. This drug can be given daily for up to 14 days.

Over 60 Years of Age: Same as 12 to 60 years of age.

Conditions Requiring Dosing Adjustments

Liver Function: Not significantly involved in the elimination of this drug.

Kidney Function: Roughly 90% of a given filgrastim dose is eliminated by the kidneys. Changes in dosing are not defined.

▷ **Dosing Instructions:** The solution in the reconstituted vial should be colorless and clear. Once your doctor or nurse has taught you how to inject the medicine:

- Make certain the solution has not expired (check the expiration date).
- Make certain you have the correct kind of syringe (insulin syringes are commonly used).
- Follow the provided patient instructions carefully.
- If you are using a syringe, make certain you inject the medicine under the skin, not into a vein.
- This medicine can also be given intravenously over a period of 15 to 30 minutes.

Usual Duration of Use: Continual use on a regular schedule for up to 2 weeks (10 to 14 days) may be needed to determine this drug's effectiveness in correcting low white blood cell (absolute neutrophil) count after chemotherapy. Bone marrow transplant patients may take still longer to respond. Long-term problems with white blood cells (such as chronic neutropenia) may require years of therapy. Long-term use requires periodic evaluation of response and dosage adjustment. Consult your physician on a regular basis.

Possible Advantages of This Drug

Effective recombinant product with few side effects.

▷ **This Drug Should Not Be Taken If**
- you have had an allergic reaction to any dosage form of it previously.
- your have a known allergy to products derived from *E. coli* (a bacteria).

▷ **Inform Your Physician Before Taking This Drug If**
- you have a history of gout or psoriasis.
- you have received chemotherapy within the last 24 hours.
- you have a history of heart problems (heart rhythm should be closely monitored).

- you have a history of leukemia (myeloid type). The safety and efficacy of this medicine is not established in that condition.
- you have a history of cancer (with myeloid characteristics). There is a possibility that this drug may act as a growth factor for these tumors. Use, however, in a small number of leukemia patients has not resulted in worsening of their leukemia.
- you are uncertain of how much filgrastim to take or how often to take it.

Possible Side Effects (natural, expected, and unavoidable drug actions)
Pain on injection.
Bone pain (up to 22% in Phase Three studies).

▷ **Possible Adverse Effects** (unusual, unexpected, and infrequent reactions)
If any of the following develop, consult your physician promptly for guidance.
Mild Adverse Effects
Allergic Reactions: Skin rash or itching—infrequent.
Mild decreases in blood pressure or increases in uric acid—case reports.
Drug-induced fever—infrequent to frequent.
Nausea and anorexia—rare.
Irritation of the eye (iridocyclitis, conjunctival erythema)—case reports.
Enlargement of the spleen: reported in patients with chronic lowering of the white blood cells (chronic neutropenia)—frequent, though asymptomatic in these patients.
Serious Adverse Effects
Allergic Reactions: Anaphylaxis—case report.
Depression of part of the heart action (ST depression)—rare to infrequent.
Sweet syndrome (acute neutrophilic dermatosis)—possible.
Worsening of psoriasis—case report.
Low oxygen in the blood (hypoxemia)—very rare.
Potential (though not yet reported) for this medicine to act as a growth factor for certain cancers (malignancies of the myeloid type)—possible.
Potential (though not yet reported) breathing problems (respiratory distress syndrome) in patients with serious (septic) infections, because white blood cells may travel to the infected area—possible.

▷ **Possible Effects on Sexual Function:**   None reported.

Possible Delayed Adverse Effects: Increased uric acid.

▷ **Adverse Effects That May Mimic Natural Diseases or Disorders**
None reported.

Natural Diseases or Disorders That May Be Activated by This Drug
Gout.

Possible Effects on Laboratory Tests
Absolute neutrophil count: increased.
Alkaline phosphatase: increased markedly.
Uric acid: increased mildly.
Lactate dehydrogenase (LDH): increased.

CAUTION
1. Bone pain may be prevented by taking acetaminophen (Tylenol, others) before this medicine is injected.
2. Call your doctor if you have chills, fever, or any other sign of infection.

3. Be certain to follow up with your laboratory testing as scheduled.
4. The solution in the vial should be clear. Do **not** inject any discolored or cloudy solution.
5. Make sure you have the correct kind of syringe before you inject this medicine.
6. This medicine can be given intravenously when it is appropriately prepared. If your doctor has instructed you on how to give yourself an injection using a syringe, the medicine should be given under the skin. Be certain you understand the technique.
7. Always change the site in which you inject this medicine, as your doctor instructed.

Precautions for Use

By Infants and Children: This medicine has been used in children with long-term lowering of white blood cell counts (chronic neutropenia) in doses of 5 to 10 mcg per kg of body mass per day.

By Those Over 60 Years of Age: No specific precautions.

▷ **Advisability of Use During Pregnancy**

Pregnancy Category: C. See Pregnancy Risk Categories at the back of this book.
Animal studies: In rabbits given 80 mcg per kg of body mass per day (very high doses), increased abortion and death of embryos were observed.
Human studies: Information from adequate studies of pregnant women is not available. Ask your doctor for help with this benefit-to-risk decision.

Advisability of Use If Breast-Feeding

Presence of this drug in breast milk: Unknown.
Ask your doctor for guidance.

Habit-Forming Potential: None.

Effects of Overdosage: No maximum tolerated dose has been identified.

Possible Effects of Long-Term Use: Enlarged spleens may occur in up to 25% of patients (splenomegaly) with severe chronic neutropenia. Skin rashes may occur in up to 6% of patients.

Suggested Periodic Examinations While Taking This Drug (at physician's discretion)

Complete blood cell counts and platelet counts should be obtained prior to chemotherapy and twice weekly during filgrastim therapy.

▷ **While Taking This Drug, Observe the Following**

Foods: No restrictions.
Beverages: No restrictions.
▷ *Alcohol:* No restrictions.
Tobacco Smoking: No interactions expected, but I advise everyone to quit smoking.
▷ *Other Drugs*

Filgrastim *taken concurrently* with
• lithium (Lithobid, others) may (in theory) result in additive release of white blood cells.
▷ *Driving, Hazardous Activities:* No restrictions presently attributed to this medicine.

Aviation Note: The use of this drug *is probably not a disqualification* for piloting. Consult a designated Aviation Medical Examiner.

Exposure to Sun: SEVERE intolerance of sunlight (photophobia) has been a treatment-limiting factor.

Occurrence of Unrelated Illness: Report development of chills, fever, or other signs or symptoms of infection immediately to your doctor.

Discontinuation: In patients receiving medicine that suppresses the bone marrow: the drug is usually stopped if a white blood cell count (absolute neutrophil count) reaches 10,000 per cubic mm after the expected lowest white blood cell count is reached, specific to the chemotherapy that was given.

In people receiving medicine that destroys the bone marrow and who subsequently have a bone marrow transplant: the drug is started as described earlier. If the white blood cell count reaches 1,000 per cubic mm, the dose is decreased to 5 mcg per kg of body mass per day. Once the white blood cell count reaches 1,000 per cubic mm for 6 consecutive days, filgrastim can be stopped.

Special Storage Instructions: This drug should be stored at 36 to 46 degrees F (2 to 8 degrees C) once it has been reconstituted. Care should be taken **not to shake** the prepared drug, as it may lose activity. Care should also be taken **not to freeze** the prepared medicine, as it will clump and lose therapeutic activity.

Observe the Following Expiration Times: Once the medicine is prepared, it is stable for 1 day (24 hours) if it is refrigerated. If the drug is stored at room temperature, it is stable for 6 hours. Medicine left at room temperature for more than 6 hours should be returned.

FINASTERIDE (fin ES tur ide)

Introduced: 1992   **Class:** 5-alpha reductase inhibitor   **Prescription:** USA: Yes   **Controlled Drug:** USA: No; Canada: No   **Available as Generic:** USA: No; Canada: No

Brand Names: Proscar, Propecia

BENEFITS versus RISKS	
Possible Benefits	*Possible Risks*
NONSURGICAL TREATMENT OF SYMPTOMATIC BENIGN PROSTATIC HYPERPLASIA. Shrinkage of prostatic tissue and increase in urine flow Increased hair growth	Impotence (small percentage) Decreased libido (small percentage) Gynecomastia

▷ **Principal Uses**

As a Single Drug Product: Uses currently included in FDA-approved labeling: Treatment of symptomatic benign prostatic hyperplasia (BPH). Maximum shrinkage of the prostate has occurred after 6 months of therapy.

Other (unlabeled) generally accepted uses: A study of 200 men showed 58% had clinically significant hair growth after 1 year of use. FDA approval as a hair-restoring agent is being sought.

How This Drug Works: Finasteride blocks an enzyme (chemical responsible for helping a chemical reaction take place) called 5-alpha reductase. This effect blocks the conversion of testosterone to dihydrotestosterone in the liver and tissues; when the dihydrotestosterone hormone is not available, the prostate shrinks. When the prostate shrinks, symptoms such as urgency and difficulty in urination improve.

Available Dosage Forms and Strengths

Finasteride (Proscar) tablets — 5 mg

How to Store

Keep at room temperature. Avoid exposure to extreme humidity.

▷ **Recommended Dosage Ranges** (Actual dosage and administration schedule must be determined for each patient individually.)

Infants and Children: Not indicated.

12 to 60 Years of Age: Symptomatic benign prostatic hyperplasia often does not occur in the younger end of this adult dosing range; however, the dose for this age range is—5 mg each day, taken by mouth.

Hair-restoring agent: 1 mg daily appears to be the appropriate dose.

Over 60 Years of Age: Same as 12 to 60 years of age, unless liver function has decreased.

Conditions Requiring Dosing Adjustments

Liver Function: Extensive metabolism occurs in the liver; however, specific guidelines for decreases in doses are not available. People with abnormal liver function tests should be followed more closely by their physicians.

Kidney Function: No dose decreases needed for mild to moderate kidney failure.

▷ **Dosing Instructions:** May be taken without regard to food. Food changes time to peak blood concentration only.

Usual Duration of Use: Use on a regular schedule for at least 6 months is needed to see this drug's peak benefit in shrinking the prostate and decreasing symptoms. Use for 1 year may be required to demonstrate hair regrowth.

Possible Advantages of This Drug

May give you symptomatic relief of benign prostatic hyperplasia (BPH) without surgery. May be more effective than other available agents in helping hair regrowth.

▷ **This Drug Should Not Be Taken If**
- you have had an allergic reaction to any dosage form of it previously.
- you are a woman or a child.

▷ **Inform Your Physician Before Taking This Drug If**
- you have a history of impaired liver function or liver disease.
- you have kidney problems of any nature.
- your sexual partner is pregnant.

Possible Side Effects (natural, expected, and unavoidable drug actions)

Usually increases testosterone levels; however, the significance of this effect is not known.

▷ **Possible Adverse Effects** (unusual, unexpected, and infrequent reactions)

If any of the following develop, consult your physician promptly for guidance.

Mild Adverse Effects
  Allergic Reactions: Skin rash, hives—rare.
  Plasma testosterone—decreased.
Serious Adverse Effects
  Allergic Reactions: Hypersensitivity reactions—case reports.

▷ **Possible Effects on Sexual Function:** Gynecomastia (most frequent adverse effect)—rare.
  Impotence, decreased libido or decreased volume of ejaculate—infrequent.
  Adverse sexual effects may resolve in more than 60% of patients who continue this medication.

Possible Delayed Adverse Effects: Not defined at present.

Possible Effects on Laboratory Tests
  Decreased PSA (prostate specific antigen).

CAUTION
  1. You should have a digital rectal examination and other examinations for prostate cancer before this medicine is started.
  2. If you have a change in liver function, inform your doctor.
  3. If your sexual partner is pregnant, avoid exposing your partner to your semen. Exposure to finasteride-containing semen may cause genital abnormalities in male offspring.

Precautions for Use
  By Infants and Children: Safety and effectiveness for infants and children are not established.
  By Those Over 60 Years of Age: No specific precautions other than changes related to decreased liver function.

▷ **Advisability of Use During Pregnancy**
  Pregnancy Category: X. See Pregnancy Risk Categories at the back of this book.
  Animal studies: When administered to pregnant rats, the male offspring developed hypospadias. The offspring experienced decreased prostatic and seminal vesicular weight, slow preputial separation, and transient nipple problems.
  Human studies: Contraindicated in women who are pregnant or who plan to become pregnant. Women who are pregnant must avoid exposure to crushed tablets and semen of a sexual partner who is on finasteride.
  Ask your physician for guidance.

Advisability of Use if Breast-Feeding
  Refrain from nursing if you have been exposed to finasteride or finasteride-containing semen.

Habit-Forming Potential: None.

Effects of Overdosage: Multiple doses of up to 80 mg per day have been taken without adverse effect.

Possible Effects of Long-Term Use: Adverse effects of long-term use are similar to short-term use effects.

Suggested Periodic Examinations While Taking This Drug (at physician's discretion)
  Patients should be monitored for signs and symptoms of hypersensitivity.
  Patients should be monitored for improvement in symptoms of BPH.

▷ **While Taking This Drug, Observe the Following**

Foods: This medicine is best taken on an empty stomach.

Beverages: No restrictions.

▷ *Alcohol:* No restrictions.

Tobacco Smoking: No interactions expected, but I advise everyone to quit smoking.

Marijuana Smoking: No interactions expected.

▷ *Other Drugs*

Finasteride may *decrease* the effects of
- theophylline (Theo-Dur, others).

▷ *Driving, Hazardous Activities:* No restrictions.

Aviation Note: No restrictions.

Exposure to Sun: No restrictions.

Special Storage Instructions

Keep at room temperature. Avoid exposure to extreme humidity.

FLUCONAZOLE (flu KOHN a zohl)

Introduced: 1985   **Class:** Antifungal (triazole)   **Prescription:** USA: Yes
Controlled Drug: USA: No; Canada: No   **Available as Generic:** USA: No; Canada: No

Brand Name: Diflucan

BENEFITS versus RISKS	
Possible Benefits	*Possible Risks*
EFFECTIVE TREATMENT AND SUPPRESSION OF CRYPTOCOCCAL MENINGITIS	Severe skin reactions Possible liver damage
EFFECTIVE TREATMENT OF *CANDIDA* INFECTIONS OF THE MOUTH, THROAT, AND ESOPHAGUS	
EFFECTIVE TREATMENT OF SYSTEMIC *CANDIDA* INFECTIONS	
EFFECTIVE SINGLE-DOSE TREATMENT OF VAGINAL YEAST INFECTIONS	

▷ **Principal Uses**

As a Single Drug Product: Uses currently included in FDA-approved labeling: (1) Treatment of *Candida* (yeast) infections of the mouth, throat, and esophagus (may be AIDS related); (2) therapy of systemic *Candida* infections—pneumonia, peritonitis, urinary tract infections (may be AIDS related).

Other (unlabeled) generally accepted uses: (1) Prevention of yeast infections in patients with low white blood cell counts or cancer, or those taking steroids; (2) treatment and suppression of cryptococcal meningitis; (3) treatment of some fungal eye infections (endophthalmitis); (4) single-dose treatment of vaginal yeast infections; (5) treatment of *Aspergillus* pneumonia;

(6) treatment of candidal urinary tract infections; (7) used to treat some fungal infections that may occur in people who have received transplanted organs.

How This Drug Works: By damaging cell walls and blocking essential cell enzymes, this drug inhibits cell growth and reproduction (with low drug concentrations) and destroys fungal cells (with high drug concentrations).

Available Dosage Forms and Strengths

> Injection — 200 mg in 100 ml and 400 mg in 200 ml
> Tablets — 50 mg, 100 mg, 150 mg, 200 mg
> Oral suspension — 50 mg/5 ml
> — 200 mg/5 ml

▷ **Recommended Dosage Ranges** (Actual dosage and administration schedule must be determined for each patient individually.)

Infants and Children: From 3 to 13 years of age: 3–6 mg per kg of body mass daily, depending on the kind and site of infection.

Cryptococcal meningitis has a recommendation for 12 mg per kg of body mass on the first day, followed by 6 mg per kg of body mass once daily for 10 to 12 weeks after the cerebrospinal fluid (CSF) culture becomes negative.

13 to 60 Years of Age: For treatment of cryptococcal meningitis: 400 mg once daily until significant improvement occurs; then 200 to 400 mg once daily for 10 to 12 weeks after the cerebrospinal fluid (CSF) culture becomes negative.

For suppression of cryptococcal meningitis: 200 mg once daily.

For treatment of *Candida* infections of mouth and throat: 200 mg on the first day; then 100 mg once daily for 2 weeks.

For treatment of *Candida* infection of the esophagus: 200 mg on the first day; then 100 mg once daily for at least 3 weeks; continue treatment for 2 weeks after all signs of infection are gone. If needed, doses up to 400 mg once daily may be used. Some patients with chronic mucocutaneous *Candida* infections have benefited from 50 mg/day of this medicine.

For treatment of systemic *Candida* infections: 400 mg once daily for at least 4 weeks; continue treatment for 2 weeks after clearance of all symptoms of infection.

For treatment of vaginal yeast infections (*Candida*): one 150-mg tablet by mouth.

Over 60 Years of Age: Same as 13 to 60 years of age. Dose must be adjusted for impaired kidneys.

Conditions Requiring Dosing Adjustments

Liver Function: This drug is a rare cause of hepatitis and should be used with caution by patients with liver compromise.

Kidney Function: In mild to moderate kidney failure, the usual dose should be given every 48 hours. In severe kidney failure, half (50%) of the usual dose should be given every 48 hours.

▷ **Dosing Instructions:**   The tablet may be crushed; may be taken with or after food to reduce stomach upset.

Usual Duration of Use: Use on a regular schedule for 2 to 4 weeks is usually needed to see this drug's benefit in controlling candidal or cryptococcal infections. Actual cures or long-term suppression often require continual treatment for many months. May be continuous therapy in AIDS patients.

Currently a "Drug of Choice"
for maintenance therapy to prevent relapse following control of AIDS-related candidal esophagitis.

▷ **This Drug Should Not Be Taken If**
- you have had an allergic reaction to it previously.
- you have active liver disease.

▷ **Inform Your Physician Before Taking This Drug If**
- you are allergic to: clotrimazole, itraconazole, ketoconazole, or miconazole.
- you have impaired liver or kidney function.
- you are taking any other drugs currently.
- you tend to have low blood potassium.

▷ **Possible Adverse Effects** (unusual, unexpected, and infrequent reactions)
If any of the following develop, consult your physician promptly for guidance.

Mild Adverse Effects
Allergic Reactions: Skin rash—rare.
Hair loss—very rare with usual doses. Reversible hair loss (alopecia) may be more common with high doses of fluconazole given for 2 months or longer.
Headache—rare.
Nausea, vomiting , stomach pain, diarrhea—frequent.

Serious Adverse Effects
Allergic Reactions: Severe dermatitis (Stevens-Johnson syndrome)—very rare. Anaphylactic reactions—case reports.
Liver toxicity—rare.
Abnormally low platelet counts: abnormal bruising/bleeding or low white blood cell counts—rare.
Seizures or adrenal suppression—case reports, rare.

▷ **Possible Effects on Sexual Function:** No conclusive reports.

Possible Delayed Adverse Effects: Liver toxicity.

▷ **Adverse Effects That May Mimic Natural Diseases or Disorders**
Possible liver reaction may suggest viral hepatitis.

Possible Effects on Laboratory Tests
Blood platelet counts: decreased.
Liver function tests: increased liver enzymes (ALT/GPT, AST/GOT, and alkaline phosphatase), increased bilirubin.
Blood potassium: lowered—rare.

Precautions for Use
By Infants and Children: Safety and effectiveness for those under 13 years of age are not established.
By Those Over 60 Years of Age: Age-related decrease in kidney function may require adjustment of dosage.

▷ **Advisability of Use During Pregnancy**
Pregnancy Category: C. See Pregnancy Risk Categories at the back of this book.
Animal studies: Rat studies revealed significant abnormalities in bone growth and development.

Human studies: Adequate studies of pregnant women are not available. Use this drug only if clearly needed. Ask your doctor for help.

Advisability of Use If Breast-Feeding
Presence of this drug in breast milk: Unknown.
Avoid drug or refrain from nursing.

Habit-Forming Potential: None.

Effects of Overdosage: Possible nausea, vomiting, diarrhea.

Possible Effects of Long-Term Use: None reported.

Suggested Periodic Examinations While Taking This Drug (at physician's discretion)
Liver and kidney function tests.

▷ **While Taking This Drug, Observe the Following**
Foods: No restrictions.
Beverages: No restrictions. May be taken with milk.
▷ *Alcohol:* No interactions expected.
Tobacco Smoking: No interactions expected, but I advise everyone to quit smoking.
▷ *Other Drugs*
Fluconazole may *increase* the effects of
- cyclosporine (Sandimmune).
- oral antidiabetic drugs (chlorpropamide, glipizide, glyburide, tolbutamide), and cause hypoglycemia; check glucose levels carefully.
- phenytoin (Dilantin, etc.), and cause phenytoin toxicity; monitor phenytoin blood levels.
- trimetrexate (Neutrexin).
- warfarin (Coumadin), and cause unwanted bleeding; monitor prothrombin times as necessary.
- zidovudine (AZT) and result in toxicity. The zidovudine dose may need to be decreased if this combination is to be continued.

The following drugs may *decrease* the effects of fluconazole
- cimetidine (Tagamet).
- rifampin (Rifadin, Rimactane, etc.).

Fluconazole *taken concurrently* with
- astemizole (Hismanal) may result in fatal toxicity to the heart.
- cisapride (Propulsid) may lead to adverse effects on the heart. DO NOT COMBINE.
- hydrochlorothiazide (Esidrix, others) may increase potassium loss.
- loratadine (Claritin) may result in increased blood levels of loratadine, but to date, toxicity to the heart has not been reported. Since blood levels may be increased if combined use is undertaken, it is prudent to decrease the dose of loratadine.
- oral hypoglycemic agents (see Antidiabetic Drugs) may result in increased lowering of blood sugar.
- terfenadine (Seldane) may result in toxicity to the heart.

▷ *Driving, Hazardous Activities:* No restrictions.
Aviation Note: The use of this drug *is probably not a disqualification* for piloting. Consult a designated Aviation Medical Examiner.
Exposure to Sun: No restrictions.

Discontinuation: Take the full course prescribed. Continual treatment for several months may be necessary. Consult your physician regarding the appropriate time to consider discontinuation.

FLUCYTOSINE (flu SI toh seen)

Other Names: 5-fluorocytosine, 5-FC

Introduced: 1977   **Class:** Antifungal   **Prescription:** USA: Yes   **Controlled Drug:**   USA: No; Canada: No   **Available as Generic:**   USA: No; Canada: No

Brand Names: Ancobon, ✦Ancotil

BENEFITS versus RISKS	
Possible Benefits	*Possible Risks*
EFFECTIVE ADJUNCTIVE TREATMENT OF CERTAIN INFECTIONS CAUSED BY *CANDIDA, CRYPTOCOCCUS* FUNGI, and *Aspergillus* Effective adjunctive treatment of chromomycosis infection	BONE MARROW DEPRESSION DRUG-INDUCED LIVER DAMAGE Peripheral neuritis

▷ **Principal Uses**

As a Single Drug Product: Uses currently included in FDA-approved labeling: (1) Treatment of endocarditis, osteomyelitis, arthritis, meningitis, pneumonia, septicemia, and urinary tract infections caused by *Candida*; (2) treatment of meningitis, pneumonia, septicemia, endocarditis, and urinary tract infections caused by *Cryptococcus*.

Other (unlabeled) generally accepted uses: (1) Treatment of disseminated candidiasis, chromomycosis, and cryptococcosis (these infections may be AIDS related); (2) treatment of general fungal infections.

Note: Flucytosine is usually used together with amphotericin B to treat disseminated fungal infections.

How This Drug Works: This drug goes into fungal cells and blocks production of RNA and DNA, thus inhibiting fungal development and reproduction.

Available Dosage Forms and Strengths

Capsules — 250 mg, 500 mg

▷ **Recommended Dosage Ranges** (Actual dosage and administration schedule must be determined for each patient individually.)

Infants and Children: 50 to 150 mg per kg of body mass, divided into four equal doses and given every 6 hours.

12 to 60 Years of Age: 50 to 150 mg per kg of body mass, divided into equal doses and given every 6 hours. In some severe infections, 250 mg per kg of body mass per day have been given.

Over 60 Years of Age: Same as 12 to 60 years of age. If kidney function is impaired, dosage reduction is mandatory.

Conditions Requiring Dosing Adjustments

Liver Function: In mild to moderate liver compromise, changes in dosage do not presently appear to be needed. Flucytosine has been associated with liver toxicity (especially with blood levels greater than 100 mcg/ml), and should be used with caution by patients with liver compromise.

Kidney Function: In mild to moderate kidney failure, the usual dose can be given every 12–24 hours. In severe kidney failure, the usual dose can be given every 24–48 hours.

▷ **Dosing Instructions:**   If a single dose requires more than one capsule, space administration over a period of 15 minutes to reduce stomach irritation and nausea. The capsule may be opened and taken with or after food.

Usual Duration of Use: Use on a regular schedule for 4 to 6 weeks is needed to see effectiveness in controlling *Candida* or cryptococcal infection. Long-term use (months to years) requires periodic physician evaluation.

▷ **This Drug Should Not Be Taken If**
  • you have had an allergic reaction to it previously.
  • you have an active blood cell or bone marrow disorder.
  • you have active liver disease.

▷ **Inform Your Physician Before Taking This Drug If**
  • you have a history of drug-induced bone marrow depression.
  • you have a history of peripheral neuritis.
  • you have impaired liver or kidney function.

Possible Side Effects (natural, expected, and unavoidable drug actions)
  None.

▷ **Possible Adverse Effects** (unusual, unexpected, and infrequent reactions)
  If any of the following develop, consult your physician promptly for guidance.

  Mild Adverse Effects
  Allergic Reactions: Skin rash, itching.
  Headache, dizziness, drowsiness, confusion, hallucinations—infrequent.
  Loss of appetite, nausea, vomiting, stomach pain, diarrhea—possible and dose related.

  Serious Adverse Effects
  Allergic Reactions: Anaphylactic reactions.
  Bone marrow depression (see Glossary): fatigue, weakness, fever, sore throat, abnormal bleeding or bruising—rare.
  Liver damage, with or without jaundice (see Glossary)—case reports.
  Peripheral neuritis (see Glossary)—possible.
  Bowel perforation or kidney damage—rare.

▷ **Possible Effects on Sexual Function:**   None reported.

▷ **Adverse Effects That May Mimic Natural Diseases or Disorders**
  Drug-induced hepatitis may suggest viral hepatitis.

Natural Diseases or Disorders That May Be Activated by This Drug
  Crohn's disease, ulcerative colitis.

Possible Effects on Laboratory Tests
  Complete blood counts: decreased red cells, hemoglobin, white cells, and platelets.
  Liver function tests: increased liver enzymes (ALT/GPT, AST/GOT, and alkaline phosphatase), increased bilirubin.
  Kidney function tests: increased blood urea nitrogen (BUN) and creatinine.
  Serum creatinine: may be falsely increased if tested by some methods.

CAUTION
1. When this drug is used alone, resistance can occur rapidly; it is usually used concurrently with amphotericin B (Abelcet) (given intravenously).

Precautions for Use
By Infants and Children: No information available.
By Those Over 60 Years of Age: If necessary, adjust dosage for age-related decrease in kidney function.

▷ **Advisability of Use During Pregnancy**
Pregnancy Category: C. See Pregnancy Risk Categories at the back of this book.
  Animal studies: Rat studies reveal drug-induced birth defects.
  Human studies: Adequate studies of pregnant women are not available.
  Use this drug only if clearly needed. Ask your physician for guidance.

Advisability of Use If Breast-Feeding
  Presence of this drug in breast milk: Yes.
  Avoid drug or refrain from nursing.

Habit-Forming Potential: None.

Effects of Overdosage: Nausea, vomiting, stomach pain, diarrhea, confusion.

Possible Effects of Long-Term Use: Bone marrow depression, liver or kidney damage.

Suggested Periodic Examinations While Taking This Drug (at physician's discretion)
  Measurement of blood levels of flucytosine.
  Complete blood cell counts.
  Liver and kidney function tests.

▷ **While Taking This Drug, Observe the Following**
Foods: No restrictions.
Beverages: No restrictions. May be taken with milk.
▷ *Alcohol:* No interactions expected.
Tobacco Smoking: No interactions expected, but I advise everyone to quit smoking.
▷ *Other Drugs*
  The following drugs may *decrease* the effects of flucytosine
  • antacids.
  • cytarabine (Cytosar).
  Flucytosine *taken concurrently* with
  • amphotericin B may result in increased risk of kidney toxicity; lipid-associated form (Abelcet) may help avoid this.
  • zidovudine (AZT) may result in additive and serious blood (hematological) toxicity.
▷ *Driving, Hazardous Activities:* This drug may cause dizziness, drowsiness, or confusion. Limit activities as necessary.
Aviation Note: The use of this drug *may be a disqualification* for piloting. Consult a designated Aviation Medical Examiner.
Exposure to Sun: Use caution—this drug may cause photosensitivity (see Glossary).
Discontinuation: This drug may be needed for an extended period of time. Your physician should decide the appropriate time to stop it.

FLUNISOLIDE (flu NIS oh lide)

Introduced: 1980   **Class:** Antiasthmatic, cortisonelike drugs   **Prescription:** USA: Yes   **Controlled Drug:** USA: No; Canada: No   **Available as Generic:** No

Brand Names: AeroBid, AeroBid-M, ✦Bronalide, Nasalide, Nasarel, ✦Rhinalar

BENEFITS versus RISKS	
Possible Benefits	*Possible Risks*
EFFECTIVE CONTROL OF SEVERE, CHRONIC BRONCHIAL ASTHMA	Yeast infections of mouth and throat (inhaler form)
	Increased susceptibility to respiratory tract infections (inhaler form)
	Localized areas of "allergic" pneumonia (inhaler form)

▷ **Principal Uses**

As a Single Drug Product: Uses currently included in FDA-approved labeling: (1) Treats chronic bronchial asthma in people who require cortisonelike drugs for asthma control. This inhalation form is better than cortisone taken by mouth (swallowed) or by injection, as it works locally on the respiratory tract; (2) treatment of various kinds of hay fever (seasonal or perennial allergic rhinitis).

Other (unlabeled) generally accepted uses: (1) Treatment of nasal polyps; (2) treatment of bronchopulmonary dysplasia; (3) may have a role in acute or chronic sinusitis in combination with an antibiotic (amoxicillin/clavulanate in one study).

How This Drug Works: By increasing cyclic AMP, this drug may increase epinephrine, which is an effective bronchodilator and antiasthmatic. An additional benefit is reduction of local allergic reaction and inflammation.

Available Dosage Forms and Strengths

Inhalation aerosol — 0.25 mg (250 mcg) per metered spray
Nasal solution — 25 mcg per actuation

▷ **Recommended Dosage Ranges** (Actual dosage and administration schedule must be determined for each patient individually.)

Infants and Children: Oral inhalation:
Up to 6 years old—not recommended.
6–15 years old—two inhalations or 500 mcg twice a day. Maximum daily dose is 1 mg.
Nasal inhalation:
Up to 6 years old—not recommended.
6–15 years old—0.25 mcg (one spray in each nostril) three times a day. Once the peak effect is seen, the dose should be reduced to the smallest dose and frequency that works. Maximum is four sprays in each nostril (200 mcg/day).
Aqueous nasal form:
Up to 6 years old—not recommended.
6–14 years old—two sprays in each nostril twice daily or one spray in each

nostril three times a day. Once the peak effect is seen, the dose should be reduced to the smallest dose and frequency that works.

15 to 60 Years of Age: Oral inhalation:

0.5 to 1 mg (two to four metered sprays) twice a day, morning and evening. Limit total daily dose to 2 mg (four inhalations twice daily). Once the peak effect is seen, the dose should be reduced to the smallest dose and frequency that works.

Nasal inhalation:

Two sprays per nostril twice daily. The dose may be increased to two sprays in each nostril three times a day (300 mcg/day). Maximum dose with this route is eight sprays in each nostril (400 mcg) daily. Once the peak effect is seen, the dose should be reduced to the smallest dose and frequency that works.

Aqueous nasal form:

Two sprays in each nostril twice daily to start. Maintenance dosing is continued with the lowest dose that is effective. This may be as low as one spray in each nostril daily.

Over 60 Years of Age: Same as 15 to 60 years of age.

Conditions Requiring Dosing Adjustments

Liver Function: Specific guidelines are not available for dosage adjustment in liver compromise.

Kidney Function: No specific changes are recommended for patients with compromised kidneys.

▷ **Dosing Instructions:** May be used as needed without regard to eating. Shake the container well before using. Carefully follow the printed patient instructions provided with the inhaler; rinse the mouth and throat (gargle) with water thoroughly after each inhalation.

Usual Duration of Use: Use on a regular schedule for 1 to 4 weeks is necessary to see effectiveness in controlling severe, chronic asthma. Long-term use requires physician supervision and guidance.

▷ **This Drug Should Not Be Taken If**
- you have had an allergic reaction to it previously.
- you are experiencing severe acute asthma or status asthmaticus that requires more intense treatment for prompt relief.
- you have a form of nonallergic bronchitis with asthmatic features.

▷ **Inform Your Physician Before Taking This Drug If**
- you are now taking or have recently taken any cortisone-related drug (including ACTH by injection; see Drug Classes) for any reason.
- you have a history of tuberculosis (inhalation form).
- you have herpes simplex infection of the eye.
- you have chickenpox.
- you have had recent surgery of the nose, have ulcers of the nose or nosebleeds—this medicine should be used cautiously until the site has healed.
- you have chronic bronchitis or bronchiectasis.
- you think you may have an active infection of any kind, especially a respiratory infection.

Possible Side Effects (natural, expected, and unavoidable drug actions)

Yeast infections (thrush) of the mouth and throat.

Unpleasant taste. Orally inhaled flunisolide can cause flu-like symptoms occasionally in people taking the drug by oral inhalation.

▷ **Possible Adverse Effects** (unusual, unexpected, and infrequent reactions)

If any of the following develop, consult your physician promptly for guidance.

Mild Adverse Effects

Allergic Reactions: Skin rash, hives, itching.

Headache, dizziness, nervousness, moodiness, insomnia, loss of smell or taste—rare to infrequent.

Aftertaste (nasal form)—frequent.

Upper respiratory infections, cough—possible.

Heart palpitation, increased blood pressure, swelling of feet and ankles (inhalation form)—possible.

Loss of appetite, indigestion, nausea, vomiting, stomach pain, diarrhea—infrequent.

Sore throat, stinging of the nose—infrequent to frequent.

Nasal irritation—infrequent to frequent (less common with the aqueous form).

Impaired sense of smell—possible.

Osteoporosis—possible with long-term use.

Serious Adverse Effects

Allergic Reaction: Localized areas of "allergic" pneumonitis (lung inflammation).

Bronchospasm, asthmatic wheezing—rare with the inhalation form.

Tachycardia or hypertension—rare with the inhalation form.

▷ **Possible Effects on Sexual Function:**   None reported.

Natural Diseases or Disorders That May Be Activated by This Drug

Cortisone-related drugs (used by inhalation) that produce systemic effects can impair immunity and lead to reactivation of "healed" or quiescent tuberculosis. People with a history of tuberculosis should be watched closely during use of cortisonelike drugs by inhalation.

Possible Effects on Laboratory Tests

None reported.

CAUTION

1. This drug does not act primarily as a brochodilator and **should not be used** for immediate relief of acute asthma.
2. If you were using any cortisone-related drugs for treatment of your asthma *before* changing to this inhaler, you may need to restart the cortisone-related drug if you are injured, have an infection, or require surgery. Be sure to tell your doctor about prior use of cortisone-related drugs taken either by mouth or by injection.
3. If severe asthma returns while using this drug, call your physician immediately so that supportive treatment can be provided as needed.
4. If you have used cortisone-related drugs in the past year, carry a card that says this has happened. During periods of stress it may be necessary to resume cortisone treatment in adequate dosage.
5. Five to ten minutes should separate the inhalation of bronchodilators

such as albuterol, epinephrine, pirbuterol, etc. (which should be used first) and the inhalation of this drug. This lets more flunisolide reach the bronchial tubes and reduces risk of adverse effects from the propellants used in the two inhalers.

6. A decongestant may be a good idea in people with blocked nasal passages. Talk with your doctor or pharmacist.

Precautions for Use
By Infants and Children: Safety and effectiveness for those under 4 years of age are not established. To obtain maximal benefit, the use of a spacer device is recommended for inhalation therapy in children.

By Those Over 60 Years of Age: People with chronic bronchitis or bronchiectasis should be watched closely for the development of lung infections.

▷ **Advisability of Use During Pregnancy**
Pregnancy Category: C. See Pregnancy Risk Categories at the back of this book.
Animal studies: Rat and rabbit studies reveal significant birth defects due to this drug.
Human studies: Adequate studies of pregnant women are not available.
Avoid drug during the first 3 months. Use infrequently and only as clearly needed during the final 6 months.

Advisability of Use If Breast-Feeding
Presence of this drug in breast milk: Unknown.
Avoid drug or refrain from nursing.

Habit-Forming Potential: With recommended dosage, a state of functional dependence (see Glossary) is not likely to develop.

Effects of Overdosage: Indications of cortisone excess (due to systemic absorption)—fluid retention, flushing of the face, stomach irritation, nervousness.

Possible Effects of Long-Term Use: Development of acne, cataracts, altered menstrual pattern. Osteoporosis.

Suggested Periodic Examinations While Taking This Drug (at physician's discretion)
Inspection of mouth and throat for evidence of yeast infection.
Check of adrenal function in people who have used cortisone-related drugs for an extended period of time before using this drug. X ray of the lungs of people with a prior history of tuberculosis. Bone mineral density testing (osteoporosis test) with long-term use.

▷ **While Taking This Drug, Observe the Following**
Foods: No specific restrictions beyond those advised by your physician.
Beverages: No specific restrictions.

▷ *Alcohol:* No interactions expected.

Tobacco Smoking: No interactions expected. However, smoking can worsen asthma and reduce the effectiveness of this drug. I advise everyone to quit smoking.

▷ *Other Drugs*
The following drugs may *increase* the effects of flunisolide
- inhalant bronchodilators—albuterol, bitolterol, epinephrine, etc.
- oral bronchodilators—aminophylline, ephedrine, terbutaline, theophylline, etc.

Flunisolide *taken concurrently* with
- stanozolol may result in increased risk of acne or edema.

▷ *Driving, Hazardous Activities:* No restrictions.

Aviation Note: The use of this drug and the disorder for which this drug is prescribed *may be disqualifications* for piloting. Consult a designated Aviation Medical Examiner.

Exposure to Sun: No restrictions.

Occurrence of Unrelated Illness: Acute infections, serious injuries, or surgical procedures can create an urgent need for cortisone-related drugs given by mouth and/or injection. Call your doctor immediately in the event of new illness or injury.

Discontinuation: If this drug has made it possible to reduce or discontinue cortisonelike drugs by mouth, *do not* stop this drug abruptly. If you must stop this drug, call your doctor promptly. Cortisone preparations and other measures may be necessary.

Special Storage Instructions: Store at room temperature. Avoid exposure to temperatures above 120 degrees F (49 degrees C). Do not store or use this inhaler near heat or open flame.

FLUOROQUINOLONE ANTIBIOTICS

Ciprofloxacin (sip roh FLOX a sin) **Levofloxacin** (leev oh FLOX a sin) **Lomefloxacin** (loh me FLOX a sin) **Norfloxacin** (nor FLOX a sin) **Ofloxacin** (oh FLOX a sin) **Sparfloxacin** (SPAR flox a sin)

Introduced: 1984, 1996, 1992, 1986, 1984, 1996, respectively**Author's Note: Information on levofloxacin (Levaquin) and sparfloxacin (Zagam) will be expanded once it is available.**   **Class:** Anti-infective, fluoroquinolone

Prescription: USA: Yes   **Controlled Drug:** USA: No   **Available as Generic:** USA: No

Brand Names: Ciprofloxacin: Ciloxan, Cipro; Lomefloxacin: Maxaquin, Norfloxacin: Noroxin, Noroxin Ophthalmic, Chibroxin; Ofloxacin: Floxin, Floxin Uropak, Ocuflox

Warning: Some physicians are using the name "Norflox" to identify this drug when issuing orders (for inpatients) or prescriptions (for outpatients). Norflox is not an accepted name for this drug in any setting for any reason. This coinage of an abbreviated name has resulted in serious medication errors— the dispensing of Norflex, the generic drug orphenadrine, a skeletal muscle relaxant. Ask your pharmacist to verify that you are getting the right drug, an anti-infective.

Warning: **Reports are being made for some drugs in this class which find tendon rupture as a rare adverse effect. Ask your doctor about limits on strenuous exercise while you are taking this medicine. A rare idiosyncratic reaction has also been reported which presents as mental confusion and disorientation. Use of these medicines after head trauma may be a risk factor. If you have suffered a fall, ask your doctor if a medicine in a different antibiotic class should be substituted. If you are taking this drug and notice a change in your thinking, call your doctor.**

BENEFITS versus RISKS	
Possible Benefits	*Possible Risks*
HIGHLY EFFECTIVE TREATMENT FOR INFECTIONS OF THE LOWER RESPIRATORY TRACT (ciprofloxacin and ofloxacin), URINARY TRACT, BONES, JOINTS, AND SKIN TISSUES due to susceptible organisms Effective treatment for some forms of bacterial gastroenteritis (diarrhea) Effective treatment for some infections of the prostate gland	Nausea, indigestion Drug-induced colitis Hallucination or seizure Tendon rupture

▷ **Principal Uses**

As a Single Drug Product: Uses currently included in FDA-approved labeling: Treats responsive infections (in adults) of: (1) the lower respiratory tract (lungs and bronchial tubes); (2) the urinary tract (kidneys, bladder, urethra [including uncomplicated gonorrhea], and prostate gland); (3) the digestive tract (small intestine and colon); (4) bones and joints (ciprofloxacin; ofloxacin—unlabeled); (5) skin and related tissues; (6) used in an ophthalmic preparation to treat bacterial conjunctivitis caused by susceptible organisms; (7) ciprofloxacin has been approved to treat mild to moderate acute sinusitis caused by *Streptococcus pneumoniae*, *Haemophilus influenzae*, or *Moraxella catarrhalis*.

Other (unlabeled) generally accepted uses: (1) Can have a role in treating cholera where the organisms are resistant to doxycycline (ciprofloxacin); (2) lessens symptoms or prevents traveler's diarrhea; (3) ciprofloxacin can be of use in treating some unusual organisms such as *Aeromonas*, cat-scratch fever, or chancroid; (4) ofloxacin may help in combination therapy of leprosy.

How These Drugs Work: These medicines block the bacterial enzyme DNA gyrase (required for DNA synthesis and cell reproduction), and arrests bacterial growth (in low concentrations) and kills bacteria (in high concentrations).

Available Dosage Forms and Strengths

Ciprofloxacin:
  Tablets — 250 mg, 500 mg, 750 mg
Ophthalmic solution — 0.3%
Lomefloxacin:
  Tablets — 400 mg
Norfloxacin:
  Tablets — 400 mg
Ophthalmic solution — 3 mg/ml
Ofloxacin:
  Tablets — 200 mg, 300 mg, 400 mg
Ophthalmic solution — 3 mg/ml

▷ **Usual Adult Dosage Range:**   Ciprofloxacin: 250 mg to 750 mg every 12 hours, depending upon the nature and severity of the infection. The total daily dosage should not exceed 1500 mg. Mild to moderate sinusitis (caused by organisms outlined above) is treated with 500 mg every 12 hours for 10 days in adults. Ophthalmic: one or two drops instilled in the eye every 2 hours while awake for 2 days, then one or two drops for 5 more days, which is given every 4 hours while awake.

Norfloxacin: Uncomplicated urinary tract infections—400 mg every 12 hours for 3 days. Complicated urinary tract infections—400 mg every 12 hours for 10 to 21 days. Total daily dosage should not exceed 800 mg. Ophthalmic dosing: one to two drops to the affected eye four times daily.

Ofloxacin: 200 mg to 400 mg every 12 hours (for 10 days for lower respiratory infections), depending upon the nature and severity of the infection. The total daily dosage should not exceed 800 mg. Ophthalmic dosing (conjunctivitis)—one to two drops every 2 to 4 hours for 2 days, then four times a day for 7 to 10 days.

Infants and Children: Lomefloxacin: Use not recommended.

18 to 60 Years of Age: Lomefloxacin: For bronchitis—400 mg daily for 10 days. For bladder infections (cystitis)—400 mg daily for 10 days. For complicated urinary tract infections—400 mg daily for 14 days. For preoperative prevention of urinary tract infection—400 mg (single dose) taken 2 to 6 hours before surgery.

Over 60 Years of Age: Lomefloxacin: Same as 18 to 60 years of age.

Note: Actual dosage and administration schedule for all these medicines must be determined for each patient individually.

Conditions Requiring Dosing Adjustments

Liver Function: Ciprofloxacin, norfloxacin: use with caution in severe liver failure. No changes for ofloxacin.

Kidney Function: Ciprofloxacin, lomefloxacin, norfloxacin, and ofloxacin **must** be decreased (or interval lengthened) in kidney compromise. For patients with moderate to severe kidney compromise, the ofloxacin dose should be decreased to 400 mg daily. For patients with moderate kidney failure, the usual ofloxacin dose can be taken every 24 hours. For patients with severe failure, one-half the usual dose should be taken every 24 hours. Since norfloxacin is a rare cause of crystalluria, patients taking the drug should drink adequate quantities of water.

Cystic Fibrosis

A loading dose for ciprofloxacin, as well as ongoing doses of 750 mg every 8 hours, is taken by cystic fibrosis patients. This dosing gives blood levels that are more aggressive versus the bacteria which usually cause infections in these patients. No changes for the other drugs are presented.

▷ **Dosing Instructions:**   Ciprofloxacin, lomefloxacin, or norfloxacin may be taken with or without food (NOT dairy products) and all may be crushed. Ofloxacin is best taken 2 hours after eating. Drink large amounts of fluids during treatment. Avoid aluminum or magnesium antacids, iron, zinc, or calcium for 2 hours before and after taking these medicines.

Usual Duration of Use: Use on a regular schedule for 7 to 14 days is needed to see these drugs' effectiveness in eradicating infection. The drugs should be continued for at least 2 days after all indications of infection have disappeared. Bone and joint infections (ciprofloxacin or ofloxacin) or prostate gland infections may be treated for 6 weeks or longer. Long-term use requires periodic evaluation of response.

Possible Advantages of These Drugs

Ciprofloxacin and ofloxacin: very broad spectrums of antibacterial activity of all currently available oral antimicrobial drugs. Highly effective in treating numerous types of infection caused by a wide spectrum of bacteria. Provide effective drug levels in the prostate gland (a difficult place to penetrate). Lomefloxacin has not had significant effects on kidney function.

▷ **These Drugs Should Not Be Taken If**
- you have had an allergic reaction to these or any quinolone drug previously.
- you are pregnant or breast-feeding.
- you have a seizure disorder that is not adequately controlled.
- these drugs have been prescribed for a person under 18 years of age.

▷ **Inform Your Physician Before Taking These Drugs If**
- you are allergic to cinoxacin (Cinobac), nalidixic acid (NegGram), or other quinolone drugs.
- you have a seizure disorder or a circulatory disorder of the brain.
- you have impaired liver or kidney function.
- you have a history of mental disorders (psychosis).
- you are taking any form of probenecid or theophylline.
- your work requires heavy manual labor. Several cases of tendon rupture have been reported with fluoroquinolone use. Heavy exercise or work may be contraindicated. Call your doctor immediately if you develop inflammation or pain in a tendon.

Possible Side Effects (natural, expected, and unavoidable drug actions)

Superinfections (see Glossary). Permanent greenish tooth discoloration if used in infants (ciprofloxacin).

▷ **Possible Adverse Effects** (unusual, unexpected, and infrequent reactions)

If any of the following develop, consult your physician promptly for guidance.

Mild Adverse Effects

Allergic Reactions: Rash, itching, localized swelling—rare.

Dizziness, headache (frequent with lomefloxacin), weakness, migraine, anxiety, abnormal vision—rare.

Nausea, diarrhea, vomiting, indigestion—rare to infrequent.

Muscle aches—case reports.

Burning feeling in the eye when the ophthalmic solutions are used—possible.

Decreased vision (with ophthalmic use)—case reports.

Serious Adverse Effects

Allergic Reactions: Anaphylaxis—case reports.

Idiosyncratic Reactions: Central nervous system stimulation—restlessness, tremor, confusion, hallucinations, seizures. One medication of this class has had instances of severe neurological compromise reported with use of the drug. Stop the medication immediately and call your doctor if you experience confusion, trouble speaking, or disorientation once taking this drug—case reports.

Kidney disease (interstitial nephritis)—case reports.

Tendon rupture—case reports.

Abnormal heart beats or palpitations—rare.

Liver toxicity—rare.

Intracranial hypertension (ciprofloxacin or ofloxacin)—case reports.

Worsening of myasthenia gravis—case reports.

▷ **Possible Effects on Sexual Function:** Vaginitis with discharge has been reported. Painful menstruation, excessive menstrual bleeding (ofloxacin only)—case reports. Lomefloxacin has case reports of intermenstrual bleeding.

Natural Diseases or Disorders That May Be Activated by These Drugs

Latent epilepsy, latent gout.

Possible Effects on Laboratory Tests

Kidney function: increased blood creatinine and urea nitrogen (BUN)—rare.

Liver function tests: increased as a sign of liver toxicity—rare.

Red and white blood cell counts: rarely decreased (norfloxacin).

Blood glucose levels: rare fluctuations.

CAUTION

1. With high doses or prolonged use, crystal formation in the kidneys may occur. This can be prevented by drinking large amounts of water, up to 2 quarts daily.
2. These drugs may decrease saliva formation, making dental cavities or gum disease more likely. Consult your dentist if dry mouth persists.
3. Strenuous exercise is NOT recommended while these medicines are being taken.
4. If a sudden change in mental status is noticed, call your doctor immediately.

Precautions for Use

By Infants and Children: Avoid the use of this drug completely. Impairs normal bone growth and development.

By Those Over 60 Years of Age: Impaired kidney function may require dosage reduction.

▷ **Advisability of Use During Pregnancy**

Pregnancy Category: C. See Pregnancy Risk Categories at the back of this book.

Animal studies: No birth defects due to this drug found in mouse or rat studies. Rabbit studies showed maternal weight loss and increased abortions (ciprofloxacin). Ofloxacin: mild skeletal defects due to this drug were found in rat studies; toxic effects on the fetus were shown in rat and rabbit studies. These drugs can impair normal bone development in immature dogs.

Human studies: Adequate studies of pregnant women are not available. However, the potential for adverse effects on fetal bone development contraindicates the use of these drugs during entire pregnancy.

Advisability of Use If Breast-Feeding

Presence of this drug in breast milk: Probably yes; ofloxacin, yes.

Avoid drug or refrain from nursing.

Habit-Forming Potential: None.

Effects of Overdosage: Confusion, headache, abdominal pain, diarrhea, liver toxicity, seizures, kidney toxicity, and hallucinations.

Possible Effects of Long-Term Use: Superinfections (see Glossary); crystal formation in kidneys.

Suggested Periodic Examinations While Taking These Drugs (at physician's discretion)
Liver function tests, urine analysis.

While Taking These Drugs, Observe the Following
Foods: Caffeine will remain in your system longer than usual. Use care in the amount of caffeine consumed. Dairy foods will decrease the effectiveness of these drugs by decreasing the amount absorbed.
Beverages: No restrictions (see note on caffeine above). May be taken with milk.
▷ *Alcohol:* No interactions expected, but since heavy alcohol intake can blunt the immune system, limit alcohol if you are ill enough to require an antibiotic.
Tobacco Smoking: No interactions expected, but I advise everyone to quit smoking.
▷ *Other Drugs*
The following drug may ***increase*** the effects of fluoroquinolones
• probenecid (Benemid).
Fluoroquinolones ***taken concurrently*** with
• azlocillin may result in toxicity.
• caffeine will result in increased caffeine levels.
• cyclosporine (Sandimmune) may result in increased risk of kidney toxicity.
• foscarnet (Foscavir) may result in an increased risk of seizures.
• phenytoin (Dilantin) may result in increased or decreased Dilantin levels.
• theophylline (Theo-Dur, others) (norfloxacin or ciprofloxacin) may lead to theophylline toxicity over time.
• warfarin (Coumadin) can result in increased risk of bleeding. More frequent INR testing is needed.
The following drugs may ***decrease*** the effects of fluoroquinolones
• antacids containing aluminum or magnesium can reduce absorption and lessen effectiveness.
• calcium supplements.
• didanosine (ciprofloxacin only).
• iron salts.
• magnesium—will decrease the therapeutic benefits.
• nitrofurantoin (Macrodantin, etc.)—may antagonize the antibacterial action in the urinary tract. Avoid this combination.
• sucralfate (Carafate).
• zinc salts.
▷ *Driving, Hazardous Activities:* May cause dizziness or impair vision. Restrict activities as necessary.
Aviation Note: The use of these drugs ***may be a disqualification*** for piloting. Consult a designated Aviation Medical Examiner.
Exposure to Sun: Some members of this class have caused photosensitivity (see Glossary). Sunglasses are advised if eyes are overly sensitive to bright light. A strong sunblock is advised for your skin.
Heavy Exercise or Exertion: Several reports have surfaced regarding tendon rupture in patients on some of the medications in this class. It is prudent to avoid heavy exercise or exertion while you are taking a fluoroquinolone.
Discontinuation: If you experience no adverse effects from these drugs, take the full course prescribed for best results. Ask your doctor when to stop treatment.

FLUOXETINE (flu OX e teen)

Introduced: 1978   **Class:** Antidepressant   **Prescription:** USA: Yes
Controlled Drug: USA: No   **Available as Generic:** USA: No
Brand Name: Prozac

BENEFITS versus RISKS	
Possible Benefits	*Possible Risks*
EFFECTIVE TREATMENT OF MAJOR DEPRESSIVE DISORDERS	Serious allergic reactions
	Conversion of depression to mania in manic-depressive (bipolar) disorders
Possibly effective in relieving the symptoms of obsessive-compulsive disorder	

▷ **Principal Uses**

As a Single Drug Product: Uses currently included in FDA-approved labeling: (1) Treatment of major forms of depression. This drug should not be used to treat the symptoms of mild and transient (reactive) depression; (2) obsessive-compulsive disorder; (3) treatment of bulimia.

Other (unlabeled) generally accepted uses: (1) refractory diabetic neuropathy; (2) may help control kleptomania; (3) can be of help in treating obesity, especially when obesity is accompanied by depression; (4) eases symptoms of panic attacks; (5) may be given only during the premenstrual period to treat premenstrual syndrome (PMS); (6) used to treat seasonal affective disorder (such as depression limited to winter months).

How This Drug Works: It slowly restores normal levels of a nerve transmitter (serotonin).

Available Dosage Forms and Strengths

Capsules — 10 mg, 20 mg
Syrup — 20 mg/5 ml

▷ **Usual Adult Dosage Range:**   Started at 20 mg as a single morning dose; if no improvement occurs after several weeks of treatment, the dose may be increased by 20 mg/day as needed and tolerated. Doses over 20 mg/day should be divided into two equal doses and taken twice daily. Maximum daily dosage is 80 mg. **Note: Actual dosage and administration schedule must be determined for each patient individually.**

Conditions Requiring Dosing Adjustments

Liver Function: The dose should be decreased or the dosing interval lengthened for patients with liver compromise. Some clinicians decrease the dose by 50% in compensated cirrhosis. This drug is also a rare cause of liver toxicity, and should be used with caution by this patient population.

Kidney Function: The dose should be decreased or the time between doses increased in severe kidney (renal) compromise.

▷ **Dosing Instructions:**   The capsule may be opened and the contents mixed with any convenient food. To make smaller doses, the contents may be mixed with orange juice or apple juice (NOT GRAPEFRUIT JUICE) and refrigerated; doses of 5–10 mg may prove effective and better tolerated.

Usual Duration of Use: Use on a regular schedule for as little as 1 to 2 weeks may reveal the beginning of improvement in depression. Up to 4 to 8 weeks may be needed to determine (1) this drug's effectiveness in relieving depression; (2) the pattern of both favorable and unfavorable effects. Since there is an active metabolite and a long half-life, it may take several weeks before the benefits of a change in dose are seen. Long-term use (months to years) requires periodic physician evaluation.

Possible Advantages of This Drug

Does not cause weight gain, a common side effect of tricyclic antidepressants. May actually cause weight loss.

Less likely to cause dry mouth, constipation, urinary retention, orthostatic hypotension (see Glossary), and heart rhythm disturbances than tricyclic antidepressants.

Does not cause Parkinson-like reactions.

▷ **This Drug Should Not Be Taken If**

• you have had an allergic reaction to any dosage form of it previously.
• you currently take or have taken within the past 14 days any monoamine oxidase (MAO) type A inhibitor (see Drug Classes).

▷ **Inform Your Physician Before Taking This Drug If**

• you have had any adverse effects from antidepressant drugs.
• you have impaired liver or kidney function.
• you have Parkinson's disease.
• you have a seizure disorder.
• you have a history of psychosis.
• you have a history of SIADH (talk with your doctor).
• you are pregnant or plan pregnancy while taking this drug.

Possible Side Effects (natural, expected, and unavoidable drug actions)

Decreased appetite, weight loss. Case reports of orthostatic hypotension (see Glossary).

▷ **Possible Adverse Effects** (unusual, unexpected, and infrequent reactions)

If any of the following develop, consult your physician promptly for guidance.

Mild Adverse Effects

Allergic Reactions: Skin rash, hives, itching—rare.

Headache, nervousness, insomnia, drowsiness, tremor, dizziness, tingling of extremities—rare.

Altered taste, nausea—frequent; vomiting, diarrhea—possible to rare.

Hair loss—case reports.

Fast heart rate (tachycardia) or palpitations—rare.

Blurred vision—infrequent.

Excessive sweating—frequent.

Serious Adverse Effects

Allergic Reactions: Serum-sickness-like syndrome: fever, weakness, joint pain and swelling, swollen lymph glands, fluid retention, skin rash and/or hives.

Drug-induced seizures—rare.

Worsening of Parkinson's disease—possible.

Intense suicidal preoccupation in severe depression that does not respond to this drug (see "Current Controversies," below)—possible.

Mania or hypomania and psychosis or hallucinations—rare.

Abnormal and excessive urination (SIADH)—case reports.
Liver toxicity—rare.

▷ **Possible Effects on Sexual Function:** Impaired erection (1.9%), inhibition of ejaculation or inhibited orgasm in men and women—case reports.

Natural Diseases or Disorders That May Be Activated by This Drug
Latent epilepsy.

Possible Effects on Laboratory Tests
Blood glucose level: decreased.
Blood sodium level: decreased.

CAUTION
1. If any skin reaction develops (rash, hives, etc.), stop this drug and inform your physician promptly.
2. If dry mouth develops and persists for more than 2 weeks, consult your dentist for help.
3. Ask your doctor or pharmacist before taking any other prescription or over-the-counter drug while taking fluoxetine.
4. If you must start any monoamine oxidase (MAO) type A inhibitor (see Drug Classes), allow an interval of 5 weeks after stopping this drug before starting the MAO inhibitor.
5. This drug should be withheld if electroconvulsive therapy (ECT, "shock" treatment) is to be used.

Precautions for Use
By Infants and Children: Safety and effectiveness for those under 12 years of age are not established.
By Those Over 60 Years of Age: Total daily dosage should not exceed 60 mg.

▷ **Advisability of Use During Pregnancy**
Pregnancy Category: B. See Pregnancy Risk Categories at the back of this book.
Animal studies: No birth defects due to this drug found in rat or rabbit studies.
Human studies: Adequate studies of pregnant women are not available.
Use this drug only if clearly needed.

Advisability of Use If Breast-Feeding
Presence of this drug in breast milk: Yes.
Avoid drug or refrain from nursing.

Habit-Forming Potential: Reports of patients using excess doses of fluoxetine or combining the drug with alcohol have surfaced. It appears possible that a euphoric effect and abuse potential exists.

Effects of Overdosage: Agitation, restlessness, excitement, nausea, vomiting, seizures.

Possible Effects of Long-Term Use: None reported.

Suggested Periodic Examinations While Taking This Drug (at physician's discretion)
None.

▷ **While Taking This Drug, Observe the Following**
Foods: No restrictions (see "Beverages" below).
Beverages: Grapefruit juice may lead to increased blood levels. AVOID IT. May be taken with milk.

▷   *Alcohol:* Does not appear to increase the central nervous system effects of fluoxetine or change the metabolism of alcohol.

Tobacco Smoking: No interactions expected, but I advise everyone to quit smoking.

▷   *Other Drugs*

Fluoxetine may ***increase*** the effects of
- diazepam (Valium).
- digitalis preparations (digitoxin, digoxin).
- phenytoin (Dilantin) by increasing the drug level.
- warfarin (Coumadin) and related oral anticoagulants. Test INR more often.

Fluoxetine ***taken concurrently*** with
- antidiabetic drugs (insulin, oral hypoglycemics) may increase the risk of hypoglycemic reactions; monitor blood sugar levels carefully.
- astemizole (Hismanal), terfenadine (Seldane), or similar drugs may result in increased terfenadine levels and risk of heart arrhythmias. **Avoid** combining.
- buspirone (Buspar) may increase underlying anxiety. **Avoid** the combination.
- carbamazepine (Tegretol) will increase the carbamazepine level. Drug levels are critical if the drugs are combined.
- clozapine (Clozaril) may result in increased levels of clozapine. The clozapine dose may need to be decreased if both medicines are to be used at the same time.
- dextromethorphan (a cough suppressant in many "DM" labeled nonprescription cough medicines) may result in visual hallucinations if these drugs are combined. **DO NOT** combine these medicines.
- haloperidol (Haldol) will increase haloperidol levels. Dosage decrease and blood levels are needed.
- ketorolac (Toradol) may result in hallucinations. **DO NOT** take these medicines at the same time.
- lithium (Lithobid, etc.) will result in increased lithium levels and increased risk of neurotoxicity. **Avoid** the combination.
- loratadine (Claritin) may result in increased loratadine levels. It may be prudent to decrease the dose if these medicines are to be combined. Unlike some of the other nonsedating antihistamines (see Drug Classes), loratadine has not (to date) resulted in abnormal heart rhythms.
- monoamine oxidase (MAO) type A inhibitor drugs may cause confusion, agitation, high fever, seizures, and dangerous elevations of blood pressure. Avoid combining these drugs.
- tryptophan will result in central nervous system toxicity. **Avoid** the combination.
- any tricyclic antidepressant (amitriptyline, nortriptyline, etc.) will result in increased antidepressant drug levels that will persist for weeks. **Avoid** the combination.
- selegiline (Eldepryl) can result in serotonin toxicity syndrome. **Avoid** this combination.
- tramadol (Ultram) may increase seizure risk. DO NOT COMBINE.

▷   *Driving, Hazardous Activities:* This drug may cause drowsiness, dizziness, impaired judgment, and delayed reaction time. Restrict activities as necessary.

Aviation Note: The use of this drug *is a disqualification* for piloting. Consult a designated Aviation Medical Examiner.

Exposure to Sun: No restrictions.

Discontinuation: Slow drug elimination makes withdrawal effects unlikely. However, call your doctor if you plan to stop this drug for any reason.

Current Controversies in Drug Management

In 1990 six patients being treated with fluoxetine experienced intense and violent suicidal preoccupation. All six had severe depression that had not responded to the use of fluoxetine for 2 to 7 weeks. For most of them, suicidal mentality persisted for 2 to 3 months after stopping the drug. Adverse publicity suggested that this may be characteristic of fluoxetine in contrast to other antidepressant drugs. A review of relevant literature on this subject reveals that the development or intensification of suicidal thoughts during treatment (regardless of the severity of depression) has been documented repeatedly for many antidepressant drugs in wide use. Suicidal thinking may emerge during treatment with any antidepressant. Recent reports establish that some patients who become suicidal while taking one antidepressant can be switched to fluoxetine and experience cessation of suicidal thinking and satisfactory relief of depression.

This is another example of the marked variability of individual response to drug therapy. The choice of a drug to treat many serious disorders remains an experiment of trial and error. Successful management requires clinical judgment (based on experience), close monitoring, and appropriate doses.

FLUPHENAZINE (flu FEN a zeen)

Introduced: 1959   **Class:** Strong tranquilizer, phenothiazines   **Prescription:** USA: Yes   **Controlled Drug:** USA: No; Canada: No   **Available as Generic:** USA: Yes; Canada: Yes

Brand Names: ✦Apo-Fluphenazine, ✦Modecate, ✦Moditen, Permitil, PMS-Fluphenazine, Prolixin

---

BENEFITS versus RISKS

Possible Benefits	*Possible Risks*
EFFECTIVE CONTROL OF ACUTE MENTAL DISORDERS	SERIOUS TOXIC EFFECTS ON BRAIN with long-term use
Beneficial effects on thinking, mood, and behavior	Liver damage with jaundice
	Blood cell disorders: abnormally low white blood cell counts

---

▷ **Principal Uses**

As a Single Drug Product: Uses currently included in FDA-approved labeling: Treatment of schizophrenia.

Other (unlabeled) currently accepted uses: (1) Combination treatment of refractory neuropathy; (2) an alternative neuroleptic drug in treating Tourette syndrome in combination with clonidine; (3) therapy of Alzheimer's disease symptoms; (4) may help control sexual aggressiveness.

How This Drug Works: By inhibiting the action of dopamine, this drug acts to correct an imbalance of nerve impulse transmissions.

Available Dosage Forms and Strengths
> Concentrate — 5 mg/ml (1% alcohol)
>   Elixir — 2.5 mg/5 ml (14% alcohol)
> Injection — 2.5 mg/ml
>   Tablets — 1 mg, 2.5 mg, 5 mg, 10 mg

▷ **Usual Adult Dosage Range:**   2.5 to 10 mg given three to four times daily. The dose is adjusted as needed and tolerated. Total daily dosage should not exceed 40 mg. **Note: Actual dosage and administration schedule must be determined for each patient individually.**

Conditions Requiring Dosing Adjustments
> *Liver Function:* Use with caution in patients with both liver and kidney compromise.
> *Kidney Function:* Use with caution in patients with compromised kidneys and livers.

▷ **Dosing Instructions:**   Regular tablets can be crushed and taken with or following meals to reduce stomach irritation. Prolonged-action tablets should be swallowed whole (not crushed). The concentrate must be diluted in 4 to 6 ounces of water, milk, fruit juice, or carbonated beverage.

Usual Duration of Use: Use on a regular schedule for several weeks is needed to determine effectiveness in controlling psychotic disorders. If not of benefit in 6 weeks, it should be stopped. Long-term use (months to years) requires periodic physician evaluation.

▷ **This Drug Should Not Be Taken If**
- you are allergic to any of the drugs bearing the brand names listed.
- you have a history of brain damage.
- you have active liver disease.
- you have cancer of the breast.
- you have an active blood dyscrasia.
- you are taking large doses of other medicines that can depress the central nervous system.
- you have a current blood cell or bone marrow disorder.

▷ **Inform Your Physician Before Taking This Drug If**
- you are allergic or sensitive to any phenothiazine (see Drug Classes).
- you have impaired liver or kidney function.
- you have any type of seizure disorder.
- you have diabetes, glaucoma, heart disease, or chronic lung disease.
- you have a history of lupus erythematosus.
- you have a history of depressed white blood cell counts of the granulocytic series (agranulocytosis).
- you have a history of neuroleptic malignant syndrome.
- you take any drug with sedative effects or will have surgery under general or spinal anesthesia.

Possible Side Effects (natural, expected, and unavoidable drug actions)
> Drowsiness (usually during the first 2 weeks), orthostatic hypotension (see Glossary), blurred vision, dry mouth, nasal congestion, constipation, impaired urination (all mild).

▷ **Possible Adverse Effects** (unusual, unexpected, and infrequent reactions)
> **If any of the following develop, consult your physician promptly for guidance.**

Mild Adverse Effects

Allergic Reactions: Skin rash, hives, itching.

Lowering of body temperature, especially in the elderly—possible.

Headache, dizziness, weakness, excitement, restlessness, unusual dreaming—infrequent.

Increased appetite and weight gain—possible.

Serious Adverse Effects

Allergic Reactions: Hepatitis with jaundice (see Glossary), usually between second and fourth week; anaphylactic reaction (see Glossary).

Idiosyncratic Reaction: Neuroleptic malignant syndrome (see Glossary)—case reports.

Impaired production of white blood cells: fever, sore throat, infections—rare.

Parkinson-like disorders (see Glossary): muscle spasms of face, jaw, neck, back—rare to infrequent and may be dose related.

Liver toxicity—case reports.

Depression or seizures—case reports.

Pituitary tumors or porphyria—case reports.

Abnormal heartbeats—rare.

▷ **Possible Effects on Sexual Function**

Decreased male libido; increased female libido.

Impaired erection—frequent; complete impotence—case reports. Inhibited male or female orgasm—frequent. Inhibited ejaculation—frequent.

Altered timing and pattern of menstruation—frequent.

Female breast enlargement and milk production (galactorrhea)—possible.

Prolonged and painful erection (priapism)—case reports. Male breast enlargement and tenderness (gynecomastia)—case reports.

May help treat sexual hyperactivity.

▷ **Adverse Effects That May Mimic Natural Diseases or Disorders**

Nervous system reactions may suggest Parkinson's disease.

Liver reactions may suggest viral hepatitis.

Reactions resembling systemic lupus erythematosus may occur.

Natural Diseases or Disorders That May Be Activated by This Drug

Latent epilepsy, glaucoma, prostatism (see Glossary).

Possible Effects on Laboratory Tests

Complete blood counts: decreased red cells, hemoglobin, white cells, and platelets; increased eosinophils (allergic reaction).

Blood sugar (glucose): decreased.

Liver function tests: increased liver enzymes (ALT/GPT, AST/GOT, and alkaline phosphatase), increased bilirubin.

Urine pregnancy tests: false positive results.

Urine screening test for drug abuse: initial test may be falsely *positive* for barbiturates; the confirmatory test will be *negative*.

CAUTION

1. Many over-the-counter medications (see Glossary) for allergies, colds, and coughs can interact unfavorably with this drug. Ask your physician or pharmacist for help before using any such medications.
2. Antacids containing aluminum and/or magnesium can prevent absorption.
3. Obtain prompt evaluation of any change or disturbance of vision.

Precautions for Use

By Infants and Children: Do not use this drug in infants under 6 months of age, or in children of any age with symptoms suggestive of Reye syndrome (see Glossary). Monitor carefully for blood cell changes.

Children with psychosis have been given 0.25 to 0.75 mg from one to four times daily.

By Those Over 60 Years of Age: Small starting doses are advisable. Increased risk of drowsiness, lethargy, constipation, lowering of body temperature (hypothermia), and orthostatic hypotension (see Glossary). This drug can enhance existing prostatism (see Glossary). You may also be more susceptible to the development of Parkinson-like reactions and/or tardive dyskinesia (see discussion of these terms in Glossary).

▷ **Advisability of Use During Pregnancy**

Pregnancy Category: C. See Pregnancy Risk Categories at the back of this book.

Animal studies: Significant birth defects reported in mice.

Human studies: Adequate studies of pregnant women are not available.

Avoid drug during the first 3 months and during the final month because of possible effects on the newborn infant.

Advisability of Use If Breast-Feeding

Presence of this drug in breast milk: Yes.

Does not usually accumulate in high enough concentrations to effect the infant. Watch the infant closely and discuss the situation with your doctor.

Habit-Forming Potential: None.

Effects of Overdosage: Marked drowsiness, weakness, tremor, agitation, unsteadiness, deep sleep, coma, convulsions.

Possible Effects of Long-Term Use: Tardive dyskinesia (see Glossary); eye changes—cataracts and pigmentation of retina; gray to violet pigmentation of skin in exposed areas, more common in women.

Suggested Periodic Examinations While Taking This Drug (at physician's discretion)

Complete blood counts.

Liver function tests, electrocardiograms.

Complete eye examinations—eye structures and vision.

Careful tongue exam for evidence of fine, involuntary, wavelike movements that could be the beginning of tardive dyskinesia.

▷ **While Taking This Drug, Observe the Following**

Foods: No restrictions.

Beverages: No restrictions. May be taken with milk.

▷ *Alcohol:* Avoid completely. Alcohol can increase phenothiazine sedation and accentuate depressant effects on brain function and blood pressure. Phenothiazines can increase the intoxicating effects of alcohol.

Tobacco Smoking: Possible increased fluphenazine removal and need for dose increase. I advise everyone to quit smoking.

Marijuana Smoking: Moderate increase in drowsiness; accentuation of orthostatic hypotension; increased risk of precipitating latent psychoses, confusing the interpretation of mental status and drug responses.

▷ *Other Drugs*

Fluphenazine may *increase* the effects of

- all atropinelike drugs, and cause nervous system toxicity.
- all sedative drugs, and cause excessive sedation.

Fluphenazine may *decrease* the effects of
- guanethidine (Ismelin, Esimil), and reduce its effectiveness in lowering blood pressure.

Fluphenazine *taken concurrently* with
- beta-blocker drugs (see Drug Classes) may cause increased effects of both drugs; watch drug effects—may need smaller doses.
- clonidine (Catapres, others) may result in an acute organic brain syndrome (disorientation, agitation, delirium). These medicines should not be combined.
- lithium (Lithobid, others) can cause increase toxicity to the nerves.
- MAO inhibitors (see Drug Classes) can cause very low blood pressure and worsening of the central nervous system and respiratory depression effects.
- oral antidiabetic drugs (see Drug Classes) may result in lower blood sugar levels than expected. Doses of the oral hypoglycemic agents may need to be decreased.
- tramadol (Ultram) may increase seizure risk. DO NOT COMBINE.
- vitamin C (ascorbic acid) may decrease the therapeutic benefits of fluphenazine.

The following drugs may *decrease* the effects of fluphenazine
- antacids containing aluminum and/or magnesium.
- benztropine (Cogentin).
- trihexyphenidyl (Artane).

▷ *Driving, Hazardous Activities:* This drug can impair mental alertness, judgment, and physical coordination. Avoid hazardous activities.

Aviation Note: The use of this drug *is a disqualification* for piloting. Consult a designated Aviation Medical Examiner.

Exposure to Sun: Use caution—some phenothiazines can cause photosensitivity (see Glossary).

Exposure to Heat: Use caution and avoid excessive heat. This drug may impair the regulation of body temperature and increase heatstroke risk.

Exposure to Cold: Use caution and dress warmly. Increased risk of hypothermia in the elderly.

Discontinuation: After long-term use, do not stop this drug suddenly. Gradual withdrawal over 2 to 3 weeks under physician supervision is needed. Do not stop this drug without your doctor's knowledge and approval. The relapse rate of schizophrenia after discontinuation is 50–60%.

FLURAZEPAM (flur AZ e pam)

Introduced: 1970   **Class:** Hypnotic, benzodiazepines   **Prescription:** USA: Yes   **Controlled Drug:** USA: C-IV*; Canada: No   **Available as Generic:** USA: Yes; Canada: Yes

Brand Names: ✦Apo-Flurazepam, Dalmane, Durapam, ✦Novo-Flupam, ✦Somnol

*See schedules of Controlled Drugs at the back of this book.

BENEFITS versus RISKS	
Possible Benefits	*Possible Risks*
EFFECTIVE HYPNOTIC	Habit-forming potential with
NO SUPPRESSION OF REM (RAPID	long-term use
EYE MOVEMENT) SLEEP	Minor impairment of mental
NO REM SLEEP REBOUND after	functions ("hangover" effect)
discontinuation	Jaundice
Wide margin of safety with	Blood cell disorder
therapeutic doses	Suppression of stage-4 sleep with
	reduced "quality" of sleep

▷ **Principal Uses**

As a Single Drug Product: Uses currently included in FDA-approved labeling: Short-term treatment of insomnia consisting of difficulty in falling asleep, frequent nighttime awakenings, and/or early morning awakenings.

Other (unlabeled) generally accepted uses: May be of benefit in patients who have undergone herniorrhaphy, in helping them sleep.

How This Drug Works: By enhancing the action of the nerve transmitter gamma-aminobutyric acid (GABA), arousal of higher brain centers is blocked and helps sleep occur.

Available Dosage Forms and Strengths

Capsules — 15 mg, 30 mg (U.S., Canada)

Tablets — 15 mg, 30 mg (Canada)

▷ **Recommended Dosage Ranges** (Actual dosage and administration schedule must be determined for each patient individually.)

Infants and Children: Up to 15 years of age—use not recommended.

15 to 60 Years of Age: Initially 15 mg at bedtime; increase to 30 mg only if needed and tolerated.

Over 60 Years of Age: Same as 15 to 60 years of age. Usually 15 mg is adequate; use higher doses with caution.

Conditions Requiring Dosing Adjustments

Liver Function: The dose **must** be decreased for patients with liver compromise. Flurazepam is also a rare cause of hepatocellular and cholestatic jaundice, and must be used as a benefit-to-risk decision for patients with compromised livers.

Kidney Function: Changes in dosage are not usually needed.

▷ **Dosing Instructions:**   The capsule may be opened and taken on an empty stomach or with food or milk. Do not stop this drug abruptly if taken for more than 4 weeks.

Usual Duration of Use: Use for 3 nights is usually needed to see this drug's benefit in relieving insomnia. If possible, this drug should be used for periods of 3 to 5 nights intermittently, repeated as needed with appropriate dosage adjustment. Avoid uninterrupted and prolonged use. Duration of use should not exceed 2 weeks without reappraisal of continued need. Newer agents may disrupt normal sleep architecture less.

▷ **This Drug Should Not Be Taken If**

• you have had an allergic reaction to it previously.

• you are pregnant.

- you have sleep apnea.
- you have acute narrow-angle glaucoma.

▷ **Inform Your Physician Before Taking This Drug If**
- you are allergic to any benzodiazepine (see Drug Classes).
- you have a history of alcoholism or drug abuse.
- you are planning pregnancy.
- you have impaired liver or kidney function.
- you are an alcoholic.
- you have a history of serious depression or mental disorder.
- you are taking other drugs with sedative effects.
- you have asthma, emphysema, epilepsy, or myasthenia gravis.

Possible Side Effects (natural, expected, and unavoidable drug actions)
"Hangover" effects on arising: drowsiness, lethargy, and unsteadiness—may be frequent in older patients.

▷ **Possible Adverse Effects** (unusual, unexpected, and infrequent reactions)
If any of the following develop, consult your physician promptly for guidance.

Mild Adverse Effects
Allergic Reactions: Skin rash, hives, burning eyes, swelling of tongue.
Dizziness, fainting, blurred vision, double vision, slurred speech, nausea, indigestion—possible to infrequent.
Ringing in the ears, increased heart rate or taste disorders—possible to case reports.

Serious Adverse Effects
Allergic Reactions: Rare liver damage with jaundice (see Glossary)—rare.
Idiosyncratic Reactions: Nervousness, talkativeness, irritability, apprehension, euphoria, excitement, hallucinations.
Bone marrow depression: impaired production of white blood cells, fever, sore throat—rare.
Sleep apnea or intraocular pressure increases—possible to infrequent.
Increased risk of hip fracture (from falls) if used in those over 60—possible.

▷ **Possible Effects on Sexual Function:**   None reported.

▷ **Adverse Effects That May Mimic Natural Diseases or Disorders**
Liver reaction with jaundice may suggest viral hepatitis.

Possible Effects on Laboratory Tests
Liver function tests: increased liver enzymes (ALT/GPT, AST/GOT, and alkaline phosphatase), increased bilirubin.
Urine sugar tests: no drug effect with Tes-Tape; false low results with Clinistix and Diastix; false positive result with Benedict's solution.
Urine screening tests for drug abuse: may be *positive*. (Test results depend upon amount of drug taken and testing method used.)

CAUTION
1. This drug should not be stopped abruptly if it has been taken continually for more than 4 weeks.
2. Some over-the-counter drug products that contain antihistamines (allergy and cold preparations, sleep aids) can cause excessive sedation.
3. Regular nightly use of any hypnotic drug should be avoided.
4. This drug is transformed by the liver into long-acting forms that can per-

sist in the body for 24 hours or more. With continual use of this drug daily, these active drug forms accumulate and produce increasing sedation. If you experience a "hangover" effect, avoid hazardous activities (driving, etc.).

Precautions for Use

By Infants and Children: Safety and effectiveness for those under 15 years of age not established.

By Those Over 60 Years of Age: Starting doses are reduced and given less often. Watch for lethargy, indifference, fatigue, weakness, unsteadiness, disturbing dreams, nightmares, and paradoxical reactions (excitement, agitation, anger, and rage.)

Because this is a long-acting benzodiazepine, it may cause residual sluggishness and unsteadiness with increased risk of falls. This drug may also increase the number of periods of sleep apnea in this age group.

▷ Advisability of Use During Pregnancy

Pregnancy Category: X. See Pregnancy Risk Categories at the back of this book.

Animal studies: No birth defects reported in rat and rabbit studies.

Human studies: Adequate studies of pregnant women are not available.

Several studies indicate an increased risk of birth defects if drugs of this class (benzodiazepines) are used during the first 3 months.

Frequent use in late pregnancy can cause the "floppy infant" syndrome in the newborn: weakness, lethargy, unresponsiveness, depressed breathing, low body temperature.

Avoid use during entire pregnancy.

Advisability of Use If Breast-Feeding

Presence of this drug in breast milk: Probably yes.

Avoid drug or refrain from nursing.

Habit-Forming Potential: This drug can produce psychological and/or physical dependence (see Glossary) if used in large doses for an extended period of time. Avoid continual use.

Effects of Overdosage: Marked drowsiness, weakness, feeling of drunkenness, staggering gait, tremor, stupor progressing to deep sleep or coma.

Possible Effects of Long-Term Use: Psychological and/or physical dependence, impaired liver function.

Suggested Periodic Examinations While Taking This Drug (at physician's discretion)

Complete blood cell counts and liver function tests during long-term use.

▷ While Taking This Drug, Observe the Following

Foods: No restrictions.

Beverages: Avoid excessive intake of caffeine-containing beverages (coffee, tea, cola) within 4 hours of taking this drug. May be taken with milk.

▷ *Alcohol:* Alcohol may increase the absorption of this drug and add to its depressant effects on the brain. It is advisable to avoid alcohol completely— throughout the day and night.

Tobacco Smoking: Heavy smoking may reduce the hypnotic action of this drug. I advise everyone to quit smoking.

Marijuana Smoking: Increased sedation and significant impairment of intellectual and physical performance.

▷   *Other Drugs*
Flurazepam may *increase* the effects of
- digoxin (Lanoxin), and cause digoxin toxicity.
- lithium (Lithobid, others) and cause additive drowsiness.
- phenytoin (Dilantin), and cause phenytoin toxicity.

Flurazepam may *decrease* the effects of
- levodopa (Sinemet, etc.), and reduce its effectiveness in treating Parkinson's disease.

Flurazepam *taken concurrently* with
- macrolide antibiotics (azithromycin, clarithromycin, dirithromycin, or erythromycin) may lead to flurazepam toxicity.
- narcotics, other benzodiazepines, phenothiazines, or antihistamines (see Drug Classes) or other medicines with sedating properties may result in additive sedation.
- ritonavir (Norvir) and perhaps other protease inhibitors (see Drug Classes) may lead to toxicity.

The following drugs may *increase* the effects of flurazepam
- cimetidine (Tagamet).
- disulfiram (Antabuse).
- isoniazid (INH, Rifamate, etc.).
- omeprazole (Prilosec).
- oral contraceptives.
- valproic acid (Depakene).

The following drugs may *decrease* the effects of flurazepam
- rifampin (Rimactane, etc.).
- theophylline (aminophylline, Theo-Dur, etc.).

▷   *Driving, Hazardous Activities:* This drug can impair mental alertness, judgment, physical coordination, and reaction time. Avoid hazardous activities accordingly.

Aviation Note: The use of this drug *is a disqualification* for piloting. Consult a designated Aviation Medical Examiner.

Exposure to Sun: No restrictions.

Exposure to Heat: Use caution until the effect of excessive perspiration is determined. Because of reduced urine volume, this drug may accumulate in the body and produce effects of overdosage.

Discontinuation: Avoid sudden discontinuation if this drug has been taken for over 4 weeks without interruption. Dosage should be tapered gradually to prevent a withdrawal syndrome that could include depression, confusion, hallucinations, tremor, seizures, muscle cramping, sweating, and vomiting.

FLURBIPROFEN (flur BI proh fen)

See the propionic acids (nonsteroidal anti-inflammatory drugs) profile for further information.

FLUTAMIDE (FLU ta mide)

Introduced: 1983 **Class:** Anticancer (antineoplastic) **Prescription:**
USA: Yes **Controlled Drug:** USA: No; Canada: No **Available as Generic:**
USA: No; Canada: No

Brand Names: ✦Euflex, Eulexin, Flutamex (Germany)

BENEFITS versus RISKS	
Possible Benefits	*Possible Risks*
EFFECTIVE ADJUNCTIVE	Rare drug-induced hepatitis
TREATMENT OF PROSTATE	Breast enlargement and tenderness
CANCER	Hot flashes

▷ **Principal Uses**

    As a Single Drug Product: Uses currently included in FDA-approved labeling:
    Treatment of metastatic prostate cancer, used concurrently with leuprolide
    (given by injection).

    Other (unlabeled) generally accepted uses: (1) There has been some isolated
    use as a 2% alcoholic gel in treating acne; (2) some early data on use in
    bulimia; (3) can help excessive hair growth in women (hirsutism).

How This Drug Works: Flutamide is an antiandrogenic drug and suppresses
the effects of the male sex hormone (testosterone, an androgen) by blocking
uptake and binding target tissues (such as the prostate gland). Used in conjunction with leuprolide, a drug that suppresses production of testosterone
by the testicles (by damping the pituitary gland's testicular stimulation).
The combination of these two drug actions—chemical castration by leuprolide and testosterone blockage by flutamide—significantly reduces hormonal stimulation of cancerous prostate tissue.

Available Dosage Forms and Strengths

    Capsules — 125 mg (U.S.)
    Tablets — 250 mg (Canada, Germany)

▷ **Recommended Dosage Ranges** (Actual dosage and administration schedule
    must be determined for each patient individually.)

    Infants and Children: Not used in this age group.
    12 to 60 Years of Age: 250 mg every 8 hours. Flutamide is to be taken concur-
    rently with leuprolide; the usual dose of leuprolide is 7.5 mg given by injec-
    tion once a month.
    Over 60 Years of Age: Same as 12 to 60 years of age.

Conditions Requiring Dosing Adjustments

    Liver Function: Use with caution by patients with liver compromise. It is also a
    rare cause of cholestatic jaundice.
    Kidney Function: Primarily eliminated by the kidneys. Use with caution in kid-
    ney compromise.

▷ **Dosing Instructions:** May be taken without regard to food. The capsule may be
    opened and the tablet may be crushed for administration.

Warning: Since this medicine is an antineoplastic agent, proper disposal (ask
your doctor) of urine or vomit MUST be undertaken.

Usual Duration of Use: Use on a regular schedule for 2 to 3 months is usually needed to see this drug's effectiveness in controlling prostate cancer. Long-term use (months to years) requires periodic physician evaluation.

Possible Advantages of This Drug
Ease of use. Less toxicity than chemotherapeutic drugs.

Currently a "Drug of Choice"
for the management of prostate cancer (in combination with leuprolide).

▷ **This Drug Should Not Be Taken If**
• you have had an allergic reaction to it previously.

▷ **Inform Your Physician Before Taking This Drug If**
• you have a history of liver disease or impaired liver function.
• you have high blood pressure (hypertension).
• you have a history of anemia, low white blood cells, or low blood platelets.
• you have a history of lupus erythematosus.

Possible Side Effects (natural, expected, and unavoidable drug actions)
Hot flashes (61%), loss of libido (with combination LHRH therapy), impotence, breast enlargement and tenderness.

▷ **Possible Adverse Effects** (unusual, unexpected, and infrequent reactions)
If any of the following develop, consult your physician promptly for guidance.
Mild Adverse Effects
Allergic Reactions: Skin rash.
Drowsiness, confusion, nervousness—rare.
Indigestion, nausea/vomiting, diarrhea—infrequent.
Blurred vision—rare.
Fluid retention (edema) of legs—possible.
Serious Adverse Effects
Drug-induced hepatitis with jaundice (see Glossary)—rare.
Low blood platelets, white blood cells, or anemia—rare.
Lupus-erythematosus-like skin rash—case reports.
Heart attack—rare.

▷ **Possible Effects on Sexual Function**
See "Possible Side Effects" above. Flutamide itself does not presently appear to change libido, sexual performance, or the ability to have an erection. Combination therapy does appear to carry the risks of these adverse effects. Swelling and tenderness of male breast tissue (gynecomastia)—may be frequent.

▷ **Adverse Effects That May Mimic Natural Diseases or Disorders**
Drug-induced hepatitis may suggest viral hepatitis.

Possible Effects on Laboratory Tests
Complete blood counts: decreased red and white cells, hemoglobin, and platelets.
Liver function tests: increased liver enzymes (ALT/GPT, AST/GOT, and alkaline phosphatase), increased bilirubin.
Sperm counts and testosterone levels: decreased.

CAUTION
1. For best results, flutamide and leuprolide should be started together and continued for the duration of therapy.

2. During combination therapy with flutamide and leuprolide, symptoms of prostate cancer (difficult urination, bone pain, etc.) may worsen temporarily; these are transient and not significant.

Precautions for Use

By Those Over 60 Years of Age: This drug is more slowly excreted. If digestive symptoms or edema are troublesome, ask your doctor about adjusting your dose.

▷ **Advisability of Use During Pregnancy**

Pregnancy Category: D. See Pregnancy Risk Categories at the back of this book.

Animal studies: Rat studies reveal malformation of bone structures and feminization of male fetuses.

Human studies: Adequate studies of pregnant women are not available.

Discuss this benefit-to-risk decision with your doctor.

Habit-Forming Potential: None.

Effects of Overdosage: Possible drowsiness, unsteadiness, nausea, vomiting.

Possible Effects of Long-Term Use: None reported.

Suggested Periodic Examinations While Taking This Drug (at physician's discretion)

Prostate-specific antigen (PSA) assays.

Complete blood cell counts.

Liver function tests.

▷ **While Taking This Drug, Observe the Following**

Foods: No restrictions.

Beverages: No restrictions. May be taken with milk.

▷ *Alcohol:* No interactions expected.

Tobacco Smoking: No interactions expected, but I advise everyone to quit smoking.

Marijuana Smoking: Animal studies have shown this combination to result in additive suppression of the immune system. The combination therefore is not advisable.

Other Drugs

Flutamide *taken concurrently* with

• influenza, pneumococcal, or yellow fever vaccine may result in blunting of immune response to the vaccine.

▷ *Driving, Hazardous Activities:* This drug may cause drowsiness. Restrict activities as necessary.

Aviation Note: The use of this drug *may be a disqualification* for piloting. Consult a designated Aviation Medical Examiner.

Exposure to Sun: This drug may cause photosensitivity (see Glossary).

Discontinuation: To be determined by your physician.

FLUTICASONE (flu TIC a zone)

Introduced: 1994 **Class:** Adrenocortical steroids **Prescription:** USA: Yes **Controlled Drug:** USA: No; Canada: No **Available as Generic:** USA: No; Canada: No

Brand Names: Cutivate, Flonase, Flovent**Author's Note: This profile focuses on the aqueous nasal form of this medicine.**

Warning: Even though this medicine is a nasal spray, there is still a remote risk of suppression of the hypothalamic pituitary adrenal (HPA) axis.

BENEFITS versus RISKS	
Possible Benefits	*Possible Risks*
EFFECTIVE, ONCE-A-DAY RELIEF OF SEASONAL ALLERGIC RHINITIS EFFECTIVE ONCE-DAILY ECZEMA TREATMENT	Reversible adrenal gland suppression Irritation of the nose

▷ **Principal Uses**
> *As a Single Drug Product:* Uses currently included in FDA-approved labeling: (1) Management of perennial and seasonal (hay fever) allergic or nonallergic rhinitis in adults or children who are 12 years of age or older; (2) the topical form is used for a variety of skin conditions from sunburn to lupus erythematosus; (3) the inhaler form was approved in 1996 for treatment of asthma; (4) the cream was recently approved for once-daily treatment of eczema.
>
> Other (unlabeled) generally accepted uses: Crohn's disease.

How This Drug Works: This medicine belongs to a new class of corticosteroids. The exact mechanism of action of this medicine is not known; however, halomethyl carbothionates have very potent anti-inflammatory and blood-vessel-contracting (vasoconstrictive) activity.

Available Dosage Forms and Strengths
> Amber glass bottle — 16 g (120 actuations) and 9 g (60 actuations)
> Cream (Germany) — 0.05 mg/g
> Inhalation powder (Germany) — 50, 100, and 250 mcg per actuation

▷ **Recommended Dosage Ranges** (Actual dosage and administration schedule must be determined for each patient individually.)
> *Infants and Children:* Safety and efficacy for those less than 12 years of age have not yet been defined.
>
> *12 to 60 Years of Age:* Nasal dosing: Started with two sprays (50 mcg in each spray) in each nostril once daily. The same dose can also be given as 100 mcg twice daily (8 A.M. and 8 P.M.). After a few days, the dose can often be decreased to 100 mcg (one spray in each nostril) daily.
>
> Inhalation for asthma: Starting dose is 88 mcg twice a day for patients who were previously treated with bronchodilators alone. Maximum daily dose is 440 mcg. Patients who required an inhaled corticosteroid previously are given 88 to 220 mcg twice daily. Maximum daily dose is 880 mcg.
>
> *Over 60 Years of Age:* Same as 12 to 60 years of age.

Conditions Requiring Dosing Adjustments
> *Liver Function:* This drug is extensively changed in the liver; however, no specific dosing changes are defined for patients with compromised livers.
>
> *Kidney Function:* No changes in dosing are needed.

▷ **Dosing Instructions:** A patient instruction sheet will always accompany this medicine. The instructions should be followed closely. Your doctor should be called if the condition worsens or does not improve.

Usual Duration of Use: Continual use on a regular schedule for several days is usually necessary to determine this drug's effectiveness in treating seasonal and perennial allergic rhinitis. Long-term use (months to years) requires periodic evaluation of response and dosage adjustment. Consult your physician on a regular basis.

Possible Advantages of This Drug
Once-a-day dosing.

▷ **This Drug Should Not Be Taken If**
- you have had an allergic reaction to any dosage form of it previously.
- you have sudden onset asthma and only have the fluticasone inhaler.

▷ **Inform Your Physician Before Taking This Drug If**
- you are already taking systemic prednisone.
- you are exposed to measles or chickenpox.
- you are uncertain of how much fluticasone to take or how often to take it.
- you take other prescription or nonprescription medicines that were not discussed with your doctor when fluticasone was prescribed.
- you have signs or symptoms of an infection in your nose.
- your skin is shrunken (atrophied) or you have acne, warts, or other skin problems (topical form).
- you have damage from an accident or surgery to your nose while you are taking this medicine.
- your allergic rhinitis does not improve or worsens.

Possible Side Effects (natural, expected, and unavoidable drug actions)
Irritation of the nose. Systemic steroid effects—possible.

▷ **Possible Adverse Effects** (unusual, unexpected, and infrequent reactions)
If any of the following develop, consult your physician promptly for guidance.
Mild Adverse Effects
Allergic Reactions: Contact dermatitis.
Nosebleeds or nasal burning—case reports to infrequent.
Dizziness or headache—rare to infrequent.
Unpleasant taste, nausea, or vomiting—rare.
Increased heart rate—case reports.
Serious Adverse Effects
Allergic Reactions: Anaphylaxis—case report.
Suppression of the hypothalamic pituitary adrenal (HPA) axis—rare.
Increased risk from viral infections—possible.
Increased pressure in the head (more likely in children)—possible.
Yeast infections of the nose—rare.
Glaucoma or cataracts—case reports (inhaled form).
Cushing's syndrome (with excessive doses or very sensitive patients)—possible.
Osteoporosis—increased risk with long-term use.

▷ **Possible Effects on Sexual Function:** None defined.

Possible Delayed Adverse Effects: Yeast infections of the nose—rare. Osteoporosis—increased risk.

▷ **Adverse Effects That May Mimic Natural Diseases or Disorders**
   None defined.

Natural Diseases or Disorders That May Be Activated by This Drug
   If systemic effects occur, the patient may be more susceptible to infections, or dormant infections may become active.

Possible Effects on Laboratory Tests
   Cortisol levels: decreased.

CAUTION
   1. Call your doctor if you are exposed to measles or chickenpox.
   2. Long-term use requires periodic evaluation for yeast infection of the nose.
   3. Call your doctor if your condition does not improve or worsens.

Precautions for Use
   By Infants and Children: Safety and effectiveness for use by those under 12 years of age have not been established for the intranasal form. Many adolescents can be started successfully with one spray in each nostril per day (100 mcg). Maximum total daily dosage should not exceed 200 mcg.
   By Those Over 60 Years of Age: No specific precautions.

▷ **Advisability of Use During Pregnancy**
   Pregnancy Category: C. See Pregnancy Risk Categories at the back of this book.
      Animal studies: High-dose studies in rats revealed fetal toxicity consistent with changes caused by other steroids.
      Human studies: Information from adequate studies of pregnant women is not available. Ask your doctor for guidance.

Advisability of Use If Breast-Feeding
   Presence of this drug in breast milk: Unknown.
   Monitor nursing infant closely and discontinue drug or nursing if adverse effects develop.

Habit-Forming Potential: Not defined.

Effects of Overdosage: Not defined.

Possible Effects of Long-Term Use: Rare nasal yeast infections.

Suggested Periodic Examinations While Taking This Drug (at physician's discretion)
   Nasal exams.

▷ **While Taking This Drug, Observe the Following**
   Foods: No restrictions.
   Beverages: No restrictions.
▷   *Alcohol:* No interactions expected.
   Tobacco Smoking: No interactions expected, but I advise everyone to quit smoking.
▷   *Other Drugs*
      Fluticasone *taken concurrently* with
      • Systemic steroids (such as prednisone) may increase the likelihood of suppression of the hypothalamic pituitary adrenal (HPA) axis.
▷   *Driving, Hazardous Activities:* This drug may cause dizziness. Restrict activities as necessary.

Aviation Note: The use of this drug *may be a disqualification* for piloting. Consult a designated Aviation Medical Examiner.

Exposure to Sun: No restrictions.

Discontinuation: This medicine should not be stopped abruptly. Talk with your doctor before stopping this drug.

FLUVASTATIN (flu va STAT in)

Introduced: 1994 **Class:** Cholesterol-reducing drug, HMG-CoA reductase inhibitor **Prescription:** USA: Yes **Controlled Drug:** USA: No; Canada: No **Available as Generic:** USA: No; Canada: No

Brand Name: Lescol

BENEFITS versus RISKS	
Possible Benefits	*Possible Risks*
EFFECTIVE REDUCTION OF TOTAL BLOOD CHOLESTEROL	Increased liver enzymes
SLOWS PROGRESSION OF CORONARY ATHEROSCLEROSIS	Muscle pain or weakness

▷ **Principal Uses**

As a Single Drug Product: Uses currently included in FDA-approved labeling: (1) Management of abnormally high cholesterol in people with type II hypercholesterolemia; (2) slows the progression of atherosclerosis in patients with coronary heart disease.

Author's Note: A study in *Clinical Therapeutics* found this agent to be the most effective for patients with high blood cholesterol.

Other (unlabeled) generally accepted uses: Not fully defined at present.

How This Drug Works: This medicine is changed (hydrolyzed) in the body to the beta-hydroxy-acid form. The beta-hydroxy-acid form inhibits an enzyme (HMG-CoA reductase) that is the (rate-controlling) enzyme in the process the body uses to make cholesterol.

Available Dosage Forms and Strengths

Tablets — 10 mg, 20 mg, 40 mg

▷ **Recommended Dosage Ranges** (Actual dosage and administration schedule must be determined for each patient individually.)

Infants and Children: Safety and efficacy for those less than 12 years of age have not yet been defined.

18 to 60 Years of Age: Dosing is started with 20 mg a day, taken with the evening meal. This dose is increased as needed and tolerated to 80 mg with each evening (24 hours apart) meal. Any needed increases are made at intervals of 4 weeks. Patients who take immunosuppressant medicines are started on 10 mg of lovastatin daily and should not receive more than 20 mg daily with the evening meal.

Over 60 Years of Age: Same as 12 to 60 years of age.

Conditions Requiring Dosing Adjustments

Liver Function: This drug is extensively changed in the liver; however, no specific dosing changes are defined for patients with compromised livers.

Kidney Function: Patients with severe kidney failure (creatinine clearance less then 30 ml/min) should be given more than 20 mg a day only with great caution.

▷ **Dosing Instructions:**   This medicine is best taken with the evening meal, as it produces the best cholesterol-lowering results or outcomes.

Usual Duration of Use: Continual use on a regular schedule for 3 to 4 weeks may be needed to determine this drug's effectiveness in helping lower low-density lipoprotein (LDL) level. Long-term use (months to years) requires periodic evaluation of response and dosage adjustment. Consult your physician on a regular basis.

Possible Advantages of This Drug
Requires once-daily dosing and has a good side-effect profile.

▷ **This Drug Should Not Be Taken If**
  • you have had an allergic reaction to any dosage form of it previously.
  • you have active liver disease.
  • you are pregnant or breast-feeding your infant.

▷ **Inform Your Physician Before Taking This Drug If**
  • you have previously taken any other drugs in this class: lovastatin (Mevacor), pravastatin (Pravachol).
  • you have a history of liver disease or impaired liver function.
  • you are not using any method of birth control, or you are planning pregnancy.
  • you regularly consume substantial amounts of alcohol.
  • you have cataracts or impaired vision.
  • you have any type of chronic muscular disorder.
  • you develop muscle pain, weakness, or soreness that is unexplained while taking this medicine.
  • you plan to have major surgery in the near future.

Possible Side Effects (natural, expected, and unavoidable drug actions)
Development of abnormal liver function tests without associated symptoms.

▷ **Possible Adverse Effects** (unusual, unexpected, and infrequent reactions)
  If any of the following develop, consult your physician promptly for guidance.
Mild Adverse Effects
  Allergic reactions: Rash.
  Headache or insomnia—infrequent.
  Indigestion, nausea, excessive gas, constipation, diarrhea—infrequent.
  Lowering of the blood pressure—possible.
Serious Adverse Effects
  Marked and persistent abnormal liver function tests with focal hepatitis (without jaundice)—case reports.
  Acute myositis (muscle pain and tenderness)—occurred rarely during long-term use.
  Rhabdomyolysis—rare.
  Cataracts (based on animal data, not reported in humans)—possible.
  Lichen planus skin rash—rare.

▷ **Possible Effects on Sexual Function:**   None reported.

Possible Delayed Adverse Effects: None reported to date. Doses of 15 to 33 times the human dose of another drug in this class given to rats caused an increase in liver cancers.

Natural Diseases or Disorders That May Be Activated by This Drug
Latent liver disease.

Possible Effects on Laboratory Tests
Blood alanine aminotransferase (ALT) enzyme level: increased (with higher doses of drug).
Blood total cholesterol, LDL cholesterol, and triglyceride levels: decreased.
Blood HDL cholesterol level: increased.

CAUTION
1. If pregnancy occurs while taking this drug, stop it immediately and consult your physician.
2. Report promptly any development of muscle pain or tenderness, especially if accompanied by fever or weakness (malaise).
3. Report promptly altered or impaired vision so that appropriate evaluation can be made.

Precautions for Use
By Infants and Children: Safety and effectiveness for those under 20 years of age are not established.
By Those Over 60 Years of Age: Inform your physician regarding any personal or family history of cataracts. Comply with all recommendations regarding periodic eye examinations. Report promptly any alterations in vision.

▷ **Advisability of Use During Pregnancy**
Pregnancy Category: X. See Pregnancy Risk Categories at the back of this book.
Animal studies: Mouse and rat studies reveal skeletal birth defects due to a closely related drug of this class.
Human studies: Adequate studies of pregnant women are not available.
This drug should be avoided during entire pregnancy.

Advisability of Use If Breast-Feeding
Presence of this drug in breast milk: Unknown.
Avoid drug or refrain from nursing.

Habit-Forming Potential: None.

Effects of Overdosage: Increased indigestion, stomach distress, nausea, diarrhea.

Possible Effects of Long-Term Use: Abnormal liver function with focal hepatitis.

Suggested Periodic Examinations While Taking This Drug (at physician's discretion)
Blood cholesterol studies: total cholesterol, HDL and LDL fractions.
Liver function tests before treatment, every 6 weeks during the first 3 months of use, every 8 weeks for the rest of the first year, and at 6-month intervals thereafter. Complete eye examination at beginning of treatment and at any time that significant change in vision occurs. Ask your physician for guidance.

▷ **While Taking This Drug, Observe the Following**
  Foods: Follow a standard low cholesterol diet.
  Beverages: No restrictions. May be taken with milk.
▷ *Alcohol:* No interactions expected. Use sparingly.
  Tobacco Smoking: No interactions expected, but I advise everyone to quit smoking.
▷ *Other Drugs*
    Fluvastatin may ***increase*** the effects of
    • digoxin (Lanoxin).
    • warfarin (Coumadin); more frequent testing of INR (prothrombin time) will be needed.
    Fluvastatin ***taken concurrently*** with
    • clofibrate (Atromid-S) or other fibrate compounds may result in increased risk of serious muscle toxicity.
    • cyclosporine (Sandimmune) can result in kidney failure and myopathy.
    • erythromycin and perhaps other macrolide antibiotics (see Drug Classes) may increase risk of muscle damage (myopathy or rhabdomyolysis).
    • gemfibrozil (Lopid) may alter the absorption and excretion of fluvastatin; these drugs should not be taken concurrently.
    • niacin may cause an increased frequency of muscle problems (myopathy) when combined with a related medicine (lovastatin). Caution is advised.
    • omeprazole (Prilosec) may increase fluvastatin levels and lead to toxicity.
    • ranitidine (Zantac) may increase peak blood levels of fluvastatin.
    The following drug may ***decrease*** the effects of fluvastatin
    • cholestyramine (Questran)—may reduce absorption of fluvastatin; take fluvastatin 1 hour before or 4 hours after cholestyramine.
▷ *Driving, Hazardous Activities:* No restrictions.
  Aviation Note: No restrictions.
  Exposure to Sun: No restrictions.
  Discontinuation: Do not stop this drug without your physician's knowledge and guidance. There may be significant increase in blood cholesterol levels following discontinuation of this drug.

FLUVOXAMINE (FLU vox a meen)

Introduced: 1995   **Class:** Antidepressant, selective serotonin reuptake inhibitor   **Prescription:** USA: Yes   **Controlled Drug:** USA: No; Canada: No   **Available as Generic:** USA: No; Canada: No

Brand Name: Luvox

Warning: **Do not** combine this medicine with terfenadine (Seldane) or astemizole (Hismanal).

BENEFITS versus RISKS	
Possible Benefits	*Possible Risks*
TREATMENT OF OBSESSIVE-COMPULSIVE DISORDER IN ADULTS TREATMENT OF OBSESSIVE-COMPULSIVE DISORDER IN CHILDREN	Nausea and vomiting (often resolves with time)

▷ **Principal Uses**

As a Single Drug Product: Uses currently included in FDA-approved labeling: Treatment of obsessive compulsive disorder in adults and children.

Other (unlabeled) generally accepted uses: (1) May have a role in helping compulsive exhibitionism; (2) can have a role in treating depression; (3) may be useful in eating problems where bingeing is a key difficulty; (4) can help panic attacks; (5) could have a role in long-standing (chronic) tension headaches.

How This Drug Works: This medicine inhibits the reuptake of the neurotransmitter 5-HT, effecting a beneficial change in the treated behaviors or conditions.

Available Dosage Forms and Strengths

Tablets — 50 mg, 100 mg

▷ **Recommended Dosage Ranges** (Actual dosage and administration schedule must be determined for each patient individually.)

Infants and Children: Safety and efficacy have recently been established in pediatrics (children and adolescents): Dosing is started with 25 mg at bedtime for 3 days. The dose is then increased by 25-mg steps every 3 to 4 days until a maximum of 200 mg is reached. If the required dose is larger than 75 mg, the total daily dose is divided into two equal doses and given twice daily.

18 to 60 Years of Age: Therapy is started with 50 mg taken at bedtime. The dose may then be increased as needed and tolerated by 50-mg intervals every 4 to 7 days to a maximum dose of 300 mg daily. The prescriber should remember that the drug may take from 4 to 14 days to begin to work. If a patient needs a daily dose greater than 100 mg, the dose should be divided in half and taken twice daily.

Over 60 Years of Age: This medicine is removed half as slowly as in younger patients. Plasma concentrations are also roughly 40% higher than in younger patients. Slower time frames for any increases beyond the starting dose and lower maintenance doses are indicated.

Conditions Requiring Dosing Adjustments

Liver Function: This drug is extensively changed by the liver. If it is used by patients with liver disease, lower starting doses, slow dose increases, and careful patient monitoring is indicated.

Kidney Function: A lower starting dose and careful patient monitoring is needed.

▷ **Dosing Instructions:**   Take this medicine exactly as prescribed and at the same time. This medicine may be taken with or without food. Call your doctor if vomiting (a possible side effect) continues for more than 2 days after you start treatment.

Usual Duration of Use: Continual use on a regular schedule for 4 to 14 days is usually necessary to determine this drug's effectiveness in helping obsessive-compulsive disorder. Long-term use (months to years) requires periodic evaluation of response and dosage adjustment. Consult your physician on a regular basis.

Possible Advantages of This Drug
Requires once-daily dosing and has a good side-effect profile.

▷ **This Drug Should Not Be Taken If**
  • you have had an allergic reaction to any dosage form of it previously.
  • you have taken or are taking terfenadine or astemizole.

▷ **Inform Your Physician Before Taking This Drug If**
  • you have continued to have a problem with vomiting 2 days after starting this medicine.
  • you feel light-headed when you get up from a sitting position.
  • you have a history of seizures.
  • you are uncertain of how much fluvoxamine to take or how often to take it.
  • you have taken a MAO inhibitor (see Drug Classes) within the last 14 days.
  • you have a history of heart problems.
  • you take other prescription or nonprescription medicines that were not discussed with your doctor when fluvoxamine was prescribed.

Possible Side Effects (natural, expected, and unavoidable drug actions)
Nausea and vomiting (usually stops after a few days of treatment).

▷ **Possible Adverse Effects** (unusual, unexpected, and infrequent reactions)
  If any of the following develop, consult your physician promptly for guidance.
  Mild Adverse Effects
  Allergic Reactions: Skin rash.
  Somnolence, headache, agitation, sleep disorders—infrequent.
  Liver toxicity—rare.
  Dry mouth, anorexia, or constipation—possible.
  Serious Adverse Effects
  Allergic Reactions: Anaphylactic reaction—case reports.
  Serious skin rash—case reports.
  Liver toxicity—rare.
  Seizures or mania—rare.
  Tourette syndrome—case reports.
  Excessive urination—rare.

▷ **Possible Effects on Sexual Function:**   Delayed or absent orgasm, failure to ejaculate—case reports.

Possible Delayed Adverse Effects: Not reported.

▷ **Adverse Effects That May Mimic Natural Diseases or Disorders**
  Not reported.

Natural Diseases or Disorders That May Be Activated by This Drug
  None defined.

Possible Effects on Laboratory Tests
  Liver function tests: increased.
  Melatonin level: increased.

CAUTION
1. This medicine has several important drug–drug interactions. Be certain to tell any health care professionals who provide care for you that you take this medicine.
2. If nausea and vomiting continue for more than 2 days after you start this medicine, call your doctor.

Precautions for Use
By Infants and Children: Safety and effectiveness for use by those under 18 years of age have not been established.
By Those Over 60 Years of Age: Lowering starting and maintenance doses are indicated.

▷ **Advisability of Use During Pregnancy**
Pregnancy Category: C. See Pregnancy Risk Categories at the back of this book.
    Animal studies: Consistent with category C.
    Human studies: Information from adequate studies of pregnant women is not available. Ask your doctor for help.

Advisability of Use If Breast-Feeding
Presence of this drug in breast milk: Yes, in small amounts.
Monitor nursing infant closely and discontinue drug or nursing if adverse effects develop.

Habit-Forming Potential: None, but a withdrawal syndrome has been reported if the medicine is stopped abruptly.

Effects of Overdosage: Nausea, vomiting, seizures.

Possible Effects of Long-Term Use: Not defined.

Suggested Periodic Examinations While Taking This Drug (at physician's discretion)
Liver function tests.

▷ **While Taking This Drug, Observe the Following**
Foods: No restrictions.
Beverages: No restrictions.
▷ *Alcohol:* No significant interaction. Ask your doctor for guidance.
Tobacco Smoking: Fluvoxamine stays in the body up to one-quarter less the time than in nonsmokers. I advise everyone to quit smoking.
Marijuana Smoking: Additive somnolence.
▷ *Other Drugs*
Fluvoxamine *taken concurrently* with
- amitriptyline (Elavil others) can result in amitriptyline toxicity.
- astemizole (Hismanal) may cause **serious heart arrhythmias**. Do not combine.
- benzodiazepines (see Drug Classes) may result in benzodiazepine toxicity.
- beta-blockers (see Drug Classes) may result in decreased drug clearance and toxicity.
- carbamazepine (Tegretol) may cause toxicity.
- cimetidine (Tagamet) may lead to toxicity.
- clomipramine (Anafranil) may cause toxicity.
- clozapine (Clozaril) can result in higher clozapine levels and toxicity.
- imipramine (Tofranil, others) may result in imipramine toxicity.
- lithium (Lithobid) can cause serotonin syndrome.

- MAO inhibitors (see Drug Classes) can cause toxicity. Do **not** combine.
- maprotiline can cause maprotiline toxicity.
- methadone may result in increased opioid effects.
- oral antidiabetic drugs (see Drug Classes) may remain in the body longer than expected, requiring a dosage decrease. This has not been reported with fluvoxamine, but has been reported with sertraline, a medicine in the same pharmacological family.
- phenytoin (Dilantin) may lead to phenytoin toxicity. Patients should be watched closely for problems walking (ataxia) or drowsiness (early toxicity signs), and their doctor notified at once if these occur.
- terfenadine (Seldane) may cause **serious heart arrhythmias**. Do not combine.
- theophylline may result in theophylline toxicity.
- tramadol (Ultram) may increase seizure risk. **Do NOT combine.**
- tryptophan may increase serotonin effects of fluvoxamine and cause severe vomiting.
- warfarin (Coumadin) can result in increased warfarin concentrations and may lead to bleeding. More frequent INR testing is needed.

▷ *Driving, Hazardous Activities:* This drug may cause drowsiness. Restrict activities as necessary.

Aviation Note: The use of this drug *is probably a disqualification* for piloting. Consult a designated Aviation Medical Examiner.

Exposure to Sun: No restrictions.

Discontinuation: A withdrawal syndrome has been reported if this medicine is abruptly stopped. The doses should be slowly tapered.

FOSINOPRIL (FOH sin oh pril)

Introduced: 1986   **Class:** Antihypertensive, ACE inhibitor   **Prescription:** USA: Yes   **Controlled Drug:** USA: No   **Available as Generic:** No
Brand Name: Monopril

BENEFITS versus RISKS	
Possible Benefits	*Possible Risks*
EFFECTIVE CONTROL OF MILD TO MODERATE HIGH BLOOD PRESSURE	Low blood pressure Allergic swelling of face, tongue, throat, vocal cords

▷ **Principal Uses**

As a Single Drug Product: Uses currently included in FDA-approved labeling: Treats mild to moderate high blood pressure, alone or in combination with other medicines.

Other (unlabeled) generally accepted uses: (1) Combination with other drugs (digoxin and diuretics) to treat congestive heart failure; (2) may help decrease enlargement of the left side of the heart; (3) reduces abnormal elimination of protein by the kidneys; (4) improves survival after a heart attack.

How This Drug Works: By blocking an enzyme system (angiotensin-converting enzyme, ACE), this drug relaxes arterial walls and lowers blood pressure. This, in turn, reduces the workload of the heart and improves its performance.

Available Dosage Forms and Strengths

Tablets — 10 mg, 20 mg

▷ **Recommended Dosage Ranges** (Actual dosage and administration schedule must be determined for each patient individually.)

Infants and Children: Dosage not established.

18 to 60 Years of Age: Hypertension: Initially 10 mg once daily. Usual maintenance dose is 20 to 40 mg daily taken in a single dose. Total daily dosage should not exceed 80 mg.

Congestive heart failure: Starting doses of 5 mg (especially for patients who are dehydrated or have kidney failure) to 10 mg have been recommended. Some studies have used once-daily dosing; however, individual dosing strategies must be used.

Over 60 Years of Age: Same as 18 to 60 years of age, but these patients may be more sensitive to fosinopril. Smaller and more gradual dose increases are prudent as needed and tolerated.

Conditions Requiring Dosing Adjustments

Liver Function: Fosinopril is a prodrug, and is changed into fosinoprilat (the active form) by the liver. It should be used with caution and in lower doses by patients with liver compromise. Fosinopril can also be a rare cause of hepatitis.

Kidney Function: This drug undergoes liver and bile (dual hepatobiliary) and kidney (renal) elimination. Patients with renal compromise (especially those with renal artery stenosis) should start on a decreased dose, and the dose should be increased slowly and only if needed.

▷ **Dosing Instructions:**   The tablet may be crushed, and taken on an empty stomach or with food, at the same time each day.

Usual Duration of Use: Use on a regular schedule for 2 to 3 weeks determines effectiveness in controlling high blood pressure. Long-term use of effective medicines and periodic physician evaluation is needed in high blood pressure.

Possible Advantages of This Drug

May (for some patients) control blood pressure effectively with one daily dose. Relatively low incidence of adverse effects. No adverse influence on asthma, cholesterol blood levels, or diabetes. Sudden withdrawal does not result in a rapid increase in blood pressure.

▷ **This Drug Should Not Be Taken If**
- you have had an allergic reaction to it previously.
- you are pregnant (final 6 months).
- you have an abnormally high level of blood potassium.

▷ **Inform Your Physician Before Taking This Drug If**
- you have had an allergic reaction (or other adverse effect) to any ACE inhibitor (see Drug Classes).
- you are planning pregnancy.
- you plan to breast-feed your baby.
- you have a history of kidney disease or impaired kidney function.
- you have scleroderma or systemic lupus erythematosus.
- you currently have a blood cell or bone marrow disorder.
- you have cerebral artery disease.

- you have any form of heart disease.
- you are taking other antihypertensives, diuretics, nitrates, or potassium supplements.
- you plan to have surgery under general anesthesia in the near future.

Possible Side Effects (natural, expected, and unavoidable drug actions)

Dizziness or orthostatic hypotension (see Glossary)—rare increased blood potassium level. Cough—infrequent.

▷ **Possible Adverse Effects** (unusual, unexpected, and infrequent reactions)

If any of the following develop, consult your physician promptly for guidance.

Mild Adverse Effects

Allergic Reactions: Skin rash, hives, itching—rare.
Headache, fatigue, drowsiness, numbness and tingling, weakness—rare.
Chest pain, palpitation—rare to infrequent.
Indigestion, nausea and vomiting or diarrhea—rare.

Serious Adverse Effects

Allergic Reactions: Swelling (angioedema) of face, tongue, and/or vocal cords—rare; can be life-threatening—case reports.
Impairment of kidney function—rare.
Decreased white blood cells—case reports.
Pancreatitis (not reported for this drug, only with members of the same chemical family)—case reports.
Symptomatic lowering of the blood pressure (hypotension)—rare.
Compromise of kidney function—more likely in those with severe congestive heart failure.

▷ **Possible Effects on Sexual Function:**   Decreased libido or abnormal swelling of male breast tissue (gynecomastia)—rare. Impotence has been reported with other members of the same pharmacological family.

Possible Effects on Laboratory Tests

Blood potassium level: increased.
Liver function tests: increased liver enzymes (ALT/GPT, AST/GOT, alkaline phosphatase), or bilirubin.
Kidney function tests: increased blood urea nitrogen (BUN) and creatinine.
May give a falsely low test for digoxin levels.

CAUTION

1. Ask your doctor if you should stop other antihypertensive drugs (especially diuretics) for 1 week before starting this drug.
2. **Inform your physician immediately if you become pregnant.** This drug should not be taken beyond the first 3 months of pregnancy.
3. ***Report promptly*** any indications of infection (fever, sore throat), or water retention (weight gain, puffiness, swollen feet or ankles).
4. Do not use a salt substitute without your physician's knowledge and approval. (Many salt substitutes contain potassium.)
5. It is best to obtain blood cell counts and urine analyses ***before*** starting this drug.

Precautions for Use

By Infants and Children: Safety and effectiveness for those under 18 years of age not established.

By Those Over 60 Years of Age: Small starting doses are advisable. Sudden and excessive lowering of blood pressure can predispose to stroke or heart attack in impaired brain circulation or coronary artery heart disease.

▷ **Advisability of Use During Pregnancy**

Pregnancy Category: C during the first 3 months (trimester). D during the second and third trimesters (fourth to ninth months). See Pregnancy Risk Categories at the back of this book.

Animal studies: Significant birth defects associated with this drug.

Human studies: The use of ACE inhibitor drugs during the final 6 months of pregnancy is known to possibly cause very serious injury and possible death to the fetus: skull and limb malformations, lung defects, and kidney failure have been reported in over 50 cases worldwide.

Avoid this drug completely during the final 6 months. During the first 3 months of pregnancy, use this drug only if clearly needed. Ask your physician for guidance.

Advisability of Use If Breast-Feeding

Presence of this drug in breast milk: Yes.

Avoid drug or refrain from nursing.

Habit-Forming Potential: None.

Effects of Overdosage: Excessive drop in blood pressure, light-headedness, dizziness, fainting.

Possible Effects of Long-Term Use: Gradual increase in blood potassium level.

Suggested Periodic Examinations While Taking This Drug (at physician's discretion)

Before starting drug: Complete blood counts; urine analysis with measurement of protein content; blood potassium level. During use of drug: Blood cell counts; measurements of blood potassium.

▷ **While Taking This Drug, Observe the Following**

Foods: Consult your physician regarding salt intake.

Nutritional Support: **Do not** take potassium supplements unless directed by your physician.

Beverages: No restrictions. May be taken with milk.

▷   *Alcohol:* Use caution—alcohol may enhance the blood-pressure-lowering effect.

Tobacco Smoking: No interactions expected, but I advise everyone to quit smoking.

▷   *Other Drugs*

Fosinopril *taken concurrently* with

- chlorpromazine (Thorazine) can cause large and undesirable decreases in blood pressure. Avoid this combination.
- cyclosporine (Sandimmune) can cause a large decrease in kidney function.
- lithium (Lithobid) causes increased lithium blood levels and toxicity; blood levels and dosage decreases are critical.
- loop diuretics—furosemide or bumetanide (Lasix, Bumex)—can cause marked lowering of blood pressure on standing (postural hypotension).
- nonsteroidal anti-inflammatory drugs (NSAIDs) such as ketorolac (Toradol) blunts benefits.
- potassium preparations (K-Lyte, Slow-K, etc.) may cause increased blood levels of potassium with risk of serious heart rhythm disturbances.

- potassium-sparing diuretics—amiloride (Moduretic), spironolactone (Aldactazide), triamterene (Dyazide)—may cause increased blood levels of potassium with risk of serious heart rhythm disturbances.

▷ *Driving, Hazardous Activities:* Usually no restrictions. Be aware of possible drops in blood pressure with resultant dizziness or faintness.

Aviation Note: The use of this drug *may be a disqualification* for piloting. Consult a designated Aviation Medical Examiner.

Exposure to Sun: Caution is advised. A similar drug of this class can cause photosensitivity.

Exposure to Heat: Caution is advised. Avoid excessive perspiring with resultant loss of body water and drop in blood pressure.

Occurrence of Unrelated Illness: Promptly report any nausea, vomiting, or diarrhea. Fluid and chemical imbalances must be corrected as soon as possible.

Discontinuation: This drug may be stopped abruptly without causing a sudden increase in blood pressure. However, you should ask your physician before stopping this drug for any reason.

FUROSEMIDE (fur OH se mide)

Introduced: 1964   **Class:** Antihypertensive, diuretic   **Prescription:** USA: Yes   **Controlled Drug:** USA: No; Canada: No   **Available as Generic:** USA: Yes; Canada: Yes

Brand Names: ✦Albert Furosemide, ✦Apo-Furosemide, Fumide MD, Furomide MD, Furocot, Furosemide-10, ✦Furoside, Lasaject, Lasimide, Lasix, ✦Lasix Special, Lo-Aqua, Luramide, Myrosemide, Ro-Semide, SK-Furosemide, ✦Uritol

BENEFITS versus RISKS	
Possible Benefits	*Possible Risks*
PROMPT, EFFECTIVE, RELIABLE DIURETIC	WATER AND ELECTROLYTE DEPLETION with excessive use
MODEST ANTIHYPERTENSIVE IN MILD TO MODERATE HYPERTENSION	Excessive potassium and magnesium loss
ENHANCES EFFECTIVENESS OF OTHER ANTIHYPERTENSIVES	Increased blood sugar level
	Increased blood uric acid level
	Decreased blood calcium level
	Liver damage
	Blood cell disorder

▷ **Principal Uses**

As a Single Drug Product: Uses currently included in FDA-approved labeling: (1) Used to increase urine and remove excessive water (edema), as in congestive heart failure or some forms of liver, lung, and kidney disease; (2) used in the treatment of high blood pressure, but usually is combined with other drugs.

Other (unlabeled) generally accepted uses: (1) Inhaled furosemide may help protect the lungs in people with asthma; (2) can have a role in helping infants with lung problems (chronic bronchopulmonary dysplasia).

How This Drug Works: By increasing the elimination of salt and water through increased urine production, this drug reduces fluid in the blood and body tissues. These changes also contribute to lowering blood pressure.

Available Dosage Forms and Strengths

Injection — 10 mg/ml

Solution — 10 mg/ml

Tablets — 20 mg, 40 mg, 80 mg

▷ **Usual Adult Dosage Range:**   As antihypertensive: 40 mg every 12 hours initially; increase dose as needed and tolerated. As diuretic: 20 to 80 mg in a single dose initially; if necessary, increase the dose by 20 to 40 mg every 6 to 8 hours. The smallest effective dose should be used, and total daily dose should not exceed 640 mg. In general, other medicines effective in treating high blood pressure should be added on before the daily oral dose is increased beyond 80 mg per day. **Note: Actual dosage and administration schedule must be determined for each patient individually.**

Conditions Requiring Dosing Adjustments

Liver Function: Larger doses may be needed for patients with liver compromise, and extreme care must be used to maintain critical electrolytes.

Kidney Function: Larger initial doses may be needed before any benefit is seen. Furosemide is also capable of causing kidney stones and protein in urine.

Cystic Fibrosis: Patients with this disease may be more sensitive to the drug, and smaller starting doses are indicated.

▷ **Dosing Instructions:**   The tablet may be crushed and taken with or following meals to reduce stomach irritation. Best taken in the morning to avoid nighttime urination.

Usual Duration of Use: Use on a regular schedule for 2 to 3 weeks is best to see effectiveness in lowering high blood pressure. Long-term use (months to years) requires periodic physician evaluation of response.

▷ **This Drug Should Not Be Taken If**
- you have had an allergic reaction to any dosage form of it previously.
- your kidneys are not making urine.

▷ **Inform Your Physician Before Taking This Drug If**
- you are allergic to any form of "sulfa" drug.
- you are pregnant or planning pregnancy.
- you have a history of kidney or liver disease.
- you have diabetes, gout, or lupus erythematosus.
- you have impaired hearing.
- you have low blood potassium or other electrolytes (talk with your doctor).
- you take any form of cortisone, digitalis, oral antidiabetic drug, or insulin.
- you plan to have surgery under general anesthesia in the near future.

Possible Side Effects (natural, expected, and unavoidable drug actions)

Light-headedness on arising from sitting or lying position (see Orthostatic Hypotension in Glossary).

Increase in blood sugar level, affecting control of diabetes.

Increase in blood uric acid level, affecting control of gout.

Decrease in blood potassium level, causing muscle weakness and cramping.

Decreased magnesium level.

▷ **Possible Adverse Effects** (unusual, unexpected, and infrequent reactions)
If any of the following develop, consult your physician promptly for guidance.

Mild Adverse Effects

Allergic Reactions: Skin rashes, hives, drug fever—case reports.

Headache, dizziness, blurred or yellow vision, ringing in ears, numbness and tingling—rare to infrequent.

Reduced appetite, indigestion, nausea, vomiting, diarrhea—possible.

Metabolic alkalosis—possible.

Serious Adverse Effects

Allergic Reactions: Hepatitis with jaundice (see Glossary), anaphylactic reaction (see Glossary), severe skin reactions—case reports.

Idiosyncratic Reaction: Fluid accumulation in lungs—case reports.

Temporary hearing loss—case reports.

Inflammation of the pancreas (severe abdominal pain)—rare.

Bone marrow depression (see Glossary): fatigue, weakness, fever, sore throat, abnormal bleeding or bruising—case reports.

Low blood pressure on standing or abnormal heartbeat (arrhythmias)—rare.

Drug-induced porphyria or excessive parathyroid gland action (hyperparathyroidism)—case reports.

Low blood potassium or magnesium—possible.

Vitamin deficiency (thiamine)—possible.

Kidney stones (calcium containing)—case reports.

Liver toxicity (cholestatic jaundice)—rare.

Skin lesions (erythema multiforme or Stevens-Johnson syndrome)—case reports.

Hip fractures (may increase risk).

▷ **Possible Effects on Sexual Function:**   Impotence using recommended dosage of 20 to 80 mg per day—infrequent.

▷ **Adverse Effects That May Mimic Natural Diseases or Disorders**
Liver reaction may suggest viral hepatitis.

Natural Diseases or Disorders That May Be Activated by This Drug
Diabetes, gout, systemic lupus erythematosus.

Possible Effects on Laboratory Tests

Complete blood counts: reduced red cells, hemoglobin, white cells, and platelets.

Blood amylase and lipase levels: increased (possible pancreatitis).

Blood sodium and chloride levels: decreased.

Blood levels of total cholesterol, LDL and VLDL cholesterol, and triglycerides: increased.

Blood glucose level: increased.

Glucose tolerance test (GTT): decreased tolerance.

Blood potassium or magnesium level: decreased.

Blood thyroid hormone (T_3 and T_4) levels: decreased.

Blood uric acid level or blood urea nitrogen (BUN): increased.

Urine sugar tests: no drug effect with Tes-Tape; false low results with Clinistix and Diastix.

CAUTION
1. Take exactly the dose that was prescribed. Increased doses can cause serious loss of sodium and potassium, with resultant loss of appetite, nausea, fatigue, weakness, confusion, and tingling in the extremities.
2. If you take a digitalis preparation (digitoxin, digoxin), ensure an adequate intake of high potassium foods to prevent potassium deficiency. (See Table 13, "High Potassium Foods," Section Six.)

Precautions for Use

By Infants and Children: Avoid overdosage that could cause serious dehydration. Significant potassium loss can occur within the first 2 weeks of drug use.

By Those Over 60 Years of Age: Small starting doses are critical. Increased risk of impaired thinking, orthostatic hypotension, potassium loss, and blood sugar increase. Overdosage and extended use of this drug can cause excessive loss of body water, thickening (increased viscosity) of the blood, and an increased tendency for the blood to clot—predisposing to stroke, heart attack, or thrombophlebitis (vein inflammation with blood clot).

▷ **Advisability of Use During Pregnancy**

Pregnancy Category: C. See Pregnancy Risk Categories at the back of this book.
Animal studies: Significant birth defects have been reported.
Human studies: Adequate studies of pregnant women are not available.
It should not be used during pregnancy unless a very serious complication occurs for which this drug is significantly beneficial. Avoid completely during the first 3 months. Ask your physician for guidance.

Advisability of Use If Breast-Feeding

Presence of this drug in breast milk: Yes.
Avoid drug or refrain from nursing.

Habit-Forming Potential: None.

Effects of Overdosage: Dry mouth, thirst, lethargy, weakness, muscle cramping, nausea, vomiting, drowsiness progressing to stupor or coma.

Possible Effects of Long-Term Use: Impaired water, salt, and potassium balance; dehydration and increased blood coagulability, with risk of blood clots. Development of diabetes in predisposed individuals.

Suggested Periodic Examinations While Taking This Drug (at physician's discretion)
Complete blood counts, measurements of blood levels of sodium, potassium, chloride, sugar, and uric acid.
Kidney and liver function tests.

▷ **While Taking This Drug, Observe the Following**

Foods: Ask your doctor about eating foods rich in potassium. If so advised, see Table 13, "High Potassium Foods," Section Six. Follow your physician's advice regarding the use of salt. Food decreases absorption of furosemide by up to 30%. Take this medicine 1 hour before or 2 hours after a meal.

Beverages: No restrictions. This drug may be taken with milk.

▷ *Alcohol:* Use with caution—alcohol may exaggerate the blood-pressure-lowering effects of this drug and cause orthostatic hypotension.

Tobacco Smoking: No interactions expected, but I advise everyone to quit smoking.

▷ *Other Drugs*

Furosemide may *increase* the effects of
- other antihypertensive drugs; dosage adjustments may be necessary to prevent excessive lowering of blood pressure.
- digoxin (Lanoxin) and result in digoxin toxicity.
- lithium (Lithobid, others), and cause lithium toxicity.

Furosemide may *decrease* the effects of
- oral antidiabetic drugs (sulfonylureas); dosage adjustments may be necessary for proper control of blood sugar.

Furosemide *taken concurrently* with
- adrenocortical steroids (see Drug Classes) may cause additive loss of potassium.
- amikacin, gentamicin, tobramycin, or other aminoglycosides may cause hearing toxicity (ototoxicity).
- cephalosporin antibiotics (see Drug Classes) may increase risk of kidney problems (nephrotoxicity).
- cholestyramine (Questran) may cause loss of furosemide effectiveness.
- clofibrate (Atromid-S) may lead to muscle stiffness and increased diuretic effects.
- colestipol (Colestid) may cause loss of furosemide effectiveness.
- cyclosporine (Sandimmune) may cause elevated uric acid levels (hyperuricemia) and gout.
- digitalis preparations (digitoxin, digoxin) requires blood tests or dose changes to maintain potassium levels and avoid heart rhythm problems.
- lomefloxacin (Maxaquin) may increase lomefloxacin levels and lead to toxicity.
- NSAIDs (see Drug Classes) may cause loss of diuretic effectiveness.
- phenytoin (Dilantin) may decrease furosemide diuretic effects.

▷ *Driving, Hazardous Activities:* Use caution until the possible occurrence of orthostatic hypotension, dizziness, or impaired vision has been determined.

Aviation Note: The use of this drug *may be a disqualification* for piloting. Consult a designated Aviation Medical Examiner.

Exposure to Sun: Use caution—this drug may cause photosensitivity (see Glossary).

Exposure to Heat: Avoid excessive perspiring, which could cause additional loss of salt and water from the body.

Heavy Exercise or Exertion: Avoid exertion that produces light-headedness, excessive fatigue, or muscle cramping. Isometric exercises—the "overload" technique for strengthening individual muscles—can raise blood pressure significantly. Ask your physician for guidance regarding participation in this form of exercise.

Occurrence of Unrelated Illness: Vomiting or diarrhea can produce a serious imbalance of important body chemistry. Ask your doctor for guidance.

Discontinuation: It may be best to discontinue this drug 5 to 7 days before major surgery. Ask your physician, surgeon, and/or anesthesiologist for guidance regarding dosage adjustment or drug withdrawal.

GANCICLOVIR (ganz EYE klo veer)

Introduced: 1995 (tablet)   **Class:** Antiviral   **Prescription:** USA: Yes
Controlled Drug: USA: No; Canada: No   **Available as Generic:** USA: No;
Canada: No

Brand Names: Cytovene, Vitrasert

Warning: The oral form of this medicine should only be used by patients who
   are not candidates for intravenous administration and in whom the risk of
   more rapid disease progression of cytomegalovirus (CMV) retinitis is outweighed by the benefit of avoiding the intravenous route.

BENEFITS versus RISKS

Possible Benefits	*Possible Risks*
Oral, intravenous, or implanted treatment of cytomegalovirus (CMV) retinitis	More rapid progression of CMV disease (capsules)
Decreased side effects with the oral form	Bone marrow suppression
Transition to an oral form following intravenous induction	

▷ **Principal Uses**

   As a Single Drug Product: Uses currently included in FDA-approved labeling: (1)
      Treatment of cytomegalovirus (CMV) retinitis; (2) prevention of CMV reti-
      nitis in a variety of patients such as liver, kidney, lung, bone marrow, and
      heart transplant patients; (3) implantation of the ocular implant into the
      diseased area. This form may work for 5 months or more; (4) prevention of
      CMV disease in patients with advanced HIV infection.

   Other (unlabeled) generally accepted uses: (1) Treatment of pediatric CMV;
      (2) may have a role in treating Epstein-Barr virus infection; (3) can have a
      role in treating leukoplakia.

How This Drug Works: This medicine is changed into an active triphosphate
   form by cells infected with cytomegalovirus. This active form interferes
   with synthesis of DNA and the ability of the virus to survive.

Available Dosage Forms and Strengths
   Capsules — 250 mg
   Intravenous — 500 mg/10 ml
   Intravitreal insert — 4.5 mg

How To Store
   The intravenous solution should be stored at 39 degrees F (4 degrees C) and
   used within 12 hours after it has been reconstituted.

▷ **Recommended Dosage Ranges** (Actual dosage and administration schedule
      must be determined for each patient individually.)

   Infants and Children: **Author's Note: This drug has potential for reproduc-
      tive toxicity and the risk of causing cancer. It is used in children only
      after careful evaluation and with extreme caution.**

   Induction: 2.5 mg per kg of body mass given intravenously three times daily.
   Maintenance: 6.5 mg per kg of body mass given intravenously once daily five
      to seven times a week.

12 to 60 Years of Age: Induction: 5 mg per kg of body mass intravenously (infused over 1 hour) every 12 hours for 14 to 21 days.

Maintenance dose: 2.1 to 6 mg per kg of body mass infused into a vein over 1 hour each day. Some centers have used 6 mg per kg of body mass given once daily 5 days per week. The maker of this drug suggests 5 mg per kg of body mass intravenously daily. If retinitis progresses, the patient can be restarted on the twice-daily-dosing approach. Maximum dose is 6 mg per kg of body mass infused over 1 hour.

Oral: Once the intravenous induction dosing has been accomplished, oral ganciclovir is given 1000 mg three times daily. Some centers have opted for 500 mg six times per day, given every 3 hours while the patient is awake. If retinitis progresses, intravenous induction therapy should be given.

Intravitreous: This device is surgically implanted and has been effective for 5 or more months.

Over 60 Years of Age: Kidney function must be checked and the dose appropriately adjusted.

Conditions Requiring Dosing Adjustments

Liver Function: The liver is only minimally involved in the elimination of this drug, and dosing changes in liver compromise are not needed.

Kidney Function: The dose **must** be decreased in kidney compromise. This adjustment is accomplished based on creatinine clearance (see Glossary):

Induction—70 ml/min or higher: 5 mg per kg of body mass every 12 hours; 50–69: 2.5 mg per kg of body mass every 12 hours; 25–49: 2.5 mg per kg of body mass every 24 hours; 10–24: 1.25 mg per kg of body mass every 24 hours; less than 10: 1.25 mg per kg of body mass three times per week.

Maintenance:—70 ml/min or higher: 5 mg per kg of body mass every 24 hours; 50–69: 2.5 mg per kg of body mass every 24 hours; 25–49: 1.25 mg per kg of body mass every 24 hours; 10–24: 0.625 mg per kg of body mass every 24 hours; less than 10: 0.625 mg per kg of body mass three times per week.

▷ **Dosing Instructions:** This medicine should be taken with food if taken by mouth (orally). It is best to take the medicine at the same time each day. Capsule form should not be opened or crushed, because you may have adverse reactions from the toxic powder. If you are taking the capsule form and your vision declines, call your doctor immediately.

Usual Duration of Use: Continual use on a regular schedule for up to 16 days is usually needed to determine this drug's effectiveness in treating retinitis. Because of a very high frequency of relapse, most centers recommend ongoing maintenance therapy. Long-term use (months to years) requires periodic evaluation of response and dosage adjustment. The new ocular implant form may work for 5 months or more. Consult your physician on a regular basis.

Possible Advantages of This Drug

Transition from the intravenous form to the oral form (if successful in treatment) offers a clear quality of life advantage.

Currently a "Drug of Choice"

for patients with kidney failure.

▷ **This Drug Should Not Be Taken If**
- you have had an allergic reaction to any dosage form of it previously.
- your absolute neutrophil count (a specific kind of white blood cell) is less than 500 per cubic mm.
- your platelet count is less than 25,000 per cubic mm.

▷ **Inform Your Physician Before Taking This Drug If**
- you think you are dehydrated (this drug is primarily removed by the kidneys).
- you have a sore throat or fever.
- you have a history of blood cell disorders.
- you are planning pregnancy.
- you are male and are planning pregnancy (attempted conception should be avoided for at least 3 months after ganciclovir therapy).
- you are uncertain of how much ganciclovir to take, how often to take it, or how to handle the intravenous solution.
- you take other prescription or nonprescription medicines that were not discussed with your doctor when ganciclovir was prescribed. This includes natural extracts or herbal remedies and "underground" therapies for AIDS.

Possible Side Effects (natural, expected, and unavoidable drug actions)
Pain at the injection site with the IV form. Possible phlebitis.

▷ **Possible Adverse Effects** (unusual, unexpected, and infrequent reactions)
If any of the following develop, consult your physician promptly for guidance.
Mild Adverse Effects
Allergic Reactions: Skin rash and itching.
Confusion, headache, nervousness, tremor, somnolence, abnormal dreams, ataxia, "pins-and-needles" sensations of the hands (paresthesias)—infrequent.
Fever—may be frequent with oral therapy.
Decreased blood glucose or potassium—rare.
Nausea, vomiting, or diarrhea—infrequent to frequent.
Serious Adverse Effects
Allergic Reactions: Anaphylactic reaction—case reports.
Bone marrow suppression—rare.
Lowered white blood cell (neutropenia) counts—frequent.
Lowered blood platelets—infrequent.
Arrhythmias—rare.
Coma, psychosis, or seizures—case reports.
Neuropathy—infrequent to frequent.
Liver toxicity—rare to infrequent.
Retinal detachment—infrequent.
This drug is a potential cancer-causing (carcinogenic) agent—no percentage defined.

▷ **Possible Effects on Sexual Function:**   Reversible infertility in men.

Possible Delayed Adverse Effects: Lowered white blood cell counts or platelets.

▷ **Adverse Effects That May Mimic Natural Diseases or Disorders**
Increased liver enzymes may mimic hepatitis.

Natural Diseases or Disorders That May Be Activated by This Drug
None defined.

Possible Effects on Laboratory Tests
Liver enzymes: increased.
Serum bilirubin or creatinine: increased.
Blood glucose, platelets, or white blood cells: decreased.

CAUTION

1. The oral form may be less effective than the intravenous form. Call your doctor immediately if your vision declines.
2. This drug can cause bone marrow suppression. Call your doctor if you develop a sore throat, start to bruise easily, or develop a fever.

Precautions for Use
By Infants and Children: Safety and effectiveness for use by those under 18 years of age have not been established. The drug has been used selectively in patients as young as 36 weeks.
By Those Over 60 Years of Age: Because of the age-related decline in kidney function, a creatinine clearance should be obtained and dosing adjusted appropriately.

▷ **Advisability of Use During Pregnancy**
Pregnancy Category: C. See Pregnancy Risk Categories at the back of this book.
Animal studies: Rabbits have developed cleft palate, exhibited poorly developed organs, and have experienced fetal death.
Human studies: Information from adequate studies of pregnant women is not available. Use of this drug during pregnancy is not recommended.

Advisability of Use If Breast-Feeding
Presence of this drug in breast milk: Unknown.
Avoid drug or refrain from nursing.

Habit-Forming Potential: None.

Effects of Overdosage: Nausea and vomiting, excessive salivation, increased liver function tests, bone marrow suppression, and kidney failure.

Possible Effects of Long-Term Use: Not defined.

Suggested Periodic Examinations While Taking This Drug (at physician's discretion)
Platelet counts and complete blood counts: every 2 days during induction and weekly thereafter. Liver function tests: monthly. Kidney function tests: every 2 weeks.
Eye (ophthalmologic) exams: weekly during induction and every 2 weeks thereafter. These exams may be needed more frequently if the optic nerve or macula of the eye is involved.

▷ **While Taking This Drug, Observe the Following**
Foods: No restrictions—the oral form should be taken with food.
Beverages: No restrictions.
▷ *Alcohol:* No restrictions; however, alcohol may blunt the immune system.
Tobacco Smoking: No interactions expected, but I advise everyone to quit smoking.
Marijuana Smoking: May increase somnolence.
▷ *Other Drugs*
Ganciclovir ***taken concurrently*** with

- amphotericin B (Fungizone) may result in increased bone marrow suppression.
- cancer chemotherapy may result in additive bone marrow suppression.
- cotrimoxazole (Septra) may result in added bone marrow suppression problems.
- cyclosporine (Sandimmune) can result in increased kidney toxicity.
- dapsone is a benefit-to-risk decision, as additive bone marrow suppression may occur.
- flucytosine (Ancobon) can cause additive bone marrow toxicity.
- imipenem/cilastatin (Primaxin) can cause seizures.
- pentamidine may result in additive bone marrow suppression.
- zidovudine (AZT) will cause a serious increase in bone marrow suppression.

The following drugs may *increase* the effects of ganciclovir
- probenecid (Benemid)—by interfering with elimination by the kidney.

▷ *Driving, Hazardous Activities:* This drug may cause somnolence. Restrict activities as necessary.

Aviation Note: The use of this drug *may be a disqualification* for piloting. Consult a designated Aviation Medical Examiner.

Exposure to Sun: Caution is advised. Photosensitivity has been reported.

Discontinuation: Talk with your doctor before stopping this medicine.

Special Storage Instructions: The intravenous form should be stored at 39 degrees F (4 degrees C).

Observe the Following Expiration Times: The intravenous form will be stamped or labeled with a specific expiration time if this has been provided by a home infusion company; it should be used within 12 hours after it has been reconstituted.

GEMFIBROZIL (jem FI broh zil)

Introduced: 1976   **Class:** Anticholesterol   **Prescription:** USA: Yes
Controlled Drug: USA: No; Canada: No   **Available as Generic:** USA: Yes;
Canada: No

Brand Names: Lopid, Gemcor

BENEFITS versus RISKS	
Possible Benefits	*Possible Risks*
EFFECTIVE REDUCTION OF TRIGLYCERIDE BLOOD LEVELS	Gallstone formation with long-term use
INCREASE IN HIGH-DENSITY LIPOPROTEIN (HDL) BLOOD LEVELS	Decreased white blood cell counts

▷ **Principal Uses**

As a Single Drug Product: Uses currently included in FDA-approved labeling: (1) Reduces abnormally high blood levels of triglycerides in Types II and IV blood lipid (fat) disorders; (2) decreases risk for developing coronary artery heart disease.

Other (unlabeled) generally accepted uses: Used by diabetics as combination therapy with oral hypoglycemic agents to further increase desirable HDLs.

How This Drug Works: Reduces blood levels of triglycerides by inhibiting their production in the liver. Decreases VLDL and LDL. Causes a larger increase in desirable HDL than clofibrate.

Available Dosage Forms and Strengths
>   Capsules — 300 mg
>   Tablets — 600 mg

▷ **Usual Adult Dosage Range:**   1200 to 1600 daily in two divided doses. The average dose is 1200 mg daily. Dose increases should be made gradually over a period of 2 to 3 months. **Note: Actual dosage and administration schedule must be determined for each patient individually.**

Conditions Requiring Dosing Adjustments
Liver Function: This drug is contraindicated in primary biliary cirrhosis and severe liver failure.
Kidney Function: For patients with moderate kidney failure, 50% of the usual dose should be taken at the usual interval. Patients with severe kidney failure should take 25% of the usual dose at the usual dosing interval.

▷ **Dosing Instructions:**   The capsule may be opened and taken 30 minutes before the morning and evening meals.

Usual Duration of Use: Use on a regular schedule for 4 to 8 weeks determines effectiveness in reducing blood levels of triglycerides. Long-term use (months to years) requires periodic physician evaluation.

▷ **This Drug Should Not Be Taken If**
- you have had an allergic reaction to it previously.
- you have biliary cirrhosis of the liver.
- you have severe kidney compromise.

▷ **Inform Your Physician Before Taking This Drug If**
- you have impaired liver or kidney function.
- you have gallbladder disease or gallstones.
- you are a diabetic.
- you have an underactive thyroid (hypothyroidism).

Possible Side Effects (natural, expected, and unavoidable drug actions)
Moderate increase in blood sugar levels.

▷ **Possible Adverse Effects** (unusual, unexpected, and infrequent reactions)
If any of the following develop, consult your physician promptly for guidance.
Mild Adverse Effects
Allergic Reactions: Skin rash, hives, itching.
Headache, dizziness, blurred vision, fatigue, muscle aches, and cramps—infrequent.
Indigestion, excessive gas, stomach discomfort, nausea, vomiting, diarrhea—rare to infrequent.
Paresthesias—very rare.
Serious Adverse Effects
Abnormally low white blood cell count: fever, chills, sore throat—rare.
Formation of gallstones with long-term use or low blood potassium—possible.

Raynaud's phenomenon—case report.

Liver toxicity—possible.

Myopathy (muscle weakness) or rhabdomyolysis (inability to walk)—case reports to rare.

▷ **Possible Effects on Sexual Function:** Decreased libido or impotence—rare to infrequent.

Natural Diseases or Disorders That May Be Activated by This Drug

Latent diabetes, latent urinary tract infections.

Possible Effects on Laboratory Tests

Complete blood counts: decreased red cells, hemoglobin, white cells, and platelets.

Blood HDL cholesterol levels: increased.

Blood triglyceride levels: decreased.

Liver function tests: increased liver enzymes (ALT/GPT, AST/GOT, and alkaline phosphatase), increased bilirubin.

CAUTION

1. Gemfibrozil is used only after diet has NOT worked to lower triglyceride levels.
2. If you used the drug clofibrate (Atromid-S) in the past, inform your physician fully regarding your experience.
3. Periodic triglyceride and cholesterol levels are critical.

Precautions for Use

By Infants and Children: Safety and effectiveness for those under 12 years of age are not established.

By Those Over 60 Years of Age: Watch for increased tendency to infection; treat all infections promptly.

▷ **Advisability of Use During Pregnancy**

Pregnancy Category: C. See Pregnancy Risk Categories at the back of this book.

Animal studies: Produces adverse effects in rabbits and rats.

Human studies: Adequate studies of pregnant women are not available.

Ask your physician for guidance.

Advisability of Use If Breast-Feeding

Presence of this drug in breast milk: Yes.

Avoid drug or refrain from nursing.

Habit-Forming Potential: None.

Effects of Overdosage: Abdominal pain, nausea, vomiting, diarrhea.

Possible Effects of Long-Term Use: Formation of gallstones.

Suggested Periodic Examinations While Taking This Drug (at physician's discretion)

Complete blood cell counts and liver function tests.

Measurements of blood levels of total cholesterol, HDL and LDL cholesterol fractions, triglycerides, and sugar.

▷ **While Taking This Drug, Observe the Following**

Foods: Follow the diet prescribed by your physician.

Beverages: No restrictions. May be taken with milk.

▷ *Alcohol:* No interactions expected.

Tobacco Smoking: No interactions expected, but I advise everyone to quit smoking.

▷   *Other Drugs*

Gemfibrozil may *increase* the effects of
- glyburide and other oral antidiabetic drugs (see Drug Classes).
- lovastatin and perhaps other HMG-CoA type medicines may increase risk of muscle damage (myopathy) if taken at the same time.
- warfarin (Coumadin), and increase the risk of bleeding. Increased frequency of INR (prothrombin time or protime) measurements and dose changes based on results are critical.

Gemfibrozil may *decrease* the effects of
- chenodiol (Chenix), reducing its benefit in gallstone therapy.

▷   *Driving, Hazardous Activities:* This drug may cause dizziness and blurred vision. Restrict activities as necessary.

Aviation Note: The use of this drug **is usually not a disqualification** for piloting. Consult a designated Aviation Medical Examiner.

Exposure to Sun: No restrictions.

Discontinuation: If triglyceride lowering does not occur after 3 months, this drug should be stopped.

GLIMEPIRIDE (glim EP er ide)

Introduced: 1996   **Class:** Antidiabetic, sulfonylureas   **Prescription:** USA: Yes   **Controlled Drug:** USA: No   **Available as Generic:** No
Brand Name: Amaryl

BENEFITS versus RISKS	
Possible Benefits	*Possible Risks*
TIGHTER CONTROL OF BLOOD SUGAR (adjunctive to appropriate diet and weight control) DECREASED RISK OF HEART DISEASE, KIDNEY DISEASE, ETC., BY ATTAINING TIGHTER CONTROL OF BLOOD SUGAR ONCE-A-DAY DOSING DECREASED RISK OF INCREASED INSULIN LEVELS DECREASED RISK OF HYPOGLYCEMIA	Allergic skin reactions Possible increased risk of heart (cardiovascular) mortality

▷ **Principal Uses**

As a Single Drug Product: Uses currently included in FDA-approved labeling: (1) Better control of mild to moderate type II diabetes mellitus (adult, maturity-onset) that does not require insulin, but is not adequately controlled by diet alone; (2) approved for combination use with insulin if diet and exercise and glimepiride are not adequate, and in secondary failures.

Other (unlabeled) generally accepted uses: None at present.

How This Drug Works: This drug (1) stimulates the secretion of insulin; (2) enhances the utilization of insulin by appropriate tissues (increased sensitivity); and (3) may bind to a different receptor site than other sulfonylureas.

Available Dosage Forms and Strengths

Tablets — 1 mg, 2 mg, 4 mg

▷ **Usual Adult Dosage Range (Actual dosage and administration schedule must be determined for each patient individually):** Treatment is started with 1 or 2 mg once daily, given with breakfast or the first meal. Once a dose of 2 mg is reached, any further dose increases should be made as needed and tolerated at 1- to 2-week intervals in increments of no more than 2 mg; the maximum daily dose is 8 mg. Typical ongoing doses have ranged from 1 to 4 mg a day. Some clinicians advocate that Type II patients with secondary failure be considered for combined glimepiride and insulin therapy. If the fasting blood sugar (glucose) is greater than 150 mg/dl and this is undertaken, 8 mg administered with the first main meal is recommended. Low-dose insulin is started, and increased as needed and tolerated on a weekly basis consistent with blood glucose measurements.

Conditions Requiring Dosing Adjustments

Liver Function: Since glimepiride is removed by the liver, it appears prudent that patients with mild liver failure should take small starting doses. Data regarding use by patients with moderate to severe compromised livers are not available, and use should probably be avoided.

Kidney Function: Patients with kidney compromise may take 1 mg of glimepiride a day. Any further dose changes should be based on results of blood sugar testing.

▷ **Dosing Instructions:** The tablet may be crushed for administration. Follow your doctor's instructions regarding dosing and diet closely. If meals are skipped after this medicine is taken, hypoglycemia may result. Be certain you know the signs and symptoms of hypoglycemia.

Usual Duration of Use: Use on a regular schedule for 1 to 2 weeks determines effectiveness in controlling diabetes. Failure to respond to maximal doses within 1 month constitutes a primary failure. Blood sugars must be measured, and your doctor will decide if the drug should be continued.

Possible Advantages of This Drug

Effective with once-daily dosing.

May be less likely to cause excessive lowering of the blood sugar (hypoglycemia).

May cause less excessive insulin in the bloodstream (hyperinsulinemia).

▷ **This Drug Should Not Be Taken If**
- you have had an allergic reaction to it previously.
- you have severe impairment of liver or kidney function.
- you have diabetic ketoacidosis (insulin is the drug of choice).
- you are pregnant or are breast-feeding your infant.

▷ **Inform Your Physician Before Taking This Drug If**
- you are allergic to other sulfonylurea drugs or to "sulfa" drugs.
- you have been experiencing prolonged vomiting.
- you do not know how to recognize or treat hypoglycemia (see Glossary).
- you have a history of congestive heart failure, peptic ulcer disease, cirrhosis of the liver, or hypothyroidism.

- you are malnourished or have a high fever or pituitary or adrenal insufficiency.

Possible Side Effects (natural, expected, and unavoidable drug actions)
Hypoglycemia will occur if drug dosage is excessive or if meals are missed or inadequate. The risk of hypoglycemia may be increased if this medicine is combined with insulin.

▷ **Possible Adverse Effects** (unusual, unexpected, and infrequent reactions)
If any of the following develop, consult your physician promptly for guidance.
Mild Adverse Effects
Allergic Reactions: Skin rash, hives, itching (may subside over time).
Headache, dizziness, or blurred vision—rare.
Nausea—rare.
Serious Adverse Effects
Allergic Reactions: None reported.
Lowering of sodium or porphyria reported with other medicines in this class—case reports.
Low blood sugar (hypoglycemia)—possible.

▷ **Possible Effects on Sexual Function:**   None reported.

▷ **Adverse Effects That May Mimic Natural Diseases or Disorders**
Increased liver enzymes may suggest viral hepatitis.

Possible Effects on Laboratory Tests
Hemoglobin A1C (glycosylated hemoglobin): trending toward normal if tight control of blood sugar has been achieved.
Blood glucose levels: decreased.
Liver function tests: increased liver enzymes (ALT/GPT, AST/GOT, and alkaline phosphatase), increased bilirubin.

CAUTION
1. This drug is only one part of a total diabetes program. It is not a substitute for a proper diet and regular exercise.
2. Over time (usually several months) this drug may not work. Periodic follow-up examinations are necessary.

Precautions for Use
By Infants and Children: Safety and effectiveness in pediatrics have not been established.
By Those Over 60 Years of Age: Use with caution, and start with 1 mg/day. Dose should be increased slowly as needed and tolerated and glucose checked often. Repeated hypoglycemia in the elderly can cause brain damage.

▷ **Advisability of Use During Pregnancy**
Pregnancy Category: C. See Pregnancy Risk Categories at the back of this book.
Human studies: Adequate studies of pregnant women are not available.
Because uncontrolled blood sugar levels during pregnancy are associated with a higher incidence of birth defects, many experts recommend that insulin instead of an oral agent be used as necessary to control diabetes during pregnancy.

Advisability of Use If Breast-Feeding
Presence of this drug in breast milk: Yes in animal data; unknown in humans.
Avoid drug or refrain from nursing.

Habit-Forming Potential: None.

Effects of Overdosage: Symptoms of mild to severe hypoglycemia: headache, light-headedness, faintness, nervousness, confusion, tremor, sweating, heart palpitation, weakness, hunger, nausea, vomiting, stupor progressing to coma.

Possible Effects of Long-Term Use: Increased frequency and severity of heart and blood vessel diseases with long-term use of this class of drugs are highly controversial and inconclusive. A direct cause-and-effect relationship (see Glossary) is tenuous. Ask your physician for help.

Suggested Periodic Examinations While Taking This Drug (at physician's discretion)
> Hemoglobin A1C, liver function tests, evaluation of heart and circulatory system, blood sugar levels.

▷ **While Taking This Drug, Observe the Following**
> *Foods:* Follow the diabetic diet prescribed by your physician.
> *Beverages:* As directed in the diabetic diet. May be taken with milk.
▷ *Alcohol:* Use with extreme caution—alcohol can prolong this drug's hypoglycemic effect. Other drugs in this class can also cause a disulfiramlike reaction (see Glossary).
> *Tobacco Smoking:* No interactions expected, but I advise everyone to quit smoking.
▷ *Other Drugs*
> The following drugs may *increase* the effects of glimepiride
> - aspirin and other salicylates.
> - cimetidine (Tagamet).
> - clofibrate (Atromid-S).
> - fenfluramine (Pondimin).
> - miconazole (Lotrimin).
> - monoamine oxidase (MAO) type A inhibitors (see Drug Classes).
> - NSAIDs (see Drug Classes).
> - probenecid (SK-Probenecid).
> - ranitidine (Zantac).
> - sulfa drugs such as Septra.
> The following drugs may *decrease* the effects of glimepiride
> - beta-blocker drugs (see Drug Classes).
> - bumetanide (Bumex).
> - conjugated estrogens (Premarin).
> - diazoxide (Proglycem).
> - ethacrynic acid (Edecrin).
> - furosemide (Lasix).
> - phenytoin (Dilantin).
> - rifampin (Rifadin, others).
> - steroids (betamethasone, prednisone, others).
> - thiazide diuretics (see Drug Classes).
> Glimepiride *taken concurrently* with
> - antacids (magnesium hydroxide containing) may result in increased risk of excessively lowered blood sugar.
> - antifungal agents (such as itraconazole or other azoles) may result in severe lowering of blood sugar.

- calcium channel blockers (see Drug Classes) may cause excessive lowering of blood glucose.
- cyclosporine (Sandimmune) may result in cyclosporine toxicity.
- warfarin (Coumadin) can cause an increased hypoglycemic effect.

▷ *Driving, Hazardous Activities:* Dosing schedule, eating schedule, and physical activities must be coordinated to prevent hypoglycemia. Know the early symptoms of hypoglycemia so you can avoid hazardous activities and take corrective measures.

Aviation Note: Diabetes *is a disqualification* for piloting. Consult a designated Aviation Medical Examiner.

Exposure to Sun: Some drugs of this class can cause photosensitivity (see Glossary).

Occurrence of Unrelated Illness: Acute infections, vomiting or diarrhea, serious injuries, and surgical procedures can worsen diabetic control and may require insulin. If any of these conditions occur, call your doctor.

Discontinuation: Because of secondary failures, the continued benefit of this drug should be evaluated every 6 months.

GLIPIZIDE (GLIP i zide)

Introduced: 1972   **Class:** Antidiabetic, sulfonylureas   **Prescription:** USA: Yes   **Controlled Drug:** USA: No   **Available as Generic:** Yes
Brand Names: Glucotrol, Glucotrol XL

BENEFITS versus RISKS	
Possible Benefits	*Possible Risks*
TIGHTER CONTROL OF BLOOD SUGAR (adjunctive to appropriate diet and weight control)	HYPOGLYCEMIA, severe and prolonged
DECREASED RISK OF HEART DISEASE, KIDNEY DISEASE, ETC., BY ATTAINING TIGHTER CONTROL OF BLOOD SUGAR	Allergic skin reactions (some severe)
	Blood cell and bone marrow disorders
	Possible increased risk of heart (cardiovascular) mortality
ONCE-A-DAY DOSING	

▷ **Principal Uses**

As a Single Drug Product: Uses currently included in FDA-approved labeling: Better control of mild to moderate type II diabetes mellitus (adult, maturity-onset) that does not require insulin, but is not adequately controlled by diet alone.

Other (unlabeled) generally accepted uses: Delay of abnormal metabolism and blood vessel disease if given early in diabetes.

How This Drug Works: This drug (1) stimulates the secretion of insulin; and (2) enhances the utilization of insulin by appropriate tissues.

Available Dosage Forms and Strengths

Tablets — 5 mg, 10 mg
Tablets, extended release — 5 mg, 10 mg

▷ **Usual Adult Dosage Range:** Initially 5 mg daily before a meal. At 3- to 7-day intervals the dose may be increased by increments of 2.5 to 5 mg daily as needed and tolerated. Total daily dosage should not exceed 40 mg. The extended-release form is started at 5 mg, taken with breakfast. If the dose needs to be increased, it is done so at 7-day intervals. Most patients have a favorable response to 10 mg daily. The maximum daily extended-release-form dose is 20 mg. **Note: Actual dosage and administration schedule must be determined for each patient individually.**

Conditions Requiring Dosing Adjustments
Liver Function: Patients with liver failure should take a starting dose of 2.5 mg, and be closely followed.
Kidney Function: Some clinicians DO NOT recommend use of glipizide in severe renal compromise. Patients should be monitored closely if the drug is used in mild to moderate renal (kidney) compromise. It is a rare cause of kidney stones.

▷ **Dosing Instructions:** If the daily maintenance dose is found to be 15 mg or more, the total dose should be divided into two equal doses—the first taken with the morning meal, the second with the evening meal. The tablet may be crushed.

Usual Duration of Use: Use on a regular schedule for 1 to 2 weeks determines effectiveness in controlling diabetes. Failure to respond to maximal doses within 1 month constitutes a primary failure. Up to 10% of those who respond initially may develop secondary failure. Blood sugars must be measured, and your doctor will decide if the drug should be continued.

Possible Advantages of This Drug
Effective with once-daily dosing.
Onset of action within 30 minutes. Near-normal insulin response to eating.
Well tolerated by the elderly diabetic.

Currently a "Drug of Choice"
for starting therapy in noninsulin-dependent diabetes when diet and weight control fail.

▷ **This Drug Should Not Be Taken If**
• you have had an allergic reaction to it previously.
• you have severe impairment of liver or kidney function.
• you have diabetic ketoacidosis.
• you are pregnant.

▷ **Inform Your Physician Before Taking This Drug If**
• you are allergic to other sulfonylurea drugs or to "sulfa" drugs.
• your diabetes has been unstable or "brittle" in the past.
• you do not know how to recognize or treat hypoglycemia (see Glossary).
• you are pregnant.
• you have a history of congestive heart failure, peptic ulcer disease, cirrhosis of the liver, bone marrow depression, hypothyroidism, or porphyria.

Possible Side Effects (natural, expected, and unavoidable drug actions)
If drug dosage is excessive or if meals are missed or inadequate, abnormally low blood sugar (hypoglycemia) will occur as a drug effect.

▷ **Possible Adverse Effects** (unusual, unexpected, and infrequent reactions)
If any of the following develop, consult your physician promptly for guidance.

Mild Adverse Effects
Allergic Reactions: Skin rash, hives, itching.
Headache, drowsiness, dizziness, fatigue, sweating—rare to infrequent.
Indigestion, nausea, vomiting, diarrhea—rare to infrequent.
Serious Adverse Effects
Allergic Reactions: Hepatitis with jaundice (see Glossary), severe skin reactions—case reports.
Idiosyncratic Reaction: Hemolytic anemia (see Glossary).
Disulfiramlike reaction (see Glossary) with concurrent use of alcohol—infrequent.
Low blood sodium or drug-induced urinary stones—possible.
Bone marrow depression (see Glossary): fatigue, weakness, fever, sore throat, abnormal bleeding or bruising—case reports.
Risk of cardiovascular mortality (based on an old study with a different drug)—possible.

▷ **Possible Effects on Sexual Function:**   None reported.

▷ **Adverse Effects That May Mimic Natural Diseases or Disorders**
Liver reactions may suggest viral hepatitis.

Possible Effects on Laboratory Tests
Complete blood counts: decreased red cells, hemoglobin, white cells, and platelets.
Blood glucose levels: decreased.
Liver function tests: increased liver enzymes (ALT/GPT, AST/GOT, and alkaline phosphatase), increased bilirubin.

CAUTION
1. This drug is only one part of a total diabetes program. It is not a substitute for a proper diet and regular exercise.
2. Over time (usually months), this drug may not work. Periodic follow-up examinations are needed.

Precautions for Use
By Infants and Children: This drug does not work in type I (juvenile, growth-onset) insulin-dependent diabetes.
By Those Over 60 Years of Age: Use with caution, and start with 2.5 mg/day. Dose should be increased slowly and glucose checked often. Repeated hypoglycemia in the elderly can cause brain damage.

▷ **Advisability of Use During Pregnancy**
Pregnancy Category: C. See Pregnancy Risk Categories at the back of this book.
Animal studies: No birth defects reported in rats and rabbits.
Human studies: Adequate studies of pregnant women are not available.
Because uncontrolled blood sugar levels during pregnancy are associated with a higher incidence of birth defects, many experts recommend that insulin (instead of an oral agent) be used as necessary to control diabetes during the entire pregnancy.

Advisability of Use If Breast-Feeding
Presence of this drug in breast milk: Unknown.
Avoid drug or refrain from nursing.

Habit-Forming Potential: None.

Effects of Overdosage: Symptoms of mild to severe hypoglycemia: headache, light-headedness, faintness, nervousness, confusion, tremor, sweating, heart palpitation, weakness, hunger, nausea, vomiting, stupor progressing to coma.

Possible Effects of Long-Term Use: Reduced thyroid function (hypothyroidism). Increased frequency and severity of heart and blood vessel diseases with long-term use of this class of drugs are highly controversial and inconclusive. A direct cause-and-effect relationship (see Glossary) is tenuous. Ask your physician for help.

Suggested Periodic Examinations While Taking This Drug (at physician's discretion)

Complete blood cell counts, liver function tests, thyroid function tests, periodic evaluation of heart and circulatory system.

▷ **While Taking This Drug, Observe the Following**

Foods: Follow the diabetic diet prescribed by your physician.

Beverages: As directed in the diabetic diet. May be taken with milk.

▷ *Alcohol:* Use with extreme caution—alcohol can prolong this drug's hypoglycemic effect. This drug can also cause a disulfiramlike reaction (see Glossary): facial flushing, sweating, palpitation.

Tobacco Smoking: No interactions expected, but I advise everyone to quit smoking.

▷ *Other Drugs*

The following drugs may ***increase*** the effects of glipizide
- acarbose (Precose) may increase risk of excessive lowering of blood sugar.
- aspirin and other salicylates.
- chloramphenicol (Chloromycetin).
- cimetidine (Tagamet).
- clofibrate (Atromid-S).
- cotrimoxazole (Septra).
- fenfluramine (Pondimin).
- magnesium (increased absorption into the body).
- monoamine oxidase (MAO) type A inhibitors (see Drug Classes).
- NSAIDs (see Drug Classes).
- ranitidine (Zantac).
- sulfa drugs such as trimethoprim/sulfamethoxazole (Septra) or erythromycin/sulfisoxazole (Pediazole).

The following drugs may ***decrease*** the effects of glipizide
- beta-blocker drugs (see Drug Classes).
- birth control pills (oral contraceptives).
- bumetanide (Bumex).
- conjugated estrogens (Premarin).
- diazoxide (Proglycem).
- ethacrynic acid (Edecrin).
- furosemide (Lasix).
- phenytoin (Dilantin).
- rifampin (Rifadin, others).
- steroids (betamethasone, prednisone, others).
- thiazide diuretics (see Drug Classes).

Glipizide *taken concurrently* with
- antacids (containing magnesium hydroxide) may result in increased risk of excessively lowered blood sugar.
- antifungal agents (such as itraconazole or other azoles) may result in severe lowering of blood sugar.
- calcium channel blockers (see Drug Classes) may cause excessive lowering of blood glucose.
- cyclosporine (Sandimmune) may result in cyclosporine toxicity.
- warfarin (Coumadin) can cause an increased hypoglycemic effect.

▷ *Driving, Hazardous Activities:* Dosing schedule, eating schedule, and physical activities must be coordinated to prevent hypoglycemia. Know the early symptoms of hypoglycemia so you can avoid hazardous activities and take corrective measures.

Aviation Note: Diabetes *is a disqualification* for piloting. Consult a designated Aviation Medical Examiner.

Exposure to Sun: Some drugs of this class can cause photosensitivity (see Glossary).

Occurrence of Unrelated Illness: Acute infections, vomiting or diarrhea, serious injuries, and surgical procedures can worsen diabetic control and may require insulin. If any of these conditions occur, call your doctor.

Discontinuation: Because of secondary failures, the continued benefit of this drug should be evaluated every 6 months.

GLYBURIDE (GLI byoor ide)

Other Name: Glibenclamide

Introduced: 1970   **Class:** Antidiabetic, sulfonylureas   **Prescription:** USA: Yes   **Controlled Drug:** USA: No; Canada: No   **Available as Generic:** Yes

Brand Names: ✦Albert-Glyburide, ✦Apo-Glyburide, DiaBeta, ✦Euglucon, ✦Gen-Glybe, Glubate, Glynase Prestab, Micronase, ✦Novo-Glyburide

BENEFITS versus RISKS	
Possible Benefits	*Possible Risks*
Helps in regulating blood sugar in noninsulin-dependent diabetes (adjunctive to appropriate diet and weight control)	HYPOGLYCEMIA, severe and prolonged Liver damage Blood cell and bone marrow disorders Allergic skin reactions (some severe) Possible increased risk of heart (cardiovascular) mortality

▷ **Principal Uses**

As a Single Drug Product: Uses currently included in FDA-approved labeling: Helps control mild to moderate type II diabetes mellitus (adult, maturity-onset) that does not require insulin, but can't be adequately controlled by diet alone.

Other (unlabeled) generally accepted uses: None.

How This Drug Works: This drug (1) stimulates the secretion of insulin, (2) decreases glucose production in the liver, and (3) enhances insulin use.

Available Dosage Forms and Strengths
Tablets — 1.25 mg, 1.5 mg, 2.5 mg, 3 mg, 5 mg, 6 mg

▷ **Usual Adult Dosage Range:** Regular-release products: 2.5 to 5 mg daily with breakfast. At 7-day intervals the dose may be increased by increments of 2.5 mg daily as needed and tolerated. Total daily dosage should not exceed 20 mg. Some patients respond to 1.25 mg daily.

Micronized products: 1.5 to 3 mg daily taken with breakfast. (Patients more sensitive to oral agents should be started at 0.75 mg daily.) Maximum dose is 12 mg daily. **Note: Actual dosage and administration schedule must be determined for each patient individually.**

Conditions Requiring Dosing Adjustments
Liver Function: Glyburide may cause catastrophic hypoglycemia (low blood sugar) if it is used by patients with liver disease. Very low starting doses should be taken and the patient closely followed. It is also a rare cause of hepatitis and cholestatic jaundice.

Kidney Function: Glyburide should be used with caution in mild renal compromise, with low initial doses and careful patient monitoring. The drug SHOULD NOT be used by patients with moderate kidney failure (creatinine clearances less than 50 ml/min) or in severe kidney failure.

▷ **Dosing Instructions:** If the daily maintenance dose is 10 mg or more, the total dose should be divided into two equal doses: the first taken with the morning meal, the second with the evening meal. The tablet may be crushed.

Usual Duration of Use: Use on a regular schedule for 1 to 2 weeks determines effectiveness in controlling diabetes. No response to peak doses in 1 month constitutes a primary failure. Up to 10% of those who respond initially may develop secondary failure. The duration of effective use can only be determined by periodic measurement of the blood sugar.

▷ **This Drug Should Not Be Taken If**
- you have had an allergic reaction to it previously.
- you have severe impairment of liver and kidney function.
- you have diabetic ketoacidosis.
- you are pregnant.

▷ **Inform Your Physician Before Taking This Drug If**
- you are allergic to other sulfonylurea drugs or to "sulfa" drugs.
- your diabetes has been unstable or "brittle" in the past.
- you do not know how to recognize or treat hypoglycemia (see Glossary).
- you have a history of problems with blood clotting or have a glucose-6-phosphate dehydrogenase (G6PD) deficiency.
- you have a history of congestive heart failure, peptic ulcer disease, cirrhosis of the liver, hypothyroidism, or porphyria.

Possible Side Effects (natural, expected, and unavoidable drug actions)
If drug dosage is excessive or food intake is delayed or inadequate, abnormally low blood sugar (hypoglycemia) will occur as a predictable drug effect.

▷ **Possible Adverse Effects** (unusual, unexpected, and infrequent reactions)
If any of the following develop, consult your physician promptly for guidance.

Mild Adverse Effects
 Allergic Reactions: Skin rash, hives, itching.
 Headache, drowsiness, dizziness, fatigue—possible.
 Indigestion, heartburn, nausea—rare.
 Bed-wetting at night (nocturnal enuresis), especially in young adults—case
 reports.
Serious Adverse Effects
 Allergic Reactions: Hepatitis with jaundice (see Glossary), severe skin reac-
 tions (exfoliative dermatitis)—case reports.
 Idiosyncratic Reaction: Hemolytic anemia (see Glossary).
 Disulfiramlike reaction with concurrent use of alcohol (see Glossary)—possi-
 ble.
 Bone marrow depression (see Glossary): fatigue, fever, sore throat, abnormal
 bleeding—case reports.
 Liver toxicity (cholestatic jaundice)—case reports.
 Blood clotting defects (coagulation)—rare.
 Cardiovascular mortality (based on an old study of a different medicine)—
 increased risk.

▷ **Possible Effects on Sexual Function:**   None reported.

▷ **Adverse Effects That May Mimic Natural Diseases or Disorders**
 Liver reactions may suggest viral hepatitis.

Possible Effects on Laboratory Tests
 Blood platelet counts: decreased.
 Blood cholesterol and triglyceride levels: decreased.
 Blood glucose levels: decreased.
 Liver function tests: increased liver enzymes (ALT/GPT, AST/GOT, and alka-
 line phosphatase).

CAUTION
 1. This drug is only part of the program for management of your diabetes. It
 is not a substitute for a proper diet and regular exercise.
 2. Over time (usually several months), this drug may not work. Periodic
 follow-up examinations are necessary.

Precautions for Use
 By Infants and Children: This drug does not work in type I (juvenile, growth-
 onset) insulin-dependent diabetes.
 By Those Over 60 Years of Age: Use with caution and start with 1.25 mg/day of
 the regular form. Dose should be slowly increased and glucose closely followed. Repeated hypoglycemia in the elderly can cause brain damage.

▷ **Advisability of Use During Pregnancy**
 Pregnancy Category: C. See Pregnancy Risk Categories at the back of this book.
 Animal studies: No birth defects reported in rats and rabbits.
 Human studies: Adequate studies of pregnant women are not available.
 Uncontrolled blood sugar levels during pregnancy are associated with a
 higher incidence of birth defects, so many experts recommend insulin (in-
 stead of an oral agent) to control diabetes during the entire pregnancy.

Advisability of Use If Breast-Feeding
 Presence of this drug in breast milk: Unknown.
 Avoid drug or refrain from nursing.

Habit-Forming Potential: None.

Effects of Overdosage: Symptoms of mild to severe hypoglycemia: headache, light-headedness, faintness, nervousness, confusion, tremor, sweating, heart palpitation, weakness, hunger, nausea, vomiting, stupor progressing to coma.

Possible Effects of Long-Term Use: Reduced thyroid gland function (hypothyroidism). Reports of increased frequency and severity of heart and blood vessel diseases associated with long-term use of this class of drugs are highly controversial and inconclusive. A direct cause-and-effect relationship (see Glossary) is tenuous. Ask your physician for guidance.

Suggested Periodic Examinations While Taking This Drug (at physician's discretion)
 Complete blood cell counts, liver function tests, thyroid function tests, periodic evaluation of heart and circulatory system.

▷ **While Taking This Drug, Observe the Following**
 Foods: Follow the diabetic diet prescribed by your physician.
 Beverages: As directed in the diabetic diet. May be taken with milk.
▷ *Alcohol:* Use with extreme caution—alcohol can exaggerate this drug's hypoglycemic effect. This drug can cause a disulfiramlike reaction (see Glossary): facial flushing, sweating, palpitation.
 Tobacco Smoking: No interactions expected, but I advise everyone to quit smoking.
▷ *Other Drugs*
 The following drugs may *increase* the effects of glyburide
 • acarbose (Precose).
 • aspirin and other salicylates.
 • chloramphenicol (Chloromycetin).
 • cimetidine (Tagamet).
 • clofibrate (Atromid-S).
 • fenfluramine (Pondimin).
 • gemfibrozil (Lopid).
 • monoamine oxidase (MAO) type A inhibitors (see Drug Classes).
 • phenylbutazone (Butazolidin).
 • ranitidine (Zantac).
 • sulfa drugs such as trimethoprim/sulfamethoxazole (Septra) or erythromycin/sulfisoxazole (Pediazole).
 The following drugs may *decrease* the effects of glyburide
 • beta-blocker drugs (see Drug Classes).
 • bumetanide (Bumex).
 • diazoxide (Proglycem).
 • ethacrynic acid (Edecrin).
 • furosemide (Lasix).
 • phenytoin (Dilantin).
 • rifampin (Rifadin, others).
 • thiazide diuretics (see Drug Classes).
 • thyroid hormones.
 Glyburide *taken concurrently* with
 • antacids (containing magnesium hydroxide) or magnesium supplements may result in increased risk of excessively lowered blood sugar.

- antifungal agents (such as itraconazole or other azoles) may result in severe lowering of blood sugar.
- enalapril (Vasotec) may enhance blood sugar lowering effect.
- MAO inhibitors (see Drug Classes) may increase risk of hyperglycemia.
- steroids (betamethasone, prednisone, others) blunts benefits.
- warfarin (Coumadin) may result in bleeding. More frequent INR (prothrombin time) testing is needed.

▷ *Driving, Hazardous Activities:* Regulate dosing, eating, and physical activities carefully to prevent hypoglycemia. Know the early symptoms of hypoglycemia so you can avoid hazardous activities and take corrective measures.

Aviation Note: Diabetes **is a disqualification** for piloting. Consult a designated Aviation Medical Examiner.

Exposure to Sun: Use caution until sensitivity has been determined. Some drugs of this class can cause photosensitivity (see Glossary).

Occurrence of Unrelated Illness: Acute infections, vomiting or diarrhea, serious injuries, and surgical procedures can worsen diabetic control and may require insulin. If any of these conditions occur, consult your physician promptly.

Discontinuation: Because of the possibility of secondary failure, it is advisable to evaluate the continued benefit of this drug every 6 months.

GUANFACINE (GWAHN fa seen)

Introduced: 1980   **Class:** Antihypertensive   **Prescription:** USA: Yes
Controlled Drug: USA: No   **Available as Generic:** USA: Yes
Brand Name: Tenex

BENEFITS versus RISKS	
Possible Benefits	*Possible Risks*
EFFECTIVE ANTIHYPERTENSIVE in mild to moderate high blood pressure	Amnesia
EFFECTIVE in high blood pressure of pregnancy	

▷ **Principal Uses**

As a Single Drug Product: Uses currently included in FDA-approved labeling: (1) Used to treat mild to moderate high blood pressure; (2) used alone or in combination to treat high blood pressure caused by kidney problems.

Other (unlabeled) generally accepted uses: (1) Heroin withdrawal; (2) may be useful in problem pregnancies; (3) could have a role in treating attention deficit hyperactivity disorder (ADHD); (4) may help some sleep disorders.

How This Drug Works: By reducing sympathetic nervous system output (by affecting brain alpha-2-receptors), this drug causes relaxation of blood vessel walls and lowering of blood pressure.

Available Dosage Forms and Strengths

Tablets — 1 mg, 2 mg

▷ **Usual Adult Dosage Range:** Initially 1 mg once daily taken at bedtime. The dose may be increased after 3 to 4 weeks to 2 mg daily, as needed and tolerated. If needed, the dose may be increased again after 3 to 4 weeks to 3 mg daily. Total daily dose may be taken in two divided doses if needed for blood pressure control. Use of up to 40 mg daily has been reported, but combination therapy is used before such doses. Usual maximum is 6 mg daily. **Note: Actual dosage and administration schedule must be determined for each patient individually.**

Conditions Requiring Dosing Adjustments
Liver Function: Should be used with caution by patients with liver compromise.
Kidney Function: Use with caution, but drug can be removed by nonkidney mechanisms.

▷ **Dosing Instructions:** Tablets may be crushed and taken without regard to eating. It is recommended that the daily dose be taken at bedtime to reduce the side effect of daytime drowsiness.

Usual Duration of Use: Continual use on a regular schedule for 4 to 6 weeks is usually necessary to determine this drug's effectiveness in controlling high blood pressure. Peak benefit may not be seen for 12 weeks. Long-term use (months to years) requires supervision and guidance. Consult your physician on a regular basis.

▷ **This Drug Should Not Be Taken If**
- you have had an allergic reaction to it previously.

▷ **Inform Your Physician Before Taking This Drug If**
- you have a circulatory disorder of the brain.
- you have angina or coronary artery disease.
- you have or have had serious emotional depression.
- you have impaired liver or kidney function.
- you are a diabetic.
- you have a history of orthostatic hypotension.
- you are taking any sedative or hypnotic drugs or an antidepressant.
- you plan to have surgery under general anesthesia in the near future.

Possible Side Effects (natural, expected, and unavoidable drug actions)
Drowsiness—frequent; dry nose and mouth—frequent; constipation—infrequent; mild lowering of blood pressure on standing (orthostatic hypotension; see Glossary).

▷ **Possible Adverse Effects** (unusual, unexpected, and infrequent reactions)
If any of the following develop, consult your physician promptly for guidance.
Mild Adverse Effects
Allergic Reactions: Skin rash, itching.
Headache, dizziness, fatigue, sedation, or insomnia—rare to infrequent.
Indigestion, nausea, diarrhea—infrequent.
Edema or leg cramps—rare.
Serious Adverse Effects
Slow heartbeat (bradycardia)—infrequent.
Liver toxicity—rare.
Amnesia—infrequent.
Rebound hypertension (if abruptly stopped).

▷ **Possible Effects on Sexual Function:**   Dose-related decreased libido, impotence—case reports.

Possible Effects on Laboratory Tests
Liver function tests: increased.
Blood sugar (glucose): increased.

CAUTION
1. *Do not stop this drug suddenly.* Sudden withdrawal can produce anxiety, nervousness, tremors, fast or irregular heart action, nausea, stomach cramps, vomiting, and rebound hypertension.
2. Hot weather and fever can reduce blood pressure significantly. Dosage adjustments may be necessary.
3. Report the development of any tendency to emotional depression.

Precautions for Use
By Infants and Children: Safety and effectiveness for use by those under 12 years of age have not been established.
By Those Over 60 Years of Age: Proceed cautiously. Pressure should be reduced without creating the risks associated with excessively low blood pressure. Watch for light-headedness, dizziness, unsteadiness, fainting, and falling. Sedation and dry mouth occur commonly in elderly users. Report promptly any changes in mood or behavior: depression, delusions, hallucinations.

▷ **Advisability of Use During Pregnancy**
Pregnancy Category: B. See Pregnancy Risk Categories at the back of this book.
Animal studies: No birth defects due to this drug reported in rat and rabbit studies.
Human studies: Adequate studies of pregnant women are not available.
Use this drug only if clearly needed. Ask your physician for guidance.

Advisability of Use If Breast-Feeding
Presence of this drug in breast milk: Probably.
Avoid drug or refrain from nursing.

Habit-Forming Potential: None.

Effects of Overdosage: Marked drowsiness, dry mouth, slow pulse, low blood pressure, vomiting, stupor progressing to coma.

Possible Effects of Long-Term Use: Development of tolerance (see Glossary) with loss of drug effectiveness.

Suggested Periodic Examinations While Taking This Drug (at physician's discretion)
Blood pressure measurements.

▷ **While Taking This Drug, Observe the Following**
Foods: Avoid excessive salt, and ask your doctor about degree of salt restriction.
Beverages: No restrictions. May be taken with milk.
▷ *Alcohol:* Use with extreme caution—can cause marked drowsiness or exaggerated reduction of blood pressure.
Tobacco Smoking: No interactions expected, but I advise everyone to quit smoking.
▷ *Other Drugs*
Guanfacine *taken concurrently* with
• amitriptyline (Elavil) and other tricyclic antidepressants (see Drug Classes) can cause decreased effectiveness as an antihypertensive.

- desipramine and other tricyclic antidepressants can cause loss of therapeutic benefits of guanfacine.
- phenobarbital can lead to loss of therapeutic effect of guanfacine.

▷ *Driving, Hazardous Activities:* Use caution. This drug can cause drowsiness and can impair mental alertness, judgment, and coordination.

Aviation Note: Hypertension (high blood pressure) *is a disqualification* for piloting. Consult a designated Aviation Medical Examiner.

Exposure to Sun: No restrictions.

Exposure to Heat: Use caution. Hot environments may reduce the blood pressure significantly; be alert to the possibility of orthostatic hypotension (see Glossary).

Heavy Exercise or Exertion: Use caution. Isometric exercises can raise blood pressure significantly. This drug may intensify the hypertensive response to isometric exercise. Ask your physician for guidance.

Occurrence of Unrelated Illness: Fever may lower blood pressure significantly. Vomiting may prevent regular use of this drug and result in acute withdrawal reactions. Call your doctor.

*Discontinuation: **Do not stop this drug suddenly.*** Withdrawal reactions occur within 2 to 7 days after the last dose. It is best to reduce dose gradually (over 3 to 4 days), with periodic monitoring of the blood pressure.

HALOPERIDOL (hal oh PER i dohl)

Introduced: 1958   **Class:** Antipsychotic; tranquilizer, strong   **Prescription:** USA: Yes   **Controlled Drug:** USA: No; Canada: No   **Available as Generic:** USA: Yes; Canada: Yes

Brand Names: ✦Apo-Haloperidol, Haldol, ✦Haldol LA, Halperon, ✦Novo-Peridol, ✦Peridol, ✦PMS-Haloperidol

BENEFITS versus RISKS	
Possible Benefits	*Possible Risks*
EFFECTIVE CONTROL OF PSYCHOSES	FREQUENT PARKINSON-LIKE side effects
BENEFICIAL EFFECTS ON THINKING, MOOD, AND BEHAVIOR	SERIOUS TOXIC EFFECTS ON BRAIN with long-term use
EFFECTIVE CONTROL OF SOME CASES OF TOURETTE SYNDROME	Rare blood cell disorders
Beneficial in management of some hyperactive children	Abnormally low white blood cell count

▷ **Principal Uses**

As a Single Drug Product: Uses currently included in FDA-approved labeling: (1) Helps control psychotic thinking and abnormal behavior associated with acute psychosis of unknown nature, acute schizophrenia, paranoid states, and the manic phase of manic-depressive disorders; (2) helps control outbursts of aggression and agitation; (3) used to treat Tourette syndrome.

Other (unlabeled) generally accepted uses: (1) Helps control refractory hiccups; (2) used to lessen delirium in LSD flashbacks and phencyclidine intoxication; (3) used as combination (adjuvant) therapy in chronic pain syndromes; (4) may be helpful in autistic patients; (5) may have a role in refractory vomiting caused by cancer chemotherapy; (6) can ease symptoms in refractory sneezing; (7) may be helpful as adjunctive therapy in stuttering.

How This Drug Works:　By interfering with a nerve impulse transmitter (dopamine) in the brain, this drug reduces anxiety and agitation, improves coherence and organization of thinking, and abolishes delusions and hallucinations.

Available Dosage Forms and Strengths
　　Concentrate — 2 mg/ml
　　　Injection — 5, 50, and 100 mg/ml
　　　　Tablets — 0.5 mg, 1 mg, 2 mg, 5 mg, 10 mg, 20 mg

▷ **Usual Adult Dosage Range:**　Initially 0.5 to 2 mg two or three times daily. Dose may be increased by 0.5 mg/day at 3- to 4-day intervals as needed and tolerated. The usual dosage range is 0.5 to 30 mg daily. The total daily dosage should not exceed 100 mg. **Note: Actual dosage and administration schedule must be determined for each patient individually.**

Conditions Requiring Dosing Adjustments
Liver Function: The dose, dosing interval, and titration interval (time to adjust the drug to desired effect) should be adjusted for liver compromise.
Kidney Function: High doses of haloperidol should be used with caution in kidney compromise.

▷ **Dosing Instructions:**　The tablet may be crushed and taken with or following food to reduce stomach irritation. The concentrate may be diluted in 2 ounces of water or fruit juice; do not add it to coffee or tea.

Usual Duration of Use:　Use on a regular schedule for several weeks determines this drug's effectiveness in controlling psychotic behavior. If it doesn't provide significant benefit in 6 weeks, it should be stopped. Long-term use requires supervision and periodic physician evaluation.

▷ **This Drug Should Not Be Taken If**
- you have had an allergic reaction to any dosage form of it previously.
- you are experiencing severe mental depression.
- you have any form of Parkinson's disease.
- you have cancer of the breast.
- you have severe active liver disease.
- you are presently experiencing central nervous system (CNS) depression due to alcohol or narcotics.
- you currently have a bone marrow or blood cell disorder.

▷ **Inform Your Physician Before Taking This Drug If**
- you are allergic or abnormally sensitive to phenothiazine drugs.
- you have a history of mental depression.
- you have any type of heart disease.
- you have impaired liver or kidney function.
- you have thyroid disease.
- you are allergic to the dye tartrazine.
- you are pregnant or are planning pregnancy.
- you have a history of neuroleptic malignant syndrome.

- you have low blood pressure, epilepsy, or glaucoma.
- you are taking any drugs with a sedative effect.
- you plan to have surgery and general or spinal anesthesia soon.

Possible Side Effects (natural, expected, and unavoidable drug actions)
Mild drowsiness, low blood pressure, blurred vision, dry mouth, constipation, marked and frequent Parkinson-like reactions (see Glossary).

▷ **Possible Adverse Effects** (unusual, unexpected, and infrequent reactions)
If any of the following develop, consult your physician promptly for guidance.
Mild Adverse Effects
Allergic Reactions: Skin rash, hives.
Dizziness, weakness, agitation, insomnia—case reports to infrequent.
Loss of appetite, indigestion, nausea, vomiting, diarrhea—case reports.
Serious Adverse Effects
Allergic Reactions: Rare liver reaction with jaundice, asthma, spasm of vocal cords.
Idiosyncratic Reactions: Neuroleptic malignant syndrome (see Glossary).
Blood cell disorders: lowered white blood cell count—rare.
Nervous system reactions: rigidity of extremities, tremors, seizures, constant movement, facial grimacing, eye-rolling, spasm of neck muscles, tardive dyskinesia (see Glossary)—case reports to infrequent.
Abnormal heartbeat (premature ventricular contractions)—possible with aggressive dosing.
Worsening of psychosis—possible.
Low blood sugar or abnormal and frequent urination (SIADH)—case reports.
Liver toxicity—possible.
Bronchospasm or myasthenia gravis—case reports.

▷ **Possible Effects on Sexual Function**
Decreased libido; impotence—infrequent to frequent; painful ejaculation; priapism (see Glossary).
Tender and enlarged breast tissue in men (gynecomastia); breast enlargement with milk production in women.
Altered timing and pattern of menstruation—case reports.

▷ **Adverse Effects That May Mimic Natural Diseases or Disorders**
Liver reaction may suggest viral hepatitis. Nervous system reactions may suggest Parkinson's disease or Reye syndrome.

Natural Diseases or Disorders That May Be Activated by This Drug
Latent epilepsy, glaucoma, diabetes.

Possible Effects on Laboratory Tests
Complete blood counts: decreased red cells, hemoglobin, and white cells; increased eosinophils.
INR (prothrombin time): decreased.
Blood cholesterol level: decreased.
Blood glucose level: increased.
Liver function tests: increased liver enzymes (ALT/GPT, AST/GOT, and alkaline phosphatase), increased bilirubin.

CAUTION
1. The smallest effective dose should be used for long-term therapy.
2. Use with extreme caution in epilepsy; can alter seizure patterns.
3. Those with lupus erythematosus or who are taking prednisone have more nervous system reactions.
4. Levodopa should **not** be used to treat Parkinson-like reactions; it can cause agitation and worsening of the psychotic disorder.
5. Obtain prompt evaluation of any change or disturbance in vision.

Precautions for Use

By Infants and Children: This drug should not be used in children under 3 years of age or 15 kg in weight. Avoid this drug in the presence of symptoms suggestive of Reye syndrome. Children are quite susceptible to nervous system reactions induced by this drug.

By Those Over 60 Years of Age: Small doses are indicated when therapy is started. This drug can cause significant changes in mood and behavior; watch for confusion, disorientation, agitation, restlessness, aggression, and paranoia. You may be more susceptible to the development of drowsiness, lethargy, orthostatic hypotension (see Glossary), hypothermia (see Glossary), Parkinson-like reactions, and prostatism (see Glossary).

▷ Advisability of Use During Pregnancy

Pregnancy Category: C. See Pregnancy Risk Categories at the back of this book.
Animal studies: Cleft palate reported in mouse studies.
Human studies: No increase in birth defects reported in 100 exposures. Adequate studies of pregnant women are not available.
Avoid during the first 3 months (trimester). Use only if clearly needed. Ask your physician for guidance.

Advisability of Use If Breast-Feeding

Presence of this drug in breast milk: Possible.
Monitor nursing infant closely and discontinue drug or nursing if adverse effects develop.

Habit-Forming Potential: Reports of recreational use have been filed. If the drug is stopped suddenly, patient may experience a withdrawal syndrome.

Effects of Overdosage: Marked drowsiness, weakness, tremor, unsteadiness, agitation, stupor, coma, convulsions.

Possible Effects of Long-Term Use: Eye damage—deposits in cornea, lens, or retina; tardive dyskinesia (see Glossary).

Suggested Periodic Examinations While Taking This Drug (at physician's discretion)
Complete blood counts, liver function tests, eye examinations, electrocardiograms.
The tongue should be watched for fine, involuntary, wavelike movements that could be the beginning of tardive dyskinesia.

▷ While Taking This Drug, Observe the Following

Foods: No restrictions.
Beverages: No restrictions. May be taken with milk.

▷ *Alcohol:* Avoid completely. Alcohol can increase the sedative action of haloperidol and accentuate its depressant effects on brain function. Haloperidol can increase the intoxicating effects of alcohol.

Tobacco Smoking: Combination with nicotine actually increased suppression of tics in Tourette syndrome in one study. I advise everyone to quit smoking.

Marijuana Smoking: Moderate increase in drowsiness; accentuation of orthostatic hypotension; increased risk of precipitating latent psychosis, confusing interpretation of mental status and of drug response.

▷ *Other Drugs*

Haloperidol may *increase* the effects of
- all drugs with sedative actions, and cause excessive sedation.
- fluvoxamine (Luvox) and result in toxicity (altered mental status, GI side effects).
- some antihypertensive drugs and cause excessive lowering of blood pressure; monitor the combined effects carefully.

Haloperidol may *decrease* the effects of
- guanethidine (Esimil, Ismelin), and reduce its antihypertensive effect.

Haloperidol *taken concurrently* with
- anticholinergic drugs (see Drug Classes) can cause additive anticholinergic effects (dry mouth, constipation, or sedation).
- beta-blocker drugs may cause excessive lowering of blood pressure.
- fluoxetine (Prozac) can result in an increased risk of haloperidol toxicity.
- lithium (Lithobid, others) may cause toxic effects on the brain and nervous system.
- MAO inhibitors (see Drug Classes) may exaggerate low blood pressure and brain (CNS) effects.
- methyldopa (Aldomet) may cause serious dementia.
- ritonavir (Norvir) and perhaps other protease inhibitors (see Drug Classes) may lead to toxicity.

The following drugs may *decrease* the effects of haloperidol
- antacids containing aluminum and/or magnesium may reduce its absorption.
- barbiturates.
- benztropine (Cogentin).
- carbamazepine (Tegretol).
- phenytoin (Dilantin).
- rifampin (Rifater, others).
- trihexyphenidyl (Artane).

▷ *Driving, Hazardous Activities:* This drug may impair mental alertness, judgment, and physical coordination. Restrict activities as necessary.

Aviation Note: The use of this drug *is a disqualification* for piloting. Consult a designated Aviation Medical Examiner.

Exposure to Sun: Use caution—this drug can cause photosensitivity.

Exposure to Heat: Use caution in hot environments. This drug may impair the regulation of body temperature and increase the risk of heatstroke.

Exposure to Cold: This drug can increase the risk of hypothermia (see Glossary) in the elderly.

Discontinuation: This drug should not be stopped abruptly following long-term use. Gradual withdrawal over a period of 2 to 3 weeks is advised. Ask your doctor for help.

HISTAMINE (H₂) BLOCKING DRUGS

Cimetidine (si MET i deen)   **Ranitidine** (ra NI te deen)   **Famotidine** (fa MOH te deen)   **Nizatidine** (ni ZA te deen)

Introduced: 1977, 1983, 1986, 1988, respectively   **Class:** Histamine (H₂) blocking drugs   **Prescription:** USA: Yes   **Controlled Drug:** USA: No; Canada: No   **Available as Generic:** USA: Yes (prescription forms); Canada: Yes

Brand Names: Cimetidine: ✢Apo-Cimetidine, ✢Enlon, ✢Novo-Cimetine, ✢Nu-Cimet, ✢Peptol, Tagamet, Tagamet HB 200 (nonprescription form); Ranitidine: Zantac, ✢Zantac-C, ✢Apo-Ranitidine, Novo-Ranidine, Nu-Ranit, Xantac 75 (nonprescription form); Famotidine: Pepcid, Pepcid AC (nonprescription form); Nizatidine: Axid, Axid AR (nonprescription form)

Warning: The brand names Zantac and Xanax are similar and can be mistaken. These are very different drugs, and can lead to serious problems. Check the color chart insert of drugs and verify that you are taking the correct drug.

BENEFITS versus RISKS

Possible Benefits	*Possible Risks*
EFFECTIVE TREATMENT OF PEPTIC ULCER DISEASE: relief of symptoms, acceleration of healing, prevention of recurrence	Drug-induced hepatitis
	Bone marrow depression (lowered white blood cells or hemoglobin)
CONTROL OF HYPERSECRETORY STOMACH DISORDERS	Confusion (particularly in compromised elderly with some of these drugs)
TREATMENT OF REFLUX ESOPHAGITIS	Low blood platelet counts
TREATMENT OF HEARTBURN	(All of the above are case report to rare effects.)
PREVENTION OF HEARTBURN (cimetidine, famotidine, and nizatidine)	

Author's Note: The nonprescription heartburn-preventing or -treating forms of these medicines have, in general because of episodic use and lower doses, side effects or adverse effects that occur even less frequently or not at all when compared to the already well-tolerated prescription forms.

▷ **Principal Uses**

As a Single Drug Product: Uses currently included in FDA-approved labeling: (1) Treatment and prevention of recurrence of peptic ulcer; (2) all are used for both duodenal and gastric ulcers; (3) cimetidine, ranitidine, and famotidine are used in conditions where extreme production (Zollinger-Ellison syndrome) of stomach acid occurs; (4) all four medications are used to control excess acid moving from the stomach into the lower throat (gastroesophageal reflux disease—GERD); (5) cimetidine is approved for use in preventing upper stomach/intestinal bleeding; (6) cimetidine, ranitidine, famotidine, and nizatidine have been used as combination treatment with antibiotics and bismuth compounds (Pepto-Bismol and others) in refractory ulcers where the organism *Helicobacter pylori* has been found; (7) cimetidine is approved to prevent ulcers caused by stress (stress ulcer prophylaxis); (8) all of these medicines are approved in nonprescription forms for treatment of heartburn. Cimetidine (Tagamet HB 200), famotidine (Pepcid AC), and nizatidine (Axid AR) are also approved for *prevention* of heartburn.

Other (unlabeled) generally accepted uses: (1) Ranitidine, famotidine, and nizatidine have been used in the prevention of upper stomach/intestinal bleeding; (2) cimetidine has been used prior to surgery to prevent aspiration pneumonitis caused by anesthesia, and ranitidine has shown some benefit here as well; (3) ranitidine and famotidine have been used to help prevent ulcers that may occur in acutely and seriously ill patients; (4) cimetidine appears to have a role in helping patients with colorectal cancer live longer, but further research is needed; (5) cimetidine also may have a role in helping recurrent and resistant warts in some children.

How These Drugs Work: These drugs block the action of histamine, and by doing this, inhibit the ability of the stomach to make acid. Once the acid production is decreased, the body is able to heal itself. Ulcers that are resistant to healing have now been shown to have an infectious component (*Helicobacter pylori*), and antibiotics combined with a histamine (H$_2$) blocking drug can work.

Available Dosage Forms and Strengths

Cimetidine:
Injection — 300 mg/2 ml
— 300 mg/50 ml (single dose in 0.9% sodium chloride)
Liquid — 300 mg/5 ml (2.8% alcohol)
Oral solution — 300 mg/5 ml
Tablets — 200 mg, 300 mg, 400 mg, 600 mg, 800 mg
— 100 mg
Tablets (nonprescription) — 200 mg
Ranitidine:
GELdose capsules — 150 mg, 300 mg
Injection — 0.5 mg/ml (single dose in 100 ml)
— 25 mg/ml (in 2-, 10-, and 40-ml vials and 2-ml syringes)
Oral solution (Canada) — 84 mg/5 ml
Syrup — 15 mg/ml (7.5% alcohol)
Tablets — 150 mg, 300 mg (effervescent)
— 150 mg
Tablets (nonprescription) — 75 mg
Famotidine:
Injection — 10 mg/ml (in 2- and 4-ml vials)
Oral suspension — 40 mg/5 ml
Tablets — 20 mg, 40 mg
Tablets (nonprescription) — 10 mg
Nizatidine:
Pulvules (capsules) — 150 mg, 300 mg
— 75 mg
Tablets (nonprescription) — 75 mg

▷ **Recommended Dosage Ranges** (Actual dosage and administration schedule must be determined for each patient individually.)

Infants and Children: Cimetidine: Routine use is not recommended in those less than 16 years old. Doses of 20 to 40 mg per kg of body mass per day have been used.

Ranitidine: For those 2 to 18 years old: 1.25 to 2 mg per kg of body mass per dose given every 12 hours, or 37.5 mg per dose.

Famotidine: 0.5 mg per kg of body mass twice a day for 8 weeks in those 6–15 years old.

Nizatidine: No data.

16 to 60 Years of Age: Peptic ulcer and hypersecretory states:

Cimetidine: 300 mg by mouth four times daily, taken with meals and at bedtime. A maintenance dose of 400 mg at bedtime is useful for some patients.

Ranitidine: 150 mg by mouth twice daily, or 300 mg at bedtime. Maintenance doses of 150 g at bedtime may be of benefit for some patients. Up to 6 g in hypersecretory states.

Famotidine: 40 mg by mouth at bedtime for 4 or up to 8 weeks. Maintenance doses of 20 mg at bedtime have been used. Up to 640 mg daily for hypersecretory states.

Nizatidine: 300 mg by mouth at bedtime, or 150 mg twice a day for up to 8 weeks. A maintenance dose of 150 mg at bedtime is useful for some patients. Not used for hypersecretory states.

Heartburn (nonprescription forms):

Cimetidine: 200 mg by mouth before eating foods or drinking liquids that cause you problems or once heartburn has started.

Ranitidine: 75 mg by mouth.

Famotidine: 10 mg by mouth before eating foods or drinking liquids that cause you problems or once heartburn has started.

Nizatidine: 75 mg up to twice daily before eating foods or drinking liquids that cause you problems or once heartburn has started.

Over 60 Years of Age: Cimetidine: Half the usual adult dose to start.

Ranitidine, famotidine, and nizatidine: Same dose as 16 to 60 years of age. All pose a risk for formation of masses (phytobezoars) of undigested vegetable fibers. Watch for nervousness, confusion, loss of appetite, stomach fullness, nausea, and vomiting.

Conditions Requiring Dosing Adjustments:

Liver Function: Cimetidine and famotidine are most dependent on the liver for elimination. Dose must be decreased in liver failure.

Kidney Function: All of these H$_2$ blockers are primarily eliminated by the kidneys. Doses **must** be decreased in moderate kidney failure.

▷ **Dosing Instructions:** Cimetidine and ranitidine should be taken immediately after meals to obtain the longest decrease in stomach acid when treating peptic ulcers. Cimetidine, ranitidine, and famotidine should be taken after meals when used in hypersecretory states.

Usual Duration of Use: Use on a regular schedule for 4 to 6 weeks usually determines effectiveness in healing active peptic ulcer disease. Long-term use (months to years) for prevention requires periodic individualized consideration by your physician. Continual use for 6 to 12 weeks is needed to heal the esophagus when cimetidine, ranitidine, famotidine, or nizatidine is used in gastroesophageal reflux disease (GERD). Since nonprescription forms are available for heartburn, if heartburn relief has not occurred in 2 hours, call your doctor, as there may be another reason for your symptoms.

Possible Advantages of These Drugs

Famotidine, ranitidine, and nizatidine offer effective treatment of peptic ulcer disease with once-daily dosing. Nonprescription forms offer relief of heartburn discomfort. Famotidine is approved for nonprescription *prevention* of heartburn.

These Drugs Should Not Be Taken If

- you have had an allergic reaction to any dosage form of it previously.

▷ Inform Your Physician Before Taking This Drug If

- you have impaired liver or kidney function.
- you have a low sperm count (cimetidine).
- you are taking any anticoagulant drug.
- you do not tolerate or should not take phenylalanine (ranitidine EFFER-dose tablets or granules).
- you have had low white blood cell counts.
- you have a history of acute porphyria (ranitidine).

Possible Side Effects (natural, expected, and unavoidable drug actions)

None reported.

▷ Possible Adverse Effects (unusual, unexpected, and infrequent reactions)

If any of the following develop, consult your physician promptly for guidance.

Mild Adverse Effects

Allergic Reactions: Skin rash and hives.

Headache: ranitidine—rare, cimetidine—rare, famotidine—infrequent, and nizatidine—frequent.

Abnormal dreams: nizatidine—rare.

Diarrhea: ranitidine, nizatidine, cimetidine, and famotidine—all rare.

Joint pain (arthralgia): cimetidine, ranitidine, and famotidine—all rare.

Depression: cimetidine—case reports.

Muscle pain: cimetidine, nizatidine, and famotidine—rare.

Serious Adverse Effects

Allergic Reactions: Cimetidine and ranitidine can be rare causes of pancreatitis and anemia. Cimetidine and nizatidine can cause exfoliative dermatitis. There have been some case reports of serious skin rashes with cimetidine, nizatidine, and famotidine.

Anaphylactic reactions: cimetidine, nizatidine—rare.

Idiosyncratic Reactions: Nervousness, confusion, hallucinations.

Liver damage—case reports.

Abnormal heart rhythm changes (slow heartbeat or atrioventricular block): cimetidine, ranitidine, famotidine, and nizatidine—case reports.

Bone marrow depression: cimetidine, ranitidine, and famotidine—rare.

Decreased platelets: cimetidine, ranitidine, and nizatidine—rare. Famotidine has been in case reports as a questionable cause.

Bronchospasm: cimetidine and ranitidine—rare; famotidine—rare and questionable.

▷ **Possible Effects on Sexual Function:** Impotence: ranitidine, famotidine, cimetidine, and nizatidine—case reports.

Decreased libido: cimetidine—rare.

Male breast enlargement (gynecomastia): nizatidine and cimetidine—case reports.

Possible Delayed Adverse Effects: Male breast enlargement (nizatidine and cimetidine).

▷ **Adverse Effects That May Mimic Natural Diseases or Disorders**

Liver changes may mimic viral hepatitis.

Possible Effects on Laboratory Tests

Blood platelet counts: may be decreased by all histamine (H$_2$) blockers.

Complete blood counts: rare white blood cell (granulocytes) decrease by cimetidine, ranitidine, and famotidine.

Urine protein tests (Multistix): false positive with ranitidine use.

Urine urobilinogen: false positive with nizatidine.

Thyroid hormones: T$_4$ and free T$_4$ are decreased with ranitidine use.

Liver enzymes (SGPT, OT, etc.): can be increased with liver damage.

Sperm count: decreased with cimetidine.

CAUTION

1. Ulcer rebound/perforation may occur if you stop these drugs abruptly when they are being used to treat ulcers.
2. Once medicines are stopped, call your doctor promptly if symptoms recur.
3. Use of these medicines and symptom relief does not absolutely remove possibility of cancer of the stomach (gastric malignancy).
4. The nonprescription forms of these medicines should NOT be used to treat ulcers.
5. Some of cimetidine is removed by hemodialysis. Redose is needed.

Precautions for Use

By Infants and Children: Cimetidine: Routine use is not recommended in those less than 16 years old. Doses of 20 to 40 mg per kg of body mass per day have been used.

Ranitidine: For those 2 to 18 years old—1.25 to 2 mg per kg of body mass per dose given every 12 hours, or 37.5 mg per dose.

Famotidine: 0.5 mg per kg of body mass twice a day for 8 weeks in those 6–15 years old.

Nizatidine: No data.

By Those Over 60 Years of Age: Increased risk of masses of partially digested vegetable fibers (phytobezoars), especially in people who can't chew well. Watch closely for decreased appetite, stomach fullness, nausea, and vomiting.

▷ **Advisability of Use During Pregnancy**

Pregnancy Category: B for cimetidine, ranitidine, and famotidine. C for nizatidine. See Pregnancy Risk Categories at the back of this book.

Animal studies: No birth defects for cimetidine, ranitidine, and famotidine. Rabbit studies of nizatidine showed heart, brain/spinal cord defects.

Human studies: Adequate studies of pregnant women are not available.

Use cimetidine, ranitidine, or famotidine only if clearly needed. Ask your doctor for advice.

Nizatidine should be avoided during the first 3 months of pregnancy. Ask your doctor for guidance.

Advisability of Use If Breast-Feeding
Presence of this drug in breast milk: Yes.
Avoid drugs or refrain from nursing.

Habit-Forming Potential: None.

Effects of Overdosage: Cimetidine (rarely documented): confusion, tachycardia, sweating, drowsiness, muscle twitching, seizures, respiratory failure, severe CNS symptoms such as coma (after 20–40 g). Nizatidine (rarely documented): increased tearing of the eyes, salivation, vomiting, and diarrhea. Ranitidine and famotidine: no documentation of overdose changes. Adverse effects of the usual dose. Symptomatic and supportive care would be indicated (nonprescription forms do not have documentation of overdoses).

Possible Effects of Long-Term Use: Rare liver damage with cimetidine, ranitidine, and nizatidine. Swelling and tenderness of breast tissue with cimetidine, ranitidine, and nizatidine.

Suggested Periodic Examinations While Taking This Drug (at physician's discretion)
Complete blood counts, liver and kidney function tests, more frequent tests of INR (prothrombin times) if an anticoagulant is also taken, and sperm counts (cimetidine).

▷ **While Taking This Drug, Observe the Following**
Foods: Protein-rich foods increase stomach acid secretion. Garlic, onions, citrus fruits, and tomatoes may also increase acid secretion. Many people know the kinds of foods that are likely to result in significant heartburn. Ask your doctor or pharmacist for help in timing the dose of a nonprescription agent for heartburn.
Nutritional Support: Diet as prescribed by your doctor.
Beverages: The caffeine in caffeine-containing beverages such as coffee, tea, and some sodas may stay in the body up to 50% longer usual with cimetidine (Tagamet) use. Milk may increase acid secretion.
▷ *Alcohol:* Stomach acidity is increased by alcohol—avoid use. Cimetidine may produce a drug interaction with higher than expected levels.
Tobacco Smoking: Smoking is a clear risk factor for peptic ulcer disease. I advise everyone to quit smoking.
Marijuana Smoking: Possible additive reduction in sperm counts with cimetidine use.
▷ *Other Drugs*
Cimetidine may **increase** the effects of
• amiodarone (Cordarone).
• amitriptyline (Elavil) and perhaps other tricyclic antidepressants (see Drug Classes). Decreased doses may be needed if the medicines are to be combined.
• benzodiazepines (Librium, etc.—see Drug Classes).

- carbamazepine (Tegretol), with increased toxicity risk. Blood levels are recommended and ongoing carbamazepine doses adjusted to blood levels.
- flecainide (Tambocor) and require dosing changes and more frequent blood level checks.
- loratadine (Claritin) by causing a large increase in blood levels. A study did NOT report any adverse effects on the heart from these levels, but since excessive blood levels of any medicine may be more likely to cause undesirable effects, it appears prudent to lower loratadine doses if these medicines are to be combined.
- meperidine (Demerol, others) and result in toxicity with potential respiratory depression and low blood pressure.
- metoprolol (Lopressor, others, and perhaps other beta-blockers—see Drug Classes) and result in very slow heartbeat and excessively low blood pressure.
- morphine (MS Contin, MSIR, others) and result in central nervous system depression and respiratory depression.
- oral anticoagulants, with increased risk of bleeding. Increased frequency of INR testing is recommended.
- phenytoin (Dilantin).
- procainamide (Procan, Pronestyl).
- propranolol (Inderal).
- quinidine (Quinaglute).
- theophylline (Theo-Dur, etc.).
- venlafaxine (Effexor).
- warfarin (Coumadin).

Ranitidine may *increase* the effects of
- diazepam (Valium).
- glipizide (Glucotrol) and perhaps other oral antidiabetic drugs (see Drug Classes).
- midazolam (Versed).
- procainamide (Procan, Pronestyl).
- theophylline (Theo-Dur, etc.).
- warfarin (Coumadin)—rarely. Increased INR testing is recommended.

Nizatidine, ranitidine, and famotidine (prescription forms) may *increase* the effects of
- amoxicillin.
- high-dose aspirin (may increase level and toxicity risk).
- pentoxifylline (Trental); however, this interaction has only been documented with cimetidine.

Nizatidine, ranitidine, and famotidine (prescription forms) may *increase* the effects of
- theophylline (Theo-Dur, others). Ongoing theophylline dosing should be based on more frequent blood levels if these medicines are to be taken together.

Cimetidine *taken concurrently* with
- most calcium channel blockers (see Drug Classes) may result in increased blood levels of the calcium channel blockers and potential toxicity. Decreased calcium-channel-blocker doses may be needed. This may also occur with other H$_2$ blockers and caution is advised.

- carmustine (BiCNU) may cause severe bone marrow depression.
- chloroquine may result in toxicity and may cause cardiac arrest.
- cisapride (Propulsid) may result in increased cisapride levels and a potential serious increase in heart rate.
- clozapine (Clozaril) may result in increased blood levels and clozapine toxicity.
- digoxin (Lanoxin) may result in changes in digoxin levels.
- oral hypoglycemic agents such as glipizide (Glucotrol), glyburide (DiaBeta, Micronase), and tolbutamide (Tolinase, others) may result in severe low blood sugars and seizures.
- paroxetine (Paxil) and perhaps other SSRI antidepressants (see Drug Classes) may result in increased blood levels of the SSRI and require dosing changes.
- pentoxifylline (Trental) may result in increases in blood levels of pentoxifylline. Pentoxifylline dose changes may be needed.
- zalcitabine (Hivid) may result in increased blood levels of zalcitabine and result in toxicity. Decreased doses of zalcitabine may be needed.

Cimetidine, ranitidine, famotidine, and nizatidine **taken concurrently with**

- antacids will result in a decreased histamine blocker level. It may be prudent to separate the dosing of these medicines (prescription forms).

Cimetidine **may decrease** the effects of

- indomethacin (Indocin) and perhaps other NSAIDs, by decreasing absorption.
- iron salts, by decreasing absorption.
- ketoconazole, itraconazole, and fluconazole.
- tetracyclines, by decreasing absorption.

Ranitidine, nizatidine, and famotidine may **decrease** the effects of

- indomethacin, by decreasing absorption.
- ketoconazole, itraconazole, and fluconazole.
- sucralfate (Carafate).

▷ *Driving, Hazardous Activities:* Use caution until the degree of confusion, dizziness, or other effect is seen.

Aviation Note: The use of these drugs (prescription forms) **may be a disqualification** for piloting. Consult a designated Aviation Medical Examiner.

Exposure to Sun: Rare and questionable association with ranitidine; use caution with sun exposure when first starting this medicine.

Occurrence of Unrelated Illness: Idiopathic thrombocytopenic purpura (ITP), a rare lowering of blood platelets, is a contraindication for use of any of these medications. Aplastic anemia, whatever the cause, may be worsened by cimetidine. If symptoms of heartburn get worse, you experience unexplained weight loss, and are over 45 years old, talk with your doctor . . . this may be an indication of stomach cancer.

Discontinuation: **Do not** stop these medicines suddenly if they are being taken for peptic ulcer disease. Ask your doctor for withdrawal instructions. Be alert to the recurrence of ulcers any time after these drugs are stopped. Recurrent or refractory ulcers may also represent an infectious disease caused by *Helicobacter pylori*. If this is the case, combination therapy with an antibiotic may be indicated.

HYDRALAZINE (hi DRAL a zeen)

Introduced: 1950   **Class:** Antihypertensive   **Prescription:** USA: Yes
Controlled Drug: USA: No; Canada: No   **Available as Generic:** USA: Yes;
Canada: No

Brand Names: Alazine, Apo-Hydralazine, Apresazide [CD], Apresoline, Apresoline-Esidrix [CD], Cam-Ap-Es, Dralserp, Dralzine, H-H-R, H.H.R., Hydroserpine [CD], Lo-Ten, Novo-Hylazin, Nu-Hydral, Ser-Ap-Es [CD], Serpasil-
Apresoline [CD], Tri-Hydroserpine, Unipres [CD]

BENEFITS versus RISKS	
Possible Benefits	*Possible Risks*
EFFECTIVE ADJUNCT IN MODERATE TO SEVERE HYPERTENSION	DRUG-INDUCED LUPUS-ERYTHEMATOSUS-LIKE SYNDROME
Possibly beneficial in the management of severe congestive heart failure	Intensification of angina pectoris Rare blood cell disorders Rare liver damage

▷ **Principal Uses**

As a Single Drug Product: Uses currently included in FDA-approved labeling: (1)
Treats (in combination with other drugs) moderate to severe high blood
pressure or hypertensive crisis; (2) therapy of hypertension caused by abnormal changes in kidney blood vessels.

Other (unlabeled) generally accepted uses: (1) Therapy for aortic or mitral
heart valve insufficiency, providing support until surgery can be performed; (2) treatment of acute congestive heart failure in combination with
dobutamine; (3) help in anorexia or cachexia; (4) therapy of high blood
pressure in pregnancy; (5) painful erections that may occur in sickle cell
disease (sickle cell priapism).

As a Combination Drug Product [CD]: Available combined with hydrochlorothiazide (a diuretic) and with reserpine (another type of antihypertensive).
When used in combination, several different types of drug action occur at
the same time and result in a more beneficial decrease in blood pressure.

How This Drug Works: By causing direct relaxation of arterial walls (mechanism unknown), this drug lowers blood pressure. The dilation of blood vessels can also help in some cases of heart failure by reducing the workload
and increasing the output of the heart. Combination therapy with a diuretic
reduces the amount of sodium and water in the body, and combination
with reserpine reduces the rate and force of contraction of the heart and
increases blood vessel expansion.

Available Dosage Forms and Strengths

Tablets — 10 mg, 25 mg, 50 mg, 100 mg

▷ **Usual Adult Dosage Range:** Hypertension: Initially 10 mg four times daily for 2
to 4 days; then increase to 25 mg four times daily for the balance of the first
week. During the second week the dose may be increased to 50 mg four
times daily if needed and tolerated. Total daily dosage should not exceed
300 mg for fast acetylators or 200 mg for slow acetylators. Ask your physi-

cian for guidance. **Note: Actual dosage and administration schedule must be determined for each patient individually.**

Conditions Requiring Dosing Adjustments

Liver Function: Hydralazine can cause hepatitis, hepatic necrosis, and noncancerous growths. It should be used with caution by patients with liver compromise.

Kidney Function: In cases of mild to moderate kidney failure the usual dose can be taken every 8 hours. In severe kidney failure and for people with slow hydralazine metabolism, the usual dose is taken every 12 to 24 hours and 200 mg per day is a maximum. This medication should be used with caution.

▷ **Dosing Instructions:**   The tablet may be crushed and the capsule [CD] may be opened, and is best taken with or following meals to help absorption and reduce stomach upset.

Usual Duration of Use: Use on a regular schedule for several weeks determines effectiveness in lowering blood pressure. Long-term use requires physician supervision.

▷ **This Drug Should Not Be Taken If**
- you have had an allergic reaction to it previously.
- you have rheumatic heart disease.
- you have coronary artery disease.
- you have a dissecting aneurysm of the aorta.
- you have mitral valvular heart disease.

▷ **Inform Your Physician Before Taking This Drug If**
- you have a history of any type of heart disease.
- you have lupus erythematosus.
- you are allergic to aspirin or yellow dyes.
- you have active angina pectoris.
- you have impaired brain circulation, or have had a stroke.
- you are subject to migraine headaches.
- you have impaired kidney function.
- you have systemic lupus erythematosus.
- you have a history of liver sensitivity to other drugs.
- you plan to have surgery under general anesthesia in the near future.

Possible Side Effects (natural, expected, and unavoidable drug actions)

Orthostatic hypotension (see Glossary), nasal congestion, constipation, delayed or impaired urination, increased heart rate of 10 to 25 beats/min, excessive lowering of blood pressure.

▷ **Possible Adverse Effects** (unusual, unexpected, and infrequent reactions)

If any of the following develop, consult your physician promptly for guidance.

Mild Adverse Effects

Allergic Reactions: Skin rash, hives, itching, drug fever.

Headache, dizziness, flushing of face, palpitation—infrequent.

Loss of appetite, nausea, vomiting, diarrhea—possible.

Taste or smell disorders—rare.

Arthritis, tremors, muscle cramps—infrequent.

Reflex tachycardia—possible.

Serious Adverse Effects

Allergic Reactions: Liver reaction, with or without jaundice. Serious skin rashes (Stevens-Johnson syndrome)—case reports.

Idiosyncratic Reactions: Behavioral changes: nervousness, confusion, emotional depression. Asthma, bleeding into lung tissue: densities found on X ray.

Syndrome resembling rheumatoid arthritis or lupus erythematosus (see Glossary)—case reports.

Intensification of coronary artery disease—possible.

Peripheral neuropathy (see Glossary): weakness, numbness, and/or pain—case reports.

Drug-induced periarteritis nodosa, porphyria, gastrointestinal bleeding, gallstones, or congestive heart failure—case reports.

Kidney problems (glomerulonephritis)—infrequent.

Bone marrow depression (see Glossary): fatigue, fever, sore throat, bleeding/bruising—case reports.

▷ **Possible Effects on Sexual Function:** Impotence and priapism (see Glossary)—case reports.

▷ **Adverse Effects That May Mimic Natural Diseases or Disorders**

Drug fever may suggest systemic infection. Liver reaction may suggest viral hepatitis. Skin and joint symptoms may suggest lupus erythematosus.

Natural Diseases or Disorders That May Be Activated by This Drug

Latent coronary artery disease.

Possible Effects on Laboratory Tests

Complete blood cell counts: decreased red cells, hemoglobin, white cells, and platelets.

Blood antinuclear antibodies (ANA): positive.

Blood cholesterol level: decreased.

Blood lupus erythematosus (LE) cells: positive.

Blood urea nitrogen (BUN) level: increased (kidney damage).

Liver function tests: increased liver enzymes (ALT/GPT, AST/GOT, and alkaline phosphatase), increased bilirubin.

CAUTION

1. Increased risk of toxicity with large doses. Follow prescribed doses exactly and keep appointments for follow-up examinations.
2. Report the development of any tendency to emotional depression.
3. May cause salt and water retention if not taken with a diuretic.
4. This drug can provoke migraine headache.

Precautions for Use

By Infants and Children: Dosage is based upon age, weight, and kidney function status. For high blood pressure: 0.75 to 1 mg per kg of body mass daily. This dose is divided into two to four equal doses and given every 6 to 12 hours. This is gradually increased as needed and tolerated to a maximum of 200 mg per day. Watch for development of a lupus-erythematosus-like reaction.

By Those Over 60 Years of Age: Low doses are indicated. Unacceptably high blood pressure should be slowly reduced, avoiding the risks associated with excessively low blood pressure. Sudden, rapid, and excessive reduction of blood pressure can predispose to stroke or heart attack. Watch for dizziness, unsteadiness, fainting, or falling. Headache, palpitation, and rapid heart rates are more common in the elderly and can mimic acute anxiety states.

▷ **Advisability of Use During Pregnancy**

Pregnancy Category: C. See Pregnancy Risk Categories at the back of this book.

Animal studies: Birth defects of head and facial bones reported in mice.

Human studies: Adequate studies of pregnant women are not available.

Avoid use during the first and final 3 months; if taken late in pregnancy, this drug can cause low blood platelets (see Glossary) in the newborn.

Advisability of Use If Breast-Feeding

Presence of this drug in breast milk: Yes.

Avoid drug or refrain from nursing.

Habit-Forming Potential: None, but sudden stopping of this medicine may result in congestive heart failure.

Effects of Overdosage: Marked light-headedness, dizziness, headache, flushing of skin, nausea, vomiting, collapse of circulation; loss of consciousness, cold and sweaty skin, weak and rapid pulse, irregular heart rhythm.

Possible Effects of Long-Term Use: An acute or subacute syndrome resembling rheumatoid arthritis or lupus erythematosus, usually seen in slow acetylators taking daily doses of over 200 mg. Tolerance to the therapeutic benefits may develop.

Suggested Periodic Examinations While Taking This Drug (at physician's discretion)

Complete blood counts, liver function tests, blood tests for evidence of lupus erythematosus.

▷ **While Taking This Drug, Observe the Following**

Foods: May decrease hydralazine absorption and lessen its therapeutic effect.

Nutritional Support: Watch for peripheral neuropathy and take pyridoxine (vitamin B_6) as needed. Ask your physician for guidance.

Beverages: No restrictions. May be taken with milk.

▷ *Alcohol:* Use with extreme caution—alcohol can exaggerate the blood-pressure-lowering effect of this drug and cause excessive reduction.

Tobacco Smoking: Avoid completely. Nicotine can contribute significantly to this drug's ability to intensify angina in susceptible patients.

▷ *Other Drugs*

Hydralazine may *increase* the effects of

• metoprolol (Lopressor) and other beta-blocking medicines.

• oxprenolol (Trasicor).

• propranolol (Inderal).

Hydralazine *taken concurrently* with

• clonidine (Catapres) may result in additive lowering of blood pressure. This may be used to therapeutic benefit.

• furosemide (Lasix) can result in decreased furosemide levels and a need to increase the dose in order to get the same therapeutic benefit if these two drugs are combined.

• nitrates (isosorbide dinitrate, others) may result in increased benefits in patients with heart failure.

• NSAIDs (see Drug Classes) may blunt hydralazine's benefit in lowering blood pressure.

▷ *Driving, Hazardous Activities:* May cause light-headedness or dizziness. Limit activities as necessary.

Aviation Note: Hypertension and the use of this drug *are disqualifications* for piloting. Consult a designated Aviation Medical Examiner.

Exposure to Sun: No restrictions.

Exposure to Heat: Caution is advised. Hot environments may reduce blood pressure significantly.

Exposure to Cold: Caution is advised. Cold environments may increase this drug's ability to cause angina in susceptible individuals.

Heavy Exercise or Exertion: Caution is advised. Exertion can increase this drug's ability to cause angina. Also, isometric exercises can raise blood pressure significantly.

HYDROCHLOROTHIAZIDE (hi droh klor oh THI a zide)

See the thiazide diuretics profile for further information.

HYDROCODONE (hi droh KOH dohn)

Other Name: Dihydrocodeinone

Introduced: 1951   **Class:** Analgesic, strong; cough suppressant; opioid

Prescription: USA: Yes   **Controlled Drug:** USA: C-III*; Canada: Yes

Available as Generic: USA: Yes; Canada: No

Brand Names: Allay [CD], Anaplex, Anexsia [CD], Anexsia 7.5 [CD], Anolor DH5, Azdone [CD], Ban-Tuss-HC [CD], ✦Biohisdex DHC [CD], ✦Biohisdine DHC [CD], Chemdal-HD [CD], Codone, Detussin [CD], DHC Plus, Dicoril, Dimetane Expectorant-DC [CD], Duocet [CD], Duratuss HD [CD], Endagen HD [CD], Endal-HD, Entuss-D, Histinex-HC [CD], Histussin HC [CD], ✦Hycodan, Hycodan [CD], ✦Hycomine [CD], Hycomine Compound [CD], Hycomine Pediatric Syrup [CD], ✦Hycomine-S [CD], Hycomine Syrup [CD], Hycotuss Expectorant [CD], Lorcet-HD [CD], Lorcet Plus [CD], Lortab [CD], Lortab ASA [CD], Medipain 5, Norcet 7 [CD], ✦Novahistex DH [CD], ✦Novahistine DH [CD], Polygesic, Protuss, ✦Robidone, T-Gesic [CD], Triaminic Expectorant DH [CD], ✦Tussaminic Expectorant DH [CD], Tussend [CD], Tussend Expectorant [CD], Tussionex [CD], Tycolet [CD], Vanex [CD], Vicodin [CD], Vicodin ES [CD], Zydone [CD]

BENEFITS versus RISKS	
Possible Benefits	*Possible Risks*
EFFECTIVE RELIEF OF MILD TO MODERATE PAIN	Mild allergic reactions—infrequent
	Nausea, constipation
EFFECTIVE CONTROL OF COUGH	Potential for addiction

▷ **Principal Uses**

As a Single Drug Product: Uses currently included in FDA-approved labeling: (1) Controls cough; (2) relieves mild to moderate pain.

*See schedules of Controlled Drugs at the back of this book.

Other (unlabeled) generally accepted uses: May be a benefit for some patients with chronic obstructive lung disease (COPD).

As a Combination Drug Product [CD]: Hydrocodone is often added to cough mixtures containing antihistamines, decongestants, and expectorants to make these "shotgun" preparations more effective in reducing cough. It is also combined with milder analgesics, such as acetaminophen and aspirin, to enhance pain relief.

How This Drug Works: Depresses some brain functions, decreasing pain perception, calming emotional responses to pain, and reducing cough reflex sensitivity.

Available Dosage Forms and Strengths

    Syrup — 5 mg/5-ml

    Tablets — 5 mg

▷ **Usual Adult Dosage Range:**   As analgesic: 5 to 10 mg every 6 hours to start and may later be reduced as needed. Maximum for pain is 40 mg. For cough: 5 mg every 6 to 8 hours as needed. Total daily dosage should not exceed 20 mg. **Note: Actual dosage and administration schedule must be determined for each patient individually.**

Conditions Requiring Dosing Adjustments

Liver Function: Use with caution by patients with severe liver compromise, with decreases in dose or longer time between doses.

Kidney Function: This drug may cause urinary retention, and a benefit-to-risk decision should be made for patients with renal (kidney) outflow problems. Up to 20% of this drug is eliminated by the kidneys. Consideration for reduced doses should be given, especially for longer-term therapy.

▷ **Dosing Instructions:**   Tablet may be crushed and taken with or following food to reduce stomach irritation or nausea.

Usual Duration of Use: As required, to control pain or cough. Continual use should not exceed 5 to 7 days without interruption and reassessment of need.

▷ **This Drug Should Not Be Taken If**

- you have had an allergic reaction to any dosage form of it previously.
- you have a lesion in your head (intracranial) that causes increased pressure.
- you are having an acute attack of asthma.

▷ **Inform Your Physician Before Taking This Drug If**

- you have had an unfavorable reaction to any narcotic drug in the past.
- you have a history of drug abuse or alcoholism.
- you have chronic lung disease with impaired breathing.
- you have impaired liver or kidney function.
- you have gallbladder disease, a seizure disorder, or an underactive thyroid gland.
- you have difficulty emptying the urinary bladder.
- you are allergic to sulfites (some preparations contain sulfites).
- you are taking any other drugs that have a sedative effect.
- you plan to have surgery under general anesthesia in the near future.

Possible Side Effects (natural, expected, and unavoidable drug actions)

Drowsiness, light-headedness, dry mouth, urinary retention, constipation.

▷ **Possible Adverse Effects** (unusual, unexpected, and infrequent reactions)
    **If any of the following develop, consult your physician promptly for
    guidance.**
    Mild Adverse Effects
    Allergic Reactions: Skin rash, hives, itching.
    Dizziness, impaired concentration, sensation of drunkenness, confusion, de-
        pression, blurred or double vision, facial flushing, sweating—infrequent to
        frequent.
    Nausea, vomiting—infrequent to frequent (may also be dose related).
    Abnormal constriction of the pupils of the eye (miosis)—possible.
    Serious Adverse Effects
    Allergic Reactions: Anaphylaxis, severe skin reactions—case reports.
    Idiosyncratic Reactions: Delirium, hallucinations, excitement, increased sen-
        sitivity to pain after the analgesic effect has worn off.
    Seizures—possible.
    Impaired breathing (respiratory depression)—dose related.
    Liver or kidney toxicity—case reports.
    Psychological and physical dependence—possible.

▷ **Possible Effects on Sexual Function:**   Blunting of sexual response or drive—
    possible.

▷ **Adverse Effects That May Mimic Natural Diseases or Disorders**
    Paradoxical behavioral disturbances may suggest psychotic disorder.

Possible Effects on Laboratory Tests
    Blood amylase and lipase levels: increased (natural side effect).
    Urine screening tests for drug abuse: ***initial*** test result may be falsely *positive*;
        confirmatory test result will be *negative*. (Test results depend upon amount
        of drug taken and testing method used.)

CAUTION
    1. Patients with asthma, chronic bronchitis, or emphysema may have sig-
        nificant respiratory problems with excessive use of this drug because of
        thickening of bronchial secretions and suppression of coughing.
    2. Combination of this drug with atropinelike drugs can increase the risk of
        urinary retention and reduced intestinal function.
    3. Do not take this drug following acute head injury.

Precautions for Use
    By Infants and Children: Do not use this drug in children under 2 years of age
        because of their vulnerability to life-threatening respiratory depression.
    By Those Over 60 Years of Age: Small doses and short-term treatment are indi-
        cated. Patients in this group may have increased susceptibility to drowsi-
        ness, dizziness, unsteadiness, falling, urinary retention, and constipation
        (often leading to fecal impaction).

▷ **Advisability of Use During Pregnancy**
    Pregnancy Category: C. See Pregnancy Risk Categories at the back of this book.
    Animal studies: Birth defects reported in hamster studies.
    Human studies: Adequate studies of pregnant women are not available. Hy-
        drocodone taken repeatedly during the final few weeks before delivery may
        cause withdrawal symptoms in the newborn infant.
    Use this drug only if clearly needed and in small, infrequent doses.

Advisability of Use If Breast-Feeding
Presence of this drug in breast milk: Unknown.
Monitor nursing infant closely and discontinue drug or nursing if adverse effects develop. Ask your physician for guidance.

Habit-Forming Potential: Psychological and/or physical dependence can develop with use of large doses for an extended period of time. True dependence is infrequent and unlikely with prudent use.

Effects of Overdosage: Drowsiness, restlessness, agitation, nausea, vomiting, dry mouth, vertigo, weakness, lethargy, stupor, coma, seizures.

Possible Effects of Long-Term Use: Psychological and physical dependence, chronic constipation.

Suggested Periodic Examinations While Taking This Drug (at physician's discretion)
Liver function tests.

▷ **While Taking This Drug, Observe the Following**
Foods: No restrictions.
Beverages: No restrictions. May be taken with milk.
▷ *Alcohol:* Use extreme caution. Hydrocodone can intensify the intoxicating effects of alcohol, and alcohol can intensify the depressant effects of hydrocodone on brain function, breathing, and circulation.
Tobacco Smoking: No interactions expected, but I advise everyone to quit smoking.
Marijuana Smoking: Increased drowsiness and pain relief; impaired mental and physical status.
▷ *Other Drugs*
Hydrocodone may ***increase*** the effects of
• other drugs with sedative effects.
• atropinelike drugs, and increase the risk of constipation and urinary retention.
Hydrocodone ***taken concurrently*** with
• cimetidine (Tagamet) may result in increased risk of breathing problems and central nervous system suppression.
• MAO inhibitors (see Drug Classes) may result in an increased effect and the need to decrease the dose of hydrocodone.
• ritonavir (Norvir) and perhaps other protease inhibitors (see Drug Classes) can lead to toxicity.
▷ *Driving, Hazardous Activities:* This drug can impair mental alertness, judgment, reaction time, and physical coordination. Avoid hazardous activities accordingly.
Aviation Note: The use of this drug ***is a disqualification*** for piloting. Consult a designated Aviation Medical Examiner.
Exposure to Sun: No restrictions.
Discontinuation: This drug is best limited to short-term use. If used for extended periods, discontinuation should be gradual to minimize withdrawal (usually mild with this drug).

HYDROXYCHLOROQUINE (hi drox ee KLOR oh kwin)

Introduced: 1967   **Class:** Antimalarial, immunosuppressant   **Prescription:** USA: Yes   **Controlled Drug:** USA: No; Canada: No   **Available as Generic:** USA: Yes; Canada: No

Brand Names: ✦Dermoplast, Plaquenil

BENEFITS versus RISKS

Possible Benefits	*Possible Risks*
EFFECTIVE PREVENTION AND TREATMENT OF CERTAIN FORMS OF MALARIA	INFREQUENT DAMAGE OF CORNEAL AND RETINAL EYE TISSUES
Possibly effective in the management of acute and chronic rheumatoid arthritis and juvenile arthritis	BONE MARROW DEPRESSION Heart muscle damage Ear damage: hearing loss, ringing in ears
Possibly effective in the management of chronic discoid and systemic lupus erythematosus	

▷ **Principal Uses**

As a Single Drug Product: Uses currently included in FDA-approved labeling: (1) Prevention and therapy of acute attacks of certain types of malaria; (2) reduces disease activity in rheumatoid arthritis; (3) suppresses disease activity in chronic discoid and systemic lupus erythematosus.

Other (unlabeled) generally accepted uses: (1) Treatment of Sjögren's syndrome; (2) treatment of refractory Lyme arthritis; (3) therapy of sarcoidosis, polymorphous light eruption, porphyria, solar urticaria, and chronic vasculitis; (4) may have a role in helping decrease steroid requirements in patients with asthma; (5) can help decrease insulin needs in patients who take an oral hypoglycemic agent with insulin; (6) part of a combination regimen in treating Weber-Christian disease.

How This Drug Works: As an anti-infective in treating malaria, it is thought that this drug impairs the function of DNA in the organisms. As an antiarthritic and anti-lupus drug, it is thought to act as a mild immunosuppressant. It accumulates in white blood cells and inhibits many enzymes involved in tissue destruction.

Available Dosage Forms and Strengths

Tablets — 200 mg

▷ **Usual Adult Dosage Range:** For malaria suppression: 400 mg once every 7 days.

For malaria treatment: (1) 800 mg as a single dose; or (2) initially 800 mg, followed by 400 mg in 6 to 8 hours; then 400 mg once a day on the second and third days.

For pediatric malaria treatment: 10 mg per kg of body mass followed in 6 hours by 5 mg per kg of body mass, with 5 mg per kg of body mass given 18 hours after the second dose; then 5 mg per kg of body mass taken 24 hours after the first dose.

For rheumatoid arthritis: Up to 6.5 mg per kg of lean body mass daily.

For lupus erythematosus: Up to 6.5 mg per kg of lean body mass daily.

Note: Actual dosage and administration schedule must be determined for each patient individually.

Conditions Requiring Dosing Adjustments

Liver Function: It should be used with caution and as a benefit-to-risk decision by patients with liver compromise or who are already taking liver-toxic drugs.

Kidney Function: Use with caution in kidney compromise.

▷ **Dosing Instructions:** Take with food or milk to reduce stomach irritation. The tablet may be crushed and mixed with jam, jelly, or gelatin for administration. Take full course of treatment as prescribed.

Note: For malaria prevention, begin medication 2 weeks before entering malarious area; continue medication while in the area and for 4 weeks after leaving the area.

For treating arthritis and lupus, take medication on a regular schedule daily; continual use for 6 months may be necessary to determine maximal benefit.

Usual Duration of Use: Use on a regular schedule for 2 weeks before exposure, during period of exposure, and 4 weeks after exposure determines this drug's effectiveness in preventing attacks of malaria. Use on a regular schedule for up to 6 months may be required to evaluate benefits in reducing rheumatoid arthritis and lupus erythematosus. If significant improvement is not achieved, this drug should be stopped. Long-term use (months to years) requires periodic physician evaluation of response and dosage adjustment.

Possible Advantages of This Drug

Considered to have less potential for retinal toxicity than chloroquine.

Currently a "Drug of Choice"

for the treatment of chronic discoid and systemic lupus erythematosus.

▷ **This Drug Should Not Be Taken If**

- you have had an allergic reaction to chloroquine or hydroxychloroquine.
- you have an active bone marrow or blood cell disorder.
- should not be used for long-term treatment in children.

▷ **Inform Your Physician Before Taking This Drug If**

- you are pregnant or planning pregnancy.
- you have had bone marrow depression or a blood cell disorder.
- you have a deficiency of glucose-6-phosphate dehydrogenase (G6PD—talk with your doctor).
- you have any disorder of the eyes, especially disease of the cornea or retina, or visual field changes.
- you have impaired hearing or ringing in the ears.
- you have a seizure disorder of any kind.
- you have a history of peripheral neuritis.
- you have low blood pressure or a heart rhythm disorder.
- you have peptic ulcer disease, Crohn's disease, or ulcerative colitis.
- you have impaired liver or kidney function.
- you have a history of porphyria.
- you have any form of psoriasis.
- you are taking antacids, cimetidine, digoxin, or penicillamine.

Possible Side Effects (natural, expected, and unavoidable drug actions)
Light-headedness (low blood pressure); blue-black discoloration of skin, fingernails, or mouth lining with long-term use.

▷ **Possible Adverse Effects** (unusual, unexpected, and infrequent reactions)
If any of the following develop, consult your physician promptly for guidance.

Mild Adverse Effects
Allergic Reactions: Skin rash, itching (more common in African-Americans).
Loss of hair color, loss of hair.
Headache, blurring of near vision (reading), ringing in ears—possible to infrequent.
Loss of appetite, nausea, vomiting, stomach cramps, diarrhea—infrequent.
Dizziness—case reports.

Serious Adverse Effects
Allergic Reactions: Severe skin rash, exfoliative dermatitis.
Idiosyncratic Reactions: Hemolytic anemia in those with glucose-6-phosphate dehydrogenase (G6PD) deficiency in red blood cells.
Emotional or psychotic mental changes; seizures—case reports.
Loss of hearing, porphyria—case reports.
Eye tissue damage, specifically cornea and retina, with significant impairment of vision—case reports.
Aplastic anemia (see Glossary): abnormally low red blood cell counts (fatigue and weakness); abnormally low white blood cell counts (fever, sore throat, infections); abnormally low platelet counts (abnormal bruising or bleeding)—case reports.

▷ **Possible Effects on Sexual Function:**   None reported.

Possible Delayed Adverse Effects: Irreversible retinal damage has developed 7 years after discontinuation of chloroquine, a closely related drug. Retinal damage is more likely to occur following high-dose and/or long-term use.

▷ **Adverse Effects That May Mimic Natural Diseases or Disorders**
Central nervous system toxicity may suggest unrelated neuropsychiatric disorder. Seizures may suggest the onset of epilepsy.

Natural Diseases or Disorders That May Be Activated by This Drug
Porphyria, psoriasis.

Possible Effects on Laboratory Tests
Complete blood cell counts: decreased red cells, hemoglobin, white cells, and platelets.
Liver function tests: increased liver enzymes (ALT/GPT, AST/GOT, and alkaline phosphatase), increased bilirubin.
Electrocardiogram: conduction abnormalities, prolonged QRS interval, T-wave changes, and heart block have all been reported for chloroquine, a closely related drug.

CAUTION
1. This drug does not prevent relapses in certain types of malaria.
2. High-dose and/or long-term use of this drug may cause irreversible retinal damage, significant visual impairment, or hearing loss due to nerve damage. Report promptly any changes in vision or hearing so appropriate evaluation can be made.

Precautions for Use

By Infants and Children: This age group is very sensitive to the effects of this drug. Dosages should be determined and therapy should be monitored by a qualified pediatrician.

By Those Over 60 Years of Age: Tolerance for this drug may be reduced. Watch for behavioral changes, low blood pressure, heart rhythm disturbances, muscle weakness, and changes in vision or hearing.

▷ **Advisability of Use During Pregnancy**

Pregnancy Category: D. See Pregnancy Risk Categories at the back of this book.

Animal studies: No information available.

Human studies: Adequate studies of pregnant women are not available. However, closely related drugs of this class are known to cause abnormal retinal pigmentation and hemorrhage, and congenital deafness in the fetus.

Avoid use during pregnancy except for the suppression or treatment of malaria.

Advisability of Use If Breast-Feeding

Presence of this drug in breast milk: Yes.

Avoid drug or refrain from nursing.

Habit-Forming Potential: None.

Effects of Overdosage: Drowsiness, headache, blurred vision, excitability, low blood pressure, seizures, coma.

Possible Effects of Long-Term Use: Irreversible eye damage (cornea and retina), hearing loss, muscle weakness, aplastic anemia.

Suggested Periodic Examinations While Taking This Drug (at physician's discretion)

Complete blood cell counts; liver and kidney function tests.

Serial blood pressure readings and electrocardiograms.

Neurological examinations for significant muscle weakness.

Complete eye examinations before starting high-dose and/or long-term treatment and every 3 to 6 months during drug use.

Hearing tests as indicated.

▷ **While Taking This Drug, Observe the Following**

Foods: No restrictions.

Beverages: No restrictions. May be taken with milk.

▷ *Alcohol:* Use sparingly to minimize stomach irritation.

Tobacco Smoking: No interactions expected, but I advise everyone to quit smoking.

▷ *Other Drugs*

Hydroxychloroquine may *increase* the effects of

• digoxin (Lanoxin), and increase its toxic potential.

• penicillamine (Cuprimine, Depen), and increase its toxic potential.

The following drug may *increase* the effects of hydroxychloroquine

• cimetidine (Tagamet).

The following drugs may *decrease* the effects of hydroxychloroquine

• magnesium salts and antacids.

▷ *Driving, Hazardous Activities:* This drug may cause light-headedness, blurred vision, or impaired hearing. Restrict activities as necessary.

Aviation Note: The use of this drug *may be a disqualification* for piloting. Consult a designated Aviation Medical Examiner.

Exposure to Sun: Use caution until sensitivity has been determined. Closely related drugs of this class may cause photosensitivity (see Glossary).

Discontinuation: This drug should be stopped and prompt evaluation should be made if any of the following develop—any changes in vision or hearing, seizures, unusual muscle weakness, indications of infection (fever, sore throat, etc.), abnormal bruising or bleeding.

HYDROXYUREA (hi DROX EE yur ia)

Introduced: 1995 (AIDS or sickle cell)   **Class:** Anti-AIDS, anticancer, anti-sickle-cell anemia   **Prescription:** USA: Yes   **Controlled Drug:** USA: No; Canada: No   **Available as Generic:** USA: No; Canada: No

Brand Name: Hydrea

Warning: This drug is a cytotoxic agent. Appropriate precautions must be taken as with other chemotherapy.

BENEFITS versus RISKS	
Possible Benefits	*Possible Risks*
COMBINATION TREATMENT OF AIDS	BONE MARROW SUPPRESSION
DECREASED SEVERITY AND FREQUENCY OF SICKLE CELL CRISES	Hepatitis
Treatment of chronic myelocytic leukemia, melanoma, and other cancers	

▷ **Principal Uses**

As a Single Drug Product: Uses currently included in FDA-approved labeling: (1) Blast crisis; (2) chronic myelogenous leukemia; (3) head and neck cancers; (4) chronic leukemias; (5) cancers of certain cell types (squamous cell).

Other (unlabeled) generally accepted uses: (1) Used to decrease the frequency and severity of sickle cell crises; (2) used to treat certain diseases of the red blood cells (polycythemia vera); (3) used in combination with didanosine to treat AIDS patients.

How This Drug Works: When used in cancer, this medicine is a cell-cycle-specific drug. It works in the S phase of mitosis. When used in AIDS patients, the exact mechanism of action is not fully understood. When used in sickle cell patients, the specific mechanism has not been identified.

Available Dosage Forms and Strengths

Capsule — 500 mg

▷ **Recommended Dosage Ranges** (Actual dosage and administration schedule must be determined for each patient individually.)

Infants and Children: Safety and effectiveness have not been defined in this age group.

18 to 60 Years of Age: All doses are decided based on ideal or actual body mass, whichever is less.

Oral dosing: usual oral doses range from 20 to 30 mg per kg of body mass per day, which is given as a single daily dose. Some centers give 80 mg per kg of body mass every third day. If a patient is in blast crisis, up to 12 g per day has been given to rapidly decrease white blood cell counts.

In the sickle cell studies: patients were started on 15 mg per kg of body mass and had their dose increased by 5 mg per kg of body mass every 12 weeks unless toxicity occurred or the maximum dose of 35 mg per kg of body mass per day was reached.

In AIDS: the protocols are still changing.

Over 60 Years of Age: Same as 18 to 60 years of age.

Conditions Requiring Dosing Adjustments

Liver Function: No changes in dosing are anticipated.

Kidney Function: The dose must be decreased for patients with kidney compromise. Decreases of up to 80% are needed in severe compromise.

▷ **Dosing Instructions:**   This medicine is best taken on an empty stomach. Call your doctor if you vomit after taking this medicine.

Usual Duration of Use: Continual use on a regular schedule for up to 16 weeks may be needed to treat cancers of the head and neck. Treatment in sickle cell disease is ongoing, using the lowest effective dose. Treatment in AIDS is yet to be defined.

Long-term use (months to years) requires periodic evaluation of response and dosage adjustment. Consult your physician on a regular basis.

Currently a "Drug of Choice"

for reducing the frequency and severity of sickle cell crises in patients with sickle cell disease.

▷ **This Drug Should Not Be Taken If**
- you have had an allergic reaction to any dosage form of it previously.
- you have severely depressed bone marrow. This is seen in very low white blood cell, platelet, or hemoglobin levels.

▷ **Inform Your Physician Before Taking This Drug If**
- you have signs or symptoms of cancer.
- you are considering pregnancy (males or females).
- you have had chemotherapy or radiation therapy previously.
- you have compromised kidneys.
- you have herpes zoster (shingles).
- you have recently been exposed to chickenpox.
- you are having unusual bruising or bleeding.
- you are unsure of how to appropriately dispose of urine or vomit.
- you are uncertain of how much hydroxyurea to take or how often to take it.
- you take other prescription or nonprescription medicines that were not discussed with your doctor when hydroxyurea was prescribed.

Possible Side Effects (natural, expected, and unavoidable drug actions)

Hair loss, painful mouth sores, sensitivity to the sun.

▷ **Possible Adverse Effects** (unusual, unexpected, and infrequent reactions)
If any of the following develop, consult your physician promptly for guidance.

Mild Adverse Effects

Allergic Reactions: Skin rash and itching.

Dizziness, disorientation, headaches, or fever—rare.

Nausea, vomiting, or diarrhea—frequent.
Difficulty urinating—rare.
Ulceration of the skin—rare.
Serious Adverse Effects
Allergic Reactions: Skin ulceration.
Idiosyncratic Reactions: Not reported.
Bone marrow depression—possible.
Convulsions or hallucinations—rare.
Hepatitis or kidney problems—rare.
Drug-induced lupus erythematosus—rare.
Lung problems (acute interstitial lung disease)—rare.

▷ **Possible Effects on Sexual Function:**   None reported.

Possible Delayed Adverse Effects: Bone marrow suppression.

▷ **Adverse Effects That May Mimic Natural Diseases or Disorders**
Liver toxicity may be similar to acute hepatitis.

Natural Diseases or Disorders That May Be Activated by This Drug
Not defined.

Possible Effects on Laboratory Tests
Liver function tests: increased.
Complete blood counts: decreases in several components.

CAUTION
1. This medicine is toxic to cells. Be certain your doctor has carefully explained how to dispose of urine or vomit.
2. Call your doctor at once if you have a seizure.
3. Both women and men should avoid conception for several months after taking this medicine.
4. Wash your hands after taking this medicine **before** you touch your eyes or your nose.

Precautions for Use
By Infants and Children: Safety and effectiveness for use by those under 18 years of age have not been established.
By Those Over 60 Years of Age: Natural declines in kidney function may require decreases in doses.

▷ **Advisability of Use During Pregnancy**
Pregnancy Category: D. See Pregnancy Risk Categories at the back of this book.
Animal studies: Causes birth defects in animals.
Human studies: Adequate studies of pregnant women are not available.
Talk with your doctor about this benefit-to-risk decision.

Advisability of Use If Breast-Feeding
Presence of this drug in breast milk: Yes.
Avoid drug or refrain from nursing.

Habit-Forming Potential: None.

Effects of Overdosage: Bone marrow depression, increased heart rate, liver cell and testicular damage.

Possible Effects of Long-Term Use: Bone marrow depression.

Suggested Periodic Examinations While Taking This Drug (at physician's discretion)
  Complete blood cell counts; dental exams.

▷ **While Taking This Drug, Observe the Following**
  Foods: No restrictions.
  Beverages: No restrictions. May be taken with milk.
▷ *Alcohol:* Do not drink alcohol.
  Tobacco Smoking: No interactions expected, but I advise everyone to quit smoking.
▷ *Other Drugs*
  Hydroxyurea *taken concurrently* with
  • amphotericin (Abelcet) may increase risk of kidney toxicity and spasm of bronchi.
  • fluorouracil (Efudil) may increase toxicity to nerves.
  • other medicines that cause bone marrow depression (see Table 5, Section Six) may lead to additive toxicity to bone marrow.
▷ *Driving, Hazardous Activities:* This drug may cause light-headedness, blurred vision, or impaired hearing. Restrict activities as necessary.
  Aviation Note: The use of this drug *may be a disqualification* for piloting. Consult a designated Aviation Medical Examiner.
  Exposure to Sun: Use caution until sensitivity has been determined. Closely related drugs of this class may cause photosensitivity (see Glossary).
  Discontinuation: This drug should be stopped and prompt evaluation should be made if any of the following develop—any changes in vision or hearing, seizures, unusual muscle weakness, indications of infection (fever, sore throat, etc.), abnormal bruising or bleeding.

IBUPROFEN (i byu PROH fen)

See the propionic acids (nonsteroidal anti-inflammatory drugs) profile for further information.

IMIPRAMINE (im IP ra meen)

Introduced: 1955   **Class:** Antidepressant   **Prescription:** USA: Yes
Controlled Drug: USA: No; Canada: No   **Available as Generic:** USA: Yes; Canada: Yes

Brand Names: Antipress, ✚Apo-Imipramine, ✚Impril, Janimine, ✚Novopramine, ✚PMS Imipramine, SK-Pramine, Tipramine, Tofranil, Tofranil-PM

```
┌─────────────────────────────────────────────────────────────────────┐
│                      BENEFITS versus RISKS                          │
│      Possible Benefits                    Possible Risks            │
│ EFFECTIVE RELIEF OF VARIOUS        ADVERSE BEHAVIORAL EFFECTS       │
│   NEUROTIC AND PSYCHOTIC           CONVERSION OF DEPRESSION TO      │
│   DEPRESSIVE STATES                  MANIA in manic-depressive      │
│ EFFECTIVE TREATMENT FOR              (bipolar) disorders            │
│   CHILDHOOD BED-WETTING           Aggravation of schizophrenia and │
│   (enuresis)                         paranoia                      │
│ Helps manage chronic, severe pain Induction of serious heart rhythm│
│ Aids cocaine withdrawal              abnormalities                 │
│ Relieves symptoms of attention deficit Abnormally low white blood cell and │
│   disorder                           platelet counts              │
│ Helps prevent panic attacks                                        │
│ Helps control binge eating and                                     │
│   purging in bulimia                                               │
└─────────────────────────────────────────────────────────────────────┘
```

▷ **Principal Uses**

As a Single Drug Product: Uses currently included in FDA-approved labeling: (1) Relieves severe emotional depression and to initiate gradual restoration of normal mood; (2) aids in the prevention of childhood bed-wetting in children over 6 years of age; (3) used to treat delusions.

Other (unlabeled) generally accepted uses: (1) Helps treat agoraphobia; (2) some case evidence of helping in treating aspermia; (3) can be of help in chronic pain syndromes; (4) eases diabetic neuropathy; (5) inappropriate emotionalism (such as pathological crying) can be controlled by this drug; (6) of use in globus hystericus; (7) may have a role in treating panic disorder; (8) can help posttraumatic stress disorder; (9) may help control retrograde ejaculation; (10) can be of adjunctive benefit in helping control schizophrenia; (11) shows some benefit in patients who fail ENT surgery or weight reduction as treatment of sleep apnea; (12) may be of help as a second-line agent in attention deficit hyperactivity disorder (ADHD).

How This Drug Works: Not completely established. It is thought that by increasing brain tissue concentrations of certain nerve impulse transmitters (norepinephrine and serotonin), this drug relieves the symptoms associated with depression. Beneficial effects in treating bed-wetting are thought to be due partially to this drug's atropinelike action.

Available Dosage Forms and Strengths

Capsules — 75 mg, 100 mg, 125 mg, 150 mg
Injection — 25 mg/2 ml
Tablets — 1g, 25 mg, 50 mg, 75 mg

▷ **Usual Adult Dosage Range:** Initially 75 mg daily, divided into three doses. Dose may be increased cautiously as needed and tolerated by 10 mg to 25 mg daily at intervals of 1 week. The usual maintenance dose is 50 mg to 150 mg every 24 hours. The total daily dosage should not exceed 200 mg for outpatient therapy. (When determined, the optimal daily requirement may be given at bedtime as a single dose.) **Note: Actual dosage and administration schedule must be determined for each patient individually.**

Conditions Requiring Dosing Adjustments

Liver Function: This drug is significantly metabolized in the liver to active and inactive metabolites. It should be used with caution and in decreased dose by patients with liver compromise. It is also a rare cause of hepatic necrosis.

Kidney Function: No changes in dosing are anticipated in kidney compromise.

▷ **Dosing Instructions:** May be taken without regard to meals. If necessary, may be taken with food to reduce stomach irritation. The capsule may be opened and the tablet may be crushed for administration. Note: Tofranil-PM capsules should not be used to treat childhood bed-wetting.

Usual Duration of Use: Continual use on a regular schedule for 3 to 4 weeks is usually necessary to determine this drug's effectiveness in relieving depression; optimal response may require 3 or more months of use. Long-term use (months to years) requires periodic evaluation of response and dosage adjustment. Consult your physician on a regular basis.

Possible Advantages of This Drug

Less likely to increase the heart rate than other tricyclic antidepressants.

Less hazardous and more easily managed than monoamine oxidase (MAO) inhibitor antidepressants.

Currently a "Drug of Choice"

for adjunctive use in treating childhood bed-wetting when organic causes for this disorder have been eliminated.

▷ **This Drug Should Not Be Taken If**

- you have had an allergic reaction to it previously.
- you are taking, or have taken within the past 14 days, any monoamine oxidase (MAO) type A inhibitor drug (see Drug Classes).
- you have had a recent heart attack (myocardial infarction).
- you have angina, abnormal heartbeats, or congestive heart failure.
- you are pregnant.

▷ **Inform Your Physician Before Taking This Drug If**

- you have had an adverse reaction to any other antidepressant drug.
- you have any type of seizure disorder.
- you have increased internal eye pressure.
- you have narrow-angle glaucoma.
- you have any type of heart disease, especially coronary artery disease or a heart rhythm disorder.
- you are subject to bronchial asthma.
- you have impaired liver or kidney function.
- you have any type of thyroid disorder or are taking thyroid medication.
- you have diabetes or sugar intolerance.
- you have prostatism (see Glossary).
- you have a history of alcoholism.
- you plan to have surgery under general anesthesia in the near future.

Possible Side Effects (natural, expected, and unavoidable drug actions)

Moderate drowsiness; abnormally low blood pressure on standing (orthostatic hypotension); light-headedness (low blood pressure); blurred vision; dry mouth (xerostomia)—frequent; constipation; impaired urination. Increased appetite, weight gain.

▷ **Possible Adverse Effects** (unusual, unexpected, and infrequent reactions)
If any of the following develop, consult your physician promptly for guidance.

Mild Adverse Effects

Allergic Reactions: Skin rash, hives, swelling of face or tongue, drug fever (see Glossary).

Headache, dizziness, nervousness, weakness, unsteadiness, tremors, fainting—possible to rare.

Sleep disturbances, ringing in the ears—case reports.

Irritation of tongue or mouth, dental cavities, altered taste, indigestion, nausea—possible.

Fluctuations of blood sugar—case reports.

Serious Adverse Effects

Allergic Reactions: Drug-induced hepatitis, with or without jaundice; anaphylactic reaction (see these terms in Glossary).

Idiosyncratic Reactions: Neuroleptic malignant syndrome (see Glossary).

Adverse behavioral effects: delirium, delusions, hallucinations, Tourette syndrome—case reports to rare.

Porphyria or abnormal urine excretion (SIADH)—rare.

Liver or kidney toxicity—rare.

Drug-induced myasthenia gravis—case reports.

Seizures, reduced control of epilepsy—possible.

Eye changes (glaucoma, ophthalmoplegia)—case reports.

Heart rhythm disturbances or spasm of blood vessels—case reports.

Abnormally low white blood cell and platelet counts: fever, sore throat, infections, abnormal bleeding or bruising—case reports.

▷ **Possible Effects on Sexual Function**

Decreased libido, increased libido (antidepressant effect)—possible.

Impaired erection or ejaculation—frequent; impotence, inhibited male orgasm—case reports to infrequent; inhibited female orgasm—may be frequent.

Male breast enlargement and tenderness, female breast enlargement with milk production, swelling of testicles—case reports.

▷ **Adverse Effects That May Mimic Natural Diseases or Disorders**

Liver toxicity may suggest viral hepatitis.

Natural Diseases or Disorders That May Be Activated by This Drug

Latent diabetes, epilepsy, glaucoma, prostatism.

Possible Effects on Laboratory Tests

Complete blood cell counts: decreased white cells and platelets; increased eosinophils (allergic reaction).

Blood glucose levels: increased and decreased (fluctuations).

Liver function tests: increased liver enzymes (ALT/GPT, AST/GOT, and alkaline phosphatase), increased bilirubin.

CAUTION

1. Look for early signs of toxicity or overdosage: confusion, agitation, rapid heart rate, heart irregularity. Measurement of the drug blood level will clarify the situation.
2. Use with caution in treating depression associated with schizophrenia. Observe closely for any deterioration of thinking or behavior.

3. It is advisable to withhold this drug if electroconvulsive therapy (ECT) is to be used to treat the depression in the near future.

Precautions for Use

By Infants and Children: Safety and effectiveness for use by those under 6 years of age have not been established. Recent experience indicates that children (6 to 12 years of age) may be more susceptible than adults to heart toxicity from this and related drugs.

Bed-wetting (enuresis): children 6 or older have been given 25 mg by mouth an hour before bedtime. Dosage and management should be supervised by a properly trained pediatrician.

By Those Over 60 Years of Age: Treatment is started with 25 mg at bedtime. Dosage may be increased gradually as needed and tolerated to 100 mg daily in divided doses. During the first 2 weeks of treatment, observe for behavioral reactions: restlessness, agitation, forgetfulness, disorientation, delusions, or hallucinations. Also observe for unsteadiness and instability that may predispose to falling. This drug may aggravate prostatism.

▷ **Advisability of Use During Pregnancy**

Pregnancy Category: D. See Pregnancy Risk Categories at the back of this book. Animal studies: Skeletal defects reported in rabbit studies. No defects reported in mouse, rat, and monkey studies.

Human studies: Information from adequate studies of pregnant women is not available. Case reports of fetal respiratory distress, convulsions.

Ask your doctor for guidance.

Advisability of Use If Breast-Feeding

Presence of this drug in breast milk: Yes, in small amounts.

Monitor nursing infant closely and discontinue drug or nursing if adverse effects develop.

Habit-Forming Potential: Psychological or physical dependence is possible. A withdrawal syndrome has been described.

Effects of Overdosage: Confusion, hallucinations, drowsiness, tremors, heart irregularity, seizures, stupor, hypothermia (see Glossary) early, fever later.

Possible Effects of Long-Term Use: Neuroleptic malignant syndrome (see Glossary): fever, fast or irregular heartbeat, fast breathing, sweating, weakness, muscle stiffness, seizures, loss of bladder control.

Suggested Periodic Examinations While Taking This Drug (at physician's discretion)

Monitoring of blood drug levels as appropriate.

Complete blood cell counts; liver and kidney function tests.

Serial blood pressure readings and electrocardiograms.

Measurement of internal eye pressure.

▷ **While Taking This Drug, Observe the Following**

Foods: No specific restrictions. May need to limit food intake to avoid excessive weight gain. Vitamin C in large doses (more than 2 g per day) may require higher imipramine doses.

Beverages: No restrictions. May be taken with milk.

▷ *Alcohol:* Avoid completely. This drug can markedly increase the intoxicating effects of alcohol; the combination can depress brain function significantly.

Tobacco Smoking: May accelerate the elimination of this drug and require increased dosage. I advise everyone to quit.

Marijuana Smoking: Increased drowsiness and mouth dryness; possible reduced effectiveness of this drug. Excessive increases in heart rate.

▷   *Other Drugs*

Imipramine may ***increase*** the effects of
- all drugs with atropinelike effects (see Drug Classes).
- all drugs with sedative effects; observe for excessive sedation.
- norepinephrine.
- phenytoin (Dilantin).
- warfarin (Coumadin) and require more frequent INR testing.

Imipramine may ***decrease*** the effects of
- clonidine (Catapres).
- guanadrel (Hylorel).
- guanethidine (Ismelin, Esimil).
- guanfacine (Tenex).

Imipramine ***taken concurrently*** with
- anticonvulsants requires careful monitoring for changes in seizure patterns and need to adjust anticonvulsant dosage.
- antihistamines (see Drug Classes) may result in urinary retention, acute glaucoma, or excessive anticholinergic actions.
- ethchlorvynol (Placidyl) may cause delirium; avoid concurrent use.
- meperidine (Demerol) may result in increased meperidine caused depression of breathing.
- monoamine oxidase (MAO) type A inhibitor drugs (see Drug Classes) may cause high fever, seizures, and excessive rise in blood pressure; avoid concurrent use of these drugs and provide periods of 14 days between administration of either.
- ritonavir (Norvir) and perhaps other protease inhibitors (see Drug Classes) may lead to toxicity.
- stimulant drugs (amphetamine, cocaine, epinephrine, phenylpropanolamine, etc.) may cause severe high blood pressure and/or high fever.
- thyroid preparations may increase the risk of heart rhythm disorders.

The following drugs may ***increase*** the effects of imipramine
- cimetidine (Tagamet).
- estrogens (various).
- fluoxetine (Prozac).
- fluvoxamine (Luvox).
- labetalol (Normodyne).
- methylphenidate (Ritalin).
- oral contraceptives.
- phenothiazines (see Drug Classes).
- quinidine(Quinaglute, others).
- ranitidine (Zantac).

The following drugs may ***decrease*** the effects of imipramine
- barbiturates (see Drug Classes).
- carbamazepine (Tegretol).
- chloral hydrate (Noctec, Somnos, etc.).
- lithium (Lithobid, Lithotab, etc.).
- reserpine (Serpasil, Ser-Ap-Es, etc.).
- vitamin C (if more than 2 g per day are taken).

▷ *Driving, Hazardous Activities:* This drug may impair mental alertness, judgment, physical coordination, and reaction time. Restrict activities as necessary.

Aviation Note: The use of this drug *is a disqualification* for piloting. Consult a designated Aviation Medical Examiner.

Exposure to Sun: Use caution until sensitivity has been determined. This drug may cause photosensitivity (see Glossary).

Exposure to Heat: Use caution. This drug can inhibit sweating and impair the body's adaptation to hot environments, increasing the risk of heatstroke. Avoid saunas.

Exposure to Cold: The elderly should use caution and avoid conditions conducive to hypothermia (see Glossary).

Exposure to Environmental Chemicals: This drug may mask the symptoms of poisoning due to handling certain insecticides (organophosphorus types). Read their labels carefully.

Discontinuation: It is advisable to discontinue this drug gradually over a period of 3 to 4 weeks. Abrupt withdrawal after prolonged use may cause nausea, vomiting, diarrhea, headache, malaise, disturbed sleep, and vivid dreaming. When this drug is stopped, it may be necessary to adjust the dosages of other drugs taken concurrently.

INDAPAMIDE (in DAP a mide)

Introduced: 1974   **Class:** Antihypertensive, diuretic   **Prescription:** USA: Yes   **Controlled Drug:** USA: No; Canada: No   **Available as Generic:** Yes

Brand Names: ✦Lozide, Lozol

BENEFITS versus RISKS	
Possible Benefits	*Possible Risks*
EFFECTIVE ONCE-A-DAY TREATMENT OF MILD TO MODERATE HYPERTENSION	Excessive loss of blood potassium or magnesium
EFFECTIVE, MILD DIURETIC	Increased blood sugar level
	Increased blood uric acid level

▷ **Principal Uses**

As a Single Drug Product: Uses currently included in FDA-approved labeling: (1) Increases urine output (diuresis) to correct fluid retention seen in congestive heart failure (edema); (2) used as starting therapy in high blood pressure (hypertension).

Other (unlabeled) generally accepted uses: (1) Helps ease the excessive elimination of calcium in the urine (hypercalciuria); (2) may help protect the heart after blood-flow problems (preserves ischemic heart from reperfusion injury).

How This Drug Works: Increases elimination of salt and water (through increased urine production). Relaxes the walls of smaller arteries and decreases pressure reactions (angiotensin II). The combined effects lower blood pressure.

Available Dosage Forms and Strengths
Tablets — 1.25 mg, 2.5 mg

▷ **Usual Adult Dosage Range:**   Hypertension: 1.25 mg per day, as a single dose in the morning. If needed, the dose may be increased to 2.5 mg/day after 4 weeks. Use in treating edema may require a starting dose of 2.5 mg. Maximum total daily dose is 5 mg. (In Canada, the total daily dosage limit is given as 2.5 mg.) **Note: Actual dose and dosing schedule must be determined for each individual patient.**

Conditions Requiring Dosing Adjustments
Liver Function: Should be use with caution and in decreased doses by patients with liver problems. Blood chemistry (electrolytes) should be closely followed.

Kidney Function: Must be stopped if kidney failure progresses after indapamide is started.

▷ **Dosing Instructions:**   The tablet may be crushed and taken with or following food to reduce stomach upset. Take in the morning to avoid nighttime urination.

Usual Duration of Use: Use on a regular schedule for 2 to 4 weeks determines peak effect in lowering blood pressure. Long-term use (months to years) requires periodic physician evaluation.

Possible Advantages of This Drug
Causes no significant increase in blood cholesterol levels.
Less likely to cause significant loss of potassium.

▷ **This Drug Should Not Be Taken If**
- you have had an allergic reaction to it previously.
- your kidneys are not making any urine.

▷ **Inform Your Physician Before Taking This Drug If**
- you are allergic to any form of "sulfa" drug.
- you are pregnant or planning pregnancy.
- you presently have an excessively low blood potassium.
- you have a history of kidney or liver disease.
- you have diabetes, gout, or lupus erythematosus.
- you take any form of cortisone, digoxin, oral antidiabetic drug, or insulin.
- you have had a sympathectomy.
- you plan to have surgery under general anesthesia in the near future.

Possible Side Effects (natural, expected, and unavoidable drug actions)
Light-headedness on arising from sitting or lying position (see Orthostatic Hypotension in Glossary). Increase in blood sugar level, affecting control of diabetes. Increase in blood uric acid level, affecting control of gout. Decrease in blood potassium level, causing muscle weakness and cramping. Low blood sodium and magnesium.

▷ **Possible Adverse Effects** (unusual, unexpected, and infrequent reactions)
If any of the following develop, consult your physician promptly for guidance.
Mild Adverse Effects
Allergic Reactions: Skin rashes, hives, itching—infrequent.
Headache, dizziness, drowsiness, weakness, lethargy, visual disturbance—case reports.

Reduced appetite, indigestion, nausea, vomiting, diarrhea—rare.
Paresthesias—rare.
Urination at night—possible, especially with evening dosing.
Serious Adverse Effects
Abnormal heartbeat (premature ventricular contractions)—rare.
Liver or kidney toxicity—rare.
Serious skin rashes (Stevens-Johnson syndrome, toxic epidermal necrolysis)—case reports.

▷ **Possible Effects on Sexual Function**
Decreased libido—infrequent; impotence—rare.

Natural Diseases or Disorders That May Be Activated by This Drug
Diabetes, gout, systemic lupus erythematosus.

Possible Effects on Laboratory Tests
Total cholesterol and LDL cholesterol levels: no effect or slightly increased.
Blood HDL cholesterol level: no effect or slightly decreased.
Blood potassium, magnesium, or sodium level: decreased.
Blood uric acid level or blood sugar (glucose): increased.

CAUTION
1. Take exactly as prescribed—excessive doses can cause excessive sodium and potassium loss, with decrease in appetite, nausea, fatigue, weakness, confusion, and tingling in the extremities.
2. If you take a digitalis preparation (digitoxin, digoxin), ensure intake of high potassium foods to help avoid digitalis toxicity. (See Table 13, "High Potassium Foods," Section Six.)

Precautions for Use
By Infants and Children: Safety and effectiveness for those under 12 years of age are not established.
By Those Over 60 Years of Age: It is best to start with small doses. You may be more susceptible to impaired thinking, orthostatic hypotension, potassium loss, and blood sugar increase. Overdosage or extended use causes excessive loss of body water, thickening (increased viscosity) of blood, and an increased tendency for the blood to clot—predisposing to stroke, heart attack, or thrombophlebitis (vein inflammation with blood clot).

▷ **Advisability of Use During Pregnancy**
Pregnancy Category: B. See Pregnancy Risk Categories at the back of this book.
Animal studies: No birth defects reported.
Human studies: Data from studies of pregnant women are not available.
This drug should not be used during pregnancy unless a very serious complication occurs for which this drug is significantly beneficial. Ask your physician for guidance.

Advisability of Use If Breast-Feeding
Presence of this drug in breast milk: Unknown.
Avoid drug or refrain from nursing.

Habit-Forming Potential: None.

Effects of Overdosage: Dry mouth, thirst, lethargy, weakness, muscle cramping, nausea, vomiting, drowsiness progressing to stupor or coma.

Possible Effects of Long-Term Use: Impaired balance of water, salt, and potassium in blood and body tissues. Development of diabetes in predisposed individuals.

Suggested Periodic Examinations While Taking This Drug (at physician's discretion)

Measurements of blood levels of sodium, potassium, chloride, sugar, and uric acid.

▷ **While Taking This Drug, Observe the Following**

Foods: Ask about a high potassium diet. If so advised, see Table 13, "High Potassium Foods," in Section Six. Follow your doctor's advice about salt use.

Beverages: No restrictions. This drug may be taken with milk.

▷ *Alcohol:* Alcohol may exaggerate the blood-pressure-lowering effects of this drug and cause orthostatic hypotension.

Tobacco Smoking: No interactions expected, but I advise everyone to quit smoking.

▷ *Other Drugs*

Indapamide may *increase* the effects of

• other antihypertensive drugs; dosage adjustments may be necessary to prevent excessive lowering of blood pressure.

• lithium (Lithobid, others), and cause lithium toxicity.

Indapamide may *decrease* the effects of

• oral antidiabetic drugs (sulfonylureas); dose adjustments may be needed for proper control of blood sugar.

Indapamide *taken concurrently* with

• digitalis preparations (digitoxin, digoxin) must be followed closely and adjustments made to prevent fluctuations of blood potassium levels and serious disturbances of heart rhythm.

• NSAIDs (see Drug Classes) may blunt the therapeutic benefit of indapamide.

The following drugs may *decrease* the effects of indapamide

• cholestyramine (Cuemid, Questran)—may interfere with its absorption.

• colestipol (Colestid)—may interfere with its absorption.

Take cholestyramine and colestipol 1 hour before any oral diuretic.

▷ *Driving, Hazardous Activities:* Use caution until the possible occurrence of orthostatic hypotension, drowsiness, dizziness, or impaired vision has been determined.

Aviation Note: The use of this drug *may be a disqualification* for piloting. Consult a designated Aviation Medical Examiner.

Exposure to Sun: No restrictions.

Exposure to Heat: Excessive perspiring could cause additional loss of salt and water.

Heavy Exercise or Exertion: Isometric exercises can raise blood pressure significantly. Ask your physician for help.

Occurrence of Unrelated Illness: Vomiting or diarrhea can produce a serious imbalance of important body chemistry. Consult your physician for guidance.

Discontinuation: It may be advisable to discontinue this drug 5 to 7 days before major surgery. Ask your physician, surgeon, and/or anesthesiologist for guidance.

INDOMETHACIN (in doh METH a sin)

See the acetic acids (nonsteroidal anti-inflammatory drugs) profile for further information.

INFLUENZA VACCINE (IN flu en za VAX ceen)

Other Names: Flu vaccine

Introduced: Specific formulation for each year   **Class:** Antiviral   **Prescription:** USA: Yes   **Controlled Drug:**   USA: No; Canada: No   **Available as Generic:**   USA: No; Canada: No

Brand Names: Fluogen, Flu-Immune, Flu-Shield, Fluzone

> **Author's Note: The three virus strains for the 1997–1998 flu season vaccines have changed from the 1996–1997 season and are: A/Bayern, A/Wuhan, and B/Beijing-like. In the U.S., manufacturers will use antigenically equal A/Johannesburg, A/Nanchang, and B/Harbin because of their growth properties.**

Warning: Since the vaccine is formulated to contain the viral strains expected to cause the most serious problems in a given year, the side effects or adverse effects may differ annually.

BENEFITS versus RISKS

Possible Benefits	*Possible Risks*
PREVENTION OF INFLUENZA CAUSED BY THE MOST SERIOUS OR PREVALENT VIRAL STRAINS IDENTIFIED FOR A GIVEN YEAR	GUILLAIN-BARRÉ SYNDROME (questionable causation) Hypersensitivity
Possible cross protection from other similar virus strains	

▷ **Principal Uses**

As a Single Drug Product: Uses currently included in FDA-approved labeling: Prevention of influenza.

Other (unlabeled) generally accepted uses: (1) Used in patients with compromised immune systems (such as HIV-positive, cancer, and bone marrow transplant patients); (2) can be of use in isolated outbreaks such as in nursing homes or military camps; (3) may decrease the number of middle ear infections in children who attend day-care centers.

How This Drug Works: This vaccine is made of purified parts of the surface of the virus, split virus, or whole virus, which has been inactivated. When it is injected, it stimulates the immune system to make antibodies. These antibodies (which are created and the production knowledge stored in immune cells roughly 2 weeks after vaccination) act to reduce disease severity or decrease the probability of infection by the expected flu viruses.

Available Dosage Forms and Strengths

Typical split virus: 15 mcg/0.5 ml of each of the three selected strains.

How To Store

This vaccine is ideally stored in the refrigerator. If this is how storage is accomplished, the outdate specified by the manufacturer is valid. If the vaccine is stored at room temperature, it is stable for up to 7 days.

▷ **Recommended Dosage Ranges** (Actual dosage and administration schedule must be determined for each patient and each flu season individually.)

Infants and Children: Those 6 to 35 months old should be given 0.25 ml of a split-dose vaccine. If this is the first vaccination, two doses should be given 1 month apart. Split dose is suggested for children because it tends to cause fewer undesirable effects. For infants and young children, the vaccine is usually given in the thigh muscle.

Children 3 to 8 years old should be given 0.5 ml of the selected split-virus vaccine. Children in this age range who have not been previously vaccinated should be given two vaccinations, 1 month apart.

Children 9 years old or older should be given a single vaccination of 0.5 ml of split-virus vaccine in the deltoid muscle.

13 to 60 Years of Age: Should be given 0.5 ml of whole or split-virus vaccine in the deltoid muscle.

Over 60 Years of Age: Same as 13 to 60 years of age.

Conditions Requiring Dosing Adjustments

Liver Function: Not involved.

Kidney Function: Not involved.

▷ **Dosing Instructions:**   Prior vaccination **does not** mean you are immune to the current year's virus strains. Some tenderness at the injection site is possible. Fever and muscular aches or pains are also possible and may be treated with acetaminophen (Tylenol, others).

Usual Duration of Use: Single vaccination confers relative immunity to the expected viral strains in 2 weeks. This does **not** confer immunity to all strains of virus capable of causing an influenzalike (flu-like) syndrome. Annual vaccination is strongly suggested.

Possible Advantages of This Drug

Allows the prevention of a viral syndrome that can cause loss of several weeks of work in younger, otherwise healthy patients or serious illness in older or compromised patients.

Currently a "Drug of Choice"

for prevention of type A influenza due to the viral strains that are of the greatest concern in the current flu season.

▷ **This Drug Should Not Be Taken If**

- you have had an allergic reaction to any dosage form of it previously.
- you are allergic to eggs (the virus is grown on eggs).
- you have an acute illness and a fever.

▷ **Inform Your Physician Before Taking This Drug If**

- you are HIV-positive.
- you have a history of blood disorders.
- you have had Guillain-Barré syndrome.
- you have a history of seizures.
- you have been receiving cancer therapy (chemotherapy).

Possible Side Effects (natural, expected, and unavoidable drug actions)

Pain at the vaccination site. Muscle aches, fever, or bothersome tiredness (malaise). This is **not** the flu. The vaccine contains viral fragments or noninfectious virus. These symptoms are a reaction to the components of the vaccine.

▷ **Possible Adverse Effects** (unusual, unexpected, and infrequent reactions)
If any of the following develop, consult your physician promptly for guidance.

Mild Adverse Effects
Allergic Reactions: Swelling and redness—possible.
Muscle aches or fever—infrequent.
Fatigue, nausea, and headache infrequent.
Vasculitis (joint pain, weakness, fever, and rash)—rare.

Serious Adverse Effects
Allergic Reactions: Anaphylactic reactions.
Low blood platelets or pericarditiscase reports.
Guillain-Barré syndrome (only reported during the 1976–1977 flu season and of questionable causation).
Kidney toxicity—case report.
Vision changes—case report.

▷ **Possible Effects on Sexual Function**
None reported.

Possible Delayed Adverse Effects: None reported.

▷ **Adverse Effects That May Mimic Natural Diseases or Disorders**
Reaction to vaccine contents may mimic the flu.

Natural Diseases or Disorders That May Be Activated by This Drug
None reported.

Possible Effects on Laboratory Tests
Hepatitis B test: false positive.
Hepatitis C test: false positive.
HTLV-1 test: false positive.

CAUTION
1. The fact that a patient has had the vaccine in the previous year does **not** confer immunity to the flu in following years.
2. The flu vaccine typically confers immunity to the virus types that are predicted to cause the most problems in a particular flu season. The vaccine does not confer immunity to all strains of virus that are capable of causing a flu-like syndrome.
3. If muscle aches or fever occur after vaccination, acetaminophen (Tylenol, others) is recommended. **Do not** take aspirin to address these symptoms if they occur after vaccination.
4. Call your doctor immediately if you develop hives, facial swelling, or difficulty breathing after the vaccination.
5. It is ALWAYS better to prevent a disease or condition than to have to treat it. Talk with your doctor or pharmacist. If you do not have a medical reason for avoiding a flu shot—get one!

Precautions for Use
By Infants and Children: Safety and effectiveness for use by those under 6 months of age have not been established.
By Those Over 60 Years of Age: The vaccine is especially **valuable** in this age group, as the effects of the flu may be devastating.

▷ **Advisability of Use During Pregnancy**
Pregnancy Category: C. See Pregnancy Risk Categories at the back of this book.
Animal studies: Animal studies have not been conducted.
Human studies: Information from adequate studies of pregnant women is not available. Ask your doctor for guidance.

Advisability of Use If Breast-Feeding
Presence of this drug in breast milk: Not defined.
Monitor nursing infant closely and contact your doctor if adverse effects develop. The CDC has **not** listed breast-feeding as a precaution against receiving this vaccine.

Habit-Forming Potential: None.

Effects of Overdosage: No specific cases reported. Treatment would be consistent with any symptoms of the patient.

Possible Effects of Long-Term Use: Not indicated for long-term use.

Suggested Periodic Examinations While Taking This Drug (at physician's discretion)
None indicated.

▷ **While Taking This Drug, Observe the Following**
Foods: No restrictions.
Beverages: No restrictions.
▷ *Alcohol:* No restrictions.
Tobacco Smoking: No interactions expected, but I advise everyone to quit smoking.
▷ *Other Drugs*
Influenza vaccine may ***increase*** the effects of
• carbamazepine (Tegretol) by decreasing the elimination of the drug.
• phenobarbital by increasing the half-life of the drug.
• theophylline (Theo-Dur, others) by increasing the blood level of the drug.
• warfarin (Coumadin) and pose an increased risk of bleeding. More frequent INR (prothrombin time or protime) testing is suggested.
Influenza vaccine ***taken concurrently*** with
• cyclosporine (Sandimmune) can cause blunting of the immune response to the vaccine.
• immunosuppressive agents (chemotherapy, corticosteroids) may be associated with an impaired or blunted immune response to the vaccine.
• methotrexate (Rheumatrex) can result in blunting of the immune response to this vaccine.
• phenytoin (Dilantin) has had variable effects on the blood levels of this drug.
▷ *Driving, Hazardous Activities:* This drug may cause excessive tiredness and muscle aches. Restrict activities as necessary.
Aviation Note: The use of this drug ***may be a short-term disqualification*** for piloting. Consult a designated Aviation Medical Examiner.
Exposure to Sun: No restrictions.
Exposure to Heat: Since this vaccine may cause short-duration fevers, it is wise to avoid hot environments for a day after vaccination.
Heavy Exercise or Exertion: A fever may result and it is wise to avoid strenuous exercise for a day after vaccination.

Special Storage Instructions: This vaccine is ideally stored in the refrigerator. If this is how storage is accomplished, the outdate specified by the manufacturer is valid.

Observe the Following Expiration Times: If the vaccine is stored at room temperature, it is stable for up to 7 days.

Author's Note: There is now a Vaccine Adverse Event Reporting System (VAERS). The toll-free number is 1–800–822–7967.

INSULIN (IN suh lin)

Introduced: 1922   **Class:** Antidiabetic   **Prescription:** USA: No
Controlled Drug: USA: No; Canada: No   **Available as Generic:** Yes

Brand Names: Humalog, Humulin BR, Humulin L, Humulin N, Humulin R, Humulin U, Humulin U Ultralente, Humulin 70/30, Humulin 30/70, Iletin I NPH, Iletin II Pork, ✤Initard, Insulatard NPH, ✤Insulin Human, ✤Insulin-Toronto, Lente Iletin I, Lente Iletin II Beef, Lente Iletin II Pork, Lente Insulin, Lente Purified Pork, Mixtard, Mixtard Human 70/30, Novolin L, Novolin N, NovolinPen, Novolin R, Novolin 30/70, Novolin 70/30, ✤Novolin-Lente, ✤Novolin-NPH, Novolin-70/30, ✤Novolin-Toronto, ✤Novolin-Ultralente, ✤Novolinset, ✤Novolinset 30/70, ✤Novolinset NPH, ✤Novolinset Toronto, NPH Iletin I, NPH Iletin II Beef, NPH Iletin II Pork, NPH Insulin, NPH Purified Pork, Protamine, Zinc & Iletin I, Protamine, Zinc & Iletin II Beef, Protamine, Zinc & Iletin II Pork, Regular Concentrated Iletin II, Regular Iletin I, Regular Iletin II Beef, Regular Iletin II Pork, Regular Iletin II U-500, Regular Insulin, Regular Purified Pork Insulin, Semilente Iletin I, Semilente Insulin, Semilente Purified Pork, Ultralente Iletin I, Ultralente Insulin, Ultralente Purified Beef, Velosulin, ✤Velosulin Cartridge, Velosulin Human

BENEFITS versus RISKS	
Possible Benefits	*Possible Risks*
EFFECTIVE CONTROL OF TYPE I (INSULIN-DEPENDENT) DIABETES MELLITUS	HYPOGLYCEMIA WITH EXCESSIVE DOSAGE
TIGHT CONTROL OF BLOOD SUGAR MAY AVOID OR DELAY DEVELOPMENT OF HIGH BLOOD PRESSURE, KIDNEY, HEART, NERVE, EYE, OR OTHER DAMAGE THAT HAPPENS WHEN BLOOD SUGAR IS OUT OF CONTROL	Infrequent allergic reactions

▷ **Principal Uses**

As a Single Drug Product: Uses currently included in FDA-approved labeling: (1) Used in diabetes mellitus that is insulin-dependent, and by people who have noninsulin-dependent diabetes who are experiencing stress such as illness; (2) used to control blood sugar in critically ill patients who are being fed by intravenous nutrient mixtures.

Other (unlabeled) generally accepted uses: (1) Controls blood sugar in pregnancy (gestational diabetes); (2) insulin in combination with glucagon has been used in alcoholic hepatitis; (3) may have a role in combination therapy with an oral hypoglycemic agent in some diabetics; (4) helps diabetic ketoacidosis; (5) can help diabetic neuropathy and retinopathy; (6) can be of help in critically ill patients with maple syrup urine disease.

How This Drug Works: Insulin helps sugar through the cell wall to the inside of the cell (by direct action on cell membranes), where it is used for energy.

Available Dosage Forms and Strengths
>   Injections — 40, 100, and 500 units per ml
> PenFil cartridges — 150 units

▷ **Usual Adult Dosage Range:**   According to individual requirements for the best regulation of blood sugar on a 24-hour basis. **Note: Actual dosage and administration schedule must be determined for each patient individually.**

Conditions Requiring Dosing Adjustments
Liver Function: Specific adjustment guidelines are not available.
Kidney Function: Caution should be used by patients with compromised kidneys. Requirements become extremely variable.
Thyrotoxicosis: Glucose utilization is typically increased and insulin requirements may actually decrease.

▷ **Dosing Instructions:**   Inject insulin subcutaneously according to the schedule prescribed by your physician. The timing and frequency of injections will vary with the type of insulin prescribed. The following table of insulin actions (according to type) will help you understand the treatment schedule prescribed for you.

Insulin Type	Action Onset	Peak	Duration
Insulin lispro	0.25 hr	0.5–1.5 hrs	3–4 hrs
Regular	0.5–1 hr	2–4 hrs	5–7 hrs
Isophane (NPH)	3–4 hrs	6–12 hrs	18–28 hrs
Regular 30%/NPH 70%	0.5 hr	4–8 hrs	24 hrs
Semilente	1–3 hrs	2–8 hrs	12–16 hrs
Lente	1–3 hrs	8–12 hrs	18–28 hrs
Ultralente	4–6 hrs	18–24 hrs	36 hrs
Protamine Zinc	4–6 hrs	14–24 hrs	36 hrs

Usual Duration of Use: In Type I insulin-dependent (juvenile-onset) diabetes mellitus, insulin therapy is usually required for life. Type II noninsulin-dependent (maturity-onset) diabetes may be controlled by oral antidiabetic drugs and/or diet, but can require insulin when you have a serious infection, injuries, burns, surgical procedures, and other physical stress. See your doctor on a regular basis.

▷ **This Drug Should Not Be Taken If**
  • the need for insulin and its dosage schedule has not been established by a qualified physician.

▷ **Inform Your Physician Before Taking This Drug If**
  • you have an insulin allergy.
  • you do not know how to recognize and treat abnormally low blood sugar (see Hypoglycemia in Glossary).

- you are pregnant.
- you take aspirin, beta-blockers, fenfluramine (Pondimin), monoamine oxidase (MAO) type A inhibitors (see Drug Classes).

Possible Side Effects (natural, expected, and unavoidable drug actions)

In stable diabetes, no side effects occur when insulin dose, diet, and physical activity are correctly balanced and maintained. In unstable ("brittle") diabetes, unexpected drops in blood sugar levels can occur, resulting in hypoglycemia (see Glossary). Weight gain.

▷ **Possible Adverse Effects** (unusual, unexpected, and infrequent reactions)

If any of the following develop, consult your physician promptly for guidance.

Mild Adverse Effects

Allergic Reactions: Local redness, swelling, and itching at site of injection, or hives—infrequent.

Taste disorders—possible.

Thinning of subcutaneous tissue at sites of injection—infrequent.

Serious Adverse Effects

Allergic Reaction: Anaphylactic reactions (see Glossary).

Severe, prolonged hypoglycemia—possible to infrequent.

Inflammation of the parotid (parotitis)—case reports.

Hemolytic anemia or porphyria—case reports.

Arrhythmias (associated with hypoglycemia) or very fast heart rate (with intravenous use)—case reports.

▷ **Possible Effects on Sexual Function**

May resolve sexual dysfunction in patients who have this prior to starting insulin therapy. May also cause decrease in libido and erectile dysfunction—case reports (may also be a result of nerve/blood vessel damage).

▷ **Adverse Effects That May Mimic Natural Diseases or Disorders**

The early signs of hypoglycemia may be mistaken for alcoholic intoxication.

Possible Effects on Laboratory Tests

Blood cholesterol level: decreased.

Blood glucose level: decreased.

Blood potassium level: decreased.

Glycosylated hemoglobin (hemoglobin A1-C): decreased.

CAUTION

1. Carry a card in your purse or wallet with a notation that you have diabetes and are taking insulin.
2. Know how to recognize hypoglycemia and how to treat it. Always carry a readily available form of sugar, such as hard candy or sugar cubes. Report all episodes of hypoglycemia to your doctor.
3. Your vision may improve during the first few weeks of insulin therapy. Postpone eye exams for eyeglasses for 6 weeks after starting insulin.
4. Insulin is absorbed more quickly or slowly depending on where it is injected. Absorption is 80% greater from the abdominal wall than from the leg, and 30% greater than from the arm. It is advisable to rotate the injection site within the same body region than from one site to another.

Precautions for Use

By Infants and Children: Insulin dosages and schedules are modified according to patient's size. Adhere strictly to the physician's prescribed routine.

By Those Over 60 Years of Age: Insulin needs may change with age. Periodic individual evaluation is needed to identify the best dose and schedule. The aging brain adapts well to higher blood sugar levels. Rigid attempts at "tight" sugar control may result in hypoglycemia that shows as confusion and abnormal behavior. Repeated hypoglycemia (especially if severe) may cause brain damage.

▷ **Advisability of Use During Pregnancy**
Pregnancy Category: B. See Pregnancy Risk Categories at the back of this book. Animal studies: Inconclusive.
Human studies: Adequate studies of pregnant women are not available. Birth defects occur two to four times more frequently in infants of diabetic mothers than in infants of mothers who do not have diabetes. The exact causes of this are not known. Insulin is the drug of choice for managing diabetes during pregnancy. To preserve the health of the mother and fetus, every effort must be made to establish the best dose of insulin necessary for "good control" and to prevent episodes of hypoglycemia.

Advisability of Use If Breast-Feeding
Presence of this drug in breast milk: No.
Insulin treatment of the mother has no adverse effect on the nursing infant. Breast-feeding may decrease insulin requirements; dosage adjustment may be necessary.

Habit-Forming Potential: None; however, cases of surreptitious insulin injection have been reported.

Effects of Overdosage: Hypoglycemia: fatigue, weakness, headache, nervousness, irritability, sweating, tremors, hunger, confusion, delirium, abnormal behavior (resembling alcoholic intoxication), loss of consciousness, seizures.

Possible Effects of Long-Term Use: Thinning of subcutaneous fat tissue at sites of insulin injection. Insulin resistance.

Suggested Periodic Examinations While Taking This Drug (at physician's discretion)
Historically, estimates of blood sugar were obtained by checking urine sugar. This method has been replaced by fingerstick testing of blood glucose. Fingerstick testing accurately reflects the blood sugar and helps ensure better control (tighter control) of blood glucose. If you are ill, increased frequency of fingerstick blood glucose testing may be indicated. Routine testing of blood sugar levels at intervals recommended by your physician is prudent.

▷ **While Taking This Drug, Observe the Following**
Foods: Follow your diabetic diet conscientiously. Do not omit snack foods in mid-afternoon or at bedtime if they help prevent hypoglycemia.
Beverages: According to prescribed diabetic diet.
▷ *Alcohol:* Used excessively, alcohol can cause severe hypoglycemia, resulting in brain damage.
Tobacco Smoking: Regular smoking can decrease insulin absorption and increase insulin requirements by 30%. It is advisable to stop smoking altogether.
Marijuana Smoking: Possible increase in blood sugar levels.

▷ *Other Drugs*
   The following drugs may *increase* the effects of insulin
   - acarbose (Precose)—by decreasing the amount of sugar that insulin has to work on.
   - aspirin and other salicylates.
   - some beta-blocker drugs (especially the nonselective ones; see Drug Classes)—may prolong insulin-induced hypoglycemia.
   - clofibrate (Atromid-S).
   - fenfluramine (Pondimin).
   - monoamine oxidase (MAO) type A inhibitors (see Drug Classes).
   - oral antidiabetic drugs (see Drug Classes)—results in additive hypoglycemia.

   The following drugs may *decrease* the effects of insulin (by raising blood sugar levels)
   - birth control pills (oral contraceptives).
   - chlorthalidone (Hygroton).
   - cortisonelike drugs (see Drug Classes).
   - furosemide (Lasix).
   - phenytoin (Dilantin, etc.).
   - thiazide diuretics (see Drug Classes).
   - thyroid preparations (various).

▷ *Driving, Hazardous Activities:* Be prepared to stop and take corrective action if hypoglycemia develops.
   Aviation Note: Diabetes and the use of this drug *are disqualifications* for piloting. Consult a designated Aviation Medical Examiner.
   Exposure to Sun: No restrictions.
   Exposure to Heat: Use caution. Sauna baths can significantly increase the rate of insulin absorption and cause hypoglycemia.
   Heavy Exercise or Exertion: Use caution. Periods of unusual or unplanned heavy physical activity will use up sugar more quickly and predispose to hypoglycemia.
   Occurrence of Unrelated Illness: Omission of meals as a result of nausea, vomiting, or injury may lead to hypoglycemia. Infections can increase insulin needs. Ask your doctor for help.
   Discontinuation: Do not stop this drug without asking your doctor. Omission of insulin may result in life-threatening coma.
   Special Storage Instructions: Keep in a cool place, preferably in the refrigerator. Protect from freezing. Protect from strong light and high temperatures when not refrigerated.
   Observe the Following Expiration Times: Do not use this drug if it is older than the expiration date on the vial. Always use fresh, "within-date" insulin.

INSULIN LISPRO (IN suh lin LIS proh)

Introduced: 1996   **Class:** Antidiabetic   **Prescription:** USA: No
Controlled Drug: USA: No; Canada: No   **Available as Generic:** No
Brand Name: Humalog

```
┌─────────────────────────────────────────────────────────────────┐
│                     BENEFITS versus RISKS                         │
│        Possible Benefits              Possible Risks              │
│   EFFECTIVE CONTROL OF TYPE I      HYPOGLYCEMIA WITH              │
│     (INSULIN-DEPENDENT)              EXCESSIVE DOSAGE             │
│     DIABETES MELLITUS              Infrequent allergic reactions  │
│   TIGHT CONTROL OF BLOOD                                          │
│     SUGAR MAY AVOID OR DELAY                                      │
│     DEVELOPMENT OF HIGH                                           │
│     BLOOD PRESSURE, KIDNEY,                                       │
│     HEART, NERVE, EYE, OR OTHER                                   │
│     DAMAGE THAT HAPPENS WHEN                                      │
│     BLOOD SUGAR IS OUT OF                                         │
│     CONTROL                                                       │
│   RAPID ABSORPTION ALLOWS                                         │
│     INJECTION JUST BEFORE                                         │
│     MEALS                                                         │
└─────────────────────────────────────────────────────────────────┘
```

▷ **Principal Uses**

As a Single Drug Product: Uses currently included in FDA-approved labeling: Used in diabetes mellitus that is insulin-dependent.

Other (unlabeled) generally accepted uses: May be helpful in some cases of resistance to insulin.

How This Drug Works: Insulin lispro helps sugar through the cell wall to the inside of the cell (by direct action on cell membranes), where it is used for energy.

Available Dosage Forms and Strengths

Injections — 100 units per ml

▷ **Usual Adult Dosage Range:**   According to individual requirements for the best regulation of blood sugar on a 24-hour basis. **Note: Actual dosage and administration schedule must be determined for each patient individually.**

Conditions Requiring Dosing Adjustments

Liver Function: Specific adjustment guidelines are not available.

Kidney Function: Caution should be used by patients with compromised kidneys. Requirements become extremely variable.

Thyrotoxicosis: Glucose utilization is typically increased and insulin requirements may actually decrease.

▷ **Dosing Instructions:**   Inject insulin subcutaneously according to the schedule prescribed by your physician. The timing and frequency of injections will vary.

Author's Note: The information in this profile will be expanded once more information becomes available on insulin lispro.

IPRATROPIUM (i pra TROH pee um)

Introduced: 1975   **Class:** Bronchodilator   **Prescription:** USA: Yes
Controlled Drug: USA: No; Canada: No   **Available as Generic:** USA: No;
Canada: No
Brand Names: Atrovent, Atrovent Nasal Spray, Combivent

BENEFITS versus RISKS	
Possible Benefits	*Possible Risks*
EFFECTIVE BRONCHODILATOR FOR TREATMENT OF CHRONIC BRONCHITIS AND EMPHYSEMA	Mild and infrequent adverse effects (see below)
EFFECTIVE TREATMENT OF RUNNY NOSE (RHINORRHEA)	
Possibly effective as adjunctive treatment in some cases of bronchial asthma	

▷ **Principal Uses**
As a Single Drug Product: Uses currently included in FDA-approved labeling: (1)
Helps prevent or relieve episodes of difficult breathing in chronic bronchitis and emphysema. Should not be used to treat acute attacks of asthma
because it takes a while to work; (2) used in nasal spray form to relieve
symptoms of runny nose (rhinorrhea) that comes from allergic or nonallergic perennial rhinitis (this includes runny nose from the common cold) in
adults and children more than 12 years old.
Other (unlabeled) generally accepted uses: None.

How This Drug Works: This drug is a derivative of atropine. Through its atropinelike (anticholinergic) action, it blocks bronchial constriction and opens
up the bronchi. In the nasal form, it keeps acetylcholine from working (antagonizes it) and decreases production and secretion of mucus.

Available Dosage Forms and Strengths
Inhalation aerosol — 14-g metered dose inhaler; 18 mcg per inhalation
Nebulizer — 250 mcg/ml solution
Nasal inhaler — 20 mcg per actuation
Nasal spray — 0.03 and 0.06%

▷ **Usual Adult Dosage Range:** Initially two inhalations (36 mcg) four times a day,
4 hours apart. If needed, the dose may be increased to four inhalations (80
mcg) at one time to get optimal relief. Maintain 4-hour intervals between
doses. Maximum daily dose is 12 inhalations (216 mcg). The nasal spray is
used as: 0.03%—two sprays (21 mcg each) in each nostril two to three times
a day for up to 4 days; 0.06%—two sprays (42 mcg each) in each nostril
three to four times a day for up to 4 days. **Note: Actual dose and dosing
schedule must be determined for each patient individually.**

Conditions Requiring Dosing Adjustments
Liver Function: Specific guidelines for dosage decreases have not been elabo-
rated.
Kidney Function: Should be used with caution by patients with bladder neck
obstructions.

▷ **Dosing Instructions:**   Carefully follow the patient instructions provided with the inhaler. Shake well before using. Many people do NOT take the time to learn the best inhaler technique for them; take the time to do this. The pump of the nasal form must be primed before the unit is used. Read the package insert carefully, and ask your pharmacist for help if you don't understand the directions that come with this medicine.

Usual Duration of Use: Inhalation form: continual use on a regular schedule for 48 to 72 hours is usually necessary to determine this drug's effectiveness. Long-term use (months to years) requires check of response and dosage adjustment. See your doctor.

Nasal spray: the nasal form does NOT relieve sneezing or nasal congestion that may happen with a cold. The nasal spray may only be used for up to 4 days.

Possible Advantages of This Drug

Inhalation form: produces a greater degree of bronchodilation than theophylline in patients with chronic bronchitis and emphysema. Causes minimal adverse effects. Repeated use does not lead to tolerance and loss of effectiveness. Suitable for long-term maintenance therapy.

Nasal spray: eases a very annoying symptom of the common cold.

Currently a "Drug of Choice"

for difficult breathing associated with chronic bronchitis and emphysema.

▷ **This Drug Should Not Be Taken If**
- you have had an allergic reaction to it previously.
- you are allergic to soybeans or peanuts (inhalation form).
- you are allergic to atropine or to aerosol propellants (fluorocarbons) (inhalation form).
- you are allergic to benzalkonium chloride or edetate disodium (nasal spray).

▷ **Inform Your Physician Before Taking This Drug If**
- you have had an adverse effect from any belladonna derivative previously.
- you have a history of glaucoma.
- you have any form of urinary retention or prostatism (see Glossary).

Possible Side Effects (natural, expected, and unavoidable drug actions)

Throat dryness, cough, irritation from aerosol—rare; blurred vision, dry mouth. Bad or bitter taste may be frequent.

▷ **Possible Adverse Effects** (unusual, unexpected, and infrequent reactions)
If any of the following develop, consult your physician promptly for guidance.
Mild Adverse Effects
Allergic Reactions: Skin rash, hives—rare.
Headache, dizziness, nervousness—rare.
Palpitations—rare.
Nosebleeds (with nasal spray)—infrequent to frequent.
Serious Adverse Effects
Allergic Reactions: Rare first-dose angioedema or bronchospasm.
Author's Note: Other than the rare allergic reactions, the nasal spray does not have any serious adverse effects.

Abnormal heartbeat (supraventricular tachycardia)—case report.
Intraocular pressure changes—rare.

▷ **Possible Effects on Sexual Function**
None reported.

Natural Diseases or Disorders That May Be Activated by This Drug
Angle-closure glaucoma, prostatism (see Glossary).

Possible Effects on Laboratory Tests
None reported.

CAUTION
1. This drug won't start to work for 5 to 15 minutes. It should **not** be used alone to treat acute attacks of asthma needing a fast result.
2. When used as combination therapy with beta-adrenergic antiasthmatic drugs (albuterol, terbutaline, metaproterenol, etc.), the beta-adrenergic aerosol should be used about 5 minutes before using ipratropium to prevent fluorocarbon toxicity.
3. When used as an adjunct to steroid or cromolyn aerosols (beclomethasone; Intal), ipratropium should be used about 5 minutes before using the steroid or cromolyn aerosol to prevent fluorocarbon toxicity.
4. Contact with the eyes can cause temporary blurring of vision.
5. Call your doctor if you are using the nasal spray and your runny nose (rhinorrhea) continues or gets worse and you develop a fever.

Precautions for Use
By Infants and Children: Safety and effectiveness for those under 12 years of age are not established.
By Those Over 60 Years of Age: Watch for possible development of prostatism and adjust dosage as necessary.

▷ **Advisability of Use During Pregnancy**
Pregnancy Category: B. See Pregnancy Risk Categories at the back of this book.
Animal studies: No drug-induced birth defects in mouse, rat, or rabbit studies.
Human studies: Adequate studies of pregnant women are not available.
Use this drug during pregnancy only if clearly needed.

Advisability of Use If Breast-Feeding
Presence of this drug in breast milk: Possibly yes, but in very small amounts.
Watch nursing infant closely and stop drug or nursing if adverse effects start.

Habit-Forming Potential: None.

Effects of Overdosage: This drug is not well absorbed into the circulation when it is taken by aerosol inhalation. No systemic effects of overdose are expected.

Possible Effects of Long-Term Use: Drying of the nose.

Suggested Periodic Examinations While Taking This Drug (at physician's discretion)
Internal eye pressure measurements if appropriate.

▷ **While Taking This Drug, Observe the Following**
Foods: No restrictions.
Beverages: No restrictions.
▷ *Alcohol:* No interactions expected.

Tobacco Smoking: No interactions expected. However, smoking should be avoided completely if you have chronic bronchitis or emphysema. I advise everyone to quit smoking.

Marijuana Smoking: Possible excessive increase in heart rate (tachycardia).

▷ *Other Drugs*

Ipratropium may *increase* the effects of
- albuterol (Proventil, others).
- other atropinelike drugs (see Drug Classes).

Ipratropium *taken concurrently* with
- cisapride (Propulsid) may lessen benefits of cisapride.
- tricyclic antidepressants (see Drug Classes) may result in additive anticholinergic effects.

▷ *Driving, Hazardous Activities:* May cause dizziness or blurred vision. Restrict activities as necessary.

Aviation Note: The use of this drug *may be a disqualification* for piloting. Consult a designated Aviation Medical Examiner.

Exposure to Sun: No restrictions.

Exposure to Cold: Inhaling cold air may cause bronchospasm and induce asthmatic breathing and cough; dosage adjustment of this drug may be necessary.

Heavy Exercise or Exertion: This drug is not considered to be consistently effective in preventing or treating exercise-induced asthma.

Discontinuation: Ask your doctor for help. Substitute medication may be advisable.

ISONIAZID (i soh NI a zid)

Other Names: Isonicotinic acid hydrazide, INH

Introduced: 1956   **Class:** Antituberculosis   **Prescription:** USA: Yes
Controlled Drug: USA: No; Canada: No   **Available as Generic:** USA: Yes; Canada: Yes

Brand Names: INH, ✶Isotamine, Laniazid, Nydrazid, P-I-N Forte [CD], ✶PMS Isoniazid, Rifamate [CD], Rifater [CD], Rimactane/INH Dual Pack [CD], Teebaconin, Teebaconin and Vitamin B-6 [CD]

BENEFITS versus RISKS	
Possible Benefits	*Possible Risks*
EFFECTIVE PREVENTION AND TREATMENT OF ACTIVE TUBERCULOSIS	ALLERGIC LIVER REACTION—RARE
	Peripheral neuropathy (see Glossary)
	Bone marrow depression (see Glossary)
	Mental and behavioral disturbances

▷ **Principal Uses**

As a Single Drug Product: Uses currently included in FDA-approved labeling: (1) Used alone to prevent the development of tuberculous infection in people who are at high risk because of exposure to infection or recent conversion of a negative tuberculin skin test to positive; (2) used **in combination** with other drugs to treat tuberculosis in a variety of body sites.

Other (unlabeled) generally accepted uses: May have a role in treating atypical mycobacteria that can be associated with Crohn's disease.

As a Combination Drug Product [CD]: Available in combination with rifampin, another antitubercular drug that works in a different way. This combination is more effective than either drug used alone. Isoniazid can cause low pyridoxine (vitamin B_6); for this reason, a combination of the two drugs is available in tablet form.

How This Drug Works: By interfering with metabolism or cell walls, this drug kills (bactericidal) or inhibits (bacteriostatic) susceptible tuberculosis organisms.

Available Dosage Forms and Strengths

Injection — 100 mg/ml

Syrup — 50 mg/5 ml

Tablets — 50 mg, 100 mg, 300 mg

▷ **Usual Adult Dosage Range:**   For prevention: 300 mg once daily (usually for 6 to 12 months). For treatment: 5 mg per kg of body mass daily. The total daily dosage should not exceed 300 mg. **Note: Actual dose and dosing schedule must be determined on an individual basis.**

Conditions Requiring Dosing Adjustments

Liver Function: This drug should **not** be used in sudden (acute) liver disease. It should be discontinued if the liver function tests become increased to three times the normal value.

Kidney Function: This drug should be used with caution in kidney compromise—it is a rare cause of nephrosis. For severe kidney failure (creatinine clearance less than 10 ml/min), the daily dose should be decreased by 50%.

▷ **Dosing Instructions:**   The tablet may be crushed and taken with food to prevent stomach irritation.

Usual Duration of Use: Use on a regular schedule for 1 year or more is often necessary, depending upon the nature of the infection. Shorter courses of intermittent high doses may work. See your doctor on a regular basis.

▷ **This Drug Should Not Be Taken If**
  • you have had an allergic reaction (especially a liver reaction) to any dosage form of it previously.
  • you have active liver disease.

▷ **Inform Your Physician Before Taking This Drug If**
  • you have serious impairment of liver or kidney function.
  • you drink an alcoholic beverage daily.
  • you are an alcoholic.
  • your are pregnant or are breast-feeding your baby.
  • you have a seizure disorder.
  • you take other drugs on a long-term basis, especially phenytoin (Dilantin).
  • you plan to have surgery under general anesthesia in the near future.

Possible Side Effects (natural, expected, and unavoidable drug actions)

Toxic fever—rare.

▷ **Possible Adverse Effects** (unusual, unexpected, and infrequent reactions)

If any of the following develop, consult your physician promptly for guidance.

Mild Adverse Effects

Allergic Reactions: Skin rash, fever, swollen glands, painful muscles and joints.

Dizziness, indigestion, nausea, vomiting.

Peripheral neuritis (see Glossary): numbness, tingling, pain, weakness in hands and/or feet—frequent in adults, rare in children (may be prevented with pyridoxine).

Serious Adverse Effects

Allergic Reactions: Drug-induced hepatitis (see Glossary): loss of appetite, nausea, fatigue, itching, dark-colored urine, yellowing of eyes and skin, hypersensitivity, meningitis—case reports.

Severe skin reactions (Stevens-Johnson syndrome, pellagra)—case reports.

Acute mental/behavioral disturbances, psychosis, impaired vision, increase in epileptic seizures—rare.

High or low blood sugars (hyperglycemia or hypoglycemia)—possible.

Porphyria or kidney toxicity—case reports.

Lupus-erythematosus-like syndrome or abnormal muscle changes (rhab-domyolysis)—case reports.

Pellagra—rare.

Bone marrow depression (see Glossary): fatigue, weakness, fever, sore throat, abnormal bleeding or bruising—case reports.

▷ **Possible Effects on Sexual Function**

Male breast enlargement and tenderness (gynecomastia)—rare.

Possible Delayed Adverse Effects: An increase in the frequency of cirrhosis of the liver has been reported.

▷ **Adverse Effects That May Mimic Natural Diseases or Disorders**

Drug-induced hepatitis may suggest viral hepatitis. Collagen vascular changes may mimic rheumatoid arthritis or systemic lupus erythematosus. Pseudolymphoma may occur.

Natural Diseases or Disorders That May Be Activated by This Drug

Latent epilepsy, systemic lupus erythematosus (questionable).

Possible Effects on Laboratory Tests

Complete blood cell counts: decreased red cells, hemoglobin, white cells, and platelets; increased eosinophils (allergic reaction).

Blood amylase level: increased (possible pancreatitis).

Blood antinuclear antibodies (ANA): positive.

Blood lupus erythematosus (LE) cells: positive.

Blood glucose level: increased (with large doses).

Liver function tests: increased liver enzymes (ALT/GPT, AST/GOT, and alka-line phosphatase), increased bilirubin.

Urine sugar tests: increased; false positive results with Benedict's solution and Clinitest.

CAUTION

1. **Recently, the FDA has required a new warning for Laniazid: "A recent report suggests an increased risk of fatal hepatitis associated with isoniazid among women, particularly Black and Hispanic women. The risk may also be increased during the postpartum period."** Increased laboratory testing is also suggested.

2. Ask your doctor about determining if you are a "slow" or "rapid" inactivator (acetylator) of isoniazid. This has a bearing on your predisposition to developing adverse effects.
3. Copper sulfate tests for urine sugar may give a false-positive test result. (Diabetics, please note.)

Precautions for Use

By Infants and Children: Use with caution in children with seizure disorders. "Slow acetylators" are more prone to adverse drug effects. It is advisable to give supplemental pyridoxine (vitamin B$_6$).

By Those Over 60 Years of Age: There is a greater incidence of liver damage in this age group, and liver status should be closely watched. Observe for any indications of an "acute brain syndrome" consisting of confusion, delirium, and seizures.

▷ **Advisability of Use During Pregnancy**

Pregnancy Category: C. See Pregnancy Risk Categories at the back of this book.
Animal studies: No birth defects reported in mice, rats, or rabbits.
Human studies: Data from adequate studies of pregnant women are not available.
If clearly needed, this drug is now used at any time during pregnancy. Ask your physician for guidance.

Advisability of Use If Breast-Feeding

Presence of this drug in breast milk: Yes.
Avoid drug or refrain from nursing.

Habit-Forming Potential: None.

Effects of Overdosage: Nausea, vomiting, dizziness, blurred vision, hallucinations, slurred speech, stupor, coma, seizures.

Possible Effects of Long-Term Use: Peripheral neuritis due to a deficiency of pyridoxine (vitamin B$_6$).

Suggested Periodic Examinations While Taking This Drug (at physician's discretion)
Complete blood cell counts, liver function tests, complete eye examinations.

▷ **While Taking This Drug, Observe the Following**

Foods: Eat the following foods cautiously until your tolerance is determined: Swiss and Cheshire cheeses, tuna fish, skipjack fish, and *Sardinella* species. These may interact with the drug to produce skin rash, itching, sweating, chills, headache, light-headedness, or rapid heart rate. Taking this drug with food also acts to decrease absorption and lessen therapeutic benefits. Some red wines and aged cheeses also contain high levels of tyramine. This may result in an undesirable increase in blood pressure if consumed. Avoid this combination.

Nutritional Support: It is advisable to take a supplement of pyridoxine (vitamin B$_6$) to prevent peripheral neuritis. Ask your physician for help.

Beverages: No restrictions. May be taken with milk.

▷ *Alcohol:* Alcohol may reduce the effectiveness of this drug and increase the risk of liver toxicity.

Tobacco Smoking: No interactions expected, but I advise everyone to quit smoking.

▷   *Other Drugs*
Isoniazid may *increase* the effects of
- carbamazepine (Tegretol), and cause toxicity.
- phenytoin (Dilantin), and cause toxicity.

The following drugs may *decrease* the effects of isoniazid
- cortisonelike drugs (see Drug Classes).

Isoniazid *taken concurrently* with
- acetaminophen (Tylenol) may increase the risk of hepatoxicity.
- antacids may decrease the absorption of this medicine. Separate antacid dosing by 2 hours from dosing of this medicine.
- BCG vaccine will result in decreased vaccine effectiveness.
- cyclosporine (Sandimmune) may blunt cyclosporine benefits.
- diazepam and perhaps other benzodiazepines (see Drug Classes) may result in increased blood levels and toxicity.
- ketoconazole, itraconazole, or related compounds may result in decreased therapeutic benefits of the antifungal.
- meperidine (Demerol) may result in excessive lowering of blood pressure.
- oral antidiabetic drugs (see Drug Classes) may result in loss of control of blood glucose.
- rifampin (Rifadin, others) can result in a serious increased risk of liver toxicity.
- theophylline may result in theophylline toxicity.
- valproic acid (Depakene) can result in isoniazid or valproic acid toxicity.
- warfarin (Coumadin) may result in increased bleeding risk. More frequent INR (prothrombin time or protime) testing is needed.

▷   *Driving, Hazardous Activities:* This drug may cause dizziness. Restrict activities as necessary.
Aviation Note: The use of this drug *may be a disqualification* for piloting. Consult a designated Aviation Medical Examiner.
Exposure to Sun: No restrictions.
Discontinuation: Long-term treatment is required. Do not stop this drug without asking your physician.

ISOSORBIDE DINITRATE (i soh SOHR bide di NI trayt)

Other Name: Sorbide nitrate

Introduced: 1959   **Class:** Anti-anginal, nitrates   **Prescription:** USA: Yes   **Controlled Drug:** USA: No; Canada: No   **Available as Generic:** USA: Yes; Canada: No

Brand Names: ✤Apo-ISDN, ✤Cedocard-SR, ✤Coradur, ✤Coronex, Dilatrate-SR, Iso-BID, Isonate, Isordil, Isordil Tembids, Isordil Titradose, Isotrate Timecelles, ✤Novosorbide, Sorbitrate-SA, Sorbitrate

Warning: The brand names Isordil and Isuprel are similar and can be mistaken for each other; this can lead to serious medication errors. These names represent very different drugs. Isordil is the generic drug isosorbide dinitrate, used to treat angina. Isuprel is the generic drug isoproterenol, used for asthma. Verify that you are taking the correct drug.

BENEFITS versus RISKS

Possible Benefits	*Possible Risks*
EFFECTIVE RELIEF AND PREVENTION OF ANGINA	Orthostatic hypotension (see Glossary)
EFFECTIVE ADJUNCTIVE TREATMENT IN SOME CASES OF CONGESTIVE HEART FAILURE	Rare skin reactions (severe peeling)

▷ **Principal Uses**

As a Single Drug Product: Uses currently included in FDA-approved labeling: (1) The sublingual (under-the-tongue) tablets and the chewable tablets are used to prevent and relieve acute attacks of anginal pain; (2) the longer-acting tablets and capsules are used to prevent the development of angina, but are not effective in relieving acute episodes of anginal pain (nitroglycerin is the drug of choice in those cases).

Other (unlabeled) generally accepted uses: (1) This drug is also used to improve heart function in selected cases of congestive heart failure; (2) can help ease the pressure in esophageal varices in alcoholics; (3) can help painful leg cramping (intermittent claudication); (4) used after a heart attack intravenously to help address congestive heart failure.

How This Drug Works: By direct action on the muscle in blood vessel walls, this drug relaxes and dilates both arteries and veins. Its beneficial effects in treating angina and heart failure are due to (1) dilation of coronary arteries and (2) dilation of systemic veins. The net effects are improved blood flow to the heart muscle and reduced workload of the heart.

Available Dosage Forms and Strengths

Capsules — 40 mg

Capsules, prolonged action — 40 mg

Tablets — 5 mg, 10 mg, 20 mg, 30 mg, 40 mg

Tablets, chewable — 5 mg, 10 mg

Tablets, prolonged action — 20 mg, 40 mg

Tablets, sublingual — 2.5 mg, 5 mg, 10 mg

▷ **Recommended Dosage Ranges** (Actual dosage and administration schedule must be determined for each patient individually.)

Infants and Children: Dosage not established.

12 to 60 Years of Age: Sublingual tablets: 5 to 10 mg dissolved under tongue every 2 to 3 hours; use for relief of acute attack and for prevention of anticipated attack.

Chewable tablets: initially 5 mg chewed to evaluate tolerance; increase dose to 5 or 10 mg every 2 to 3 hours as needed and tolerated. Use for relief of acute attack and for prevention of anticipated attack.

Tablets: 5 to 20 mg four times daily to prevent acute attack; usual dose is 10 to 40 mg four times daily.

Prolonged-action capsules and tablets: 40 mg to start, then 40–80 mg every 8 to 12 hours as needed to prevent acute attacks.

The total daily dosage should not exceed 120 mg.

Author's Note: Dosing for all forms is set up to give a 12-hour nitrate-free period in order to avoid tolerance to the therapeutic benefits of this medicine.

Over 60 Years of Age: Same as 12 to 60 years of age; however, excessive lowering of the blood pressure on standing (postural hypotension) may be more likely in this population.

Conditions Requiring Dosing Adjustments

Liver Function: This drug should be used with caution and in decreased doses by patients with liver compromise, as increased blood levels will occur.

Kidney Function: No specific dosing changes are needed for compromised kidneys. This drug can discolor (brown to black) urine.

▷ **Dosing Instructions:**   Capsules and tablets to be swallowed are best taken on an empty stomach to achieve maximal blood levels. Regular tablets may be crushed for administration; prolonged-action capsules and tablets should be taken whole, NOT chewed.

Usual Duration of Use: Use on a regular schedule for 3 to 7 days is needed to (1) identify this drug's peak effect in preventing or relieving acute anginal pain, and (2) to find the optimal dosage schedule. Long-term use (months to years) requires physician supervision.

▷ **This Drug Should Not Be Taken If**
 • you have had an allergic reaction to any dosage form of it previously.
 • you have severe anemia.
 • you have increased intraocular pressure.
 • you have suffered trauma to the head.
 • you have an overactive thyroid gland.
 • you have abnormal growth of the heart muscle (hypertrophic cardiomyopathy).
 • you have had a very recent heart attack (myocardial infarction) and have elevated blood pressure or very rapid heart rate (tachycardia).

▷ **Inform Your Physician Before Taking This Drug If**
 • you have had an unfavorable response to other nitrate drugs or vasodilators in the past.
 • you have a history of low blood pressure.
 • you have any form of glaucoma.
 • you have had a cerebral hemorrhage recently.
 • you are pregnant or are planning pregnancy.
 • you are allergic to the dye tartrazine.
 • you have a glucose-6-phosphate dehydrogenase (G6PD) deficiency (ask your doctor).

Possible Side Effects (natural, expected, and unavoidable drug actions)
Flushing of face, throbbing in head, palpitation, rapid heart rate, orthostatic hypotension (see Glossary).

▷ **Possible Adverse Effects** (unusual, unexpected, and infrequent reactions)
If any of the following develop, consult your physician promptly for guidance.

Mild Adverse Effects
Allergic Reaction: Skin rash.
Headache (may be severe and persistent)—infrequent to frequent; dizziness, fainting—possible.
Nausea, vomiting—possible.
Urine discoloration—possible and not clinically significant.

Serious Adverse Effects

Allergic Reaction: Severe dermatitis with peeling of skin—case reports.

Transient ischemic attacks (TIAs) in presence of impaired circulation within the brain: dizziness, fainting, impaired vision or speech, localized numbness or weakness—possible.

Anemia (in those with G6PD deficiency)—possible.

Abnormal heart rates or conduction—case reports.

Abnormally low blood pressure on standing (postural hypotension)—possible.

Tolerance—possible with 24-hour use (daily 12-hour drug-free period is used to prevent this).

▷ **Possible Effects on Sexual Function**

None reported.

▷ **Adverse Effects That May Mimic Natural Diseases or Disorders**

Spells of low blood pressure (due to this drug) may mimic late-onset epilepsy.

Possible Effects on Laboratory Tests

None reported.

CAUTION

1. Tolerance (see Glossary) to long-acting forms of nitrates may cause sublingual tablets of nitroglycerin to be less effective in relieving acute anginal attacks. Anti-anginal effectiveness is restored after 1 week of abstinence from long-acting nitrates. Daily 12-hour periods without use of the drug are needed.
2. Many over-the-counter (OTC) medications for allergies, colds, and coughs contain drugs that may counteract the desired drug effects. Ask your physician or pharmacist for help before using such medications.

Precautions for Use

By Those Over 60 Years of Age: Small starting doses are advisable. You may be more susceptible to the development of low blood pressure and associated "blackout" spells, fainting, and falling. Throbbing headaches and flushing may be more apparent.

▷ **Advisability of Use During Pregnancy**

Pregnancy Category: C. See Pregnancy Risk Categories at the back of this book.

Animal studies: No information available.

Human studies: Adequate studies of pregnant women are not available.

Use this drug only if clearly needed.

Advisability of Use If Breast-Feeding

Presence of this drug in breast milk: Unknown.

If this drug is thought to be necessary, monitor the nursing infant for low blood pressure and poor feeding.

Habit-Forming Potential: None.

Effects of Overdosage: Headache, dizziness, marked flushing of face and skin, vomiting, weakness, fainting, difficult breathing, coma.

Possible Effects of Long-Term Use: Development of tolerance with temporary loss of effectiveness at recommended doses. Development of abnormal hemoglobin (red blood cell pigment).

Suggested Periodic Examinations While Taking This Drug (at physician's discretion)

Measurement of internal eye pressure. Red cell counts and hemoglobin tests.

▷ **While Taking This Drug, Observe the Following**

Foods: Oral doses are best taken on an empty stomach to insure quick absorption.

Beverages: No restrictions. May be taken with milk.

▷ *Alcohol:* Use extreme caution and avoid alcohol completely in the presence of any side effects or adverse effects of this drug. Alcohol may exaggerate the blood-pressure-lowering effect of this drug.

Tobacco Smoking: Nicotine can reduce the benefits of this drug. Avoid all forms of tobacco.

Marijuana Smoking: Possible reduced effectiveness of this drug; mild to moderate increase in angina; possible changes in electrocardiogram, confusing interpretation.

▷ *Other Drugs*

Isosorbide dinitrate *taken concurrently* with

- antihypertensive drugs may cause excessive lowering of blood pressure; dosage adjustments may be necessary.
- hydralazine (Apresoline) may work well to help control angina.
- propranolol (Inderal) can help improve exercise time without angina.

▷ *Driving, Hazardous Activities:* Usually no restrictions. This drug may cause dizziness or spells of low blood pressure. Restrict activities as necessary.

Aviation Note: Coronary artery disease *is a disqualification* for piloting. Consult a designated Aviation Medical Examiner.

Exposure to Sun: No restrictions.

Exposure to Heat: Use caution. Hot environments can cause significant drop in blood pressure.

Exposure to Cold: Cold environments can increase the need for this drug and limit its benefits.

Heavy Exercise or Exertion: This drug may improve your ability to be more active without anginal pain. Use caution and avoid excessive exertion.

Discontinuation: It is advisable to gradually withdraw this drug after long-term use. Dose and frequency of prolonged-action dosage forms should be reduced gradually over a period of 4 to 6 weeks.

ISOSORBIDE MONONITRATE (i soh SOHR bide mon oh NI trayt)

Introduced: 1983   **Class:** Anti-anginal, nitrates   **Prescription:** USA: Yes   **Controlled Drug:** USA: No   **Available as Generic:** USA: No

Brand Names: Elan (Italy), Elantan, Imdur, Ismo, Monoket

BENEFITS versus RISKS	
Possible Benefits	*Possible Risks*
EFFECTIVE PREVENTION OF ANGINA	Orthostatic hypotension (see Glossary)
	Headache

▷ **Principal Uses**

As a Single Drug Product: Uses currently included in FDA-approved labeling: To reduce the frequency and severity of recurrent angina; not effective in acute anginal pain.

Other (unlabeled) generally accepted uses: (1) May have a role in treating congestive heart failure (intravenous); (2) can help in decreasing the number of attacks and time spent in silent myocardial ischemia; (3) may be of help in heart attacks (myocardial infarction).

How This Drug Works: By direct action on the muscle in blood vessel walls, this drug relaxes and dilates both arteries and veins. Beneficial effects in treating angina are due to (1) dilation of coronary arteries, and (2) dilation of systemic veins. The net effects are improved blood flow to the heart muscle and reduced workload of the heart.

Available Dosage Forms and Strengths
> Capsules, sustained release — 60 mg—50 mg (Italy)
> Tablets — 10 mg, 20 mg
> Tablets, sustained release — 30 mg, 60 mg, 120 mg

▷ **Recommended Dosage Ranges** (Actual dosage and administration schedule must be determined for each patient individually.)
Infants and Children: Dosage not established.
12 to 60 Years of Age: Regular release: 20 mg (one tablet), taken twice daily. Take the first tablet on arising; take the second tablet 7 hours later. Do not take additional doses during the balance of the day. Total daily dosage should not exceed 40 mg.
Author's Note: Dosing is set up to give a 12-hour nitrate-free period in order to avoid tolerance to the therapeutic benefits of this medicine.
Sustained release: 30 mg (one half-tablet) or 60 mg (a whole tablet) once daily, taken in the morning when you get up. Total daily dose should not exceed 240 mg.
Over 60 Years of Age: Same as 12 to 60 years of age.

Conditions Requiring Dosing Adjustments
Liver Function: This drug should be used with caution by patients with liver compromise; however, no specific guidelines for dosage reduction are available.
Kidney Function: No dosing changes are recommended in renal compromise. Isosorbide mononitrate may turn the urine brown to black in color.

▷ **Dosing Instructions:**   The tablet may be crushed and is preferably taken on an empty stomach to achieve the best blood levels. Sustained-release forms should not be chewed or crushed.

Usual Duration of Use: Use on a regular schedule for 3 to 7 days determines this drug's effectiveness in preventing episodes of acute anginal pain. Long-term use (months to years) requires physician supervision.

Possible Advantages of This Drug
Designed to provide the best possible prevention of acute angina with minimal development of tolerance (loss of effectiveness—see Glossary). The nitrate-free interval during the evening and night prevents the development of tolerance.

▷ **This Drug Should Not Be Taken If**
• you have had an allergic reaction to it previously.
• you have had a very recent heart attack (myocardial infarction) and your heart is beating quickly (tachycardia) or your blood pressure is excessively high.

- you currently have congestive heart failure or a severe anemia.
- your thyroid is overactive.
- you have a hypertrophic cardiomyopathy.

▷ **Inform Your Physician Before Taking This Drug If**
- you have had an unfavorable response to other nitrate drugs or vasodilators in the past.
- you have a history of low blood pressure.
- you have had a cerebral hemorrhage recently.
- you are pregnant or are planning pregnancy, or you are breast-feeding your baby.
- you have any form of glaucoma.

Possible Side Effects (natural, expected, and unavoidable drug actions)
Flushing of face, throbbing in head, palpitation, rapid heart rate, orthostatic hypotension (see Glossary).

▷ **Possible Adverse Effects** (unusual, unexpected, and infrequent reactions)
If any of the following develop, consult your physician promptly for guidance.
Mild Adverse Effects
Allergic Reactions: Skin rash, itching—infrequent.
Headache—frequent, but decreases over time.
Dizziness, fainting, or blurred vision—possible.
Nausea, vomiting, or bad breath (halitosis)—possible.
Urine discoloration—possible and not clinically significant.
Serious Adverse Effects
Transient ischemic attacks (TIAs) in presence of impaired circulation within the brain: dizziness, fainting, impaired vision or speech, localized numbness or weakness—possible.
Bone marrow depression—infrequent and of uncertain relationship.
Anemia (in patients with glucose-6-phosphate dehydrogenase G6PD deficiency)—possible.
Abnormally low blood pressure—possible.
Abnormal heartbeat—case reports.
Tolerance—possible with 24-hour use (daily 12-hour drug-free period is used to prevent this).

▷ **Possible Effects on Sexual Function**
Decreased libido and impotence—infrequent.

▷ **Adverse Effects That May Mimic Natural Diseases or Disorders**
Spells of low blood pressure with fainting (due to this drug) may be mistaken for late-onset epilepsy.

Possible Effects on Laboratory Tests
Liver function tests: increased.

CAUTION
1. Take this drug exactly as prescribed. If headaches are frequent or troublesome, call your doctor. Aspirin or acetaminophen may be taken to relieve headaches.
2. Many over-the-counter (OTC) medications for allergies, colds, and coughs contain drugs that may counteract the desired effects of this drug. Ask your doctor or pharmacist for help before using such medications.

Precautions for Use

By Those Over 60 Years of Age: Small starting doses are advisable. Increased risk of low blood pressure and associated "blackout" spells, fainting, and falling. Throbbing headaches and flushing may be more apparent.

▷ **Advisability of Use During Pregnancy**

Pregnancy Category: Ismo: C. Imdur: B. See Pregnancy Risk Categories at the back of this book.

Animal studies: Rat and rabbit studies reveal embryo deaths due to large doses of Ismo. Rat and rabbit studies did not reveal embryo deaths from Imdur.

Human studies: Adequate studies of pregnant women are not available.

Use this drug only if clearly needed. Ask your physician for guidance.

Advisability of Use If Breast-Feeding

Presence of this drug in breast milk: Unknown.

If this drug is thought to be necessary, watch the nursing infant for low blood pressure and poor feeding.

Habit-Forming Potential: None.

Effects of Overdosage: Headache, dizziness, marked flushing of face and skin, vomiting, weakness, fainting, difficult breathing, coma.

Possible Effects of Long-Term Use: Development of abnormal hemoglobin (red blood cell pigment).

Suggested Periodic Examinations While Taking This Drug (at physician's discretion)

Measurement of internal eye pressure.

▷ **While Taking This Drug, Observe the Following**

Foods: No restrictions.

Beverages: No restrictions. May be taken with milk.

▷ *Alcohol:* Use extreme caution. Avoid alcohol completely in the presence of any side effects or adverse effects of this drug. Alcohol may exaggerate the blood-pressure-lowering effect of this drug.

Tobacco Smoking: Nicotine can reduce the effectiveness of this drug. Avoid all forms of tobacco.

Marijuana Smoking: Possible reduced effectiveness of this drug; mild to moderate increase in angina; possible changes in electrocardiogram, confusing interpretation.

▷ *Other Drugs*

Isosorbide mononitrate *taken concurrently* with

- antihypertensive drugs may cause excessive lowering of blood pressure; dosage adjustments may be necessary.
- calcium-channel-blocking drugs (see Drug Classes) may cause marked orthostatic hypotension (see Glossary).
- hydralazine (Apresoline) may work well to help control angina.
- propranolol (Inderal) can help improve exercise time without angina.

▷ *Driving, Hazardous Activities:* Usually no restrictions. This drug may cause dizziness or spells of low blood pressure. Restrict activities as necessary.

Aviation Note: Coronary artery disease *is a disqualification* for piloting. Consult a designated Aviation Medical Examiner.

Exposure to Sun: No restrictions.

Exposure to Heat: Use caution. Hot environments can cause significant drop in blood pressure.

Exposure to Cold: Cold environments can increase the need for this drug and limit its effectiveness.

Heavy Exercise or Exertion: This drug may improve your ability to be more active without anginal pain. Use caution and avoid excessive exertion.

Discontinuation: It is best to withdraw this drug gradually (over a period of 2 to 4 weeks) after long-term use.

ISOTRETINOIN (i soh TRET i noin)

Introduced: 1979 **Class:** Antiacne **Prescription:** USA: Yes **Controlled Drug:** USA: No; Canada: No **Available as Generic:** Yes
Brand Name: Accutane

BENEFITS versus RISKS	
Possible Benefits	*Possible Risks*
EFFECTIVE TREATMENT OF SEVERE CYSTIC ACNE	MAJOR BIRTH DEFECTS
Treatment of other skin conditions	Initial worsening of acne (transient)
	Inflammation of lips
	Dry skin, nose, and mouth
	Musculoskeletal discomfort
	Corneal opacities

▷ **Principal Uses**

As a Single Drug Product: Uses currently included in FDA-approved labeling: (1) Reserved to treat severe, disfiguring nodular and cystic acne that has failed to respond to all other forms of therapy. ***It should not be used to treat mild forms of acne.*** (2) It is also used to treat some less common conditions of the skin that are due to disorders of keratin production.

Other (unlabeled) generally accepted uses: (1) May be helpful in refractory hypertrophic lupus erythematosus; (2) can help control resistant oral leukoplakia; (3) used in Apert's syndrome facial treatment; (4) used adjunctively to surgery in some cervical cancers; (5) treats mycosis fungoides; (6) eases symptoms in Darier's disease; (7) may have a role in treating dysplastic nevi; (8) eases symptoms of Grover's disease; (9) can help treat the abnormal gum growth (gingival hyperplasia) that can occur with phenytoin therapy; (10) treats severe and refractory rosacea; (11) has been combined with interferon alpha treatment in squamous cell skin cancer.

How This Drug Works: By an unknown action, this drug reduces the size of sebaceous glands and inhibits sebum (skin oil) production. This helps to correct the major feature of acne and its complications.

Available Dosage Forms and Strengths

Capsules — 10 mg, 20 mg, 40 mg

▷ **Usual Adult Dosage Range:** Starting dose is based on the patient's weight and severity of acne; the usual dose is 0.5 to 2 mg per kg of body mass daily, taken in two divided doses for 15 to 20 weeks. After weeks of treatment, the dose should be adjusted according to response of the acne and the development of adverse effects. **Note: Actual dosage and administration schedule must be determined for each patient individually.**

Conditions Requiring Dosing Adjustments

Liver Function: The dose should be decreased when isotretinoin is used by patients with compromised livers.

Kidney Function: Isotretinoin should be used with caution in kidney compromise.

▷ **Dosing Instructions:** Begin treatment only on the second or third day of your next normal menstrual period. Take with meals (morning and evening) to achieve optimal blood levels. The capsule should not be opened for administration.

Usual Duration of Use: Use on a regular schedule for 15 to 20 weeks best determines effectiveness in clearing or improving severe cystic acne. The drug may be stopped earlier if the total cyst count is reduced by more than 70%. If a repeat course of treatment is necessary, it should not be started for 2 months. Long-term use (months to years) requires physician supervision.

▷ **This Drug Should Not Be Taken If**
- you have had an allergic reaction to it previously.
- you are allergic to parabens, preservatives used in this drug product.
- you are pregnant or planning pregnancy.

▷ **Inform Your Physician Before Taking This Drug If**
- you have had an allergic reaction to any form of vitamin A in the past.
- you routinely take a nonprescription form of vitamin A.
- you have diabetes mellitus.
- you are considering giving blood (you will NOT be eligible for 1 month after the last isotretinoin dose).
- you have a cholesterol or triglyceride disorder.
- you are considering having a child.
- you wear contact lenses (your tolerance for these may decrease while you take this medicine).
- you have a history of liver or kidney disease.

Possible Side Effects (natural, expected, and unavoidable drug actions)

Frequent dryness of the nose and mouth, inflammation of the lips, dryness of the skin with itching, peeling of the palms and soles. Dose-related increase in triglycerides.

▷ **Possible Adverse Effects** (unusual, unexpected, and infrequent reactions)

If any of the following develop, consult your physician promptly for guidance.

Mild Adverse Effects

Allergic Reaction: Skin rash—may resemble pityriasis rosea.

Thinning of hair, conjunctivitis, intolerance of contact lenses, decreased night vision, muscular and joint aches, headache, fatigue, indigestion—infrequent.

Serious Adverse Effects

Depression—case reports to infrequent.

Skin infections, worsening of arthritis, inflammatory bowel disorders—case reports.

Abnormal acceleration of bone development in children—possible.

Development of opacities in the cornea of the eye—possible.

Reduced red blood cell and white blood cell counts; increased blood platelet count—infrequent.

Seizures—case reports.

Kidney toxicity, liver toxicity, or pancreatitis—rare.

Abnormal blood glucose control—infrequent.

Increased pressure within the head (headache, visual disturbances, nausea/vomiting)—case reports.

▷ **Possible Effects on Sexual Function**

Decreased male or female libido—possible.

Ejaculatory failure—case report.

Decreased vaginal secretions—possible.

Altered timing and pattern of menstruation—case reports.

Possible Effects on Laboratory Tests

Complete blood cell counts: infrequently decreased red cells and white cells.

Sedimentation rate: increased.

Blood total cholesterol, LDL cholesterol, VLDL cholesterol, and triglyceride levels: increased.

Blood HDL cholesterol levels: decreased.

Blood thyroid hormones (T_3, T_4, and free T_4 index): decreased.

Liver function tests: infrequently increased liver enzymes (ALT/GPT, AST/GOT, and alkaline phosphatase), increased bilirubin.

Blood calcium level: increased.

Protein in the urine: positive though infrequent.

CAUTION

1. This drug should not be used to treat mild forms of acne.
2. Worsening of your acne may occur during the first few weeks of treatment; this will subside with continued use of the drug.
3. Do not take any other form of vitamin A while taking this drug. (Check contents of multiple vitamin preparations.)
4. Women with potential for pregnancy should have a ***blood*** pregnancy test within 2 weeks before taking this drug and should use two effective forms of contraception simultaneously during its use. Contraception should be continued until normal menstruation resumes after discontinuing this drug.
5. This drug may cause increased blood levels of cholesterol and triglycerides.
6. If repeated courses of this drug are prescribed, wait a minimum of 2 months between courses before resuming medication.

Precautions for Use

By Infants and Children: Long-term use (6 to 12 months) may cause abnormal acceleration of bone growth and development. Your physician can monitor this possibility by periodic X-ray examination of long bones.

▷ **Advisability of Use During Pregnancy**

Pregnancy Category: X. See Pregnancy Risk Categories at the back of this book.

Animal studies: Birth defects of skull, brain, and vertebral column found in rats; skeletal birth defects found in rabbits.

Human studies: Adequate studies of pregnant women are not available. How-

ever, many serious birth defects (thought to be due to this drug) have been reported. These include major abnormalities of the head, brain, heart, blood vessels, and hormone-producing glands.
Avoid this drug completely during entire pregnancy.

Advisability of Use If Breast-Feeding
Presence of this drug in breast milk: Unknown.
Avoid drug or refrain from nursing.

Habit-Forming Potential: None.

Effects of Overdosage: Increased blood pressure, lethargy, nausea, vomiting, mild gastrointestinal bleeding, elevated blood calcium, hallucinations, and psychosis.

Suggested Periodic Examinations While Taking This Drug (at physician's discretion)
Complete blood cell counts, including platelet counts.
Measurements of blood cholesterol and triglyceride levels. Complete eye examinations.
Liver and kidney function tests.

▷ **While Taking This Drug, Observe the Following**
Foods: Increases absorption and may be a good mechanism to maintain blood levels.
Beverages: No restrictions.
▷ *Alcohol:* A disulfiramlike reaction was described in one case report.
Tobacco Smoking: No interactions expected, but I advise everyone to quit smoking.
▷ *Other Drugs*
Isotretinoin *taken concurrently* with
• carbamazepine (Tegretol) may cause subtherapeutic carbamazepine levels.
• minocycline may increase risk of severe headache, papilledema, and visual changes.
• tetracyclines may cause increased risk of pseudotumor cerebri.
▷ *Driving, Hazardous Activities:* No restrictions.
Exposure to Sun: Caution: this drug can cause photosensitivity (see Glossary).

ISRADIPINE (is RA di peen)

Introduced: 1984   **Class:** Antihypertensive, calcium channel blocker
Prescription: USA: Yes   **Controlled Drug:** USA: No   **Available as Generic:** USA: No

Brand Name: DynaCirc

Controversies in Medicine: Medicines in this class have been subject to much conflicting data. There have also been several FDA hearings held on the calcium-channel-blocker class. **Amlodipine became the first calcium channel blocker to be FDA approved as safe for use in treating hypertension or angina in patients who also have congestive heart failure**. More recent data found the long-acting forms of calcium channel blockers to be safe and effective.

+---+
| **BENEFITS versus RISKS** |
| |
| *Possible Benefits*   *Possible Risks* |
| EFFECTIVE TREATMENT OF MILD   Headache |
| TO MODERATE HYPERTENSION   Dizziness |
| Fluid retention |
| Palpitations |
+---+

▷ **Principal Uses**

As a Single Drug Product: Uses currently included in FDA-approved labeling: (1) Treats mild to moderate hypertension, alone or in combination with thiazide-type diuretics; (2) treats hypertension in pregnancy.

Other (unlabeled) generally accepted uses: (1) Treatment of chronic, stable angina; (2) combination therapy of congestive heart failure; (3) may help prevent progression of early lesions in atherosclerosis; (4) could have a role in treating premature labor.

How This Drug Works: By blocking passage of calcium through cell walls (which is necessary for the function of nerve and muscle tissue), this drug inhibits the contraction of coronary arteries and peripheral arterioles. As a result of these effects, this drug promotes dilation of the coronary arteries (anti-anginal effect); reduces the degree of contraction of peripheral arterial walls, resulting in relaxation and consequent lowering of blood pressure. This further reduces the workload of the heart and helps prevent angina.

Available Dosage Forms and Strengths

Capsules — 2.5 mg, 5 mg

▷ **Usual Adult Dosage Range:** Hypertension: Initially 2.5 mg twice daily, 12 hours apart, for a trial period of 2 to 4 weeks. If needed, the dose may be increased by 5 mg per day at intervals of 2 to 4 weeks. The usual maintenance dose is 5 to 10 mg daily. The total daily dosage should not exceed 20 mg. **Note: Actual dose and dosing schedule must be determined for each patient individually.**

Conditions Requiring Dosing Adjustments

Liver Function: Specific guidelines for dosage reduction are not available, yet empiric decreases in dosing are prudent for patients with compromised livers.

Kidney Function: Use with caution in kidney compromise. Initial dose should be 2.5 mg twice a day.

▷ **Dosing Instructions:** May be taken with or following food to reduce stomach irritation. The capsule may be opened, mixed with food, and swallowed promptly.

Usual Duration of Use: Use on a regular schedule for 2 to 4 weeks determines this drug's effectiveness in controlling hypertension or in reducing the frequency and severity of angina. The smallest effective dose should be used for long-term (months to years) therapy. Periodic physician evaluation is essential.

Possible Advantages of This Drug

Does not cause orthostatic hypotension (see Glossary). No adverse effects on heart or kidney function. No adverse effects on blood cholesterol levels.

▷ **This Drug Should Not Be Taken If**
  • you have had an allergic reaction to it previously.
  • you have symptomatic low blood pressure (hypotension).
  • you have advanced narrowing of the aorta.
  • you have severe problems in the left side of your heart (left ventricular dysfunction).

▷ **Inform Your Physician Before Taking This Drug If**
  • you have had an unfavorable response to any calcium-channel-blocker drug in the past (see Drug Classes).
  • you are currently taking any beta-blocker drug (see Drug Classes).
  • you are taking any drugs that lower blood pressure.
  • you have a history of congestive heart failure, heart attack, or stroke.
  • you are subject to disturbances of heart rhythm.
  • you have muscular dystrophy or myasthenia gravis.
  • you develop a skin reaction while taking this drug.
  • you have impaired liver or kidney function.
  • you plan to have surgery under general anesthesia in the near future.

Possible Side Effects (natural, expected, and unavoidable drug actions)
  Rapid heart rate—rare.
  Swelling of the feet and ankles, cough, flushing and sensation of warmth—infrequent.
  Small weight loss—possible.

▷ **Possible Adverse Effects** (unusual, unexpected, and infrequent reactions)
  If any of the following develop, consult your physician promptly for guidance.
  Mild Adverse Effects
  Allergic Reactions: Skin rash, hives, itching—rare.
  Headache—frequent; dizziness, weakness—infrequent; nervousness, blurred vision—rare.
  Decreased skin sensation—rare.
  Palpitation, shortness of breath—infrequent.
  Indigestion, nausea, vomiting, constipation—infrequent.
  Cramps in legs and feet—rare.
  Increased urination—rare.
  Abnormal growth of the gums (gingival hyperplasia)—frequent with some drugs in the same class.
  Serious Adverse Effects
  Allergic Reactions: Erythema multiforme, exfoliative dermatitis—case reports.
  Heart rhythm disturbances—infrequent.
  Increased frequency or severity of angina (when therapy is started or dose increased)—possible.
  Marked drop in blood pressure with fainting—rare.
  Low white blood cell counts—rare.

▷ **Possible Effects on Sexual Function**
  Decreased libido, impotence (less than 1%).

▷ **Adverse Effects That May Mimic Natural Diseases or Disorders**
  Flushing and warmth may resemble menopausal "hot flashes."

Possible Effects on Laboratory Tests
White blood cell counts: decreased (less than 1% of users).
Liver function tests: increased enzyme levels—infrequent.
Electrocardiogram: slight increase in QT interval.

CAUTION
1. If you are monitoring your own blood pressure, check it just before each dose and 2 to 3 hours after each dose. This will detect excessive fluctuations between high and low readings.
2. Tell all physicians and dentists who treat you that you take this drug. Note the use of this drug on your personal identification card.
3. Nitroglycerin and other nitrate drugs may be used as needed to relieve acute episodes of angina pain. However, if your angina attacks are becoming more frequent or intense, notify your physician promptly.

Precautions for Use
By Infants and Children: Safety and effectiveness for those under 18 years of age are not established.
By Those Over 60 Years of Age: Usually well tolerated by this age group. However, watch for weakness, dizziness, fainting, and falling. Take necessary precautions to prevent injury.

▷ Advisability of Use During Pregnancy
Pregnancy Category: C. See Pregnancy Risk Categories at the back of this book.
Animal studies: Embryo and fetal toxicity reported in small animals, but no birth defects due to this drug.
Human studies: Adequate studies of pregnant women are not available.
Avoid this drug during the first 3 months. Use during the final 6 months only if clearly needed. Ask your physician for guidance.

Advisability of Use If Breast-Feeding
Presence of this drug in breast milk: Unknown.
Avoid drug or refrain from nursing.

Habit-Forming Potential: None.

Effects of Overdosage: Weakness, light-headedness, fainting, fast pulse, low blood pressure, shortness of breath, flushed and warm skin, tremors, and abnormal heartbeats.

Possible Effects of Long-Term Use: None reported.

Suggested Periodic Examinations While Taking This Drug (at physician's discretion)
Evaluations of heart function, including electrocardiograms; measurements of blood pressure in supine, sitting, and standing positions.

▷ While Taking This Drug, Observe the Following
Foods: No restrictions. Avoid excessive salt intake.
Beverages: No restrictions. May be taken with milk.
▷ *Alcohol:* Use caution. Alcohol may exaggerate the drop in blood pressure in some people.
Tobacco Smoking: Nicotine may reduce the effectiveness of this drug. I advise everyone to quit smoking.
Marijuana Smoking: Possible reduced effectiveness; mild to moderate increase in angina; possible changes in electrocardiogram, confusing interpretation.

▷ *Other Drugs*

Isradipine ***taken concurrently*** with

- antifungals (triazoles) such as fluconazole, itraconazole, or ketoconazole may lead to toxicity.
- beta-blocker drugs or digitalis preparations (see Drug Classes) may affect heart rate and rhythm adversely. Careful monitoring by your physician is needed if these drugs are taken concurrently.
- carbamazepine (Tegretol) has resulted in decreased blood levels of carbamazepine with calcium channel blockers from the same pharmacological family. Caution is advised.
- digoxin (Lanoxin) may increase blood levels. Laboratory testing of blood levels should be performed more often if these drugs are combined.
- magnesium, especially in doses used in premature labor, can cause very low and abnormal blood pressure.
- phenytoin (Dilantin) may result in loss of isradipine's effectiveness. Caution is advised.
- propranolol (Inderal, others) can result in increased blood levels of isradipine and excessive lowering of blood pressure and slowing of the heart.
- rifampin (Rifadin, others) may result in a decreased therapeutic benefit from isradipine.
- ritonavir (Norvir) and perhaps other protease inhibitors (see Drug Classes) can lead to toxicity.

▷ *Driving, Hazardous Activities:* Usually no restrictions. This drug may cause drowsiness or dizziness. Restrict activities as necessary.

Aviation Note: Coronary artery disease and hypertension ***are disqualifications*** for piloting. Consult a designated Aviation Medical Examiner.

Exposure to Sun: No restrictions.

Exposure to Heat: Caution is advised. Hot environments can exaggerate the blood-pressure-lowering effects of this drug. Observe for light-headedness or weakness.

Heavy Exercise or Exertion: This drug may improve your ability to be more active without resulting angina pain. Use caution and avoid excessive exercise that could impair heart function in the absence of warning pain.

Discontinuation: Do not stop this drug abruptly. Ask your doctor about gradual withdrawal. Watch for the development of rebound angina.

KETOCONAZOLE (kee toh KOHN a zohl)

Introduced: 1981 **Class:** Antifungal **Prescription:** USA: Yes **Controlled Drug:** USA: No; Canada: No **Available as Generic:** USA: No; Canada: No

Brand Name: Nizoral

BENEFITS versus RISKS

Possible Benefits	*Possible Risks*
EFFECTIVE TREATMENT OF THE FOLLOWING FUNGUS INFECTIONS: Blastomycosis, candidiasis, chromomycosis, coccidioidomycosis, histoplasmosis, paracoccidioidomycosis, tinea (ringworm)	SERIOUS DRUG-INDUCED LIVER DAMAGE (1 in 10,000) Allergic reactions Low blood platelets and anemia
Beneficial short-term treatment of advanced prostate cancer	
Beneficial auxiliary treatment of Cushing's syndrome	

▷ **Principal Uses**

As a Single Drug Product: Uses currently included in FDA-approved labeling: (1) Treatment of lung and systemic blastomycosis; (2) treatment of *Candida* (yeast) infections of the skin, mouth, throat, and esophagus (may be AIDS-related); (3) treatment of systemic *Candida* infections—pneumonia, peritonitis, urinary tract infections (may be AIDS-related); (4) auxiliary treatment of chromomycosis; (5) treatment of lung and systemic coccidioidomycosis; (6) treatment of lung and systemic histoplasmosis; (7) treatment of para-coccidioidomycosis; (8) treatment of tinea infections of the body, groin (jock itch), and feet (athlete's foot); (9) therapy of tinea versicolor (pityriasis).

Other (unlabeled) generally accepted uses: (1) Treatment of *Candida* infections of the vulva and vagina; (2) short-term treatment of prostate cancer; (3) treatment of Cushing's syndrome (excessive adrenal hormones); (4) treatment of systemic sporotrichosis; (5) topical treatment of fungal dandruff; (6) therapy of fungal infections of the toenails; (7) designated as an orphan drug in therapy for kidney toxicity caused by cyclosporine; (8) treats visceral leishmaniasis.

How This Drug Works: As an antifungal: By damaging cell walls and impairing critical cell enzymes, this drug inhibits cell growth and reproduction (with low drug levels) and destroys fungal cells (with high drug concentrations).

In treating prostate cancer: This drug decreases testosterone (male hormone) levels—prostate cancer cells need testosterone to grow.

In treating Cushing's syndrome: This drug suppresses the excessive production of adrenal corticosteroid hormones.

Available Dosage Forms and Strengths

Cream — 2% (for local application to *Candida* or tinea skin infections)

Shampoo — 2%

Oral suspension — 100 mg/5 ml (Canada)

Tablets — 200 mg (U.S. and Canada)

▷ **Recommended Dosage Ranges** (Actual dosage and administration schedule must be determined for each patient individually.)

Infants and Children: Up to 2 years of age: Dosage not established.

Over 2 years of age: 3.3 to 6.6 mg per kg of body mass, once daily; the dosage depends upon the nature of the infection.

12 to 60 Years of Age: For fungus infections—200 to 400 mg once daily; 800 mg maximum daily dose.

For prostate cancer—400 mg three times daily; 1200 mg maximum daily dose.

For Cushing's syndrome—600 to 1200 mg once daily; total daily dosage should not exceed 1200 mg.

Over 60 Years of Age: Same as 12 to 60 years of age.

Conditions Requiring Dosing Adjustments

Liver Function: The dose should be empirically decreased for patients with liver compromise.

Kidney Function: Decreased doses are not needed in kidney compromise.

Achlorhydria (lack of acid in the stomach): This medicine requires an acid environment in the stomach to be absorbed. Talk with your doctor about making a dilute acid solution to drink prior to taking the tablet form.

▷ **Dosing Instructions:**   The tablet may be crushed and is best taken with or after food to enhance absorption and reduce stomach irritation. Do not take with antacids. Take the full course prescribed.

Usual Duration of Use: Use on a regular schedule for 2 to 4 weeks determines effectiveness in controlling fungal infections. Actual cures or long-term suppression often require continual treatment for many months. Periodic physician evaluation of response and dosage adjustment are essential.

▷ **This Drug Should Not Be Taken If**
- you have had an allergic reaction to it previously.
- you have active liver disease.
- you take astemizole or terfenadine.

▷ **Inform Your Physician Before Taking This Drug If**
- you are allergic to related antifungal drugs: clotrimazole, fluconazole, itraconazole, or miconazole.
- you have a history of liver disease or impaired liver function.
- you take loratadine. Heart problems have not been reported as with other nonsedating antihistamines, but the blood level does increase if the drugs are combined; the dose of loratadine may need to be decreased.
- you have a history of adrenal gland problems (adrenal insufficiency).
- you have a history of low blood platelets or anemia.
- you have a history of alcoholism.
- you have a deficiency of stomach hydrochloric acid.
- you are taking any other drugs currently.

Possible Side Effects (natural, expected, and unavoidable drug actions)

Suppression of testosterone and adrenal corticosteroid hormone production (more pronounced with high drug doses).

▷ **Possible Adverse Effects** (unusual, unexpected, and infrequent reactions)
If any of the following develop, consult your physician promptly for guidance.

Mild Adverse Effects

Allergic Reactions: Skin rash, hives, itching—rare.

Headache, dizziness, drowsiness, photophobia—infrequent.

Nausea (helped by taking with meals) and vomiting, stomach pain, diarrhea—rare.

Increased blood pressure—possible.

Hair loss or ringing in the ears—case reports.

Muscle and joint aches—infrequent.

Serious Adverse Effects

Allergic Reactions: Anaphylactic reaction (see Glossary).

Severe liver toxicity: loss of appetite, nausea, yellow skin or eyes, dark urine, light-colored stools (see jaundice in Glossary)—rare.

Suppression of the adrenal gland or low thyroid function—case reports.

Mental depression—rare.

Hemolytic anemia or abnormally low platelet counts (abnormal bruising or bleeding)—rare.

▷ **Possible Effects on Sexual Function**

Decreased testosterone blood levels: reduced sperm counts, decreased libido, impotence, male breast enlargement and tenderness (gynecomastia).

Altered menstrual patterns—case reports.

Possible Delayed Adverse Effects: Deficiency of adrenal corticosteroid hormones (cortisone related); this could be serious during stress resulting from illness or injury.

▷ **Adverse Effects That May Mimic Natural Diseases or Disorders**

Drug-induced liver reaction may suggest viral hepatitis.

Possible Effects on Laboratory Tests

Complete blood cell counts: decreased red cells, white cells, and platelets.

Liver function tests: increased liver enzymes (ALT/GPT, AST/GOT, and alkaline phosphatase), increased bilirubin.

Thyroid function tests: decreased—rare.

Adrenal corticosteroid blood levels: decreased.

Testosterone blood levels: decreased.

Precautions for Use

By Infants and Children: Safety and effectiveness for those under 2 years of age are not established.

By Those Over 60 Years of Age: No information is available. It is advisable to avoid high doses.

▷ **Advisability of Use During Pregnancy**

Pregnancy Category: C. See Pregnancy Risk Categories at the back of this book.

Animal studies: Rat studies revealed significant embryo toxicity and birth defects due to this drug.

Human studies: Adequate studies of pregnant women are not available.

Use this drug only if clearly needed. Ask your physician for guidance.

Advisability of Use If Breast-Feeding

Presence of this drug in breast milk: Yes.

Avoid drug or refrain from nursing.

Habit-Forming Potential: None.

Effects of Overdosage: Possible nausea, vomiting, diarrhea.

Possible Effects of Long-Term Use: Suppression of adrenal corticosteroid hormone production, requiring replacement therapy during periods of stress.

Suggested Periodic Examinations While Taking This Drug (at physician's discretion)

Liver function tests should be obtained BEFORE long-term therapy is started, and checked monthly during treatment.

Sperm counts.

▷ **While Taking This Drug, Observe the Following**

Foods: No restrictions.

Beverages: No restrictions. May be taken with milk.

▷ *Alcohol:* Avoid completely. Alcohol can cause a disulfiramlike reaction (see Glossary). In addition, alcohol may cause liver toxicity.

Tobacco Smoking: No interactions expected, but I advise everyone to quit smoking.

▷ *Other Drugs*

Ketoconazole may *increase* the effects of

- cortisonelike drugs (prednisone, etc.).
- cyclosporine (Sandimmune).
- oral antidiabetic drugs (see Drug Classes) and result in very low blood sugars.
- nonsedating antihistamines such as astemizole (Hismanal) and terfenadine (Seldane), and may cause large increases in blood levels and result in serious heart rhythm problems. DO NOT COMBINE.
- loratadine (Claritin)—this is also a nonsedating antihistamine, but **HAS NOT** been associated with heart rhythm problems when combined with ketoconazole. The blood level does appear to increase, and lower doses of loratadine are prudent if these medicines are to be combined.
- protease inhibitors (see Drug Classes).
- quinidine (Quinaglute) and cause toxicity. Blood levels are needed.
- sucralfate (Carafate) may decrease the blood levels of ketoconazole.
- warfarin (Coumadin) and cause bleeding. Increased testing of INR (prothrombin time or protime) are needed.

Ketoconazole may *decrease* the effects of

- amphotericin B (Abelcet).
- didanosine (Videx).
- theophyllines (aminophylline, Theo-Dur, etc.).

The following drugs may *decrease* the effects of ketoconazole

- antacids; if needed, take antacids 2 hours after ketoconazole.
- histamine (H_2) blocking drugs: cimetidine, famotidine, nizatidine, ranitidine. If needed, take 2 hours after ketoconazole.
- isoniazid (Laniazid, Nydrazid, etc.).
- rifampin (Rifadin, Rifater, Rimactane, etc.).

Ketoconazole *taken concurrently* with

- cisapride (Propulsid) can lead to serious heart toxicity. DO NOT COMBINE.
- miconazole (Monistat) may increase the blood levels of ketoconazole or miconazole.
- phenytoin (Dilantin) may change the levels of both drugs.
- trimexate (Neutrexin) may lead to toxicity.

▷ *Driving, Hazardous Activities:* This drug may cause dizziness or drowsiness. Restrict activities as necessary.

Aviation Note: The use of this drug *may be a disqualification* for piloting. Consult a designated Aviation Medical Examiner.

Exposure to Sun: This drug may cause photophobia; wear sunglasses if appropriate.

Discontinuation: Take the full course prescribed. Continual treatment for several months may be needed. Ask your doctor when the drug should be stopped.

KETOPROFEN (kee toh PROH fen)

See the propionic acids (nonsteroidal anti-inflammatory drugs) profile for further information.

LABETALOL (la BET a lohl)

Introduced: 1978   **Class:** Antihypertensive, alpha- and beta-adrenergic blocker   **Prescription:** USA: Yes   **Controlled Drug:** USA: No; Canada: No   **Available as Generic:** No
Brand Names: Normodyne, Normozide [CD], Trandate, Trandate HCT [CD]

BENEFITS versus RISKS	
Possible Benefits	*Possible Risks*
EFFECTIVE, WELL-TOLERATED ANTIHYPERTENSIVE in mild to moderate high blood pressure	CONGESTIVE HEART FAILURE in advanced heart disease
PROLONGS LIFE AFTER A HEART ATTACK	Worsening of angina in coronary heart disease (if drug is abruptly withdrawn)
	Masking of low blood sugar (hypoglycemia) in drug-treated diabetes
	Liver toxicity

▷ **Principal Uses**

As a Single Drug Product: Uses currently included in FDA-approved labeling: (1) Therapy of mild to moderate high blood pressure; (2) treats hypertension in pregnancy; (3) useful in hypertension and angina.

Other (unlabeled) generally accepted uses: (1) Combination therapy of hypertension in heart attacks (acute MI)—beta-blockers have also been shown to decrease the risk of repeat heart attacks, limit the size of the original heart attack damage, and help control arrhythmias; (2) treatment of cocaine overdose; (3) therapy of phobic anxiety reactions; (4) treatment of angina; (5) therapy of pheochromocytoma, a tumor that releases compounds that increase blood pressure.

As a Combination Drug Product [CD]: This drug has been combined with hydrochlorothiazide (a thiazide diuretic) to attack high blood pressure through the combination benefit of two different medicines.

How This Drug Works: By blocking part of the sympathetic nervous system, this drug
• reduces the rate and contraction force of the heart, thus lowering the ejection pressure of blood leaving the heart.

- reduces the degree of contraction of blood vessel walls, resulting in their expansion and lowering of blood pressure.

Available Dosage Forms and Strengths
Injection — 5 mg/ml
Tablets — 100 mg, 200 mg, 300 mg

▷ **Usual Adult Dosage Range:** Initially 100 mg twice daily, 12 hours apart; the dose may be increased by 100 mg twice daily every 2 to 3 days as needed to reduce blood pressure. The usual maintenance dose is 200 to 400 mg twice daily. Maximum daily dose is 2400 mg daily, given as 800 mg three times daily. **Note: Actual dose and dosing schedule must be determined individually.**

Conditions Requiring Dosing Adjustments
Liver Function: The dose **must** be decreased for patients with compromised livers. The average dose for patients with long-standing liver disease is about half that of patients with healthy livers. It is also a rare cause of severe liver (hepatocellular) injury.
Kidney Function: Decreased doses are not thought to be needed in kidney compromise.

▷ **Dosing Instructions:** The tablet may be crushed and is best taken at the same times daily, ideally following morning and evening meals. Do not abruptly stop this drug.

Usual Duration of Use: Use on a regular schedule for 10 to 14 days determines effectiveness in lowering blood pressure. Long-term use (months to years) of this drug will be determined by your individual response to an overall treatment program (weight reduction, salt restriction, smoking cessation, etc.).

Possible Advantages of This Drug
Decreases blood pressure more rapidly than other beta-blocker drugs. Can be used to treat hypertensive emergencies.

▷ **This Drug Should Not Be Taken If**
- you have had an allergic reaction to it previously.
- you have active bronchial asthma.
- you have congestive heart failure.
- you are in cardiogenic shock.
- you have an abnormally slow heart rate or a serious form of heart block.

▷ **Inform Your Physician Before Taking This Drug If**
- you have had an adverse reaction to any beta-blocker drug (see Drug Classes).
- you have a history of serious heart disease.
- you have a history of hay fever (allergic rhinitis), asthma, chronic bronchitis, or emphysema.
- you have a history of overactive thyroid function (hyperthyroidism).
- you have a history of low blood sugar (hypoglycemia).
- you have sporadic cramping of the leg muscles (intermittent claudication).
- you have a history of spasms of the bronchi of the lungs.
- you have impaired liver or kidney function.
- you have intermittent claudication.
- you have diabetes or myasthenia gravis.

- you take any form of digitalis, quinidine, or reserpine, or any calcium-channel-blocker drug (see Drug Classes).
- you plan to have surgery under general anesthesia in the near future.

Possible Side Effects (natural, expected, and unavoidable drug actions)
Lethargy and fatigability—frequent; light-headedness in upright position (see Orthostatic Hypotension in Glossary).

▷ **Possible Adverse Effects** (unusual, unexpected, and infrequent reactions)
If any of the following develop, consult your physician promptly for guidance.
Mild Adverse Effects
Allergic Reactions: Skin rash, itching.
Headache, drowsiness, dizziness—frequent; scalp tingling (during early treatment)—possible.
Vivid dreams, nightmares, depression—infrequent.
Urine retention, difficulty urinating—case reports.
Indigestion, nausea, diarrhea—infrequent.
Joint and muscle discomfort, fluid retention (edema)—rare.
Serious Adverse Effects
Allergic Reactions: Anaphylaxis—case reports.
Chest pain, shortness of breath, precipitation of congestive heart failure—possible.
Induction of bronchial asthma (in asthmatic individuals)—possible.
Lichen planus—case reports.
Muscle toxicity (toxic myopathy, worsening of intermittent claudication)—possible.
Drug-induced systemic lupus erythematosus—rare.
Aggravation of myasthenia gravis—case reports.
Liver damage with jaundice—rare and often reversible.

▷ **Possible Effects on Sexual Function**
Impotence, inhibited ejaculation, prolonged erection following orgasm (related to higher doses), Peyronie's disease (see Glossary)—rare to infrequent.
Decreased vaginal secretions (with low doses), inhibited female orgasm (higher doses)—possible.

Possible Effects on Laboratory Tests
Blood potassium or glucose: slight increase.
Liver function tests: rare increases.

CAUTION
1. ***Do not stop this drug suddenly*** without the knowledge and help of your doctor. Carry a note or wear a labetalol drug-identification bracelet.
2. Ask your physician or pharmacist before using nasal decongestants, which are usually present in over-the-counter cold preparations and nose drops. These can cause sudden increases in blood pressure if combined with labetalol.
3. Report the development of any tendency to emotional depression.

Precautions for Use
By Infants and Children: Safety and effectiveness for those under 12 years of age are not established. However, if this drug is used, watch for low blood sugar (hypoglycemia) during periods of reduced food intake.

By Those Over 60 Years of Age: Proceed **cautiously** with all antihypertensive drugs. Therapy should be started with small doses, with frequent checks of blood pressure. Sudden, rapid, or excessive lowering of blood pressure can increase stroke or heart attack risk. Watch for dizziness, unsteadiness, tendency to fall, confusion, hallucinations, depression, or urinary frequency.

▷ **Advisability of Use During Pregnancy**

Pregnancy Category: C. See Pregnancy Risk Categories at the back of this book.
Animal studies: No significant increase in birth defects found in rats or rabbits; some increase in fetal deaths reported.
Human studies: Adequate studies of pregnant women are not available.
Use this drug only if clearly needed. Ask your physician for guidance.

Advisability of Use If Breast-Feeding

Presence of this drug in breast milk: Yes, in very small amounts.
Avoid drug or refrain from nursing.

Habit-Forming Potential: None.

Effects of Overdosage: Weakness, slow pulse, low blood pressure, fainting, cold and sweaty skin, congestive heart failure, possible coma, and convulsions.

Possible Effects of Long-Term Use: Reduced heart reserve and eventual heart failure in susceptible individuals with advanced heart disease.

Suggested Periodic Examinations While Taking This Drug (at physician's discretion)

Measurements of blood pressure, evaluation of heart function.

▷ **While Taking This Drug, Observe the Following**

Foods: May increase the absorption of labetalol and result in a larger than expected blood level. Patients taking this medicine should also avoid excessive salt intake.

Beverages: No restrictions. May be taken with milk.

▷ *Alcohol:* Use with caution. Alcohol may exaggerate this drug's ability to lower blood pressure and may increase its mild sedative effect.

Tobacco Smoking: Nicotine may reduce this drug's effectiveness. I advise everyone to quit smoking.

▷ *Other Drugs*

Labetalol may **increase** the effects of
- oral antidiabetic drugs (see Drug Classes) and prolong recovery from any hypoglycemia (low blood sugar) that may occur.
- other antihypertensive drugs and cause excessive lowering of blood pressure. Dosage adjustments may be necessary.

Labetalol **taken concurrently** with
- amiodarone (Cordarone) may result in extremely slow heart rates and cardiac arrest.
- cimetidine (Tagamet) can cause elevated labetalol levels and low blood pressure or heart rate.
- clonidine (Catapres) must be closely watched for rebound high blood pressure if clonidine is withdrawn while labetalol is still being taken.
- epinephrine may result in severe increases in blood pressure.
- fluvoxamine (Luvox) may result in excessive lowering of blood pressure or excessive slowing of the heart.

- imipramine and other tricyclic antidepressants may result in increases in antidepressant blood levels and toxicity.
- insulin must be watched for development of hypoglycemia (see Glossary).
- NSAIDs (see Drug Classes) may result in blunting of the therapeutic effects of labetalol.
- phenothiazines (see Drug Classes) may cause additive lowering of the blood pressure.
- ritodrine (Yutopar) may blunt the beneficial effects of ritodrine.

▷ *Driving, Hazardous Activities:* Use caution until the full extent of fatigue, dizziness, and blood pressure change has been determined.

Aviation Note: The use of this drug *is a disqualification* for piloting. Consult a designated Aviation Medical Examiner.

Exposure to Sun: No restrictions.

Exposure to Heat: Caution is advised. Hot environments can lower the blood pressure and exaggerate the effects of this drug.

Exposure to Cold: Caution is advised. Cold environments can increase blood flow problems in the extremities that may occur with beta-blocker drugs. The elderly should take precautions to prevent hypothermia (see Glossary).

Heavy Exercise or Exertion: It is advisable to avoid exertion that produces light-headedness, excessive fatigue, or muscle cramping. The use of this drug may intensify the hypertensive response to isometric exercise.

Occurrence of Unrelated Illness: Fever can lower blood pressure and require decreased doses. Nausea or vomiting may interrupt scheduled doses. Ask your doctor for help.

Discontinuation: If possible, gradual reduction of dose over a period of 2 to 3 weeks is recommended—otherwise rebound increases in blood pressure may occur. Ask your physician for specific guidance.

LAMIVUDINE (LAMB iv u deen)

Introduced: 1995   **Class:** Antiviral, anti-retroviral, reverse transcriptase inhibitor, nucleoside analog   **Prescription:** USA: Yes   **Controlled Drug:** USA: No   **Available as Generic:** No

Brand Name: Epivir

BENEFITS versus RISKS	
Possible Benefits	*Possible Risks*
IMPRESSIVE SUPPRESSION OF VIRAL LOAD WHEN USED IN COMBINATION THERAPY TREATING AIDS	DECREASED WHITE BLOOD CELL COUNTS
	Peripheral neuropathy
DOES NOT LEAD TO SUPPRESSION OF THE BONE MARROW	Pancreatitis
EFFECTIVE TREATMENT OF HEPATITIS B INFECTION	

▷ **Principal Uses**

As a Single Drug Product: Uses currently included in FDA-approved labeling: (1) Used to treat HIV infection. Used in combination because of possible resistance. This medicine was one of the three drugs used together that resulted in decrease of HIV virus levels to undetectable amounts. (2) Recently approved for combination use with zidovudine (AZT) in reducing the risk of disease progression and death in AIDS patients.

Author's Note: *The Panel on Clinical Practices for Treatment of HIV Infection Report* **says that the preferred regimen is: Two nucleoside analogs and one potent protease inhibitor. Single-agent therapy (with the exception of AZT use in preventing HIV transmission from mother to fetus) was rejected by the panel.**

Other (unlabeled) generally accepted uses: Pending FDA approval for use in treating hepatitis B. One significant study found that single-agent therapy with lamivudine cleared hepatitis B virus from the blood of some of the test patients.

How This Drug Works: This medicine is a potent reverse transcriptase inhibitor and, as such, interferes with the ability of the HIV virus to create genetic material. The exact mechanism of action in treating hepatitis B is not clear.

Available Dosage Forms and Strengths

Solution — 10 mg/ml

Tablets — 150 mg

▷ **Recommended Dosage Ranges:** (Actual dosage and administration schedule must be determined for each patient individually.)

Infants and Children: 3 months to 12 years old: 4 mg per kg of body mass twice daily (300 mg maximum a day).

12 to 65 Years of Age: Usual dose is 150 mg twice daily.

Adults weighing less than 110 lb or 50 kg: 2 mg per kg of body mass twice daily.

Over 65 Years of Age: Not studied in those over 65.

Conditions Requiring Dosing Adjustments

Liver Function: Metabolism is a minor (less than 5% of a given dose) route of elimination.

Kidney Function: Up to 70% of a given dose is removed by the kidneys. Those with creatinine clearances (see Glossary) of 5 to 14 ml/min should take a first dose of 150 mg and then 50 mg once daily.

▷ **Dosing Instructions:**   Lamivudine tablets and solution can be taken without regard to meals. A solution is available for patients who can't swallow the tablets.

Usual Duration of Use: Measurement of viral load (burden) and/or CD4 counts are now used by many clinicians to decide the effectiveness of treatment and help in the decision to continue or change medications.

Possible Side Effects (natural, expected, and unavoidable drug actions)

Paresthesias and/or peripheral neuropathy (12% in a study in children taking lamivudine monotherapy).

▷ **Possible Adverse Effects** (unusual, unexpected, and infrequent reactions)

If any of the following develop, consult your physician promptly for guidance.

Mild Adverse Effects
   Skin rash—infrequent.
   Headache—frequent; dizziness—infrequent.
   Sleep disorders—infrequent to frequent.
   Nausea, vomiting, or diarrhea—infrequent to frequent.
   Cough—frequent.
   Muscle aches—infrequent.
Serious Adverse Effects
   Lowered white blood cell counts—infrequent in adults, frequent in pediatrics.
   Pancreatitis (more common in children receiving lamivudine monotherapy)—infrequent.
   Seizures—case reports.

▷ **Possible Effects on Sexual Function**
   None reported.

Possible Delayed Adverse Effects: Anemia or lowering of white blood cell counts. Pancreatitis, peripheral neuropathy.

▷ **Adverse Effects That May Mimic Natural Diseases or Disorders**
   Seizures may suggest the possibility of epilepsy.

Possible Effects on Laboratory Tests
   Complete blood cell counts: decreased red cells. Increased amylase and lipase (if pancreatitis occurs).

CAUTION
   1. This drug is **not** a cure for AIDS or AIDS-related complex, nor does it protect completely against other infections or complications. Follow your physician's instructions and take all medications exactly as prescribed.
   2. This drug does not reduce the risk of transmitting AIDS to others through sexual contact or contamination of the blood. The use of an effective condom is mandatory. Needles for drug administration should not be shared.

Precautions for Use
   By Infants and Children: Patients from 3 months to 12 years old are dosed on a mg-per-kg-of-body-mass basis.
   By Those Over 60 Years of Age: Impaired kidney function requires dosage reduction.

▷ **Advisability of Use During Pregnancy**
   Pregnancy Category: C. See Pregnancy Risk Categories at the back of this book.
   Animal studies: Rat and rabbit studies reveal no birth defects.
   Human studies: Adequate studies of pregnant women are not available. Your physician should call 1–800–722–9292, ext. 38465, if the decision is made to use this medicine while you are pregnant.

Advisability of Use If Breast-Feeding
   Presence of this drug in breast milk: Unknown.
   Refrain from nursing (HIV may be transferred via breast milk).

Habit-Forming Potential: None.

Effects of Overdosage: Nausea, vomiting, diarrhea, bone marrow depression.

Possible Effects of Long-Term Use: Anemia and loss of white blood cells.
   Pancreatitis or peripheral neuropathy.

Suggested Periodic Examinations While Taking This Drug (at physician's discretion)

> Complete blood cell counts before starting treatment until tolerance is established.

> Periodic CD4 counts or measurements of viral load are needed, and undesirable changes are indicators that treatment is failing and demand change of antiretroviral therapy.

> Amylase and lipase.

> Check for peripheral neuropathy.

▷ **While Taking This Drug, Observe the Following**

Foods: No restrictions.

Beverages: No restrictions. May be taken with milk.

▷ *Alcohol:* No interactions expected.

Tobacco Smoking: No interactions expected, but I advise everyone to quit smoking.

▷ *Other Drugs*

Lamivudine *taken concurrently* with

- indinavir (Crixivan) and zidovudine (AZT) resulted in undetectable HIV in some AIDS patients.
- other medicines capable of causing pancreatitis may result in increased pancreatitis risk.
- other medicines capable of lowering white or red cell counts may cause additive risks.
- trimexate (Mexate) may cause additive blood (hematological) toxicity.

▷ *Driving, Hazardous Activities:* This drug may cause dizziness or fainting. Restrict activities as necessary.

Aviation Note: The use of this drug *is a disqualification* for piloting. Consult a designated Aviation Medical Examiner.

Exposure to Sun: No restrictions.

Discontinuation: Do not stop this drug without your physician's knowledge and guidance.

LAMOTRIGINE (la MOH tri jean)

Introduced: 1995   **Class:** Anticonvulsant, phenyltriazine   **Prescription:** USA: Yes   **Controlled Drug:** USA: No; Canada: No   **Available as Generic:** USA: No

Brand Name: Lamictal

BENEFITS versus RISKS	
Possible Benefits	*Possible Risks*
EFFECTIVE MANAGEMENT OF SEIZURES THAT RESIST THERAPY	Rashes
	Changes in vision
	Dizziness
INCREASE IN SEIZURE-FREE DAYS	

▷ **Principal Uses**

As a Single Drug Product: Uses currently included in FDA-approved labeling: Adjunctive combination therapy of partial seizures in adults who have not responded to treatment with other medicines.

Other (unlabeled) generally accepted uses: (1) May have a role in treating epilepsy in children that has not responded to more established treatment; (2) could have a role in treating status epilepticus; (3) of use in treating Lennox-Gastaut syndrome.

How This Drug Works: The exact mechanism of action is not known, but animal models appear to show that this medicine blocks voltage-dependent sodium channels. This causes a decreased amount of glutamate and aspartate transmitters, and a decreased likelihood of seizures.

Available Dosage Forms and Strengths

Tablets — 25 mg, 100 mg, 150 mg, 200 mg

▷ **Recommended Dosage Ranges:** (Actual dosage and administration schedule must be determined for each patient individually.)

Infants and Children: Safety and efficacy in those less than 16 years old have not been established. Some researchers used lamotrigine in treating intractable epilepsy: 2 to 15 mg per kg of body mass divided into two equal doses and given every 12 hours.

16 to 65 Years of Age: In patients receiving medicines known to interact (phenytoin, primidone, carbamazepine, or phenobarbital): the starting dose is 50 mg a day for 2 weeks, and then 50 mg twice a day as needed or tolerated, with increases as needed and tolerated of 100 mg a day every week. Most patients end up taking 300–500 mg a day divided into two equal doses. Some centers have used doses as high as 700 mg a day. Patients only taking valproic acid may need still lower doses, but studies have not been done.

Over 65 Years of Age: Same dosing as 16 to 65 (single-dose pharmacokinetics were similar to younger adults). Few patients over 65 were included during premarketing studies, so specific statements can't presently be made.

Conditions Requiring Dosing Adjustments

Liver Function: This drug is primarily glucuronidated in the liver, but guidelines are not available for adjusting the dose in liver failure. Specific studies in this population have not been made.

Kidney Function: Most of this medicine is removed by the kidneys, but guidelines for decreasing the dose or interval are not available. Use with caution; decreased doses are suggested.

▷ **Dosing Instructions:**   Take this medicine exactly as prescribed. Food does not affect how much medicine gets into your body. Talk with your doctor immediately if you develop a rash with swollen lymph glands and fever.

Usual Duration of Use: Use on a regular schedule for 3 months in children with resistant seizures may be needed to see the peak benefits. Long-term use (months to years) of this drug will be determined by your individual response to therapy and requires periodic physician followup.

Possible Advantages of This Drug

Generally well-tolerated medicine, effective where single medicines have failed.

▷ **This Drug Should Not Be Taken If**
- you have developed a rash with swollen lymph glands while taking this medicine.
- you are allergic to this medicine or ones similar to it.

▷ **Inform Your Physician Before Taking This Drug If**
- you develop a rash.
- you do not understand how much or how often to take this medicine.

Possible Side Effects (natural, expected, and unavoidable drug actions)
Somnolence.
Weight gain.

▷ **Possible Adverse Effects** (unusual, unexpected, and infrequent reactions)
If any of the following develop, consult your physician promptly for guidance.

Mild Adverse Effects
Allergic Reactions: Skin rash (should be reported to your doctor), itching—infrequent.
Dizziness and headache—most common adverse effects.
Problems coordinating movements (ataxia)—infrequent.
Nausea and vomiting—dose related.
Blurred vision—dose related.

Serious Adverse Effects
Allergic Reactions: Anaphylaxis—case reports.
Serious rashes (Stevens-Johnson syndrome, toxic epidermal necrolysis)—case reports.
Hostility—rare.
Lowered blood platelets (thrombocytopenia) or sudden (acute) liver (hepatic) failure—case reports.
Disseminated intravascular coagulation—rare.
Blood in the urine—infrequent.
Peripheral neuropathy—rare and of questionable cause.
Sudden unexplained death (SUDEP). The rate of SUDEP was similar to that of another agent also tested, and appears to be a population effect—case reports.

▷ **Possible Effects on Sexual Function**
None reported.

Possible Effects on Laboratory Tests
Blood levels of interacting medicines may be changed.

CAUTION
1. **DO NOT** stop this medicine suddenly, as seizures may occur.

Precautions for Use
By Infants and Children: This medicine is approved for add-on therapy in children over 16 years of age.
By Those Over 60 Years of Age: No specific changes.

▷ **Advisability of Use During Pregnancy**
Pregnancy Category: C. See Pregnancy Risk Categories at the back of this book.
Animal studies: No evidence of drug-related changes were found in mice or rabbits that were given up to 1.2 times the human dose.
Human studies: This medicine has been shown to cause toxicity to the mother

and, because of this, toxicity to the fetus. Adequate studies of pregnant women are not available. Discuss the benefits-to-risk balance with your doctor.

Advisability of Use If Breast-Feeding
Presence of this drug in breast milk: Probably yes.
Avoid drug or refrain from nursing.

Habit-Forming Potential: None.

Effects of Overdosage: Sleepiness, changes in muscular reflexes, coma. Keep a seizure diary to check for decrease in seizure frequency.

Possible Effects of Long-Term Use: Weight gain.

Suggested Periodic Examinations While Taking This Drug (at physician's discretion)
Examinations for nystagmus, muscular coordination.

▷ **While Taking This Drug, Observe the Following**
Foods: No restrictions.
Beverages: No restrictions. May be taken with milk.
▷   *Alcohol:* Avoid alcohol use, unless you discuss this with your doctor.
Tobacco Smoking: No interactions expected, but I advise everyone to quit smoking.
▷   *Other Drugs*
Lamotrigine *taken concurrently* with
- long-standing use of acetaminophen (Tylenol, others) may result in decreases in blood levels of this medicine and a potential decrease in seizure control. Periodic use should not cause problems.
- carbamazepine (Tegretol) may increase the removal of lamotrigine from the body and require dosing adjustments.
- phenobarbital may result in a faster removal of lamotrigine from the body and require dosing changes.
- phenytoin (Dilantin) may result in a faster removal of lamotrigine from the body and require dosing changes.
- primidone (Mysoline) may result in a faster removal of lamotrigine from the body and require dosing changes.
- valproic acid (Depakene) may result in slower removal of lamotrigine from the body and require decreases in lamotrigine doses in order to avoid toxicity.
▷   *Driving, Hazardous Activities:* Use caution until the full extent of fatigue, dizziness, or coordination or vision changes have been determined.
Aviation Note: The use of this drug *is a disqualification* for piloting. Consult a designated Aviation Medical Examiner.
Exposure to Sun: No restrictions.
Exposure to Heat: Use caution; muscular coordination problems may be worsened by excessive heat.
Discontinuation: DO NOT stop this medicine abruptly without talking with your doctor first. Abrupt discontinuation of lamotrigine without first starting another antiseizure medicine may result in seizures.

LANSOPRAZOLE (lan SO pra sole)

Introduced: 1995   **Class:** Antiulcer, proton pump inhibitor   **Prescription:** USA: Yes   **Controlled Drug:** USA: No; Canada: No   **Available as Generic:** USA: No; Canada: No

Brand Name: Prevacid

BENEFITS versus RISKS

Possible Benefits	*Possible Risks*
VERY EFFECTIVE TREATMENT OF CONDITIONS ASSOCIATED WITH EXCESSIVE PRODUCTION OF STOMACH (GASTRIC) ACID: ZOLLINGER-ELLISON SYNDROME, MASTOCYTOSIS, ENDOCRINE ADENOMA	Liver enzyme increases Protein in the urine
VERY EFFECTIVE TREATMENT OF REFLUX ESOPHAGITIS	
VERY EFFECTIVE TREATMENT OF DUODENAL ULCER	
EFFECTIVE MAINTENANCE THERAPY OF HEALED DUODENAL ULCERS	

▷ **Principal Uses**

As a Single Drug Product: Uses currently included in FDA-approved labeling: (1) Used to treat duodenal ulcers; (2) treats erosive esophagitis; (3) used in syndromes (such as Zollinger-Ellison) where excessive amounts of stomach acid are produced; (4) recently approved for use in maintenance of healed duodenal ulcers.

Other (unlabeled) generally accepted uses: (1) Treatment of stomach (gastric) ulcers; (2) helps refractory reflux esophagitis.

How This Drug Works: This drug inhibits a specific enzyme system (the H/K adenosine triphosphate) in the stomach (parietal cells) lining and stops the production of stomach acid. By doing this it eliminates the principal cause of ulcers or esophagitis and also creates an environment conducive to healing.

Available Dosage Forms and Strengths

Capsules — 15 mg, 30 mg

▷ **Recommended Dosage Ranges** (Actual dosage and administration schedule must be determined for each patient individually.)

Infants and Children: Not studied in this age group.

18 to 60 Years of Age: For duodenal ulcer: 15 mg daily, taken before a meal. Some patients require 30 mg daily. Four weeks of therapy are indicated. For maintenance therapy of healed duodenal ulcers: 15 mg once daily.

For erosive esophagitis: 30 mg daily, taken before a meal. Up to 8 weeks of treatment can be given. If healing does not occur, an additional 8 weeks may be considered.

For excessive acid production syndromes: dosing is started at 60 mg daily.

The dose is increased as needed and tolerated. Doses up to 90 mg twice daily have been used. Once the condition is under control, the dose is usually reduced in stepwise fashion to 30 mg a day.

Helicobacter pylori: 30 mg twice daily days 1–7, colloidal bismuth subcitrate 120 mg four times daily days 4–7, tetracycline 500 mg four times daily days 4–7, and metronidazole 500 mg three times daily days 4–7.

Over 60 Years of Age: Same as 18 to 60 years of age.

Conditions Requiring Dosing Adjustments

Liver Function: The manufacturer strongly suggests a dose of 15 mg daily for people with significant liver problems.

Kidney Function: No dosing changes are needed.

▷ **Dosing Instructions:**   The capsules contain enteric-coated granules that protect the medicine in the stomach's acid. Take the capsules whole. Some studies have found that lansoprazole **taken in the morning** worked the best in controlling stomach acid. If swallowing is a problem, some patients have been able to take this drug by opening a capsule and sprinkling the intact granules into applesauce. Take this medicine exactly as prescribed.

Usual Duration of Use: Use on a regular schedule for 7 days resulted in a 90–94% decrease in stimulated acid release. Patients with stomach (gastric) or duodenal ulcers had a decrease in symptoms in about 1 week—this DOES NOT mean that the ulcer is gone. Especially with the new indication for maintenance of healing of duodenal ulcers, therapy may be ongoing. People with reflux esophagitis had significant decreases in heartburn after 7 to 28 days. Some esophagitis patients needed a second 8-week course to bring symptoms under control. Long-term use requires periodic physician followup.

▷ **This Drug Should Not Be Taken If**
  • you are allergic to the medicine or any of its components.

▷ **Inform Your Physician Before Taking This Drug If**
  • you have a history of liver disease.
  • you smoke and expect to continue smoking (worsens acid secretion).

Possible Side Effects (natural, expected, and unavoidable drug actions)
  Increased serum gastrin levels (clinical significance is unknown).

▷ **Possible Adverse Effects** (unusual, unexpected, and infrequent reactions)
  If any of the following develop, consult your physician promptly for guidance.
  Mild Adverse Effects
  Allergic reactions: Skin rash.
  Headache, dizziness, or tiredness—infrequent.
  Diarrhea or nausea—infrequent.
  Ringing in the ears—rare.
  Serious Adverse Effects
  Allergic Reaction: Not defined.
  Protein in the urine—rare.
  Liver toxicity or low blood platelets—rare and of questionable cause.

▷ **Possible Effects on Sexual Function**
  None reported.

▷ **Adverse Effects That May Mimic Natural Diseases or Disorders**
  Drug-induced liver reaction may suggest viral hepatitis.

Possible Effects on Laboratory Tests
Liver function tests: increased.

CAUTION
1. Follow your doctor's advice as to how long to take this medicine.
2. This drug effectively treats ulcers, but does not preclude the chance of cancer of the stomach.

Precautions for Use
By Infants and Children: Not indicated in this age group.
By Those Over 60 Years of Age: This medicine may cause dizziness. Use caution until you've seen the effects it has on you.

▷ **Advisability of Use During Pregnancy**
Pregnancy Category: B. See Pregnancy Risk Categories at the back of this book.

Advisability of Use If Breast-Feeding
Presence of this drug in breast milk: Unknown.
Avoid drug or refrain from nursing.

Habit-Forming Potential: None.

Effects of Overdosage: Possible nausea, vomiting, dizziness, lethargy, and abdominal pain.

Possible Effects of Long-Term Use: Serum gastrin levels are increased by this medicine, but the clinical significance is not known. Presently it is indicated for a maximum of two 8-week courses in erosive esophagitis. Maintenance of healed ulcers will further define effects of longer-term treatment.

Suggested Periodic Examinations While Taking This Drug (at physician's discretion)
Complete blood counts, liver function tests.

▷ **While Taking This Drug, Observe the Following**
Foods: Lansoprazole is best taken on an empty stomach. Follow your doctor's instructions regarding the types of foods you eat.
Beverages: No restrictions.
▷ *Alcohol:* No specific interactions; however, alcohol stimulates the secretion of stomach acid and may lessen the therapeutic benefits of this medicine.
Tobacco Smoking: Smoking can stimulate stomach acid and lessen benefits of this drug. I advise everyone to quit smoking.
▷ *Other Drugs*
Lansoprazole *taken concurrently* with
- sucralfate (Carafate) may decrease lansoprazole absorption. Separate doses by 2 hours.
- theophylline (Theo-Dur, others) may decrease blood theophylline level, requiring dosing adjustments.
▷ *Driving, Hazardous Activities:* Caution: this medicine may cause drowsiness. Limit activities as necessary.
Aviation Note: The use of this drug **may be a disqualification** for piloting. Consult a designated Aviation Medical Examiner.
Exposure to Sun: No restrictions.
Discontinuation: Talk with your doctor before stopping this medicine for any reason. Taking the medicine for a shorter time than needed may result in incomplete ulcer healing and continuation of the original problem.

LEVODOPA (lee voh DOH pa)

Introduced: 1967   **Class:** Anti-parkinsonism   **Prescription:** USA: Yes
Controlled Drug: USA: No; Canada: No   **Available as Generic:** USA: Yes; Canada: No

Brand Names: Bendopa, Dopar, Larodopa, ✦Prolopa [CD], Sinemet [CD]

BENEFITS versus RISKS

Possible Benefits	*Possible Risks*
EFFECTIVE SYMPTOM RELIEF IN IDIOPATHIC PARKINSON'S DISEASE	Emotional depression, confusion, abnormal thinking and behavior
Helpful in parkinsonism after encephalitis	Abnormal involuntary movements
Roughly 6-month benefit in parkinsonism after manganese poisoning	Heart rhythm disturbance
	Urinary bladder retention
	Induction of peptic ulcer
	Blood abnormalities: hemolytic anemia, reduced white blood cell count

---

▷ **Principal Uses**

As a Single Drug Product: Uses currently included in FDA-approved labeling: Treats major types of Parkinson's disease: paralysis agitans ("shaking palsy" of unknown cause), the type that follows encephalitis, parkinsonism that develops with aging (associated with hardening of the brain arteries), and the parkinsonism that follows poisoning by carbon monoxide or manganese.

Other (unlabeled) generally accepted uses: (1) May have a limited role in treating catatonic stupor; (2) can improve conscious level in coma caused by liver failure; (3) can help restless leg or periodic limb movements in sleep; (4) could be helpful in treating severe congestive heart failure.

As a Combination Drug Product [CD]: This drug is available in combination with carbidopa, a chemical that prevents the breakdown of levodopa before it reaches its site of action. The addition of carbidopa reduces levodopa requirements by 75%, and also decreases the frequency and severity of adverse effects.

How This Drug Works: Levodopa enters the brain tissue and is converted to dopamine. After sufficient dosage, this corrects the dopamine deficiency (thought to be the cause of parkinsonism) and restores a more normal brain chemistry. Carbidopa blocks an enzyme (decarboxylase) that degrades levodopa before it reaches the brain. This allows a lower dose to have a greater benefit. Products containing carbidopa also have fewer adverse effects.

Available Dosage Forms and Strengths

Capsules — 100 mg, 250 mg, 500 mg
Tablets — 100 mg, 250 mg, 500 mg
Sinemet tablets — 10–100 mg, 25–100 mg, 25–250 mg
Sinemet CR, sustained-release tablets — 25–100 mg, 50–200 mg

▷ **Usual Adult Dosage Range:**   Initially 250 mg two to four times daily. Dose may be increased by increments of 100 to 750 mg at 3- to 7-day intervals as needed and tolerated. Total dosage should not exceed 8000 mg daily. If the combination drug Sinemet is used, the total levodopa requirement will be considerably less. For someone who has not taken levodopa before (levodopa naive and using the sustained-release form): one 50–200 tablet twice daily, no more frequently than every 6 hours while awake. The dose is then increased as needed and tolerated by either daily or every-other-day dosing of one tablet, to a maximum of eight tablets daily. **Note: Actual dosage and administration schedule must be determined for each patient individually.**

Conditions Requiring Dosing Adjustments
Liver Function: Dosing changes are not indicated in liver compromise.
Kidney Function: Possible urine retention requires that patients with urine out-flow problems should be closely watched. No dose decreases are needed in kidney failure.
Intestinal Parasites: A report of large increases in doses needed by patients with *Strongyloides stercoralis* has been filed. Cure of this intestinal parasite allowed the levodopa dose to be decreased by 33%.

▷ **Dosing Instructions:**   Tablet may be crushed and is best taken with or following carbohydrate foods to reduce stomach upset. When possible, don't take this drug with high-protein foods. Sustained-release tablet (Sinemet CR) may be cut in half, but it should not be crushed or chewed. The last daily dose should be taken before 7 P.M. in order to avoid problems with normal sleeping patterns. "Drug holidays" (periods when no medicine is taken) are controversial, and not all patients benefit from this approach to therapy.

Usual Duration of Use: Use on a regular schedule for 3 to 6 weeks determines effectiveness in relieving the major symptoms of parkinsonism. Maximal effectiveness may require continual use for 6 months. Long-term use (months to years) requires physician supervision and periodic evaluation.

Possible Advantages of This Drug
The slow-release formulation of Sinemet CR allows a 25 to 50% reduction in dosing frequency. The wearing-off phenomenon and end-of-dose failure seen with standard Sinemet may be reduced or eliminated.

▷ **This Drug Should Not Be Taken If**
- you are allergic to any of the drugs bearing the brand names listed.
- you have narrow-angle glaucoma (inadequately controlled).
- you have a history of melanoma.
- you are taking, or have taken within the past 14 days, any monoamine oxidase (MAO) type A inhibitor drug (see Drug Classes).

▷ **Inform Your Physician Before Taking This Drug If**
- you have diabetes, epilepsy, heart disease, high blood pressure, or chronic lung disease.
- you have impaired liver or kidney function.
- you have problems making blood (hematopoiesis).
- you have had a heart attack and have some abnormal heart rhythms.
- you have a history of depression or other mental illness.

- you have a history of peptic ulcer disease or malignant melanoma.
- you plan to have surgery under general anesthesia in the near future.

Possible Side Effects (natural, expected, and unavoidable drug actions)
Fatigue, lethargy.
Altered taste, offensive body odor.
Orthostatic hypotension (see Glossary).
Pink- to red-colored urine, which turns black on exposure to air (of no significance).
Gout.

▷ **Possible Adverse Effects** (unusual, unexpected, and infrequent reactions)
If any of the following develop, consult your physician promptly for guidance.
Mild Adverse Effects
Allergic Reactions: Skin rash, itching.
Headache, dizziness, numbness, insomnia, nightmares, blurred or double vision—infrequent.
Nausea and vomiting—frequent; dry mouth, difficult swallowing, gas, diarrhea, constipation—infrequent.
Decreased taste sensation—possible.
Loss of hair—case reports.
Serious Adverse Effects
Idiosyncratic Reactions: Hemolytic anemia (see Glossary). Neuroleptic malignant syndrome (see Glossary), high blood pressure—case reports.
Confusion, hallucinations, paranoia, depression—infrequent to frequent; psychotic episodes, seizures—rare.
Congestive heart failure—rare.
Mania or seizures—rare.
Abnormal involuntary movements of the head, face, and extremities—frequent.
Disturbances of heart rhythm—infrequent, low blood pressure—rare.
Development of peptic ulcer, gastrointestinal bleeding—case reports.
Urinary bladder retention—case reports.
Low white blood cell count: increased infection risk, sore throat (transient, but may require you to stop this medicine until the condition clears), or low blood platelets—case reports to rare.

▷ **Possible Effects on Sexual Function**
Increased males or female libido—infrequent; inhibited ejaculation, priapism (see Glossary), postmenopausal bleeding—all rare.

▷ **Adverse Effects That May Mimic Natural Diseases or Disorders**
Mental reactions may resemble idiopathic psychosis.

Natural Diseases or Disorders That May Be Activated by This Drug
Latent peptic ulcer, gout.

Possible Effects on Laboratory Tests
Complete blood cell counts: occasionally decreased white cells; occasionally increased eosinophils (without symptoms).
Blood thyroxine (T_4) level: increased.
Urine sugar tests: no effect with Tes-Tape; false negative with Clinistix; false positive with Clinitest.

Urine ketone tests: false positive with Ketostix and Phenistix.
Blood uric acid, growth hormone: increased.
Blood potassium or sodium: may be decreased.

CAUTION

1. It is best to begin treatment with small doses, increasing gradually until desired response is achieved.
2. As improvement occurs, avoid excessive and hurried activity (often causes falls and injury).

Precautions for Use

By Infants and Children: This drug can cause precocious puberty in prepubertal boys. Watch for hypersexual behavior and premature growth of genital organs.

By Those Over 60 Years of Age: Therapy should start with half the usual adult dose; dose increases should be made in small increments as needed and tolerated. Watch for significant behavioral changes: depression or inappropriate elation, acute confusion, agitation, paranoia, dementia, nightmares, and hallucinations. Abnormal involuntary movements may also occur.

▷ **Advisability of Use During Pregnancy**

Pregnancy Category: C. See Pregnancy Risk Categories at the back of this book.
Animal studies: Significant birth defects reported in rodent studies.
Human studies: Adequate studies of pregnant women are not available.
Avoid use of drug during the first 3 months. Use only if clearly needed during the final 6 months.

Advisability of Use If Breast-Feeding

Presence of this drug in breast milk: Yes.
Avoid drug or refrain from nursing.

Habit-Forming Potential: None.

Effects of Overdosage: Muscle twitching, spastic closure of eyelids, nausea, vomiting, diarrhea, weakness, fainting, confusion, agitation, hallucinations.

Possible Effects of Long-Term Use: Development of abnormal involuntary movements involving the head, face, mouth, and extremities. May be reversible and gradually subside as the drug is withdrawn.

Suggested Periodic Examinations While Taking This Drug (at physician's discretion)

Complete blood cell counts; measurements of internal eye pressure; blood pressure measurements in lying, sitting, and standing positions.

▷ **While Taking This Drug, Observe the Following**

Foods: Insofar as possible, do not take concurrently with protein foods; proteins compete for absorption.

Nutritional Support: If taken alone (without carbidopa), watch for tingling of the extremities (peripheral neuritis). Small (10 mg or less) doses of pyridoxine (vitamin B_6) may help. Larger doses can decrease the effectiveness of levodopa. If taking Sinemet, supplemental pyridoxine is not required. Rare reports of vitamin C (ascorbic acid) decreasing nausea and other side effects have been made.

Beverages: No restrictions. May be taken with milk.

▷   *Alcohol:* No interactions expected.

Tobacco Smoking: No interactions expected, but I advise everyone to quit smoking.

Marijuana Smoking: Increased fatigue and lethargy; possible accentuation of orthostatic hypotension (see Glossary).

▷ *Other Drugs*

Levodopa *taken concurrently* with

- benzodiazepines (see Drug Classes) may blunt the therapeutic benefit of levodopa.
- bromocriptine (Parlodel) may result in decreased blood levels of bromocriptine.
- clonidine (Catapres) can result in decreased therapeutic benefit of levodopa. Avoid this combination.
- fentanyl/droperidol (Innovar) can cause muscular rigidity.
- isoniazid (INH) may cause flushing, worsening of symptoms, or increased blood pressure. DO NOT COMBINE.
- monoamine oxidase (MAO) type A inhibitor drugs (see Drug Classes) can cause a dangerous rise in blood pressure and body temperature. Do not combine these drugs.
- phenothiazines (see Drug Classes) may blunt therapeutic benefits of levodopa. DO NOT combine.
- reserpine (Naquival, others) may blunt the therapeutic benefits of levodopa. Avoid this combination.
- risperidone (Risperdal) can blunt the therapeutic benefits of levodopa. Avoid this combination.
- tricyclic antidepressants (see Drug Classes) may decrease the therapeutic effect of levodopa.

The following drugs may *decrease* the effects of levodopa

- chlordiazepoxide (Librium) or other benzodiazepines (see Drug Classes).
- iron salts.
- papaverine (Cerespan, Pavabid, Vasospan, etc.).
- phenytoin (Dilantin, etc.).
- pyridoxine (vitamin B_6).

▷ *Driving, Hazardous Activities:* May cause dizziness, impaired vision, and orthostatic hypotension. Restrict activities as necessary.

Aviation Note: Parkinson's disease *is a disqualification* for piloting. Consult a designated Aviation Medical Examiner.

Exposure to Sun: No restrictions.

Exposure to Heat: Use caution. This drug can cause flushing and excessive sweating and predispose to heat exhaustion.

Occurrence of Unrelated Illness: Dark-colored skin lesions should be evaluated carefully by your doctor, as they may be malignant melanoma. White blood cell counts should be closely followed if you develop an infection.

LEVOTHYROXINE (lee voh thi ROX een)

Other Names: L-thyroxine, thyroxine, T-4

Introduced: 1953   **Class:** Thyroid hormones   **Prescription:** USA: Yes
Controlled Drug: USA: No; Canada: No   **Available as Generic:** USA: Yes;
Canada: No

Brand Names: Armour Thyroid, ✦Eltroxin, Euthroid [CD], L-Thyroxine, Le-
vothroid, Levoxine, Synthroid, Synthrox, Syroxine, Thyroid USP, Thyrolar
[CD]

BENEFITS versus RISKS

Possible Benefits	*Possible Risks*
EFFECTIVE REPLACEMENT THERAPY IN STATES OF THYROID HORMONE DEFICIENCY (HYPOTHYROIDISM) EFFECTIVE TREATMENT OF SIMPLE GOITER, CHRONIC THYROIDITIS, AND THYROID GLAND CANCER	Intensification of angina in presence of coronary artery disease Drug-induced hyperthyroidism (with excessive dosage) Spasm of the coronary vessels

---

▷ **Principal Uses**

As a Single Drug Product: Uses currently included in FDA-approved labeling: (1)
Replacement therapy to correct thyroid deficiency (drug induced, hypothyroidism, cretinism, myxedema); (2) treatment of simple (nonendemic) goiter and benign thyroid nodules; (3) treatment of Hashimoto's thyroiditis;
(4) adjunctive prevention and treatment of thyroid cancer.

Other (unlabeled) generally accepted uses: (1) Helps amenorrhea caused by
(secondary to) low thyroid function; (2) may be helpful in helping fetal lung
tissue mature in babies expected to be premature; (3) treatment of Grave's
disease.

As a Combination Drug Product [CD]: This thyroid hormone is available in combination with the other principal thyroid hormone, liothyronine, in a
preparation (generic name: liotrix) that resembles the natural hormone
material produced by the thyroid gland.

How This Drug Works: By altering cellular chemistry that stores energy in an
inactive (reserve) form, this drug makes more energy available and increases the rate of cellular metabolism of all tissues throughout the body.
Thyroid hormones are essential to normal growth and development, especially the development of the infant's brain and nervous system.

Available Dosage Forms and Strengths

Injections — 100 mcg/ml, 200 mcg/ml, 500 mcg/ml
Tablets — 0.0125 mg, 0.025 mg, 0.05 mg, 0.075 mg, 0.088 mg, 0.1 mg,
0.112 mg, 0.125 mg, 0.037 mg, 0.15 mg, 0.175 mg, 0.2 mg, 0.3
mg

▷ **Recommended Dosage Ranges** (Actual dosage and administration schedule
must be determined for each patient individually.)

Infants and Children: Up to 6 months of age—8 to 10 mcg per kg of body mass, in a single daily dose.

6 to 12 months of age—6 to 8 mcg per kg of body mass, in a single daily dose.

1 to 5 years of age—5 to 6 mcg per kg of body mass, in a single daily dose.

6 to 12 years of age—4 to 5 mcg per kg of body mass, in a single daily dose.

Over 12 years of age—2 to 3 mcg per kg of body mass, in a single daily dose, until the usual adult daily dose is reached: 150 to 200 mcg.

12 to 60 Years of Age: Start at 0.05 mg as a single daily dose; increase by 0.025 to 0.05 mg at intervals of 2 to 3 weeks as needed and tolerated. Usual maintenance dose is 0.17 mg/day. Total daily dosage should not exceed 0.3 mg. If response is not seen at this level, absorption problems or misunderstanding in taking the medicine should be evaluated.

Over 60 Years of Age: Initially 0.0125 to 0.025 mg as a single daily dose; increase gradually at intervals of 3 to 4 weeks, as needed and tolerated. The usual maintenance dose is approximately 0.075 mg daily.

Author's Note: A recent University of California Medical Center at San Francisco study found the generic to be as effective as the brand name and saving 50% of the cost of brand name drug therapy.

Conditions Requiring Dosing Adjustments

Liver Function: Dosing changes are not indicated for patients with liver compromise.

Kidney Function: Dosing changes are not indicated in kidney compromise.

▷ **Dosing Instructions:** The tablets may be crushed and are best taken in the morning on an empty stomach to ensure maximal absorption and uniform results.

Usual Duration of Use: Use on a regular schedule for 4 to 6 weeks determines effectiveness in correcting the symptoms of thyroid deficiency. Long-term use (months to years, possibly for life) requires physician supervision.

Currently a "Drug of Choice"
for the treatment of hypothyroidism.

▷ **This Drug Should Not Be Taken If**
- you have had an allergic reaction to it previously.
- you are recovering from a heart attack; ask your doctor for help.
- you have an adrenal insufficiency that has not been corrected.
- you are using it to lose weight and your thyroid function is normal (no deficiency).

▷ **Inform Your Physician Before Taking This Drug If**
- you have high blood pressure, any form of heart disease, or diabetes.
- you have a history of Addison's disease or adrenal gland deficiency.
- you are taking any antiasthmatic medications.
- you are taking an anticoagulant.

Possible Side Effects (natural, expected, and unavoidable drug actions)
None if dosage is adjusted correctly.

▷ **Possible Adverse Effects** (unusual, unexpected, and infrequent reactions)
If any of the following develop, consult your physician promptly for guidance.

Mild Adverse Effects

    Allergic Reactions: Skin rash, hives.

    Headache in sensitive people, even with proper dosage adjustment—may be frequent.

Serious Adverse Effects

    Increased frequency or intensity of angina in people with coronary artery disease—possible.

    Spasm of the arteries that supply blood to the heart—rare.

    Seizures, pseudotumor cerebri, drug-induced porphyria, or myasthenia gravis—case reports to rare.

    Decrease in IgA immune concentration—rare.

    May be a part of the development of osteoporosis. Bone mineral density testing is recommended.

    Note: Other adverse effects are manifestations of excessive dosage. See "Effects of Overdosage" below.

▷ **Possible Effects on Sexual Function**

    Altered menstrual pattern during dosage adjustments.

    Possibly beneficial in treating impaired sexual function that is associated with true hypothyroidism.

Natural Diseases or Disorders That May Be Activated by This Drug

    Latent coronary artery insufficiency (angina), diabetes.

Possible Effects on Laboratory Tests

    Prothrombin time: increased (when taken concurrently with warfarin).

    Blood total cholesterol, HDL and LDL cholesterol levels: decreased.

    Blood triglyceride levels: no effect.

    Blood glucose level: increased.

    Blood thyroid hormone levels: increased T_3, T_4, and free T_4.

    Blood thyroid-stimulating hormone (TSH) level: decreased.

CAUTION

    1. Careful supervision of individual response is needed to identify correct dosage. Do not change dosing without asking your physician.

    2. This drug should not be used to treat nonspecific fatigue, obesity, infertility, or slow growth. Such use is inappropriate and could be harmful.

Precautions for Use

    By Infants and Children: Thyroid-deficient children often require higher doses than adults. Transient hair loss may occur during the early months of treatment. Follow the child's response to thyroid therapy by periodic measurements of bone age, growth, and mental and physical development.

    By Those Over 60 Years of Age: Usually requirements for thyroid hormone replacement are about 25% lower than in younger adults. Watch closely for any indications of toxicity.

▷ **Advisability of Use During Pregnancy**

    Pregnancy Category: A. See Pregnancy Risk Categories at the back of this book.

    Animal studies: Cataract formation reported in rat studies. Other defects reported in rabbit and guinea pig studies.

    Human studies: Thyroid hormones do not reach the fetus (cross the placenta) in significant amounts. Clinical experience has shown that appropriate use of thyroid hormones causes no adverse effects on the fetus.

    Use this drug only if clearly needed and with carefully adjusted dosage.

Advisability of Use If Breast-Feeding
> Presence of this drug in breast milk: Yes, in minimal amounts.
> Breast-feeding is considered safe with correctly adjusted dosage.

Habit-Forming Potential: None.

Effects of Overdosage: Headache, sense of increased body heat, nervousness, increased sweating, hand tremors, insomnia, rapid and irregular heart action, diarrhea, muscle cramping, weight loss, heart attack.

Possible Effects of Long-Term Use: Bone loss (osteoporosis) in the lumbar vertebrae (spine).

Suggested Periodic Examinations While Taking This Drug (at physician's discretion)
> Measurement of thyroid hormone levels in blood. Bone mineral density testing.

▷ **While Taking This Drug, Observe the Following**

Foods: Enteral formulas for nutrition support that contain soybeans may increase the fecal elimination of thyroxine.

Beverages: No restrictions.

▷ *Alcohol:* No interactions expected.

Tobacco Smoking: No interactions expected, but I advise everyone to quit smoking.

▷ *Other Drugs*

Levothyroxine may ***increase*** the effects of
- warfarin (Coumadin), and increase the risk of bleeding; decreased anticoagulant dosage is usually needed. More frequent INR testing (prothrombin time or protime) are needed.

Levothyroxine may ***decrease*** the effects of
- digoxin (Lanoxin), when correcting hypothyroidism; a larger dose of digoxin may be needed.

Levothyroxine ***taken concurrently*** with
- antacids may cause decreased levothyroxine absorption and a decreased therapeutic effect.
- all antidiabetic drugs (insulin and oral hypoglycemic agents) may require an increased dose to obtain proper control of blood sugar levels.
- benzodiazepines (Librium and others) can enhance the toxic or therapeutic effects of both drugs.
- conjugated estrogens (Premarin) may require an increased levothyroxine dose.
- tricyclic antidepressants (see Drug Classes) may cause an increase in activity of both drugs.

The following drugs may ***decrease*** the effects of levothyroxine
- cholestyramine (Cuemid, Questran)—may reduce its absorption; intake of the two drugs should be separated by 5 hours.
- colestipol (Colestid).
- iron salts—by decreasing absorption.
- lovastatin (Mevacor).
- phenytoin (Dilantin)—can increase levothyroxine clearance.
- sodium polystyrene sulfonate (Kayexalate).
- sucralfate (Carafate).

▷ *Driving, Hazardous Activities:* No restrictions.

Aviation Note: The use of this drug *is probably not a disqualification* for piloting. Consult a designated Aviation Medical Examiner.

Exposure to Sun: No restrictions.

Exposure to Heat: This drug may decrease individual tolerance to warm environments, increasing discomfort due to heat. Consult your physician if you develop symptoms of overdosage during the warm months of the year.

Heavy Exercise or Exertion: Use caution if you have angina (coronary artery disease). This drug may increase the frequency or severity of angina during physical activity.

Discontinuation: This drug must be taken continually on a regular schedule to correct thyroid deficiency. Do not stop it without consulting your physician.

LIOTHYRONINE (li oh THI roh neen)

Other Names: Triiodothyronine, T-3

Introduced: 1956   **Class:** Thyroid hormone   **Prescription:** USA: Yes
Controlled Drug: USA: No; Canada: No   **Available as Generic:** USA: Yes; Canada: No

Brand Names: Armour Thyroid, Cyronine, Cytomel, Euthroid [CD], Thyroid USP, Thyrolar [CD]

BENEFITS versus RISKS	
Possible Benefits	*Possible Risks*
EFFECTIVE REPLACEMENT THERAPY IN STATES OF THYROID HORMONE DEFICIENCY (HYPOTHYROIDISM) EFFECTIVE TREATMENT OF SIMPLE GOITER, CHRONIC THYROIDITIS, AND THYROID GLAND CANCER	Intensification of angina in presence of coronary artery disease Drug-induced hyperthyroidism (with excessive dosing) Rapid heartbeat Heart attack

▷ **Principal Uses**

As a Single Drug Product: Uses currently included in FDA-approved labeling: (1) Replacement therapy to correct thyroid deficiency (hypothyroidism); (2) treatment of simple (nonendemic) goiter and benign thyroid nodules; (3) treatment of Hashimoto's thyroiditis; (4) adjunctive prevention and treatment of thyroid cancer; (5) therapy of cretinism; (6) used to help diagnose different kinds of thyroid problems.

Other (unlabeled) generally accepted uses: (1) Can help infertility caused by low thyroid function; (2) thyroid replacement of choice for thyroid cancer.

As a Combination Drug Product [CD]: This thyroid hormone is available in combination with the other principal thyroid hormone, levothyroxine, in a preparation (generic name: liotrix) that resembles the natural hormone material produced by the thyroid gland.

How This Drug Works: By altering cellular chemistry that stores energy reserves, this drug makes more energy available and increases cellular metabolism in all tissues of the body. Thyroid hormones are essential to normal growth and development, especially the development of the infant's brain and nervous system.

Available Dosage Forms and Strengths

Injection — 10 mcg/ml
Tablets — 5 mcg, 25 mcg, 50 mcg

▷ **Recommended Dosage Ranges** (Actual dosage and administration schedule must be determined for each patient individually.)

Infants and Children: Infants several months old may need 20 mcg a day. When they reach 1 year, 50 mcg a day may be needed. Children more than 3 years old may need the full adult dose.

12 to 60 Years of Age: For mild hypothyroidism—initially 25 mcg daily; increase by 12.5 to 25 mcg every 1 to 2 weeks as needed and tolerated. The usual maintenance dose is 20 to 75 mcg daily.

For severe hypothyroidism—initially 2.5 to 5 mcg daily; increase by 5 to 10 mcg at intervals of 1 to 2 weeks. When a dose of 25 mcg is reached, increase by 12.5 to 25 mcg at intervals of 1 to 2 weeks, as needed and tolerated. The usual maintenance dose is 50 to 100 mcg daily.

For simple goiter—initially 5 mcg daily; increase by 5 to 10 mcg at intervals of 1 to 2 weeks. When a dose of 25 mcg is reached, increase by 12.5 to 25 mcg at intervals of 1 week, as needed and tolerated. The usual maintenance dose is 50 to 100 mcg daily.

Over 60 Years of Age: Initially 5 mcg as a single daily dose; increase by 5 mcg at intervals of 1 to 2 weeks, as needed and tolerated. The usual maintenance dose is 12.5 to 37.5 mcg daily.

Conditions Requiring Dosing Adjustments

Liver Function: Dosing changes are not indicated for patients with liver compromise.

Kidney Function: Dosing changes are not indicated in renal compromise. Caution should be used when increasing the dose of this medicine by those with kidney problems.

▷ **Dosing Instructions:**   The tablets may be crushed and are preferably taken in the morning on an empty stomach to ensure maximal absorption and uniform results.

Usual Duration of Use: Use on a regular schedule for 2 to 4 days determines effectiveness in correcting the symptoms of thyroid deficiency. Long-term use (months to years, possibly for life) requires physician supervision.

▷ **This Drug Should Not Be Taken If**
- you have had an allergic reaction to it previously.
- you are recovering from a heart attack; ask your doctor for guidance.
- you have an uncorrected adrenal cortical deficiency.
- you are using it to lose weight and your thyroid function is normal (no deficiency).

▷ **Inform Your Physician Before Taking This Drug If**
- you have high blood pressure, any form of heart disease, or diabetes.
- you have a history of Addison's disease or adrenal gland deficiency.
- you are taking any antiasthmatic medications.
- you take digoxin.
- you are taking an anticoagulant.

Possible Side Effects (natural, expected, and unavoidable drug actions)
None if dosage is adjusted correctly.

▷ **Possible Adverse Effects** (unusual, unexpected, and infrequent reactions)
If any of the following develop, consult your physician promptly for guidance.

Mild Adverse Effects
Allergic Reactions: Skin rash, hives.
Headache in sensitive individuals, even with proper dosage adjustment—may be frequent.
Rapid heart rate (tachycardia)—possible.
Hair loss—case reports.

Serious Adverse Effects
Allergic Reactions: Erythema, bullae, and papules.
Increased frequency or intensity of angina or abnormal heartbeat—possible.
Lowering of blood pressure—rare.
Heart attack—rare.
Osteoporosis: bone mineral density testing is recommended—possible increased risk.
Hyperthyroidism—possible with improper dosing.
Drug fever or drug-induced myasthenia gravis—case reports.
Note: Other adverse effects are manifestations of excessive dosage. See "Effects of Overdosage" below.

▷ **Possible Effects on Sexual Function**
Altered menstrual pattern during dosage adjustments.
Possibly beneficial in treating impaired sexual function that is associated with true hypothyroidism.

Natural Diseases or Disorders That May Be Activated by This Drug
Latent coronary artery insufficiency (angina), diabetes.

Possible Effects on Laboratory Tests
Prothrombin time: increased (when taken concurrently with warfarin).
Blood total cholesterol, HDL and LDL cholesterol levels: decreased.
Blood triglyceride levels: no effect.
Blood glucose level: increased.
Blood thyroid hormone levels: increased T_3.
Blood thyroid-stimulating hormone (TSH) level: decreased.

CAUTION
1. Careful supervision of individual response is needed to identify correct dose. Do not change dosing schedule without asking your doctor.
2. This drug should not be used to treat nonspecific fatigue, obesity, infertility, or slow growth. Such use is inappropriate and could be harmful.

Precautions for Use
By Infants and Children: **Not** recommended for treatment of this age group. It must reach the brain and nervous system, and this drug may not do that. Levothyroxine is the drug of choice to treat thyroid deficiency in infants and children.
By Those Over 60 Years of Age: Requirements for thyroid hormone replacement are usually about 25% lower than in younger adults. Watch closely for any toxicity.

▷ **Advisability of Use During Pregnancy**
Pregnancy Category: A. See Pregnancy Risk Categories at the back of this book.
Animal studies: No information available.
Human studies: Thyroid hormones do not reach the fetus (cross the placenta) in significant amounts. Clinical experience has shown that appropriate use of thyroid hormones causes no adverse effects on the fetus.
Use this drug only if clearly needed and with carefully adjusted dosage.

Advisability of Use If Breast-Feeding
Presence of this drug in breast milk: Yes, in minimal amounts.
Breast-feeding is considered safe with correctly adjusted dosage.

Habit-Forming Potential: None.

Effects of Overdosage: Headache, sense of increased body heat, nervousness, increased sweating, hand tremors, insomnia, rapid and irregular heart action, diarrhea, muscle cramping, weight loss, heart attack.

Possible Effects of Long-Term Use: Bone loss (osteoporosis) in the lumbar vertebrae (spine). Bone mineral density testing is recommended.

Suggested Periodic Examinations While Taking This Drug (at physician's discretion)
Measurement of thyroid hormone levels in blood.

▷ **While Taking This Drug, Observe the Following**
Foods: No restrictions.
Beverages: No restrictions.
▷ *Alcohol:* No interactions expected.
Tobacco Smoking: No interactions expected, but I advise everyone to quit smoking.
▷ *Other Drugs*
Liothyronine may *increase* the effects of
• warfarin (Coumadin), and increase the risk of bleeding; more frequent INR (prothrombin time or protime) tests are needed.
Liothyronine may *decrease* the effects of
• digoxin (Lanoxin) when correcting hypothyroidism; a larger dose of digoxin may be needed.
Liothyronine *taken concurrently* with
• all antidiabetic drugs (insulin and oral hypoglycemic agents) may require an increased dose to obtain proper control of blood sugar.
• estrogens (including birth control pills and Premarin) may require increased doses of liothyronine.
• monoamine oxidase inhibitors (MAO inhibitors—see Drug Classes) may increase the therapeutic benefits of the antidepressant.
• tricyclic antidepressants (see Drug Classes) may cause an increase in the activity of both drugs; watch for signs of toxicity.
The following drugs may *decrease* the effects of liothyronine
• cholestyramine (Cuemid, Questran), and perhaps other cholesterol-lowering resins, may reduce its absorption; intake of the two drugs should be separated by 5 hours.
▷ *Driving, Hazardous Activities:* No restrictions.
Aviation Note: The use of this drug *is probably not a disqualification* for piloting. Consult a designated Aviation Medical Examiner.

Exposure to Sun: No restrictions.

Exposure to Heat: This drug may decrease individual tolerance to warm environments, increasing discomfort due to heat. Consult your physician if you develop symptoms of overdosage during the warm months of the year.

Heavy Exercise or Exertion: Use caution if you have angina (coronary artery disease). This drug may increase the frequency or severity of angina during physical activity.

Discontinuation: This drug must be taken continually on a regular schedule to correct thyroid deficiency. Do not stop it without consulting your physician.

LISINOPRIL (li SIN oh pril)

Introduced: 1988   **Class:** Antihypertensive, ACE inhibitor   **Prescription:** USA: Yes   **Controlled Drug:** USA: No; Canada: No   **Available as Generic:** No

Brand Names: Prinivil, Prinzide [CD], Zestoretic [CD], Zestril

<table>
<tr><td colspan="2" align="center">BENEFITS versus RISKS</td></tr>
<tr><td align="center">*Possible Benefits*</td><td align="center">*Possible Risks*</td></tr>
<tr><td>EFFECTIVE CONTROL OF MILD TO SEVERE HIGH BLOOD PRESSURE
IMPROVES PATIENT SURVIVAL AFTER A HEART ATTACK</td><td>Headache, dizziness, fatigue
Low blood pressure
Allergic swelling of face, tongue, throat, vocal cords
Kidney compromise
Possible lowering of white blood cell counts</td></tr>
</table>

▷ **Principal Uses**

As a Single Drug Product: Uses currently included in FDA-approved labeling: (1) Treats high blood pressure. Mild to moderate usually responds to low doses; severe high blood pressure may require higher doses and concurrent use of a thiazide or other class of antihypertensive drug; (2) helps improve survival in congestive heart failure; (3) the first drug in this class approved by the FDA to help improve survival and symptoms after a heart attack in hemodynamically stable patients.

Other (unlabeled) generally accepted uses: (1) May slow or reduce atherosclerosis; (2) helps patients with some kidney problems (nephrotic syndrome); (3) can be of marked help in preventing migraines.

As a Combination Drug Product [CD]: Combined with the diuretic hydrochlorothiazide to enhance antihypertensive action.

How This Drug Works: By blocking certain enzyme systems, this drug helps relax arterial walls throughout the body and lowers the resistance to blood flow that causes high blood pressure. This, in turn, reduces the workload of the heart and improves its performance.

Available Dosage Forms and Strengths

Tablets — 5 mg, 10 mg, 20 mg, 40 mg

Prinzide, Zestoretic — 20 mg lisinopril with 12.5 or 25 mg of hydrochlorothiazide

▷ **Recommended Dosage Ranges** (Actual dosage and administration schedule must be determined for each patient individually.)

Infants and Children: Dosage not established.

12 to 60 Years of Age: Initially 10 mg once daily for those not taking a diuretic; 5 mg once daily for those taking a diuretic. Usual maintenance dose is 20 to 40 mg daily, taken in a single dose. Maximum total daily dosage is 80 mg. After a heart attack in patients who are hemodynamically stable: 5 mg may be given within 24 hours after symptoms started. If this dose is tolerated, a repeat dose is given 24 hours later and then increased to 10 mg a day. Therapy continues for at least 6 weeks.

Over 60 Years of Age: Exercise tolerance was improved by 2.5 to 20 mg daily. Any needed dose increases should be made at longer intervals between adjustments.

Conditions Requiring Dosing Adjustments

Liver Function: The liver is minimally involved in the elimination of this drug.

Kidney Function: Patients with moderate kidney failure should be started on 5 mg daily. In severe kidney failure, the patient can take 2.5 mg of lisinopril daily. This drug is contraindicated in kidney blood flow problems (renal artery stenosis).

▷ **Dosing Instructions:**   The tablet may be crushed and taken on an empty stomach or with food, at same time each day.

Usual Duration of Use: Use on a regular schedule for several weeks determines effectiveness in controlling high blood pressure. The proper treatment of high blood pressure usually requires the long-term use of effective medications.

Possible Advantages of This Drug

Controls blood pressure effectively with one daily dose.

Relatively low incidence of adverse effects.

No adverse influence on asthma, cholesterol blood levels, or diabetes.

Sudden withdrawal does not result in a rapid increase in blood pressure.

▷ **This Drug Should Not Be Taken If**
- you have had an allergic reaction to it previously.
- you currently have a blood cell or bone marrow disorder.
- you are pregnant.
- you have an abnormally high level of blood potassium.

▷ **Inform Your Physician Before Taking This Drug If**
- you have a history of kidney disease or impaired kidney function.
- you have myasthenia gravis or a specific autoimmune disease.
- you have scleroderma or systemic lupus erythematosus.
- you have cerebral artery disease.
- you are taking another drug that can suppress the immune system.
- you have any form of heart disease.
- you are breast-feeding your infant.
- you have swelling of the face, glottis, or tongue. Call your doctor immediately.

- you have a history of elevated potassium.
- you are taking other antihypertensives, diuretics, nitrates, or potassium supplements.
- you plan to have surgery under general anesthesia in the near future.

Possible Side Effects (natural, expected, and unavoidable drug actions)

Dizziness, orthostatic hypotension (see Glossary)—rare; increased blood potassium level.

Feeling of a scalded mouth has been reported with other medicines in this class. Cough.

▷ **Possible Adverse Effects** (unusual, unexpected, and infrequent reactions)

If any of the following develop, consult your physician promptly for guidance.

Mild Adverse Effects

Allergic Reactions: Skin rash, psoriasis, or itching—rare.

Headache, fatigue, numbness and tingling—rare; weakness—rare; insomnia—possible. (Headache responds to acetaminophen.)

Blurred vision—rare.

Ringing in the ears—rare.

Joint pain with positive ANA titer—case reports.

Chest pain or palpitation—rare.

Indigestion, nausea, vomiting, or diarrhea—rare to infrequent.

Taste disturbances—possible.

Serious Adverse Effects

Allergic Reactions: Swelling (angioedema) of face, tongue, and/or vocal cords—rare; can be life-threatening—case reports.

Purpura—rare.

Heart attack (myocardial infarction)—case report.

Impairment of kidney or liver function—case reports.

Bone marrow depression—case reports.

Neutropenia—infrequent except in vascular collagen disease or kidney failure.

Abnormal heartbeat—rare.

Hyperkalemia, hyperuricemia, and gout—rare.

Hyperthermia, arthralgia, and positive ANA titer—rare.

Pancreatitis—case reports.

▷ **Possible Effects on Sexual Function**

Decreased libido, impotence, swelling and tenderness of male breast tissue—all rare.

Possible Effects on Laboratory Tests

Blood potassium or uric acid: increased.

ANA titer: positive.

CAUTION

1. Ask your doctor if you should stop other antihypertensive drugs (especially diuretics) for 1 week before starting this drug.
2. **Report promptly** any signs of infection (fever, sore throat), or water retention (weight gain, puffiness, swollen feet or ankles).
3. Do not use a salt substitute without your physician's knowledge and approval. (Many salt substitutes contain potassium.)
4. It is advisable to obtain blood cell counts and urine analyses **before** starting this drug.

Precautions for Use

By Infants and Children: Safety and effectiveness for use by those in this age group have not been established.

By Those Over 60 Years of Age: Small starting doses are indicated. Sudden and excessive lowering of blood pressure can predispose to stroke or heart attack in those with impaired brain circulation or coronary artery heart disease.

▷ **Advisability of Use During Pregnancy**

Pregnancy Category: D during the first 3 months of pregnancy. D during the second and third trimester. See Pregnancy Risk Categories at the back of this book.

Animal studies: No birth defects found in mouse or rat studies. Impaired bone formation found in rabbit studies.

Human studies: May cause fetal or neonatal injury or death. May cause fetal death or injury if used during the final 6 months of pregnancy. Discuss this with your doctor.

Advisability of Use If Breast-Feeding

Presence of this drug in breast milk: Unknown.

Avoid drug or refrain from nursing.

Habit-Forming Potential: None.

Effects of Overdosage: Excessive drop in blood pressure, light-headedness, dizziness, fainting.

Possible Effects of Long-Term Use: Gradual increase in blood potassium level.

Suggested Periodic Examinations While Taking This Drug (at physician's discretion)

Before starting drug: complete blood cell counts; urine analysis with measurement of protein content; blood potassium level.

During use of drug: blood cell counts; measurements of blood potassium. ANA titer.

▷ **While Taking This Drug, Observe the Following**

Foods: Consult your physician regarding salt intake.

Nutritional Support: **Do not** take potassium supplements unless directed by your physician.

Beverages: No restrictions. May be taken with milk.

▷ *Alcohol:* Use caution until combined effect has been determined. Alcohol may enhance the blood-pressure-lowering effect of this drug.

Tobacco Smoking: No interactions expected, but I advise everyone to quit smoking.

▷ *Other Drugs*

Lisinopril *taken concurrently* with

- acetaminophen may increase blood pressure (single study and nonclinical degree).
- allopurinol (Zyloprim): increased risk of hypersensitivity.
- chlorpromazine (Thorazine) may cause low blood pressure.
- cyclosporine (Sandimmune) can cause acute kidney (renal) failure.
- interferons (alpha and beta) may greatly increase risk of blood problems. DO NOT combine.
- lithium (Lithobid, others) may cause lithium toxicity.

- loop diuretics (bumetanide—Bumex) increases effect of both drugs.
- NSAIDs (see Drug Classes) can cause blunting of the therapeutic effects of lisinopril.
- potassium preparations (K-Lyte, Slow-K, etc.) may cause increased blood levels of potassium with risk of serious heart rhythm disturbances.
- potassium-sparing diuretics—amiloride (Moduretic), spironolactone (Aldactazide), triamterene (Dyazide)—may cause increased blood levels of potassium with risk of serious heart rhythm disturbances.

▷ *Driving, Hazardous Activities:* Usually no restrictions. Be aware of possible drops in blood pressure with resultant dizziness or faintness.

Aviation Note: The use of this drug *may be a disqualification* for piloting. Consult a designated Aviation Medical Examiner.

Exposure to Sun: Caution is advised. A similar drug of this class can cause photosensitivity.

Exposure to Heat: Caution is advised. Avoid excessive perspiring with resultant loss of body water and drop in blood pressure.

Occurrence of Unrelated Illness: Report promptly any disorder that causes nausea, vomiting, or diarrhea. Fluid and chemical imbalances must be corrected as soon as possible.

Discontinuation: This drug may be stopped abruptly without causing a sudden increase in blood pressure. However, ask your doctor before stopping this drug for any reason.

LITHIUM (LITH i um)

Introduced: 1949 **Class:** Antidepressant **Prescription:** USA: Yes
Controlled Drug: USA: No; Canada: No **Available as Generic:** USA: Yes; Canada: No

Brand Names: ✦Carbolith, Cibalith-S, ✦Duralith, Eskalith, Eskalith CR, Lithane, ✦Lithizine, Lithobid, Lithonate, Lithotabs

BENEFITS versus RISKS	
Possible Benefits	*Possible Risks*
RAPID REVERSAL OF ACUTE MANIA	VERY NARROW MARGIN OF TREATMENT
STABILIZATION OF MOOD	POTENTIALLY FATAL TOXICITY with inadequate monitoring
Prevention of recurrent depression in "responders"	Infrequent induction of diabetes mellitus, hypothyroidism
	Diabetes-insipidus-like syndrome (excessive dilute urine without sugar)

▷ **Principal Uses**

As a Single Drug Product: Uses currently included in FDA-approved labeling: (1) Management of bipolar disorder. Promptly corrects acute mania, and also reduces frequency and severity of recurrent manic-depressive mood swings; (2) used to treat mania; (3) helps control mania.

Other (unlabeled) generally accepted uses: (1) May be helpful in chronic hair pulling (trichotillomania); (2) can help prevent cluster headaches; (3) may help control aggressive behavior; (4) can have a role in treating Fanconi's aplastic anemia; (5) could have an adjunctive role in treating AIDS patients who have low platelet and white blood cells; (6) may help patients who have mood problems that also affects their sex drive.

How This Drug Works: It is thought that lithium changes the way nerve signals are transmitted and interpreted, influencing emotional status and behavior.

Available Dosage Forms and Strengths

Capsules — 150 mg, 300 mg, 600 mg
Syrup — 8 mEq/5 ml
Tablets — 300 mg
Tablets, prolonged action — 300 mg, 450 mg

▷ **Usual Adult Dosage Range:**   First day: 900 to 1200 mg per day; this is divided into three equal doses. This dose is then increased as needed and tolerated by 300-mg increments to attain a blood level of 1–1.5 mmol/L. The usual maintenance dose is 1200 to 1800 mg daily taken in three divided doses. The total daily dosage should not exceed 3600 mg. **Note: Actual dose and dosing schedule must be determined for each patient individually.**

Conditions Requiring Dosing Adjustments

Liver Function: The liver is minimally involved in the elimination of lithium.

Kidney Function: Frequent and careful monitoring and decreased dosing must be provided. Doses are usually decreased and blood levels obtained more often. In moderate to severe kidney failure (creatinine clearance of 10–50 ml/min), 50–75% of the usual dose is taken. In severe kidney failure, 25–50% of the usual dose is taken.

▷ **Dosing Instructions:**   The capsules may be opened and regular tablets crushed and taken with or after meals to reduce stomach upset. The prolonged-action tablets should be swallowed whole and not altered.

Usual Duration of Use: Use on a regular schedule for 1 to 3 weeks determines effectiveness in correcting acute mania; several months of continual treatment may be required to correct depression. Long-term use (months to years) requires physician supervision and periodic evaluation.

Currently a "Drug of Choice"

for the treatment of acute mania in bipolar manic-depressive disorders.

▷ **This Drug Should Not Be Taken If**
- you have had an allergic reaction to any dosage form of it previously.
- you have uncontrolled diabetes or uncorrected hypothyroidism.
- you are breast-feeding your infant.
- you will be unable to comply with the need for regular monitoring of lithium blood levels.
- you have severe kidney failure.

▷ **Inform Your Physician Before Taking This Drug If**
- you have a history of a schizophreniclike thought disorder.
- you have any type of organic brain disease, or a history of grand mal epilepsy.
- you have diabetes, heart disease, hypothyroidism, or impaired kidney function.

- you are on a salt-restricted diet.
- you are pregnant or planning pregnancy.
- you are taking any diuretic drug or a cortisonelike steroid preparation.
- you plan to have surgery under general anesthesia in the near future.

Possible Side Effects (natural, expected, and unavoidable drug actions)
Increased thirst and urine volume in 60% of initial users and in 20% of long-term users.
Weight gain in first few months of use.
Drowsiness and lethargy in sensitive individuals. Metallic taste.
Increased white blood cells—**not** a sign of infection, but an effect of lithium.
Tremor (fine)—frequent (may respond to a beta-blocker).

▷ **Possible Adverse Effects** (unusual, unexpected, and infrequent reactions)
If any of the following develop, consult your physician promptly for guidance.
Mild Adverse Effects
Allergic Reactions: Skin rashes, generalized itching.
Skin dryness, loss of hair—case reports.
Headache, joint pain, dizziness, weakness, blurred vision, ringing in ears, unsteadiness—infrequent.
Nausea, vomiting, diarrhea—frequent.
Metallic taste—possible.
Edema—possible.
Serious Adverse Effects
"Blackout" spells, confusion, stupor, slurred speech, spasmodic movements of extremities, epilepticlike seizures—case reports to rare.
Abnormal fixed eye position (oculogyric crisis)—case reports.
Abnormal changes in heart rate, rhythm, and wave forms—frequent.
Loss of bladder or rectal control—infrequent.
Diabetes-insipidus-like syndrome: excessive dilute urine—infrequent to frequent.
Abnormal movements (may be a sign of toxicity)—rare.
Cerebellar atrophy or neuroleptic malignant syndrome—case reports.
Inflammation of the heart muscle (myocarditis)—case reports.
Pseudotumor cerebri, myasthenia gravis, or systemic lupus erythematosus—case reports.
Low thyroid function or abnormally high thyroid function—possible to case reports.
Elevated blood calcium or blood sugar—rare.
Porphyria or inflammation of the parotid gland—case reports.
Seizures—case reports and certainly with toxicity.
Drug-induced low potassium—possible.

▷ **Possible Effects on Sexual Function**
Decreased libido (blood level of 0.7 to 0.9 mEq/L)—case reports; inhibited erection (0.6 to 0.8 mEq/L)—frequent; male infertility; female breast swelling with milk production—case reports.

▷ **Adverse Effects That May Mimic Natural Diseases or Disorders**
Painful discoloration and coldness of the hands and feet may resemble Raynaud's phenomenon.

Natural Diseases or Disorders That May Be Activated by This Drug

Diabetes mellitus may be worsened. Psoriasis may be intensified. Myasthenia gravis may be induced (one case).

Possible Effects on Laboratory Tests

White blood cell and platelet counts: increased.

Blood alkaline phosphatase (bone isoenzyme): markedly increased in 66% of users.

Blood cholesterol level: increased.

Blood parathyroid hormone level: increased.

Blood thyroid-stimulating hormone (TSH) level: increased.

Blood thyroid hormone (T_3 and T_4) levels: decreased.

Blood uric acid level: decreased.

Blood bromide, calcium, or glucose levels: increased.

Blood potassium level: increased or decreased.

CAUTION

1. The blood level required for this drug to work is close to the level that can cause toxic effects. Periodic blood lithium levels are mandatory. Follow instructions about drug dosage and periodic blood tests.

2. Lithium should be stopped at the first signs of toxicity: drowsiness, sluggishness, unsteadiness, tremor, muscle twitching, vomiting, or diarrhea.

3. The major causes of lithium toxicity are:

- accidental overdose (may be due to inadequate blood level checks)
- impaired kidney function
- salt restriction
- inadequate fluid intake, dehydration
- concurrent use of diuretics
- intercurrent illness
- childbirth (rapid decrease in kidney clearance of lithium)
- initiation of treatment with a new drug

4. Over-the-counter preparations that contain iodides (some cough products and vitamin–mineral supplements) should be avoided because of the added antithyroid effect when taken with lithium.

Precautions for Use

By Infants and Children: Safety and effectiveness for those under 12 years of age are not established. Follow your physician's instructions exactly.

By Those Over 60 Years of Age: Treatment should start with a "test" dose of 75 to 150 mg daily. Observe closely for early indications of toxic effects, especially if on a low-salt diet and using diuretics. Increased risk of parkinsonian reactions (abnormal gait and movements); coma can develop without warning symptoms.

▷ **Advisability of Use During Pregnancy**

Pregnancy Category: D. See Pregnancy Risk Categories at the back of this book.

Animal studies: Cleft palate reported in mice; eye, ear, and palate defects reported in rats.

Human studies: Adequate studies of pregnant women are not available. However, cardiovascular defects and goiter in newborn infants (of mothers using lithium) have been reported. If the infant's blood level of lithium approaches the toxic range before delivery, the newborn may suffer the "floppy infant" syndrome: weakness, lethargy, unresponsiveness, low body temperature, weak cry, and poor feeding ability.

Avoid use of drug during the first 3 months. Use only if clearly necessary during the final 6 months. Monitor mother's blood lithium levels carefully to avoid possible toxicity.

Advisability of Use If Breast-Feeding
Presence of this drug in breast milk: Yes, in significant amounts.
Avoid drug or refrain from nursing.

Habit-Forming Potential: None.

Effects of Overdosage: Drowsiness, weakness, lack of coordination, nausea, vomiting, diarrhea, muscle spasms, blurred vision, dizziness, staggering gait, slurred speech, confusion, stupor, coma, cerebellar atrophy, seizures.

Possible Effects of Long-Term Use: Hypothyroidism (5%), goiter, reduced sugar tolerance, diabetes-insipidus-like syndrome, serious kidney damage.

Suggested Periodic Examinations While Taking This Drug (at physician's discretion)
Regular determinations of blood lithium levels are absolutely essential.
Time to sample blood for lithium level: 12 hours after evening dose, or in the morning, just before next dose. Therapeutic range: 0.8 to 1.5 mEq/L (acute) and 0.6 to 1.2 (maintenance).
Periodic evaluation of thyroid gland size and function.
Complete blood cell counts; kidney function tests.

▷ **While Taking This Drug, Observe the Following**
Foods: Maintain a normal diet; **do not** restrict your use of salt.
Beverages: No restrictions. Drink at least 8 to 12 glasses of liquids daily. This drug may be taken with milk.
▷ *Alcohol:* Use with caution. May have an increased intoxicating effect. Avoid alcohol completely if any symptoms of lithium toxicity develop.
Tobacco Smoking: Lithium may increase sensitivity to nicotine. I advise everyone to quit smoking.
Marijuana Smoking: Possible increase in apathy, lethargy, drowsiness, or sluggishness; accentuation of lithium-induced tremor; possible increased risk of precipitating psychotic behavior.
▷ *Other Drugs*
Lithium may *increase* the effects of
• tricyclic antidepressants (see Drug Classes).
Lithium *taken concurrently* with
• ACE inhibitors such as captopril (Capoten) may increase lithium levels by as much as three times the level prior to combination therapy.
• calcium channel blockers (see Drug Classes) such as diltiazem may cause neurotoxicity or psychosis.
• carbamazepine (Tegretol) may result in neurotoxicity.
• chlorpromazine (Thorazine, etc.) and other phenothiazines (see Drug Classes) may result in decreased lithium or phenothiazine therapeutic effects.
• clozapine (Clozaril) may result in serious agranulocytosis, delirium, and neuroleptic malignant syndrome. Do not combine these medicines.
• diazepam (Valium) may cause hypothermia.
• fludrocortisone (Florinef) may result in loss of the mineralocorticoid benefits of fludrocortisone.
• fluoxetine (Prozac) may result in neurotoxicity.

- fluvoxamine (Luvox) may result in increased lithium levels and toxicity.
- haloperidol (Haldol) or with other neuroleptics may result in decreased beneficial effects from both medicines.
- methyldopa (Aldomet, etc.) is usually well tolerated; however, it may cause a severe neurotoxic reaction in susceptible individuals. These combinations should be used very cautiously.
- metronidazole (Flagyl) may lead to lithium toxicity.
- monoamine oxidase inhibitors (MAO inhibitors—see Drug Classes) may result in the serotonin syndrome and potential fatality.
- nicotine (Nicorette gum or nicotine patches) may cause supersensitivity to nicotine.
- verapamil (Calan, Isoptin) may cause unpredictable effects; both lithium toxicity and decreased lithium blood levels have been reported.

The following drugs may **increase** the effects of lithium

- bumetanide (Bumex).
- ethacrynic acid (Edecrin).
- fluoxetine (Prozac).
- furosemide (Lasix, etc.).
- indomethacin (Indocin).
- piroxicam (Feldene) or any nonsteroidal anti-inflammatory drug (NSAID— see Drug Classes).
- thiazide diuretics (see Drug Classes).

The following drugs may **decrease** the effects of lithium

- acetazolamide (Diamox, etc.).
- sodium bicarbonate.
- theophylline (Theo-Dur, etc.) and related drugs.

▷ *Driving, Hazardous Activities:* This drug may impair mental alertness, judgment, physical coordination, and reaction time. Restrict activities as necessary.

Aviation Note: The use of this drug *is a disqualification* for piloting. Consult a designated Aviation Medical Examiner.

Exposure to Sun: No restrictions.

Exposure to Heat: Excessive sweating can cause significant depletion of salt and water and resultant lithium toxicity. Avoid sauna baths.

Occurrence of Unrelated Illness: Fever, sweating, vomiting, or diarrhea can result in significant alterations of blood and tissue lithium concentrations. Close monitoring of your physical condition and blood lithium levels is needed to prevent serious toxicity.

Discontinuation: Sudden discontinuation does not cause withdrawal symptoms. Avoid premature discontinuation; some individuals may require continual treatment for up to a year to achieve maximal response. Discontinuation by "responders" may result in recurrence of either mania or depression. Lithium should be discontinued if symptoms of brain toxicity appear or if an uncorrectable diabetes-insipidus-like syndrome develops.

LOMEFLOXACIN (loh me FLOX a sin)

Author's Note: See the new fluoroquinolone antibiotics profile for more information.

LOPERAMIDE (loh PER a mide)

Introduced: 1977   **Class:** Antidiarrheal   **Prescription:** USA: Yes
Controlled Drug: USA: No; Canada: No   **Available as Generic:** Yes

Brand Names: Anti-Diarrheal, Imodium, Imodium AD, Kaopectate 1-D, Maalox A/D, Pepto Diarrhea Control

BENEFITS versus RISKS	
Possible Benefits	*Possible Risks*
EFFECTIVE RELIEF OF INTESTINAL CRAMPING AND DIARRHEA	Drowsiness Constipation Induction of toxic megacolon

▷ **Principal Uses**

As a Single Drug Product: Uses currently included in FDA-approved labeling: (1) Control of cramping and diarrhea associated with acute gastroenteritis and chronic enteritis and colitis; (2) used to reduce the volume of discharge from ileostomies.

Other (unlabeled) generally accepted uses: (1) Used in irritable bowel syndrome that has failed to respond to dietary supplements; (2) combination therapy of traveler's diarrhea; (3) decreases unformed stools in *Shigella* diarrhea.

How This Drug Works: This drug acts directly on the nerve supply of the gastrointestinal tract, decreases secretions, and helps relieve cramping and diarrhea.

Available Dosage Forms and Strengths

Capsules — 2 mg
Liquid — 1 mg/5 ml (5.25% alcohol)—0.2 mg/5 ml (4.07% alcohol)
Tablets — 2 mg

▷ **Usual Adult Dosage Range:** For acute diarrhea: 4 mg initially, then 2 mg after each unformed stool until diarrhea is controlled. Chronic diarrhea: 4 to 8 mg daily in divided doses, taken 8 to 12 hours apart. Maximum daily dosage is 16 mg.

Pediatric dosing: NOT recommended for children under 2 years old. 2 to 5 year olds can be given 1 mg three times a day on the first day (13–20 kg); 6 to 8 year olds can have 2 mg twice daily on the first day (20–30 kg); 8–12 years old can have 2 mg three times daily (greater than 30 kg). Follow-up doses on the next day are 1 mg per 10 kg of body mass, up to the maximum daily doses on day 1. If diarrhea persists, call your doctor. **Note: Actual dosage and administration schedule must be determined for each patient individually.**

Conditions Requiring Dosing Adjustments

Liver Function: Dosing adjustments for patients with liver compromise are not needed. Half of a given dose is removed unchanged in the feces.

Kidney Function: Changes in dosing are not indicated in kidney compromise.

▷ **Dosing Instructions:** The capsule may be opened and taken on an empty stomach or with food if stomach upset occurs.

Usual Duration of Use: Use on a regular schedule for 48 hours determines effectiveness in controlling acute diarrhea; continual use for 10 days may be needed to evaluate its effectiveness in controlling chronic diarrhea. If diarrhea persists, consult your physician.

▷ **This Drug Should Not Be Taken If**
- you have had an allergic reaction to it previously.
- it is prescribed for a child under 2 years of age.

▷ **Inform Your Physician Before Taking This Drug If**
- you have a history of liver disease or impaired liver function.
- you have regional enteritis or ulcerative colitis.
- you develop swelling (distention) of the abdomen while taking this medicine.
- you have acute dysentery.

Possible Side Effects (natural, expected, and unavoidable drug actions)
Drowsiness, constipation.

▷ **Possible Adverse Effects** (unusual, unexpected, and infrequent reactions)
If any of the following develop, consult your physician promptly for guidance.

Mild Adverse Effects
Allergic Reaction: Skin rash.
Fatigue, dizziness—rare.
Reduced appetite, cramps, dry mouth, nausea, vomiting, stomach pain, bloating—infrequent.

Serious Adverse Effects
"Toxic megacolon" (distended, immobile colon with fluid retention) may develop while treating acute ulcerative colitis—possible.
Necrotizing enterocolitis or paralytic ileus—rare.

▷ **Possible Effects on Sexual Function**
None reported.

Possible Effects on Laboratory Tests
None reported.

CAUTION
1. Do not exceed recommended doses.
2. If treating chronic diarrhea, promptly report development of bloating, abdominal distention, nausea, vomiting, constipation, or abdominal pain.

Precautions for Use
By Infants and Children: Do not use in those under 2 years of age. Follow your physician's instructions exactly regarding dosage. Watch for drowsiness, irritability, personality changes, and altered behavior.
By Those Over 60 Years of Age: Small starting doses are needed, as you may be more sensitive to the sedative and constipating effects of this drug.

▷ **Advisability of Use During Pregnancy**
Pregnancy Category: B. See Pregnancy Risk Categories at the back of this book.
Animal studies: No birth defects found in rat and rabbit studies.
Human studies: Adequate studies of pregnant women are not available.
Use sparingly and only if clearly needed. Ask your physician for guidance.

Advisability of Use If Breast-Feeding
Presence of this drug in breast milk: Small, clinically insignificant amounts.
Talk with your doctor about the benefits versus risks of using this medicine
and nursing.

Habit-Forming Potential: Physical dependence has occurred in monkeys, but
there have been no reports in humans.

Effects of Overdosage: Drowsiness, lethargy, depression, dry mouth.

Possible Effects of Long-Term Use: None identified.

Suggested Periodic Examinations While Taking This Drug (at physician's discretion)
Decreased frequency of stools within 48 hours.

▷ **While Taking This Drug, Observe the Following**
Foods: No restrictions. Follow prescribed diet.
Beverages: No restrictions, other than your doctor's recommendations regard-
ing diet.
▷ *Alcohol:* Use with caution. This drug may increase the depressant action of alco-
hol on the brain.
Tobacco Smoking: No interactions expected.
▷ *Other Drugs*
No significant drug interactions reported.
▷ *Driving, Hazardous Activities:* This drug may cause drowsiness or dizziness. Re-
strict activities as necessary.
Aviation Note: The use of this drug *is a disqualification* for piloting. Consult a
designated Aviation Medical Examiner.
Exposure to Sun: No restrictions.

LORATADINE (lor AT a deen)

Introduced: 1992   **Class:** Antihistamines, nonsedating **Author's Note: See
the new minimally sedating antihistamines profile for further information.**

LORAZEPAM (lor A za pam)

Introduced: 1977   **Class:** Mild tranquilizer, benzodiazepines   **Prescription:** USA: Yes   **Controlled Drug:** USA: C-IV*; Canada: No   **Available as
Generic:** USA: Yes; Canada: Yes

Brand Names: ✦Apo-Lorazepam, Ativan, Lorazepam Intensol, ✦Novo-Loraze-
pam, ✦Nu-Loraz

*See schedules of Controlled Drugs at the back of this book.

```
┌─────────────────────────────────────────────────────────────────────┐
│                         BENEFITS versus RISKS                         │
│        Possible Benefits              Possible Risks                  │
│   RELIEF OF ANXIETY AND         Habit-forming potential with          │
│      NERVOUS TENSION               prolonged use                      │
│   NOT CHANGED SIGNIFICANTLY     Minor impairment of mental            │
│      INTO ACTIVE DRUG FORMS IN     functions                          │
│      THE LIVER                  Blood cell, movement, or liver        │
│   Wide margin of safety with       disorders                         │
│      therapeutic doses          Dose-related respiratory depression   │
│                                 Withdrawal symptoms if abruptly       │
│                                    stopped                            │
└─────────────────────────────────────────────────────────────────────┘
```

▷ **Principal Uses**

As a Single Drug Product: Uses currently included in FDA-approved labeling: (1) Helps treat anxiety; (2) used to relieve insomnia; (3) used in surgical cases to help in delivering effective anesthesia; (4) used intravenously as a sedative.

Other (unlabeled) generally accepted uses: (1) Used to help prevent the severe symptoms of alcohol detoxification (delirium tremens or DT); (2) used under the tongue to treat serial seizures in children; (3) can be used to promote amnesia in patients who must take chemotherapy and have suffered vomiting.

How This Drug Works: This drug attaches to a specific site (GABA-A receptor) in the brain and enables gamma-aminobutyric acid to inhibit activity of nervous tissue. Drugs in this class also reduce the time it takes to fall asleep and the number of times people awaken during the night.

Available Dosage Forms and Strengths

Tablet — 0.5 mg, 1 mg, 2 mg
Sublingual tablet — 0.5 mg, 1 mg, 2 mg
Oral solution — 2 mg/ml
Injection — 2 mg/ml, 4 mg/ml

▷ **Recommended Dosage Ranges** (Actual dose and dosing schedule must be determined for each patient individually.)

Infants and Children: Safety and effectiveness in those under 18 years of age are not established. Has been used in 1- to 4-mg doses under the tongue for treatment of serial seizures in children.

18 to 60 Years of Age: Sedation and anxiety: therapy is started with 1 to 2 mg per day in two to three divided doses. Doses may be increased as needed and tolerated to the usual maintenance dose of 2 to 6 mg daily in divided doses. The maximum dose is 10 mg daily in two to three divided doses.

Insomnia: 2 to 4 mg at bedtime.

Over 60 Years of Age: Sedation and anxiety: therapy is started with 0.5 to 1 mg in divided doses. The initial dose should **not** exceed 2 mg daily.

Insomnia: 0.5 to 1 mg at bedtime.

Conditions Requiring Dosing Adjustments

Liver Function: The dose **must** be decreased in liver compromise, and the drug should **not** be used in liver failure. Use of the lowest effective dose is recommended by those with mild to moderate liver failure.

Kidney Function: The drug should **not** be used in kidney failure. In mild to moderate kidney compromise, the dose **must** be decreased, and the lowest effective dose is recommended.

▷ **Dosing Instructions:**   The tablet may be crushed and taken on an empty stomach or with milk or food. Do **not** stop this drug abruptly if it has been taken for more than 4 weeks.

Usual Duration of Use: Use on a regular schedule for 3 to 5 days usually determines effectiveness in relieving moderate anxiety or insomnia. Continual use should be limited to 1 to 3 weeks. Consult your physician on a regular basis.

Possible Advantages of This Drug
More direct elimination and lack of active forms may be of benefit in the elderly. Increased lipid solubility is of benefit when the drug is used to treat acute alcohol withdrawal.

▷ **This Drug Should Not Be Taken If**
• you have had an allergic reaction to any dosage form or any component of the dose previously.
• you have a primary depression or psychosis.
• you have excessively low blood pressure.
• you have narrow-angle glaucoma.

▷ **Inform Your Physician Before Taking This Drug If**
• you are allergic to any benzodiazepine (see Drug Classes).
• you have a history of alcoholism or drug abuse.
• you are prone to respiratory depression.
• you are pregnant or planning pregnancy.
• you have impaired liver or kidney function.
• you have a history of low white blood cell counts.
• you have asthma, emphysema, epilepsy, or myasthenia gravis.
• you take other prescription or nonprescription medicines that were not discussed with your doctor when lorazepam was prescribed.

Possible Side Effects (natural, expected, and unavoidable drug actions)
Sedation, "hangover" effects on the day following bedtime use.

▷ **Possible Adverse Effects** (unusual, unexpected, and infrequent reactions)
If any of the following develop, consult your physician promptly for guidance.
Mild Adverse Effects
Allergic Reactions: Rashes, hives—rare.
Dizziness, amnesia, insomnia, fainting, confusion, blurred vision, slurred speech, constipation, and sweating—infrequent.
Ringing in the ears (associated with withdrawal), decreased hearing ability—infrequent.
Serious Adverse Effects
Allergic Reactions: Liver damage with jaundice (see Glossary)—case reports.
Low white blood cell counts (leukopenia)—rare.
Paradoxical excitement and rage—case reports.
Low blood pressure—rare.
Hallucinations (transient)—rare.
Porphyria, seizures, or abnormal body movements—case reports.
Respiratory depression—dose related.

▷ **Possible Effects on Sexual Function**

Decreased male libido or impotence—case reports.

Possible Effects on Laboratory Tests

White blood cell counts: decreased.

Liver function tests: increased SGPT, SGOT, and LDH.

CAUTION

1. This drug should **not** be stopped abruptly if it has been taken continually for more than 4 weeks.
2. Over-the-counter medicines with antihistamines can cause excessive sedation if taken with lorazepam.
3. Lorazepam should **not** be combined with alcohol. This combination will worsen adverse mental and coordination decreases, and increase lorazepam levels.

Precautions for Use

By Infants and Children: Safety and effectiveness for those under 18 years of age are not established. Lorazepam has been used under the tongue in children with serial seizures.

By Those Over 60 Years of Age: Small doses are indicated. Watch for lethargy, fatigue, weakness, and paradoxical agitation, anger, hostility, and rage.

▷ **Advisability of Use During Pregnancy**

Pregnancy Category: D. See Pregnancy Risk Categories at the back of this book.

Animal studies: Cleft palate has been reported in mice; skeletal defects in rats with similar drugs in this class.

Human studies: Adequate studies of pregnant women are not available.

Frequent use in late pregnancy can result in "floppy infant" syndrome in the newborn: weakness, lethargy, depressed breathing, and low body temperature.

Avoid use during the entire pregnancy

Advisability of Use If Breast-Feeding

Presence of this drug in breast milk: Yes.

Avoid drug or refrain from nursing.

Habit-Forming Potential: This drug can cause psychological and/or physical dependence (see Glossary).

Effects of Overdosage: Marked drowsiness, weakness, feeling of drunkenness, staggering gait, depression of breathing, stupor progressing to coma.

Possible Effects of Long-Term Use: Psychological or physical dependence, rare liver toxicity.

Suggested Periodic Examinations While Taking This Drug (at physician's discretion)

Liver function tests and complete blood cell counts.

▷ **While Taking This Drug, Observe the Following**

Foods: No restrictions.

Beverages: Avoid excessive caffeine-containing beverages: coffee, tea, and cola.

▷ *Alcohol:* Avoid this combination. Alcohol increases depression of mental function, further worsens coordination, and causes increased lorazepam levels.

Tobacco Smoking: Heavy smoking may reduce the calming action of this drug. I advise everyone to quit smoking.

Marijuana Smoking: Additive drowsiness, and impaired physical performance.

▷   *Other Drugs*
Lorazepam *taken concurrently* with
- clozapine (Clozaril) may result in marked sedation and muscular incoordination.
- heparin may result in increased effects of lorazepam (increased free fraction).
- lithium (Lithobid, others) may result in a lowering of body temperature (hypothermic reaction).
- oxycodone (Percocet, others) and other central nervous system depressants may result in additive CNS or respiratory depression.
- phenytoin (Dilantin) may result in altered phenytoin or lorazepam levels.

The following drugs may *increase* the effects of lorazepam
- macrolide antibiotics (see Drug Classes).
- probenecid (Benemid)—may result in a 50% increased lorazepam level. Decreased lorazepam doses or an increased time between doses is indicated.
- valproic acid (Depakene). Decreased doses or an increased time between doses may be needed.

The following drugs may *decrease* the effects of lorazepam
- birth control pills (oral contraceptives).
- caffeine, amphetamines, or other stimulants.
- theophylline (Theo-Dur, others).

▷   *Driving, Hazardous Activities:* This drug can impair alertness and coordination. Restrict activities as necessary.

Aviation Note: The use of this drug *is a disqualification* for piloting. Consult a designated Aviation Medical Examiner.

Exposure to Sun: No restrictions.

Discontinuation: Do **not** stop this drug suddenly if it has been taken for over 4 weeks. Consult your doctor about a gradual tapering of dosage.

LOSARTAN (loh SAR tan)

Introduced: 1995   **Class:** Angiotensin II antagonist   **Prescription:** USA: Yes   **Controlled Drug:** USA: No; Canada: No   **Available as Generic:** USA: No; Canada: No

Brand Names: Cozaar, Hyzaar

BENEFITS versus RISKS	
Possible Benefits	*Possible Risks*
EFFECTIVE CONTROL OF HIGH BLOOD PRESSURE	Generally well tolerated
DECREASED NUMBER OF DEATHS FROM CONGESTIVE HEART FAILURE	
Decreased cough versus ACE inhibitors	

▷ **Principal Uses**
As a Single Drug Product: Uses currently included in FDA-approved labeling: (1) Treatment of high blood pressure; (2) decreases abnormal size of the left ventricle (left ventricular hypertrophy).

Other (unlabeled) generally accepted uses: **The ELITE study compared lo-sartan to an ACE inhibitor (in patients over 65 with ejection fraction mean of 30%) and found a significant decrease in all-cause death in treating congestive heart failure.**

As a Combination Drug Product [CD]: This drug has been combined with hydro-chlorothiazide in a new fixed-dosage form. The drug is called Hyzaar, and it contains 12.5 mg of hydrochlorothiazide and 50 mg of losartan. These drugs work to complement each other, making the combination a more effective antihypertensive.

How This Drug Works: This drug and its active metabolite block the effects of angiotensin II by binding to a specific site (the AT1) receptor. This helps the blood vessels stay more open and thereby controls blood pressure. This drug and its metabolite also block the secretion of aldosterone.

Available Dosage Forms and Strengths
  Tablet — 25 mg, 50 mg

▷ **Recommended Dosage Ranges** (Actual dosage and administration schedule must be determined for each patient individually.)
  Infants and Children: Not recommended for use in this age group.
  18 to 60 Years of Age: A starting dose of 50 mg daily is used. If the blood pressure response is not sufficient, the same dose may be divided into two equal doses and given twice daily. The dose may also be increased as needed and tolerated and taken in two divided doses daily. Peak effects may not be seen for 3 to 6 weeks before dosing changes are made. The maximum daily dose is 100 mg.
  Over 60 Years of Age: Patients who are dehydrated or have a decreased intravas-cular volume should take 25 mg once daily as a starting dose.

Conditions Requiring Dosing Adjustments
  Liver Function: This drug is extensively changed (metabolized) in the liver to an active metabolite. The starting dose should be 25 mg. Dosing is then in-creased as needed and tolerated at weekly intervals. The fixed-dose drug Hyzaar should not be used by patients with liver failure.
  Kidney Function: No dosing changes appear to be needed. The fixed-dose com-bination Hyzaar should not be used by patients with creatinine clearances (see Glossary) less than 30 ml/min.

▷ **Dosing Instructions:**   Food slows the absorption of losartan, but does not de-crease the total absorption of this medicine.

Usual Duration of Use: Continual use on a regular schedule for 3 to 6 weeks is usually necessary to determine this drug's effectiveness in controlling high blood pressure. Long-term use (months to years) requires periodic evalua-tion of response and dosage adjustment. Consult your physician on a regu-lar basis.

Possible Advantages of This Drug
  A completely new mechanism of action.
  Appears to avoid the cough effect typical of ACE inhibitors.

▷ **This Drug Should Not Be Taken If**
  • you have had an allergic reaction to any dosage form of it previously.
  • you are pregnant.

▷ **Inform Your Physician Before Taking This Drug If**
  • you have a history of liver or kidney disease.
  • you have a history of circulation problems in the brain.
  • you are breast-feeding your infant.
  • you have a history of aspirin or penicillin allergy.
  • you have a history of disease in the blood vessels that supply the heart (coronary artery disease).
  • you are uncertain of how much losartan to take or how often to take it.

Possible Side Effects (natural, expected, and unavoidable drug actions)
  Taste disorders.

▷ **Possible Adverse Effects** (unusual, unexpected, and infrequent reactions)
  If any of the following develop, consult your physician promptly for guidance.
  Mild Adverse Effects
  Allergic Reactions: Skin rash.
  Dizziness, headache, or sleep disturbances—infrequent.
  Fatigue or muscle cramps—infrequent.
  Diarrhea—infrequent.
  Serious Adverse Effects
  Allergic Reactions: Not defined.
  Swelling of the face and lips (angioedema)—case reports.
  Taste disturbances—possible.
  Migraine headaches—rare.
  Gout—rare and of questionable cause.
  Liver toxicity—case reports.
  Dose-related increase in blood potassium (hyperkalemia).
  Anemia—case reports and of minimal clinical significance.

▷ **Possible Effects on Sexual Function**
  Decreased libido, impotence—both rare and of questionable causation.

Possible Delayed Adverse Effects: None reported.

▷ **Adverse Effects That May Mimic Natural Diseases or Disorders**
  Increases in liver function tests may mimic infectious hepatitis.

Natural Diseases or Disorders That May Be Activated by This Drug
  None reported.

Possible Effects on Laboratory Tests
  Liver function tests: increased.

CAUTION
  1. This drug should **not** be taken during pregnancy.

Precautions for Use
  By Infants and Children: Safety and effectiveness for use by those under 18 years of age have not been established.
  By Those Over 60 Years of Age: People in this age group may be more sensitive to the effects of medicines that lower blood pressure. Lower starting doses are indicated for patients who are dehydrated.

▷ **Advisability of Use During Pregnancy**
  Pregnancy Category: C in the first 3 months, D in the fourth month through birth. See Pregnancy Risk Categories at the back of this book.

Animal studies: Rat studies have produced kidney toxicity and death in fetuses.

Human studies: Information from adequate studies of pregnant women is not available. If pregnancy is detected, this medicine should be stopped as soon as possible.

Advisability of Use If Breast-Feeding

Presence of this drug in breast milk: Unknown, but expected.

Avoid drug or refrain from nursing.

Habit-Forming Potential: None.

Effects of Overdosage: Severe decreases in blood pressure. Increased heart rate.

Possible Effects of Long-Term Use: Not defined.

Suggested Periodic Examinations While Taking This Drug (at physician's discretion)

Periodic checks of blood pressure and liver function tests.

▷ **While Taking This Drug, Observe the Following**

Foods: Follow the diet that your doctor has prescribed.

Nutritional Support: Specific measures are not indicated.

Beverages: Avoid excessive caffeine intake.

▷ *Alcohol:* Alcohol may intensify the blood-pressure-lowering effects of this medicine. Ask your doctor for guidance.

Tobacco Smoking: No interactions expected, but I advise everyone to quit smoking.

Marijuana Smoking: May increase the blood-pressure-lowering effects of this drug.

▷ *Other Drugs*

Losartan *taken concurrently* with

• moxonidine (Cynt, available in Germany) may result in additive lowering of blood pressure.

▷ *Driving, Hazardous Activities:* This drug may cause confusion. Restrict activities as necessary.

Aviation Note: The use of this drug *may be a disqualification* for piloting. Consult a designated Aviation Medical Examiner.

Exposure to Sun: Caution is advised. Isolated cases of photosensitivity have been reported.

Exposure to Heat: Caution: excessive sweating (perspiration) may lead to dehydration and an excessive blood-pressure-lowering effect of this drug.

Discontinuation: Talk with your doctor before stopping this medicine for any reason.

LOVASTATIN (loh vah STA tin)

Introduced: 1987   **Class:** Anticholesterol   **Prescription:** USA: Yes
Controlled Drug: USA: No   **Available as Generic:** USA: No; Canada: No
Brand Name: Mevacor

```
┌─────────────────────────────────────────────────────────────────────┐
│                      BENEFITS versus RISKS                           │
│        Possible Benefits                    Possible Risks           │
│   EFFECTIVE REDUCTION OF TOTAL    Drug-induced hepatitis (without    │
│      BLOOD CHOLESTEROL               jaundice)                       │
│   SLOWS PROGRESSION OF            Drug-induced myositis (muscle      │
│      CORONARY ATHEROSCLEROSIS        inflammation)                   │
│                                   Drug-induced stomach ulceration    │
└─────────────────────────────────────────────────────────────────────┘
```

▷ **Principal Uses**

As a Single Drug Product: Uses currently included in FDA-approved labeling: (1) Reduces abnormally high total blood cholesterol levels in people with type II hypercholesterolemia. Should not be used until nondrug methods have proven to be inadequate; (2) recently approved for use in **slowing the progression** of coronary (heart) atherosclerosis in patients with coronary heart disease. It also showed a reduction in the number of heart attacks.

Other (unlabeled) generally accepted uses: (1) May help decrease hypercholesterolemia in cholesterol ester storage disease prior to liver transplant; (2) could have a role in helping blue toe syndrome (peripheral atheroembolism); (3) could help lower cholesterol in secondary hyperlipidemia; (4) may help (low dose) in the nephrotic syndrome; (5) could help hyperlipidemia in transplant recipients.

How This Drug Works: This drug is converted in the body to mevinolinic acid, which inhibits the liver enzyme that starts to make cholesterol. It decreases low-density lipoproteins (LDL), the fraction of total blood cholesterol that increases the risk of coronary heart disease. This drug also increases high-density lipoproteins (HDL), the cholesterol fraction that is thought to reduce the risk of heart disease.

Available Dosage Forms and Strengths

Tablets — 10 mg, 20 mg, 40 mg

▷ **Usual Adult Dosage Range:** Initially 20 mg once a day with the evening meal. Dose may be increased up to 40 mg twice a day as needed and tolerated. Dosage adjustments should be made at 4-week intervals. Limited data support low-dose therapy, where some patients responded to 20 mg as a single evening dose. Maximum daily dosage should not exceed 80 mg. **Note: Actual dose and dosing schedule must be determined for each patient individually.**

Conditions Requiring Dosing Adjustments

Liver Function: This drug should be used with caution by patients with liver compromise. 83% of a dose is removed in the feces.

Kidney Function: Great caution should be used in considering doses above 20 mg per day for patients with severe kidney problems (creatinine clearance less than 30 ml/min).

▷ **Dosing Instructions:** Take with food, preferably with the evening meal for maximal effectiveness. Highest rates of cholesterol production occur between midnight and 5 A.M. Tablet may be crushed.

Usual Duration of Use: Use on a regular schedule for 4 to 6 weeks determines effectiveness in reducing blood levels of total and LDL cholesterol. Long-term use (months to years) requires periodic physician evaluation of response.

Possible Advantages of This Drug: Recent studies indicate that this drug is more effective and better tolerated than other drugs currently available for reducing total and LDL cholesterol. Its long-term effects are yet to be determined.

▷ **This Drug Should Not Be Taken If**
- you have had an allergic reaction to it previously.
- you have active liver disease.
- you are pregnant or breast-feeding.

▷ **Inform Your Physician Before Taking This Drug If**
- you have a history of liver disease or impaired liver function.
- you have had peptic ulcer disease or upper gastrointestinal bleeding.
- you are not using any method of birth control, or you are planning pregnancy.
- you have a history of kidney compromise.
- you regularly consume substantial amounts of alcohol.
- you have cataracts or impaired vision.
- you have any type of chronic muscular disorder.

Possible Side Effects (natural, expected, and unavoidable drug actions)
Development of abnormal liver function tests without associated symptoms.

▷ **Possible Adverse Effects** (unusual, unexpected, and infrequent reactions)
If any of the following develop, consult your physician promptly for guidance.
Mild Adverse Effects
Allergic Reactions: Skin rash, itching.
Headache, insomnia, dizziness, blurred vision, altered taste—rare to infrequent.
Indigestion, stomach pain, nausea, excessive gas, constipation, diarrhea—infrequent.
Muscle cramps or pain—infrequent.
Impaired sense of smell—possible.
Serious Adverse Effects
Marked and persistent abnormal liver function tests with focal hepatitis (without jaundice) after 1 year of use—rare.
Acute myopathy (muscle pain and tenderness) or rhabdomyolysis—case reports.
Cataracts were a concern based on some early data; however, long-term information fails to demonstrate any adverse effect on the lens of the eye.
Neuropathy or systemic-lupus-erythematosus-like syndrome—case reports.

▷ **Possible Effects on Sexual Function**
None reported.

Possible Delayed Adverse Effects: Myopathy.

Natural Diseases or Disorders That May Be Activated by This Drug
Latent liver disease.

Possible Effects on Laboratory Tests
Blood alanine aminotransferase (ALT) enzyme level: increased (with higher doses of drug).
Blood total cholesterol, LDL cholesterol, and triglyceride levels: decreased.
Blood HDL cholesterol level: increased.

CAUTION
1. Stop the drug immediately and call your doctor if you become pregnant.
2. Promptly report development of unexplained muscle pain or tenderness.
3. Call your doctor right away if altered or impaired vision happens.

Precautions for Use

By Infants and Children: Safety and effectiveness for those under 20 years of age are not established.

By Those Over 60 Years of Age: Tell your doctor about any personal or family history of cataracts. Comply with periodic eye examinations. Promptly report any alterations in vision.

▷ **Advisability of Use During Pregnancy**

Pregnancy Category: X. See Pregnancy Risk Categories at the back of this book.

Animal studies: Mouse and rat studies reveal skeletal birth defects due to this drug.

Human studies: Adequate studies of pregnant women are not available.

This drug should be avoided during entire pregnancy.

Advisability of Use If Breast-Feeding

Presence of this drug in breast milk: Probably yes.

Avoid drug or refrain from nursing.

Habit-Forming Potential: None.

Effects of Overdosage: Increased indigestion, stomach distress, nausea, diarrhea.

Possible Effects of Long-Term Use: Abnormal liver function with focal hepatitis. Studies in rats with three to four times the human dose have resulted in increases in hepatocellular carcinoma (cancer). Clinical significance in humans is not known.

Suggested Periodic Examinations While Taking This Drug (at physician's discretion)

Blood cholesterol studies: total cholesterol, HDL and LDL fractions.

Liver function tests every 4 to 6 weeks during the first 15 months of use and periodically thereafter.

Complete eye examination at beginning of treatment and periodically thereafter. Ask your physician for guidance.

▷ **While Taking This Drug, Observe the Following**

Foods: Follow a standard low cholesterol diet.

Beverages: No restrictions. May be taken with milk.

▷   *Alcohol:* No interactions expected. Use sparingly.

Tobacco Smoking: No interactions expected, but I advise everyone to quit smoking.

▷   *Other Drugs*

Lovastatin *taken concurrently* with
- clofibrate (Atromid-S, others) may result in a severe rhabdomyolysis.
- cyclosporine (Sandimmune) can cause a severe myopathy.
- erythromycin (E.E.S.) and perhaps other macrolide antibiotics (azithromycin, clarithromycin, or dirithromycin) may result in severe rhabdomyolysis.
- gemfibrozil (Lopid) may cause myopathy.
- niacin (various) can cause myopathy.

- warfarin may result in bleeding. Increased frequency of INR (prothrombin time or protime) testing is suggested.

▷ *Driving, Hazardous Activities:* This drug may cause dizziness or impaired vision. Restrict activities as necessary.

Aviation Note: The use of this drug *may be a disqualification* for piloting. Consult a designated Aviation Medical Examiner.

Exposure to Sun: No restrictions.

Discontinuation: Do not stop this drug without your physician's knowledge and guidance.

MACROLIDE ANTIBIOTICS (ma KRO lied)

Azithromycin (a zith roh MY sin)   **Clarithromycin** (KLAR ith roh my sin)
Erythromycin (er ith roh MY sin)

Introduced: 1991, 1991, 1952, respectively   **Class:** Anti-infective, antibiotic, macrolide antibiotic   **Prescription:** USA: Yes   **Controlled Drug:** USA: No; Canada: No   **Available as Generic:** Azithromycin: No; clarithromycin: no; erythromycin: yes

Brand Names: Azithromycin: Zithromax; Clarithromycin: Biaxin; Erythromycin: AK-Mycin Ophthalmic, Akne-Mycin, ✦Apo-Erythro Base, ✦Apo-Erythro E-C, ✦Apo-Erythro-ES, ✦Apo-Erythro-S, A/T/S, Benzamycin [CD], C-Solve 2, E.E.S., E.E.S. 200, E.E.S. 400, Emgel, E-Mycin, E-Mycin Controlled Release, E-Mycin E, E-Mycin 333, Eramycin, ✦Erybid, ERYC, Erycette, Eryderm, Erygel, Erymax, Erypar, EryPed, Ery-Tab, Erythrocin, ✦Erythromid, E-Solve 2, ETS-2%, Ilosone, Ilotycin, ✦Novorythro, PCE, Pediamycin, ✦Pediazole [CD], ✦PMS-Erythromycin, Robimycin, Sans-Acne, SK-Erythromycin, Staticin, ✦Stievamycin, T-Stat, Wyamycin E, Wyamycin S

BENEFITS versus RISKS	
Possible Benefits	*Possible Risks*
EFFECTIVE TREATMENT OF INFECTIONS due to susceptible microorganisms	Allergic reactions, mild and infrequent
	Liver reaction (most common with erythromycin estolate)
	Mild gastrointestinal symptoms
	Drug-induced colitis
	Superinfections

▷ **Principal Uses**

As a Single Drug Product: Uses currently included in FDA-approved labeling: Treatment of (1) skin and skin structure infections (such as acne and *Streptococcus*); (2) upper and lower respiratory tract infections, including "strep" throat, diphtheria, and several types of pneumonia; (3) gonorrhea and syphilis; (4) amebic dysentery (erythromycin); (5) Legionnaire's disease (erythromycin); (6) long-term prevention of recurrences of rheumatic fever (erythromycin). Effective use requires the precise identification of the causative organism and determination of its sensitivity to a macrolide antibiotic; (7) treatment of mycoplasmal pneumonia; (8) listeriosis; (9) neonatal conjunctivitis (erythromycin); (10) treatment of ear infections (otitis media) (azithromycin, erythromycin); (11) treatment of AIDS-related *Mycobacterium avium-intracellulare complex* (azithromycin or clarithromycin); (12) azithromycin treats *Chlamydia trachomatis* urethritis; (13) therapy of *Helicobacter pylori* duodenal ulcers in combination with omeprazole (clarithromycin).

Author's Note: A recent Agency for Health Care Policy and Research (AHCPR) study found that most patients who were 60 or younger obtained the same outcomes and significantly reduced costs when erythromycin was used to treat community-acquired pneumonia.

Other (unlabeled) generally accepted uses: (1) Treatment of early Lyme disease (erythromycin; azithromycin is an alternative drug); (2) erythromycin helps sterilize the bowel before surgical procedures; (3) may help threatened preterm labor if the cause is *Ureaplasma* organisms (erythromycin); (4) helps impetigo (erythromycin); (5) treatment of *Helicobacter pylori* (7-day course of azithromycin); (6) azithromycin or clarithromycin are second choice for Legionnaire's disease; may treat some heart attacks.

How These Drugs Work: They prevent growth and multiplication of susceptible organisms by interfering with their formation of essential proteins.

Available Dosage Forms and Strengths

Azithromycin:

Capsules —	250 mg
Oral suspension —	100 mg/5 ml—200 mg/5 ml

Clarithromycin:

Tablets —	250 mg, 500 mg
Oral suspension granules —	125 mg, 250 mg

Erythromycin:

Capsules —	125 mg, 250 mg
Capsules, enteric coated —	125 mg, 250 mg
Drops —	100 mg/ml
Eye ointment —	5 mg/g
Gel —	2%
Oral suspension —	125 mg/5 ml, 250 mg/5 ml
Skin ointment —	2%
Tablets —	250 mg, 500 mg
Tablets, chewable —	125 mg, 200 mg, 250 mg
Tablets, delayed release —	250 mg, 333 mg
Tablets, dispersible (Canada) —	500 mg
Tablets, enteric coated —	250 mg, 333 mg, 500 mg
Tablets, film coated —	250 mg, 500 mg
Topical solution —	1.5%, 2%

▷ **Usual Adult Dosage Range:**   Erythromycin: 250 to 500 mg every 6 hours, according to nature and severity of infection. Total daily dosage should not exceed 4 g. For endocarditis prophylaxis (stearate oral form): 1 g 2 hours before procedure and 500 mg 6 hours later. Pediatrics: oral erythromycin is usually given at a dose of 30 to 50 mg per kg of body mass per day and is divided into three or four doses.

Infants and Children: Azithromycin: Otitis media: 10 mg per kg of body mass as a single dose on the first day (up to 500 mg), followed by 5 mg per kg of body mass (up to 250 mg) on days 2–5. Pharyngitis: 12 mg per kg of body mass (up to 500 mg) daily for 5 days.

Clarithromycin: Used to treat otitis media (caused by *Haemophilus influenzae*, *M. catarrhalis*, or *Strep. pneumoniae*) in children: the dose is 7.5 mg per kg of body mass twice daily, up to a maximum of 500 mg twice a day for 10 days. For *Mycobacterium avium-intracellulare complex* infections in children: the dose is 7.5 mg per kg of body mass twice daily, to a maximum of 500 mg twice a day. If this dose is successful, therapy is continued for life.

12 to 60 Years of Age: Clarithromycin: For pharyngitis/tonsillitis—250 mg every 12 hours for 10 days. For maxillary sinusitis—500 mg every 12 hours for 14 days. For acute bronchitis—250 to 500 mg every 12 hours for 7 to 14 days. For pneumonia—250 mg every 12 hours for 7 to 14 days. For skin infections—250 mg every 12 hours for 7 to 14 days.

16 to 60 Years of Age: Azithromycin: For pharyngitis/tonsillitis, bronchitis, pneumonia, and skin infections—500 mg as a single dose on the first day, then 250 mg once daily on days 2–4 for a total dose of 1.5 g. For *Helicobacter pylori*: 500 mg daily for 7 days. For nongonococcal urethritis and cervicitis—a single 1 g (1000 mg) dose.

Over 60 Years of Age: Azithromycin: Same as 16 to 60 years of age. If liver or kidney function is limited, the dose must be reduced.

Clarithromycin: Same as 12 to 60 years of age. Dose must be reduced in kidney compromise. **Note: Actual dosage and administration schedule must be determined for each patient individually.**

Conditions Requiring Dosing Adjustments

Liver Function: These drugs are metabolized in the liver, and will accumulate in patients with liver compromise. Decreased doses may be needed. They should be used with caution by patients with biliary tract disease. Clarithromycin does not need to be adjusted for patients with liver problems if kidney function is normal.

Kidney Function: No dosing changes are needed for azithromycin. The dose of clarithromycin **must be decreased** or **the time between doses (dosing interval) prolonged** for patients with compromised kidneys. Patients with severe kidney failure can take 50–75% of the usual erythromycin dose at the usual time. Azithromycin and erythromycin are rare causes of interstitial nephritis (inflammation of a specific part of the kidney).

▷ **Dosing Instructions:** Nonenteric-coated preparations should be taken 1 hour before or 2 hours after eating. Enteric-coated preparations may be taken without regard to food. Azithromycin may be better tolerated if taken with food. Do not take azithromycin with antacids containing aluminum or magnesium. Regular uncoated capsules may be opened and tablets may be crushed for administration; coated and prolonged-action preparations should be swallowed whole. Ask your pharmacist for guidance.

Usual Duration of Use: Use on a regular schedule for 3 to 5 days is necessary to determine this drug's effectiveness in controlling infections. For streptococcal infections: not less than 10 consecutive (5 consecutive for azithromycin) days (without interruption) to reduce the possibility of developing rheumatic fever or glomerulonephritis. The duration of use should not exceed the time required to eliminate the infection.

Possible Advantages of This Drug

Azithromycin and clarithromycin: Broader spectrum of infectious microorganism coverage; equivalent to erythromycin, some penicillins, and some cephalosporins. Effective with fewer doses (only one dose for azithromycin and two for clarithromycin). Azithromycin and clarithromycin are very well tolerated; infrequent and minor adverse effects.

▷ **These Drugs Should Not Be Taken If**
- you have had an allergic reaction to any form of erythromycin previously.
- you have active liver disease (erythromycin estolate form).
- you are pregnant or planning pregnancy (some forms).
- you are allergic to *para*-aminobenzoic-acid-type anesthetics (intramuscular form of erythromycin).
- you are taking terfenadine (Seldane) or astemizole (Hismanal).

▷ **Inform Your Physician Before Taking This Drug If**
- you have a history of a previous "reaction" to any macrolide antibiotic.
- you are allergic by nature: hay fever, asthma, hives, eczema.
- you have a blood disorder.
- you have an abnormal heart rhythm.
- you have a history of porphyria.
- you have a history of kidney disorder.
- you have myasthenia gravis.
- you have a hearing disorder.
- you have a history of low blood platelets (some macrolides).
- you have taken the estolate form of erythromycin previously.

Possible Side Effects (natural, expected, and unavoidable drug actions)

Superinfections (see Glossary).

▷ **Possible Adverse Effects** (unusual, unexpected, and infrequent reactions)

If any of the following develop, consult your physician promptly for guidance.

Mild Adverse Effects

Allergic Reactions: Skin rash, hives, itching—rare.

Nausea, vomiting, diarrhea, abdominal cramping—infrequent.

Headache—rare.

Drug-induced increased liver enzymes (see Jaundice in Glossary)—rare.

Serious Adverse Effects

Allergic Reaction: Anaphylactic reaction (see Glossary)—rare.

Idiosyncratic Reactions: Liver reaction: nausea, vomiting, fever, jaundice (usually, but not exclusively, associated with erythromycin estolate).

Decreased white blood cells (erythromycin)—rare.

Lowered blood platelets (clarithromycin)—case report.

Abnormal heart rhythm—rare.

Worsening of myasthenia gravis—case reports.

Low body temperature (hypothermia)—rare.

Pseudomembranous colitis—rare.

Pancreatitis (erythromycin)—rare.

Kidney problems (interstitial nephritis) (azithromycin, erythromycin)—case reports.

Hearing loss (ototoxicity)—case reports.

▷ **Possible Effects on Sexual Function:**   None reported.

▷ **Adverse Effects That May Mimic Natural Diseases or Disorders**
Liver toxicity may resemble acute gallbladder disease or viral hepatitis.

Possible Effects on Laboratory Tests
Complete blood cell counts: white cells may increase or decrease; eosinophils increased (allergic reaction); platelets decreased.
INR (prothrombin time): increased (drug taken concurrently with warfarin).
Liver function tests: liver enzymes increased (ALT/GPT, AST/GOT, and alkaline phosphatase), increased bilirubin.

CAUTION
1. Take the **full dosage prescribed** to help prevent resistant bacteria.
2. If you have a history of liver disease or impaired liver function, avoid any form of erythromycin estolate.
3. If diarrhea develops and continues for more than 24 hours, consult your physician promptly.

Precautions for Use
By Infants and Children: Watch allergic children closely for indications of developing allergy to this drug. Observe also for evidence of gastrointestinal irritation. Dosing based on body mass is critical.
By Those Over 60 Years of Age: Watch for itching reactions in the genital and anal regions, often due to yeast superinfections. Observe also for evidence of hearing loss. Report such developments promptly. If liver or kidney function is impaired, dosage decreases must be considered.

▷ **Advisability of Use During Pregnancy**
Pregnancy Category: C for clarithromycin. B for others. See Pregnancy Risk Categories at the back of this book.
Animal studies: Studies of rats are inconclusive for erythromycin. Monkey, rabbit, and rat studies have shown problems in pregnancy outcomes and fetal development.
Human studies: Information from adequate studies of pregnant women is not available.
Generally thought to be safe during entire pregnancy, *except for erythromycin estolate*; this form of erythromycin can cause toxic liver reactions during pregnancy and should be avoided. Clarithromycin should be avoided unless no other antibiotic option is available.

Advisability of Use If Breast-Feeding
Presence of this drug in breast milk: Yes for others; clarithromycin unknown. Watch nursing infant closely and discontinue drug or nursing if adverse effects develop.

Habit-Forming Potential: None.

Effects of Overdosage: Possible nausea, vomiting, hallucinations (clarithromycin), diarrhea, and abdominal discomfort.

Possible Effects of Long-Term Use: Superinfections (see Glossary).

Suggested Periodic Examinations While Taking This Drug (at physician's discretion)
Liver function tests if the erythromycin estolate form is used. Complete blood counts to measure response of infection.

▷ **While Taking This Drug, Observe the Following**

> *Foods:* New formulation absorption is decreased by more than 70% (especially high-fat meals) and effectiveness may be seriously compromised for erythromycin. Azithromycin and clarithromycin are not affected.

> *Beverages:* Avoid fruit juices and carbonated beverages for 1 hour after taking any nonenteric-coated preparation of erythromycin. May be taken with milk.

▷   *Alcohol:* Avoid if you have impaired liver function or are taking the estolate form.

> *Tobacco Smoking:* No interactions expected, but I advise everyone to quit smoking.

▷   *Other Drugs*

> These medicines may ***increase*** the effects of
> - benzodiazepines (see Drug Classes).
> - carbamazepine (Tegretol), and cause toxicity.
> - digoxin (Lanoxin), and cause toxicity.
> - ergotamine (Cafergot, Ergostat, etc.), and cause impaired circulation to extremities.
> - methylprednisolone (Medrol) and prednisone, and cause excess steroid effects.
> - tacrolimus (Prograf).
> - theophylline (aminophylline, Theo-Dur, etc.), and cause toxicity.
> - warfarin (Coumadin), and increase the risk of bleeding.

> These medicines may ***decrease*** the effects of
> - clindamycin.
> - lincomycin.
> - penicillins.

> These medicines ***taken concurrently*** with
> - astemizole (Hismanal) may cause serious arrhythmias.
> - birth control pills (oral contraceptives) can cause loss of effectiveness and result in pregnancy.
> - cisapride (Propulsid) (clarithromycin only) may lead to cisapride toxicity.
> - cyclosporine (Sandimmune) may result in cyclosporine toxicity.
> - dihydroergotamine and other ergot derivatives can lead to increased levels and ergot toxicity.
> - disopyramide may cause heart (cardiac) arrhythmias.
> - loratadine (Claritin) may result in increased loratadine levels, but they do not appear to cause the serious arrythmias of some of the other nonsedating antihistamines. Since loratadine levels may be increased, it may be prudent to decrease loratadine doses while taking erythromycin.
> - lovastatin can cause rhabdomyolysis (serious muscle damage).
> - midazolam (and probably other benzodiazepines—see Drug Classes) may lead to excessive central nervous system depression.
> - nevirapine (Viramune) may lead to nevirapine toxicity.
> - ritonavir (Norvir) and perhaps other protease inhibitors (see Drug Classes) may lead to toxicity.
> - terfenadine (Seldane) can cause cardiac (heart) arrhythmias.
> - triazolam may cause toxicity.
> - trimexate (Mexate) decrease trimexate metabolism and can lead to toxicity.
> - valproic acid (Depakene, Depakote) can lead to toxic blood levels.

- zidovudine (AZT) may lead to decreased levels and lack of zidovudine effectiveness.

▷ *Driving, Hazardous Activities:* This drug may cause nausea and/or diarrhea. Restrict activities as necessary.

Aviation Note: The use of this drug **may be a disqualification** for piloting. Consult a designated Aviation Medical Examiner.

Exposure to Sun: Use caution; some medicines in this class have caused increased sensitivity to the sun (photosensitivity).

Special Storage Instructions: Keep liquid forms refrigerated.

Observe the Following Expiration Times: Freshly mixed oral suspension—14 days. Premixed oral suspension—18 months. Ask your pharmacist for help.

MAPROTILINE (ma PROH ti leen)

Introduced: 1974   **Class:** Antidepressant   **Prescription:** USA: Yes
Controlled Drug: USA: No; Canada: No   **Available as Generic:**   Yes
Brand Name: Ludiomil

BENEFITS versus RISKS	
Possible Benefits	*Possible Risks*
EFFECTIVE RELIEF OF ALL TYPES OF DEPRESSION	ADVERSE BEHAVIORAL EFFECTS CONVERSION OF DEPRESSION TO MANIA in manic-depressive (bipolar) disorders
	Irregular heart rhythms
	Liver toxicity with jaundice
	Seizures with therapeutic doses
	Low white blood cells

Author's Note: Because use of this medicine has declined in favor of newer medicines, the information in this profile has been abbreviated.

MECLOFENAMATE (me kloh fen AM ayt)

See the fenamates (nonsteroidal anti-inflammatory drugs) profile for further information.

MEDROXYPROGESTERONE (me DROX e proh jess te rohn)

Introduced: 1959   **Class:** Female sex hormones, progestins   **Prescription:** USA: Yes   **Controlled Drug:**   USA: No; Canada: No   **Available as Generic:**   Yes

Brand Names: Amen, Curretab, Cycrin, Depo-Provera, Premphase, Prempro, Provera

BENEFITS versus RISKS	
Possible Benefits	*Possible Risks*
EFFECTIVE TREATMENT OF ABSENT OR ABNORMAL MENSTRUATION due to hormone imbalance	Thrombophlebitis
	Pulmonary embolism
	Liver reaction with jaundice
	Drug-induced birth defects
EFFECTIVE CONTRACEPTION when given by injection	
Useful adjunctive therapy in selected cases of uterine and kidney cancer	

▷ **Principal Uses**

As a Single Drug Product: Uses currently included in FDA-approved labeling: (1) Used to initiate and regulate menstruation and correct abnormal patterns of menstrual bleeding caused by hormonal imbalance (and not by organic disease); (2) used in combination to treat metastatic, inoperable, or recurrent endometrial carcinoma; (3) treatment of renal cell carcinoma; (4) used as a contraceptive injected into the muscle once every 3 months; (5) helps dysfunctional uterine bleeding.

Other (unlabeled) generally accepted uses: (1) Used as a part of combination therapy in breast, refractory prostate, lung, and ovarian cancers; (2) therapy of endometriosis; (3) used in osteoporosis to help increase bone mineral density; (4) helps abnormal hair growth in women (hirsutism); (5) can help breast pain (mastodynia); (6) used in combination with estrogen to help symptoms of menopause; (7) can be of use in pelvic congestion and pickwickian syndrome; (8) may help severe PMS; (9) can be of use in male hypersexuality.

How This Drug Works: By inducing and maintaining a lining in the uterus that resembles pregnancy, this drug can prevent uterine bleeding until it is withdrawn. By suppressing the release of the pituitary gland hormone that induces ovulation, and by stimulating the secretion of mucus by the uterine cervix (to resist the passage of sperm), this drug can prevent pregnancy.

Available Dosage Forms and Strengths

Injection — 150 mg (single-dose vials)
— 100, 150, and 400 mg/ml
Tablets — 2.5 mg, 5 mg, 10 mg

▷ **Usual Adult Dosage Range:** To initiate menstruation: 5 to 10 mg daily for 5 to 10 days, started at any time.

To correct abnormal bleeding: 5 to 10 mg daily for 5 to 10 days, started on the 16th or 21st day of the menstrual cycle. Withdrawal bleeding usually begins within 3 to 7 days after stopping the drug.

As a contraceptive: Intramuscular injections of 150 mg every 3 months are needed.

Note: Actual dosage and administration schedule must be determined for each patient individually.

Conditions Requiring Dosing Adjustments

Liver Function: This drug should be used with caution, and the dose empirically decreased, by patients with liver compromise.

Kidney Function: The kidneys are not involved in the elimination of this medication.

▷ **Dosing Instructions:** The tablet may be crushed and taken on an empty stomach or with food to prevent nausea.

Usual Duration of Use: Use on a regular schedule for two or three menstrual cycles determines effectiveness in correcting abnormal patterns of menstrual bleeding. Consult your physician on a regular basis.

▷ **This Drug Should Not Be Taken If**
- you have had an allergic reaction to it previously.
- you are pregnant.
- you have experienced a missed abortion.
- you have seriously impaired liver function.
- you have a history of cancer of the breast or reproductive organs.
- you have a history of thrombophlebitis, embolism, or stroke.
- you have abnormal and unexplained vaginal bleeding.

▷ **Inform Your Physician Before Taking This Drug If**
- you have impaired kidney function.
- you have any of the following disorders: asthma, diabetes, emotional depression, epilepsy, heart disease, migraine headaches.

Possible Side Effects (natural, expected, and unavoidable drug actions)
Fluid retention, weight gain, changes in menstrual timing and flow, spotting between periods.

▷ **Possible Adverse Effects** (unusual, unexpected, and infrequent reactions)
If any of the following develop, consult your physician promptly for guidance.
Mild Adverse Effects
Allergic Reactions: Skin rash, hives, itching.
Fatigue, weakness, nausea—infrequent.
Acne, excessive hair growth—case reports.
Serious Adverse Effects
Liver toxicity with jaundice (see Glossary): yellow eyes/skin, dark-colored urine, light-colored stools—possible.
Thrombophlebitis (inflammation of a vein with blood clot formation): pain or tenderness in thigh or leg, with or without swelling of the foot, ankle, or leg—case reports.
Pulmonary embolism (movement of blood clot to lung): sudden shortness of breath, chest pain, cough, bloody sputum—case reports.
Stroke (blood clot in the brain): sudden headache, weakness or paralysis of any part of the body—possible.
Retinal thrombosis (blood clot in the eye): sudden impairment or loss of vision—case reports.
Drug-induced pseudotumor cerebri—possible.
Pneumonitis, especially in patients who have received radiation therapy—case reports.

▷ **Possible Effects on Sexual Function**
Altered timing and pattern of menstruation. Female breast tenderness and secretion. Decreased vaginal secretions. Infertility—case reports.

▷ **Adverse Effects That May Mimic Natural Diseases or Disorders**
Liver toxicity may suggest viral hepatitis.

Possible Effects on Laboratory Tests

Blood total cholesterol, HDL cholesterol, LDL cholesterol, and triglyceride levels: decreased.

Glucose tolerance test (GTT): decreased.

CAUTION

1. There is an increased risk of birth defects in children whose mothers take this drug during the first 4 months of pregnancy.
2. Inform your physician promptly if you think you may be pregnant.
3. This drug should not be used as a test for pregnancy.

Precautions for Use

By Infants and Children: Not used in this age group.

By Those Over 60 Years of Age: Used as adjunctive therapy in cancer of the breast, uterus, prostate, and kidney. Watch for excessive fluid retention.

▷ **Advisability of Use During Pregnancy**

Pregnancy Category: D. See Pregnancy Risk Categories at the back of this book.

Animal studies: Genital defects reported in rat and rabbit studies; masculinization of the female rodent fetus; various defects in chick embryos and rabbits.

Human studies: In a study of 1,016 pregnancies, oral doses of 80–120 mg daily used from the 5th–7th week of pregnancy up to the 18th week were not associated with teratogenic effects. Other data show masculinization of the female genitals: enlargement of the clitoris, fusion of the labia. Increased risk of heart, nervous system, and limb defects when used in the second and third trimesters of pregnancy.

The drug is used as a benefit-to-risk decision in the first 3 months of pregnancy. Avoid this drug completely during the final 6 months of pregnancy.

Advisability of Use If Breast-Feeding

Presence of this drug in breast milk: Yes.

Avoid drug or refrain from nursing.

Habit-Forming Potential: None.

Effects of Overdosage: Nausea, vomiting, fluid retention, breast enlargement and discomfort, abnormal vaginal bleeding.

Possible Effects of Long-Term Use: There has been considerable controversy regarding use of this drug and cancer. The most recent large patient studies do not show an increased relative risk that is statistically significant.

Suggested Periodic Examinations While Taking This Drug (at physician's discretion)

Regular examinations (every 6 to 12 months) of the breasts and reproductive organs (pelvic examination of the uterus and ovaries, including Pap smear).

▷ **While Taking This Drug, Observe the Following**

Foods: No restrictions.

Beverages: No restrictions.

▷ *Alcohol:* No interactions expected.

Tobacco Smoking: I advise everyone to quit smoking.

▷ *Other Drugs*

The following drugs may *decrease* the effects of medroxyprogesterone
- rifampin (Rifadin, Rimactane, etc.) may hasten its elimination.

Medroxyprogesterone *taken concurrently* with
- digitoxin may result in slightly higher than expected digoxin levels.

- ritonavir (Norvir) and perhaps other protease inhibitors (see Drug Classes) may lead to toxicity.
- tamoxifen (Nolvadex) may result in blunting of the therapeutic benefits of tamoxifen.
- warfarin (Coumadin) may increase warfarin effects. Increased lab INR (prothrombin time or protime) testing is needed.

▷ *Driving, Hazardous Activities:* Usually no restrictions. Ask your doctor about your individual risk and for guidance regarding specific restrictions.

Aviation Note: The use of this drug **may be a disqualification** for piloting. Consult a designated Aviation Medical Examiner.

Exposure to Sun: No restrictions.

MEFENAMIC ACID (me FEN am ik a sid)

See the fenamates (nonsteroidal anti-inflammatory drugs) profile for further information.

MEPERIDINE (me PER i deen)

Other Name: Pethidine

Introduced: 1939   **Class:** Strong analgesic, opioids   **Prescription:** USA: Yes   **Controlled Drug:** USA: C-II*; Canada: Yes   **Available as Generic:** Yes

Brand Names: Demerol, Demerol APAP [CD], Mepergan, Pethadol

BENEFITS versus RISKS	
Possible Benefits	*Possible Risks*
EFFECTIVE RELIEF OF MODERATE TO SEVERE PAIN	POTENTIAL FOR HABIT FORMATION (DEPENDENCE)
	Weakness, fainting
	Disorientation, hallucinations
	Interference with urination

▷ **Principal Uses**

As a Single Drug Product: Uses currently included in FDA-approved labeling: Used by mouth or injection to relieve moderate to severe pain of any cause. Other (unlabeled) generally accepted uses: (1) Used to treat fevers caused by amphotericin B; (2) can help porphyrias; (3) eases postanesthesia chills; (4) used for sickle cell disease pain.

As a Combination Drug Product [CD]: This drug is available in combination with acetaminophen (Demerol APAP) to create a dosage form that utilizes two pain relievers, and also reduces fever.

How This Drug Works: Acting primarily as a depressant of certain brain functions, this drug suppresses the perception of pain and calms the emotional response to pain.

*See schedules of Controlled Drugs at the back of this book.

Available Dosage Forms and Strengths

    Injection — 10 mg/ml, 25 mg/ml, 50 mg/ml, 75 mg/ml, 100 mg/ml

     Syrup — 50 mg/5 ml teaspoonful

     Tablets — 50 mg, 100 mg

▷ **Usual Adult Dosage Range:**   Taken by mouth: 50 to 150 mg every 3 to 4 hours to relieve pain. The usual dose is 100 mg. The total daily dosage should not exceed 900 mg. **Note: Actual dosage and dosing schedule must be determined for each patient individually.**

    Author's Note: The old "as-needed" dosing has been replaced by scheduled (such as every 4 hours) dosing because it can keep pain from happening, rather than trying to treat it after a pain medicine blood level has gotten low enough to allow pain to return.

Conditions Requiring Dosing Adjustments

    Liver Function: The initial dose should be the same in liver compromise; however, subsequent doses should be decreased by 50% or the dosing interval doubled. Some clinicians report that doses of 25 to 50 mg have produced acceptable effects in some patients with severe liver disease.

    Kidney Function: Patients with mild to moderate kidney failure should take 75% of the usual dose at the usual interval. Patients with severe kidney failure should take 50% of the usual dose at the usual time. **Multiple doses should be avoided** as a toxic (normeperidine) metabolite may accumulate and can cause severe central nervous system reactions.

▷ **Dosing Instructions:**   The tablet may be crushed and taken with or following food to reduce stomach irritation or nausea. The syrup may be diluted in 4 ounces of water to reduce the numbing effect on the tongue and mouth tissues.

Usual Duration of Use: As required to control pain. Current pain therapy often uses timed or scheduled doses to prevent pain rather than treat it. Continual use should not exceed 5 to 7 days without interruption and reassessment of need.

▷ **This Drug Should Not Be Taken If**

- you have had an allergic reaction to any dosage form of it previously.
- you are having an acute attack of asthma.
- you have increased intracranial pressure (talk with your doctor).
- you have an abnormal heart rhythm (atrioventricular flutter).
- you have a history of convulsions or seizures.
- you have a history of kidney failure and multiple doses are scheduled.
- you have significant respiratory depression.
- you are taking, or have taken within the past 14 days, any monoamine oxidase (MAO) type A inhibitor drug (see Drug Classes).

▷ **Inform Your Physician Before Taking This Drug If**

- you have a history of drug abuse or alcoholism.
- you have impaired liver or kidney function.
- you have a history of asthma, epilepsy, or glaucoma.
- you are taking any other drugs that have a sedative effect.
- you plan to have surgery under general anesthesia in the near future.

Possible Side Effects (natural, expected, and unavoidable drug actions)

    Drowsiness, light-headedness, weakness, euphoria, dry mouth, urinary retention, constipation. Dose-related respiratory depression.

▷ **Possible Adverse Effects** (unusual, unexpected, and infrequent reactions)
If any of the following develop, consult your physician promptly for guidance.

Mild Adverse Effects

Allergic Reactions: Skin rash, hives, itching.

Headache, dizziness, impaired concentration, sensation of drunkenness, confusion, depression, blurred or double vision—infrequent, but can be dose related.

Facial flushing, sweating, heart palpitation—case reports.

Nausea, vomiting—infrequent to frequent and can be dose related.

Serious Adverse Effects

Allergic Reactions: Anaphylactic reactions.

Drop in blood pressure, causing severe weakness and fainting—case reports and dose related.

Disorientation, hallucinations, unstable gait, tremor, muscle twitching—possible, case reports.

Drug-induced myasthenia gravis—case reports.

Urinary retention—possible.

Kidney failure—rare.

Seizures, especially in patients with kidney failure who are given multiple doses (normeperidine accumulation)—case reports.

▷ **Possible Effects on Sexual Function:**   Blunting of sexual response. Retrograde ejaculation.

▷ **Adverse Effects That May Mimic Natural Diseases or Disorders**
Paradoxical behavioral disturbances may suggest psychotic disorder.

Possible Effects on Laboratory Tests

Blood alanine aminotransferase (ALT) and aspartate aminotransferase (AST) levels: increased (natural side effects).

Blood amylase and lipase levels: increased (natural side effects).

CAUTION

1. If you have asthma, chronic bronchitis, or emphysema, excessive use of this drug may cause significant respiratory difficulty, thickening of bronchial secretions, and suppression of coughing.

2. The concurrent use of this drug with atropinelike drugs can increase the risk of urinary retention and reduced intestinal function.

3. Do not take this drug following acute head injury.

Precautions for Use

By Infants and Children: Do not use this drug in infants under 1 year of age because of their vulnerability to life-threatening respiratory depression.

By Those Over 60 Years of Age: Small doses initially and slow increases as needed and tolerated. Limit use to short-term treatment only if possible. There may be increased risk of drowsiness, dizziness, unsteadiness, falling, urinary retention, and constipation (often leading to fecal impaction).

▷ **Advisability of Use During Pregnancy**

Pregnancy Category: B; D if used in higher doses or for a longer period of time, especially when the baby is due to be born. See Pregnancy Risk Categories at the back of this book.

Animal studies: Significant birth defects reported in hamster studies.

Human studies: Adequate studies of pregnant women are not available. However, no significant increase in birth defects was found in 1,100 drug exposures.

Avoid during the first 3 months. Use sparingly and in small doses during the final 6 months only if clearly needed, as it has clear effects on the breathing capabilities of the infant.

Advisability of Use If Breast-Feeding

Presence of this drug in breast milk: Yes.

Avoid drug or refrain from nursing.

Habit-Forming Potential: This drug can cause psychological and physical dependence (see Glossary).

Effects of Overdosage: Marked drowsiness, confusion, tremors, convulsions, stupor leading to coma.

Possible Effects of Long-Term Use: Psychological and physical dependence, chronic constipation.

Suggested Periodic Examinations While Taking This Drug (at physician's discretion)

Should assess bowel status if prone to constipation.

▷ **While Taking This Drug, Observe the Following**

Foods: No restrictions.

Beverages: No restrictions. May be taken with milk.

▷ *Alcohol:* Opioid analgesics can intensify the intoxicating effects of alcohol, and alcohol can intensify the depressant effects of opioids on brain function, breathing, and circulation. Alcohol is best avoided.

Tobacco Smoking: No interactions expected, but I advise everyone to quit smoking.

Marijuana Smoking: Increase in drowsiness and pain relief; impairment of mental and physical performance.

▷ *Other Drugs*

Meperidine may *increase* the effects of

- atropinelike drugs, and increase the risk of constipation and urinary retention.
- other drugs with sedative effects.

Meperidine *taken concurrently* with

- acyclovir (Zovirax) may increase risk of nerve toxicity.
- cimetidine (Tagamet), famotidine (Pepcid), nizatidine (Axid), ranitidine (Zantac), and omeprazole (Prilosec) can increase alkalinity of the stomach and may result in increased meperidine levels and toxicity.
- intravenous acyclovir (Zovirax) can result in kidney and nerve problems.
- monoamine oxidase (MAO) type A inhibitor drugs (see Drug Classes) can cause the equivalent of an acute narcotic overdose: unconsciousness, severe breathing depression, slowed heart action and circulation. Can also cause excitability, convulsions, high fever, and rapid heart action.
- phenothiazines (see Drug Classes) can cause excessive and prolonged depression of brain functions, breathing, and circulation.
- phenytoin (Dilantin) can result in decreased therapeutic effects of meperidine.

- ritonavir (Norvir) and perhaps other protease inhibitors (see Drug Classes) may lead to toxicity.
- tricyclic antidepressants (amitriptyline, others) may result in worsening of meperidine's respiratory depression side effect.

▷ *Driving, Hazardous Activities:* This drug can impair mental alertness, judgment, reaction time, and physical coordination. Avoid hazardous activities.

Aviation Note: The use of this drug *is a disqualification* for piloting. Consult a designated Aviation Medical Examiner.

Exposure to Sun: No restrictions.

Discontinuation: This drug is best limited to short-term use. If used for extended periods of time, discontinuation should be gradual to minimize withdrawal effects.

MERCAPTOPURINE (mer kap toh PYUR een)

Other Names: 6-mercaptopurine, 6-MP

Introduced: 1960   **Class:** Anticancer (antineoplastic), immunosuppressant
Prescription: USA: Yes   **Controlled Drug:** USA: No; Canada: No   **Available as Generic:** USA: No; Canada: No

Brand Name: Purinethol

BENEFITS versus RISKS	
Possible Benefits	*Possible Risks*
EFFECTIVE TREATMENT OF CERTAIN ACUTE AND CHRONIC LEUKEMIAS AND LYMPHOMAS	BONE MARROW DEPRESSION (see Glossary)
Effective treatment of polycythemia vera	DRUG-INDUCED LIVER DAMAGE
Possibly effective treatment of Crohn's disease and ulcerative colitis	Rare gastrointestinal ulceration
Possibly effective treatment of severe psoriatic arthritis	

▷ **Principal Uses**

As a Single Drug Product: Uses currently included in FDA-approved labeling: Combination treatment of (1) acute lymphocytic leukemia; (2) acute non-lymphocytic leukemia.

Other (unlabeled) generally accepted uses: Treatment of (1) inflammatory bowel diseases (Crohn's disease and ulcerative colitis); (2) certain cases of severe psoriatic arthritis; (3) may help in cases of autoimmune hepatitis.

How This Drug Works: This drug interferes with specific stages of cell reproduction (tissue growth) by inhibiting the formation of DNA and RNA.

Available Dosage Forms and Strengths

Tablets — 50 mg

▷ **Recommended Dosage Ranges** (Actual dosage and administration schedule must be determined for each patient individually.)

Infants and Children: For leukemia—2.5 mg per kg of body mass (to the nearest

25 mg) daily (roughly 50 mg for the average 5-year-old), in single or divided doses. If the platelets and white blood cell counts do not fall, and clinical improvement is not acceptable after 4 weeks of the induction dosing, the dose may be increased to 5 mg per kg of body mass per day. If there is still no response, some centers give mercaptopurine as 75 mg per square meter on days 29–42. This is combined with vincristine, prednisone, and methotrexate. Maintenance therapy then occurs as in adult dosing.

12 to 60 Years of Age: For leukemia—Induction: initially 2.5 mg per kg of body mass (to the nearest 25 mg) daily, in single or divided doses, for 4 weeks. If the white blood cell or platelet counts do not fall and there is no clinical improvement, the dose may be increased as needed and tolerated to 5 mg per kg of body mass daily. For maintenance, 1.5 to 2.5 mg per kg of body mass daily.

For inflammatory bowel disease—1.5 mg per kg of body mass daily. The dose is subsequently adjusted to keep the platelet count above 100,000 and the white blood cell count above 4,500.

Over 60 Years of Age: Same as 12 to 60 years of age.

Conditions Requiring Dosing Adjustments

Liver Function: This drug should be used with caution and in decreased doses by patients with liver compromise. It is also a rare cause of liver hepatoxicity.

Kidney Function: The dose should be decreased for patients with renal (kidney) compromise to avoid accumulation of this drug. It is a rare cause of drug crystals in urine.

TPMT Negatives: Some patients do not have an enzyme called thiopurine methyltransferase (TPMT). The mercaptopurine dose is decreased by 10% for these patients.

▷ **Dosing Instructions:**   The tablet may be crushed and taken with or following food to reduce stomach upset.

Usual Duration of Use: Use on a regular schedule for 4 to 6 weeks determines effectiveness in inducing remission in leukemia; continual use for 2 to 3 months determines benefit in treating inflammatory bowel disease. Long-term use (months to years) requires periodic physician evaluation.

▷ **This Drug Should Not Be Taken If**
- you have had an allergic reaction to it previously.
- you have a solid tumor or lymphoma (this drug is **not** indicated).
- you have leukemia that has spread to the central nervous system.
- you are pregnant. (Ask your physician for guidance.)

▷ **Inform Your Physician Before Taking This Drug If**
- you have a history of drug-induced bone marrow depression.
- you have impaired liver or kidney function.
- you are not using any contraception.
- you have gout.
- you are taking allopurinol (the mercaptopurine dose must be reduced).
- you have inflammatory bowel disease.
- you do not understand the steps needed to dispose of any vomit or urine.
- you have been exposed recently to chickenpox or herpes zoster (shingles).
- you are taking any of the following drugs: allopurinol, probenecid, sulfinpyrazone, anticoagulants, immunosuppressants.

Possible Side Effects (natural, expected, and unavoidable drug actions)

Bone marrow depression (see Glossary). Abnormally increased blood uric acid levels; possible urate kidney stones, hyperpigmentation of the skin. Possible drug fever.

▷ **Possible Adverse Effects** (unusual, unexpected, and infrequent reactions)

If any of the following develop, consult your physician promptly for guidance.

Mild Adverse Effects

Allergic Reactions: Skin rash, itching, joint pain—case reports.

Headache, weakness—infrequent.

Loss of appetite, mouth and lip sores, nausea, vomiting, diarrhea—infrequent.

Serious Adverse Effects

Liver damage with jaundice (see Glossary)—infrequent.

Kidney damage: fever, cloudy or bloody urine—rare.

Pancreatitis (especially in patients taking this medicine for inflammatory bowel disease)—infrequent.

Gastrointestinal ulceration: stomach pain, bloody or black stools.

Increased cancer risk (carcinogen): one case report of cancer in a patient with bowel disease—possible.

▷ **Possible Effects on Sexual Function:**   Suppression of sperm production. Cessation of menstruation—case reports.

Possible Delayed Adverse Effects: Bone marrow depression may not be apparent during early treatment.

▷ **Adverse Effects That May Mimic Natural Diseases or Disorders**

Drug-induced liver damage may suggest viral hepatitis.

Natural Diseases or Disorders That May Be Activated by This Drug

Latent gout, peptic ulcer disease, inflammatory bowel disease.

Possible Effects on Laboratory Tests

Complete blood cell counts: decreased red cells, hemoglobin, white cells, and platelets.

Blood glucose levels: falsely increased with SMA testing.

Blood uric acid levels: increased.

Liver function tests: increased enzymes (ALT/GPT, AST/GOT, and alkaline phosphatase) or bilirubin.

Kidney function tests: increased blood urea nitrogen (BUN) and creatinine.

Sperm counts: decreased.

CAUTION

1. Comply fully with all requests for periodic laboratory tests.
2. Call your doctor at the first sign of infection or abnormal bleeding or bruising.
3. Inform your physician promptly if you become pregnant.
4. It is best to avoid immunizations while taking this drug, and to avoid contact with people who have recently taken oral poliovirus vaccine.

Precautions for Use

By Infants and Children: No specific problems anticipated.

By Those Over 60 Years of Age: Increased risk of bone marrow depression. Periodic blood counts are mandatory.

▷ **Advisability of Use During Pregnancy**
Pregnancy Category: D. See Pregnancy Risk Categories at the back of this book.
Animal studies: Rat studies reveal toxic effects on the embryo.
Human studies: Adequate studies of pregnant women are not available. This drug is known to cause abortions and premature births.
Avoid drug during entire pregnancy if possible. Use a nonhormonal method of contraception.

Advisability of Use If Breast-Feeding
Presence of this drug in breast milk: Unknown.
Avoid drug or refrain from nursing.

Habit-Forming Potential: None.

Effects of Overdosage: Headache, dizziness, abdominal pain, nausea.

Possible Effects of Long-Term Use: Development of new malignant diseases.

Suggested Periodic Examinations While Taking This Drug (at physician's discretion)
Complete blood cell counts. Blood uric acid levels.
Liver and kidney function tests.

▷ **While Taking This Drug, Observe the Following**
Foods: No restrictions.
Beverages: No restrictions. Drink liquids liberally, up to 2 quarts daily.
▷ *Alcohol:* Avoid completely.
Tobacco Smoking: No interactions expected, but I advise everyone to quit smoking.
▷ *Other Drugs*
Mercaptopurine may ***decrease*** the effects of
• warfarin (Coumadin); the INR (prothrombin time or protime) should be checked more frequently.
The following drug may ***increase*** the effects of mercaptopurine
• allopurinol (Zyloprim). Doses must be reduced to 33% or even as low as 25% of the usual dose if these two medicines are to be combined.
Mercaptopurine ***taken concurrently*** with
• amphotericin B (Abelcet) may increase risk of kidney toxicity or spasm of the bronchi.
• methotrexate (Mexate) can result in mercaptopurine toxicity.
▷ *Driving, Hazardous Activities:* No restrictions.
Aviation Note: The use of this drug ***may be a disqualification*** for piloting. Consult a designated Aviation Medical Examiner.
Exposure to Sun: No restrictions.
Discontinuation: To be determined by your physician.

MESALAMINE (me SAL a meen)

Other Names: Mesalazine, 5-aminosalicylic acid, 5-ASA

Introduced: 1982   **Class:** Bowel anti-inflammatory   **Prescription:** USA: Yes   **Controlled Drug:**   USA: No; Canada: No   **Available as Generic:** USA: No; Canada: No

Brand Names: Asacol, Pentasa, Rowasa, ✦Salofalk

> | **BENEFITS versus RISKS** | |
> | --- | --- |
> | *Possible Benefits* | *Possible Risks* |
> | EFFECTIVE SUPPRESSION OF INFLAMMATORY BOWEL DISEASE | Allergic Reactions: Acute intolerance syndrome, drug-induced kidney damage |

▷ **Principal Uses**

As a Single Drug Product: Uses currently included in FDA-approved labeling: Treatment of active mild to moderate ulcerative colitis, proctosigmoiditis, and proctitis.

Other (unlabeled) generally accepted uses: (1) May help improve semen quality that had been damaged by prior sulfasalazine treatment; (2) can ease canker sores (aphthous ulcers); (3) has a steroid-sparing effect in Crohn's disease; (4) used to maintain remission in ulcerative colitis.

How This Drug Works: This drug suppresses the formation of prostaglandins (and related compounds), tissue substances that induce inflammation, tissue destruction, and diarrhea, the main problems in ulcerative colitis and proctitis.

Available Dosage Forms and Strengths

Capsules, controlled release — 250 mg
Rectal suspension — 4 g per 60-ml unit
Suppositories — 250 mg (Canada) and 500 mg (U.S. and Canada)
Tablets, delayed release — 250 mg, 400 mg, 500 mg

▷ **Recommended Dosage Ranges** (Actual dosage and administration schedule must be determined for each patient individually.)

Infants and Children: Dosage not established.

12 to 60 Years of Age: Rectal suspension—4 g (as a retention enema) every night for 3 to 6 weeks.

Suppositories—500 mg (inserted into rectum) two or three times daily.

Tablets—400 to 800 mg (one or two tablets by mouth) three times daily for 6 weeks. The total daily dose should not exceed 2400 mg.

Over 60 Years of Age: Same as 12 to 60 years of age.

Conditions Requiring Dosing Adjustments

Liver Function: Specific guidelines for dosage adjustment in liver compromise are not available. The drug is changed by the liver and colon wall to Ac-5-ASA.

Kidney Function: This drug should be used with caution in kidney compromise.

▷ **Dosing Instructions:**   Rectal suspension—Use as a retention enema at bedtime. If possible, empty the rectum before inserting suspension; try to retain the suspension all night.

Tablets—Best taken with 8 ounces of water on an empty stomach, 1 hour before or 2 hours after eating. However, it may be taken with or following food to reduce stomach upset. The sustained-release tablet should be swallowed whole without alteration.

Usual Duration of Use: Use on a regular schedule for 1 to 3 weeks determines effectiveness in controlling ulcerative colitis. Long-term use (months to years) requires supervision and periodic physician evaluation.

Possible Advantages of This Drug

Does not cause bone marrow or blood cell disorders.

Does not inhibit sperm production or function.

▷ **This Drug Should Not Be Taken If**

- you have had an allergic reaction to it previously.
- you have severely impaired kidney function.
- you have a known sulfite allergy. (Rectal suspension should NOT be used.)
- you have active ulcer disease.

▷ **Inform Your Physician Before Taking This Drug If**

- you are allergic to aspirin (or other salicylates), olsalazine, or sulfasalazine.
- you are allergic by nature: history of hay fever, asthma, hives, eczema.
- you have impaired liver or kidney function.
- you have a history of a blood clotting (coagulation) disorder.
- you have a history of low white blood cell counts.
- you are taking other medicines that effect the bone marrow. Discuss this with your doctor.
- you are currently taking sulfasalazine (Azulfidine).

Possible Side Effects (natural, expected, and unavoidable drug actions)

Anal irritation (with use of rectal suspension or suppositories). Flu-like syndrome with oral mesalamine use.

▷ **Possible Adverse Effects** (unusual, unexpected, and infrequent reactions)

If any of the following develop, consult your physician promptly for guidance.

Mild Adverse Effects

Allergic Reactions: Skin rash.

Headache (may be dose related), hair loss—rare.

Blurred vision, ringing in the ears—possible.

Paresthesias, neck and joint pain, dizziness, cough—infrequent.

Nausea, stomach pain, excessive gas—infrequent.

Serious Adverse Effects

Allergic Reactions: Acute intolerance syndrome: fever, skin rash, severe headache, severe stomach pain, bloody diarrhea.

Kidney damage (nephrosis, interstitial nephritis)—rare.

Peripheral neuropathy—rare.

Pancreatitis, peptic ulcers, or hepatitis—rare.

Low white blood cell or platelet counts or anemia—rare.

Myocarditis, pericarditis, or pericardial effusions—rare.

▷ **Possible Effects on Sexual Function:**   Oligospermia and infertility has been reported with other forms of mesalamine, but NOT with the oral form.

Possible Effects on Laboratory Tests

Increased liver function tests.

CAUTION

1. Report promptly any signs of acute intolerance syndrome. Stop taking drug.
2. Shake the rectal suspension thoroughly before administering.
3. This medicine is a salicylate and as such is a cousin of aspirin. Avoid taking this medicine in combination with other medicines or during other conditions in which aspirin is contraindicated.

Precautions for Use

By Infants and Children: Safety and effectiveness by those under 12 years of age are not established.

By Those Over 60 Years of Age: None.

▷ **Advisability of Use During Pregnancy**

Pregnancy Category: B. See Pregnancy Risk Categories at the back of this book.

Animal studies: No drug-induced birth defects found in rat or rabbit studies.

Human studies: Adequate studies of pregnant women are not available.

Use this drug only if clearly needed. Ask your physician for guidance.

Advisability of Use If Breast-Feeding

Presence of this drug in breast milk: Yes.

Avoid drug or refrain from nursing.

Habit-Forming Potential: None.

Effects of Overdosage: Headache, dizziness, nausea, vomiting, abdominal cramping.

Possible Effects of Long-Term Use: None reported.

Suggested Periodic Examinations While Taking This Drug (at physician's discretion)

Kidney function tests, urinalysis.

▷ **While Taking This Drug, Observe the Following**

Foods: Decreased mesalamine levels. Follow prescribed diet.

Beverages: No restrictions. May be taken with milk.

▷ *Alcohol:* No interactions expected.

Tobacco Smoking: No interactions expected, but I advise everyone to quit smoking.

▷ *Other Drugs:* Mercaptopurine *taken concurrently* with

- alendronate (Fosamax) may increase stomach or intestinal upset risks (because of salicylate).
- varicella vaccine (Varivax) may result in Reye syndrome. Avoid taking this medicine for 6 weeks following varicella vaccine.

▷ *Driving, Hazardous Activities:* No restrictions.

Aviation Note: The use of this drug *is probably not a disqualification* for piloting. Consult a designated Aviation Medical Examiner.

Exposure to Sun: No restrictions.

METAPROTERENOL (met a proh TER e nohl)

Other Name: Orciprenaline

Introduced: 1964   **Class:** Antiasthmatic, bronchodilator   **Prescription:** USA: Yes   **Controlled Drug:**   USA: No; Canada: No   **Available as Generic:** Yes

Brand Names: Alupent, Arm-a-Med, Dey-Dose, Dey-Lute, Metaprel, Prometa

```
┌─────────────────────────────────────────────────────────────────────────┐
│                        BENEFITS versus RISKS                              │
│        Possible Benefits                     Possible Risks               │
│   VERY EFFECTIVE RELIEF OF          Increased blood pressure              │
│     BRONCHOSPASM                    Fine hand tremor                      │
│                                     Fast heart rate                       │
│                                     Irregular heart rhythm (with excessive│
│                                       use)                                │
└─────────────────────────────────────────────────────────────────────────┘
```

▷ **Principal Uses**

As a Single Drug Product: Uses currently included in FDA-approved labeling: (1) Relieves acute bronchial asthma and reduces the frequency and severity of chronic, recurrent asthmatic attacks; (2) used to relieve reversible bronchospasm associated with chronic bronchitis and emphysema; (3) eases symptoms in obstructive bronchial disease.

Other (unlabeled) generally accepted uses: Has been used in threatened abortion.

How This Drug Works: This drug acts to dilate those bronchial tubes that are in sustained constriction, thereby increasing the size of the airway and improving the ability to breathe.

Available Dosage Forms and Strengths

Oral suspension — 10 mg/5 ml
Powder for inhalation — 0.65 mg per inhalation
Solution for nebulizer — 0.4%, 0.6%, 5%
Syrup — 10 mg/5 ml
Tablets — 10 mg, 20 mg

▷ **Usual Adult Dosage Range:**   Inhaler: two or three inhalations as often as every 3 to 4 hours; do not exceed 12 inhalations daily.

Hand nebulizer: 5 to 15 inhalations every 4 hours; do not exceed 40 inhalations daily.

Syrup and tablets: 20 mg up to every 6 to 8 hours. **Note: Actual dosage and administration schedule must be determined for each patient individually.**

Conditions Requiring Dosing Adjustments

Liver Function: Specific guidelines for dosing adjustment for patients with liver compromise are not usually indicated.

Kidney Function: Dosing changes are not indicated in kidney compromise.

▷ **Dosing Instructions:**   May be taken on empty stomach or with food or milk. Tablets should not be crushed for administration. For aerosol and nebulizer, follow the written instructions carefully. Do not overuse. If symptoms are not controlled with the most frequent dosing allowed, call your doctor immediately.

Usual Duration of Use: According to individual requirements. Do not use beyond the time necessary to terminate episodes of asthma.

▷ **This Drug Should Not Be Taken If**

• you have had an allergic reaction to any dosage form of it previously.
• you currently have an irregular heart rhythm.
• you are taking, or have taken within the past 2 weeks, any monoamine oxidase (MAO) type A inhibitor drug (see Drug Classes).

▷ **Inform Your Physician Before Taking This Drug If**
- you are overly sensitive to other sympathetic stimulant drugs.
- you currently use epinephrine (Adrenalin, Primatene Mist, etc.) to relieve asthmatic breathing.
- you have any type of heart or circulatory disorder, especially high blood pressure or coronary heart disease.
- you have diabetes or an overactive thyroid gland (hyperthyroidism).
- you are taking any form of digitalis or any stimulant drug.

Possible Side Effects (natural, expected, and unavoidable drug actions)
Aerosol—dryness or irritation of mouth or throat, altered taste.
Tablet—nervousness, palpitation.

▷ **Possible Adverse Effects** (unusual, unexpected, and infrequent reactions)
If any of the following develop, consult your physician promptly for guidance.
Mild Adverse Effects
Headache, dizziness, restlessness, insomnia, fine tremor of hands—possible, infrequent.
Increased sweating; muscle cramps in arms and legs—case reports.
Nausea, heartburn, vomiting—possible.
Serious Adverse Effects
Rapid or irregular heart rhythm, intensification of angina, increased blood pressure—possible.
Hallucinations and psychosis—rare.
Paradoxical spasm of the bronchi (bronchospasm)—rare.

▷ **Possible Effects on Sexual Function:**   None reported.

Natural Diseases or Disorders That May Be Activated By This Drug
Latent coronary artery disease, diabetes, or high blood pressure.

Possible Effects on Laboratory Tests
Urine sugar tests: positive (unreliable results with Benedict's solution).

CAUTION
1. Combined use of this drug by aerosol inhalation with beclomethasone aerosol (Beclovent, Vanceril) may increase the risk of toxicity due to fluorocarbon propellants. Use this aerosol 20 to 30 minutes *before* beclomethasone aerosol, as this will reduce the risk of toxicity and enhance the penetration of beclomethasone.
2. *Avoid excessive use of aerosol inhalation.* Excessive or prolonged use of this drug by inhalation can reduce its effectiveness and cause serious heart rhythm disturbances, including cardiac arrest.
3. Do not combine this drug with epinephrine. These two drugs may be used alternately if an interval of 4 hours is allowed between doses.
4. If you do not respond to your usually effective dose, ask your doctor for help. Do not increase the size or frequency of the dose without your physician's approval.

Precautions for Use
By Infants and Children: Safety and effectiveness of the aerosol and nebulized solution are not established for children under 12 years of age. Oral dosing in children less than 6 years old: 1.3 to 2.6 mg per kg of body mass per day, divided into equal doses and given three to four times a day. In children 6 to

9 years old or less than 60 pounds: 10 mg per dose three to four times a day. Children more than 9 years old or over 60 pounds are given 20 mg three or four times a day.

Safety and effectiveness of the syrup and tablet are not established for children under 6 years of age.

By Those Over 60 Years of Age: Avoid excessive and continual use. If acute asthma is not relieved promptly, other drugs will have to be tried. Watch for nervousness, palpitations, irregular heart rhythm, and muscle tremors. Use with extreme caution if you have hardening of the arteries, heart disease, or high blood pressure.

▷ **Advisability of Use During Pregnancy**

Pregnancy Category: C. See Pregnancy Risk Categories at the back of this book. Animal studies: Significant birth defects reported in rabbit studies.

Human studies: Adequate studies of pregnant women are not available.

Avoid use during first 3 months. Use during the final 6 months only if clearly needed.

Advisability of Use If Breast-Feeding

Presence of this drug in breast milk: Unknown.

Avoid drug or refrain from nursing.

Habit-Forming Potential: None.

Effects of Overdosage: Nervousness, palpitation, rapid heart rate, sweating, headache, tremor, vomiting, chest pain.

Possible Effects of Long-Term Use: Loss of effectiveness. See "CAUTION" above.

Suggested Periodic Examinations While Taking This Drug (at physician's discretion)

Blood pressure measurements, evaluation of heart status.

▷ **While Taking This Drug, Observe the Following**

Foods: No restrictions.

Beverages: Avoid excessive use of caffeine-containing beverages: coffee, tea, cola, chocolate.

▷ *Alcohol:* No interactions expected.

Tobacco Smoking: No interactions expected, but I advise everyone to quit smoking.

▷ *Other Drugs*

Metaproterenol *taken concurrently* with

- albuterol (Proventil, others) may result in increased heart (cardiovascular) side effects.
- monoamine oxidase (MAO) type A inhibitor drugs may cause excessive increase in blood pressure and undesirable heart stimulation.
- phenothiazines (see Drug Classes) may blunt the central effects of this medicine.

▷ *Driving, Hazardous Activities:* Usually no restrictions. Use caution if excessive nervousness or dizziness occurs.

Aviation Note: The use of this drug *is a disqualification* for piloting. Consult a designated Aviation Medical Examiner.

Exposure to Sun: No restrictions.

Heavy Exercise or Exertion: Use caution. Excessive exercise can induce asthma in sensitive individuals.

METFORMIN (met FOR min)

Introduced: 1995 **Class:** Antidiabetes drug, oral; biguanide **Prescription: USA:** Yes **Controlled Drug: USA:** No; Canada: No **Available as Generic: USA:** No; Canada: No

Brand Name: Glucophage

Warning: Avoid excessive alcohol intake with this drug. Alcohol can cause lactic acidosis, a condition that metformin can also rarely cause. All oral hypoglycemic agents may carry the risk of increased cardiovascular death, based on a 1975 study of tolbutamide and phenformin.

BENEFITS versus RISKS

Possible Benefits	*Possible Risks*
EFFECTIVE GLUCOSE CONTROL	LACTIC ACIDOSIS
WITHOUT INSULIN INJECTIONS	Possible anemia with long-term use
MAY BE USED CONCURRENTLY	
WITH A SULFONYLUREA	
DOES NOT LEAD TO WEIGHT GAIN	
TAKEN BY MOUTH, VERSUS	
INJECTION OF INSULIN	
Usually avoids excessive lowering of	
blood sugar	
Favorable effects on lipids	

▷ **Principal Uses**

As a Single Drug Product: Uses currently included in FDA-approved labeling: (1) Used in combination with diet restrictions to treat noninsulin-dependent diabetes; (2) can be combined with a sulfonylurea (see Drug Classes) for those patients who do not have an adequate response to diet restrictions plus a sulfonylurea.

Other (unlabeled) generally accepted uses: (1) May be used as single-agent therapy to overcome insulin resistance; (2) could help nondiabetic, obese women with high blood pressure in helping improve blood pressure and lipid profile; (3) may have a role in insulin-dependent diabetics in helping decrease their insulin requirements.

How This Drug Works: This biguanide decreases sugar (glucose) production in the liver. It also increases sensitivity of the body to insulin.

Available Dosage Forms and Strengths

Tablets — 500 mg, 850 mg

▷ **Recommended Dosage Ranges** (Actual dosage and administration schedule must be determined for each patient individually.)

Infants and Children: Not approved for use in this population.

12 to 60 Years of Age: Dosing is started at 500 mg twice daily. It is best to take this medicine with the morning and evening meal. Typical effective dosages are 850 mg twice daily. Maximum dose is 850 mg three times daily.

Over 60 Years of Age: Lower doses are used. Some patients may have acceptable blood sugar control with as little as 500 mg daily. If this dose is used, it should be taken with the morning meal. The dose may be slowly increased as needed and tolerated.

Conditions Requiring Dosing Adjustments

Liver Function: This drug should **not** be used by patients with liver compromise. This is a risk factor for lactic acidosis.

Kidney Function: This drug should **not** be used by patients who have kidney problems (renal dysfunction) defined as females with steady-state creatinine levels greater than 1.4 or males with steady-state creatinine levels greater than 1.5.

▷ **Dosing Instructions:** This drug should be taken with the morning and evening meal if it has been prescribed on a twice-daily basis.

Usual Duration of Use: Continual use on a regular schedule for a week is usually necessary to determine this drug's effectiveness in establishing tight glucose control. A month of continuous use will be needed before an effect on glycosylated hemoglobin (a measure of past success of glucose control) is seen. Long-term use (months to years) requires periodic evaluation of response and dosage adjustment. Consult your physician on a regular basis.

Possible Advantages of This Drug

Does not lead to weight gain.

Can be used (because of its mechanism of action) in combination with a sulfonylurea.

Can be used to overcome insulin resistance.

Does not cause excessive lowering of blood sugar (hypoglycemia) when used as monotherapy.

Currently a "Drug of Choice"

for treatment of hyperglycemia in the elderly.

▷ **This Drug Should Not Be Taken If**

- you have had an allergic reaction to any dosage form of it or related medicines previously.
- you have impaired kidneys (serum creatinine greater than 1.4 for females or 1.5 for males).
- you have liver disease.
- you have a serious infection (increases risk of lactic acidosis).
- you are an alcoholic.
- you have a heart or lung insufficiency (increased lactic acidosis risk).
- you are going to have a radiology test that uses iodinated contrast media (ask your doctor).
- you have chronic metabolic acidosis or ketoacidosis.
- you are breast-feeding your infant.

▷ **Inform Your Physician Before Taking This Drug If**

- you are planning to have surgery soon.
- you have a history of megaloblastic anemia.
- you have seen another physician and a diagnosis of ketoacidosis has been made.
- you are uncertain of how much metformin to take or how often to take it.

Possible Side Effects (natural, expected, and unavoidable drug actions)

Lactic acidosis—rare.

▷ **Possible Adverse Effects** (unusual, unexpected, and infrequent reactions)

If any of the following develop, consult your physician promptly for guidance.

Mild Adverse Effects
Allergic Reactions: Rash.
Metallic taste—case reports.
Anorexia, nausea, vomiting, or diarrhea—up to 30% when started, then they often subside.
Headache, nervousness, dizziness, or tiredness—infrequent.
Serious Adverse Effects
Allergic Reactions: Not reported.
Idiosyncratic Reactions: None reported.
Lactic acidosis—rare.
Lowered vitamin B_{12} levels and resultant anemia (megaloblastic)—rare.
Drug-induced porphyria—case reports.
All oral hypoglycemic agents carry a label indicating that they may increase risk of cardiovascular death (based on a 1975 study of tolbutamide and phenformin)—possible.

▷ **Possible Effects on Sexual Function:**   None reported.

Possible Delayed Adverse Effects: Low vitamin B_{12} levels and anemia (megaloblastic).

▷ **Adverse Effects That May Mimic Natural Diseases or Disorders**
Acidosis may mimic ketoacidosis, which is seen in diabetics.

Natural Diseases or Disorders That May Be Activated by This Drug
None reported.

Possible Effects on Laboratory Tests
Blood glucose: decreased.

CAUTION
1. This drug may cause lactic acidosis. Ask your doctor for signs or symptoms that may occur.
2. Drugs in this class (phenformin) or tolbutamide were reported to increase risk of cardiovascular death. Although there is no data to support that effect for this medicine, patients should be closely followed.

Precautions for Use
By Infants and Children: Safety and effectiveness for use by those under 18 years of age have not been established.
By Those Over 60 Years of Age: Smaller starting doses (500 mg daily) are indicated. People in this age group tend to have an age-related decline in kidney function as well as a more compromised ability to tolerate lower blood sugar levels.

▷ **Advisability of Use During Pregnancy**
Pregnancy Category: B. See Pregnancy Risk Categories at the back of this book.
Animal studies: No birth defects in rats at two times the typical human dose.
Human studies: Information from adequate studies of pregnant women is not available. The manufacturer does not recommend the use of this drug in pregnancy. Insulin is still considered the drug of choice to control blood sugar in pregnancy.

Advisability of Use If Breast-Feeding
Presence of this drug in breast milk: Yes.
Avoid drug or refrain from nursing.

Habit-Forming Potential: None.

Effects of Overdosage: Nausea and vomiting, pulmonary edema, hemorrhage from the stomach, lactic acidosis, seizures, intractable lowering of the blood pressure, coma.

Possible Effects of Long-Term Use: Lowering of vitamin B_{12} and resultant anemia (megaloblastic). Possible malabsorption of folic acid and amino acids.

Suggested Periodic Examinations While Taking This Drug (at physician's discretion)
Vitamin B_{12} levels, tests of kidney and liver function.

▷ **While Taking This Drug, Observe the Following**
Foods: No restrictions.
Nutritional Support: Diet as prescribed by your doctor.
Beverages: No restrictions.
▷ *Alcohol:* Use with extreme caution. Alcohol worsens the effect of metformin on lactate. Avoid alcohol in excessive amounts.
Tobacco Smoking: No interactions expected, but I advise everyone to quit smoking.
Marijuana Smoking: May worsen dizziness.
▷ *Other Drugs*
Metformin may ***increase*** the effects of
- insulin in the sense that the lowering of blood sugar will be increased. This may be used to therapeutic advantage in some insulin-dependent diabetics.

Metformin ***taken concurrently*** with
- ACE inhibitors (see Drug Classes) may increase lowering of blood sugar to an undesirable extent.
- beta-blockers (see Drug Classes) may slow recovery from any hypoglycemia that occurs and can also block symptoms of low blood sugar.
- contract media for certain X-ray studies may increase risk of lactic acidosis. Metformin should not be combined with these agents. Some clinicians substitute a different agent to control blood sugar, stop the metformin 48 hours before the X ray, then stop the substituted agent and restart metformin once kidney function is tested and found to be normal.
- itraconazole or other azole antifungal agents can result in severe lowering of the blood sugar.
- thyroid hormones (see Drug Classes) can result in blunting of metformin's therapeutic effect.

The following drugs may ***increase*** the effects of metformin
- cimetidine (Tagamet)— may result in toxicity.
- oral antidiabetic drugs (see Drug Classes). This effect may be used to therapeutic advantage.

▷ *Driving, Hazardous Activities:* This drug may cause drowsiness or dizziness. Restrict activities as necessary.
Aviation Note: Diabetes ***is a disqualification*** for piloting. Consult a designated Aviation Medical Examiner.
Exposure to Sun: Use caution. Some medicines that are similar in chemical structure can cause increased sensitivity to the sun.
Heavy Exercise or Exertion: Heavy exercise will tend to use up sugar faster than

usual. This drug will have an effect on lowering the blood sugar. Be alert to the symptoms of low blood sugar.

Occurrence of Unrelated Illness: Infections or other illness may still require use of insulin to achieve acceptable blood sugar control.

Discontinuation: Periodic physician evaluations of the continued benefit of this medicine are needed.

METHOTREXATE (meth oh TREX ayt)

Other Names: Amethopterin, MTX

Introduced: 1948   **Class:** Anticancer drugs, anti-psoriasis   **Prescription:** USA: Yes   **Controlled Drug:** USA: No; Canada: No   **Available as Generic:** Yes

Brand Names: Abitrexate, Folex, Folex PFS, Mexate, Mexate AQ, Rheumatrex Dose Pack

BENEFITS versus RISKS	
Possible Benefits	*Possible Risks*
EFFECTIVE TREATMENT OF SOME CASES OF SEVERE DISABLING PSORIASIS	GASTROINTESTINAL ULCERATION AND BLEEDING
EFFECTIVE TREATMENT OF CERTAIN ADULT AND CHILDHOOD CANCERS	MOUTH AND THROAT ULCERATION
PREVENTION OF REJECTION OF BONE MARROW TRANSPLANTS	SEVERE BONE MARROW DEPRESSION
USEFUL IN RHEUMATOID ARTHRITIS and related disorders	DAMAGE TO LUNGS, LIVER, OR KIDNEYS
	Loss of hair

▷ **Principal Uses**

As a Single Drug Product: Uses currently included in FDA-approved labeling: (1) Combination therapy of acute lymphocytic leukemia; (2) combination therapy of various types of adult and childhood cancer; (3) severe and widespread forms of disabling psoriasis that have failed to respond to all standard treatment procedures; (4) various types of both adult and childhood cancer; (5) used to prevent rejection of transplanted bone marrow; (6) used in the treatment of connective tissue disorders such as rheumatoid arthritis and related conditions. Its use in rheumatoid arthritis is restricted to the treatment of selected adults with severe active disease that has failed to respond to conventional therapy.

Other (unlabeled) generally accepted uses: (1) Used in a variety of neoplastic syndromes in combination therapy; (2) may have a role in helping decrease steroid use in steroid-dependent asthma; (3) helps lessen neutropenia in Felty's syndrome; (4) used in combination with misoprostol to cause abortion; (5) can be of help in chronic granulomatous hepatitis of unknown cause (idiopathic).

How This Drug Works: By interfering with the normal utilization of folic acid in tissue cell reproduction, this drug retards abnormally rapid tissue growth (as in psoriasis and cancer).

Available Dosage Forms and Strengths

Injections — 2.5 mg/ml, 10 mg/ml, 25 mg/ml
Powder, intrathecal cryodessicated — 20 mg, 50 mg, 100 mg
Injections, preservative free — 25 mg/ml, 50 mg/ml, 100 mg/ml, 250 mg/ml
Tablets — 2.5 mg

▷ **Usual Adult Dosage Range**

For psoriasis (alternate schedules): (1) 10 to 50 mg once a week; (2) 2.5 to 5 mg every 12 hours for three doses, or every 8 hours for four doses, once a week, up to a maximum of 30 mg/week; (3) 2.5 mg/day for 5 days, followed by 2 days without drug, with gradual increase in dosage to a maximum of 6.25 mg/day.

For rheumatoid arthritis (alternate schedules): (1) single oral dose of 7.5 mg once weekly; (2) divided doses of 2.5 mg every 12 hours for three doses per week. Dosage may be increased gradually as needed and tolerated. Do not exceed a weekly dose of 20 mg.

For acute lymphocytic leukemia (ALL): Induction: 3.3 mg per square meter in combination with corticosteroid treatment is usually taken daily for 4 to 6 weeks. Maintenance: a total weekly dose of 30 mg per square meter is given as two divided oral or intramuscular injections. Some centers also use 2.5 mg per kg of body mass intravenously every 14 days.

Note: Actual dosage and administration schedule must be determined for each patient individually.

Conditions Requiring Dosing Adjustments

Liver Function: This drug should be used with caution and in decreased dose by patients with liver compromise. One researcher used some laboratory tests as a guide: when the dose is due, if the bilirubin is less than 3 mg % and the AST (SGOT) is less than 180 IU, 100% of the scheduled dose can be given. If the bilirubin is 3.1 to 5.0 mg % or AST is greater then 180 IU, 75% of the scheduled dose should be given. If the bilirubin is greater than 5.0 mg %, the dose SHOULD NOT be given.

Kidney Function: Methotrexate should be used as a result of a benefit-to-risk decision. Increased systemic adverse effects may occur if this medication is used by patients with compromised kidneys. This drug should **not** be taken by patients with severe kidney failure (creatinine clearances less than 10 ml/min). For patients with moderate kidney failure, 50% of the usual dose should be taken in the usual dosing interval.

▷ **Dosing Instructions:**   The tablet may be crushed and taken with food to reduce stomach irritation. Drink at least 2 to 3 quarts of liquids daily. Many clinicians who give methotrexate to their patients to treat rheumatoid arthritis also give folic acid in order to minimize methotrexate toxicity.

Usual Duration of Use: Use on a regular schedule for several weeks determines benefit in reducing the severity and extent of psoriasis. Response in rheumatoid arthritis usually begins after 3 to 6 weeks of treatment. When a favorable response has been achieved, the dosage should be reduced to the smallest amount that will maintain acceptable improvement. Long-term use (months to years) requires physician supervision.

▷ **This Drug Should Not Be Taken If**
- you have had an allergic reaction to it previously.
- you currently have, or have had a recent exposure to, either chickenpox or shingles (herpes zoster).
- you are pregnant or planning pregnancy in the near future, and you are taking this drug to treat psoriasis or rheumatoid arthritis.
- you are breast-feeding your infant.
- you have alcoholic liver disease.
- you have an immune deficiency.
- you have fluid in the pleura of the lung (pleural effusions).
- you have active liver disease, peptic ulcer, regional enteritis, or ulcerative colitis.
- your white blood cell count is less than 3,000 or your platelet count is less than 100,000.
- you are making very small amounts of urine or your creatinine clearance (see Glossary) is less than 40 ml/min.
- you currently have a blood cell or bone marrow disorder.

▷ **Inform Your Physician Before Taking This Drug If**
- you have a chronic infection of any kind.
- you do not understand how to handle vomit or urine while taking chemotherapy.
- you have impaired liver or kidney function.
- you have a history of bone marrow impairment of any kind, especially drug-induced bone marrow depression.
- you are dehydrated.
- you have a history of gout, peptic ulcer disease, regional enteritis, or ulcerative colitis.

Possible Side Effects (natural, expected, and unavoidable drug actions)
The following are due to the pharmacological actions of this drug. **Report such developments to your physician promptly.**

Sores on the lips, in the mouth or throat; vomiting; intestinal cramping; diarrhea (may be bloody); painful urination; bloody urine. Reduced resistance to infection, fatigue, weakness, fever, abnormal bleeding or bruising (bone marrow depression).

▷ **Possible Adverse Effects** (unusual, unexpected, and infrequent reactions)
If any of the following develop, consult your physician promptly for guidance.

Mild Adverse Effects
Allergic Reactions: Skin rash, hives, itching.
Headache, drowsiness, blurred vision, conjunctivitis—infrequent.
Loss of appetite, nausea, vomiting—infrequent to frequent.
Muscle pain—rare.
Loss of hair, loss of skin pigmentation, acne—infrequent.
Impaired sense of smell or taste—possible.

Serious Adverse Effects
Allergic Reactions: Drug-induced pneumonia: cough, chest pain, shortness of breath. Anaphylaxis.
Nervous system toxicity: speech disturbances, paralysis, seizures—infrequent.

Liver toxicity with jaundice (see Glossary)—case reports.

Kidney toxicity: reduced urine volume, kidney failure—more likely with higher doses.

Colitis or toxic megacolon—case report.

Tumor lysis syndrome: uric acid nephropathy; very low potassium, magnesium, and calcium—possible.

Fluid buildup in the lung pleura (pleural effusion)—possible.

Immune suppression and subsequent infection with *Pneumocystis carinii* pneumonia—possible.

Severe skin reactions (toxic epidermal necrolysis)—case reports.

Chromosomal damage (from occupational exposure)—possible.

▷ **Possible Effects on Sexual Function:**   Altered timing and pattern of menstruation. Swelling and tenderness of the male breast tissue (gynecomastia)—case reports.

Possible Delayed Adverse Effects: Some reports suggest that methotrexate therapy may contribute to the later development of secondary cancers. Other studies have not confirmed this.

Possible Effects on Laboratory Tests

Complete blood cell counts: decreased red cells, hemoglobin, white cells, and platelets.

Blood uric acid level: increased.

Liver function tests: increased liver enzymes (ALT/GPT, AST/GOT, and alkaline phosphatase) or bilirubin.

Kidney function tests: increased blood urea nitrogen (BUN) level; increased urine creatinine.

Fecal occult blood test: positive.

Sperm count: decreased.

CAUTION

1. This drug must be monitored carefully by a qualified physician. Request the Patient Package Insert (Rheumatrex Dose Pack) and read it thoroughly.
2. When methotrexate is used to treat rheumatoid arthritis, folic acid can minimize toxicity.
3. Appropriate laboratory examinations, performed before and during the use of this drug, are mandatory.
4. Women with potential for pregnancy should have a pregnancy test before taking this drug and should use an effective form of contraception during its use and for 8 weeks following its discontinuation.
5. Live-virus vaccines should be avoided during use of this drug. Live-virus vaccines could actually produce infection rather than stimulate an immune response.

Precautions for Use

By Those Over 60 Years of Age: Careful evaluation of kidney function should be made before starting treatment and during the entire course of therapy.

▷ **Advisability of Use During Pregnancy**

Pregnancy Category: X. See Pregnancy Risk Categories at the back of this book.

Animal studies: Skull and facial defects reported in mice.

Human studies: This drug is known to cause fetal deaths and birth defects. Its use during pregnancy to treat psoriasis or rheumatoid arthritis cannot be justified.

Advisability of Use If Breast-Feeding
Presence of this drug in breast milk: Yes.
Avoid drug or refrain from nursing.

Habit-Forming Potential: None.

Effects of Overdosage: The side effects and adverse effects listed above develop earlier and with greater severity.

Possible Effects of Long-Term Use: Liver compromise (fibrosis and cirrhosis) occurs in 3–5% of long-term users (35 to 49 months).

Suggested Periodic Examinations While Taking This Drug (at physician's discretion)
Complete blood cell counts, liver and kidney function tests, blood uric acid levels, chest X-ray examinations.

▷ **While Taking This Drug, Observe the Following**
Foods: Avoid highly seasoned foods that could be irritating. Between courses of treatment, eat liberally of the following foods: beef, chicken, lamb and pork liver, asparagus, navy beans, kale, and spinach. Any food will reduce the peak methotrexate level obtained.

Beverages: No restrictions. This drug may be taken with milk.

▷ *Alcohol:* Avoid completely.

Tobacco Smoking: No interactions expected, but I advise everyone to quit smoking.

Marijuana Smoking: May cause additional impairment of immunity.

▷ *Other Drugs*
Methotrexate may *decrease* the effects of
• digoxin (Lanoxin).
• phenytoin (Dilantin).
The following drugs may *increase* the effects of methotrexate and enhance its toxicity
• aspirin and other salicylates.
• NSAIDs (see Drug Classes).
• probenecid (Benemid).
Methotrexate *taken concurrently* with
• bismuth subsalicylate (Pepto-Bismol, others) may result in methotrexate toxicity.
• carbenicillin (Geocillin, others) may lead to methotrexate toxicity.
• cholestyramine (Questran, others) and other cholesterol-lowering resins may result in decreased methotrexate effectiveness.
• cotrimoxazole (Bactrim) may result in lowering of all blood cells (pancytopenia).
• cyclosporine (Sandimmune) can result in increased toxicity from both drugs. This combination should be avoided.
• etretinate (Tegison) results in increased liver toxicity.
• pneumococcal or smallpox vaccine may result in decreased immune response to the vaccine.
• sulfa drugs such as sulfamethoxazole can result in increased hematological toxicity.

- thiazide diuretics (see Drug Classes) may increase risk of myelosuppression.
- theophylline (Theo-Dur, others) may result in theophylline toxicity. Decreased theophylline doses may be needed.
- yellow fever vaccine can result in blunted response and benefit from the vaccine.

▷ *Driving, Hazardous Activities:* This drug may cause drowsiness, dizziness, or blurred vision. Restrict activities as necessary.

Aviation Note: The use of this drug *is a disqualification* for piloting. Consult a designated Aviation Medical Examiner.

Exposure to Sun: Use caution—this drug can cause photosensitivity. Avoid ultraviolet lamps.

METHYCLOTHIAZIDE (METH i kloh thi a zide)

See the thiazide diuretics profile for further information.

METHYLPHENIDATE (meth il FEN i dayt)

Introduced: 1956   **Class:** Amphetaminelike drug, anti-attention-deficit-disorder drug   **Prescription:** USA: Yes   **Controlled Drug:** USA: C-II*; Canada: Yes   **Available as Generic:** USA: Yes; Canada: Yes

Brand Names: ✦PMS-Methylphenidate, Ritalin, Ritalin-SR

BENEFITS versus RISKS	
Possible Benefits	*Possible Risks*
EFFECTIVE CONTROL OF NARCOLEPSY	POTENTIAL FOR SERIOUS PSYCHOLOGICAL DEPENDENCE
USEFUL AS ADJUNCTIVE TREATMENT IN THE ATTENTION-DEFICIT DISORDERS OF CHILDHOOD	SUPPRESSION OF GROWTH IN CHILDHOOD (recovers when medicine is stopped)
Useful in treatment of mild to moderate depression	Abnormal behavior
Useful in some cases of emotional withdrawal in the elderly	Rare blood cell disorders

▷ **Principal Uses**

As a Single Drug Product: Uses currently included in FDA-approved labeling: (1) Treats narcolepsy—recurrent spells of uncontrollable drowsiness and sleep; (2) attention-deficit disorders of childhood, formerly known as the hyperactive child syndrome, with minimal brain damage and minimal brain dysfunction.

Other (unlabeled) generally accepted uses: (1) Treatment of mild to moderate depression; (2) management of apathetic and withdrawal states in the elderly; (3) combination therapy of chronic pain, particularly cancer pain; (4) could have a role in helping autism.

*See schedules of Controlled Drugs at the back of this book.

How This Drug Works: This activates the brainstem, improves alertness and concentration, and increases learning ability and attention span.

Available Dosage Forms and Strengths

Tablets — 5 mg, 10 mg, 20 mg

Tablets, prolonged action — 20 mg

▷ **Usual Adult Dosage Range:**   Narcolepsy: 10 to 60 mg daily. This is divided into equal doses and given two to three times daily. Ideally, this is given 30 minutes before meals.

Pediatric dosing: Children over 6 years old: regular-release form—5 mg before breakfast and lunch (twice daily). This dose is increased as needed and tolerated at weekly intervals to a maximum recommended dose of 60 mg. **Note: Actual dosage and administration schedule must be determined for each patient individually.**

Conditions Requiring Dosing Adjustments

Liver Function: Should be used with caution and in decreased dose by patients with liver compromise.

Kidney Function: The kidney does not appear to be involved in the elimination of this drug.

▷ **Dosing Instructions:**   The regular tablet may be crushed and taken 30 to 45 minutes before meals. The prolonged-action tablet should be taken whole, not crushed.

Usual Duration of Use: Use on a regular schedule for 3 to 4 weeks determines effectiveness in controlling the symptoms of narcolepsy or improving the behavior of attention-deficit children. If there is no improvement after this time, the drug should be stopped. Long-term use (months to years) requires physician supervision and periodic evaluation.

▷ **This Drug Should Not Be Taken If**
- you have had an allergic reaction to it previously.
- you have glaucoma (inadequately treated).
- you have Tourette syndrome.
- you are experiencing a period of severe anxiety, nervous tension, or emotional depression.

▷ **Inform Your Physician Before Taking This Drug If**
- you have high blood pressure, angina, or epilepsy.
- you are taking, or have taken within the past 14 days, any monoamine oxidase (MAO) type A inhibitor drug (see Drug Classes).

Possible Side Effects (natural, expected, and unavoidable drug actions)

Nervousness, insomnia. Reduced appetite. Growth suppression (the medicine is often stopped in the summer to allow a growth spurt to compensate).

▷ **Possible Adverse Effects** (unusual, unexpected, and infrequent reactions)

If any of the following develop, consult your physician promptly for guidance.

Mild Adverse Effects

Allergic Reactions: Skin rash, hives, drug fever, joint pains—possible.

Headache, dizziness, rapid and forceful heart palpitation—infrequent.

Nausea, abdominal discomfort—infrequent.

Stuttering and hallucinations—case reports.

Serious Adverse Effects

Allergic Reactions: Severe skin reactions, extensive bruising (allergic destruction of platelets)—case reports.

Idiosyncratic Reactions: Abnormal patterns of behavior.

Porphyria or muscle damage (rhabdomyolysis)—rare.

Liver toxicity (associated with intravenous abuse of the drug)—possible.

Low red blood cell or white blood cell counts—case reports and of questionable causation.

▷ **Possible Effects on Sexual Function:**   None reported.

Natural Diseases or Disorders That May Be Activated by This Drug

Latent epilepsy.

Possible Effects on Laboratory Tests

Blood platelet counts: decreased—rare.

White and red blood cell counts: decreased—rare.

CAUTION

1. This drug should be used ONLY AFTER a careful assessment by a qualified specialist is made. True attention deficit disorder requires careful assessment to differentiate it from behavior problems arising from family tensions or other conditions that do not require Ritalin therapy.
2. Careful dosage adjustments on an individual basis are mandatory.
3. Paradoxical reactions (see Glossary) can occur, causing aggravation of initial symptoms for which this drug was prescribed.

Precautions for Use

By Infants and Children: Safety and effectiveness for those under 6 years of age are not established. If this drug is not beneficial in managing an attention deficit disorder after a trial of 1 month, it should be stopped. During long-term use, monitor the child for normal growth and development.

By Those Over 60 Years of Age: Start with small doses. Those in this group may be at increased risk for nervousness, agitation, insomnia, high blood pressure, angina, or disturbance of heart rhythm.

▷ **Advisability of Use During Pregnancy**

Pregnancy Category: B. See Pregnancy Risk Categories at the back of this book.

Animal studies: No birth defects found in mouse studies.

Human studies: Adequate studies of pregnant women are not available.

Use this drug only if clearly needed. Ask your physician for guidance.

Advisability of Use If Breast-Feeding

Presence of this drug in breast milk: Unknown.

Avoid drug or refrain from nursing.

Habit-Forming Potential: This drug can produce tolerance and cause serious psychological dependence (see Glossary), a potentially dangerous characteristic of amphetaminelike drugs (see Drug Classes).

Effects of Overdosage: Headache, vomiting, agitation, tremors, muscle twitching, dry mouth, sweating, fever, confusion, hallucinations, seizures, coma.

Possible Effects of Long-Term Use: Suppression of growth (in weight and/or height) has been reported in children during long-term use of this drug. Many patients are taken off the medicine during summer school vacations.

Suggested Periodic Examinations While Taking This Drug (at physician's discretion)
Complete blood cell counts, blood pressure measurements.

▷ **While Taking This Drug, Observe the Following**
Foods: Avoid foods rich in tyramine (see Glossary); this drug in combination with tyramine may cause an excessive rise in blood pressure.
Beverages: Avoid beverages prepared from meat or meat extracts. This drug may be taken with milk.
▷ *Alcohol:* Avoid beer, Chianti wines, and vermouth (may have high tyramine contents).
Tobacco Smoking: No interactions expected, but I advise everyone to quit smoking.
▷ *Other Drugs*
Methylphenidate may *increase* the effects of
• tricyclic antidepressants (see Drug Classes), and enhance their toxic effects.
Methylphenidate may *decrease* the effects of
• guanethidine (Ismelin), and impair its ability to lower blood pressure.
Methylphenidate *taken concurrently* with
• anticonvulsants may cause a significant change in the pattern of epileptic seizures; dosage adjustments may be necessary for proper control.
• monoamine oxidase (MAO) type A inhibitor drugs (see Drug Classes) may cause a significant rise in blood pressure. Avoid the concurrent use of these drugs.
• morphine may be used to great therapeutic benefit to increase alertness, especially if high doses of morphine must be used.
• tricyclic antidepressants may result in undesirable increases in blood pressure.
▷ *Driving, Hazardous Activities:* This drug may cause dizziness or drowsiness. Restrict activities as necessary.
Aviation Note: The use of this drug *is a disqualification* for piloting. Consult a designated Aviation Medical Examiner.
Exposure to Sun: No restrictions.
Discontinuation: If it has been necessary to use this drug for an extended period of time, do not discontinue it abruptly. Careful supervision is necessary during withdrawal to prevent severe depression and erratic behavior.

METHYLPREDNISOLONE (meth il pred NIS oh lohn)

Introduced: 1957   **Class:** Cortisonelike drugs   **Prescription:** USA: Yes
Controlled Drug: USA: No; Canada: No   **Available as Generic:** USA: Yes; Canada: Yes

Brand Names: A-Methapred, Depmedalone-40, Depmedalone-80, Depo-Medrol, Enpak Refill, Mar-Pred 40, Medrol, ✤Medrol Acne Lotion, Medrol Enpak, ✤Medrol Veriderm Cream, Meprolone, ✤Neo-Medrol Acne Lotion, ✤Neo-Medrol Veriderm, Solu-Medrol

```
┌─────────────────────────────────────────────────────────────┐
│                    BENEFITS versus RISKS                      │
│     Possible Benefits              Possible Risks             │
│  EFFECTIVE RELIEF OF          Use exceeding 2 weeks is associated │
│    SYMPTOMS IN A WIDE VARIETY   with many adverse effects:     │
│    OF INFLAMMATORY AND        ALTERED MOOD AND                │
│    ALLERGIC DISORDERS           PERSONALITY                   │
│  EFFECTIVE                    CATARACTS, GLAUCOMA             │
│    IMMUNOSUPPRESSION in        HYPERTENSION                   │
│    selected benign and malignant  OSTEOPOROSIS               │
│    disorders                  ASEPTIC BONE NECROSIS          │
│                               INCREASED SUSCEPTIBILITY TO    │
│                                 INFECTIONS                    │
│                               (See "Possible Adverse Effects" and │
│                                 "Possible Effects of Long-Term Use" │
│                                 below.)                       │
└─────────────────────────────────────────────────────────────┘
```

▷ **Principal Uses**

As a Single Drug Product: Uses currently included in FDA-approved labeling: (1) Treats a wide variety of allergic and inflammatory conditions. Used most commonly in the management of serious skin disorders, asthma, regional enteritis, multiple sclerosis, lupus erythematosus, ulcerative colitis, and all types of major rheumatic disorders including bursitis, tendonitis, and most forms of arthritis; (2) helps treat low platelet counts of unknown cause (idiopathic thrombocytopenic purpura); (3) shock due to adrenal gland insufficiency—addisonian shock; (4) adjunctive role in anaphylactic shock.

Other (unlabeled) generally accepted uses: (1) Treatment of refractory anemia; (2) therapy of chronic obstructive pulmonary disease; (3) combination treatment of acute nonlymphoblastic leukemia; (4) combination therapy of severe vomiting caused by chemotherapy; (5) helps prevent rejection of transplanted organs; (6) combination therapy of *Pneumocystis carinii* pneumonia in AIDS patients; (7) helps treat bone cysts in children; (8) has a role in treating croup; (9) can help symptoms in Still's disease; (10) used by intramuscular injection to treat polymyalgia rheumatica; (11) used to help control cancer pain, especially where inflammation is involved.

How This Drug Works: Anti-inflammatory effect is due to its ability to block normal defensive functions of certain white blood cells. Immunosuppressant effect is attributed to a reduced production of lymphocytes and antibodies.

Available Dosage Forms and Strengths

Injection, solution — 1 g per vial, 40 mg per vial, 125 mg per vial, 500 mg per vial

Injection, suspension — 40 mg/ml, 80 mg/ml

Ointment — 0.25%, 1%

Retention enema — 40 mg per bottle

Tablets — 2 mg, 4 mg, 8 mg, 16 mg, 24 mg, 32 mg

▷ **Usual Adult Dosage Range:** 4 to 48 mg daily as a single dose or in divided doses. This dose is adjusted depending on the condition being treated and the individual response. **Note: Actual dosage and administration schedule must be determined for each patient individually.**

Conditions Requiring Dosing Adjustments

Liver Function: Specific dosage adjustments in liver compromise are not defined. This drug is a rare cause of liver changes (hepatomegaly).

Kidney Function: This drug can worsen existing kidney compromise. A benefit-to-risk decision must be made regarding the use of methylprednisolone by these patients.

Obesity: The amount of time this medicine stays in the body is extended in obese patients. Dosing should be calculated based on ideal body weight.

▷ **Dosing Instructions:**   The tablet may be crushed and taken with or following food to prevent stomach irritation, preferably in the morning.

Usual Duration of Use: For sudden (acute) disorders: 4 to 10 days. For long-standing (chronic) disorders: according to individual requirements. Duration of use should not exceed the time necessary to obtain adequate symptomatic relief in acute self-limiting conditions, or the time required to stabilize a chronic condition and permit gradual withdrawal. Because of its intermediate duration of action, this drug is appropriate for alternate-day administration. See your physician on a regular basis.

▷ **This Drug Should Not Be Taken If**
- you have had an allergic reaction to any dosage form of it previously.
- you have active peptic ulcer disease.
- you have had recent bowel surgery where an anastomosis was performed.
- you have a premature infant and the injection form is ordered (contains benzyl alcohol).
- you have an active eye infection caused by the herpes simplex virus.
- you have active tuberculosis.

▷ **Inform Your Physician Before Taking This Drug If**
- you have had an adverse reaction to any cortisonelike drug in the past.
- you have a history of peptic ulcer disease, thrombophlebitis, or tuberculosis.
- you have diabetes, glaucoma, high blood pressure, deficient thyroid function, or myasthenia gravis.
- you have been exposed to measles or chickenpox.
- you plan to have surgery of any kind in the near future.
- you have liver compromise.

Possible Side Effects (natural, expected, and unavoidable drug actions)

Increased appetite, weight gain, retention of salt and water, excretion of potassium, increased susceptibility to infection. Decreased wound healing. Adrenal gland suppression. Growth retardation with chronic use in children. Increased eye pressure (intraocular). Easy bruising (ecchymosis).

▷ **Possible Adverse Effects** (unusual, unexpected, and infrequent reactions)

If any of the following develop, consult your physician promptly for guidance.

Mild Adverse Effects

Allergic Reaction: Skin rash.
Headache, dizziness, insomnia—infrequent.
Acid indigestion, abdominal distention—infrequent.
Muscle cramping, weakness, and joint pain—possible.
Acne, excessive growth of facial hair—case reports.

Serious Adverse Effects
Allergic Reactions: Anaphylaxis.
Mental and emotional disturbances of serious magnitude—case reports.
Reactivation of latent tuberculosis, *Pneumocystis carinii* pneumonia—case reports.
Development of peptic ulcer—case reports.
Seizures—possible.
Toxic megacolon—case reports.
Liver or kidney compromise—rare.
Blindness, cataracts—case reports.
Changes in white blood cell counts—possible.
Cushing's syndrome with chronic use (central obesity, buffalo hump, and moon-shaped face)—possible.
Osteoporosis, osteonecrosis—possible with long-term use.
Increased blood sugar (hyperglycemia)—possible and dose related.
Muscle changes (myopathy) or pancreatitis—case reports.
Increased blood pressure—case reports.
Abnormal heartbeat (arrythmias)—case reports.
Development of inflammation of the pancreas—case reports.
Thrombophlebitis (inflammation of a vein with the formation of blood clot): pain or tenderness in thigh or leg, with or without swelling of the foot, ankle, or leg—case reports.
Pulmonary embolism (movement of a blood clot to the lung): sudden shortness of breath, pain in the chest, coughing, bloody sputum—case reports.

▷ **Possible Effects on Sexual Function:** Altered timing and pattern of menstruation—infrequent.

▷ **Adverse Effects That May Mimic Natural Diseases or Disorders**
Pattern of symptoms and signs resembling Cushing's syndrome.

Natural Diseases or Disorders That May Be Activated by This Drug
Latent diabetes, glaucoma, peptic ulcer disease, tuberculosis.

Possible Effects on Laboratory Tests
Blood amylase and lipase levels: increased (possible pancreatitis).
Glucose tolerance test (GTT): decreased.
Blood potassium or testosterone level: decreased.

CAUTION
1. It is best to carry an identification card that says you are taking this drug, if your course of treatment is to exceed 1 week.
2. You have an increased risk of severe infection from viral illnesses such as measles or chickenpox. Try to avoid being exposed, and call your doctor if exposure occurs.
3. Growth and development of children receiving chronic steroids should be carefully followed.
4. Do not stop this drug abruptly after long-term treatment.
5. If vaccination against measles, rabies, smallpox, or yellow fever is required, discontinue this drug 72 hours before vaccination and do not resume it for at least 14 days after vaccination.
6. Dermatitis around the mouth may occur. Talk with your doctor if this happens.

Precautions for Use

By Infants and Children: Avoid prolonged use if possible. During long-term use, watch for suppression of normal growth. Intracranial pressure may increase. Long-term use may increase risk for adrenal gland deficiency during stress for as long as 18 months after the drug is stopped.

By Those Over 60 Years of Age: Cortisonelike drugs should be used very sparingly after 60 and only when the disorder under treatment is unresponsive to adequate trials of unrelated drugs. Avoid prolonged use of this drug. Continual use (even in small doses) can increase the severity of diabetes, enhance fluid retention, raise blood pressure, weaken resistance to infection, induce stomach ulcer, and accelerate the development of cataract and osteoporosis.

▷ **Advisability of Use During Pregnancy**

Pregnancy Category: C. See Pregnancy Risk Categories at the back of this book.

Animal studies: Birth defects reported in mice, rats, and rabbits.

Human studies: Adequate studies of pregnant women are not available.

Avoid completely during the first 3 months. Limit use during the final 6 months as much as possible. If used, the infant should be examined for possible deficiency of adrenal gland function.

Advisability of Use If Breast-Feeding

Presence of this drug in breast milk: Yes.

Avoid drug or refrain from nursing.

Habit-Forming Potential: Use of this drug over an extended period of time may produce a state of functional dependence (see Glossary). In the treatment of asthma and rheumatoid arthritis, the dose should be kept as small as possible and withdrawal should be attempted after periods of reasonable improvement. Such procedures may reduce the degree of "steroid rebound"—the return of symptoms as the drug is withdrawn.

Effects of Overdosage: Fatigue, muscle weakness, stomach irritation, acid indigestion, excessive sweating, facial flushing, fluid retention, swelling of extremities, increased blood pressure.

Possible Effects of Long-Term Use: Increased blood sugar (possible diabetes), increased fat deposits on the trunk of the body ("buffalo hump"), rounding of the face ("moon face"), thinning and fragility of skin, loss of texture and strength of bones (osteoporosis, aseptic necrosis), cataracts, glaucoma, retarded growth and development in children.

Suggested Periodic Examinations While Taking This Drug (at physician's discretion)

Measurements of blood pressure, blood sugar, and potassium levels.

Complete eye examinations at regular intervals. Chest X ray if history of tuberculosis.

Determination of the rate of development of the growing child to detect retardation of normal growth.

Bone mineral density testing to assess osteoporosis and fracture risk.

▷ **While Taking This Drug, Observe the Following**

Foods: No interactions expected. Ask your physician regarding need to restrict salt intake or eat potassium-rich foods. During long-term use of this drug, it is advisable to eat a high-protein diet.

Nutritional Support: During long-term use, take a vitamin supplement. During wound repair, take a zinc supplement.

Beverages: No restrictions. Drink all forms of milk liberally.

▷ *Alcohol:* No interactions expected. Use caution if you are prone to peptic ulcer disease.

Tobacco Smoking: Nicotine increases the blood levels of naturally produced cortisone and related hormones. I advise everyone to quit smoking.

Marijuana Smoking: May cause additional impairment of immunity.

▷ *Other Drugs*

Methylprednisolone may ***decrease*** the effects of
- insulin and require higher doses.
- isoniazid (INH, Niconyl, etc.).
- salicylates (aspirin, sodium salicylate, etc.).

Methylprednisolone ***taken concurrently*** with
- amphotericin B (Fungizone) may result in increased potassium loss.
- carbamazepine (Tegretol) may result in decreased methylprednisolone effectiveness.
- cholestyramine (Questran) may decrease the amount of medicine that is absorbed into your body.
- cyclosporine (Sandimmune) can result in increased steroid levels and cyclosporine toxicity.
- ketoconazole (Nizoral) may increase blood levels of methylprednisolone and result in toxicity (abnormal heartbeats or psychiatric reactions).
- loop diuretics such as furosemide (Lasix) or bumetanide (Bumex) may result in increased risk of potassium loss.
- NSAIDs may cause increased risk of ulceration of the stomach or intestine.
- oral anticoagulants (warfarin—Coumadin) may either increase or decrease their effectiveness; consult your physician regarding the need for prothrombin time testing and dosage adjustment.
- oral antidiabetic drugs (see Drug Classes) or insulin may result in loss of control of blood sugar and require higher doses or more frequent dosing of oral hypoglycemics or insulin in order to control blood sugar.
- primidone (Mysoline) may lead to increased metabolism of methylprednisolone and decreased therapeutic benefits of methylprednisolone.
- rifampin (Rifadin, others) may lead to increased metabolism of methylprednisolone and decreased therapeutic benefits of methylprednisolone.
- ritonavir (Norvir) and perhaps other protease inhibitors (see Drug Classes) may change therapeutic benefits of methylpredisolone.
- thiazide diuretics (see Drug Classes) can result in additive potassium loss.
- theophylline (Theo-Dur) results in variable changes in blood levels. More frequent theophylline blood levels are indicated.
- vaccines (such as flu or pneumococcal) may result in a blunting of the immune response to the vaccine.

The following drugs may ***decrease*** the effects of methylprednisolone
- antacids—may reduce its absorption.
- barbiturates (Amytal, Butisol, phenobarbital, etc.).
- phenytoin (Dilantin, etc.).
- rifampin (Rifadin, Rimactane, etc.).

▷ *Driving, Hazardous Activities:* Usually no restrictions. Be alert to the rare occurrence of dizziness.

Aviation Note: The use of this drug **may be a disqualification** for piloting. Consult a designated Aviation Medical Examiner.

Exposure to Sun: No restrictions.

Occurrence of Unrelated Illness: This drug may decrease resistance to infection. Tell your doctor if you develop an infection of any kind. It may also reduce your body's ability to respond to stress of acute illness, injury, or surgery. Keep your physician fully informed of any significant changes in your state of health.

Discontinuation: After extended use of this drug, do **not** stop it abruptly. Ask your doctor for help regarding gradual withdrawal. For a period of 2 years after discontinuing this drug, it is essential in the event of illness, injury, or surgery that you inform attending medical personnel that you have used this drug. The period of impaired response to stress following the use of cortisonelike drugs may last for 1 to 2 years.

METHYSERGIDE (meth i SER jide)

Introduced: 1961   **Class:** Anti-migraine drug   **Prescription:** USA: Yes
Controlled Drug: USA: No; Canada: No   **Available as Generic:** USA: No; Canada: No

Brand Name: Sansert

BENEFITS versus RISKS	
Possible Benefits	*Possible Risks*
EFFECTIVE PREVENTION OF MIGRAINE AND CLUSTER HEADACHES	FIBROSIS (SCARRING) INSIDE CHEST AND ABDOMINAL CAVITIES, OF HEART AND LUNG TISSUES, ADJACENT TO MAJOR BLOOD VESSELS AND INTERNAL ORGANS (see "Effects of Long-Term Use" below) Aggravation of hypertension, coronary artery disease, and peripheral vascular disease

▷ **Principal Uses**

As a Single Drug Product: Uses currently included in FDA-approved labeling: Prevention of frequent and/or disabling vascular headaches (migraine and cluster neuralgia) that have not responded to other conventional treatment. Other (unlabeled) generally accepted uses: May have a role in therapy of some strokes.

How This Drug Works: By blocking the inflammatory and vasoconstrictor effects of serotonin, this drug prevents blood vessel constriction that initiates vascular headaches.

Available Dosage Forms and Strengths

Tablets — 2 mg

▷ **Recommended Dosage Ranges** (Actual dosage and administration schedule must be determined for each patient individually.)

Infants and Children: Use of this drug is not recommended.

12 to 60 Years of Age: 2 to 6 mg daily, in divided doses with meals. A medication-free period of 3 to 4 weeks after every 6-month course of methysergide is necessary.

Over 60 Years of Age: 2 to 4 mg daily, in divided doses. Use very cautiously, with frequent monitoring for adverse effects.

Conditions Requiring Dosing Adjustments

Liver Function: This drug should not be used by patients with liver compromise.

Kidney Function: This drug should not be used by patients with renal compromise.

▷ **Dosing Instructions:**   The tablet may be crushed and taken with food or milk to reduce stomach irritation. Limit continual (uninterrupted) use to 6 months; avoid drug completely for a period of 4 weeks between courses.

Usual Duration of Use: Use on a regular schedule for 3 weeks usually determines effectiveness in preventing recurrence of vascular headache. If significant benefit does not occur during this trial, this drug should be stopped. Long-term use (months to years) requires periodic physician evaluation.

▷ **This Drug Should Not Be Taken If**
- you have had an allergic reaction to it previously.
- you are pregnant.
- you currently have a severe infection.
- you have any of the following conditions:
    angina pectoris
    Buerger's disease
    cellulitis of the lower legs
    chronic lung disease
    connective tissue (collagen) disease
    coronary artery disease
    hardening of the arteries (arteriosclerosis)
    heart valve disease
    high blood pressure (significant hypertension)
    kidney disease or significantly impaired kidney function
    liver disease or significantly impaired liver function
    active peptic ulcer disease
    peripheral vascular disease
    phlebitis of any kind
    Raynaud's disease or phenomenon

▷ **Inform Your Physician Before Taking This Drug If**
- you have had an adverse reaction to *any other form of ergot*.
- you have a history of peptic ulcer disease.

Possible Side Effects (natural, expected, and unavoidable drug actions)

Fluid retention, weight gain. Impaired circulation to the extremities (peripheral ischemia).

▷ **Possible Adverse Effects** (unusual, unexpected, and infrequent reactions)

If any of the following develop, consult your physician promptly for guidance.

Mild Adverse Effects

Allergic Reactions: Skin rashes, flushing of the face, transient loss of scalp hair.

Dizziness, drowsiness, agitation, unsteadiness, altered vision—infrequent to frequent.

Heartburn, nausea, vomiting, diarrhea—infrequent.

Transient muscle and joint pains—infrequent.

Serious Adverse Effects

Idiosyncratic Reactions: Nightmares, hallucinations, acute mental disturbances.

Fibrosis (scar tissue formation) involving the chest and/or abdominal cavities, heart valves, lungs, kidneys, major blood vessels—case reports.

Spasm and narrowing of coronary and peripheral arteries: anginal chest pain; cold and painful extremities; leg cramps on walking—case reports.

Hemolytic anemia (see Glossary) or abnormally low white blood cell counts—case reports.

Heart attack (myocardial infarction)—case reports.

▷ **Possible Effects on Sexual Function:**   Fibrosis of penile tissues—case reports.

▷ **Adverse Effects That May Mimic Natural Diseases or Disorders**

Swelling of the hands, lower legs, feet, and ankles (peripheral edema) may suggest heart or kidney dysfunction.

Natural Diseases or Disorders That May Be Activated by This Drug

Latent coronary artery insufficiency (angina), Buerger's disease, Raynaud's disease, peptic ulcer disease.

Possible Effects on Laboratory Tests

Complete blood cell counts: decreased white cells (lymphocytes).

Stomach hydrochloric acid: increased.

Kidney function tests: increased blood urea nitrogen (BUN).

CAUTION

1. Continual use is limited to 6 months. Gradual dose reduction is prudent during last 2 to 3 weeks of each course to prevent headache rebound. Omit drug for a period of 4 to 6 weeks before resuming. This "drug-free" period is mandatory to reduce risk of fibrosis of internal tissues.

2. Promptly report fatigue, fever, chest pain, difficult breathing, stomach or flank pain, changes in pattern of urination.

3. This drug is useful only for prevention of recurring vascular headaches; NOT recommended for treatment of acute attacks of headache. It is ineffective and should not be used for tension headaches.

Precautions for Use

By Infants and Children: Use of this drug is not recommended.

By Those Over 60 Years of Age: The age-related changes in blood vessels, circulatory functions, and kidney function can make you more susceptible to the serious adverse effects of this drug. See the list of diseases and disorders above that are contraindications to the use this drug. Ask your doctor for help.

▷ **Advisability of Use During Pregnancy**

Pregnancy Category: X. See Pregnancy Risk Categories at the back of this book.

Animal studies: No information is available.

Human studies: Adequate studies of pregnant women are not available. The manufacturer states that this drug is contraindicated during entire pregnancy.

Advisability of Use If Breast-Feeding
Presence of this drug in breast milk: Yes.
Avoid drug or refrain from nursing.

Habit-Forming Potential: None.

Effects of Overdosage: Nausea, vomiting, stomach pain, diarrhea, dizziness, excitement, cold hands and feet.

Possible Effects of Long-Term Use: Formation of scar tissue (fibrosis) inside chest cavity and/or abdominal cavity, on heart valves, in lung tissues, and surrounding major blood vessels and internal organs. This potentially dangerous reaction requires close and continual medical supervision while taking this drug.

Suggested Periodic Examinations While Taking This Drug (at physician's discretion)
Careful examination at regular intervals (6 to 12 months) for scar tissue formation or circulatory complications. Complete blood cell counts. Kidney function tests.

▷ **While Taking This Drug, Observe the Following**
Foods: No restrictions except foods you are allergic to. Some vascular headaches are due to food allergy.
Beverages: No restrictions.
▷ *Alcohol:* No interactions expected. Observe closely to determine if alcoholic beverages can initiate a migrainelike headache.
Tobacco Smoking: Avoid completely.
▷ *Other Drugs*
Methysergide *taken concurrently* with
• beta-blocker drugs (see Drug Classes) may result in hazardous constriction of peripheral arteries; monitor the combined effects of these drugs on circulation in the extremities.
▷ *Driving, Hazardous Activities:* This drug may cause dizziness, drowsiness, or impaired vision. Restrict activities as necessary.
Aviation Note: The use of this drug *is a disqualification* for piloting. Consult a designated Aviation Medical Examiner.
Exposure to Sun: No restrictions.
Exposure to Cold: Use caution. Cold environments may increase the occurrence of reduced circulation (blood flow) to the extremities.
Discontinuation: If this drug has been taken for an extended period of time, do not stop it abruptly. Gradual withdrawal (dosage reduction) over 2 to 3 weeks can prevent the development of rebound vascular headaches.

METOCLOPRAMIDE (met oh KLOH pra mide)

Introduced: 1973   **Class:** Gastrointestinal drug, antinausea (antiemetic)
Prescription: USA: Yes   **Controlled Drug:** USA: No; Canada: No   **Available as Generic:** Yes
Brand Names: ✦Apo-Metoclop, ✦Clopra, ✦Emex, ✦Maxeran, Maxolon, Octamide, Reclomide, Reglan

```
                         BENEFITS versus RISKS
        Possible Benefits                    Possible Risks
EFFECTIVE STOMACH STIMULANT       Sedation and fatigue
  FOR CORRECTING DELAYED          Parkinson-like reactions
  EMPTYING                        Tardive dyskinesia
Symptomatic relief in reflux
  esophagitis
Relief of nausea and vomiting
  associated with migraine headache
```

▷ **Principal Uses**

As a Single Drug Product: Uses currently included in FDA-approved labeling: (1) Helps stomach retention (gastroparesis) associated with diabetes; (2) acid reflux from the stomach into the esophagus (esophagitis); (3) nausea and vomiting associated with migraine headaches; (4) nausea and vomiting induced by anticancer drugs; (5) helps decrease the time needed to place a tube in the intestine; (6) used prior to cesarean section to decrease post-delivery nausea or vomiting.

Other (unlabeled) generally accepted uses: (1) Used as a preparatory drug in stomach hemorrhage; (2) may help gastrointestinal symptoms in anorexia nervosa; (3) eases drug-induced slowed functioning of the intestine (adynamic ileus); (4) decreases the frequency of accumulations of food in the stomach (bezoars); (5) can be of benefit in migraine attacks.

How This Drug Works: This drug inhibits relaxation of the stomach muscles and enhances the stimulation of the parasympathetic nervous system that is responsible for stomach muscle contractions. This action accelerates emptying of the stomach into the intestine.

Available Dosage Forms and Strengths

Injection — 5 mg/ml, 10 mg/ml
Solution — 10 mg/ml
Syrup — 5 mg/5 ml
Tablets — 5 mg, 10 mg

▷ **Usual Adult Dosage Range:** 10 mg taken 30 minutes before breakfast, lunch, and dinner and at bedtime (four times a day). The total daily dose should not exceed 0.5 mg per kg of body mass. **Note: Actual dosage and administration schedule must be determined for each patient individually.**

Conditions Requiring Dosing Adjustments

Liver Function: Specific dosage adjustments in liver compromise are not defined. It appears to be safe for use by these patients.

Kidney Function: For patients with moderate kidney failure, 75% of the usual dose can be taken at the usual dosing interval. In severe kidney failure, 50%

of the usual dose can be taken at the usual dosing interval. A benefit-to-risk decision must be made regarding the use of metoclopramide by these patients.

▷ **Dosing Instructions:**   Take tablet or syrup 30 minutes before each meal and at bedtime. The tablet may be crushed for administration.

Usual Duration of Use: Use on a regular schedule for 5 to 7 days determines benefit in accelerating stomach emptying and relieving symptoms of heartburn, fullness, and belching. Long-term use (months to years) requires physician supervision.

▷ **This Drug Should Not Be Taken If**
- you have had an allergic reaction to it previously.
- you have a seizure disorder of any kind.
- you have active gastrointestinal bleeding.
- you are taking, or have taken within the last 14 days, an MAO inhibitor (see Drug Classes).
- you are taking tricyclic antidepressants.
- you have a pheochromocytoma (adrenaline-producing tumor).

▷ **Inform Your Physician Before Taking This Drug If**
- you are allergic or overly sensitive to procaine or procainamide.
- you have impaired liver or kidney function.
- you have Parkinson's disease.
- you have epilepsy.
- you have high blood pressure.
- you have a history of depression.
- you are taking: atropinelike drugs, antipsychotics, or opioid analgesics (see Drug Classes).

Possible Side Effects (natural, expected, and unavoidable drug actions)
Drowsiness and lethargy, breast tenderness and swelling, milk production.

▷ **Possible Adverse Effects** (unusual, unexpected, and infrequent reactions)
If any of the following develop, consult your physician promptly for guidance.
Mild Adverse Effects
Allergic Reaction: Skin rash. Mild decreases in blood pressure.
Headache, dizziness, restlessness, depression, insomnia—infrequent.
Dry mouth, nausea, diarrhea, constipation—infrequent to frequent.
Urinary retention or incontinence—possible.
Serious Adverse Effects
Idiosyncratic Reactions: Neuroleptic malignant syndrome (see Glossary), bronchospastic reactions in asthmatics.
Parkinson-like reactions (see Glossary) or tardive dyskinesia (see Glossary)—case reports.
Abnormal fixed positioning of the eyes (oculogyric crisis)—case reports.
Severe decrease in white blood cells (agranulocytosis)—case reports.
Abnormal heartbeat—possible.
Severe increases in blood pressure (hypertensive crisis)—case reports.
Drug-induced porphyria—case reports.

▷ **Possible Effects on Sexual Function**

Decreased libido, impaired erection, decreased sperm count, sustained painful erection (priapism). Altered timing and pattern of menstruation, galactorrhea—case reports to infrequent.

Possible Effects on Laboratory Tests

Blood lithium level: increased.

Blood thyroid-stimulating hormone (TSH) level: increased.

Precautions for Use

By Infants and Children: Watch for development of Parkinson-like reactions soon after starting therapy. Use of the smallest effective dose can minimize such reactions. For diabetic gastroparesis, 0.5 mg per kg of body mass per day, divided into three equal doses given every 8 hours has been used. Children less than 6 years old should NOT receive single doses more than 0.1 mg per kg of body mass.

By Those Over 60 Years of Age: Parkinson-like reactions and tardive dyskinesias are more likely to occur with the use of high doses over an extended period of time. The smallest effective dose should be identified and used only when clearly needed.

▷ **Advisability of Use During Pregnancy**

Pregnancy Category: B. See Pregnancy Risk Categories at the back of this book.

Animal studies: No birth defects found due to this drug.

Human studies: Adequate studies of pregnant women are not available.

Use this drug only if clearly needed.

Advisability of Use If Breast-Feeding

Presence of this drug in breast milk: Yes.

Avoid drug or refrain from nursing.

Habit-Forming Potential: None.

Effects of Overdosage: Marked drowsiness, confusion, muscle spasms, jerking movements of head and face, tremors, shuffling gait.

Possible Effects of Long-Term Use: Parkinson-like reactions may appear within several months of use. Tardive dyskinesias usually occur after a year of continual use; they may persist after this drug is discontinued.

Suggested Periodic Examinations While Taking This Drug (at physician's discretion)

During long-term use, observe for the development of fine, wormlike movements on the surface of the tongue; these may be the first indications of an emerging tardive dyskinesia.

▷ **While Taking This Drug, Observe the Following**

Foods: No restrictions.

Beverages: No restrictions. May be taken with milk.

▷ *Alcohol:* Combined effects can result in excessive sedation and marked intoxication. Alcohol is best avoided.

Tobacco Smoking: No interactions expected, but I advise everyone to quit smoking.

▷ *Other Drugs*

Metoclopramide may **decrease** the effects of

• cimetidine (Tagamet).

• digoxin (slow-dissolving dosage forms), and reduce its effectiveness.

Metoclopramide *taken concurrently* with
- acetaminophen may increase the absorption of this drug. Decreased doses are prudent if chronic acetaminophen use will continue with metoclopramide therapy.
- cyclosporine (Sandimmune) may result in increased cyclosporine levels and toxicity.
- major antipsychotic drugs (phenothiazines, thiothixenes, haloperidol, etc.) may increase the risk of developing Parkinson-like reactions.
- morphine (slow release) may result in faster onset and increased sedation.
- penicillin may result in decreased therapeutic benefits of the antibiotic. Increased doses may be needed.
- quinidine (Quinaglute, others) may result in decreased therapeutic benefits from quinidine. Increased blood level testing and adjustment of dosing to levels is indicated.

The following drugs may *decrease* the effects of metoclopramide
- atropinelike drugs.
- opioid analgesics (see Drug Classes).

▷ *Driving, Hazardous Activities:* This drug may cause drowsiness and dizziness. Restrict activities as necessary.

Aviation Note: The use of this drug *may be a disqualification* for piloting. Consult a designated Aviation Medical Examiner.

Exposure to Sun: No restrictions.

METOLAZONE (me TOHL a zohn)

See the thiazide diuretics profile for further information.

METOPROLOL (me TOH proh lohl)

Introduced: 1974   **Class:** Antihypertensive, beta-adrenergic blocker
Prescription: USA: Yes   **Controlled Drug:** USA: No; Canada: No   **Available as Generic:** Yes

Brand Names: ✦Apo-Metoprolol, ✦Betaloc, ✦Co-Betaloc [CD], Lopressor, Lopressor Slow-Release, Lopressor HCT [CD], Lopressor OROS, ✦Novo-Metoprol, ✦Nu-Metop, Toprol, Toprol XL

BENEFITS versus RISKS	
Possible Benefits	*Possible Risks*
EFFECTIVE, WELL-TOLERATED ANTIHYPERTENSIVE in mild to moderate high blood pressure	CONGESTIVE HEART FAILURE in advanced heart disease
MAY HELP REDUCE DEATH FROM HEART ATTACKS	Worsening of angina in coronary heart disease (abrupt withdrawal)
	Masking of low blood sugar (hypoglycemia) in drug-treated diabetes
	Provocation of asthma (with high doses)

▷ **Principal Uses**

As a Single Drug Product: Uses currently included in FDA-approved labeling: (1) Treatment of mild to moderately severe high blood pressure. May be used alone or with other antihypertensive drugs, such as diuretics; (2) helps reduce the frequency and severity of angina; (3) used to reduce the risk of a second heart attack.

Other (unlabeled) generally accepted uses: (1) May help reduce symptoms of pathology of the heart muscle (dilated cardiomyopathy); (2) can be a second-line drug in treating panic attacks; (3) may decrease operative blood loss and perioperative arrhythmias in elective hysterectomy; (4) used to decrease pressure in the eye (intraocular pressure) in open-angle glaucoma.

How This Drug Works: By blocking certain actions of the sympathetic nervous system, this drug

- reduces the rate, contraction force, and ejection pressure of the heart.
- reduces contraction of blood vessel walls, resulting in expansion and lowering of blood pressure.
- prolongs the conduction time of nerve impulses through the heart, of benefit in the management of certain heart rhythm disorders.

Available Dosage Forms and Strengths

Injection — 1 mg/ml

Tablets — 50 mg, 100 mg

Tablets, prolonged action — 50 mg, 100 mg, 200 mg

▷ **Usual Adult Dosage Range:** Initially 50 mg once or twice daily (12 hours apart). The dose may be increased gradually at intervals of 7 to 10 days as needed and tolerated, up to 300 mg/day. For maintenance, 100 mg twice a day. The total daily dose should not exceed 450 mg. **Note: Actual dosage and administration schedule must be determined for each patient individually.**

Conditions Requiring Dosing Adjustments

Liver Function: This drug should be used with caution by patients with liver compromise.

Kidney Function: The kidneys are minimally involved in the elimination of this drug.

▷ **Dosing Instructions:** The regular tablet may be crushed and taken without regard to eating. Prolonged-action forms should be swallowed whole (not altered). Do not discontinue this drug abruptly.

Usual Duration of Use: Use on a regular schedule for 10 to 14 days determines effectiveness in lowering blood pressure. The long-term use of this drug (months to years) will be determined by your response to an overall treatment program (weight reduction, salt restriction, smoking cessation, etc.). Consult your physician on a regular basis.

Currently a "Drug of Choice"

for initiating treatment of hypertension with a single drug, especially for those subject to bronchial asthma or diabetes.

▷ **This Drug Should Not Be Taken If**

- you have had an allergic reaction to it previously.
- you have congestive heart failure.
- you have had a heart attack and your heart rate is less than 45 beats/min.

- you have an abnormally slow heart rate or a serious form of heart block.
- you are taking, or have taken within the past 14 days, any monoamine oxidase (MAO) type A inhibitor drug (see Drug Classes).

▷ **Inform Your Physician Before Taking This Drug If**
- you have had an adverse reaction to any beta-blocker drug in the past (see Drug Classes).
- you have a history of serious heart disease.
- you have a history of hay fever (allergic rhinitis), asthma, chronic bronchitis, or emphysema. People with bronchial asthma should generally not take beta-blockers. This drug is somewhat selective for the heart, and may be used by asthmatics with great caution.
- you have a history of overactive thyroid function (hyperthyroidism).
- you have a history of low blood sugar (hypoglycemia).
- you have impaired liver or kidney function.
- you have diabetes or myasthenia gravis.
- you currently take digitalis, quinidine, or reserpine, or any calcium-channel-blocker drug (see Drug Classes).
- you have a history of poor circulation to the extremities (peripheral vascular disease).
- you have a history of periodic cramps of your legs (intermittent claudication).
- you plan to have surgery under general anesthesia in the near future.

Possible Side Effects (natural, expected, and unavoidable drug actions)
Lethargy and fatigability, cold extremities, slow heart rate, light-headedness in upright position (see Orthostatic Hypotension in Glossary). Abnormally slow heartbeat (bradycardia).

▷ **Possible Adverse Effects** (unusual, unexpected, and infrequent reactions)
If any of the following develop, consult your physician promptly for guidance.
Mild Adverse Effects
Allergic Reactions: Skin rash, itching.
Worsening of psoriasis—case reports.
Headache, fatigue, dizziness, insomnia, abnormal dreams—infrequent.
Indigestion, nausea, vomiting, constipation, diarrhea—infrequent.
Eye and joint pain—case reports.
Joint and muscle discomfort, fluid retention (edema)—possible.
Serious Adverse Effects
Mental depression, hallucinations, anxiety—infrequent.
Chest pain, shortness of breath, precipitation of congestive heart failure—case reports.
Induction of bronchial asthma (in asthmatic patients)—possible.
Rebound hypertension—if the drug is abruptly stopped.
Precipitation of myasthenia gravis—case reports.
Carpal tunnel syndrome—case reports.
Low or high blood sugar (hypoglycemia or hyperglycemia)—possible.
Liver compromise (hepatitis)—case reports.

▷ **Possible Effects on Sexual Function:** Decreased libido (four times more common in men); impaired erection (less common with this drug than with most other beta-blockers); Peyronie's disease (see Glossary)—case reports.

Possible Effects on Laboratory Tests

Blood HDL cholesterol level: decreased.
Blood LDL and VLDL cholesterol level: decreased.
Blood glucose level: increased.
Blood triglyceride levels: increased.

CAUTION

1. ***Do not stop this drug suddenly*** without the knowledge and help of your physician. Carry a note with you that says you take this drug.
2. Ask your doctor or pharmacist before using nasal decongestants usually present in over-the-counter cold preparations and nose drops. These may cause increases in blood pressure when used with beta-blockers.
3. Report the development of any tendency to emotional depression.

Precautions for Use

By Infants and Children: Safety and effectiveness for use by those under 12 years of age have not been established. However, if this drug is used, observe for the development of low blood sugar (hypoglycemia) during periods of reduced food intake.

By Those Over 60 Years of Age: Proceed *cautiously* with all antihypertensive drugs. Unacceptably high blood pressure should be reduced slowly, to avoid the risks associated with excessively low blood pressure. Therapy should be started with small doses, and the blood pressure checked often. Sudden, rapid, and excessive reduction of blood pressure can predispose to stroke or heart attack. Watch for dizziness, unsteadiness, tendency to fall, confusion, hallucinations, depression, or urinary frequency.

▷ **Advisability of Use During Pregnancy**

Pregnancy Category: C. See Pregnancy Risk Categories at the back of this book.
Animal studies: No significant increase in birth defects due to this drug.
Human studies: Adequate studies of pregnant women are not available.
Use this drug only if clearly needed. Ask your physician for guidance.

Advisability of Use If Breast-Feeding

Presence of this drug in breast milk: Yes, in large amounts.
Avoid drug or refrain from nursing.

Habit-Forming Potential: None.

Effects of Overdosage: Weakness, slow pulse, low blood pressure, fainting, cold and sweaty skin, congestive heart failure, possible coma, and convulsions.

Possible Effects of Long-Term Use: Reduced heart reserve and eventual heart failure in susceptible individuals with advanced heart disease.

Suggested Periodic Examinations While Taking This Drug (at physician's discretion)

Measurements of blood pressure, evaluation of heart function.

▷ **While Taking This Drug, Observe the Following**

Foods: The peak drug concentration and therefore the peak effect of this drug will increase if it is taken with food. Avoid excessive salt intake.

Beverages: No restrictions. May be taken with milk.

▷ *Alcohol:* Use with caution. Alcohol may exaggerate this drug's ability to lower the blood pressure and may increase its mild sedative effect.

Tobacco Smoking: Nicotine may reduce this drug's benefit in treating high blood pressure. I advise everyone to quit smoking.

▷ *Other Drugs*

Metoprolol may *increase* the effects of
- other antihypertensive drugs, causing excessive lowering of blood pressure. Dosage adjustments may be necessary.
- reserpine (Ser-Ap-Es, etc.), and cause sedation, depression, slowing of the heart rate, and lowering of the blood pressure.
- verapamil (Calan, Isoptin), and cause excessive depression of heart function; monitor this combination closely.

Metoprolol *taken concurrently* with
- amiodarone (Cordarone) may result in extremely slow heartbeat and cardiac arrest. NOT ADVISED.
- clonidine (Catapres) requires close monitoring for rebound high blood pressure if clonidine is withdrawn while metoprolol is still being taken.
- fluoxetine (Prozac) may cause metoprolol toxicity.
- fluvoxamine (Luvox) may lead to metoprolol toxicity.
- insulin requires close monitoring to avoid undetected hypoglycemia (see Glossary).
- lidocaine can lead to lidocaine toxicity (cardiac arrest).
- nifedipine (Adalat, Procardia, others) may result in heart failure.
- oral antidiabetic drugs (see Drug Classes) can result in prolonged hypoglycemia if it occurs.
- phenothiazines (see Drug Classes) can result in low blood pressure or toxicity due to the phenothiazine.
- quinidine (Quinaglute, others) can lead to abnormally slow heartbeat and shortness of breath.
- ritonavir (Norvir) and perhaps other protease inhibitors (see Drug Classes) may cause toxicity.
- tocainide (Tonocard) may lead to depressed contraction ability of the heart (myocardial contractility).
- venlafaxine (Effexor) may lead to metabolic changes and toxic blood levels of both medicines.

The following drugs may *increase* the effects of metoprolol
- birth control pills (oral contraceptives).
- cimetidine (Tagamet).
- diltiazem (Cardizem).
- MAO inhibitors (see Drug Classes).
- methimazole (Tapazole).
- propylthiouracil (Propacil).

The following drugs may *decrease* the effects of metoprolol
- barbiturates (phenobarbital, etc.).
- indomethacin (Indocin) and possibly other aspirin substitutes, or NSAIDs, may impair metoprolol's antihypertensive effect.
- rifampin (Rifadin, Rimactane).

▷ *Driving, Hazardous Activities:* Use caution until the full extent of drowsiness, lethargy, and blood pressure change has been determined.

Aviation Note: The use of this drug *is a disqualification* for piloting. Consult a designated Aviation Medical Examiner.

Exposure to Sun: No restrictions.

Exposure to Heat: Caution is advised. Hot environments can lower the blood pressure and exaggerate the effects of this drug.

Exposure to Cold: Caution is advised. Cold environments can increase circulatory deficiency in the extremities that may occur with this drug. The elderly should take precautions to prevent hypothermia (see Glossary).

Heavy Exercise or Exertion: It is advisable to avoid exertion that produces light-headedness, excessive fatigue, or muscle cramping. The use of this drug may intensify the hypertensive response to isometric exercise.

Occurrence of Unrelated Illness: Fever can lower the blood pressure and require adjustment of dosage. Nausea or vomiting may interrupt the regular dosage schedule. Ask your doctor for help.

Discontinuation: It is advisable to avoid sudden discontinuation of this drug in all situations. If possible, gradual reduction of dose over a period of 1 to 2 weeks is recommended. Ask your physician for specific guidance.

METRONIDAZOLE (me troh NI da zohl)

Introduced: 1960   **Class:** Anti-infective   **Prescription:** USA: Yes
Controlled Drug: USA: No; Canada: No   **Available as Generic:** Yes

Brand Names: ✦Apo-Metronidazole, Femazole, Flagyl, Flagystatin, Lagyl, Metizol, MetroGel, Metro IV, Metryl, ✦Neo-Tric, ✦Novo-Nidazole, Protostat, SK Metronidazole, ✦Trikacide

BENEFITS versus RISKS	
Possible Benefits	*Possible Risks*
EFFECTIVE TREATMENT FOR *TRICHOMONAS* INFECTIONS, AMEBIC DYSENTERY, AND GIARDIASIS, and some anaerobic bacterial infections	Superinfection with yeast organisms Peripheral neuropathy Abnormally low white blood cell count (transient) Colitis
Effective local treatment for rosacea	Aggravation of epilepsy

▷ **Principal Uses**

As a Single Drug Product: Uses currently included in FDA-approved labeling: (1) Treats *Trichomonas* infections of the vaginal canal and cervix and of the male urethra; (2) also used to treat amebic dysentery and liver abscess, *Giardia* infections of the intestine, and serious infections caused by certain strains of anaerobic bacteria; (3) treats *Gardnerella* infections of the vagina; (4) treatment of rosacea with local application of a gel dosage form; (5) used in therapy of pseudomembranous colitis; (6) has a role in treating bed sores (decubitis ulcers); (7) can help prevent infection (prophylaxis) in gynecological, appendectomy, or colorectal surgery.

Other (unlabeled) generally accepted uses: (1) Combination therapy with gentamicin in treating intra-abdominal infections; (2) combination antibiotic treatment of duodenal ulcers caused by *Helicobacter pylori*; (3) can help treat infections caused by *Giardia lamblia*; (4) used to help heal the lesions in Crohn's disease.

How This Drug Works: By interacting with DNA, this drug destroys essential components (nucleus) that are needed for life and growth of infecting organisms.

Available Dosage Forms and Strengths
Capsules — 375 mg
Gel — 0.75%
Injection — 500 mg/100 ml
Tablets — 250 mg, 500 mg
Vaginal cream — 10%

▷ **Usual Adult Dosage Range:**   For trichomoniasis: 1-day course—2 g as a single dose, or 1 g for two doses 12 hours apart. 7-day course—250 mg three times a day for 7 consecutive days. (The 7-day course is preferred.)
For amebiasis: 500 to 750 mg three times a day for 5 to 10 consecutive days.
For giardiasis: 2 g once daily for 3 days; or 250 to 500 mg three times a day for 5 to 7 days.
The total daily dosage should not exceed 4 g (4000 mg).
Note: Actual dosage and administration schedule must be determined for each patient individually.

Conditions Requiring Dosing Adjustments
Liver Function: The dose should be decreased by one-third in mild to moderate liver compromise. It should not be used in severe liver compromise.
Kidney Function: In severe kidney failure, 50% of the normal dose can be taken at the usual dosing interval. A benefit-to-risk decision must be made for these patients, as there is a risk of systemic lupus erythematosus (SLE) from the metabolites of this drug.

▷ **Dosing Instructions:**   The tablet may be crushed and taken with or following food to reduce stomach irritation.

Usual Duration of Use: Use on a regular schedule as outlined is needed to ensure effectiveness. Do not repeat the course of treatment without your physician's approval.

▷ **This Drug Should Not Be Taken If**
• you have had an allergic reaction to it or any the parabens contained in the gel form previously.
• you are pregnant.
• you currently have a bone marrow or blood cell disorder.
• you have any type of central nervous system disorder, including epilepsy.

▷ **Inform Your Physician Before Taking This Drug If**
• you have a history of any type of blood cell disorder, especially one induced by drugs.
• you have a history of seizures or peripheral neuropathy.
• you have impaired liver or kidney function.
• you have a history of alcoholism.
• you are pregnant or breast-feeding.

Possible Side Effects (natural, expected, and unavoidable drug actions)
A sharp, metallic, unpleasant taste. Dark discoloration of the urine (of no clinical significance).
Superinfection (see Glossary) by yeast organisms in the mouth or vagina. Pseudomembranous colitis.

▷ **Possible Adverse Effects** (unusual, unexpected, and infrequent reactions)
If any of the following develop, consult your physician promptly for guidance.

Mild Adverse Effects
> Allergic Reactions: Skin rash, hives, flushing, itching.
> Headache, dizziness, incoordination, unsteadiness, incontinence—infrequent.
> Loss of appetite, nausea, vomiting, abdominal cramps, diarrhea—infrequent.
> Irritation of mouth and tongue, possibly due to yeast infection—possible.

Serious Adverse Effects
> Idiosyncratic Reactions: Abnormal behavior; confusion; depression; Herxheimer's reaction—sweating, diarrhea, vomiting,
> Scalding urination, joint pain, and itching—case reports.
> Peripheral neuropathy (see Glossary)—case reports.
> Abnormally low white blood cell count (transient): fever, sore throat, infections—case reports.
> Disulfiram-type reaction (nausea, vomiting) if alcoholic beverages are consumed—possible.
> Seizures—case reports.
> Drug-induced pneumonitis, porphyria, or pancreatitis—case reports.
> Hemolytic-uremic syndrome—case reports.

▷ **Possible Effects on Sexual Function:** Decreased libido; decreased vaginal secretions (difficult or painful intercourse)—case reports.

Possible Delayed Adverse Effects: Studies have shown that this drug can cause cancer in mice and possibly in rats. Two researchers concluded that the carcinogenic risk is low in doses used to treat episodic vaginitis. Follow your physician's instructions exactly. Avoid unnecessary or prolonged use.

▷ **Adverse Effects That May Mimic Natural Diseases or Disorders**
> Behavioral changes may suggest spontaneous psychosis.

Natural Diseases or Disorders That May Be Activated by This Drug
> Latent yeast infections.

Possible Effects on Laboratory Tests
> White blood cell counts: decreased.
> INR (prothrombin time): increased.
> Blood theophylline levels: falsely increased by some methods.

CAUTION
> 1. Troublesome and persistent diarrhea can develop. If diarrhea persists for more than 24 hours, stop this drug and call your physician.
> 2. Stop this drug immediately if you develop any signs of toxic effects on the brain or nervous system: confusion, irritability, dizziness, incoordination, unsteady stance or gait, muscle jerking or twitching, numbness or weakness in the extremities.

Precautions for Use
> *By Infants and Children:* Avoid use in those with a history of bone marrow or blood cell disorders.
> *By Those Over 60 Years of Age:* Natural changes in the skin may predispose to yeast infections in the genital and anal regions. Report the development of rashes and itching promptly.

▷ **Advisability of Use During Pregnancy**
> *Pregnancy Category:* B. See Pregnancy Risk Categories at the back of this book.
> Animal studies: No birth defects reported in rat studies. However, this drug is known to cause cancer in mice and possibly in rats.

Human studies: No increase in birth defects reported in 206 exposures to this drug during the first 3 months. However, information from adequate studies of pregnant women is not available.

The manufacturer advises against the use of this drug during the first 3 months. Use during the final 6 months is not advised unless it is absolutely essential to the mother's health.

Advisability of Use If Breast-Feeding
Presence of this drug in breast milk: Yes.
Avoid drug or refrain from nursing.

Habit-Forming Potential: None.

Effects of Overdosage: Weakness, stomach irritation, nausea, vomiting, confusion, disorientation.

Possible Effects of Long-Term Use: None reported. Avoid long-term use.

Suggested Periodic Examinations While Taking This Drug (at physician's discretion)
Complete blood cell counts.

▷ **While Taking This Drug, Observe the Following**
Foods: No restrictions.
Beverages: No restrictions. May be taken with milk.
▷ *Alcohol:* A disulfiramlike reaction has been reported (see Glossary). It is NOT advisable to drink alcohol while taking metronidazole.
Tobacco Smoking: No interactions expected, but I advise everyone to quit smoking.
▷ *Other Drugs*
Metronidazole may *increase* the effects of
• warfarin (Coumadin, etc.), and cause abnormal bleeding. The INR (prothrombin time or protime) should be monitored closely, especially during the first 10 days of concurrent use.
Metronidazole *taken concurrently* with
• antacids may decrease absorption of metronidazole.
• birth control pills (oral contraceptives) may block the effectiveness of contraception and result in pregnancy.
• cholestyramine (Questran) or other cholesterol-lowering resins may decrease metronidazole absorption and lower its therapeutic effect.
• cotrimoxazole or other sulfa drugs may result in a disulfiramlike effect.
• cyclosporine (Sandimmune) can lead to cyclosporine toxicity.
• disulfiram (Antabuse) may cause severe emotional and behavioral disturbances.
• lithium (Lithobid, others) can cause lithium toxicity.
• phenytoin (Dilantin) may result in increased blood levels of phenytoin. More frequent blood level testing is needed, and the phenytoin dose should be adjusted to blood levels.
▷ *Driving, Hazardous Activities:* This drug may cause dizziness or incoordination. Restrict activities as necessary.
Aviation Note: The use of this drug *may be a disqualification* for piloting. Consult a designated Aviation Medical Examiner.
Exposure to Sun: No restrictions.

MEXILETINE (mex IL e teen)

Introduced: 1973   **Class:** Antiarrhythmic   **Prescription:** USA: Yes
Controlled Drug: USA: No; Canada: No   **Available as Generic:** No
Brand Name: Mexitil

BENEFITS versus RISKS	
Possible Benefits	*Possible Risks*
EFFECTIVE TREATMENT IN SELECTED HEART RHYTHM DISORDERS	NARROW TREATMENT RANGE FREQUENT ADVERSE EFFECTS WORSENING OF SOME ARRHYTHMIAS Rare seizures, liver injury, and reduced white blood cell count

▷ **Principal Uses**

As a Single Drug Product: Uses currently included in FDA-approved labeling: Helps correct premature beats that arise in the ventricles (lower heart chambers) which are resistant (refractory) to other agents.

Other (unlabeled) generally accepted uses: (1) May have a role in reducing symptoms in diabetic nerve damage (neuropathy); (2) has shown some benefit in combination therapy of Wolf-Parkinson-White syndrome.

How This Drug Works: By slowing the transmission of electrical impulses throughout the conduction system of the heart, this drug assists in restoring normal heart rate and rhythm in selected types of arrhythmia.

Available Dosage Forms and Strengths

Capsules — 150 mg, 200 mg, 250 mg

▷ **Usual Adult Dosage Range:** A loading dose of 400 mg is given, followed by 200 mg every 8 hours. Dose can be increased at intervals of 2 to 3 days, as needed and tolerated in 50- or 100-mg steps, to a maximum total daily dose of 1200 mg. Measurement of drug blood levels is advised (when available) to determine the optimal dose and schedule. **Note: Actual dosage and administration schedule must be determined for each patient individually.**

Conditions Requiring Dosing Adjustments

Liver Function: In liver compromise, the dose should be decreased by one-fourth to one-third. Blood levels should be obtained at prudent intervals.

Kidney Function: Dose should be decreased and blood levels obtained more frequently in severe kidney failure.

▷ **Dosing Instructions:** The capsule may be opened and taken with food or antacid to reduce stomach irritation. Take at same times each day to obtain uniform results.

Usual Duration of Use: Use on a regular schedule for 1 to 2 weeks determines effectiveness in correcting or preventing responsive rhythm disorders. Long-term use requires physician supervision.

▷ **This Drug Should Not Be Taken If**

- you have had an allergic reaction to it previously.
- you have second- or third-degree heart block (determined by electrocardiogram), uncorrected by a pacemaker.

▷ **Inform Your Physician Before Taking This Drug If**
- you have had adverse reactions to other antiarrhythmic drugs in the past.
- you have a history of heart disease of any kind, especially "heart block" or heart failure.
- you have impaired liver function.
- you have Parkinson's disease.
- you are prone to low blood pressure or have a seizure disorder of any kind.
- you take any form of digitalis, a potassium supplement, or any diuretic drug that can cause potassium loss (ask your physician).

Possible Side Effects (natural, expected, and unavoidable drug actions)
Nervousness, light-headedness. Unpleasant taste.

▷ **Possible Adverse Effects** (unusual, unexpected, and infrequent reactions)
If any of the following develop, consult your physician promptly for guidance.
Mild Adverse Effects
Allergic Reaction: Skin rash.
Headache, dizziness, visual disturbance, fatigue, weakness, tremor—infrequent.
Loss of appetite, indigestion, nausea, vomiting, constipation, diarrhea, abdominal pain—rare.
Serious Adverse Effects
Idiosyncratic Reactions: Depression, confusion, amnesia, hallucinations, seizures—all rare.
Drug-induced heart rhythm disorders: shortness of breath, palpitations, chest pain, swelling—rare.
Myelofibrosis or systemic lupus erythematosus—case reports.
Seizures—case reports.
Ataxia and confusion—may be frequent.
Congestive heart failure and sinus arrest—rare.
Urinary retention—possible.
Liver damage with jaundice (see Glossary)—case reports.
Low white blood cell or platelet counts: fever, sore throat, abnormal bleeding/bruising—case reports.

▷ **Possible Effects on Sexual Function:**   Decreased libido, impotence—rare.

▷ **Adverse Effects That May Mimic Natural Diseases or Disorders**
Liver toxicity may suggest viral hepatitis.

Natural Diseases or Disorders That May Be Activated by This Drug
Latent epilepsy.

Possible Effects on Laboratory Tests
Blood white cell and platelet counts: decreased.
Liver function tests: increased liver enzymes (ALT/GPT, AST/GOT) increased in less than 1% of users.

CAUTION
1. Thorough evaluation of your heart function (including electrocardiograms) is necessary prior to using this drug.
2. Periodic evaluation of your heart function is needed to determine your response to this drug. Some individuals may experience worsening of their heart rhythm disorder and/or deterioration of heart function. Close monitoring of heart rate, rhythm, and overall performance is essential.

3. Dosage must be adjusted carefully for each individual. Do not change your dosage without the knowledge and supervision of your physician.
4. Do not take any other antiarrhythmic drug while taking this drug unless you are directed to do so by your physician.
5. Carry a card noting that you are taking this drug. Inform all attending medical personnel that you are taking this drug, especially if you require surgery of any kind.

Precautions for Use

By Infants and Children: Safety and effectiveness for those under 12 years of age are not established. Initial use of this drug requires hospitalization and supervision by a qualified cardiologist.

By Those Over 60 Years of Age: Reduced liver function may require reduction in dosage. Watch carefully for light-headedness, dizziness, unsteadiness, and tendency to fall.

▷ Advisability of Use During Pregnancy

Pregnancy Category: C. See Pregnancy Risk Categories at the back of this book.
Animal studies: No birth defects reported in mice, rats, or rabbits. However, an increased rate of fetal resorption was found.
Human studies: Adequate studies of pregnant women are not available.
Avoid during first 3 months. Use this drug only if clearly needed. Ask your physician for guidance.

Advisability of Use If Breast-Feeding

Presence of this drug in breast milk: Yes.
Avoid drug or refrain from nursing.

Habit-Forming Potential: None.

Effects of Overdosage: Impaired urination, constipation, marked drop in blood pressure, abnormal heart rhythms, congestive heart failure, dizziness, incoordination, seizures.

Possible Effects of Long-Term Use: None reported.

Suggested Periodic Examinations While Taking This Drug (at physician's discretion)

Electrocardiograms, complete blood cell counts, liver function tests, mexiletine blood levels.

▷ While Taking This Drug, Observe the Following

Foods: No restrictions. Ask your physician regarding need for salt restriction.
Beverages: No restrictions. May be taken with milk.
▷   *Alcohol:* Use caution. Alcohol can increase the blood-pressure-lowering effects of this drug.
Tobacco Smoking: Nicotine irritate the heart, reducing drug effectiveness. I advise everyone to quit smoking.
▷   *Other Drugs*
Mexiletine may *increase* the effects of
- antihypertensive drugs, and cause excessive lowering of blood pressure.
- beta-blocker drugs (see Drug Classes).
- disopyramide (Norpace).
- theophylline (Theo-Dur, others), leading to theophylline toxicity and seizures.

Mexiletine **taken concurrently** with
- ritonavir (Norvir) and perhaps other protease inhibitors (see Drug Classes) may lead to toxicity.

The following drugs may **decrease** the effects of mexiletine
- phenytoin (Dilantin, etc.).
- rifampin (Rifadin, Rimactane).

▷ *Driving, Hazardous Activities:* This drug may cause weakness, dizziness, or blurred vision. Restrict activities as necessary.

Aviation Note: The use of this drug **may be a disqualification** for piloting. Consult a designated Aviation Medical Examiner.

Exposure to Sun: No restrictions.

Occurrence of Unrelated Illness: Vomiting, diarrhea, or dehydration can affect this drug's action adversely. Report such developments promptly.

Discontinuation: This drug should not be stopped abruptly following long-term use. Ask your physician for guidance regarding gradual dose reduction.

MIBEFRADIL (mi BEF rah dill)

Introduced: 1997 **Class:** Antihypertensive, calcium channel blocker
Prescription: USA: Yes **Controlled Drug:** USA: No; Canada: No **Available as Generic:** No

Brand Name: Posicor

> **Author's Note: This medicine was approved in June 1997. Early reports show a very favorable adverse effect profile versus other available calcium channel blockers used to treat high blood pressure and angina. This profile will be expanded once further information becomes available.**

MIGLITOL (MIG lit all)

Introduced: 1997 **Class:** Antidiabetic, alpha-glucosidase inhibitor
Prescription: USA: Yes **Controlled Drug:** USA: No; Canada: No **Available as Generic:** No

Brand Name: Glyset

> **Author's Note: This medicine appears similar to acarbose. This profile will be expanded once more information about comparative benefits of miglitol versus acarbose are known.**

MINIMALLY SEDATING ANTIHISTAMINES

Astemizole (a STEM ah zohl) **Cetirizine** (sa TEER a zeen) **Fenofaxadine** (fen oh FAX a deen) **Loratadine** (lor AT a deen) **Terfenadine** (ter FEN a deen)

Introduced: 1982, 1996, 1996, 1992, 1977, respectively **Class:** Antihistamines, minimally sedating **Prescription:** USA: Yes **Controlled Drug:** USA: No; Canada: No **Available as Generic:** U.S.: Astemizole: Yes; cetirizine: no; fexofenadine: no; loratadine: yes; terfenadine: yes; Canada: Same as U.S.

Brand Names: Astemizole: Hismanal; Cetirizine: Zyrtec; Fexofenadine: Allegra; Loratadine: ✦Chlor-Tripolon ND [CD], Claritin, Claritin D [CD], ✦Claritin Extra [CD]; Terfenadine: Seldane, Seldane-D

Author's Note: Terfenadine has been identified for removal from the market by the FDA. Some other drugs in this class have some life-threatening drug interactions. Loratadine also interacts with some antibiotics and antifungals, but HAS NOT shown the same effect on the heart (in some studies of otherwise healthy young and subsequently older subjects), but does undergo an increased blood level if combined with these medicines. It would appear prudent to decrease the dose of loratadine if it is to be combined with these medicines. Current FDA labeling DOES NOT require a warning found in package inserts for some other nonsedating antihistamines.

```
                        BENEFITS versus RISKS
        Possible Benefits                    Possible Risks
EFFECTIVE AND LONG-LASTING        RARE HEART RHYTHM
  RELIEF OF ALLERGIC RHINITIS       DISTURBANCES (HAVE
EFFECTIVE RELIEF OF SOME            OCCURRED AS A DRUG
  ALLERGIC SKIN DISORDERS           INTERACTION EFFECT OR AS A
MINIMAL DROWSINESS                  DRUG EFFECT) (astemizole,
MINOR TO NO ANTICHOLINERGIC         fexofenadine, loratadine, or
  SIDE EFFECTS                      terfenadine)
                                   Low white blood cell count
                                     (leukopenia) (1.4% of fexofenadine
                                     patients)
                                   Slight atropinelike effects (some
                                     medicines in this class)
                                   Mild sedation or fatigue
```

▷ **Principal Uses**

As a Single Drug Product: Uses currently included in FDA-approved labeling: (1) Used to treat non-nasal and nasal symptoms of seasonal allergic rhinitis (hay fever); (2) helps ease symptoms of rhinitis; (3) used to treat swellings of unknown origin (chronic urticaria) (cetirizine, loratadine); (4) helps ease symptoms of pollen-induced asthma (astemizole, cetirizine, loratadine, terfenadine).

Other (unlabeled) generally accepted uses: (1) Lichen nitidus lesions (astemizole); (2) can help control chronic vertigo (astemizole); (3) chronic idiopathic urticaria (astemizole, loratadine); (4) food allergies (cetirizine).

How This Drug Works: Medications in this class block the action of histamine, thereby stopping the development of symptoms (that are caused by histamine), such as swelling and itching of the eyes.

Available Dosage Forms and Strengths

Astemizole:

Tablets — 10 mg
Oral suspension (Canada only) — 2 mg/ml

Cetirizine:

Tablets — 5 mg, 10 mg

Fexofenadine:

Capsules — 60 mg

Loratadine:

Tablets — 10 mg

Tablets, repeat action (Claritin-D [CD]) — 5 mg loratadine, 120 mg pseudoephedrine

Tablets, extended release (Claritin-D 24-hour) — 10 mg loratadine, 240 mg pseudoephedrine

Terfenadine:

Caplets (Canada) — 120 mg

Tablets — 60 mg

Tablets (D-(R) Extended Release) — 60 mg (immediate-release terfenadine)—10 mg (immediate-release pseudoephedrine)—110 mg (extended-release pseudoephedrine)

Oral suspension (Canada) — 6 mg/ml

▷ **Recommended Dosage Ranges** (Actual dosage and administration schedule must be determined for each patient individually.)

Infants and Children: **Safety and efficacy in those less than 12 years old have not been established for all of these medicines.**

12 to 60 Years of Age: Astemizole: 10 mg per day. This is also the maximum daily dose.

Cetirizine: The starting dose is 5 mg (depending on severity, may be 10 mg) and is increased as needed and tolerated to a maximum of 20 mg daily.

Fexofenadine: 60 mg twice daily.

Loratadine: A single 10-mg (of the nonrepeat action, noncombination product) tablet is taken once daily. Loratadine/pseudoephedrine (5 mg/120 mg) (nonrepeat action): One tablet twice daily. Loratadine/pseudoephedrine (10 mg/240 mg) (repeat action): One tablet daily.

Terfenadine: 60 mg twice daily. This is also the maximum dose. Terfenadine extended release (D): One tablet twice daily.

Over 60 Years of Age: Fexofenadine, loratadine (Claritin-D and Claritin-D 24-hour forms) are NOT recommended for those over 60, and cetirizine may be more slowly removed from the body by patients in this age range. Consideration should be given to a lower dose or less frequent dosing if symptoms of accumulation of this drug occur. Terfenadine (Seldane-D form) is not recommended for those over 60.

Conditions Requiring Dosing Adjustments

Liver Function: Astemizole: Use with caution in liver disease. Dosing guidelines are not available.

Cetirizine: A 5-mg dose is recommended.

Fexofenadine: Dosing changes do not appear to be needed.

Loratadine: Patients with liver compromise take a dose of 10 mg (of the nonrepeat action, noncombination product) every other day.

Terfenadine: NOT used in these patients. FATAL abnormal heartbeats can result.

Kidney Function: Astemizole: No dosing changes appear to be needed.

Cetirizine: Patients with moderate kidney decline (creatinine clearance 11–31 ml/min) may take 5 mg daily.

Fexofenadine: A daily dose of 60 mg once daily is recommended.

Loratadine: Patients with moderate kidney failure (creatinine clearance of less than 30 ml/min) should take a starting dose of 10 mg (of the nonrepeat action, noncombination product) every other day.

Terfenadine: Dosing changes do not appear to be needed.

▷ **Dosing Instructions:** Astemizole and loratadine are best taken on an empty stomach. The other medicines in this class may be taken with food. Extended-release forms of these medicines should never be crushed.

Usual Duration of Use: Although all of these medicines may go to work immediately, continual use on a regular schedule for up to 1 day (terfenadine or fexofenadine), up to 2 days (astemizole or cetirizine), and up to 3 days for (loratadine) may be necessary to see substantial improvement in allergic symptoms. Long-term use (months to years) requires periodic evaluation of response and dosage adjustment. See your doctor on a regular basis.

Possible Advantages of These Drugs

Less sedating than previously available antihistamines. Once-daily dosing for some agents in this class. Some medicines in this class do not interact with certain antifungals and macrolide antibiotics (see Drug Classes), or do interact but do not appear to cause side effects on the heart or change the safety profile. Cetirizine has NOT had ANY case reports of QTC prolongation. Tachyphylaxis or tolerance may be less likely to occur to these medicines than with earlier agents.

Currently "Drugs of Choice"

for patients who must take antihistamine-type medicines and require the best possible balance of symptom relief and minimal sedation.

▷ **These Drugs Should Not Be Taken If**

• you have had an allergic reaction to any dosage form of or any of the ingredients in it previously.
• you are presently being tested (using skin tests) for allergies.
• you are taking medicines that prolong the QT interval, such as quinidine, pentamidine, disopyramide, or others (for astemizole, cetirizine, fexofenadine, and terfenadine).
• you have urinary retention, liver disease, severe disease of the arteries of the heart (coronary artery disease), or narrow-angle glaucoma (loratadine or terfenadine combination products that contain pseudoephedrine).

▷ **Inform Your Physician Before Taking These Drugs If**

• you have asthma.
• you are at risk for drowsiness or fainting (syncope).
• you have a history of a heart rhythm disorder.
• you are taking other medicines (especially antifungal or macrolide antibiotics). Blood levels of loratadine or fexofenadine may be increased. Decreases in loratadine and fexofenadine doses may be prudent. Terfenadine and astemizole should NOT be combined with these medicines.
• you have a history of liver or kidney compromise.

Possible Side Effects (natural, expected, and unavoidable drug actions)

Dry nose, mouth, or throat, somnolence (drowsiness): cetirizine—frequent, fexofenadine—rare, loratadine—infrequent, terfenadine—infrequent.

▷ **Possible Adverse Effects** (unusual, unexpected, and infrequent reactions)
If any of the following develop, consult your physician promptly for guidance.

Mild Adverse Effects

Allergic Reactions: Skin rash, itching.
Headache, fatigue, or dizziness—infrequent.
Dry mouth—possible to infrequent.
Leg cramps, muscle aches (astemizole or loratadine)—rare.
Increased urination (terfenadine)—case reports.
Fast heart rate (tachycardia) (loratadine)—rare.
Prolonged QTc interval (fexofenadine)—case report.
Lowering of the blood pressure (loratadine)—rare.
Vision changes (loratadine or terfenadine)—rare.

Serious Adverse Effects

Allergic Reactions: Anaphylaxis (astemizole or loratadine)—rare.
Idiosyncratic Reactions: Not reported.
Serious heart rhythm disorders: astemizole or terfenadine—rare; loratadine—case report.
Tachycardia—rare.
Lowering of the white blood cell count (fexofenadine)—rare.
Abnormal liver function (loratadine or terfenadine)—case reports.
Depression, confusion, paresthesias—rare.
Passing out (syncope)—rare.

▷ **Possible Effects on Sexual Function:** Vaginitis, painful menses (dysmenorrhea), breast enlargement or breast pain (loratadine)—case reports. Menstrual disorders (loratadine, fexofenadine, terfenadine)—case reports.
Galactorrhea (loratadine or terfenadine)—case reports.
Impotence (loratadine)—case reports.

Possible Delayed Adverse Effects: None reported.

▷ **Adverse Effects That May Mimic Natural Diseases or Disorders**
Increased liver enzymes may mimic hepatitis of infectious origin.

Natural Diseases or Disorders That May Be Activated by This Drug
None reported.

Possible Effects on Laboratory Tests
Skin tests for allergies will be blunted and less diagnostic.
Liver function tests: may be increased (loratadine or terfenadine).
White blood cell counts: decreased (leukopenia) (fexofenadine)—rare in clinical trials.

CAUTION

1. Loratadine does interact with some antifungals and some macrolide antibiotics—but appears to be free of the heart (cardiac) effects, even though blood levels of loratadine may increase if it is taken with these interacting medicines. Talk to your doctor or pharmacist before taking any medicines that were not discussed when loratadine was prescribed.
2. Some of these medicines HAVE LIFE-THREATENING DRUG INTERACTIONS. Talk to your doctor or pharmacist BEFORE combining any prescription, nonprescription, or herbal remedies with medicines in this class.
3. Report dizziness, heart palpitation, or chest pain promptly when using any of these medicines.

Precautions for Use

By Infants and Children: Safety and effectiveness for use by those under 12 years of age have not been established.

By Those Over 60 Years of Age: Smaller starting and maintenance doses are needed. Longer dosing intervals may be needed as well.

▷ **Advisability of Use During Pregnancy**

Pregnancy Category: B (cetirizine, loratadine); C (fexofenadine, terfenadine). See Pregnancy Risk Categories at the back of this book.

Animal studies: No birth defects reported.

Human studies: Information from adequate studies of pregnant women is not available.

These medicines should be used during pregnancy only if clearly needed. Discuss the benefits versus risks with your doctor.

Advisability of Use If Breast-Feeding

Presence of this drug in breast milk: No data (cetirizine, fexofenadine); expected (astemizole, terfenadine); yes (loratadine).

Ask your doctor for guidance regarding stopping the drug or stopping nursing (astemizole, cetirizine, fexofenadine, or loratadine). Avoid drug or stop nursing (terfenadine).

Habit-Forming Potential: None.

Effects of Overdosage: With overdoses greater than 10 mg (40–80 mg): tachycardia, somnolence, and headache (loratadine).

Usual antihistamine protocols (cetirizine or fexofenadine).

Possible life-threatening heart rhythm problems (astemizole or terfenadine).

Possible Effects of Long-Term Use: None defined.

Suggested Periodic Examinations While Taking This Drug (at physician's discretion)

Examination for relief of the condition(s) being treated. Electrocardiogram (ECG), especially for those with heart conditions.

▷ **While Taking This Drug, Observe the Following**

Foods: Astemizole and loratadine are best taken on an empty stomach.

Beverages: Grapefruit juice may lead to increased blood levels of terfenadine and lead to toxicity. Water is the best liquid to take with medicines in this class.

▷ *Alcohol:* May cause excessive drowsiness (central nervous system depression).

Tobacco Smoking: No interactions expected, but I advise everyone to quit smoking.

Marijuana Smoking: May cause additive drowsiness or lethargy.

▷ *Other Drugs*

These medicines *taken concurrently* with

- cimetidine (Tagamet) may produce a significant increase in loratadine blood levels. No serious drug effects have been reported, but since in general the frequency of adverse effects increases with increasing blood levels, it appears prudent to decrease the dose of loratadine if these medicines are to be taken at the same time because of possible loratadine toxicity. The loratadine dose should certainly be decreased if increased frequency of adverse effects occur if these medicines are combined in usual doses. Terfenadine and astemizole may also react.

- fluoxetine (Prozac) produced a serious heart rhythm problem in a patient taking terfenadine—do NOT combine these medicines. Caution is advised for the other drugs in this class.
- fluvoxamine (Luvox) may result in increased blood levels of terfenadine, astemizole, cetirizine, or loratadine. Caution is advised.
- indinavir (Crixivan) and perhaps ritonavir, saquinavir, or nelfinavir may decrease metabolism of astemizole or terfenadine, and should NEVER be combined. Loratadine levels may be increased, and doses may need to be lowered. Other minimally sedating antihistamines may also be affected.
- itraconazole (and perhaps other similarly structured antifungals such as ketoconazole) should NEVER be combined with astemizole or terfenadine. These drugs may cause increased blood levels of loratadine. Although no serious heart rhythm toxicity has been reported to date with this medicine, caution is advised, and it appears prudent to lower the dose of loratadine if these medicines are to be combined.
- macrolide antibiotics such as azithromycin, clarithromycin, or erythromycin—astemizole or terfenadine must never be combined with these medicines. Although no serious heart rhythm toxicity has been reported to date with loratadine, caution is advised as excessive blood levels of any medicine may increase the risk of adverse effects. It appears prudent to lower the dose of loratadine if these medicines are to be combined.
- medicines that prolong the QT interval—should be avoided in combination use (such as disopyramide, ibutilide, others). Cetirizine is the only medicine in this class without any reports of QTc interval changes.
- paroxetine (Paxil) may inhibit the enzymes needed to remove astemizole, cetirizine, loratadine, or terfenadine. Caution is advised.
- quinidine (Quinaglute, others) may result in a change in the effect of quinidine and result in undesirable effects on the heart. Caution is advised.
- sotalol (Betapace) may cause additive adverse effects (QT interval prolongation) on the heart by these medicines. This combination is not recommended.
- theophylline (Theo-Dur, others) may decrease cetirizine clearance. This combination should be avoided.
- zafirlukast (Accolate)—if combined with terfenadine may decrease zafirlukast levels and blunt the therapeutic benefits of zafirlukast (and perhaps zileuton—Zyflo).

▷ *Driving, Hazardous Activities:* Although these medicines are much less likely than earlier antihistamines to cause drowsiness, caution should be used until your individual reaction to these medicines is determined. Restrict activities as necessary.

Aviation Note: The use of these drugs *are probably not a disqualification* for piloting. Consult a designated Aviation Medical Examiner.

Exposure to Sun: Rare cases of photosensitivity have been reported with some medicines (astemizole, loratadine) in this class. Use caution.

MINOXIDIL (min OX i dil)

Introduced: 1972   **Class:** Antihypertensive, hair growth stimulant
Prescription: USA: Yes   **Controlled Drug:** USA: No; Canada: No   **Available as Generic:** Yes
Brand Names: Alostil, Loniten, Minodyl, Minoximen, Rogaine
  Author's Note: Rogaine treatment for baldness is now available without a prescription.

BENEFITS versus RISKS	
Possible Benefits	*Possible Risks*
POTENT, LONG-ACTING ANTIHYPERTENSIVE	EXCESSIVE BODY HAIR GROWTH SALT AND WATER RETENTION
EFFECTIVE IN CASES OF SEVERE HYPERTENSION, ACCELERATED AND MALIGNANT HYPERTENSION	Excessively rapid heart rate Aggravation of angina Local scalp irritation (topical use)
Moderately effective in treating male pattern baldness	

▷ **Principal Uses**

As a Single Drug Product: Uses currently included in FDA-approved labeling: (1) Treatment of severe high blood pressure that cannot be controlled by conventional therapy; (2) the treatment of female androgenic baldness or male pattern baldness; (3) effective in patients with high blood pressure and kidney failure.

Other (unlabeled) generally accepted uses: Supportive therapy in hair transplants.

How This Drug Works: (1) Directly relaxes constricted muscles in the walls of small arteries, and permits expansion of the arteries and lowering of blood pressure. (2) The drug may act directly on the hair follicle, and also may increase the size of previously closed small blood vessels in the scalp (improve blood flow) and restore small hair follicles to normal size and activity.

Available Dosage Forms and Strengths
  Tablets — 2.5 mg, 10 mg
 Topical solution — 2%

▷ **Usual Adult Dosage Range:** For hypertension: Initially 5 mg once a day. The dose is then gradually increased as needed and tolerated to 10 mg, 20 mg, then 40 mg every 24 hours, taken in one or two divided doses daily. The usual maintenance dose is 10 to 40 mg daily. The total daily dosage should not exceed 50 mg.

For male pattern baldness: Apply thinly 1 ml of topical solution to the balding area of the scalp twice daily. The total daily dosage should not exceed 2 ml. **Note: Actual dosage and administration schedule must be determined for each patient individually.**

Conditions Requiring Dosing Adjustments

Liver Function: This drug is metabolized (90%) in the liver. It should be used with caution by patients with liver compromise.

Kidney Function: In moderate kidney failure, the dose should be decreased empirically.

▷ **Dosing Instructions:** For hypertension: Tablets may be crushed and taken with or following food to prevent nausea. Take at the same time each day.

For baldness: ***The topical solution is for external, local use only; it is not to be swallowed.*** Begin application at the center of the bald area; apply thinly to cover the entire area. The scalp and hair must be dry at the time of application. Follow instructions carefully.

Usual Duration of Use: Use on a regular schedule for 3 to 7 days usually determines effectiveness in controlling severe hypertension. Continual use of the topical solution for at least 4 months is necessary to determine its ability to promote hair growth. Long-term use (months to years) of both dosage forms requires physician supervision.

▷ **This Drug Should Not Be Taken If**
- you have had an allergic reaction to it previously.
- you are known to have a pheochromocytoma (an adrenaline-producing tumor).
- you have pulmonary hypertension due to mitral valve stenosis.

▷ **Inform Your Physician Before Taking This Drug If**
- you are pregnant or planning pregnancy.
- you are breast-feeding your infant.
- you have had a heart attack.
- you have existing blood vessel disease in your head (cerebrovascular disease).
- you have a history of coronary artery disease or impaired heart function.
- you have a history of stroke or impaired brain circulation.
- you have impaired liver or kidney function.

Possible Side Effects (natural, expected, and unavoidable drug actions)
Increased heart rate, fluid retention with weight gain, excessive hair growth on face, arms, legs, and back (frequent).

▷ **Possible Adverse Effects** (unusual, unexpected, and infrequent reactions)
If any of the following develop, consult your physician promptly for guidance.

Mild Adverse Effects
Allergic Reactions: Skin rash. Localized dermatitis at site of application of topical solution—rare.
Headache, dizziness, fainting—rare.
Nausea, increased thirst—infrequent.
Hair growth, and changes in hair color—case reports.
Weight gain—possible.
Mild increase in liver enzymes—infrequent.

Serious Adverse Effects
Allergic Reactions: Serious skin rash (Stevens-Johnson syndrome).
Idiosyncratic Reaction: Fluid formation around the heart (pericardial effusion).
Development of angina pectoris; high blood pressure in the lungs (pulmonary hypertension)—case reports.
Systemic lupus erythematosus—case reports.
Low white blood cells or platelets—rare and transient.

Author's Note: Topical use of this medicine for hair growth may avoid most of these adverse effects.

▷ **Possible Effects on Sexual Function:**   Male breast tenderness (gynecomastia)—case reports. Some data to support that this drug balances male ability to ejaculate and have a healthy sex drive may have been blunted by other drugs that treat high blood pressure.

Natural Diseases or Disorders That May Be Activated by This Drug
Latent coronary artery disease with symptomatic angina.

Possible Effects on Laboratory Tests
Blood HDL cholesterol level: increased.
Blood LDL cholesterol level: decreased.

CAUTION
1. Long-term use for hypertension usually requires the concurrent use of an effective diuretic to counteract salt and water retention.
2. The long-term use of this drug for hypertension may require concurrent use of a beta-blocker drug to control excessive acceleration of the heart.
3. It is best to avoid combining this drug and guanethidine; the combination can cause severe orthostatic hypotension (see Glossary).
4. Consult your physician regarding the advisability of using a "no-salt-added" diet.
5. Little of this drug is absorbed into the general circulation when the topical solution is applied to the scalp. However, some systemic effects have been reported. Inform your physician promptly if you experience any unusual symptoms while using the topical solution.

Precautions for Use
By Infants and Children: Dosage schedules should be determined by a qualified pediatrician. In children under 12 years old: starting dose is 0.1 to 0.2 mg per kg of body mass in a single dose. The dose is then increased as needed and tolerated by 0.1 to 0.2 mg per kg of body mass per day steps at 3-day intervals. Children over 12 are given the adult dose. Monitor closely for salt and water retention.
By Those Over 60 Years of Age: Treatment with small doses and a limit of total daily dose to 75 mg is indicated. Headache, palpitation, and rapid heart rate due to this drug are more common in this age group and can mimic acute anxiety states. Observe for dizziness, unsteadiness, fainting, and falling.

▷ **Advisability of Use During Pregnancy**
Pregnancy Category: C. See Pregnancy Risk Categories at the back of this book.
Animal studies: No birth defects reported in rats or rabbits. However, studies did reveal decreased fertility and increased fetal deaths.
Human studies: Adequate studies of pregnant women are not available.
Avoid during the first 3 months. Use only if clearly needed during the final 6 months.

Advisability of Use If Breast-Feeding
Presence of this drug in breast milk: Yes.
Avoid drug or refrain from nursing.

Habit-Forming Potential: None.

Effects of Overdosage: Headache, dizziness, weakness, nausea, marked low blood pressure, weak and rapid pulse, loss of consciousness.

Possible Effects of Long-Term Use: Excessive growth of body hair occurs in 80% of users after 1 to 2 months of continual treatment for hypertension. Close to 100% of users will experience this effect after 1 year of continual treatment. This may be accompanied by darkening of the skin and coarsening of facial features.

Suggested Periodic Examinations While Taking This Drug (at physician's discretion)
Body weight measurement for insidious gain due to water retention.
Electrocardiographic and echocardiographic heart examinations.

▷ **While Taking This Drug, Observe the Following**
Foods: Avoid excessive salt and heavily salted foods.
Beverages: No restrictions. May be taken with milk.
▷ *Alcohol:* Use with extreme caution. Alcohol can exaggerate the blood-pressure-lowering effects of this drug.
Tobacco Smoking: Best avoided. Nicotine can contribute significantly to angina. I advise everyone to quit smoking.
▷ *Other Drugs*
Minoxidil may *increase* the effects of
• all other antihypertensive drugs; careful dosage adjustments are mandatory.
Minoxidil *taken concurrently* with
• guanethidine (Ismelin, Esimil) may cause severe orthostatic hypotension; avoid this combination.
• NSAIDs may blunt the therapeutic benefit of minoxidil.
• vitamin E may reverse hair growth.
▷ *Driving, Hazardous Activities:* This drug may cause dizziness and fatigue. Restrict activities as necessary.
Aviation Note: The use of this drug *is a disqualification* for piloting. Consult a designated Aviation Medical Examiner.
Exposure to Sun: No restrictions.
Discontinuation: This drug should not be stopped abruptly. If it is to be discontinued, consult your physician regarding gradual reduction in dosage and appropriate replacement with other drugs for the management of hypertension. Following discontinuation of the topical solution, the pretreatment pattern of baldness may return within 3 to 4 months.

MIRTAZAPINE (mur TAZ a peen)

Introduced: 1996   **Class:** Antidepressant, piperazinoazepine, norepinephrine serotonin reuptake inhibitor   **Prescription:** USA: Yes   **Controlled Drug:** USA: No; Canada: No   **Available as Generic:** USA: No; Canada: No

Brand Name: Remeron

BENEFITS versus RISKS	
Possible Benefits	*Possible Risks*
EFFECTIVE TREATMENT OF DEPRESSION	Sleepiness
	Weight gain
BENEFICIAL ACTION ON TWO NERVE TRANSMITTERS	Lowering of white blood cells

▷ **Principal Uses**

As a Single Drug Product: Uses currently included in FDA-approved labeling: Treatment of depression.

Other (unlabeled) generally accepted uses: None at present.

How This Drug Works: This drug works to increase two nerve transmitters (norepinephrine as well as serotonin) that are thought to be low or lowered in cases of depression.

Available Dosage Forms and Strengths

Tablets — 15 mg, 30 mg

▷ **Usual Adult Dosage Range**

For treatment of depression: 15 to 45 mg at bedtime. **Note: Actual dosage and administration schedule must be determined for each patient individually.**

Author's Note: Because this medicine has only been recently approved, information in this profile will be expanded in the next edition of this book.

MISOPROSTOL (mi soh PROH stohl)

Introduced: 1987   **Class:** Gastrointestinal drug (ulcer preventive)   **Prescription:** USA: Yes   **Controlled Drug:** USA: No; Canada: No   **Available as Generic:** USA: No; Canada: No

Brand Names: Arthrotec, Cytotec

BENEFITS versus RISKS	
Possible Benefits	*Possible Risks*
EFFECTIVE PREVENTION OF STOMACH ULCERATION WHILE TAKING ANTI-INFLAMMATORY DRUGS	INCREASED RISK OF ABORTION (if used during pregnancy)
	Diarrhea (transient)
Effective treatment of duodenal ulcer	Neuropathy

▷ **Principal Uses**

As a Single Drug Product: Uses currently included in FDA-approved labeling: Prevents development of stomach ulcers during long-term use of anti-inflammatory drugs as therapy for arthritis and related conditions.

Other (unlabeled) generally accepted uses: (1) Used (in Canada and other countries) for treatment of active duodenal ulcer unrelated to use of anti-inflammatory drugs; (2) has some use in inducing abortions; (3) used in combination with cyclosporine or prednisone to decrease transplanted organ rejection; (4) may have a benefit in helping ripen the cervix in preparation for a vaginal delivery.

How This Drug Works: This drug protects the lining of the stomach and duode-num and prevents ulceration due to anti-inflammatory drugs by: (1) replac-ing tissue prostaglandins that are depleted by anti-inflammatory drugs; (2) inhibiting the secretion of stomach acid; (3) increasing the local production of bicarbonate (to neutralize acids) and mucus (to protect stomach and duodenal tissues). The combined effects prevent new ulcer formation and promote healing of existing ulcer(s).

Available Dosage Forms and Strengths
Tablets — 100 mcg, 200 mcg

Conditions Requiring Dosing Adjustments
Liver Function: Specific dosage adjustments in liver compromise are not de-fined.
Kidney Function: The dose of misoprostol should be decreased if it is used by patients with compromised kidneys and is not well tolerated.

▷ **Usual Adult Dosage Range**
For prevention of stomach ulcer—200 mcg four times daily with food, taken concurrently during the use of any anti-inflammatory drug (see Antiar-thritic or NSAIDs Drug Classes).
For treatment of duodenal ulcer—200 mcg four times daily for 4 to 8 weeks.
Note: Actual dosage and administration schedule must be determined for each patient individually.

▷ **Dosing Instructions:**   The tablet may be crushed and taken with each of three daily meals; take the last (fourth) dose of the day with food at bedtime.

Usual Duration of Use: For prevention of stomach ulcer, use is recommended for the entire period of anti-inflammatory drug use. For treatment of duo-denal ulcer, continual use on a regular schedule for 4 weeks is recom-mended; if ulcer healing is not complete, a second course of 4 weeks is advised. Long-term use (months to years) requires periodic physician eval-uation of response and dosage adjustment.

Possible Advantages of This Drug: Significantly more effective than histamine (H_2) blocking drugs (cimetidine, famotidine, nizatidine, ranitidine) or su-cralfate in preventing the development of stomach ulcers.

▷ **This Drug Should Not Be Taken If**
• you have had an allergic reaction to it previously.
• you are allergic to any type of prostaglandin.
• you are pregnant or breast-feeding.
• you are not able or willing to use effective contraception (oral contracep-tives or intrauterine device) while taking this drug.

▷ **Inform Your Physician Before Taking This Drug If**
• you have a history of peptic ulcer disease or Crohn's disease.
• you have inflammatory bowel disease.
• you have impaired kidney function.
• you have a seizure disorder.

Possible Side Effects (natural, expected, and unavoidable drug actions)
Diarrhea (14–40% of users), usually beginning after 13 days of use and sub-siding spontaneously after 8 days.
Abortion (miscarriage) of pregnancy (11% of users); this is often incomplete and accompanied by serious uterine bleeding that may require hospitaliza-tion and urgent treatment.

▷ **Possible Adverse Effects** (unusual, unexpected, and infrequent reactions)
If any of the following develop, consult your physician promptly for guidance.

Mild Adverse Effects
Allergic Reaction: Skin rash.
Headache, dizziness—infrequent.
Ringing in the ears—case reports.
Passing out (syncope)—rare.
Abdominal pain, indigestion, nausea, vomiting, flatulence, constipation—rare to infrequent.

Serious Adverse Effects
Allergic Reactions: Anaphylaxis—rare.
Anemia and low blood platelets—rare.
Blood in the urine—rare.
Bronchospasm—rare.
Neuropathy—rare.
Abortion (if taken while pregnant).

▷ **Possible Effects on Sexual Function:** Menstrual irregularity, menstrual cramps, heavy menstrual flow, spotting between periods—all rare.
Postmenopausal vaginal bleeding; this may require further evaluation.
Reduced libido and impotence—rare and causal relationship not established.

▷ **Natural Diseases or Disorders That May Be Activated by This Drug**
Latent epilepsy.

Possible Effects on Laboratory Tests
Mild increase in liver function enzymes.

CAUTION
1. Do not take this drug if you are pregnant. It can cause abortion.
2. Do not make this drug available to others who may be pregnant or who may become pregnant.
3. If this drug is prescribed, it is advisable that you have a negative serum pregnancy test within 2 weeks before starting treatment.
4. Start taking this drug only on the second or third day of your next normal menstrual period.
5. Initiate effective contraceptive measures when you begin to take this drug. Discuss the use of oral contraceptives or intrauterine devices with your physician.
6. Should you become pregnant, stop the drug immediately and call your doctor.

Precautions for Use
By Infants and Children: Safety and effectiveness for those under 18 years of age not established.
By Those Over 60 Years of Age: This drug is usually well tolerated by this age group. However, some forms of prostaglandins can cause drops in blood pressure; watch for light-headedness or faintness that may indicate low blood pressure. Report any such development to your physician.

▷ **Advisability of Use During Pregnancy**
Pregnancy Category: X. See Pregnancy Risk Categories at the back of this book.
Animal studies: No birth defects due to this drug found in rat or rabbit studies.

Human studies: Information from studies of pregnant women confirms that this drug can cause abortion, sometimes incomplete; unpassed products of conception can cause life-threatening complications.
Avoid this drug completely.

Advisability of Use If Breast-Feeding
Presence of this drug in breast milk: Unknown.
Avoid drug or refrain from nursing.

Habit-Forming Potential: None.

Effects of Overdosage: Abdominal pain, diarrhea, fever, drowsiness, weakness, tremor, convulsions, difficult breathing.

Possible Effects of Long-Term Use: Unknown at this time.

Suggested Periodic Examinations While Taking This Drug (at physician's discretion)
Monitoring for accidental pregnancy.

▷ **While Taking This Drug, Observe the Following**
Foods: High-fat meals may reduce peak blood concentration.
Beverages: No restrictions. May be taken with milk.
▷   *Alcohol:* No interactions expected. However, alcohol can promote the development of stomach ulcer and reduce the effectiveness of this drug.
Tobacco Smoking: No interactions expected. Nicotine is conducive to stomach ulcers. I advise everyone to quit smoking.
▷   *Other Drugs*
Misoprostol *taken concurrently* with
• antacids that contain magnesium may increase the risk of diarrhea; avoid this combination. Antacids in general may decrease misoprostol absorption and lessen its therapeutic benefits.
• indomethacin and some other NSAIDs may result in decreased NSAID levels.
▷   *Driving, Hazardous Activities:* This drug may cause dizziness, light-headedness, stomach pain, or diarrhea. Restrict activities as necessary.
Aviation Note: The use of this drug *may be a disqualification* for piloting. Consult a designated Aviation Medical Examiner.
Exposure to Sun: No restrictions.
Discontinuation: This drug should be taken as combination therapy while you are taking antiarthritic/anti-inflammatory drugs that can cause stomach ulceration. Call your doctor if you have reason to stop it prematurely.

MOLINDONE (moh LIN dohn)

Introduced: 1971   **Class:** Strong tranquilizer, antipsychotic   **Prescription:** USA: Yes   **Controlled Drug:** USA: No; Canada: No   **Available as Generic:** No

Brand Name: Moban

```
┌─────────────────────────────────────────────────────────────────┐
│                      BENEFITS versus RISKS                        │
│        Possible Benefits              Possible Risks              │
│  EFFECTIVE TREATMENT OF SOME    NARROW TREATMENT MARGIN           │
│    CASES OF ACUTE AND CHRONIC     SERIOUS TOXIC EFFECTS ON        │
│    SCHIZOPHRENIA                    BRAIN:                        │
│  May be effective in schizophrenia that   Parkinson-like reactions │
│    has not responded to other drugs   severe restlessness        │
│                                       abnormal involuntary movements │
│                                       tardive dyskinesias         │
│                                 Liver toxicity, jaundice          │
│                                 Atropinelike side effects         │
└─────────────────────────────────────────────────────────────────┘
```

▷ **Principal Uses**

As a Single Drug Product: Uses currently included in FDA-approved labeling: (1) Helps manage acute and chronic schizophrenia to control thought disorder, disorientation, hallucinations, perceptual distortions, and hostility; (2) may have a small role in helping relieve depression.

Other (unlabeled) generally accepted uses: May be of help in children with conduct disorders.

How This Drug Works: Acts on nerve transmitters (serotonin and dopamine) to restore the activity in the reticular activating system of the brain, and improve distorted patterns of thinking and behavior.

Available Dosage Forms and Strengths

Concentrate — 20 mg/ml
    Tablets — 5 mg, 10 mg, 25 mg, 50 mg, 100 mg

▷ **Usual Adult Dosage Range:**   Initially 50 to 75 mg daily in three or four divided doses; dose may be increased gradually in 3 days to 100 mg/day as needed and tolerated. For maintenance: mild psychosis—5 to 15 mg, three or four times daily; moderate psychosis—10 to 25 mg three or four times daily; severe psychosis—up to 225 mg/day, in three or four divided doses. The total daily dosage should not exceed 225 mg. **Note: Actual dosage and administration schedule must be determined for each patient individually.**

Conditions Requiring Dosing Adjustments

Liver Function: Specific dosage adjustments in liver compromise are not defined. This drug should be used with caution by patients with liver compromise, as it is a rare cause of liver toxicity (hepatoxicity).

Kidney Function: The kidney is minimally (3%) involved in the elimination of molindone.

▷ **Dosing Instructions:**   The tablet may be crushed and taken with food or milk to reduce stomach irritation. The liquid concentrate may be diluted with water, milk, fruit juice, or carbonated beverages.

Usual Duration of Use: Use on a regular schedule for 3 to 6 weeks is usually necessary to determine this drug's effectiveness in controlling the features of schizophrenia. Long-term use (months to years) requires supervision and periodic evaluation by your physician. Consult your physician on a regular basis.

▷ **This Drug Should Not Be Taken If**
- you have had an allergic reaction to it previously.
- you have acute alcoholic intoxication.

▷ **Inform Your Physician Before Taking This Drug If**
- you are taking any drugs that have sedative effects.
- you use alcohol excessively.
- you have any type of seizure disorder.
- you are pregnant or breast-feeding.
- you have a history of neuroleptic malignant syndrome.
- you have any type of glaucoma.
- you have Parkinson's disease or an enlarged prostate gland.
- you have impaired liver or kidney function.
- you have a history of breast cancer.

Possible Side Effects (natural, expected, and unavoidable drug actions)

Drowsiness, dry mouth, nasal congestion, constipation, impaired urination. Parkinson-like reactions (see Glossary). Lowering of blood pressure on standing (orthostatic hypotension), weight gain.

▷ **Possible Adverse Effects** (unusual, unexpected, and infrequent reactions)

If any of the following develop, consult your physician promptly for guidance.

Mild Adverse Effects

Allergic Reactions: Skin rash.

Headache, dizziness, blurred vision, lethargy, insomnia, depression, euphoria, ringing in ears—infrequent.

Rapid heartbeat, low blood pressure, fainting—case reports.

Loss of appetite, indigestion, nausea—possible

Temporary lowering or increase in white blood cells—case reports.

Serious Adverse Effects

Allergic Reactions: Liver reaction with jaundice—rare, questionable.

Idiosyncratic Reactions: Neuroleptic malignant syndrome (see Glossary).

Spasms of face and neck muscles, involuntary movements of extremities, severe restlessness—case reports.

Development of tardive dyskinesia (see Glossary)—case reports.

Lowering of the seizure threshold—possible.

Muscle damage (rhabdomyolysis) or liver toxicity—rare.

▷ **Possible Effects on Sexual Function**

Increased libido.

Male breast enlargement and tenderness; painful and extended erections.

Female breast enlargement with milk formation.

Altered timing and pattern of menstruation.

▷ **Adverse Effects That May Mimic Natural Diseases or Disorders**

Parkinson-like reactions may be mistaken for naturally occurring Parkinson's disease.

Rare liver reaction may suggest viral hepatitis.

Possible Effects on Laboratory Tests

Liver function enzymes: increased.

Blood urea nitrogen: increased.

CAUTION
1. This drug may alter the pattern of epileptic seizures and require dosage adjustments of anticonvulsant drugs.
2. Obtain prompt evaluation of any change or disturbance of vision.
3. There is a very narrow margin between the effective therapeutic dose and the dose that can cause Parkinson-like reactions. Inform your physician promptly if suggestive symptoms develop.

Precautions for Use

By Infants and Children: Safety and effectiveness for those under 12 years of age are not established.

By Those Over 60 Years of Age: Start treatment with small doses. This drug can aggravate existing prostatism (see Glossary). You may be more susceptible to the development of Parkinson-like reactions or tardive dyskinesia. Report any suggestive symptoms promptly.

▷ Advisability of Use During Pregnancy

Pregnancy Category: C. See Pregnancy Risk Categories at the back of this book. Animal studies: No birth defects reported in mice, rats, or rabbits.
Human studies: Adequate studies of pregnant women are not available.
Because of its inherent toxicity for brain tissue, avoid use during pregnancy if possible.

Advisability of Use If Breast-Feeding

Presence of this drug in breast milk: Unknown.
Avoid drug or refrain from nursing.

Habit-Forming Potential: None.

Effects of Overdosage: Marked drowsiness, weakness, tremor, agitation, impaired stance and gait, stupor progressing to coma, possible seizures.

Possible Effects of Long-Term Use: Development of tardive dyskinesia.

Suggested Periodic Examinations While Taking This Drug (at physician's discretion)

Complete blood cell counts, liver function tests.

▷ While Taking This Drug, Observe the Following

Foods: No restrictions.
Beverages: No restrictions. May be taken with milk.
▷   *Alcohol:* Avoid completely. Alcohol can increase the sedative action of this drug and enhance its depressant effects on brain function. Also, this drug can increase the intoxicating effects of alcohol.
Tobacco Smoking: No interactions expected, but I advise everyone to quit smoking.
▷   *Other Drugs*
Molindone may ***increase*** the effects of
- all drugs containing atropine or having atropinelike effects (see Drug Classes).
- all drugs with sedative effects, and cause excessive sedation.

Molindone ***taken concurrently*** with
- antiepileptic drugs (anticonvulsants) may require close monitoring for changes in seizure patterns and need for dosage adjustments.
- monoamine oxidase (MAO) inhibitors (see Drug Classes) may result in serious increases in temperature or convulsions. Some patients who do not

respond to either medicine may be able to take both at the same time without this effect, but data are limited.

▷ *Driving, Hazardous Activities:* This drug may cause dizziness and drowsiness. Restrict activities as necessary.

Aviation Note: The use of this drug *is a disqualification* for piloting. Consult a designated Aviation Medical Examiner.

Exposure to Sun: No restrictions as far as photosensitivity.

Exposure to Heat: Use caution and avoid excessive heat as much as possible. This drug may impair the regulation of body temperature and increase the risk of heatstroke.

Discontinuation: Do not stop taking this drug suddenly after long-term use. Ask your physician for guidance regarding gradual dosage reduction and withdrawal.

MORPHINE (MOR feen)

Other Name: MS (morphine sulfate)

Introduced: 1806 **Class:** Strong analgesic, opioids **Prescription:** USA: Yes **Controlled Drug:** USA: C-II*; Canada: Yes **Available as Generic:** Yes

Brand Names: Astramorph, Astramorph PF, Duramorph, ✦Epimorph, Kadian, Infumorph, ✦Morphine H.P., ✦Morphitec, ✦M.O.S., ✦M.O.S.-S.R., MS Contin, MS-IR, OMS Concentrate, Opium Tincture, Oramorph SR, Paregoric, RMS Uniserts, Roxanol, Roxanol 100, Roxanol SR✦Statex

BENEFITS versus RISKS	
Possible Benefits	*Possible Risks*
EFFECTIVE RELIEF OF MODERATE TO SEVERE PAIN	POTENTIAL FOR HABIT FORMATION (DEPENDENCE) Respiratory depression Disorientation, hallucinations Interference with urination Constipation

▷ **Principal Uses**

As a Single Drug Product: Uses currently included in FDA-approved labeling: Given by mouth, suppository, or injection to relieve moderate to severe pain of: (1) Heart attack, cancer, operations, fluid on the lungs, and other causes; (2) it is also used as an adjunct to anesthesia.

Other (unlabeled) generally accepted uses: (1) Therapy of pain in sickle cell crisis; (2) used in patient-controlled analgesia pumps to fight pain.

How This Drug Works: Acting primarily as a depressant of certain brain functions, this drug suppresses the perception of pain and calms the emotional response to pain.

*See schedules of Controlled Drugs at the back of this book.

Available Dosage Forms and Strengths

Injection — 0.5 mg/ml, 1 mg/ml, 2 mg/ml, 4 mg/ml, 5 mg/ml, 8 mg/ml, 10 mg/ml, 15 mg/ml, 25 mg/ml, 50 mg/ml

Oral solution — 20 mg/ml; 10 mg/5 ml, 20 mg/5 ml, 100 mg/5 ml

Suppositories — 5 mg, 10 mg, 20 mg, 30 mg

Syrup — 1 mg/ml, 5 mg/ml, 10 mg/ml, 20 mg/ml, 50 mg/ml (50 mg/ml Canada only)

Tablets — 5 mg, 10 mg, 15 mg, 25 mg, 30 mg, 50 mg

Tablets, soluble — 10 mg, 15 mg, 30 mg

Tablets, sustained release — 15 mg, 30 mg, 60 mg, 100 mg, 200 mg

Tablets, extended sustained release — 20 mg, 50 mg, 100 mg

▷ **Recommended Dosage Ranges** (Actual dosage and administration schedule must be determined for each patient individually.)

Infants and Children: 0.1 to 0.2 mg per kg of body mass every 4 hours. Single dose should not exceed 15 mg.

12 to 60 Years of Age: By injection—5 to 20 mg every 4 hours.

By mouth (regular solution, syrup, and tablets)—10 to 30 mg every 4 hours.

By mouth (sustained-release forms)—30 mg every 8 to 12 hours.

By mouth (Kadian brand extended sustained-release form)—once daily.

By suppository—10 to 30 mg every 4 hours.

Over 60 Years of Age: Same as 12 to 60 years of age, using the lower end of the range initially; increase dose cautiously, as needed and tolerated.

Author's Note: Previous editions have included as-needed or PRN notations by doses. Current pain treatment theory calls for timed or scheduled dosing. This tends to prevent pain, rather than allowing pain to recur and then having to be treated. Some clinicians will use timed dosing immediately after surgery and then revert to as-needed dosing once the most severe period of pain has passed.

Conditions Requiring Dosing Adjustments

Liver Function: The dose and frequency **must** be adjusted (decreased) with liver compromise.

Kidney Function: The dose and frequency should be adjusted in renal compromise.

▷ **Dosing Instructions:** The regular tablet may be crushed and taken with or following food to reduce stomach irritation or nausea. The sustained-release tablet should be swallowed whole; do not break it in half, crush it, or chew it. The oral liquid may be mixed with fruit juice to improve taste.

Usual Duration of Use: As required to control pain. For short-term, self-limiting conditions, continual use should not exceed 5 to 7 days without interruption and reassessment of need. For the long-term management of severe chronic pain, it is advisable to determine an optimal fixed-dosage schedule.

▷ **This Drug Should Not Be Taken If**

- you have had an allergic reaction to any dosage form of it previously.
- you are having an acute attack of asthma.
- you have acute respiratory depression.

▷ **Inform Your Physician Before Taking This Drug If**
- you are taking, or have taken within the past 14 days, any monoamine oxidase (MAO) type A inhibitor drug (see Drug Classes).
- you are taking atropinelike drugs, antihypertensives, metoclopramide (Reglan), or zidovudine (AZT).
- you are taking any other drugs that have a sedative effect.
- you have a history of drug abuse or alcoholism.
- you have impaired liver or kidney function.
- you have prostate gland enlargement (see Prostatism in Glossary).
- you have a history of asthma, emphysema, epilepsy, gallbladder disease, or inflammatory bowel disease.
- you have a tendency toward constipation.
- you have a history of head injury.
- you have a history of sickle cell anemia.
- you have a history of low blood pressure.
- you plan to have surgery under general anesthesia in the near future.

Possible Side Effects (natural, expected, and unavoidable drug actions)

Drowsiness, light-headedness, weakness, euphoria, dry mouth, urinary retention, dose-related constipation. Miosis or pinpoint pupils.

▷ **Possible Adverse Effects** (unusual, unexpected, and infrequent reactions)

If any of the following develop, consult your physician promptly for guidance.

Mild Adverse Effects

Allergic Reactions: Skin rash, hives, itching (especially if the intravenous form is injected too quickly).

Headache, dizziness, impaired concentration, sensation of drunkenness, confusion, depression, blurred or double vision—infrequent to frequent and may be dose related.

Facial flushing, sweating, heart palpitation—possible.

Nausea, vomiting—possible and may be dose related.

Spasm of the biliary tract—possible.

Urine retention—possible.

Serious Adverse Effects

Allergic Reactions: Swelling of throat or vocal cords, spasm of larynx or bronchial tubes.

Hallucinations, psychosis—infrequent.

Drop in blood pressure, causing severe weakness and fainting—possible.

Disorientation, hallucinations, unstable gait, tremor, muscle twitching—possible.

Drug-induced myasthenia gravis or porphyria—case reports.

Respiratory depression—dose related.

Seizures—possible.

▷ **Possible Effects on Sexual Function:** Reduced libido and/or potency.

Amenorrhea and disruption of ovulation—case reports.

▷ **Adverse Effects That May Mimic Natural Diseases or Disorders**

Paradoxical behavioral disturbances may suggest psychotic disorder.

Possible Effects on Laboratory Tests

Blood amylase and lipase levels: increased (natural side effects).

Liver function tests: increased liver enzymes (ALT/GPT, AST/GOT, and alkaline phosphatase), increased bilirubin.

Urine screening tests for drug abuse: may be **positive**. (Test results depend upon amount of drug taken and testing method used.)

CAUTION

1. If you have asthma, chronic bronchitis, or emphysema, excessive use of this drug may cause significant respiratory difficulty, thickening of bronchial secretions, and suppression of coughing.
2. Taking this drug with atropinelike drugs can increase the risk of urinary retention and reduced intestinal function.
3. Do not take this drug following acute head injury.

Precautions for Use

By Infants and Children: Use very cautiously in infants under 2 years of age because of their vulnerability to life-threatening respiratory depression. Watch for any indication of paradoxical excitement in this age group.

By Those Over 60 Years of Age: Small doses and short-term use are indicated. There may be increased risk of drowsiness, dizziness, unsteadiness, falling, urinary retention, and constipation (often leading to fecal impaction).

▷ Advisability of Use During Pregnancy

Pregnancy Category: C. See Pregnancy Risk Categories at the back of this book.
Animal studies: Significant skeletal birth defects reported in mouse and hamster studies.

Human studies: Adequate studies of pregnant women are not available. However, no significant increase in birth defects was found in 448 exposures to this drug.

Avoid during the first 3 months. Use sparingly and in small doses during the final 6 months only if clearly needed.

Advisability of Use If Breast-Feeding

Presence of this drug in breast milk: Yes.
Avoid drug or refrain from nursing.

Habit-Forming Potential: This drug can cause psychological and physical dependence (see Glossary).

Effects of Overdosage: Marked drowsiness, dizziness, confusion, restlessness, depressed breathing, tremors, convulsions, stupor progressing to coma.

Possible Effects of Long-Term Use: Psychological and physical dependence, chronic constipation.

Suggested Periodic Examinations While Taking This Drug (at physician's discretion)
None.

▷ While Taking This Drug, Observe the Following

Foods: No restrictions.

Beverages: No restrictions. May be taken with milk.

▷ *Alcohol:* Alcohol is best avoided. Opioid analgesics can intensify the intoxicating effects of alcohol, and alcohol can intensify the depressant effects of opioids on brain function, breathing, and circulation.

Tobacco Smoking: No interactions expected, but I advise everyone to quit smoking.

Marijuana Smoking: Increase in drowsiness and pain relief; impairment of mental and physical performance.

▷ *Other Drugs*

Morphine may *increase* the effects of
- antihypertensives, and cause excessive lowering of blood pressure.
- atropinelike drugs, and increase the risk of constipation and urinary retention.
- other drugs with sedative effects.

Morphine may *decrease* the effects of
- metoclopramide (Reglan).

Morphine *taken concurrently* with
- benzodiazepines (see Drug Classes) may result in increased risk of respiratory depression.
- cimetidine (Tagamet) may result in morphine toxicity.
- fluoxetine (Prozac) may antagonize morphine's pain-relieving effect.
- hydroxyzine (Vistaril) can increase pain relief, but carries the risk of increased respiratory depression.
- monoamine oxidase (MAO) type A inhibitor drugs (see Drug Classes) may cause the equivalent of an acute narcotic overdose: unconsciousness; severe depression of breathing, heart rate, and circulation. A variation can be excitability, convulsions, high fever, and rapid heart action.
- phenothiazines (see Drug Classes) may cause excessive and prolonged depression of brain functions, breathing, and circulation.
- zidovudine (AZT) may increase the toxicity of both drugs; avoid concurrent use.

▷ *Driving, Hazardous Activities:* This drug can impair mental alertness, judgment, reaction time, and physical coordination. Avoid hazardous activities.

Aviation Note: The use of this drug *is a disqualification* for piloting. Consult a designated Aviation Medical Examiner.

Exposure to Sun: No restrictions.

Discontinuation: It is advisable to limit this drug to short-term use. Longer-term use requires gradual tapering (decreasing) of doses to minimize possible effects of withdrawal: body aches, fever, sweating, nervousness, trembling, weakness, runny nose, sneezing, rapid heart rate, nausea, vomiting, stomach cramps, diarrhea.

MUPIROCIN (myu PEER oh sin)

Introduced: 1987   **Class:** Antibiotic, topical   **Prescription:** USA: Yes
Controlled Drug: USA: No; Canada: No   **Available as Generic:** USA: No; Canada: No

Brand Names: Bactroban, Bactroban Nasal

BENEFITS versus RISKS

Possible Benefits	*Possible Risks*
EFFECTIVE TOPICAL TREATMENT OF *STAPHYLOCOCCUS* AND *STREPTOCOCCUS* SKIN INFECTIONS	Skin irritation
EFFECTIVE ERADICATION OF *STAPHYLOCOCCUS AUREUS* FROM THE NOSE	

▷ **Principal Uses**

As a Single Drug Product: Uses currently included in FDA-approved labeling: (1) Used to treat skin infections caused by staphylococcal and streptococcal infections such as ecthyma or impetigo; (2) the new intranasal form is specifically formulated to kill *Staphylococcus aureus* bacteria that have colonized the nasal passages.

Other (unlabeled) generally accepted uses: (1) Used in burns where resistant *Staphylococcus aureus* is causing infection; (2) helps prevent opportunistic infections of venous access devices such as intravascular cannulas; (3) treats cellulitis caused by Gram-positive organisms; (4) has been used in some specific situations in skin surgery to prevent infections; (5) has recently been used to eradicate vaginal *Staphylococcus* infections.

How This Drug Works: This drug binds to a specific enzyme (isoleucyl transfer-RNA synthetase) and stops susceptible bacteria from being able to make critical proteins.

Available Dosage Forms and Strengths

Intranasal form — 2%

Topical ointment — 2%—20 mg/g (Canada)

▷ **Recommended Dosage Ranges** (Actual dosage and administration schedule must be determined for each patient individually.)

Infants and Children: Not indicated in infants.

Children 5 to 15 years old: Apply a thin coat of the 2% ointment to the infection site three times daily for 3 to 5 consecutive days.

16 to 60 Years of Age: 2% ointment: Apply three times daily for 5 to 14 days. Some more involved or extensive infections have been treated for longer periods. If the infection in question has not resolved after the initial course of the ointment, the site should be evaluated by a physician and systemic antibiotics or other treatment considered.

Intranasal: One-half of the ointment from the single-use tube of this new form of mupirocin is applied into one nostril and the other half is applied to the second nostril, twice daily in the morning and evening for 5 consecutive days.

Over 60 Years of Age: Same as 16 to 60 years of age.

Conditions Requiring Dosing Adjustments

Liver Function: This ointment is not usually systemically absorbed to an appreciable extent. If the ointment is applied to an extensive skin area, metabolism of the active antibiotic does occur in the liver, yet there are no existing guidelines for dosage adjustments.

Kidney Function: A substance in this formulation (polyethylene glycol) may be toxic to the kidneys if the ointment is applied over an extensive burn or wound area.

▷ **Dosing Instructions:** This medicine should be applied as a thin film or as described by your doctor. Call your doctor if the condition has not improved or worsens during the course of treatment. Do **not** combine this medicine with other ointments or treatments unless your doctor has prescribed this approach.

Usual Duration of Use: Continual use on a regular schedule for several days is usually necessary to determine this drug's effectiveness in treating skin infections. Long-term use (months to years) requires periodic physician evaluation. Consult your physician on a regular basis.

Possible Advantages of This Drug
Effective topical treatment of skin infections.

▷ **This Drug Should Not Be Taken If**
- you have had an allergic reaction to any dosage form of it previously.
- you have extensive burns or open wounds.

▷ **Inform Your Physician Before Taking This Drug If**
- several days have passed since this medicine has been prescribed and there has been no change or worsening of the wound.
- pain at the site of the infection increases.
- you are uncertain of how much mupirocin to apply or how often to apply it.

Possible Side Effects (natural, expected, and unavoidable drug actions)
Irritation at the site of infection secondary to the polyethylene glycol component.

▷ **Possible Adverse Effects** (unusual, unexpected, and infrequent reactions)
If any of the following develop, consult your physician promptly for guidance.
Mild Adverse Effects
Allergic Reactions: Skin rash and irritation at the infection site.
Soreness, stinging, or pain at the infection site—possible.
Serious Adverse Effects
Allergic Reactions: Not defined, as the medicine is not appreciably absorbed.
If this medicine is applied to an extensive skin area, polyethylene glycol may be absorbed and cause kidney toxicity—possible.

▷ **Possible Effects on Sexual Function:** Not reported.

Possible Delayed Adverse Effects: This medicine is indicated for short-term use.

▷ **Adverse Effects That May Mimic Natural Diseases or Disorders**
None reported.

Natural Diseases or Disorders That May Be Activated by This Drug
None reported.

Possible Effects on Laboratory Tests
None reported.

CAUTION
1. Do not apply this medicine to an area of skin larger than what your doctor prescribed.

Precautions for Use

By Infants and Children: Safety and effectiveness for use by those under 5 years of age have not been established.

By Those Over 60 Years of Age: No special changes are needed.

▷ **Advisability of Use During Pregnancy**

Pregnancy Category: B. See Pregnancy Risk Categories at the back of this book.
Animal studies: No fetal problems defined.
Human studies: Information from adequate studies of pregnant women is not available.

Advisability of Use If Breast-Feeding

Presence of this drug in breast milk: Unknown.
Avoid drug or refrain from nursing.

Habit-Forming Potential: None.

Effects of Overdosage: If this medicine is applied to an extensive area of skin, excessive amounts of polyethylene glycol may be absorbed and cause kidney toxicity.

Possible Effects of Long-Term Use: None defined.

Suggested Periodic Examinations While Taking This Drug (at physician's discretion)

None.

▷ **While Taking This Drug, Observe the Following**

Foods: No restrictions.
Beverages: No restrictions.
▷ *Alcohol:* No restrictions.
Tobacco Smoking: No interactions expected, but I advise everyone to quit smoking.
▷ *Other Drugs*

Mupirocin **taken concurrently** with

• other medications that are toxic to the kidneys may result in additive kidney toxicity if mupirocin is applied to a large area of skin.

Aviation Note: The use of this drug **does not appear to be a restriction** for piloting. Consult a designated Aviation Medical Examiner.

Exposure to Sun: No restrictions.

NABUMETONE (na BYU me tohn)

See the acetic acids (nonsteroidal anti-inflammatory drugs) profile for further information.

NADOLOL (NAY doh lohl)

Introduced: 1976   **Class:** Anti-anginal, antihypertensive, beta-blocker
Prescription: USA: Yes   **Controlled Drug:** USA: No; Canada: No   **Available as Generic:** Yes
Brand Names: ✦Apo-Nadol, Corgard, Corzide [CD]

BENEFITS versus RISKS	
Possible Benefits	*Possible Risks*
EFFECTIVE, WELL-TOLERATED ANTIHYPERTENSIVE for mild to moderate high blood pressure EFFECTIVE ANTI-ANGINAL DRUG IN CLASSICAL CORONARY ARTERY DISEASE with moderate to severe angina	CONGESTIVE HEART FAILURE in advanced heart disease Provocation of asthma (in predisposed patients) Masking of hypoglycemia in drug-dependent diabetes Worsening of angina following abrupt withdrawal

▷ **Principal Uses**

As a Single Drug Product: Uses currently included in FDA-approved labeling: (1) Treats moderate high blood pressure; (2) helps prevent attacks of effort-induced angina. Should not be used in Prinzmetal's vasospastic angina.

Other (unlabeled) generally accepted uses: (1) Helps prevent hemorrhage from bulging veins (esophageal varices) in cirrhosis; (2) may have an adjunctive role in helping prevent and reduce migraine severity; (3) may have a role in helping prevent death after a heart attack (myocardial infarction); (4) may help ease tremor in patients taking lithium; (5) helps decrease risk of ruptured blood vessels in the esophagus (esophageal varices) in patients with cirrhosis.

As a Combination Drug Product [CD]: This drug is available in combination with bendroflumethiazide, a mild diuretic antihypertensive drug. This combination product is more effective and more convenient for long-term use.

How This Drug Works: By blocking certain actions of the sympathetic nervous system, this drug
- reduces the rate and contraction force of the heart, lowering oxygen requirements of the heart muscle, and reducing ejection pressure of the blood leaving the heart, consequently reducing the frequency of angina and lowering blood pressure.
- reduces the degree of contraction of blood vessel walls, resulting in expansion and consequent lowering of blood pressure.
- prolongs conduction time of nerve impulses through the heart, of benefit in the management of certain heart rhythm disorders.

Available Dosage Forms and Strengths

Tablets — 20 mg, 40 mg, 80 mg, 120 mg, 160 mg

▷ **Usual Adult Dosage Range:**   For hypertension: Initially 40 mg daily in one dose; this may be increased gradually as needed and tolerated, up to 320 mg daily. The usual maintenance dose is 80 to 320 mg daily. The total daily dosage should not exceed 320 mg. For angina: Initially 40 mg daily in one dose; increase gradually at intervals of 3 to 7 days up to 240 mg daily. The usual maintenance dose is 80 to 240 mg/24 hours. The total daily dose should not exceed 240 mg.

Note: Actual dosage and administration schedule must be determined for each patient individually.

Conditions Requiring Dosing Adjustments

Liver Function: The liver is not significantly involved in the elimination of this medication.

Kidney Function: For patients with moderate kidney failure, the usual dose should be taken every 24 to 36 hours. For patients with severe kidney failure, the dose can be taken every 40 to 60 hours.

▷ **Dosing Instructions:**   The tablet may be crushed and taken without regard to eating. Do not stop this drug abruptly.

Usual Duration of Use: Use on a regular schedule for 10 to 14 days determines this drug's effectiveness in lowering blood pressure and preventing angina. The long-term use of this drug (months to years) will be determined by your response to an overall treatment program (weight reduction, salt restriction, smoking cessation, etc.). Consult your physician on a regular basis.

Possible Advantages of This Drug
Does not reduce blood flow to the kidney.
Can be used concurrently with other drugs that may reduce blood flow to the kidney (such as most anti-inflammatory aspirin substitutes).

▷ **This Drug Should Not Be Taken If**
- you have had an allergic reaction to it previously.
- you have congestive heart failure.
- you have an abnormally slow heart rate or a serious form of heart block.
- you are subject to bronchial asthma.
- you are presently experiencing seasonal hay fever.
- you are taking, or have taken within the past 14 days, any monoamine oxidase (MAO) type A inhibitor drug (see Drug Classes).

▷ **Inform Your Physician Before Taking This Drug If**
- you have had an adverse reaction to any beta-blocker (see Drug Classes).
- you have a history of serious heart disease.
- you have a history of hay fever (allergic rhinitis), asthma, chronic bronchitis, or emphysema.
- you have a history of overactive thyroid function (hyperthyroidism).
- you have a history of low blood sugar (hypoglycemia).
- you have impaired liver or kidney function.
- you have diabetes or myasthenia gravis.
- you are pregnant or breast-feeding your infant.
- you have difficulty with blood circulation to the periphery (peripheral vascular disease).
- you are currently taking any form of digitalis, quinidine, or reserpine, or any calcium-channel-blocker drug (see Drug Classes).
- you plan to have surgery under general anesthesia in the near future.

Possible Side Effects (natural, expected, and unavoidable drug actions)
Lethargy and fatigability, cold extremities, slow heart rate, light-headedness in upright position (see Orthostatic Hypotension in Glossary).

▷ **Possible Adverse Effects** (unusual, unexpected, and infrequent reactions)
If any of the following develop, consult your physician promptly for guidance.
Mild Adverse Effects
Allergic Reactions: Skin rash, itching, drug fever.
Headache, dizziness, vivid dreaming, visual disturbances, ringing in ears, slurred speech, paresthesias—case reports to infrequent.
Hair loss and sweating—case reports to infrequent.

Cough, indigestion, nausea, vomiting, diarrhea, abdominal pain—infrequent.

Increased blood potassium—possible.

Numbness and tingling of extremities—case reports.

Serious Adverse Effects

Allergic Reactions: Facial swelling, anaphylaxis.

Chest pain, shortness of breath, precipitation of congestive heart failure—possible.

Intensification of heart block or severe slowing of the heart—case reports and may be dose related.

Bronchospasm—rare.

Carpal tunnel syndrome or pancreatitis—case reports.

Induction of bronchial asthma (in asthmatic individuals)—possible and dose related.

Masking of warning indications of acute hypoglycemia in drug-treated diabetes—possible.

May precipitate cramping when walking (intermittent claudication)—possible.

Excessively low blood pressure—possible.

▷ **Possible Effects on Sexual Function:**   Decreased libido, impotence, impaired erection—case reports to frequent.

▷ **Adverse Effects That May Mimic Natural Diseases or Disorders**

Impaired circulation to the extremities may resemble Raynaud's phenomenon.

Natural Diseases or Disorders That May Be Activated by This Drug

Bronchial asthma, Prinzmetal's variant (vasospastic) angina, latent Raynaud's disease, myasthenia gravis (questionable).

Possible Effects on Laboratory Tests

Blood HDL cholesterol level: decreased.

Blood VLDL cholesterol level: increased.

Blood triglyceride levels: increased.

CAUTION

1. ***Do not stop this drug suddenly*** without the knowledge and help of your doctor. Carry a note which states that you are taking this drug.
2. Ask your physician or pharmacist **before** using nasal decongestants, which are usually present in over-the-counter cold preparations and nose drops. These can cause rapid blood pressure increases when combined with beta-blocker drugs.
3. Report the development of any tendency to emotional depression.

Precautions for Use

By Infants and Children: Safety and effectiveness for those under 12 years of age are not established. However, if this drug is used, observe for the development of low blood sugar (hypoglycemia) during periods of reduced food intake.

By Those Over 60 Years of Age: Unacceptably high blood pressure should be reduced without creating the risks associated with excessively low blood pressure. Small doses and frequent blood pressure checks are needed. Sudden, rapid, and excessive reduction of blood pressure can predispose to stroke or heart attack. Watch for dizziness, unsteadiness, tendency to fall, confusion, hallucinations, depression, or urinary frequency.

▷ **Advisability of Use During Pregnancy**

Pregnancy Category: C. See Pregnancy Risk Categories at the back of this book.

Animal studies: No significant increase in birth defects due to this drug, but embryotoxicity reported in rabbits.

Human studies: Adequate studies of pregnant women are not available.

Avoid use during the first 3 months if possible. Use this drug only if clearly needed. Ask your physician for guidance.

Advisability of Use If Breast-Feeding

Presence of this drug in breast milk: Yes, in large amounts.

Avoid drug or refrain from nursing.

Habit-Forming Potential: None.

Effects of Overdosage: Weakness, slow pulse, low blood pressure, fainting, cold and sweaty skin, congestive heart failure, possible coma, and convulsions.

Possible Effects of Long-Term Use: Reduced heart reserve and eventual heart failure in susceptible individuals with advanced heart disease.

Suggested Periodic Examinations While Taking This Drug (at physician's discretion)

Measurements of blood pressure, evaluation of heart function.

▷ **While Taking This Drug, Observe the Following**

Foods: No restrictions. Avoid excessive salt intake.

Beverages: No restrictions. May be taken with milk.

▷ *Alcohol:* Use with caution. Alcohol may exaggerate this drug's ability to lower blood pressure and may increase its mild sedative effect.

Tobacco Smoking: Nicotine may reduce this drug's effectiveness. I advise everyone to quit smoking.

▷ *Other Drugs*

Nadolol may *increase* the effects of

- other antihypertensive drugs, and cause excessive lowering of blood pressure. Dosage adjustments may be necessary.
- reserpine (Ser-Ap-Es, etc.), and cause sedation, depression, slowing of the heart rate, and lowering of blood pressure.
- verapamil (Calan, Isoptin) or other calcium channel blockers (see Drug Classes), and cause excessive depression of heart function; monitor this combination closely.

Nadolol may *decrease* the effects of

- ritodrine (Yutopar).
- theophyllines (Aminophyllin, Theo-Dur, etc.), and reduce their effectiveness in treating asthma.

Nadolol *taken concurrently* with

- amiodarone (Cordarone) can cause severe slowing of the heart and potentially stop the heart (cardiac arrest).
- antacids containing aluminum can block absorption of this medicine and lessen therapeutic nadolol effects.
- clonidine (Catapres) requires close monitoring for rebound high blood pressure if clonidine is withdrawn while nadolol is still being taken.
- epinephrine can cause serious hypertension and slowing of the heart, and should anaphylaxis occur, epinephrine resistance.

- ergot derivatives (see Drug Classes) can cause decreased blood flow to the extremities (peripheral ischemia).
- insulin requires close monitoring to avoid undetected hypoglycemia (see Glossary).
- lidocaine can lead to lidocaine toxicity (depressed heart function, cardiac arrest).
- oral antidiabetic drugs (see Drug Classes) can cause slowed recovery from any hypoglycemia that may occur.

The following drugs may *decrease* the effects of nadolol

- indomethacin (Indocin) and possibly other "aspirin substitutes," or NSAIDs—may impair nadolol's antihypertensive effect.

▷ *Driving, Hazardous Activities:* Use caution until the full extent of drowsiness, lethargy, and blood pressure change has been determined.

Aviation Note: The use of this drug *is a disqualification* for piloting. Consult a designated Aviation Medical Examiner.

Exposure to Sun: No restrictions.

Exposure to Heat: Caution is advised. Hot environments can lower blood pressure and exaggerate the effects of this drug.

Exposure to Cold: Caution is advised. Cold environments can enhance the circulatory deficiency in the extremities that may occur with this drug. The elderly should take precautions to prevent hypothermia (see Glossary).

Heavy Exercise or Exertion: It is advisable to avoid exertion that produces light-headedness, excessive fatigue, or muscle cramping. The use of this drug may intensify the hypertensive response to isometric exercise.

Occurrence of Unrelated Illness: Fever that accompanies systemic infections can lower blood pressure and require dose decreases. Nausea or vomiting may interrupt the regular dosage schedule. Ask your physician for guidance.

Discontinuation: It is advisable to avoid sudden discontinuation of this drug in all situations. If possible, gradual reduction of dose over a period of 2 to 3 weeks is recommended. Ask your physician for specific guidance.

NAFARELIN (NAF a re lin)

Introduced: 1984   **Class:** Hormones, miscellaneous   **Prescription:** USA: Yes   **Controlled Drug:** USA: No; Canada: No   **Available as Generic:** USA: No

Brand Name: Synarel

BENEFITS versus RISKS	
Possible Benefits	*Possible Risks*
VERY EFFECTIVE TREATMENT OF ENDOMETRIOSIS	Symptoms of estrogen deficiency (during treatment)
	Masculinizing effects (during treatment)
	Loss of bone density
	Lowering of the white blood cell count

▷ **Principal Uses**

As a Single Drug Product: Uses currently included in FDA-approved labeling: (1) Treats endometriosis: reduction in the size and activity of endometrial implants within the pelvis; relief of pelvic pain associated with menstruation; (2) also used to treat precocious puberty due to excessive production of gonadotropic hormones.

Other (unlabeled) generally accepted uses: (1) Intranasal dosing helps control abnormal hair growth in women; (2) can be injected below the skin (subcutaneously) to help benign prostatic hyperplasia; (3) may be used before surgery to help decrease size of some tumors (myomas).

How This Drug Works: This drug stimulates the pituitary gland to secrete two additional hormones that regulate production of estrogen by the ovaries. Initially this drug causes an increase in the production of estrogen, but with continued use the high levels of estrogen suppress (via a feedback mechanism) hormones that stimulate the ovary, and thus estrogen production is significantly reduced. The implants of endometrium (from the lining of the uterus) that are attached to the pelvic wall are stimulated by the cyclic rise and fall of estrogen that accompanies menstruation. As a result of suppressing estrogen production, the displaced endometrial tissue (endometriosis) becomes dormant; the conditions responsible for premenstrual and menstrual pain are no longer active.

Available Dosage Forms and Strengths

Nasal solution — 2 mg/ml (10-ml bottle)

▷ **Usual Adult Dosage Range:**   Endometriosis: Pregnancy MUST be excluded prior to starting therapy, then treatment starts with 400 mcg daily. Spray one dose of 200 mcg into one nostril in the morning and one dose of 200 mcg into the other nostril in the evening, 12 hours apart. Begin treatment between days 2 and 4 of the menstrual cycle. If regular menstruation persists after 2 months of treatment, the dose may be increased to 800 mcg daily: one spray into each nostril (a total of two sprays, 400 mcg) in the morning and again in the evening.

Note: Actual dosage and administration schedule must be determined for each patient individually.

Conditions Requiring Dosing Adjustments

Liver Function: The liver plays a minor role in the elimination of this medication.

Kidney Function: Specific guidelines are not available for dosing. Decreases may be needed in kidney compromise.

▷ **Dosing Instructions:**   Carefully read and follow the patient instructions provided with this drug. The solution is to be sprayed directly into the nostrils; it is not to be swallowed. Time the start of therapy and daily dosing exactly as directed. A nasal decongestant (spray or drops) should not be used for at least 30 minutes after dosing the nafarelin spray; earlier use could impair absorption of nafarelin.

Usual Duration of Use: Use on a regular schedule for 2 to 3 months usually determines effectiveness in relieving endometriosis symptoms. The standard course of treatment is limited to 6 months. After 6 months of treatment, 60% of users are free of symptoms, 32% have mild symptoms, 7% have moderate symptoms, and 1% have severe symptoms. Six months after stopping this drug, of the 60% who obtain complete relief, 50% remain free of symptoms, 33% have mild symptoms, and 17% have moderate symptoms. If symptoms of endometriosis recur following a 6-month course of treatment and a repeat course is considered, it is advisable to measure bone density before retreatment is started.

Possible Advantages of This Drug
Causes fewer masculinizing effects than danazol.
Less tendency than danazol to increase blood cholesterol levels.
Unlike danazol, this drug does not cause abnormally low HDL cholesterol levels or abnormally high LDL cholesterol levels.

Currently a "Drug of Choice"
for the management of symptoms associated with endometriosis.

▷ **This Drug Should Not Be Taken If**
- you have had an allergic reaction to it previously.
- you are pregnant or breast-feeding.
- you have abnormal vaginal bleeding of unknown cause.

▷ **Inform Your Physician Before Taking This Drug If**
- you have used this drug, danazol, or similar drugs previously.
- you are taking any type of estrogen, progesterone, or oral contraceptive.
- you are planning pregnancy in the near future.
- you have a family history of osteoporosis.
- you use alcohol or tobacco regularly.
- you have a history of low white blood cells.
- you are using anticonvulsants or cortisonelike drugs.
- you are subject to allergic or infectious rhinitis and use nasal decongestants frequently.

Possible Side Effects (natural, expected, and unavoidable drug actions)
Effects due to reduced estrogen production: hot flashes (90%), headaches, emotional lability, insomnia. Masculinizing effects: acne, muscle aches, fluid retention, increased skin oil, weight gain, excessive hair growth—rare.

▷ **Possible Adverse Effects** (unusual, unexpected, and infrequent reactions)
If any of the following develop, consult your physician promptly for guidance.
Mild Adverse Effects
Allergic Reactions: Skin rash, hives—rare.
Nasal irritation—frequent.
Vaginal dryness—infrequent to frequent.
Depression—rare.
Serious Adverse Effects
Loss of vertebral bone density: at completion of 6 months of treatment, bone density decreases an average of 8.7% and bone mass decreases an average of 4.3%; partial recovery during the posttreatment period restores bone density loss to 4.9% and bone mass loss to 3.3%.
Lowering of the white blood cell count—case reports.
Transient prostate enlargement—possible.

▷ **Possible Effects on Sexual Function**
Decreased libido, vaginal dryness, reduced breast size—infrequent to frequent.
Uterine bleeding—case reports.

Impotence occurred in most men who had used this drug for prostate problems.

Galactorrhea—case reports.

Natural Diseases or Disorders That May Be Activated by This Drug

Worsening of or increased progression of osteoporosis.

Possible Effects on Laboratory Tests

Blood testosterone level: decreased in men with benign enlargement of prostate gland.

Blood progesterone: decreased to less than 4 ng/ml.

Alkaline phosphatase: increased.

Serum estrone: decreased.

CAUTION

1. With continual use of this drug in proper dosage, menstruation will cease. If regular menstruation persists, call your doctor. Dosage adjustment may be necessary.
2. Use this drug consistently on a regular basis. Missed doses can result in breakthrough bleeding and ovulation.
3. It is advisable to avoid pregnancy during the course of treatment. Use a nonhormonal method of birth control; do not use oral contraceptives. Inform your physician promptly if you think you may be pregnant.
4. If you need to use nasal decongestant sprays or drops, delay their use for at least 30 minutes after the intranasal spray of nafarelin.

Precautions for Use

By Infants and Children: Safety and effectiveness for those under 18 years of age are not established.

By Those Over 60 Years of Age: If used for prostatism, impotence is a common side effect. Depression and hot flashes were also often reported.

▷ **Advisability of Use During Pregnancy**

Pregnancy Category: X. See Pregnancy Risk Categories at the back of this book.

Animal studies: Major fetal abnormalities and increased fetal deaths due to this drug have been demonstrated in rat studies.

Human studies: Adequate studies of pregnant women are not available.

Avoid this drug during entire pregnancy.

Advisability of Use If Breast-Feeding

Presence of this drug in breast milk: Unknown.

Avoid drug or refrain from nursing.

Habit-Forming Potential: None.

Effects of Overdosage: No significant effects expected.

Possible Effects of Long-Term Use: Continual use should be limited to 6 months. If repeated courses of treatment are considered, determination of bone density and mass should be made to assess possible bone loss, predisposition to osteoporosis, and possible therapy.

Suggested Periodic Examinations While Taking This Drug (at physician's discretion)

Blood cholesterol and triglyceride profiles.

Bone density and mass measurements.

▷ **While Taking This Drug, Observe the Following**

Foods: No restrictions.

Beverages: No restrictions.

▷   *Alcohol:* No interactions expected.
  Tobacco Smoking: No interactions expected, but I advise everyone to quit smoking.
▷   *Other Drugs*
  The following drugs will *decrease* the effects of nafarelin
  • birth control pills (oral contraceptives).
  • estrogens.
▷   *Driving, Hazardous Activities:* No restrictions.
  Aviation Note: The use of this drug *is not a disqualification* for piloting. Consult a designated Aviation Medical Examiner for confirmation.
  Exposure to Sun: No restrictions.
  Discontinuation: Normal ovarian function (ovulation, menstruation, etc.) is usually restored within 4 to 8 weeks after discontinuation of this drug.
  Special Storage Instructions: Store in an upright position at room temperature. Protect from light.

NALTREXONE (nahl TREX ohn)

Introduced: 1995   **Class:** Antialcoholism, opioid antagonist   **Prescription:** USA: Yes   **Controlled Drug:** USA: No; Canada: No   **Available as Generic:** USA: No; Canada: No

Brand Names: Trexan, ReVia

Warning: This medication can cause liver damage if taken in excessive doses. If abdominal pain, white stools, or yellowing of the eyes or skin occurs, call your doctor immediately.

BENEFITS versus RISKS	
Possible Benefits	*Possible Risks*
CONTROL OF CRAVING FOR ALCOHOL	LIVER DAMAGE IF EXCESSIVE DOSES TAKEN
PART OF AN EFFECTIVE COMBINATION APPROACH TO ALCOHOLISM	
ONCE-DAILY DOSING	

▷ **Principal Uses**
  As a Single Drug Product: Uses currently included in FDA-approved labeling: (1) Used as part of a comprehensive program to help alcohol dependence; (2) used to treat narcotic addiction.
    Other (unlabeled) generally accepted uses: (1) May help women with a specific type of cessation of menstruation (hypothalamic amenorrhea); (2) could have a role in treating Tourette syndrome.
  How This Drug Works: (1) In helping addiction to narcotics, this medicine acts as an antagonist to the effects of opioid medicines and blocks the effects or perceived benefit of the drug to the addicted patient. (2) Exact mechanism of action in alcohol addiction is unknown. It may interfere with the body's own opioids that may be released in response to drinking alcoholic beverages. If the effect of the body's own opioids (endogenous) is blocked, the craving for alcohol is thereby thought to be reduced.

Available Dosage Forms and Strengths
Tablets — 50 mg

▷ **Recommended Dosage Ranges** (Actual dosage and administration schedule must be determined for each patient individually.)
Infants and Children: Not indicated.
18 to 60 Years of Age: 50 mg daily. The best results are gained when this medicine is used as part of a comprehensive approach to curbing alcohol use.
Over 60 Years of Age: Same as 12 to 60 years of age.

Conditions Requiring Dosing Adjustments
Liver Function: This drug is extensively metabolized in the liver and is contraindicated in acute hepatitis or liver failure.
Kidney Function: Metabolites of this drug are removed by the kidneys, but specific guidelines for dosing changes are not available.

▷ **Dosing Instructions:**   If there is any question of opioid dependence, a Narcan challenge test must be performed. Naltrexone is almost completely absorbed after oral dosing. This medicine may be taken with or without food.

Usual Duration of Use: Continual use on a regular schedule for 12 weeks is usually necessary to determine this drug's effectiveness in treating alcoholism. This drug should be a part of a comprehensive alcohol treatment program. Long-term use (months to years) requires periodic evaluation of response and dosage adjustment. Consult your physician on a regular basis.

Possible Advantages of This Drug
Actually decreases the craving for alcohol.

▷ **This Drug Should Not Be Taken If**
• you have had an allergic reaction to any dosage form of it previously.
• you have liver failure or acute hepatitis.
• you are in opioid withdrawal.
• you are physically dependent on narcotics.

▷ **Inform Your Physician Before Taking This Drug If**
• you have a history of viral hepatitis.
• you are planning surgery or a diagnostic procedure requiring anesthesia.
• you are uncertain of how much naltrexone to take or how often to take it.
• you take other prescription or nonprescription medicines that were not discussed with your doctor when naltrexone was prescribed.

Possible Side Effects (natural, expected, and unavoidable drug actions)
None.

▷ **Possible Adverse Effects** (unusual, unexpected, and infrequent reactions)
If any of the following develop, consult your physician promptly for guidance.
Mild Adverse Effects
Allergic Reactions: Rash.
Oily skin, itching, hair loss—case reports.
Nosebleeds—possible.
Joint and muscle pain—infrequent.
Anorexia, weight loss, fatigue, nervousness—case reports.
Sleep disturbances—infrequent.
Depression—case reports.

Serious Adverse Effects

Allergic Reactions: None reported.

Idiosyncratic Reactions: None reported.

Liver toxicity (hepatocellular injury)—case reports.

Precipitation of acute withdrawal syndrome in patients dependent on narcotics.

Suicidal ideation—case reports.

Abnormal platelet function (idiopathic thrombocytopenic purpura)—case reports.

▷ **Possible Effects on Sexual Function:**   Delayed ejaculation—infrequent.

Possible Delayed Adverse Effects: None reported.

▷ **Adverse Effects That May Mimic Natural Diseases or Disorders**

Liver problems may mimic acute hepatitis.

Natural Diseases or Disorders That May Be Activated by This Drug

None.

Possible Effects on Laboratory Tests

Liver function tests: increased.

CAUTION

1. The therapeutic dose and doses that can cause liver damage are fairly close. Make certain that you understand how much and how often to take this medicine.
2. Self-administration of any narcotic drug may be fatal.

Precautions for Use

By Infants and Children: Safety and effectiveness for use by those under 18 years of age have not been established.

By Those Over 60 Years of Age: None.

▷ **Advisability of Use During Pregnancy**

Pregnancy Category: C. See Pregnancy Risk Categories at the back of this book.

Animal studies: This drug has been shown to be embryocidal in rats and rabbits at roughly 140 times the typical human dose.

Human studies: Information from adequate studies of pregnant women is not available. Ask your doctor for help with this benefit-to-risk decision.

Advisability of Use If Breast-Feeding

Presence of this drug in breast milk: Unknown.

Avoid drug or refrain from nursing.

Habit-Forming Potential: None.

Effects of Overdosage: Human subjects who received over 800 mg daily for a week showed no adverse effects.

Possible Effects of Long-Term Use: None defined.

Suggested Periodic Examinations While Taking This Drug (at physician's discretion)

Liver function tests.

▷ **While Taking This Drug, Observe the Following**

Foods: No restrictions.

Beverages: No restrictions.

▷ *Alcohol:* Obviously not recommended, as this medication is part of a combination approach to help problem drinkers.

Tobacco Smoking: No interactions expected, but I advise everyone to quit smoking.

Marijuana Smoking: Should not be attempted.

▷ *Other Drugs*

Naltrexone *taken concurrently* with

- narcotic medicines may result in a severe reaction.
- other drugs that are toxic to the liver may result in increased risk of liver toxicity.
- thioridazine (Mellaril) may result in somnolence and lethargy.

▷ *Driving, Hazardous Activities:* This drug may cause fatigue. Restrict activities as necessary.

Aviation Note: Alcoholism *is a disqualification* for piloting. Consult a designated Aviation Medical Examiner.

Exposure to Sun: No restrictions.

Discontinuation: Do not stop this medicine without the knowledge of your doctor.

NAPROXEN (na PROX en)

See the propionic acids (nonsteroidal anti-inflammatory drugs) profile for further information.

NEDOCROMIL (na DOK ra mil)

Introduced: 1992   **Class:** Antiasthmatic, preventive   **Prescription:** USA: Yes   **Controlled Drug:** USA: No; Canada: No   **Available as Generic:** USA: No; Canada: No

Brand Name: Tilade

BENEFITS versus RISKS	
Possible Benefits	*Possible Risks*
EFFECTIVE PREVENTION OF RECURRENT ASTHMA	Acute bronchospasm—rare
Prevention of exercise-induced asthma	Taste disorder

▷ **Principal Uses**

As a Single Drug Product: Uses currently included in FDA-approved labeling: (1) Maintenance therapy of mild to moderate bronchial asthma; (2) has a steroid-sparing effect that may allow reduction or even elimination of oral steroids; (3) helps manage asthmatic bronchitis.

Other (unlabeled) generally accepted uses: (1) May have a role in helping ease allergic rhinitis; (2) can help vernal conjunctivitis when instilled as an eyedrop; (3) may help exercise-induced asthma.

How This Drug Works: This drug inhibits the release of inflammatory chemical mediators such as histamine, prostaglandins, and leukotrienes that cause bronchial constriction and inflammation seen in acute asthma.

Available Dosage Forms and Strengths
Inhaler — 16.2-g canister
Solution for inhalation — 2 mg per actuation

▷ **Recommended Dosage Ranges** (Actual dosage and administration schedule must be determined for each patient individually.)
Infants and Children: Safety and efficacy are not established.
12 to 60 Years of Age: Two puffs (inhalations) four times daily, to provide a total of 14 mg per day.
Over 60 Years of Age: Same as 12 to 60 years of age.

Conditions Requiring Dosing Adjustments
Liver Function: Adjustments in dose in liver compromise are not defined.
Kidney Function: Adjustments in dose in kidney compromise are not defined.

▷ **Dosing Instructions:** Follow the instructions on the leaflet provided in the medication box carefully. Nedocromil use must be continued, even when you are symptom-free.

Usual Duration of Use: Use on a regular schedule for a week usually determines effectiveness in helping prevent acute asthma. Long-term use (months to years) requires periodic physician evaluation of response and dosage adjustment.

Possible Advantages of This Drug
Usually well tolerated. Rare serious adverse effects.

▷ **This Drug Should Not Be Taken If**
• you have had an allergic reaction to any dosage form of it previously.
• you are having an acute asthma attack.

▷ **Inform Your Physician Before Taking This Drug If**
• you have impaired kidney function.
• you have angina or a heart rhythm disorder.
• you are uncertain of how to take nedocromil or how often to take it.

Possible Side Effects (natural, expected, and unavoidable drug actions)
Unpleasant taste. Mild throat irritation or hoarseness. May be lessened by taking a few swallows of water after each inhalation.

▷ **Possible Adverse Effects** (unusual, unexpected, and infrequent reactions)
If any of the following develop, consult your physician promptly for guidance.
Mild Adverse Effects
Allergic Reactions: Skin rash, hives.
Headache, dizziness—rare.
Unpleasant taste or cough—infrequent.
Nausea or vomiting—rare.
Serious Adverse Effects
Allergic Reactions: Anaphylactic reaction, allergic pneumonitis (allergic reaction of the lung tissue).
Bronchospasm—case reports.

▷ **Possible Effects on Sexual Function:** None reported.

Possible Delayed Adverse Effects: Pneumonitis—case reports.

Possible Effects on Laboratory Tests
Liver function tests: increased ALT.

CAUTION

1. This drug does **not** act as a bronchodilator and should not be used for immediate relief of acute asthma.
2. If use of this drug has allowed you to stop taking a cortisone-related drug, you may need to resume the cortisone-related drug if you are injured, must stop taking nedocromil, have an infection, or need surgery.
3. If severe asthma returns, contact your doctor promptly.
4. If you use a bronchodilator drug by inhalation, it is best to take it about 5 minutes before inhaling nedocromil.

Precautions for Use

By Infants and Children: Safety and effectiveness for those under 12 years of age are not established.

By Those Over 60 Years of Age: This drug does not work in therapy of chronic bronchitis or emphysema.

▷ **Advisability of Use During Pregnancy**

Pregnancy Category: B. See Pregnancy Risk Categories at the back of this book.
    Animal studies: Rat, mouse, and rabbit studies show no impairment of fertility or harm to the fetus.
    Human studies: Adequate studies of pregnant women are not available.
    Ask your doctor for guidance.

Advisability of Use If Breast-Feeding

Presence of this drug in breast milk: Unknown.
    Avoid drug or refrain from nursing.

Habit-Forming Potential: None.

Effects of Overdosage: Head shaking, tremor, and salivation were seen in dogs given high doses.

Suggested Periodic Examinations While Taking This Drug (at physician's discretion)

Sputum analysis and X ray if pneumonitis suspected.
    Liver function tests.

▷ **While Taking This Drug, Observe the Following**

Foods: No restrictions.

Beverages: Avoid all beverages to which you may be allergic.

▷ *Alcohol:* No interaction expected.

Tobacco Smoking: No interaction expected, but I advise everyone to quit smoking.

▷ *Other Drugs*

Nedocromil may make it possible to reduce the dose or frequency of use of cortisonelike drugs. Ask your doctor for guidance.
    There are no known adverse drug interactions at present.

▷ *Driving, Hazardous Activities:* This drug may cause dizziness. Restrict activities as necessary.

Aviation Note: The use of this drug *may be a disqualification* for piloting. Consult a designated Aviation Medical Examiner.

Exposure to Sun: No restrictions.

Heavy Exercise or Exertion: This drug may enable you to partake in exercise. Ask your doctor for guidance.

Discontinuation: If this drug has made it possible to reduce or stop cortisonelike drugs, and you must stop nedocromil, you may have to resume the cortisonelike drug as well as other measures to control asthma.

NEFAZODONE (na FAZ oh dohn)

Introduced: 1994   **Class:** Antidepressant, other   **Prescription:** USA:
Yes   **Controlled Drug:** USA: No; Canada: No   **Available as Generic:**
USA: No; Canada: No

Brand Name: Serzone

BENEFITS versus RISKS	
Possible Benefits	*Possible Risks*
EFFECTIVE TREATMENT OF DEPRESSION	Dizziness
	Mild blood pressure changes on standing
Fewer cardiovascular side effects than older agents	
Minimal anticholinergic side effects	
Decreased sedation versus other medicines used for depression	

▷ **Principal Uses**

As a Single Drug Product: Uses currently included in FDA-approved labeling: Treatment of major depression.

Other (unlabeled) generally accepted uses: May have a role in pain management.

How This Drug Works: This antidepressant is unique in that it:
- blocks the reuptake of a specific nerve-transmitting chemical (5-HT).
- acts as a 5-HT$_2$ antagonist.

Because of this unique mechanism of action, this drug has fewer cardiovascular and anticholinergic side effects than previously available agents.

Available Dosage Forms and Strengths

Tablets — 100 mg, 150 mg, 200 mg, 250 mg

▷ **Recommended Dosage Ranges** (Actual dosage and administration schedule must be determined for each patient individually.)

Infants and Children: Not indicated.

18 to 60 Years of Age: The starting dose for this medicine is 200 mg daily. This is taken as 100 mg in the morning and 100 mg in the evening. The dose is increased as needed and tolerated in 100-mg increments with at least 1 week separating any dose increase. The maximum dose is 600 mg daily.

Over 60 Years of Age: Dosing in this population starts with 100 mg daily in two divided doses. The medicine is then increased (at a slower rate than in younger patients) as needed and tolerated.

Conditions Requiring Dosing Adjustments

Liver Function: The dose should be decreased for patients with liver compromise.

Kidney Function: No specific dosing changes are presently identified.

▷ **Dosing Instructions:**   Food delays the absorption and decreases total absorption, but this effect is not believed to be clinically significant. Water is expected to be the safest liquid to take this medicine with. Grapefruit juice may have an action on some liver enzymes (cytochrome P450), which help remove (metabolize) this medicine. Avoid taking with grapefruit juice until all data are in.

Usual Duration of Use: Continual use on a regular schedule for 4 to 5 weeks usually determines effectiveness in treating depression. Long-term use (months to years) requires periodic evaluation of response, dosage adjustment, and physician follow-up.

Possible Advantages of This Drug

Two different mechanisms of action and decreased side effects versus other available agents.

▷ **This Drug Should Not Be Taken If**
- you have had an allergic reaction to any dosage form of it previously.
- you are taking astemizole or terfenadine.
- you are taking an MAO inhibitor (see Drug Classes).

▷ **Inform Your Physician Before Taking This Drug If**
- you take a triazolobenzodiazepine such as triazolam or alprazolam.
- you have a history of seizure disorder.
- you have a history of heart disease.
- you are uncertain of how much nefazodone to take or how often to take it.
- you take other medicines that were not discussed with your doctor when nefazodone was prescribed.

Possible Side Effects (natural, expected, and unavoidable drug actions)

Dry mouth, blurred vision, or constipation. Lowered blood pressure on standing (postural hypotension).

▷ **Possible Adverse Effects** (unusual, unexpected, and infrequent reactions)

If any of the following develop, consult your physician promptly for guidance.

Mild Adverse Effects

Allergic Reactions: Skin rash.

Nausea, ringing in the ears—possible.

Headache, dizziness, and tremor—infrequent.

Insomnia, confusion, and agitation—rare.

Slowed heart rate—case report.

Serious Adverse Effects

Allergic Reactions: Not defined.

Idiosyncratic Reactions: Not identified.

Activation of mania—one case report.

Seizures—rare.

▷ **Possible Effects on Sexual Function:**   Impotence, absence of orgasm, or abnormal ejaculation have all been rarely reported. Priapism has been reported with a structurally similar drug.

Possible Delayed Adverse Effects: None reported.

▷ **Adverse Effects That May Mimic Natural Diseases or Disorders**

None reported.

Natural Diseases or Disorders That May Be Activated by This Drug

None reported.

Possible Effects on Laboratory Tests

Hematocrit: decreased.

CAUTION

1. Risk of suicide is present in depressed patients. Small quantities of this medicine should be dispensed at a time when therapy is started. Appropriate suicide precautions should be taken.

2. This medicine **must not** be taken with an MAO inhibitor; there MUST be an interval of 14 days between when an MAO inhibitor is stopped and before nefazodone is started.

Precautions for Use

By Infants and Children: Safety and effectiveness for use by those under 18 years of age have not been established.

By Those Over 60 Years of Age: Lower starting doses and more gradual increases in dose are indicated.

▷ **Advisability of Use During Pregnancy**

Pregnancy Category: C. See Pregnancy Risk Categories at the back of this book.

Animal studies: Increased rat pup mortality was seen when doses five times the typical human dose were used.

Human studies: Information from adequate studies of pregnant women is not available. Ask your doctor for guidance.

Advisability of Use If Breast-Feeding

Presence of this drug in breast milk: Unknown.

Avoid drug or refrain from nursing.

Habit-Forming Potential: None defined at present, but not expected.

Effects of Overdosage: Nausea, vomiting, and somnolence.

Possible Effects of Long-Term Use: None reported.

Suggested Periodic Examinations While Taking This Drug (at physician's discretion)

Periodic checks of heart rate.

▷ **While Taking This Drug, Observe the Following**

Foods: No restrictions.

Beverages: No restrictions.

▷ *Alcohol:* This combination is not recommended.

Tobacco Smoking: No interactions expected, but I advise everyone to quit smoking.

Marijuana Smoking: Increased somnolence.

▷ *Other Drugs*

Nefazodone may *increase* the effects of

- alprazolam (Xanax) and potentially other benzodiazepines (see Drug Classes).
- digoxin (Lanoxin). Increased blood level checks are suggested.
- haloperidol (Haldol).
- triazolam (Halcion).

Nefazodone *taken concurrently* with

- acebutolol (Sectral) and perhaps other beta-blockers may result in decreased acebutolol levels and increased nefazodone metabolites.
- astemizole (Hismanal) can cause serious heart toxicity.
- clozapine (Clozaril) may result in clozapine toxicity since the P450 system in the liver is involved in removing clozapine from the liver.
- dextromethorphan (cough medicines with DM on the label) may result in dextromethorphan toxicity since the P450 system in the liver is involved in removing dextromethorphan from the liver.
- MAO inhibitors (see Drug Classes) may cause serious toxicity. Do not combine.
- phenytoin (Dilantin) may result in increased phenytoin levels. More fre-

quent phenytoin blood level checks are needed, and dosing should be adjusted to blood level results.

- terfenadine (Seldane) may cause serious heart rhythm problems.
- tricyclic antidepressants (see Drug Classes) may result in increased tricyclic antidepressant levels and toxicity.

▷ *Driving, Hazardous Activities:* This drug may cause somnolence. Restrict activities as necessary.

Aviation Note: The use of this drug *is a disqualification* for piloting. Consult a designated Aviation Medical Examiner.

Exposure to Sun: Use caution—photosensitivity is possible.

Discontinuation: Do not stop this medication without discussing this with your doctor.

NEOSTIGMINE (nee oh STIG meen)

Introduced: 1931   **Class:** Antimyasthenic   **Prescription:** USA: Yes
Controlled Drug: USA: No; Canada: No   **Available as Generic:** USA: Yes; Canada: Yes
Brand Names: Prostigmin, ✚PMS-Neostigmine, Viaderm-K.C.

BENEFITS versus RISKS	
Possible Benefits	*Possible Risks*
MODERATELY EFFECTIVE TREATMENT OF OCULAR AND MILD FORMS OF MYASTHENIA GRAVIS (symptomatic relief of muscle weakness) Eases postoperative bowel slowing or block (paralytic ileus)	Cholinergic crisis (overdose): excessive salivation, nausea, vomiting, stomach cramps, diarrhea, shortness of breath (asthmalike wheezing), weakness

▷ **Principal Uses**

As a Single Drug Product: Uses currently included in FDA-approved labeling: (1) Treats ocular and milder forms of myasthenia gravis by providing temporary relief of muscle weakness and fatigability; (2) reverses depression of bowel function that may occur after surgery; (3) used to ease symptoms of bladder instability.

Other (unlabeled) generally accepted uses: Used to reverse neuromuscular blockade caused by atracurium.

How This Drug Works: This drug inhibits cholinesterase, the enzyme that destroys acetylcholine. This results in higher levels of acetylcholine, the nerve transmitter that facilitates the stimulation of muscular activity. The net effects are increased muscle strength and endurance.

Available Dosage Forms and Strengths

Injection — 0.25 mg/ml, 0.5 mg/ml, 1.0 mg/ml
Tablets — 15 mg

▷ **Usual Adult Dosage Range:** Initially: 15 mg every 3 to 4 hours; adjust dosage as needed and tolerated. Maintenance: up to 300 mg daily; the average dose is 75 to 150 mg daily. **Note: Actual dosage and administration schedule must be determined for each patient individually.**

Conditions Requiring Dosing Adjustments
> *Liver Function:* Neostigmine should be used with caution by patients with compromised livers.
>
> *Kidney Function:* Half of a given dose of neostigmine is eliminated unchanged by the kidney; however, specific guidelines for decreasing doses are not available.

▷ **Dosing Instructions:**   The tablet may be crushed and taken with food or milk. Larger portions of the daily maintenance dosage should be timed according to the pattern of fatigue and weakness.

Usual Duration of Use: Use on a regular schedule (with dosage adjustment) for 10 to 14 days determines effectiveness in relieving the symptoms of myasthenia gravis. Long-term use (months to years) requires periodic physician evaluation.

▷ **This Drug Should Not Be Taken If**
- you have had an allergic reaction to it previously.
- you are known to be allergic to bromide compounds.
- you have an obstruction in your urinary tract or intestine.

▷ **Inform Your Physician Before Taking This Drug If**
- you have any type of seizure disorder.
- you are subject to heart rhythm disorders or bronchial asthma.
- you have recurrent urinary tract infections.
- you have prostatism (see Glossary).
- you plan to have surgery under general anesthesia in the near future.

Possible Side Effects (natural, expected, and unavoidable drug actions)
> Small pupils, watering of eyes, slow pulse, excessive salivation, nausea, vomiting, stomach cramps, diarrhea, urge to urinate, increased sweating.

▷ **Possible Adverse Effects** (unusual, unexpected, and infrequent reactions)
> **If any of the following develop, consult your physician promptly for guidance.**
>
> *Mild Adverse Effects*
> Allergic Reactions: Skin rash.
> Nervousness, anxiety, unsteadiness, muscle cramps or twitching—infrequent.
>
> *Serious Adverse Effects*
> Confusion, slurred speech, seizures, difficult breathing (asthmatic wheezing)—infrequent.
> Increased muscle weakness or paralysis—variable.
> Excessive vomiting or diarrhea may induce abnormally low blood potassium levels (hypokalemia). This will accentuate muscle weakness.
> Abnormally slow heartbeat (bradycardia)—rare.
> Drug-induced porphyria—case reports.

▷ **Possible Effects on Sexual Function:**   None reported.

▷ **Adverse Effects That May Mimic Natural Diseases or Disorders**
> Seizures may suggest the possibility of epilepsy.

Natural Diseases or Disorders That May Be Activated by This Drug
> Latent bronchial asthma.

Possible Effects on Laboratory Tests

None reported.

CAUTION

1. Certain drugs can block the action of this drug and reduce its effectiveness in treating myasthenia gravis (see "Other Drugs" below). Ask your physician before starting any new drug, prescription or over-the-counter.

2. Dosing must be carefully individualized. Variations in response may occur from time to time. Because generalized muscle weakness is a major symptom of both myasthenia crisis (underdosage) and cholinergic crisis (overdosage), it may be difficult to recognize the correct cause. As a rule, weakness that begins within 1 hour after taking this drug probably represents overdosage; weakness that begins 3 or more hours after taking this drug is probably due to underdosage. Observe these time relationships and inform your physician.

3. In long-term therapy, watch for development of resistance to the drug's therapeutic action (loss of effectiveness). Ask your doctor about the advisability of stopping this drug for a few days to see if responsiveness can be restored.

Precautions for Use

By Infants and Children: Dosage and administration schedule must be modified if kidney function is severely impaired.

By Those Over 60 Years of Age: The natural decline of kidney function with aging may require smaller doses to prevent accumulation of this drug to toxic levels.

▷ **Advisability of Use During Pregnancy**

Pregnancy Category: C. See Pregnancy Risk Categories at the back of this book.
Animal studies: No information available.
Human studies: Adequate studies of pregnant women are not available.
There are no reports of birth defects due to the use of this drug during pregnancy. However, there are reports of significant muscular weakness in 20% of newborn infants whose mothers had taken this drug during pregnancy. Ask your physician for guidance.

Advisability of Use If Breast-Feeding

Presence of this drug in breast milk: Probably not.
Monitor nursing infant closely and discontinue drug or nursing if adverse effects develop.

Habit-Forming Potential: None.

Effects of Overdosage: Generalized muscular weakness, blurred vision, very small pupils, slow heart rate, difficult breathing (wheezing), excessive salivation, nausea, vomiting, stomach cramps, diarrhea, muscle cramps or twitching. This syndrome constitutes the cholinergic crisis.

Possible Effects of Long-Term Use: Development of tolerance (see Glossary) with loss of therapeutic benefit.

Suggested Periodic Examinations While Taking This Drug (at physician's discretion)

Assessment of drug effectiveness and dosage schedule for best results.

▷ **While Taking This Drug, Observe the Following**

Foods: No restrictions.
Beverages: No restrictions. May be taken with milk.

▷ *Alcohol:* Use caution. Weakness and unsteadiness may be accentuated.

   Tobacco Smoking: No interactions expected, but I advise everyone to quit smoking.

▷ *Other Drugs*

   The following drugs may ***decrease*** the effects of neostigmine

   * atropine (belladonna).
   * clindamycin (Cleocin).
   * guanadrel (Hylorel).
   * guanethidine (Esimil, Ismelin).
   * procainamide (Procan SR, Pronestyl).
   * quinidine (Cardioquin, Duraquin, etc.).
   * quinine (Quinamm).

   Neostigmine ***taken concurrently*** with

   * edrophonium may cause cholinergic crisis in patients with myasthenic weakness.
   * hydrocortisone or other adrenocortical steroids (see Drug Classes) can cause decreased neostigmine benefits.
   * physostigmine can result in additive adverse effects.

▷ *Driving, Hazardous Activities:* This drug may cause blurred vision, confusion, or generalized weakness. Restrict activities as necessary.

   Aviation Note: The use of this drug ***is a disqualification*** for piloting. Consult a designated Aviation Medical Examiner.

   Exposure to Sun: No restrictions.

   Exposure to Heat: Use caution: this may cause excessive sweating and increased weakness.

   Exposure to Environmental Chemicals: Avoid excessive exposure (inhalation, skin contamination) to the insecticides Baygon, Diazinon, and Sevin. These can accentuate potential toxicity of this drug.

   Discontinuation: Do not stop this drug abruptly without your doctor's knowledge and help.

NIACIN (NI a sin)

Other Names: Nicotinic acid, vitamin B_3

Introduced: 1937   **Class:** Anticholesterol, vasodilator   **Prescription:** USA: Tablets and liquid—no; capsules—yes   **Controlled Drug:** USA: No; Canada: No   **Available as Generic:** USA: Yes; Canada: Yes

Brand Names: ✤Antivert [CD], Endur-Acin, Niac, Niacels, Niacin TR, Niacor, Nia-Bid, Niaplus, Nicobid, Nico-400, Nicolar, Nicotinex, ✤Novoniacin, SK-Niacin, Slo-Niacin, Span-Niacin-150, Tega-Span, Tri-B3

BENEFITS versus RISKS

Possible Benefits	*Possible Risks*
EFFECTIVE REDUCTION OF TOTAL CHOLESTEROL, LOW-DENSITY CHOLESTEROL, AND TRIGLYCERIDES IN TYPES II, III, IV, AND V CHOLESTEROL DISORDERS	Activation of peptic ulcer Drug-induced hepatitis Aggravation of diabetes or gout
Specific prevention and treatment of pellagra (niacin-deficiency disease)	

▷ **Principal Uses**

As a Single Drug Product: Uses currently included in FDA-approved labeling: (1) Certain patterns of abnormally high blood levels of cholesterol and triglycerides; (2) pellagra, a niacin (vitamin B_3) deficiency disorder characterized by dementia, dermatitis, and diarrhea; (3) therapy of Hartnup disease.

Other (unlabeled) generally accepted uses: (1) Therapy of certain types of vertigo and tinnitus (ringing in the ears); (2) may help decrease diarrhea in patients with cholera; (3) treatment of chilblains.

As a Combination Drug Product [CD]: In Canada this drug is combined with meclizine to enhance its effectiveness in the treatment of motion sickness and vertigo.

How This Drug Works

It is thought that it may inhibit the initial production of triglycerides and impair the conversion of fatty tissue to cholesterol and triglycerides.

This drug corrects the specific deficiency of vitamin B_3 that is responsible for the symptoms of pellagra.

This drug causes direct dilation of peripheral blood vessels in the skin of the face and neck; for this reason it has been used to increase the blood flow to the inner ear in an attempt to relieve some types of vertigo and ringing in the ears. The effectiveness of this application is questionable.

Available Dosage Forms and Strengths

Capsules, prolonged action — 125 mg, 250 mg, 300 mg, 400 mg, 500 mg

Oral solution — 50 mg/5 ml

Tablets — 20 mg, 25 mg, 50 mg, 100 mg, 500 mg

Tablets, prolonged action — 150 mg, 250 mg, 500 mg, 750 mg

▷ **Usual Adult Dosage Range**

For cholesterol disorders: Initially 100 mg three times daily. Dose may be increased in increments of 300 mg daily at intervals of 4 to 7 days as needed and tolerated. The usual maintenance dose is 1 to 2 g three times daily. The total daily dosage should not exceed 6 to 9 g.

For niacin deficiency: 10 to 20 mg daily.

For treatment of pellagra: 50 mg 3 to 10 times daily.

Note: Actual dosage and administration schedule must be determined for each patient individually.

Conditions Requiring Dosing Adjustments

Liver Function: This drug is metabolized in the liver and is contraindicated in liver disease.

Kidney Function: Specific guidelines for adjustment of dosing are not available.

▷ **Dosing Instructions:** Take with or immediately following meals to prevent stomach irritation. Also take one-half of an adult's aspirin tablet or one children's aspirin tablet with each dose of niacin to help prevent facial flushing and itching. Dosage should be increased very slowly over 2 to 3 months as needed. The prolonged-action form of niacin is preferable to improve tolerance. The regular tablet may be crushed for administration, but the prolonged-action capsules and tablets should not be altered.

Usual Duration of Use: Use on a regular schedule for 3 to 5 weeks determines benefit in reducing levels of cholesterol and triglycerides. Long-term use (months to years) requires periodic physician evaluation.

Currently a "Drug of Choice"
for initiating treatment of elevated LDL cholesterol and VLDL triglycerides.

▷ **This Drug Should Not Be Taken If**
- you have had an allergic reaction to it previously.
- you have active peptic ulcer disease or inflammatory bowel disease.
- you have active liver disease.

▷ **Inform Your Physician Before Taking This Drug If**
- you are prone to low blood pressure.
- you have a heart rhythm disorder of any kind.
- you have a history of peptic ulcer disease, inflammatory bowel disease, liver disease, jaundice, or gallbladder disease.
- you have diabetes or gout.

Possible Side Effects (natural, expected, and unavoidable drug actions)
Flushing, itching, tingling, and feeling of warmth, usually in the face and neck. Sensitive individuals may experience orthostatic hypotension (see Glossary).

▷ **Possible Adverse Effects** (unusual, unexpected, and infrequent reactions)
If any of the following develop, consult your physician promptly for guidance.
Mild Adverse Effects
Allergic Reactions: Skin rash, itching, hives.
Headache, dizziness, faintness, impaired vision—infrequent.
Indigestion, nausea, vomiting, diarrhea—infrequent.
Flushing and tingling—infrequent to frequent.
Dryness of skin, grayish-black pigmentation of skin folds—infrequent.
Serious Adverse Effects
Drug-induced hepatitis with jaundice (see Glossary): yellow eyes and skin, dark-colored urine, light-colored stools—case reports.
Worsening of diabetes and gout—possible.
Development of heart rhythm disorders—case reports.
Myopathy or peptic ulcers—case reports.
Abnormal blood sugar—possible.

▷ **Possible Effects on Sexual Function:** None reported.

▷ **Adverse Effects That May Mimic Natural Diseases or Disorders**
Liver reactions may suggest viral hepatitis.

Natural Diseases or Disorders That May Be Activated by This Drug
Latent diabetes, gout, inflammatory bowel disease, or peptic ulcer.

Possible Effects on Laboratory Tests
Complete blood cell counts: decreased eosinophils and lymphocytes.
Blood total cholesterol, LDL cholesterol, and triglyceride levels: decreased.
Blood HDL cholesterol level: increased.
Blood glucose level: increased.
Glucose tolerance test (GTT): decreased.
Blood uric acid level: increased.
Liver function tests: increased enzymes (ALT/GPT, AST/GOT, alkaline phosphatase) or bilirubin.
Urine sugar tests: inaccurate test results with Benedict's solution.

CAUTION
1. Large doses may cause increases in blood levels of sugar and uric acid. Diabetics or gout patients should monitor their status regularly.
2. Periodic measurements of blood cholesterol and triglyceride levels are essential for monitoring response and determining the need for changes in dosage or medication.
3. Recent reports indicate that the prolonged-action dosage forms of niacin may be more likely to cause liver damage than the rapidly absorbed (crystalline) forms. Ask your doctor which is the most appropriate dosage form and schedule for you.

Precautions for Use
By Infants and Children: Safety and effectiveness for use of large doses by those under 12 years of age have not been established.
By Those Over 60 Years of Age: Observe for the possible development of low blood pressure (light-headedness, dizziness, faintness) and heart rhythm disorders.

▷ Advisability of Use During Pregnancy
Pregnancy Category: C. See Pregnancy Risk Categories at the back of this book.
Animal studies: Significant birth defects due to this drug were found in chicks.
Human studies: Adequate studies of pregnant women are not available.
Use this drug only if clearly needed. Avoid completely during the first 3 months.

Advisability of Use If Breast-Feeding
Presence of this drug in breast milk: Unknown.
Avoid drug or refrain from nursing.

Habit-Forming Potential: None.

Effects of Overdosage: Generalized flushing, nausea, vomiting, stomach cramps, diarrhea, weakness, fainting.

Possible Effects of Long-Term Use: Increased blood levels of sugar and uric acid; liver damage.

Suggested Periodic Examinations While Taking This Drug (at physician's discretion)
Measurements of blood levels of total cholesterol, HDL and LDL cholesterol fractions, triglycerides, sugar, and uric acid.
Liver function tests.

▷ While Taking This Drug, Observe the Following
Foods: Follow the low-cholesterol diet prescribed by your physician.
Beverages: No restrictions. May be taken with milk.

▷ *Alcohol:* Use with caution. Alcohol used with large doses of this drug may cause excessive lowering of blood pressure. There has been one case report of delirium.

Tobacco Smoking: May increase risk of flushing and dizziness. I advise everyone to quit smoking.

▷ *Other Drugs*

Niacin may *increase* the effects of
- some antihypertensive drugs, and cause excessive lowering of blood pressure.

Niacin may *decrease* the effects of
- antidiabetic drugs (insulin and oral antidiabetic drugs; see Drug Classes), by raising the level of blood sugar.
- probenecid (Benemid) and sulfinpyrazone (Anturane), by raising the level of blood uric acid.

Niacin *taken concurrently* with
- isoniazid (INH) may result in decreased niacin levels and require increased niacin dosing.
- lovastatin and other HMG-CoA-type cholesterol-lowering drugs may result in reversible muscle problems (myopathy or rhabdomyolysis).
- nicotine (particularly transdermal) may result in increased risk of flushing and dizziness.

▷ *Driving, Hazardous Activities:* This drug may cause dizziness and faintness. Restrict activities as necessary.

Aviation Note: The use of this drug *may be a disqualification* for piloting. Consult a designated Aviation Medical Examiner.

Exposure to Sun: No restrictions.

Discontinuation: Do not stop this drug without your physician's knowledge and guidance. Abrupt withdrawal may be followed by excessive increase in blood cholesterol and triglyceride levels.

NICARDIPINE (ni KAR de peen)

Introduced: 1984　**Class:** Anti-anginal, antihypertensive, calcium channel blocker　**Prescription:** USA: Yes　**Controlled Drug:** USA: No; Canada: No　**Available as Generic:** USA: No

Brand Names: Cardene, Cardene SR

Controversies in Medicine: Medicines in this class have been subject to much conflicting data. There have also been several FDA hearings held on the calcium-channel-blocker class. **More recent data found the long-acting forms of calcium channel blockers to be safe and effective.**

BENEFITS versus RISKS	
Possible Benefits	*Possible Risks*
EFFECTIVE PREVENTION OF CLASSICAL ANGINA OF EFFORT	Increase in angina upon starting treatment
EFFECTIVE TREATMENT OF HYPERTENSION	Water retention, ankle swelling

▷ **Principal Uses**

As a Single Drug Product: Uses currently included in FDA-approved labeling: (1) Treats classical angina-of-effort (due to atherosclerotic disease of the coronary arteries) or angina caused by spasm of the coronary arteries; (2) mild to moderate hypertension.

Other (unlabeled) generally accepted uses: (1) Combination therapy in preventing recurrence of stroke; (2) may have a role in helping correct congestive heart failure; (3) can help refractory (not responding to nonsteroidal anti-inflammatory drugs) menstrual pain; (4) may help decrease the frequency and severity of migraine attacks; (5) can halt the progression of atherosclerosis; (6) lowers postoperative hypertension; (7) may prevent vessel spasm in some kinds of vascular surgery; (8) could have a role in treating some premature labor.

How This Drug Works: By blocking passage of calcium through certain cell walls (which is necessary for the function of nerve and muscle tissue), this drug inhibits the contraction of coronary arteries and peripheral arterioles. As a result of these effects, this drug

- promotes dilation of the coronary arteries (anti-anginal effect).
- reduces the degree of contraction of peripheral arterial walls, resulting in lowering of blood pressure. This further reduces the workload of the heart during exertion and helps prevent of angina.

Available Dosage Forms and Strengths

Capsules — 20 mg, 30 mg
Injection — 2.5 mg/ml
SR Capsules — 30 mg, 45 mg, 60 mg

▷ **Usual Adult Dosage Range:**   Initially 20 mg three times daily, 6 to 8 hours apart. Dose may be increased gradually at 3-day intervals (as needed and tolerated) up to 40 mg three times daily. The total daily dosage should not exceed 120 mg. The sustained-release form is started at 30 mg twice daily and is increased as needed and tolerated to 60 mg twice daily. **Note: Actual dosage and administration schedule must be determined for each patient individually.**

Conditions Requiring Dosing Adjustments

Liver Function: The dose should be started at 20 mg twice a day. If the dose must be increased, it should be slowly advanced and taken twice a day.

Kidney Function: For patients with moderate kidney failure, the starting dose should be 20 mg twice daily. If the dose is increased, it should be titrated slowly, and the twice-daily dosing interval retained. Nicardipine can cause urine retention, and should be a benefit-to-risk decision for patients with urine outflow problems.

▷ **Dosing Instructions:**   May be taken with or following food to reduce stomach irritation, but not a high-fat meal, as total absorption may be reduced by 20 to 30%. The capsule should be swallowed whole (not altered).

Usual Duration of Use: Use on a regular schedule for 2 to 4 weeks determines this drug's benefit in reducing the frequency and severity of angina or controlling hypertension. For long-term use (months to years), the smallest effective dose should be used. Physician supervision and periodic evaluation are essential.

Possible Advantages of This Drug
> Does not impair heart function or cause heart rhythm abnormalities.
> Can be used safely with beta-blockers, digoxin, diuretics, and nitrate.

▷ **This Drug Should Not Be Taken If**
- you have had an allergic reaction to it previously.
- you have advanced aortic stenosis.

▷ **Inform Your Physician Before Taking This Drug If**
- you have had an adverse reaction to any calcium channel blocker (see Drug Classes).
- you currently take any form of digitalis or a beta-blocker drug (see Drug Classes).
- you are taking any drugs that lower blood pressure.
- you are taking cimetidine (Tagamet) or cyclosporine (Sandimmune).
- you have a history of congestive heart failure, heart attack, or stroke.
- you have a history of circulation impairment to the fingers.
- you have Duchenne muscular dystrophy.
- you are subject to disturbances of heart rhythm.
- you have impaired liver or kidney function.

Possible Side Effects (natural, expected, and unavoidable drug actions)
> Rapid heart rate, swelling of the feet and ankles, flushing and sensation of warmth. Marked drop in blood pressure with fainting—rare.

▷ **Possible Adverse Effects** (unusual, unexpected, and infrequent reactions)
If any of the following develop, consult your physician promptly for guidance.
Mild Adverse Effects
Allergic Reaction: Skin rash—rare.
Headache, dizziness, weakness, nervousness, insomnia, or ringing in the ears (tinnitus); blurred vision, confusion, increased urination—rare to infrequent.
Palpitation, shortness of breath—rare.
Indigestion, nausea, vomiting, constipation—all rare.
Joint and muscle pain, cough—rare.
Abnormal growth (hyperplasia) of the gums—rare.
Serious Adverse Effects
Allergic Reactions: None reported.
Increased frequency or severity of angina when starting therapy or after an increase in dose—possible.
Difficult urination—rare.
Liver toxicity—rare.
Decreased white blood cell counts reported with medicines in the same class (agranulocytosis).

▷ **Possible Effects on Sexual Function:** Impotence—rare.

▷ **Adverse Effects That May Mimic Natural Diseases or Disorders**
> Flushing and warmth may resemble menopausal "hot flushes." Increased liver enzymes may resemble infectious hepatitis.

Possible Effects on Laboratory Tests
> Liver function tests: elevated (1%).

CAUTION
1. If you are checking your own blood pressure, check it just before each dose and 1 to 2 hours after each dose to obtain an accurate picture of the drug's effect.
2. Be sure to tell all health care providers who provide care for you that you take this drug. Note the use of this drug on your card of personal identification.
3. You may use nitroglycerin and other nitrate drugs as needed to relieve acute episodes of angina pain. However, if you detect that your angina attacks are becoming more frequent or intense, call your doctor promptly.

Precautions for Use
By Infants and Children: Safety and effectiveness for those under 18 years of age are not established.
By Those Over 60 Years of Age: Usually well tolerated; however, watch for development of weakness, dizziness, fainting, and falling. Take necessary precautions to prevent injury. Report promptly any changes in your pattern of thirst and urination.

▷ **Advisability of Use During Pregnancy**
Pregnancy Category: C. See Pregnancy Risk Categories at the back of this book.
Animal studies: Embryo and fetal toxicity reported in small animals, but no birth defects due to this drug.
Human studies: Adequate studies of pregnant women are not available.
Avoid this drug during the first 3 months. Use during the final 6 months only if clearly needed. Ask your physician for guidance.

Advisability of Use If Breast-Feeding
Presence of this drug in breast milk: Probably yes.
Avoid drug or refrain from nursing.

Habit-Forming Potential: None.

Effects of Overdosage: Weakness, light-headedness, fainting, fast pulse, low blood pressure, shortness of breath, flushed and warm skin, tremors.

Possible Effects of Long-Term Use: None reported.

Suggested Periodic Examinations While Taking This Drug (at physician's discretion)
Evaluations of heart function, including electrocardiograms; measurements of blood pressure in supine, sitting, and standing positions.

▷ **While Taking This Drug, Observe the Following**
Foods: Food decreases the amount of this drug that is absorbed. It is also prudent to avoid excessive salt intake.
Beverages: No restrictions. May be taken with milk.
▷ *Alcohol:* Use with caution until combined effects have been determined. Alcohol may exaggerate the drop in blood pressure experienced by some individuals.
Tobacco Smoking: Nicotine may reduce the effectiveness of this drug. I advise everyone to quit smoking.
Marijuana Smoking: Possible reduced effectiveness of this drug; mild to moderate increase in angina; possible changes in electrocardiogram, confusing interpretation.

▷ *Other Drugs*
   Nicardipine may *increase* the effects of
   • cyclosporine (Sandimmune), and cause kidney toxicity.
   Nicardipine *taken concurrently* with
   • amiodarone (Cordarone) may result in cardiac arrest.
   • beta-blocker drugs or digitalis preparations (see Drug Classes) may affect
     heart rate and rhythm adversely. Careful monitoring by your physician is
     necessary if these drugs are taken concurrently.
   • magnesium may cause worsening of neuromuscular blockade and further
     lowering of blood pressure.
   • nonsteroidal anti-inflammatory agents (NSAIDs—see Drug Classes) may
     blunt the therapeutic effects of nicardipine.
   • phenytoin (Dilantin) may result in phenytoin toxicity or decreased efficacy
     of nicardipine.
   • rifampin (Rifadin, others) has caused loss of control of blood pressure with
     some other calcium channel blockers. Caution is advised if these medicines
     are combined.
   The following drug may *increase* the effects of nicardipine
   • cimetidine (Tagamet).
▷ *Driving, Hazardous Activities:* Usually no restrictions. This drug may cause
     drowsiness or dizziness. Restrict activities as necessary.
   Aviation Note: Coronary artery disease and hypertension *are disqualifications*
     for piloting. Consult a designated Aviation Medical Examiner.
   Exposure to Sun: No restrictions.
   Exposure to Heat: Caution is advised. Hot environments can exaggerate the
     blood-pressure-lowering effects of this drug. Observe for light-headedness
     or weakness.
   Heavy Exercise or Exertion: This drug may improve your ability to be more ac-
     tive without resulting angina pain. Use caution and avoid excessive exercise
     that could impair heart function in the absence of warning pain.
   Discontinuation: Do not stop this drug abruptly. Ask your doctor about gradual
     withdrawal. Watch for possible development of rebound angina.

NICOTINE (NIK oh teen)

Introduced: 1992, 1996, 1997   **Class:** Smoking cessation adjunct, nicotine
replacement therapy   **Prescription:** USA: Both Nicorettes (2 and 4 mg) are
now available without a prescription for those over 18 years old. Nicotine patches
are FDA approved for nonprescription use. The nicotine inhaler and nasal spray
are **only available with a prescription.** **Controlled Drug:** USA: No; Canada:
No   **Available as Generic:** USA: No; Canada: No

Brand Names: Habitrol, Nicoderm, Nicorette, Nicorette DS, Nicotrol, Nicotrol
    Inhaler, Nicotrol NS, Prostep

```
┌─────────────────────────────────────────────────────────────┐
│                    BENEFITS versus RISKS                      │
│      Possible Benefits              Possible Risks            │
│   EFFECTIVE REDUCTION OF      Aggravation of existing angina, │
│     NICOTINE CRAVING AND        heart rhythm disorders,       │
│     WITHDRAWAL EFFECTS when      hypertension,                │
│   used adjunctively in          insulin-dependent diabetes,   │
│   smoking-cessation treatment    peptic ulcer, and vascular   │
│   programs                       diseases                     │
│                                Increased risk of abortion (if │
│                                  used during pregnancy)       │
└─────────────────────────────────────────────────────────────┘
```

▷ **Principal Uses**

As a Single Drug Product: Uses currently included in FDA-approved labeling: Nicotine chewing gum, nicotine transdermal systems, inhaler, and nasal spray are used adjunctively in behavior modification programs to help cigarette smokers who wish to stop smoking.

Other (unlabeled) generally accepted uses: Some European data studying combination gum and patch use appear to show an increased success rate. The technique used the gum to halt "breakthrough" cigarette cravings. The thinking is that the craving resulted from an insufficient nicotine level provided by the patch, and that the gum provided a short-term increase which stopped the craving. This may also apply to add-on use of other more immediate-release products.

How This Drug Works: By providing an alternate source of nicotine (for nicotine-dependent smokers), the appropriate use of these drug products can reduce nicotine craving and lessen smoking withdrawal effects such as irritability, nervousness, headache, fatigue, sleep disturbances, and drowsiness.

Available Dosage Forms and Strengths

Nicotine chewing gum tablets (newly nonprescription in the U.S.)

Nicorette — 2 mg (U.S., Canada)—4 mg (Canada)

Nicorette DS — 4 mg (U.S., Canada)

Inhaler — 10 mg per cartridge

Nasal spray — 10 mg/ml (10-ml bottle)

Transdermal systems — 16-hour systems (U.S. only): 5 mg, 10 mg, 15 mg—24-hour systems: 7 mg (U.S., Canada), 11 mg (U.S.), 14 mg (U.S., Canada), 21 mg (U.S., Canada), 22 mg (U.S.).

How to Store

Store nicotine gum at room temperature and protect from light. Store nicotine patches at room temperature and be especially careful to avoid exposing the patches to temperatures greater than 86 degrees F (30 degrees C). Do not store unpouched. Once opened, patches should be used promptly because they may lose their strength.

▷ **Recommended Dosage Ranges** (Actual dosage and administration schedule must be determined for each patient individually.)

Infants and Children: Avoid use completely in children. Avoid accidental exposure to patches.

12 to 60 Years of Age: For chewing gum tablets: Initially one piece every hour while awake (10 to 12 pieces daily); supplement with one additional piece if and when needed to control urge to smoke. Total daily dosage should not exceed 30 pieces (60 mg).

For inhaler form: Information is pending. Once available, this profile will be updated.

Nasal spray: Two sprays, one in each nostril. Starting dose is usually two to four sprays each hour. Maximum is 5 doses per hour (5 mg) and 40 doses per day (40 mg or 80 sprays). It should be used for a maximum of 3 months.

For transdermal systems: Dosage depends upon patient characteristics and product used.

For those weighing 100 lb or more, smoking 10 or more cigarettes daily, and *without* cardiovascular disease:

Using a 16-hour system (Nicotrol)—initially one 15 mg patch applied for 16 hours daily for 4 to 12 weeks. For those who have abstained from smoking, reduce dose to one 10-mg patch applied for 16 hours daily for the next 2 to 4 weeks; then to one 5-mg patch applied for 16 hours daily for the following 2 to 4 weeks. Using a 24-hour system: Habitrol, Nicoderm—initially one 21-mg patch applied daily for 4 to 8 weeks. For those who have abstained from smoking, reduce dose to one 14-mg patch daily for the next 2 to 4 weeks; then to one 7-mg patch daily for the following 2 to 4 weeks. Prostep—initially one 22-mg patch applied daily for 4 to 8 weeks. For those who have abstained from smoking, reduce dose to one 11-mg patch daily for 2 to 4 weeks.

For those weighing less than 100 lb, smoking less than 10 cigarettes daily, or *with* cardiovascular disease:

Using a 24-hour system: Habitrol, Nicoderm—Initially one 14-mg patch applied daily for 4 to 8 weeks. For those who have abstained from smoking, reduce dose to one 7-mg patch daily for the next 2 to 4 weeks. Prostep—Initially one 11-mg patch applied daily for 4 to 8 weeks.

Over 60 Years of Age: Same as 12 to 60 years of age.

Conditions Requiring Dosing Adjustments

Liver Function: Consideration must be given to decreasing the starting dose if the liver is compromised.

Kidney Function: Doses are decreased in severe kidney compromise.

Cardiovascular Disease: See above.

▷ **Dosing Instructions: Carefully follow the manufacturer's directions provided with each product.**

For chewing gum: Limit use to one piece of gum at a time. This product is much harder than typical chewing gum. Chew each piece slowly and intermittently for 30 minutes. A tingling of your gum tissue or peppery taste usually indicates release of a sufficient amount of nicotine. Try to gradually reduce the number of pieces chewed each day by using it only when there is an urge to smoke. During participation in a smoking-cessation program, always have the gum available as a defense against smoking.

For transdermal systems: Apply a new patch at the same time each day. Do not alter the patch in any way. Apply the patch to the upper arm or body where the skin is clean, dry, and free of hair, oil, scars, and irritation of any kind; alternate sites of application. Press the patch firmly in place for 10 seconds; ensure good contact throughout. Wash your hands when you have finished applying the patch. Replace patches that are dislodged by showering, bathing, or swimming.

For spray: DO NOT swallow, inhale, or sniff when spraying the spray.

For the inhaler: Information is pending.

Usual Duration of Use: Use on a regular schedule for 2 to 3 months determines effectiveness in achieving lasting cessation of smoking. Nicotine chewing gum should not be used for more than 6 months; transdermal systems should not be used for more than 20 weeks. The nasal spray form should be used no longer than 3 months. The inhaler form should NOT be used for more than 6 months. Long-term use requires periodic physician evaluation of response and dosage adjustment.

Possible Advantages of These Drugs

Provides control and flexibility of gradual nicotine withdrawal for use in supervised smoking-cessation programs.

Currently a "Drug of Choice"

for people who are motivated to stop smoking but find it difficult to stop abruptly. Since many forms are now available without a prescription, be sure to talk with your doctor or pharmacist about how to most effectively use these medicines.

▷ This Drug Should Not Be Taken If

- you have had an allergic reaction to any dosage form of it previously.
- you have severe or uncontrolled or a pattern of worsening angina (physician's discretion).
- you have uncontrolled, life-threatening heart rhythm disorders (physician's discretion).
- you have had a recent heart attack (physician's discretion).

▷ Inform Your Physician Before Taking This Drug If

- you have any form of angina (coronary heart disease).
- you have had a heart attack at any time.
- you are subject to heart rhythm disorders.
- you have insulin-dependent diabetes.
- you have hypertension (high blood pressure).
- you have hyperthyroidism (overactive thyroid function).
- you have a pheochromocytoma (adrenaline-producing tumor).
- you have a history of esophagitis or peptic ulcer disease.
- you have a history of Buerger's disease or Raynaud's phenomenon.
- you currently have any dental problems or skin disorders.
- you have a history of kidney or liver disease.
- you have an increase in cardiovascular effects while you are taking this medicine.
- you have already taken a 3-month course of the patch from another doctor.
- you think you are pregnant or plan to become pregnant.
- you are uncertain of how much or how often to take this medicine.

Possible Side Effects (natural, expected, and unavoidable drug actions)

For chewing gum: mouth or throat irritation; injury to teeth or dental repairs. For transdermal systems: redness, itching, or burning at site of application (mild and transient). For nasal spray: runny nose, nasal irritation. For inhaler: information is pending.

▷ Possible Adverse Effects (unusual, unexpected, and infrequent reactions)

If any of the following develop, consult your physician promptly for guidance.

Mild Adverse Effects

Allergic Reactions: Skin rash, hives, itching, local or generalized swellings.

Headache, light-headedness, dizziness, drowsiness, irritability, nervousness, insomnia, joint pain, muscle aches, abnormal dreams—possible to infrequent and some may be dose related.

Rapid heartbeat, palpitation, increased sweating—infrequent to frequent, dose related.

Increased or decreased appetite, nausea, dry mouth, indigestion, constipation, or diarrhea—infrequent.

Serious Adverse Effects

Irregular heart rhythms, chest pain (angina), edema—infrequent.

See "Effects of Overdosage" below.

Stroke—case report.

▷ **Possible Effects on Sexual Function:**   There are some data questioning an effect on sperm, but a distinct demonstration of an effect is lacking.

Natural Diseases or Disorders That May Be Activated by This Drug

Latent angina, atrial fibrillation, hypertension, peptic ulcer disease, temporomandibular joint (TMJ) disorder (by chewing gum).

Possible Effects on Laboratory Tests

Free fatty acids (FFA blood level): increased.

Blood glucose: increased.

Prothrombin time (INR): decreased.

Urine screening test for drug abuse: no effect.

CAUTION

1. For these drug products to be safe and effective, **it is mandatory that all smoking be stopped immediately at the beginning of drug treatment**.

2. Extended use of chewing gum may cause damage to mouth tissues and teeth, loosen fillings and stick to dentures, and initiate or aggravate temporomandibular joint (TMJ) dysfunction.

3. Smoking cessation and the use of these drug products can result in increased blood levels of insulin (in insulin-dependent diabetics); dosage reduction of insulin may be necessary to prevent hypoglycemic reactions.

4. If you are taking any of the following drugs, consult your physician regarding the need to reduce their dosage while participating in a smoking cessation program: aminophylline, oxtriphylline, theophylline, beta-blocker drugs, propoxyphene, oxazepam, prazosin, pentazocine, imipramine.

5. If you are taking any of the following drugs, consult your physician regarding the need to increase their dosage while participating in a smoking cessation program: isoproterenol, phenylephrine.

6. Used patches should be folded in half with the adhesive sides sealed together; place them in the original pouch or aluminum foil and dispose of them promptly; keep out of reach of children and animals.

7. Use of antacids such as Tums prior to chewing nicotine gum can increase the amount of nicotine absorbed from the gum.

8. Habitrol patches have only been shown to be effective when they are part of a complete smoking cessation program that includes counseling.

9. The Centers for Disease Control (CDC) has many excellent publications

available to give you more information on stopping smoking. Call 1–800–232–1311 for more information.

Precautions for Use

By Infants and Children: Safety and effectiveness for those under 12 years of age are not established.

By Those Over 60 Years of Age: Because of the increased possibility of cardiovascular disorders in this age group, treatment should be cautiously started. Watch closely for adverse effects.

▷ **Advisability of Use During Pregnancy**

Pregnancy Category: For nicotine chewing gum: X. For nicotine transdermal systems and nasal spray: D. See Pregnancy Risk Categories at the back of this book. Inhaler category is not assigned as yet.

Animal studies: Impaired fertility found in mouse, rat, and rabbit studies. Birth defects found in high-dose studies of mice.

Human studies: Adequate studies of pregnant women are not available. However, it is known that cigarette smoking during pregnancy may cause low birth weight, increased risk of abortion, and increased risk of newborn death.

The use of these drug products is not recommended during pregnancy.

Advisability of Use If Breast-Feeding

Presence of this drug in breast milk: Yes.

Avoid drug or refrain from nursing.

Habit-Forming Potential: The prolonged use of these drug products may perpetuate the physical dependence of nicotine-dependent smokers. Patches should have the lowest potential for dependence. Potential exists for abuse of nonprescription forms of this medicine.

Effects of Overdosage: Nausea, vomiting, increased salivation, stomach cramps, diarrhea, headache, dizziness, impaired vision and hearing, weakness, confusion, fainting, difficult breathing, seizures.

Possible Effects of Long-Term Use: Perpetuation of nicotine dependence.

Suggested Periodic Examinations While Taking This Drug (at physician's discretion)

Evaluation of patient's ability to abstain from smoking.

Evaluation of patient's blood pressure and heart function.

▷ **While Taking This Drug, Observe the Following**

Foods: No restrictions.

Beverages: No restrictions.

▷ *Alcohol:* May cause an increase in cardiovascular effects.

Tobacco Smoking: Avoid all forms of tobacco completely.

Marijuana Smoking: Avoid completely.

▷ *Other Drugs*

Nicotine may ***increase*** the effects of

• adenosine.

• niacin (flushing and dizziness).

The following drugs may ***increase*** the effects of nicotine

• antacids such as Tums used prior to chewing nicotine-containing gum may increase the absorption of nicotine from the gum.

• cimetidine (Tagamet).

• lithium (Lithobid).

• ranitidine (Zantac).

Nicotine *taken concurrently* with
- niacin (Nicobid, others) can cause severe facial flushing.

▷ *Driving, Hazardous Activities:* This drug may cause dizziness or drowsiness. Restrict activities as necessary.

Aviation Note: The use of this drug *may be a disqualification* for piloting. Consult a designated Aviation Medical Examiner.

Exposure to Sun: No restrictions.

Exposure to Cold: Use caution until tolerance is determined. Cold environments may enhance the vasospastic action of nicotine.

Heavy Exercise or Exertion: Patients with angina, coronary artery disease, or hypertension should use this drug with caution.

Discontinuation: As soon as a lasting cessation of smoking has been achieved, these drugs should be gradually reduced in dosage and then discontinued. Continual use of the chewing gum or inhaler should not exceed 6 months, the nasal spray form no longer than 3 months, and the transdermal system no more than 20 weeks.

Special Storage Instructions: Store nicotine gum at room temperature and protect from light. Store nicotine patches at room temperature and be especially careful to avoid exposing the patches to temperatures greater than 86 degrees F (30 degrees C). Do not store unpouched. Once opened, patches should be used promptly because they may lose their strength.

NIFEDIPINE (ni FED i peen)

Introduced: 1972   **Class:** Anti-anginal, antihypertensive, calcium channel blocker   **Prescription:** USA: Yes   **Controlled Drug:** USA: No; Canada: No   **Available as Generic:** Yes

Brand Names: Adalat, Adalat CC, ✦Adalat P.A., ✦Adalat FT, ✦Apo-Nifed, ✦Gen-Nifedipine, ✦Novo-Nifedin, ✦Nu-Nifed, Procardia, Procardia XL

Controversies in Medicine: Medicines in this class have been subject to much conflicting data. There have also been several FDA hearings held on the calcium-channel-blocker class. More recent data found the **long-acting forms** of calcium channel blockers to be safe and effective.

BENEFITS versus RISKS	
Possible Benefits	*Possible Risks*
EFFECTIVE PREVENTION OF BOTH MAJOR TYPES OF ANGINA	Rare increase in angina upon starting treatment
EFFECTIVE TREATMENT OF HYPERTENSION (sustained-release form only)	Rare precipitation of congestive heart failure
	Rare anemia and low white blood cell counts
	Very rare drug-induced hepatitis
	Fainting

▷ **Principal Uses**

As a Single Drug Product: Uses currently included in FDA-approved labeling: (1) Treats angina pectoris due to coronary artery spasm (Prinzmetal's variant angina) that occurs spontaneously and is not associated with exertion; and (2) classical angina-of-effort (due to atherosclerotic disease of the coronary arteries) in people who have not responded to or cannot tolerate the nitrates and beta-blocker drugs customarily used to treat this disorder (sustained-release form); (3) used to treat mild to moderate hypertension (extended-release forms).

Author's Note: A retrospective chart review has found the immediate-release form of this medicine IS NOT recommended for use in treating hypertension, acute myocardial infarction (heart attack), hypertensive crisis, and some forms of unstable angina.

Other (unlabeled) generally accepted uses: (1) Treatment of symptoms associated with Raynaud's phenomenon; (2) may stop the progression of atherosclerosis; (3) can have a role in treating congestive heart failure; (4) therapy of pulmonary hypertension; (5) helps decrease risk of heart attack after coronary artery bypass grafting; (6) could have a role in some neurologically based pain disorders; (7) may have a role in treating tardive dyskinesia; (8) can help urticaria of unknown cause; (9) therapy of achalasia or esophageal spasm; (10) helps intractable hiccups; (11) helps amaurosis fugax; (12) has a role in helping abnormal reactions to cold (chilblains).

How This Drug Works: By blocking passage of calcium through certain cell walls (which is necessary for the function of nerve and muscle tissue), this drug slows the spread of electrical activity through the heart and inhibits the contraction of coronary arteries and peripheral arterioles. As a result of these combined effects, this drug

- prevents spontaneous spasm of coronary arteries (Prinzmetal's angina).
- reduces the rate and contraction force of the heart during exertion, decreasing oxygen requirements of the heart muscle and reducing the occurrence of effort-induced angina (classical angina pectoris).
- reduces the degree of contraction of peripheral arterial walls, resulting in their relaxation and consequent lowering of blood pressure. This further reduces the workload of the heart during exertion and helps prevent angina.

Available Dosage Forms and Strengths

> Capsules — 5 mg (Canada), 10 mg (U.S. and Canada), 20 mg (U.S.)
> Tablets — 10 mg, 20 mg (Canada)
> Tablets, extended release — 10 mg, 20 mg (Canada), 30 mg, 60 mg, 90 mg (U.S.)
> Tablets, sustained release — 30 mg, 60 mg, 90 mg

▷ **Recommended Dosage Ranges** (Actual dosage and administration schedule must be determined for each patient individually.)

Infants and Children: Dosage not established.

12 to 60 Years of Age: Extended-release form for high blood pressure: Initially 30 mg once daily. Dose may be increased gradually at 7- to 14-day intervals (as needed and tolerated) up to 60 mg. Maximum total daily dosage should not exceed 90 mg.

For hypertension: Initially a single 30-mg or 60-mg sustained-release tablet taken once daily. Gradually increased as a single daily dose if needed.

Sublingual for hypertensive crisis: **The immediate-release form of this medicine IS NOT recommended for use in treating hypertension, acute myocardial infarction (heart attack), hypertensive crisis, and some forms of unstable angina.**

Over 60 Years of Age: Same as 12 to 60 years of age. **Nifedipine immediate-release use by those over 71 has been associated with almost a fourfold increase in risk for all-cause death when compared to ACE inhibitors, beta-blockers, or other calcium channel blockers.**

Conditions Requiring Dosing Adjustments
Liver Function: Specific dosage adjustments in liver compromise are not defined, and the dose should be empirically decreased. This drug is also a rare cause of liver toxicity (allergic hepatitis), and should be used with caution by patients with compromised livers. It is also a potential cause of portal hypertension, and should not be used by patients with portal hypertension.
Kidney Function: For patients with compromised kidneys, nifedipine is a benefit-to-risk decision, as it can lead to kidney toxicity.

▷ **Dosing Instructions:**   May be taken with or following food to reduce stomach irritation. The capsule should be swallowed whole (not altered). The sustained-release tablet should be taken whole (not altered).

Usual Duration of Use: Use on a regular schedule for 2 to 4 weeks determines effectiveness in reducing the frequency and severity of angina and in controlling hypertension. For long-term use (months to years), the smallest effective dose should be used. Supervision and periodic physician evaluation are essential.

Possible Advantages of This Drug
The sustained-release form of this drug permits effective once-a-day treatment for both angina and hypertension.

▷ **This Drug Should Not Be Taken If**
- you have had an allergic reaction to it previously.
- you have active liver disease.
- you are over 71 and have been prescribed the immediate-release form of nifedipine.
- you have low blood pressure—systolic pressure below 90.
- you have significant narrowing of your aorta (aortic stenosis). Ask your doctor.

▷ **Inform Your Physician Before Taking This Drug If**
- you have had an adverse response to any calcium channel blocker.
- you currently take any form of digitalis or a beta-blocker drug (see Drug Classes).
- you are taking any drugs that lower blood pressure.
- you have a history of congestive heart failure, heart attack, or stroke.
- you are subject to disturbances of heart rhythm.
- you have cardiomyopathy (nonobstructive) or aortic stenosis.
- you have impaired liver or kidney function.
- you have abnormal circulation to your fingers.
- you have atrial fibrillation.
- you have developed a dermatological condition while taking this medicine.
- you have diabetes or Duchenne muscular dystrophy.
- you have a history of drug-induced liver damage.

Possible Side Effects (natural, expected, and unavoidable drug actions)
Low blood pressure, rapid heart rate, swelling of the feet and ankles, flushing and sensation of warmth, sweating.

▷ **Possible Adverse Effects** (unusual, unexpected, and infrequent reactions)

If any of the following develop, consult your physician promptly for guidance.

Mild Adverse Effects

Allergic Reactions: Skin rash, hives, itching, fever.

Headache, dizziness, weakness, nervousness, blurred vision, eye pain, or swelling around eyes—infrequent.

Pedal edema—frequent.

Depression—rare.

Abnormal growth of the gums (gingival hyperplasia)—rare.

Taste disturbances—possible.

Ringing in the ears (tinnitus)—case reports.

Sleep disturbances or bed-wetting—case reports.

Increased or decreased blood potassium—possible.

Palpitation, shortness of breath, wheezing, cough—infrequent.

Impaired sense of smell—possible.

Heartburn, nausea, taste disturbances, cramps, diarrhea—rare.

Tremors, muscle cramps—possible.

Serious Adverse Effects

Allergic Reaction: Drug-induced hepatitis—very rare; drug eruptions and erysipelaslike reactions, and exfoliative dermatitis or erythema multiforme.

Idiosyncratic Reactions: Joint stiffness and inflammation.

Increased frequency or severity of angina on initiation of treatment or following an increase in dose.

Abnormal muscle movements (myoclonus)—case reports.

Kidney toxicity or pulmonary edema—case reports.

Bezoars—rare (seen with sustained-release forms).

Acute psychosis—case report.

Worsening of circulation to the fingers—possible.

Marked drop in blood pressure with fainting—possible.

Low white blood cells, platelets, and hemoglobin—case reports.

▷ **Possible Effects on Sexual Function:**   Altered timing and pattern of menstruation; excessive menstrual bleeding.

Tenderness and swelling of male breast tissue (gynecomastia)—case reports.

▷ **Adverse Effects That May Mimic Natural Diseases or Disorders**

An allergic rash and swelling of the legs may resemble erysipelas.

Drug-induced hepatitis may suggest viral hepatitis.

Transient increases in liver function tests may suggest infectious hepatitis.

Possible Effects on Laboratory Tests

Bleeding time: increased.

Liver function tests: transient increases.

Blood total cholesterol level: no effect in those under 60 years old; decreased in those over 60 years old.

Blood HDL cholesterol level: no effect, or increased.

Blood LDL and VLDL cholesterol levels: no effect.

Blood triglyceride levels: no effect, or decreased.

CAUTION
1. Be sure to tell all health care providers you consult that you are taking this drug. Note the use of this drug on your personal identification card.
2. You may use nitroglycerin and other nitrate drugs as needed to relieve acute angina pain. However, if your angina attacks are becoming more frequent or intense, call your doctor.

Precautions for Use
By Infants and Children: Safety and effectiveness for those under 12 years of age are not established.
By Those Over 60 Years of Age: You may be more susceptible to the development of weakness, dizziness, fainting, and falling. Take necessary precautions to prevent injury. Report promptly any changes in your pattern of thirst and urination.

▷ **Advisability of Use During Pregnancy**
Pregnancy Category: C. See Pregnancy Risk Categories at the back of this book.
Animal studies: Embryo and fetal deaths reported in mice, rats, and rabbits; birth defects reported in rats.
Human studies: Adequate studies of pregnant women are not available.
Avoid this drug during the first 3 months. Use during the final 6 months only if clearly needed. Ask your physician for guidance.

Advisability of Use If Breast-Feeding
Presence of this drug in breast milk: Yes.
Avoid drug or refrain from nursing.

Habit-Forming Potential: None.

Effects of Overdosage: Weakness, light-headedness, fainting, fast pulse, low blood pressure, shortness of breath, flushed and warm skin, tremors.

Possible Effects of Long-Term Use: None reported.

Suggested Periodic Examinations While Taking This Drug (at physician's discretion)
Evaluations of heart function, including electrocardiograms; measurements of blood pressure in supine, sitting, and standing positions.

▷ **While Taking This Drug, Observe the Following**
Foods: Do not eat grapefruit for an hour after taking this medicine. It is also prudent to avoid excessive salt intake.
Beverages: Grapefruit juice may greatly increase the absorption (bioavailability) of nifedipine and result in an exaggerated therapeutic effect. Water is the best liquid to take this medicine with. May be taken with milk.
▷ *Alcohol:* Use with caution. Alcohol may exaggerate the drop in blood pressure experienced by some people.
Tobacco Smoking: Nicotine may reduce the effectiveness of this drug. I advise everyone to quit smoking.
Marijuana Smoking: Possible reduced effectiveness of this drug; mild to moderate increase in angina; possible changes in electrocardiogram, confusing interpretation.
▷ *Other Drugs*
Nifedipine *taken concurrently* with
• amiodarone (Cordarone) may cause the heart to stop.
• beta-blocker drugs or digitalis preparations (see Drug Classes) may affect

heart rate and rhythm adversely. Careful monitoring by your physician is necessary if these drugs are taken concurrently.

- cyclosporine (Sandimmune) can lead to nifedipine toxicity.
- digoxin (Lanoxin) may lead to digoxin toxicity.
- diltiazem (Cardizem) may lead to nifedipine toxicity.
- magnesium can cause additive lowering of the blood pressure.
- oral antidiabetic drugs (see Drug Classes) or insulin may result in loss of glucose control.
- phenytoin (Dilantin) can cause phenytoin toxicity.
- rifampin (Rifadin) can decrease nifedipine's effectiveness.
- theophylline can reduce the therapeutic benefits of nifedipine and may lead to theophylline toxicity as well.
- vincristine (Oncovin) can cause vincristine toxicity.

The following drugs may *increase* the effects of nifedipine

- cimetidine (Tagamet).
- quinidine (Quinaglute, others) can lead to nifedipine toxicity as well as decreased quinidine effectiveness.
- ranitidine (Zantac).

▷ *Driving, Hazardous Activities:* Usually no restrictions. This drug may cause drowsiness or dizziness. Restrict activities as necessary.

Aviation Note: Coronary artery disease *is a disqualification* for piloting. Consult a designated Aviation Medical Examiner.

Exposure to Sun: Caution—rare cases of phototoxicity have been reported.

Exposure to Heat: Caution is advised. Hot environments can exaggerate the blood-pressure-lowering effects of this drug. Observe for light-headedness or weakness.

Heavy Exercise or Exertion: This drug may improve your ability to be more active without resulting angina pain. Use caution and avoid excessive exercise that could impair heart function in the absence of warning pain.

Discontinuation: Do not stop this drug abruptly. Consult your physician regarding gradual withdrawal. Observe for the possible development of rebound angina.

NITROGLYCERIN (ni troh GLIS er in)

Introduced: 1847   **Class:** Anti-anginal, nitrates   **Prescription:** USA: Yes   **Controlled Drug:** USA: No; Canada: No   **Available as Generic:** Yes

Brand Names: Deponit, Minitran Transdermal Delivery System, Nitro-Bid, Nitrocap TD, Nitrocine Transdermal, Nitrocine Timecaps, Nitrodisc, Nitro-Dur, Nitro-Dur II, Nitrogard, ✦Nitrogard-SR, Nitroglyn, Nitrol, ✦Nitrol TSAR Kit, Nitrolin, Nitrolingual Spray, Nitrong, ✦Nitrong SR, Nitrospan, ✦Nitrostabilin, Nitrostat, Nitro Transdermal System, NTS Transdermal Patch, Transderm-Nitro✦Tridil

BENEFITS versus RISKS	
Possible Benefits	*Possible Risks*
EFFECTIVE RELIEF AND PREVENTION OF ANGINA	Orthostatic hypotension with and without fainting
EFFECTIVE ADJUNCTIVE TREATMENT IN SELECTED CASES OF CONGESTIVE HEART FAILURE	Skin rash—rare Altered hemoglobin with large doses—very rare Low blood platelets—rare

▷ **Principal Uses**

As a Single Drug Product: Uses currently included in FDA-approved labeling: (1) Treatment of symptomatic coronary artery disease. The rapid-action forms are used to relieve acute attacks of anginal pain at their onset. The sustained-action forms are used to prevent the development of angina; (2) helps improve breathing difficulty caused by heart failure (left ventricle); (3) intravenous nitroglycerin is used in surgery to control blood pressure; (4) helps relieve congestive heart failure after heart attacks.

Other (unlabeled) generally accepted uses: (1) May help ease spasms of the Oddi's sphincter; (2) topical use may help in impotence; (3) can help reduce the extent of heart damage if given following a heart attack (myocardial infarction); (4) helps relax cocaine-constricted heart arteries; (5) eases the pain of peripheral neuropathy; (6) may be of help in easing esophageal problems (achalasia); (7) when the anal sphincter does not work correctly, this drug can help reduce the muscle pressure and ease constipation; (8) nitroglycerin in combination with vasopressin may be of use in stopping bleeding esophageal varices; (9) can help loss of vision that has been caused by a clot in the retinal artery; (10) if ergot medications (see Drug Classes) have shut down circulation to the extremities, nitroglycerin can open up the circulation; (11) used to delay contractions in order to rotate an abnormally positioned fetus; (12) may help diabetics with nerve damage (diabetic neuropathy).

How This Drug Works: By direct action on the muscles in blood vessel walls, this drug relaxes and dilates both arteries and veins. Its beneficial effects in angina are due to two mechanisms of action: (1) dilation of narrowed coronary arteries; (2) dilation of veins in the general circulation, with consequent reduction of the volume and pressure of blood entering the heart. The net effects are improved blood supply to the heart muscle and reduced workload for the heart. Both actions reduce the frequency and severity of angina.

Available Dosage Forms and Strengths

Canisters, translingual spray — 13.8 g (200 doses), 0.4 mg per metered dose

Capsules, prolonged action — 2.5 mg, 2.6 mg, 6.5 mg, 9 mg

Ointment — 2%

Tablets, buccal — 1 mg, 2 mg, 3 mg

Tablets, prolonged action — 2.6 mg, 6.5 mg, 9 mg

Tablets, sublingual — 0.15 mg, 0.3 mg, 0.4 mg, 0.6 mg

Transdermal systems — 2.5 mg, 5 mg, 7.5 mg, 10 mg, 15 mg (all per 24 hours)

▷ **Usual Adult Dosage Range:**   According to dosage form:

> Sublingual spray—One metered spray (0.4 mg) under tongue every 3 to 5 minutes, up to three doses within 15 minutes, to relieve acute angina. To prevent angina, one spray taken 5 to 10 minutes before exertion.
>
> Sublingual tablets—0.15 to 0.6 mg dissolved under tongue at 5-minute intervals to relieve acute angina.
>
> Prolonged-action tablets—2.5 mg at 6- to 8-hour intervals to prevent angina.
>
> Ointment—0.5 inch or 7.5 mg applied in a thin, even layer of uniform size to hairless skin at 3- to 4-hour intervals to prevent angina.
>
> Buccal tablets—1 to 2 mg every 4 to 5 hours placed between cheek and gum.
>
> Transdermal patches—5-square-cm to 30-square-cm patch applied to hairless skin once every 24 hours to prevent angina.
>
> **Note: Actual dosage and administration schedule must be determined for each patient individually.**
>
> **Author's Note: In order to avoid tolerance to the therapeutic effects of this medicine, a nitrate-free interval of 12 hours daily is recommended: 24-hour patches are removed after having been applied for 12 hours; dosing of ointment is interrupted for 12 hours a day; oral sustained-release formulations are dosed to give a 6- to 12-hour nitrate-free interval.**

Conditions Requiring Dosing Adjustments

> *Liver Function:* Specific dosage adjustments in liver compromise are not defined.
>
> *Kidney Function:* Specific guidelines for dosing changes are not available. This drug can discolor urine.

▷ **Dosing Instructions:**   Dosage forms to be swallowed are best taken when stomach is empty (1 hour before or 2 hours after eating) to obtain maximal blood levels. Tablets should not be crushed for administration. Capsules may be opened, but the contents should not be crushed or chewed before swallowing.

Usual Duration of Use: Use on a regular schedule for 3 to 5 days is often needed to determine effectiveness in preventing and relieving acute anginal attacks. Individual dosage adjustments will be necessary for optimal results. Long-term use (months to years) requires physician supervision.

▷ **This Drug Should Not Be Taken If**

- you have had an allergic reaction to it previously.
- you are severely anemic.
- you have had recent head trauma.
- you have had a heart attack and have an increased heart rate or increased blood pressure.
- you have hyperthyroidism.
- you have increased intraocular pressure.
- you have abnormal growth of the heart muscle in response to vascular disease (hypertrophic cardiomyopathy).
- you have closed-angle glaucoma (inadequately treated).

▷ **Inform Your Physician Before Taking This Drug If**

- you have had an unfavorable response to other nitrate drugs in the past.
- you have low blood pressure.
- you have problems absorbing medicines (malabsorption syndromes) or excessive action of your stomach (gastric hypermotility).

- you have any form of glaucoma.
- you have had recent bleeding in your head.

Possible Side Effects (natural, expected, and unavoidable drug actions)
Flushing of face, headaches (50%), orthostatic hypotension (see Glossary), rapid heart rate, palpitation.

▷ **Possible Adverse Effects** (unusual, unexpected, and infrequent reactions)
If any of the following develop, consult your physician promptly for guidance.

Mild Adverse Effects
Allergic Reactions: Skin rash.
Throbbing headaches (may be severe and persistent), dizziness, fainting—possible.
Nausea, vomiting, taste disorders—infrequent.

Serious Adverse Effects
Allergic Reactions: Severe skin reactions with peeling.
Idiosyncratic Reaction: Methemoglobinemia—case reports.
Abnormally slow heartbeat (bradycardia)—rare.
Low blood supply to the head (transient ischemic attacks)—case reports.
Increased intracranial pressure—rare.

▷ **Possible Effects on Sexual Function**
Correction of impotence (one report following sublingual use). Preventive use of nitroglycerin prior to sexual activity has been recommended to eliminate or reduce the risk of angina. Consult your physician for guidance.

▷ **Adverse Effects That May Mimic Natural Diseases or Disorders**
Hypotensive spells (sudden drops in blood pressure) due to this drug may be mistaken for late-onset epilepsy.

Possible Effects on Laboratory Tests
Blood platelet count: decreased—very rare.
Bleeding time: prolonged.

CAUTION
1. This drug can provoke migraine headaches in susceptible individuals.
2. Patients with impaired brain circulation (cerebral arteriosclerosis) have increased risk of transient ischemic attacks—periods of temporary speech impairment, paralysis, numbness, etc.
3. Tolerance to long-acting forms of nitrates will happen in most patients after 24 hours of continuous use. A nitrate-free interval of 10 hours usually restores effectiveness.
4. Many over-the-counter (OTC) drug products for allergies, colds, and coughs contain drugs that may counteract the desired effects of this drug. Ask your physician or pharmacist for help before using any such medications.

Precautions for Use
By Infants and Children: Limited usefulness and experience in this age group. Dosage schedules are not established.
By Those Over 60 Years of Age: Begin treatment with small doses and increase dose cautiously as needed and tolerated. You may be more susceptible to the development of flushing, throbbing headache, dizziness, "blackout" spells, fainting, and falling.

▷ **Advisability of Use During Pregnancy**
Pregnancy Category: C. See Pregnancy Risk Categories at the back of this book.
Animal studies: No information available.
Human studies: Adequate studies of pregnant women are not available.
Use this drug only if clearly needed. Ask your physician for guidance.

Advisability of Use If Breast-Feeding
Presence of this drug in breast milk: Unknown.
Watch nursing infant closely and discontinue drug or nursing if adverse effects develop.

Habit-Forming Potential: None.

Effects of Overdosage: Throbbing headache, dizziness, marked flushing, nausea, vomiting, abdominal cramps, confusion, delirium, paralysis, seizures, circulatory collapse.

Possible Effects of Long-Term Use: The development of tolerance (see Glossary) and the temporary loss of effectiveness.

Suggested Periodic Examinations While Taking This Drug (at physician's discretion)
Measurements of blood pressure and internal eye pressures.
Evaluation of hemoglobin.

▷ **While Taking This Drug, Observe the Following**
Foods: No restrictions.
Beverages: No restrictions. May be taken with milk.
▷ *Alcohol:* Avoid alcohol completely. This combination may result in severe lowering of blood pressure. There is a potential for collapse of the circulation and pumping effectiveness of the heart.
Tobacco Smoking: Nicotine can reduce the effectiveness of this drug. I advise everyone to quit smoking.
Marijuana Smoking: Possible reduced effectiveness of this drug; mild to moderate increase in angina; possible changes in the electrocardiogram, confusing interpretation.
▷ *Other Drugs*
Nitroglycerin *taken concurrently* with
• acetylcysteine (NAC) may reverse tolerance to the intravenous form of this medicine.
• antihypertensive drugs may cause excessive lowering of blood pressure. Careful dosage adjustments may be necessary.
• dihydroergotamine or similar ergot medicines (see Drug Classes) may result in ergotamine toxicity.
• diltiazem (Cardizem) can result in abnormally low blood pressure when used with the sustained-release form of nitroglycerin.
• heparin can result in decreased therapeutic benefit of heparin.
• isosorbide dinitrate (Isordil) or mononitrate (Ismo) may result in decreased nitroglycerin therapeutic benefits.
The following drugs may *increase* the effects of nitroglycerin
• aspirin in analgesic doses (500 mg or more), and perhaps other NSAIDs.
▷ *Driving, Hazardous Activities:* Usually no restrictions. This drug may cause dizziness or faintness. Restrict activities as necessary.
Aviation Note: Coronary artery disease *is a disqualification* for piloting. Consult a designated Aviation Medical Examiner.

Exposure to Sun: No restrictions.

Exposure to Heat: Hot environments can cause significant lowering of blood pressure.

Exposure to Cold: Cold environments can increase the need for this drug and limit its effectiveness.

Heavy Exercise or Exertion: This drug can increase your tolerance for exercise. Use good judgment regarding excessive exertion in the absence of anginal pain.

Discontinuation: Do not stop this drug abruptly after long-term use. It is advisable to reduce the dose (of the prolonged-action dosage forms) gradually over a period of to 6 weeks. Observe for rebound angina.

Special Storage Instructions: For sublingual tablets, to prevent loss of strength:
- keep tablets in the original glass container.
- do not transfer tablets to a plastic or metallic container (such as a pillbox).
- do not place absorbent cotton, paper (such as the prescription label), or other material inside the container.
- do not store other drugs in the same container.
- close the container tightly immediately after each use.
- store at room temperature.

NIZATIDINE (ni ZA te deen)

See the histamine (H_2) blocking drug profile for more information.

NORFLOXACIN (nor FLOX a sin)

See the new fluoroquinolone antibiotics profile for more information.

NORTRIPTYLINE (nor TRIP ti leen)

Introduced: 1963   **Class:** Antidepressant   **Prescription:** USA: Yes
Controlled Drug: USA: No; Canada: No   **Available as Generic:** USA: Yes; Canada: No

Brand Names: Aventyl, Pamelor

BENEFITS versus RISKS	
Possible Benefits	*Possible Risks*
EFFECTIVE RELIEF OF ENDOGENOUS DEPRESSION	ADVERSE BEHAVIORAL EFFECTS: confusion, disorientation, hallucinations, delusions
Possibly beneficial in other depressive disorders	CONVERSION OF DEPRESSION TO MANIA in manic-depressive (bipolar) disorders
Possibly beneficial in the management of some types of chronic, severe pain	Aggravation of schizophrenia
	Irregular heart rhythms
	Rare blood cell abnormalities

▷ **Principal Uses**

As a Single Drug Product

Uses currently included in FDA-approved labeling: Relieves symptoms associated with spontaneous (endogenous) depression. This drug should be used only when a diagnosis of a true, primary depression of significant degree has been established. It should not be used to treat the symptoms of mild and transient (reactive) depression that may be associated with many life situations in the absence of a bona fide affective illness.

Other (unlabeled) generally accepted uses: (1) Used in conjunction with other drugs to manage chronic, severe pain associated with such conditions as cancer, migraine headache, severe arthritis, peripheral neuropathy, AIDS, etc.; (2) helps decrease the frequency of bed-wetting; (3) may have a role in helping severe PMS; (4) can help attention deficit hyperactivity disorder (ADHD); (5) may have a role in helping ringing in the ears (tinnitus).

How This Drug Works: It is thought that this drug relieves depression by slowly restoring to normal levels certain constituents of brain tissue (norepinephrine and serotonin) that transmit nerve impulses.

Available Dosage Forms and Strengths

Capsules — 10 mg, 25 mg, 50 mg, 75 mg

Oral solution — 10 mg/5 ml (4% alcohol)

▷ **Usual Adult Dosage Range:**   Initially 25 mg three or four times daily. Dose may be increased cautiously as needed and tolerated by 10 to 25 mg daily at intervals of 1 week. Usual maintenance dose is 50 to 100 mg daily. Total dose should not exceed 150 mg daily. When the optimal requirement is determined, it may be taken at bedtime as one dose. **Note: Actual dosage and administration schedule must be determined for each patient individually.**

Conditions Requiring Dosing Adjustments

Liver Function: Specific dosage adjustments in liver compromise are not defined; however, the patient should be closely followed and levels obtained. This drug is also a rare cause of hepatoxicity, and should be used with caution by patients with compromised livers.

Kidney Function: Specific dosing changes in renal compromise are not usually needed. Nortriptyline can cause a decrease in urine outflow, and should be a benefit-to-risk decision for patients with urine outflow problems.

▷ **Dosing Instructions:**   The capsule may be opened and may be taken without regard to meals.

Usual Duration of Use: Some benefit may be apparent within 1 to 2 weeks, but adequate response may require continual use for 3 months or longer. Long-term use should not exceed 6 months without physician evaluation regarding the need for continuation of the drug.

Possible Advantages of This Drug

Causes less daytime sedation.

Causes fewer atropinelike side effects.

Causes orthostatic hypotension infrequently (see Glossary).

▷ **This Drug Should Not Be Taken If**

• you have had an allergic reaction to it previously.

• you are taking, or have taken within the past 14 days, any monoamine oxidase (MAO) type A inhibitor drug (see Drug Classes).

- you are recovering from a recent heart attack.
- you have narrow-angle glaucoma.

▷ **Inform Your Physician Before Taking This Drug If**
- you are allergic or sensitive to any other tricyclic antidepressant (see Drug Classes).
- you have a history of diabetes, epilepsy, glaucoma, heart disease, prostate gland enlargement, or overactive thyroid function.
- you plan to have surgery under general anesthesia in the near future.
- you have a history of bone marrow suppression.
- you have a history of low blood pressure.

Possible Side Effects (natural, expected, and unavoidable drug actions)
Light-headedness, drowsiness, blurred vision, dry mouth, constipation, impaired urination (see Prostatism in Glossary). Fluctuation of blood sugar levels.

▷ **Possible Adverse Effects** (unusual, unexpected, and infrequent reactions)
If any of the following develop, consult your physician promptly for guidance.
Mild Adverse Effects
Allergic Reactions: Skin rash, hives, swelling of face or tongue, drug fever (see Glossary).
Headache, dizziness, memory problems, weakness, fainting, unsteady gait, tremors, blurred vision, hearing toxicity—rare to infrequent.
Peculiar taste, weight gain, cavities (dental caries), irritation of mouth, nausea—infrequent.
Serious Adverse Effects
Allergic Reactions: Hepatitis, with or without jaundice (see Glossary).
Confusion, disorientation, hallucinations, delusions—case reports.
Aggravation of paranoid psychoses and schizophrenia; seizures—possible.
Heart palpitation and irregular rhythm—case reports.
Bone marrow depression (see Glossary): fatigue, weakness, fever, sore throat, abnormal bleeding or bruising—case reports.
Drug-induced porphyria or excessive urination, leading to sodium loss—case reports.
Peripheral neuritis (see Glossary)—numbness, tingling, pain, weak arms and legs—case reports.
Parkinson-like disorders (see Glossary)—usually mild and infrequent; more likely to occur in the elderly.

▷ **Possible Effects on Sexual Function:**   Decreased libido, increased libido (antidepressant effect), male impotence, inhibited female orgasm, male and female breast enlargement, milk production, swelling of testicles—case reports.

▷ **Adverse Effects That May Mimic Natural Diseases or Disorders**
Liver toxicity may suggest viral hepatitis.

Natural Diseases or Disorders That May Be Activated by This Drug
Latent diabetes, epilepsy, glaucoma, prostatism.

Possible Effects on Laboratory Tests
White blood cell and platelet counts: decreased.
Blood glucose levels: increased and decreased (fluctuations).

Liver function tests: increased liver enzymes (ALT/GPT, AST/GOT, and alkaline phosphatase), increased bilirubin.

CAUTION

1. Dose must be individualized. Report for follow-up evaluation and laboratory tests as directed by your physician.
2. It is advisable to withhold this drug if electroconvulsive therapy (ECT, "shock" treatment) is to be used to treat your depression.

Precautions for Use

By Infants and Children: The manufacturer's labeling says that safety and effectiveness for children have not been established.

By Those Over 60 Years of Age: Usual dosage is 30 to 50 mg daily in divided doses. During the first 2 weeks of treatment, watch for confusion, agitation, forgetfulness, delusions, disorientation, and hallucinations. Reduction of dosage or discontinuation may be necessary. Unsteadiness may predispose to falling and injury. This drug can increase the degree of impaired urination associated with prostate gland enlargement (prostatism).

▷ Advisability of Use During Pregnancy

Pregnancy Category: D. See Pregnancy Risk Categories at the back of this book.
Animal studies: Results are inconclusive.
Human studies: No defects reported in 21 exposures to amitriptyline, a closely related drug. Adequate studies of pregnant women are not available for this drug.
Avoid use of drug during first 3 months. Use during final 6 months only if clearly needed. Ask your physician for guidance.

Advisability of Use If Breast-Feeding

Presence of this drug in breast milk: Yes, in small amounts.
Monitor nursing infant closely and discontinue drug or nursing if adverse effects develop: excessive drowsiness and failure to feed.

Habit-Forming Potential: Psychological or physical dependence is rare and unexpected.

Effects of Overdosage: Confusion, hallucinations, marked drowsiness, heart palpitations, dilated pupils, tremors, stupor, deep sleep, coma, convulsions.

Suggested Periodic Examinations While Taking This Drug (at physician's discretion)
Complete blood cell counts, liver function tests, serial blood pressure readings, and electrocardiograms.

▷ While Taking This Drug, Observe the Following

Foods: No restrictions. This drug may increase the appetite and cause excessive weight gain.
Beverages: No restrictions. May be taken with milk.
▷ *Alcohol:* Avoid completely. This drug can markedly increase the intoxicating effects of alcohol and accentuate its depressant action on brain function.
Tobacco Smoking: May hasten elimination of drug. Higher doses may be necessary. I advise everyone to quit smoking.
▷ *Other Drugs*
Nortriptyline may ***increase*** the effects of
- atropinelike drugs (see Drug Classes).
- dicumarol, and increase the risk of bleeding.

- epinephrine (Adrenalin).
- phenytoin (Dilantin) by increasing blood levels.
- warfarin (Coumadin) and require more frequent INR (prothrombin time or protime) testing and dosing adjustments based on laboratory results.

Nortriptyline may *decrease* the effects of
- clonidine (Catapres).
- ephedrine (Primatene tablets).
- guanethidine (Ismelin).

Nortriptyline *taken concurrently* with
- activated charcoal will decrease and almost block absorption (useful in overdose situations).
- benzodiazepines (see Drug Classes) may result in additive sedation.
- disulfiram (Antabuse) may cause acute dementia: confusion, disorientation, hallucinations.
- fluconazole (Diflucan) may result in large increases in nortriptyline levels and result in toxic reactions.
- lithium (Lithobid) may pose an increased risk of neurotoxicity in elderly patients.
- monoamine oxidase (MAO) inhibitor drugs may cause high fever, delirium, and convulsions (see Drug Classes).
- nifedipine (Adalat, others) may result in inhibition of nortriptyline's antidepressant effects.
- norepinephrine can cause a serious increase in blood pressure, abnormal heart rhythms, and fast heart rate. Avoid this combination.
- phenothiazines (see Drug Classes) can result in increased phenothiazine levels and toxicity as well as additive anticholinergic problems.
- thyroid preparations may impair heart rhythm and function. Ask your physician for guidance regarding adjustment of thyroid dose.
- venlafaxine (Effexor) may result in nortriptyline or venlafaxine toxicity.

The following drugs may *increase* the effects of nortriptyline
- cimetidine (Tagamet), and cause nortriptyline toxicity.
- fluoxetine (Prozac).
- quinidine (Quinaglute, etc.), and cause nortriptyline toxicity.
- sertraline (Zoloft).

The following drugs may *decrease* the effects of nortriptyline
- ascorbic acid (vitamin C) in high doses.
- barbiturates (see Drug Classes), and reduce its effectiveness.
- carbamazepine (Tegretol).
- conjugated estrogens.
- rifampin (Rifadin).

▷ *Driving, Hazardous Activities:* This drug may impair mental alertness, judgment, physical coordination, and reaction time. Avoid hazardous activities.

Aviation Note: The use of this drug *is a disqualification* for piloting. Consult a designated Aviation Medical Examiner.

Exposure to Sun: Use caution—this drug may cause photosensitivity (see Glossary).

Exposure to Heat: This drug can inhibit sweating and impair the body's adaptation to hot environments, increasing the risk of heatstroke. Avoid saunas.

Exposure to Cold: The elderly should use caution and avoid conditions conducive to hypothermia (see Glossary).

Discontinuation: It is best to slowly discontinue this drug. Abrupt withdrawal after long-term use can cause headache, malaise, and nausea.

OFLOXACIN (oh FLOX a sin)

See the new fluoroquinolone antibiotics profile for more information.

OLANZAPINE (oh LAN za pean)

Introduced: 1996   **Class:** Antipsychotic; tranquilizer, major; thienobenzodiazepine   **Prescription:** USA: Yes   **Controlled Drug:** USA: No; Canada: No   **Available as Generic:** USA: No; Canada: No
Brand Name: Zyprexa

BENEFITS versus RISKS	
Possible Benefits	*Possible Risks*
EFFECTIVE SHORT-TERM CONTROL OF ACUTE MENTAL DISORDERS: beneficial effects on thinking, mood, and behavior Relief of anxiety, agitation, and tension	POSSIBLE TARDIVE DYSKINESIA (SERIOUS TOXIC BRAIN EFFECT with long-term use) RARE NEUROLEPTIC MALIGNANT SYNDROME Orthostatic hypotension (see Glossary) Increased liver enzymes

▷ **Principal Uses**

As a Single Drug Product: Uses currently included in FDA-approved labeling: Helps manage thinking problems and other difficulties seen in psychosis. Other (unlabeled) generally accepted uses: None at present.

Author's Note: A recent study presented at the American Psychiatric Association found olanzapine to be more effective than risperidone.

How This Drug Works: This medicine inhibits the action of two primary nerve transmitters (dopamine and serotonin) in certain brain centers, and acts to correct an imbalance of nerve impulse transmissions thought to be responsible for certain mental disorders. It also works at histamine, muscarinic, GABA, BZD, and adrenergic sites.

Available Dosage Forms and Strengths

Tablets — 5 mg

▷ **Recommended Dosage Ranges** (Actual dosage and administration schedule must be determined for each patient individually.)

Infants and Children: Dosage not established.

18 to 60 Years of Age: Dosing is started with 5 to 10 mg daily. If the 5-mg dose is used, the dose may be increased to a maximum of 10 mg as needed and tolerated.

Author's Note: Since *gender* data is now FDA required for new approvals, it must be noted that the drug is removed (cleared) 30% slower in women than in men. Therefore effects (both desirable and undesir-

able) caused by the medicine may last longer in women (dose to dose)
than in men.

Over 60 Years of Age: 5 mg of olanzapine is taken.

Conditions Requiring Dosing Adjustments

Liver Function: The drug is highly metabolized in the liver, and although the manufacturer does not have recommendations for dosing changes, smaller doses and close patient monitoring appear prudent.

Kidney Function: Only a small amount is removed by the kidneys, and dosing changes are not thought to be needed.

Seizure Disorders: Seizures happened in 0.9% of patients during clinical trials of olanzapine. Olanzapine should be used with caution by seizure patients. Dose decreases are not defined at present.

▷ **Dosing Instructions:**   The tablet may be crushed and taken with food. It is best to take this medicine at the same time every day.

Usual Duration of Use: Use on a regular schedule for at least 1 week is required to reach steady-state levels, and hence determines effectiveness. Clinical trials that led to FDA approval were conducted for 6 weeks. Use beyond 6 weeks requires physician supervision and was not studied in clinical trials.

Possible Advantages of This Drug

Effective reversal of symptoms of psychosis while acting at different sites than previously available agents.

▷ **This Drug Should Not Be Taken If**
- you have had an allergic reaction to it previously.
- you have had neuroleptic malignant syndrome.

▷ **Inform Your Physician Before Taking This Drug If**
- you have a seizure disorder.
- your liver is compromised.
- you have constitutionally low blood pressure or are taking medicine to treat high blood pressure.
- you have severe liver disease.
- you have a history of breast cancer.
- you are taking any drug with sedative effects.
- you tend to be constipated.
- you plan to have surgery under general or spinal anesthesia in the near future.
- you have problems swallowing.

Possible Side Effects (natural, expected, and unavoidable drug actions)

Orthostatic hypotension (see Glossary), drowsiness.

▷ **Possible Adverse Effects** (unusual, unexpected, and infrequent reactions)

If any of the following develop, consult your physician promptly for guidance.

Mild Adverse Effects

Allergic Reactions: Skin rash, itching—rare.

Drowsiness, agitation, insomnia, and dizziness—frequent.

Headache, drowsiness—rare; depression—rare; dizziness—rare to infrequent.

Fast heart rate (tachycardia)—infrequent.

Weight gain, constipation, or cough—infrequent.

Serious Adverse Effects
Allergic Reactions: Hair loss—rare.
Abnormal movements (appears to be dose related)—infrequent.
Drug-induced increased liver enzymes—rare.
Difficulty swallowing (dysphagia)—case reports.
Tardive dyskinesia has been reported with other agents.
Neuroleptic malignant syndrome has been reported with other agents.

▷ **Possible Effects on Sexual Function:** Impotence, abnormal ejaculation, or menstrual changes—infrequent.

▷ **Adverse Effects That May Mimic Natural Diseases or Disorders**
Nervous system reactions may suggest true Parkinson's disease.
Liver reactions may suggest viral hepatitis.

Possible Effects on Laboratory Tests
Prolactin levels: increased.
Liver function tests: increased liver enzymes (ALT/GPT, AST/GOT, and alkaline phosphatase).

CAUTION
1. Other medicines (nonprescription or prescription) that can cause drowsiness or central nervous system effects may react unfavorably with this medicine. Talk with your doctor or pharmacist before combining any medicines.
2. Since this medicine can cause orthostatic hypotension, some high blood pressure (antihypertensive) medicines may have a greater than expected effect if taken with olanzapine.

Precautions for Use
By Infants and Children: Safety and effectiveness for those under 18 years of age are not established.
By Those Over 60 Years of Age: Lower starting doses should be taken; caution is advised regarding drowsiness, dizziness, and orthostatic hypotension, since olanzapine can cause changes in the ability of the body to regulate changes in temperature, and this regulation may be less intact in older patients to begin with. You may also be more susceptible to Parkinson-like reactions and/or tardive dyskinesia (see Glossary). Discuss early indications of these reactions with your doctor, as progression of these reactions may lead to symptoms that are not reversible.

▷ **Advisability of Use During Pregnancy**
Pregnancy Category: C. See Pregnancy Risk Categories at the back of this book.
Animal studies: Rat and mouse studies reveal increased mammary gland adenomas (when the animals were given 0.5 and 2 times the mg-per-square-meter human dose) respectively. Increased numbers of nonviable fetuses were seen in one rat study using nine times the maximum human dose.
Human studies: Adequate studies of pregnant women are not available.
Use of this drug is a benefit-to-risk decision. Ask your doctor for guidance.

Advisability of Use If Breast-Feeding
Presence of this drug in breast milk: Yes in rats; unknown in humans.
Avoid drug or refrain from nursing.

Habit-Forming Potential: None.

Effects of Overdosage: Reports of 67 overdoses were made during clinical trials. The patient who took the largest dose had drowsiness and slurred speech.

Possible Effects of Long-Term Use: None defined as yet.

Suggested Periodic Examinations While Taking This Drug (at physician's discretion)

Liver function tests. Careful inspection of the tongue for early evidence of fine, involuntary, wavelike movements that could be the beginning of tardive dyskinesia. Sitting and standing blood pressure checks may be advisable when therapy is started to assess orthostatic hypotension.

▷ **While Taking This Drug, Observe the Following**
Foods: No restrictions. Follow prescribed diet.
Beverages: No restrictions. May be taken with milk.
▷ *Alcohol:* Avoid completely.
Tobacco Smoking: Olanzapine is removed from the body up to 40% faster in people who smoke compared to those who do not. Recommendations for dosing changes are not available. I advise everyone to quit smoking.
Marijuana Smoking: Expected to cause an increase in drowsiness; accentuation of orthostatic hypotension; increased risk of precipitating latent psychoses, confusing the interpretation of mental status and drug responses.
▷ *Other Drugs:* Olsalazine **taken concurrently** with
- any sedative drugs (prescription and nonprescription) can cause excessive sedation.
- any medicine that has central nervous system activity may result in additive effects.
- any medicine that can cause liver damage may result in additive liver problems.
- activated charcoal will decrease absorption of olanzapine. (May be of use in overdoses.)
- benzodiazepines (see Drug Classes) may magnify the orthostatic hypotension problem caused by olanzapine.
- carbamazepine (Tegretol) causes up to a 50% increase in removal of olanzapine from the body. Dosing increases in olanzapine appear prudent.
▷ *Driving, Hazardous Activities:* This drug may cause drowsiness or dizziness. Restrict activities as necessary.
Aviation Note: The use of this drug **may be a disqualification** for piloting. Consult a designated Aviation Medical Examiner.
Exposure to Sun: No problems reported.
Exposure to Heat: This medicine can cause problems in regulating body temperature (core temperature homeostasis). If you work or are frequently in a hot environment, be careful to replace enough fluids to avoid dehydration.
Heavy Exercise or Exertion: Since this medicine may cause problems in temperature regulation, caution is advised.
Discontinuation: Do not stop this medicine without first talking to your doctor.

OLSALAZINE (ohl SAL a zeen)

Introduced: 1987   **Class:** Bowel anti-inflammatory   **Prescription:**
USA: Yes   **Controlled Drug:** USA: No; Canada: No   **Available as Generic:**
USA: No; Canada: No

Brand Name: Dipentum

BENEFITS versus RISKS	
Possible Benefits	*Possible Risks*
EFFECTIVE SUPPRESSION OF INFLAMMATORY BOWEL DISEASE	RARE BONE MARROW DEPRESSION (see Glossary) Drug-induced hepatitis Occasional aggravation of ulcerative colitis

▷ **Principal Uses**

As a Single Drug Product: Uses currently included in FDA-approved labeling: Used to maintain remission of chronic ulcerative colitis and proctitis.

Other (unlabeled) generally accepted uses: Has a role in treatment of active ulcerative colitis.

How This Drug Works: This drug suppresses the formation of prostaglandins (and related compounds), tissue substances that induce inflammation, tissue destruction, and diarrhea—the main features of ulcerative colitis and proctitis.

Available Dosage Forms and Strengths

Capsules — 250 mg
Tablets (in Canada only) — 500 mg

▷ **Recommended Dosage Ranges** (Actual dosage and administration schedule must be determined for each patient individually.)

Infants and Children: Dosage not established.

12 to 60 Years of Age: 500 mg twice daily, morning and evening.

Over 60 Years of Age: Same as 12 to 60 years of age.

Conditions Requiring Dosing Adjustments

Liver Function: Dosage adjustments do not appear to be needed in liver compromise. This drug rarely causes liver toxicity (granulomatous hepatitis), and should be used with caution by patients with liver problems.

Kidney Function: Some of the metabolites of olsalazine are eliminated by the kidneys. There is potential for kidney damage by one of these compounds, and the drug should be a benefit-to-risk decision by patients with compromised kidneys.

▷ **Dosing Instructions:** The capsule may be opened and taken with food, preferably with breakfast and dinner.

Usual Duration of Use: Use on a regular schedule for 1 to 3 weeks determines effectiveness in controlling the symptoms of ulcerative colitis. Long-term use (months to years) requires physician supervision.

Possible Advantages of This Drug

Does not inhibit sperm production or cause infertility.

▷ **This Drug Should Not Be Taken If**
- you have had an allergic reaction to it previously.
- you have severely impaired kidney function.
- you are allergic to aspirin.

▷ **Inform Your Physician Before Taking This Drug If**
- you are allergic to aspirin (or other salicylates), mesalamine, or sulfasalazine.
- you are allergic by nature: history of hay fever, asthma, hives, eczema.
- you have impaired kidney function.
- you have severe liver disease.
- you are currently taking sulfasalazine (Azulfidine).

Possible Side Effects (natural, expected, and unavoidable drug actions)
None.

▷ **Possible Adverse Effects** (unusual, unexpected, and infrequent reactions)
If any of the following develop, consult your physician promptly for guidance.

Mild Adverse Effects
Allergic Reactions: Skin rash, itching—rare.
Headache, drowsiness, depression, dizziness—rare.
Loss of appetite, indigestion, nausea, vomiting, stomach pain, diarrhea—rare to infrequent.
Paresthesias or blurred vision—rare.
Joint aches and pains—infrequent.

Serious Adverse Effects
Allergic Reactions: Dermatitis, hair loss—rare.
Bone marrow depression (see Glossary): fatigue, fever, sore throat, abnormal bleeding/bruising—case reports.
Drug-induced hepatitis (see Glossary), pericarditis, pancreatitis, or kidney damage—rare.
Spasm of the bronchi of the lung—rare.

▷ **Possible Effects on Sexual Function:**   Impotence, excessive menstrual flow—case reports.

Possible Effects on Laboratory Tests
Complete blood cell counts: decreased red cells, hemoglobin, white cells, and platelets; increased eosinophils.
Liver function tests: increased liver enzymes (ALT/GPT, AST/GOT, and alkaline phosphatase), increased bilirubin.
Urinalysis: red blood cells and protein present.

CAUTION
1. Report promptly any signs of infection or unusual bleeding or bruising.
2. Report promptly any indications of active or intensified ulcerative colitis: abdominal cramping, bloody diarrhea, fever.

Precautions for Use
By Infants and Children: Safety and effectiveness for those under 12 years of age are not established.
By Those Over 60 Years of Age: None.

▷ **Advisability of Use During Pregnancy**
  Pregnancy Category: C. See Pregnancy Risk Categories at the back of this book.
    Animal studies: Rat studies reveal toxic effects on the fetus, retarded bone
      development, and impaired development of internal organs.
    Human studies: Adequate studies of pregnant women are not available.
    Use this drug only if clearly needed. Ask your physician for guidance.

Advisability of Use If Breast-Feeding
  Presence of this drug in breast milk: Controversial, has caused diarrhea in
    some infants.
  Avoid drug or refrain from nursing.

Habit-Forming Potential: None.

Effects of Overdosage: Headache, dizziness, nausea, vomiting, abdominal
  cramping.

Possible Effects of Long-Term Use: Bone marrow depression (impaired production of blood cells).

Suggested Periodic Examinations While Taking This Drug (at physician's dis-
    cretion)
  Complete blood cell counts.
  Liver function tests.
  Kidney function tests, urinalysis.

▷ **While Taking This Drug, Observe the Following**
  Foods: No restrictions. Follow prescribed diet.
  Beverages: No restrictions. May be taken with milk.
▷ *Alcohol:* No interactions expected.
  Tobacco Smoking: No interactions expected, but I advise everyone to quit smok-
    ing.
▷ *Other Drugs:* Olsalazine **taken concurrently** with
      • varicella vaccine (Varivax) may result in an increased risk of Reye syn-
        drome. This drug should be avoided for 6 weeks after the vaccine is given.
▷ *Driving, Hazardous Activities:* This drug may cause drowsiness or dizziness. Re-
    strict activities as necessary.
  Aviation Note: The use of this drug **may be a disqualification** for piloting. Con-
    sult a designated Aviation Medical Examiner.
  Exposure to Sun: Use caution—this drug can cause photosensitization (see
    Glossary).

OMEPRAZOLE (oh MEH pra zohl)

Introduced: 1986   **Class:** Proton pump inhibitor   **Prescription:** USA:
Yes   **Controlled Drug:** USA: No; Canada: No   **Available as Generic:**
USA: No; Canada: No

Brand Names: Prilosec✦Losec

BENEFITS versus RISKS

Possible Benefits	*Possible Risks*
VERY EFFECTIVE TREATMENT OF CONDITIONS ASSOCIATED WITH EXCESSIVE PRODUCTION OF GASTRIC ACID: Zollinger-Ellison syndrome, mastocytosis, endocrine adenoma	Rare aplastic anemia Rare liver failure
VERY EFFECTIVE TREATMENT OF REFLUX ESOPHAGITIS, GASTRIC AND DUODENAL ULCERS	
EFFECTIVE IN COMBINATION WITH CLARITHROMYCIN in treatment of *Helicobacter pylori* infections	

▷ **Principal Uses**

As a Single Drug Product: Uses currently included in FDA-approved labeling: (1) Inhibits stomach acid formation in: acute and chronic gastritis, reflux esophagitis, gastroesophageal reflux disease, Zollinger-Ellison syndrome, mastocytosis, endocrine adenomas, and active duodenal ulcer; (2) approved for long-term use in erosive esophagitis; (3) approved for combination (with clarithromycin—Biaxin) in patients with positive *Helicobacter pylori* cultures; (4) helps in the short-term treatment of active and benign stomach (gastric) ulcers.

Other (unlabeled) generally accepted uses: (1) Used to help gastric ulcers; (2) may have a role in treating severe bleeding of the stomach (hemorrhagic gastritis).

How This Drug Works: Inhibits a specific enzyme system (proton pump H/K ATPase) in the stomach lining, stopping production of stomach acid and thereby (1) eliminates a principal cause of the condition under treatment, and (2) creates an environment conducive to healing.

Available Dosage Forms and Strengths

Capsules, delayed release — 20 mg

▷ **Usual Adult Dosage Range:** Reflux esophagitis: 20 mg once daily for 4 to 8 weeks.

Excessive stomach acid conditions: 60 mg once daily for as long as necessary.

Gastric and duodenal ulcer: 20 mg once daily for 4 to 8 weeks.

In extreme conditions, doses of 120 mg three times a day have been used.- **Note: Actual dosage and administration schedule must be determined for each patient individually.**

Conditions Requiring Dosing Adjustments

Liver Function: Dosing adjustments are not defined, however, patients should be monitored closely.

Kidney Function: Dosage adjustments do not appear to be needed.

▷ **Dosing Instructions:** Take immediately before eating, preferably the morning meal. The capsule should be swallowed whole without opening; the contents should not be crushed or chewed. This drug may be taken concurrently with antacids if they are needed to relieve stomach pain.

Usual Duration of Use: Use on a regular schedule for 2 to 3 weeks determines benefit in suppressing stomach acid production. Long-term use (months to years) requires periodic physician evaluation of response.

Possible Advantages of This Drug
Effectively inhibits acid secretion at all times: basal conditions (stomach empty and at rest) and following food, alcohol, smoking, or other stimulants. More effective than histamine (H_2) receptor blocking drugs in treating severe reflux esophagitis and refractory duodenal ulcer.

Currently a "Drug of Choice"
for the short-term treatment of severe reflux esophagitis and the long-term treatment of Zollinger-Ellison syndrome and erosive esophagitis.

▷ **This Drug Should Not Be Taken If**
  • you have had an allergic reaction to it previously.
  • you have a currently active bone marrow or blood cell disorder.

▷ **Inform Your Physician Before Taking This Drug If**
  • you have a history of liver disease or impaired liver function.
  • your history includes any bone marrow or blood cell disorder, especially a drug-induced one.
  • you take any anticoagulant medication, or diazepam (Valium) or phenytoin (Dilantin, etc.).

Possible Side Effects (natural, expected, and unavoidable drug actions)
Acid in the stomach actually works to protect it from some bacterial infections. Since omeprazole is so effective in decreasing acid, it may increase the likelihood of infection by *Campylobacter*. This organism causes gastroenteritis. Symptoms may include mucousy, loose stools and fever. Talk with your doctor if you start to develop these symptoms while taking omeprazole.

▷ **Possible Adverse Effects** (unusual, unexpected, and infrequent reactions)
  If any of the following develop, consult your physician promptly for guidance.
  Mild Adverse Effects
  Allergic Reactions: Skin rash—rare; itching.
  Headache, dizziness, muscle pain, or ringing in ears; drowsiness, paresthesias, weakness—rare to infrequent.
  Indigestion, nausea, vomiting, diarrhea, constipation—rare to infrequent.
  Serious Adverse Effects
  Allergic Reactions: Rare allergic kidney damage (interstitial nephritis).
  Bone marrow depression: fatigue, fever, sore throat, infections, abnormal bleeding/bruising—case reports.
  Liver damage with jaundice (see Glossary)—case reports.
  Chest pain or angina—case reports.
  Half-facial pain—case reports.
  Yeast infection (*Candida*) of the esophagus—possible.
  Kidney inflammation (interstitial nephritis)—case reports.

Possible Effects on Sexual Function
Drug-induced male breast enlargement and tenderness (gynecomastia) has been rarely reported.

▷ **Adverse Effects That May Mimic Natural Diseases or Disorders**

Persistent infection or bruising may be bone marrow depression; blood counts are advisable.

Liver reactions may suggest viral hepatitis.

Possible Effects on Laboratory Tests

Complete blood cell counts: decreased red cells, hemoglobin, white cells, and platelets.

Blood glucose level: decreased.

Liver function tests: increased liver enzymes (ALT/GPT, AST/GOT, and alkaline phosphatase), increased bilirubin.

CAUTION

1. Take this drug for exactly as long as your doctor prescribed. Do not extend its use without your physician's guidance.
2. Report promptly any indications of infection.
3. Tell your doctor if you plan to take any other medications (prescription or over-the-counter) while taking omeprazole.
4. Acid in the stomach actually works to protect it from some bacterial infections. Since omeprazole is so effective in decreasing acid, it may increase the likelihood of infection by *Campylobacter*. This organism causes gastroenteritis. Symptoms may include mucousy, loose stools and fever. Talk with your doctor if you start to develop these symptoms while taking omeprazole.
5. Although this drug effectively treats ulcers, it does not preclude the possibility of cancer of the stomach.

Precautions for Use

By Infants and Children: Safety and effectiveness for those under 12 years of age are not established.

By Those Over 60 Years of Age: Slower elimination of this drug makes it possible to achieve satisfactory response with smaller doses; this reduces the risk of adverse effects. Limit the daily dose to 20 mg if possible.

▷ **Advisability of Use During Pregnancy**

Pregnancy Category: C. See Pregnancy Risk Categories at the back of this book.

Animal studies: No drug-induced birth defects found in rats; drug-induced embryo and fetal toxicity were demonstrated in rats and rabbits.

Human studies: Adequate studies of pregnant women are not available.

Avoid use if possible. Use only if clearly necessary and for the shortest possible time.

Advisability of Use If Breast-Feeding

Presence of this drug in breast milk: Unknown.

Avoid drug or refrain from nursing.

Habit-Forming Potential: None.

Effects of Overdosage: Possible drowsiness, dizziness, lethargy, abdominal pain, nausea.

Possible Effects of Long-Term Use: Some long-term (2-year) studies in rats revealed the development of drug-induced carcinoid tumors in the stomach. To date, long-term use of this drug (more than 5 years) in humans has not revealed any drug-induced tumor potential. Pending more studies of long-term human use, it is advisable to limit the use of this drug to the shortest duration possible.

Suggested Periodic Examinations While Taking This Drug (at physician's discretion)
Complete blood cell counts.

▷ **While Taking This Drug, Observe the Following**
Foods: No restrictions.
Beverages: No restrictions. May be taken with milk.
▷ *Alcohol:* No interactions expected. However, alcohol is best avoided; it stimulates the secretion of stomach acid.
Tobacco Smoking: Smoking may stimulate the secretion of stomach acid. I advise everyone to quit smoking.
▷ *Other Drugs*
Omeprazole may ***increase*** the effects of
- anticoagulants (warfarin, etc.) and increase the risk of bleeding.
- clonazepam (Klonopin) and some other benzodiazepines (see Drug Classes), and lead to benzodiazepine toxicity.
- cyclosporine (Sandimmune) by increasing its level (decreased levels also reported).
- diazepam (Valium) and cause excessive sedation.
- digoxin (Lanoxin) and lead to toxicity.
- phenytoin (Dilantin, etc.) and cause phenytoin toxicity.
- warfarin (Coumadin) and lead to bleeding. More frequent INR (prothrombin time or protime) testing is needed. Warfarin doses should be adjusted according to laboratory results.
Omeprazole may ***decrease*** the effects of
- amoxicillin (various).
- ampicillin (various).
- iron preparations.
- ketoconazole (Nizoral).
▷ *Driving, Hazardous Activities:* This drug may cause drowsiness and dizziness. Limit activities as necessary.
Aviation Note: The use of this drug ***may be a disqualification*** for piloting. Consult a designated Aviation Medical Examiner.
Exposure to Sun: No restrictions.
Discontinuation: The duration of use will vary according to the condition under treatment and individual patient response. Premature discontinuation could result in incomplete healing or prompt recurrence of symptoms.

ONDANSETRON (on DAN sa tron)

Introduced: 1993   **Class:** Antiemetic, 5-HT$_3$ antagonist   **Prescription:** USA: Yes   **Controlled Drug:** USA: No; Canada: No   **Available as Generic:** USA: No; Canada: No

Brand Name: Zofran

```
┌─────────────────────────────────────────────────────────────────┐
│                   BENEFITS versus RISKS                           │
│    Possible Benefits              Possible Risks                  │
│  EFFECTIVE ORAL TREATMENT     Bronchospasm                        │
│    AND RELIEF OR PREVENTION   Grand mal seizures                  │
│    OF SEVERE VOMITING         Liver toxicity                      │
│                               Heart rate and rhythm changes       │
│                               Low potassium                       │
│                               (All rare)                          │
└─────────────────────────────────────────────────────────────────┘
```

▷ **Principal Uses**

As a Single Drug Product: Uses currently included in FDA-approved labeling: (1) Prevention of nausea and vomiting associated with initial and repeat courses of chemotherapy; (2) treatment or prevention of postoperative nausea and vomiting; (3) prevention or treatment of emesis (vomiting) caused by radiation therapy.

Other (unlabeled) generally accepted uses: (1) Helps patients keep from vomiting medicines used to treat drug overdoses; (2) may have a role in treating schizophrenia; (3) some panic attack data.

How This Drug Works: Ondansetron antagonizes 5-HT$_3$ receptors. It appears to block vomiting by blocking serotonin (a chemical causing vomiting) at 5-HT$_3$ receptors.

Available Dosage Forms and Strengths

Intravenous — 2 mg/ml

Oral solution — 4 mg/5 ml

Tablets — 4 mg, 8 mg

How To Store

Keep at room temperature. Avoid exposing this medicine to extreme humidity.

▷ **Recommended Dosage Ranges** (Actual dosage and administration schedule must be determined for each patient individually.)

Infants and Children: Little information is available regarding use in those less than 4 years old.

4 to 11 Years of Age: Vomiting from chemotherapy: one (4-mg) tablet given three times by mouth daily. The method and frequency is the same as for adults.

12 to 60 Years of Age: One 8-mg tablet taken three times a day. The first dose should be taken 30 minutes before the start of the emetogenic chemotherapy. Subsequent doses should be taken 8 hours after the first dose. Further doses of 8 mg every 12 hours are taken for 1–2 days after chemotherapy is finished.

Over 60 Years of Age: Same as 12 to 60 years of age.

Conditions Requiring Dosing Adjustments

Liver Function: Maximum dose for people with severe liver failure is 8 mg per day.

Kidney Function: Studies have not been conducted on patients with impaired kidneys. The decision to use ondansetron must be made by your physician. Only 5 to 10% of the drug is removed unchanged by the kidneys. Based on this small involvement of the kidneys, no changes are expected to be needed with short-term use.

▷ **Dosing Instructions:** May be taken on an empty stomach.

Usual Duration of Use: Since chemotherapy can cause vomiting long after it has been given, continual use on a regular schedule for 3 days is usually necessary.

Possible Advantages of This Drug
Effective oral prevention of severe vomiting caused by some kinds of chemotherapy that have been poorly controlled by earlier agents.

Currently a "Drug of Choice"
for control of vomiting secondary to emetogenic (likely to cause vomiting) cancer chemotherapy.

▷ **This Drug Should Not Be Taken If**
- you have had an allergic reaction to any dosage form of it previously.

▷ **Inform Your Physician Before Taking This Drug If**
- you have a history of liver disease.
- you have a history of kidney disease.
- you have a history of alcoholism.
- you are unsure of how much to take or how often to take ondansetron.

Possible Side Effects (natural, expected, and unavoidable drug actions)
Constipation, sedation.

▷ **Possible Adverse Effects** (unusual, unexpected, and infrequent reactions)
If any of the following develop, consult your physician promptly for guidance.
Mild Adverse Effects
Allergic Reactions: Skin rash—rare.
Headache—frequent; dizziness and light-headedness, constipation, diarrhea, dry mouth—infrequent.
Serious Adverse Effects
Allergic Reactions: Anaphylaxis—rare.
Extrapyramidal reactions (abnormal body movements) or seizures—case reports.
Bronchospasm—rare.
Angina, tachycardia, arrhythmias—all rare.
Hypokalemia (low potassium)—rare.

▷ **Possible Effects on Sexual Function:** None reported.

Possible Delayed Adverse Effects: None reported.

▷ **Adverse Effects That May Mimic Natural Diseases or Disorders**
Changes in liver enzymes may mimic hepatitis; however, specific antibodies will not be present. Bronchospasm may mimic asthma.

Natural Diseases or Disorders That May Be Activated by This Drug
Epilepsy, asthma.

Possible Effects on Laboratory Tests
Liver function tests: Transient increases in SGPT, SGOT, and bilirubin.

CAUTION
1. Even though you do not feel an urge to vomit, continue ondansetron for the prescribed length of therapy. The vomit-causing effect of cancer chemotherapy or radiation therapy continues after the medicine or radiation has been given.

Precautions for Use

By Infants and Children: Safety and effectiveness for those under 3 years of age are not established.

By Those Over 60 Years of Age: Same as for general adult population.

▷ **Advisability of Use During Pregnancy**

Pregnancy Category: B. See Pregnancy Risk Categories at the back of this book.

Animal studies: Drug and its metabolites pass into the milk. No adverse effects on gestation, postnatal development, or reproductive performance has been observed in rats.

Human studies: Adequate studies of pregnant women are not available.

Ask your physician for guidance.

Advisability of Use If Breast-Feeding

Presence of this drug in breast milk: This medicine is excreted in the milk of rats; however, human data is not available. Caution should be used if this medicine is to be used by nursing mothers.

Habit-Forming Potential: None.

Effects of Overdosage: Doses 10 times greater than recommended have not resulted in illness.

Possible Effects of Long-Term Use: Not indicated for long-term use.

Suggested Periodic Examinations While Taking This Drug (at physician's discretion)

Observe for vomiting occurrence and frequency.

▷ **While Taking This Drug, Observe the Following**

Foods: No restrictions.

Beverages: No restrictions.

▷ *Alcohol:* Additive sedation and potential additive urge to vomit if alcohol is taken in large doses. Alcohol abuse that has led to liver problems may limit the total dose which can be taken.

Tobacco Smoking: No direct clinical interactions; I advise everyone to quit smoking.

Marijuana Smoking: May induce additive sedation and provide additive antiemetic effects.

▷ *Other Drugs*

The following drugs may *increase* the effects of ondansetron

- allopurinol (Zyloprim).
- cimetidine (Tagamet).
- disulfiram (Antabuse).
- fluconazole (Diflucan).
- isoniazid (Nydrazid).
- macrolide antibiotics (erythromycin, azithromycin, clarithromycin, dirithromycin).
- metronidazole (Flagyl).
- monoamine oxidase inhibitor antidepressants (MAO inhibitors—Nardil).
- ritonavir (Norvir) and perhaps other protease inhibitors (see Drug Classes).

The following drugs may *decrease* the effects of ondansetron

- barbiturates.
- carbamazepine (Tegretol).
- phenylbutazone (Butazolidin, Azolid).

- phenytoin (Dilantin).
- rifampin (Rifadin) and rifabutin (Mycobutin).
- tolbutamide (Orinase).

▷ *Driving, Hazardous Activities:* This drug may cause drowsiness and dizziness. Restrict activities as necessary.

Aviation Note: The use of this drug ***may be a disqualification*** for piloting. Consult a designated Aviation Medical Examiner.

Exposure to Sun: No restrictions.

Discontinuation: Ondansetron may be stopped after you've completed the prescribed course (usually 3 days) of therapy.

Special Storage Instructions: Keep at room temperature. Avoid exposing this medicine to extreme humidity.

ORAL CONTRACEPTIVES (OR al kon tra SEP tivs)

Other Names: Estrogens/progestins, OCs, birth control pills

Introduced: 1956   **Class:** Female sex hormones   **Prescription:** USA: Yes   **Controlled Drug:** USA: No; Canada: No   **Available as Generic:** USA: Yes, in some forms; Canada: No

Brand Names: Brevicon, Demulen, Desogen, Enovid, Genora, Gestodene, Jenest 28, Levlen, Loestrin, Lo/Ovral, Micronor*, ♣Minestrin 1/20, Min-Ovral, Modicon, NEE, Nelova, Nelova 1/50 M, Nelova 10/11, Norcept-E 1/35, Nordette, Norethin 1/35E, Norethin 1/50M, Norinyl, Norlestrin, Nor-Q.D.*, Ortho Cyclen, Ortho Tri-Cyclen, Ortho-Novum, Ovcon, Ovral, Ovrette*, ♣Synphasic, Tri-Levlen, Tri-Norinyl, Triphasil, Triquilar, Zovia

BENEFITS versus RISKS	
Possible Benefits	*Possible Risks*
HIGHLY EFFECTIVE FOR CONTRACEPTIVE PROTECTION	SERIOUS, LIFE-THREATENING THROMBOEMBOLIC DISORDERS in susceptible individuals
Moderately effective as adjunctive treatment in management of excessive menses and endometriosis	Hypertension
	Fluid retention
	Intensification of migrainelike headaches and fibrocystic breast changes
	Accelerated growth of uterine fibroid tumors
	Drug-induced hepatitis with jaundice
	Benign liver tumors—rare

▷ **Principal Uses**

As a Single Drug Product: Uses currently included in FDA-approved labeling: (1) Prevention of conception. The "Mini-Pill" contains only one component, a progestin. This has been shown to be slightly less effective than the combination of estrogen and progestin in preventing pregnancy; (2) used in cases where women do not make enough hormones (female hypogonadism); (3)

*"Mini-Pill" type, contains progestin only.

helps decrease excessive blood flow at menstruation (hypermenorrhea); (4) of use in endometriosis as the combination mestranol and norethynodrel.

Other (unlabeled) generally accepted uses: (1) May be of benefit in abnormal hair growth in women (hirsutism); (2) some combination forms can have a protective effect against osteoporosis.

As a Combination Drug Product [CD]: Uses currently included in FDA-approved labeling: (1) Most oral contraceptives consist of a combination of an estrogen and a progestin. These products are the most effective form of medicinal contraception available; (2) they are sometimes used to treat menstrual irregularity, excessively heavy menstrual flow, and endometriosis.

Other (unlabeled) generally accepted uses: (1) Gestodene has been reported to inhibit certain breast cancer cell lines. Clinical studies are needed; (2) may have a protective effect against osteoporosis; (3) triphasic oral contraceptives can help in the prevention or treatment of menopause symptoms.

Author's Note: Recent research linked the number of times a woman ovulates to increased risk of ovarian cancer. This finding was associated with a P-53 gene, which may account for as much as 50% of ovarian cancer. Since birth control pills decrease the number of times that women ovulate, they may have a role in helping prevent cancer in people found to carry the P-53 gene. Further research is required.

How This Drug Works: When estrogen and progestin are taken in sufficient dosage and on a regular basis, the blood and tissue levels of these hormones increase to resemble those that occur during pregnancy. This results in suppression of the two pituitary gland hormones that normally cause ovulation (the formation and release of an egg by the ovary). In addition, these drugs may (1) alter the cervical mucus so that it resists the passage of sperm, and (2) alter the lining of the uterus so that it resists implantation of the egg (if ovulation occurs).

Available Dosage Forms and Strengths

Tablets — Several combinations of synthetic estrogens and progestins in varying strengths; see the package label of the brand prescribed.

▷ **Usual Adult Dosage Range:**   Start with the first tablet on the fifth day after the onset of menstruation. Follow with one tablet daily (taken at the same time each day) for 21 consecutive days. Resume treatment on the eighth day following the last tablet taken during the preceding cycle. The schedule is to take the drug daily for 3 weeks and to omit it for 1 week. For the Mini-Pill (progestin only), initiate treatment on the first day of menstruation and take one tablet daily, every day, throughout the year (no interruption). **Note: Actual dosage and administration schedule must be determined for each patient individually.**

Conditions Requiring Dosing Adjustments

Liver Function: This drug should **NOT** be taken if you have liver disease.

Kidney Function: Oral contraceptives are not significantly eliminated by the kidneys.

▷ **Dosing Instructions:**   The tablets may be crushed and taken with or after food to reduce stomach upset. To ensure regular (every day) use and uniform blood levels, it is best to take the tablet at the same time daily.

Usual Duration of Use: According to individual needs and circumstances. Long-term use (months to years) requires physician supervision and evaluation every 6 months.

▷ **This Drug Should Not Be Taken If**
- you have had an allergic reaction to any dosage form of it.
- you have a history of thrombophlebitis, embolism, heart attack, or stroke.
- you have breast cancer.
- you have active liver disease, seriously impaired liver function, or a history of liver tumor.
- you have diabetes and have developed circulatory disease.
- you have high blood pressure.
- you have not had any periods (amenorrhea).
- you have abnormal and unexplained vaginal bleeding.
- you have sickle cell disease.
- you are pregnant.

▷ **Inform Your Physician Before Taking This Drug If**
- you have had an adverse reaction to any oral contraceptive.
- you have a history of cancer of the breast or reproductive organs.
- you have fibrocystic breast changes, uterine fibroid tumors, endometriosis, migrainelike headaches, epilepsy, asthma, elevated lipids, prolapse of the mitral valve of the heart, heart disease, high blood pressure, gallbladder disease, diabetes, or porphyria.
- you are over 40. This was an age-related limit previously, but current thinking says that use of these medicines may occur as a benefit-to-risk decision.
- you smoke tobacco on a regular basis.
- you plan to have surgery in the near future.

Possible Side Effects (natural, expected, and unavoidable drug actions)
Fluid retention, weight gain, "breakthrough" bleeding (spotting in middle of menstrual cycle), altered menstrual pattern, lack of menstruation (during and following cessation of drug), increased susceptibility to yeast infection of the genital tissues. Tannish pigmentation of the face.

▷ **Possible Adverse Effects** (unusual, unexpected, and infrequent reactions)
If any of the following develop, consult your physician promptly for guidance.
Mild Adverse Effects
Allergic Reactions: Skin rash, hives, itching.
Headache, nervous tension, irritability, accentuation of migraine headaches—infrequent to frequent.
Rise in blood pressure (in some people)—possible.
Nausea, perhaps with vomiting—frequent (related to estrogen) and may ease if taken with evening meals.
Reduced tolerance to contact lenses or impaired color vision: blue tinge to objects, blue halo around lights—possible.
Serious Adverse Effects
Allergic Reactions: Anaphylaxis, erythema multiforme and nodosum (skin reactions), loss of scalp hair.
Idiosyncratic Reactions: Joint and muscle pains.
Emotional depression—infrequent to frequent.

Eye changes: optic neuritis, retinal thrombosis, altered curvature of the cornea, cataracts—possible.

Gallbladder disease, benign liver tumors, jaundice—case reports.

Enlargement of uterine fibroid tumors—possible.

Abnormal glucose tolerance (hyperglycemia)—frequent in people with pregnancy (gestational) diabetes.

Thrombophlebitis (inflammation of a vein with formation of blood clot): pain or tenderness in thigh or leg, with or without swelling of foot or leg—increased risk, especially with high estrogen doses.

Drug-induced porphyria or worsening of systemic lupus erythematosus (SLE)—case reports.

Esophageal ulcers (especially if the medicine is taken lying down with no water)—case reports.

Stroke (blood clot in brain): headaches, blackout, sudden weakness or paralysis of any part of the body, severe dizziness, altered vision, slurred speech, inability to speak—possible increased risk.

Heart attack (blood clot in coronary artery): sudden pain in chest, neck, jaw, or arm; weakness; sweating; nausea—increased risk.

Liver cancer—increased risk with long-term use.

▷ **Possible Effects on Sexual Function**

Altered character of menstruation; midcycle spotting—may be frequent.

Increased or decreased libido—possible.

Breast enlargement and tenderness with milk production—possible.

Absent menstruation and infertility (temporary) after discontinuation of drug.

Possible Delayed Adverse Effects: Estrogens taken during pregnancy can predispose the female child to the later development of cancer of the vagina or cervix following puberty. Nonpregnant use does not increase breast cancer.

▷ **Adverse Effects That May Mimic Natural Diseases or Disorders**

Liver reactions may suggest viral hepatitis.

Natural Diseases or Disorders That May Be Activated by This Drug

Latent hypertension, diabetes mellitus, acute intermittent porphyria, lupus-erythematosus-like syndrome.

Possible Effects on Laboratory Tests

Blood lupus erythematosus (LE) cells: positive.

Blood clotting time or INR: decreased.

Blood amylase and lipase levels: increased (very rare pancreatitis).

Blood total cholesterol, HDL, LDL, and VLDL cholesterol levels: usually no effects; some variability, depending upon estrogen and progestin content of preparation used.

Blood triglyceride levels: no effect to increased, depending upon estrogen and progestin content of preparation used.

Blood glucose level: increased.

Blood thyroid-stimulating hormone (TSH) level: no effect.

Blood thyroid hormone levels: T_3 and T_4 increased; free T_4 either no effect or decreased.

Liver function tests: increased liver enzymes (ALT/GPT, AST/GOT, alkaline phosphatase) and bilirubin.

CAUTION

1. Serious adverse effects due to these drugs are a very low risk. However, any unusual development should be reported and evaluated promptly.
2. Studies indicate that women over 30 years of age who smoke and use oral contraceptives are at significantly greater risk of having a serious cardiovascular event than are nonusers.
3. The risk of thromboembolism increases with the amount of estrogen in the product and the age of the user. Low-estrogen combinations are advised.
4. It is advisable to discontinue these drugs 1 month prior to elective surgery to reduce the risk of postsurgical thromboembolism.
5. Investigate promptly any alteration or disturbance of vision that occurs during the use of these drugs.
6. Investigate promptly the nature of recurrent, persistent, or severe headaches that develop while taking these drugs.
7. Observe for significant change of mood. Discontinue this drug if depression develops.
8. Certain commonly used drugs may reduce the effectiveness of oral contraceptives. Some of these are listed in the category of "Other Drugs" below.
9. Diarrhea lasting more than a few hours (and occurring during the days the drug is taken) can prevent adequate absorption of these drugs and impair their effectiveness as contraceptives.
10. If two consecutive menstrual periods are missed, ask your doctor if you should get a pregnancy test. Do not continue to use these drugs until you know whether you are pregnant.
11. **Many antibiotics may stop the effectiveness of birth control pills** (oral contraceptives). If your doctor prescribes an antibiotic, ask whether a different method of birth control is needed.

▷ **Advisability of Use During Pregnancy**

Pregnancy Category: X. See Pregnancy Risk Categories at the back of this book.

Animal studies: Genital defects reported in mice and guinea pigs; cleft palate reported in rodents.

Human studies: Information from studies of pregnant women indicates that estrogens can masculinize the female fetus. In addition, limb defects and heart malformations have been reported.

It is now known that estrogens taken during pregnancy can predispose the female child to the development of cancer of the vagina or cervix following puberty.

Avoid these drugs completely during entire pregnancy.

Advisability of Use If Breast-Feeding

Presence of these drugs in breast milk: Yes, in minute amounts (ethinyl estradiol or norethindrone). These drugs may suppress milk formation if started early after delivery.

Breast-feeding is considered to be safe during the use of oral contraceptives.

Habit-Forming Potential: None.

Effects of Overdosage: Headache, drowsiness, nausea, vomiting, fluid retention, abnormal vaginal bleeding, breast enlargement and discomfort.

Possible Effects of Long-Term Use: High blood pressure, gallbladder disease with stones, accelerated growth of uterine fibroid tumors, absent menstruation, and impaired fertility after discontinuation of drug.

Suggested Periodic Examinations While Taking This Drug (at physician's discretion)
Regular (every 6 months) evaluation of the breasts and pelvic organs, including Pap smears. Liver function tests as indicated.

▷ **While Taking This Drug, Observe the Following**
Foods: Avoid excessive use of salt if fluid retention occurs. Excessive vitamin C may increase risk of failure.
Beverages: No restrictions. May be taken with milk.
▷ *Alcohol:* No interactions expected.
Tobacco Smoking: Studies indicate that heavy smoking (15 or more cigarettes daily) while taking oral contraceptives significantly increases the risk of heart attack (coronary thrombosis). Heavy smoking should be considered a contraindication to the use of oral contraceptives. I advise everyone to quit smoking.
▷ *Other Drugs*
Oral contraceptives may *increase* the effects of
• cyclosporine (Sandimmune) and cause toxicity.
• metoprolol (Lopressor), and cause excessive beta-blocker effects.
• prednisolone and prednisone, and cause excessive cortisonelike effects.
• some benzodiazepines (see Drug Classes), and cause excessive sedation.
• theophyllines (Theo-Dur, others), and increase the risk of toxic effects.
Oral contraceptives *taken concurrently* with
• antibiotics (such as amoxicillin or ampicillin) can seriously impair effectiveness and allow pregnancy to occur.
• antidiabetic drugs (oral hypoglycemic agents) may cause unpredictable fluctuations of blood sugar.
• ascorbic acid (vitamin C) may result in increased levels of ethinyl estradiol, and breakthrough bleeding if the vitamin C is stopped.
• tricyclic antidepressants (Elavil, Sinequan, etc.) may enhance their adverse effects and reduce their antidepressant effectiveness.
• troleandomycin (TAO) may increase occurrence of liver toxicity and jaundice.
• warfarin (Coumadin) may cause unpredictable alterations of prothrombin activity. More frequent INR (prothrombin time or protime) testing is needed, and warfarin dosing should be adjusted to laboratory test results.
The following drugs may *decrease* the effects of oral contraceptives (and impair their effectiveness)
• barbiturates (phenobarbital, etc.; see Drug Classes).
• carbamazepine (Tegretol).
• griseofulvin (Fulvicin, etc.).
• nevirapine (Viramune).
• penicillins (ampicillin, penicillin V).
• phenytoin (Dilantin).
• primidone (Mysoline).
• rifampin (Rifadin, Rimactane).

- ritonavir (Norvir) and perhaps other protease inhibitors (see Drug Classes).
- tetracyclines (see Drug Classes).

▷ *Driving, Hazardous Activities:* Usually no restrictions. Consult your physician for assessment of individual risk and for guidance regarding specific restrictions.

Aviation Note: Usually no restrictions. However, watch for the rare occurrence of disturbed vision and restrict activities accordingly. Consult a designated Aviation Medical Examiner.

Exposure to Sun: Use caution—these drugs can cause photosensitivity (see Glossary).

Discontinuation: Do not stop this drug if "breakthrough" bleeding occurs. If spotting or bleeding continues, call your doctor. A higher-estrogen pill may be required. Remember: Omitting this drug for only 1 day may allow pregnancy to occur. It is best to avoid pregnancy for 3 to 6 months after stopping these drugs; aborted fetuses from women who became pregnant within 6 months after discontinuation reveal significantly increased chromosome abnormalities.

OXAPROZIN (OX a proh zin)

See the propionic acids (nonsteroidal anti-inflammatory drugs) profile for further information.

OXICAMS
(Nonsteroidal Anti-Inflammatory Drugs)

Piroxicam (peer OX i kam)

Introduced: 1978   **Class:** Mild analgesic, anti-inflammatory   **Prescription:** USA: Yes   **Controlled Drug:** USA: No; Canada: No   **Available as Generic:** Yes

Brand Names: ✦Apo-Piroxicam, Feldene, ♣Novo-Pirocam, ✦Nu-Pirox

BENEFITS versus RISKS	
Possible Benefits	*Possible Risks*
EFFECTIVE RELIEF OF MILD TO MODERATE PAIN AND INFLAMMATION	Gastrointestinal pain, ulceration, and bleeding
	Drug-induced hepatitis—rare
	Rare kidney damage
	Mild fluid retention
	Reduced white blood cell and platelet counts

▷ **Principal Uses**

As a Single Drug Product: Uses currently included in FDA-approved labeling: Relieves mild to moderately severe pain and inflammation associated with (1) rheumatoid arthritis, (2) osteoarthritis.

Other (unlabeled) generally accepted uses: (1) Treats the morning and evening pain associated with ankylosing spondylitis; (2) helps relieve the pain and inflammation of acute gout; (3) used to treat terminal cancer pain in combination with doxepin; (4) may have a role in easing temporal arteritis; (5) effective in painful menstruation (primary dysmenorrhea); (6) second-line therapy in acute gout.

How This Drug Works: This drug suppresses the formation of prostaglandins (and related compounds), chemicals involved in the production of inflammation and pain.

Available Dosage Forms and Strengths

Capsules — 10 mg, 20 mg
Rectal suppository — 10 mg, 20 mg

▷ **Usual Adult Dosage Range:** As antiarthritic: 10 mg twice daily, 12 hours apart; or 20 mg once daily. The total daily dosage should not exceed 40 mg, and then for no more than 5 days. **Note: Actual dosage and administration schedule must be determined for each patient individually.**

Conditions Requiring Dosing Adjustments

Liver Function: This drug should be used with caution and in decreased dose by patients with liver compromise.

Kidney Function: Piroxicam should be used with caution in renal compromise, and kidney function followed closely. The kidney is a minor path of removal of this medicine.

▷ **Dosing Instructions:** Take with or following food to prevent stomach irritation. Take with a full glass of water and remain upright (do not lie down) for 30 minutes. The capsule may be opened for administration.

Usual Duration of Use: Use on a regular schedule for 2 weeks usually determines effectiveness in relieving the discomfort of arthritis. Long-term use (months to years) requires physician supervision and periodic evaluation.

▷ **This Drug Should Not Be Taken If**
- you have had an allergic reaction to it previously.
- you are subject to asthma or nasal polyps caused by aspirin.
- you have active peptic ulcer disease or any form of gastrointestinal bleeding.
- you have a bleeding disorder or a blood cell disorder.
- you have active liver disease.
- you have severe impairment of kidney function.

▷ **Inform Your Physician Before Taking This Drug If**
- you are allergic to aspirin or to other aspirin substitutes.
- you have a history of peptic ulcer disease, regional enteritis, or ulcerative colitis.
- you have a history of any type of bleeding disorder.
- you have impaired liver or kidney function.
- you develop signs or symptoms of pancreatitis while taking this medicine (talk with your doctor).
- you have high blood pressure or a history of heart failure.
- you take acetaminophen, aspirin or other aspirin substitutes, anticoagulants, oral antidiabetic drugs.
- you plan to have surgery of any type in the near future.

Possible Side Effects (natural, expected, and unavoidable drug actions)
Fluid retention (weight gain), prolongation of bleeding time.

▷ **Possible Adverse Effects** (unusual, unexpected, and infrequent reactions)
If any of the following develop, consult your physician promptly for guidance.

Mild Adverse Effects
Allergic Reactions: Skin rash, itching, spontaneous bruising.
Headache, dizziness, hair loss, altered or vision, ringing in ears, drowsiness, fatigue, paresthesias, inability to concentrate—rare to infrequent.
Indigestion, nausea, vomiting, abdominal pain, diarrhea—infrequent to frequent.

Serious Adverse Effects
Esophagitis or active peptic ulcer, stomach or intestinal bleeding—possible and more likely in elderly.
Drug-induced liver or kidney damage—rare to infrequent.
Serious skin damage (toxic epidermal necrolysis)—case reports.
Pancreatitis—rare.
Bone marrow depression (see Glossary): abnormal bleeding or bruising—case reports.
Blood clotting problems—dose and half-life related.
Increased blood potassium or decreased sodium—case reports.

▷ **Possible Effects on Sexual Function:**   None reported.

Possible Delayed Adverse Effects: Mild anemia due to "silent" blood loss from the stomach.

▷ **Adverse Effects That May Mimic Natural Diseases or Disorders**
Liver reaction may suggest viral hepatitis.

Natural Diseases or Disorders That May Be Activated by This Drug
Peptic ulcer disease, ulcerative colitis. This drug may hide symptoms of gout.

Possible Effects on Laboratory Tests
Red blood cell count and hemoglobin level: decreased.
Bleeding time: increased.
Blood uric acid level: increased.
Liver function tests: increased liver enzymes (ALT/GPT, AST/GOT, and alkaline phosphatase), increased bilirubin.
Kidney function tests: blood creatinine and urea nitrogen (BUN) levels increased; urine analysis positive for red blood cells, casts, and increased protein content (kidney damage).
Fecal occult blood test: positive.

CAUTION
1. The smallest effective dose should always be used.
2. This drug may hide early signs of infection. Tell your doctor if you think you are developing an infection.

Precautions for Use
By Infants and Children: Indications and dose recommendations for those under 12 years of age are not established.
By Those Over 60 Years of Age: Small doses are advisable until tolerance is determined. Observe for any indications of liver or kidney toxicity, fluid retention, dizziness, confusion, impaired memory, stomach bleeding, or constipation.

▷ **Advisability of Use During Pregnancy**

Pregnancy Category: B. D in the final 3 months of pregnancy. See Pregnancy Risk Categories at the back of this book.

Animal studies: No birth defects reported due to this drug.

Human studies: Adequate studies of pregnant women are not available.

The manufacturer does not recommend the use of this drug during pregnancy.

Advisability of Use If Breast-Feeding

Presence of this drug in breast milk: Yes.

Avoid drug or refrain from nursing.

Habit-Forming Potential: None.

Effects of Overdosage: Possible drowsiness, dizziness, ringing in the ears, nausea, vomiting, indigestion.

Possible Effects of Long-Term Use: Development of anemia due to "silent" bleeding from the gastrointestinal tract.

Suggested Periodic Examinations While Taking This Drug (at physician's discretion)

Complete blood cell counts, liver and kidney function tests.

Complete eye examinations if vision is altered in any way.

Hearing examinations if ringing in the ears or hearing loss develops.

▷ **While Taking This Drug, Observe the Following**

Foods: No restrictions.

Beverages: No restrictions. May be taken with milk.

▷ *Alcohol:* Use with caution. Both alcohol and piroxicam can irritate the stomach lining, and can increase the risk of stomach ulceration and/or bleeding.

Tobacco Smoking: No interactions expected, but I advise everyone to quit smoking.

▷ *Other Drugs*

Piroxicam may *increase* the effects of

- acetaminophen (Tylenol, etc.), and increase the risk of kidney damage; avoid prolonged use of this combination.
- adrenocortical steroids (see Drug Classes) may result in additive stomach irritation.
- anticoagulants (Coumadin, etc.), and increase the risk of bleeding; more frequent INR (prothrombin time or protime) testing is needed and dosing should then be adjusted accordingly.
- lithium (Lithobid, others) can lead to lithium toxicity.
- methotrexate (Mexate) may lead to methotrexate toxicity.

Piroxicam *taken concurrently* with the following drugs may increase the risk of bleeding; avoid these combinations:

- aspirin.
- antihypertensives such as thiazides (see Drug Classes) and others will blunt their therapeutic benefits.
- beta-blockers (atenolol and others)—can decrease the effectiveness of the beta-blocker.
- cholestyramine (Questran).
- dipyridamole (Persantine).
- indomethacin (Indocin).
- sulfinpyrazone (Anturane).
- valproic acid (Depakene).

Piroxicam *taken concurrently* with
- ritonavir (Norvir) and perhaps other protease inhibitors (see Drug Classes) can lead to toxicity.
- thiazide diuretics (see Drug Classes) may blunt their therapeutic benefits.

▷ *Driving, Hazardous Activities:* This drug may cause drowsiness or dizziness. Restrict activities as necessary.

Aviation Note: The use of this drug *may be a disqualification* for piloting. Consult a designated Aviation Medical Examiner.

Exposure to Sun: This drug may cause photosensitivity (see Glossary). Use caution.

OXTRIPHYLLINE (ox TRY fi lin)

Other Names: Choline theophyllinate, theophylline cholinate

Introduced: 1965   **Class:** Antiasthmatic, bronchodilator, xanthines
Prescription: USA: Yes   **Controlled Drug:** USA: No; Canada: No   **Available as Generic:** Yes

Brand Names: ✤Apo-Oxtriphylline, Choledyl, Choledyl Delayed-Release, Choledyl SA, ✤Novotriphyl

Author's Note: This medicine is converted to 64% theophylline by the body. See the theophylline profile for further information.

OXYCODONE (ox ee KOH dohn)

Introduced: 1950   **Class:** Analgesic, strong; opioids   **Prescription:** USA: Yes   **Controlled Drug:** USA: C-II*; Canada: No   **Available as Generic:** USA: Yes; Canada: No

Brand Names: ✤Endocet [CD], ✤Endodan [CD], ✤Oxycocet [CD], ✤Oxycodan [CD], Oxycontin, Percocet [CD], ✤Percocet-Demi [CD], Percodan [CD], Percodan-Demi [CD], Roxicet, Roxicodone, Roxilox, Roxiprin [CD], SK-Oxycodone, ✤Supeudol, Tylox [CD]

BENEFITS versus RISKS	
Possible Benefits	*Possible Risks*
EFFECTIVE RELIEF OF MODERATE TO SEVERE PAIN	POTENTIAL FOR HABIT FORMATION (DEPENDENCE)
	Sedative effects
	Mild allergic reactions—infrequent
	Nausea, constipation

▷ **Principal Uses**

As a Single Drug Product: Uses currently included in FDA-approved labeling: Used in tablet and suppository form (Canada) to relieve moderate to severe pain.

Other (unlabeled) generally accepted uses: None.

*See schedules of Controlled Drugs at the back of this book.

As a Combination Drug Product [CD]: Oxycodone is available in combinations with acetaminophen and with aspirin. These milder pain relievers are added to enhance the analgesic effect and reduce fever when present.

How This Drug Works: Acting primarily as a depressant of certain brain functions, this drug suppresses pain perception and calms the emotional response to pain.

Available Dosage Forms and Strengths

Solution — 5 mg/5 ml
Suppositories — 10 mg, 20 mg (Canada)
Tablets — 5 mg, 10 mg (Canada)
Tablets — 2.44 mg, 4.88 mg (in combination drugs)

▷ **Usual Adult Dosage Range:** Percodan is taken as one tablet (5 mg) every 6 hours. Current pain theory says that pain medicines should be scheduled; for example, given every 4 hours. The outdated "wait until it hurts" method tended to result in suffering. May be increased to 10 mg every 4 hours if needed for severe pain. The total daily dosage should not exceed 60 mg. Oxycontin is a sustained-release formulation and is taken every 12 hours. **Note: Actual dosage and administration schedule must be determined for each patient individually.**

Conditions Requiring Dosing Adjustments

Liver Function: Dosage adjustments should be empirically made in liver failure.
Kidney Function: Dosage adjustment does not appear to be needed. Some combination products contain aspirin, which may be contraindicated in kidney failure.

▷ **Dosing Instructions:** The tablet may be crushed and taken with or following food to reduce stomach upset or nausea.

Usual Duration of Use: As required to control pain. Continual use should not exceed 5 to 7 days without interruption and reassessment of need.

▷ **This Drug Should Not Be Taken If**
• you have had an allergic reaction to any dosage form of it previously.
• you are having an acute attack of asthma.
• Patients allergic to aspirin should **not** be given Percodan.

▷ **Inform Your Physician Before Taking This Drug If**
• you have had an unfavorable reaction to any narcotic drug in the past.
• you have had a head injury with increased pressure (intracranial) in the head.
• you have a history of drug abuse or alcoholism.
• you have chronic lung disease with impaired breathing.
• you have impaired liver or kidney function.
• you have gallbladder disease, a seizure disorder, or an underactive thyroid gland.
• you have difficulty emptying the urinary bladder.
• you are taking any other drugs that have a sedative effect.
• you plan to have surgery under general anesthesia in the near future.

Possible Side Effects (natural, expected, and unavoidable drug actions)
Drowsiness, light-headedness, dry mouth, urinary retention, constipation.

▷ **Possible Adverse Effects** (unusual, unexpected, and infrequent reactions)
  If any of the following develop, consult your physician promptly for guidance.
  Mild Adverse Effects
  Allergic Reactions: Skin rash, hives, itching.
  Idiosyncratic Reactions: Skin rash and itching when combined with dairy products (milk or cheese).
  Dizziness, sensation of drunkenness, depression, blurred or double vision—dose related.
  Nausea, vomiting—may be dose related.
  Serious Adverse Effects
  Impaired breathing: use with caution in chronic lung disease—variable and can be dose related.
  Abnormal body movements, if the drug is abruptly stopped.

▷ **Possible Effects on Sexual Function:**   Blunted sexual responses—case reports.

Possible Effects on Laboratory Tests
  Urine screening tests for drug abuse: test result may be falsely **positive**; *confirmatory* test result may be **negative**. (Test results depend upon amount of drug taken and testing method used.)

CAUTION
  1. If you have asthma, chronic bronchitis, or emphysema, excessive use of this drug may cause significant respiratory difficulty, thickening of bronchial secretions, and suppression of coughing.
  2. The concurrent use of this drug with atropinelike drugs can increase the risk of urinary retention and reduced intestinal function.
  3. Do not take this drug following acute head injury.

Precautions for Use
  By Infants and Children: Do not use this drug in children under 2 years of age because of their vulnerability to life-threatening respiratory depression.
  By Those Over 60 Years of Age: Small starting doses and short-term therapy are indicated. There may be increased susceptibility to the development of drowsiness, dizziness, unsteadiness, falling, urinary retention, and constipation (often leading to fecal impaction).

▷ **Advisability of Use During Pregnancy**
  Pregnancy Category: C. See Pregnancy Risk Categories at the back of this book.
  Animal studies: No information available.
  Human studies: Adequate studies of pregnant women are not available. Oxycodone taken repeatedly during the final few weeks before delivery may cause withdrawal symptoms in the newborn infant.
  Use this drug only if clearly needed and in small, infrequent doses.

Advisability of Use If Breast-Feeding
  Presence of this drug in breast milk: Unknown.
  Avoid drug or refrain from nursing.

Habit-Forming Potential: Psychological and/or physical dependence can develop.

Effects of Overdosage: Drowsiness, restlessness, agitation, nausea, vomiting, dry mouth, vertigo, weakness, lethargy, stupor, coma, seizures.

Possible Effects of Long-Term Use: Psychological and physical dependence, chronic constipation.

Suggested Periodic Examinations While Taking This Drug (at physician's discretion)
  None.

▷ **While Taking This Drug, Observe the Following**
  Foods: No restrictions.
  Beverages: No restrictions. May be taken with milk.
▷ *Alcohol:* Oxycodone can intensify the intoxicating effects of alcohol, and alcohol can intensify the depressant effects of oxycodone on brain function, breathing, and circulation. Combined use is best avoided.
  Tobacco Smoking: No interactions expected, but I advise everyone to quit smoking.
  Marijuana Smoking: Increase in drowsiness and pain relief; impairment of mental and physical performance.
▷ *Other Drugs*
    Oxycodone may *increase* the effects of
    • atropinelike drugs, and increase the risk of constipation and urinary retention.
    • other drugs with sedative effects (see Drug Classes for benzodiazepines, tricyclic antidepressants, antihistamines, MAO inhibitors, phenothiazines, and opioid drugs (narcotics)).
    Oxycodone *taken concurrently* with
    • ritonavir (Norvir) and perhaps other protease inhibitors (see Drug Classes) may lead to toxicity.
▷ *Driving, Hazardous Activities:* This drug can impair mental alertness, judgment, reaction time, and physical coordination. Avoid hazardous activities accordingly.
  Aviation Note: The use of this drug *is a disqualification* for piloting. Consult a designated Aviation Medical Examiner.
  Exposure to Sun: No restrictions.
  Discontinuation: It is best to limit this drug to short-term use. If extended use is needed, discontinuation should be gradual to minimize possible effects of withdrawal.

PAROXETINE (pa ROCKS a teen)

Introduced: 1993   **Class:** Antidepressant, other   **Prescription:** USA: Yes   **Controlled Drug:** USA: No; Canada: No   **Available as Generic:** USA: No; Canada: No

Brand Name: Paxil

```
┌──────────────────────────────────────────────────────────────────┐
│                      BENEFITS versus RISKS                         │
│        Possible Benefits              Possible Risks               │
│   EFFECTIVE CONTROL OF           Withdrawal symptoms               │
│     DEPRESSION                   Abnormal ejaculation in males     │
│   Fewer adverse effects than tricyclic                            │
│     antidepressants                                                │
│   Helps control obsessive-compulsive                              │
│     disorder and panic disorder                                    │
└──────────────────────────────────────────────────────────────────┘
```

▷ **Principal Uses**

> *As a Single Drug Product:* Uses currently included in FDA-approved labeling: (1) Treatment of depression; (2) helps control obsessive-compulsive disorder; (3) helps control panic attacks.
>
> Other (unlabeled) generally accepted uses: (1) Can have a role in diabetic nerve pain (neuropathy); (2) helps long-standing (chronic) daily headaches; (3) can help premature ejaculation.

How This Drug Works: This phenylpiperidine antidepressant inhibits the uptake of a chemical important in mood (serotonin). When more of this chemical is available in the brain, a positive impact on thinking is often realized.

Available Dosage Forms and Strengths

> Capsules — 20 mg, 30 mg

▷ **Recommended Dosage Ranges** (Actual dosage and administration schedule must be determined for each patient individually.)

> *Infants and Children:* Not indicated.
>
> *18 to 60 Years of Age:* Depression: The usual starting dose is 20 mg, taken in the morning. Dose can then be increased as needed and tolerated in 10-mg intervals to a maximum of 50 mg daily.
>
> Obsessive-compulsive disorder: Started with 20 mg daily with increases as in depression to a usual benefit at 40 mg per day. Maximum here is 60 mg daily.
>
> *Over 60 Years of Age:* The starting dose in this population is 10 mg daily. The maximum dose is 40 mg daily.

Conditions Requiring Dosing Adjustments

> *Liver Function:* Starting dose is 10 mg and the maximum dose is 40 mg daily. Drug levels may be needed.
>
> *Kidney Function:* The starting dose and maximum dose are the same as those used by patients with liver compromise.

▷ **Dosing Instructions:**   The absorption of this medicine is not changed by food.

Usual Duration of Use: Continual use on a regular schedule for 14 days is usually necessary to determine this drug's effectiveness in treating depression. Long-term use (months to years) requires periodic evaluation of response and dosage adjustment. Consult your physician on a regular basis.

Possible Advantages of This Drug

> Fewer side effects than tricyclic antidepressants.

▷ **This Drug Should Not Be Taken If**

- you have had an allergic reaction to any dosage form of it previously.
- you are currently taking, or have taken within the last 14 days, any MAO inhibitor (see Drug Classes) medication.

▷ **Inform Your Physician Before Taking This Drug If**
- you are pregnant or breast-feeding.
- you have a history of mania or seizures.
- you take diuretics or typically drink little water.
- you have a history of liver or kidney disease.
- you take other prescription or nonprescription medicines that were not discussed with your doctor when paroxetine was prescribed.

Possible Side Effects (natural, expected, and unavoidable drug actions)
Lowered blood pressure and fainting upon standing (postural hypotension). Sedation.

▷ **Possible Adverse Effects** (unusual, unexpected, and infrequent reactions)
If any of the following develop, consult your physician promptly for guidance.
Mild Adverse Effects
Allergic Reactions: Skin rash and itching.
Headache, nervousness, or insomnia—infrequent to frequent.
Palpitations—infrequent.
Loss of appetite, nausea, taste disorders, or constipation—infrequent to frequent.
Tingling of the hands (paresthesias)—infrequent.
Sweating—frequent.
Dizziness, blurred vision—infrequent to frequent.
Serious Adverse Effects
Allergic Reactions: Not reported.
Idiosyncratic Reactions: None reported.
Abnormal movements or positioning of the mouth or face—infrequent.
Seizures—rare.
Liver toxicity—rare and of questionable causation.

▷ **Possible Effects on Sexual Function:** Galactorrhea.
Abnormal ejaculation—infrequent to frequent; inability to achieve orgasm, impotence, or sexual dysfunction—infrequent; prolonged and painful erection (priapism)—rare.

Possible Delayed Adverse Effects: None reported.

▷ **Adverse Effects That May Mimic Natural Diseases or Disorders**
Increased liver enzymes may mimic early hepatitis.

Natural Diseases or Disorders That May Be Activated by This Drug
None reported.

Possible Effects on Laboratory Tests
Liver function tests: increased.

CAUTION
1. Take this medicine as prescribed and do not stop taking it without talking with your doctor.

Precautions for Use
By Infants and Children: Safety and effectiveness for use by those under 18 years of age have not been established.
By Those Over 60 Years of Age: Lower starting and maximum doses are indicated.

▷ **Advisability of Use During Pregnancy**

Pregnancy Category: B. See Pregnancy Risk Categories at the back of this book.
Animal studies: Reproduction studies in rabbits or rats using doses of up to 10 times the typical human dose have not revealed any fetal changes.
Human studies: Information from adequate studies of pregnant women is not available.
Ask your doctor for guidance.

Advisability of Use If Breast-Feeding

Presence of this drug in breast milk: Yes, in small amounts.
Ask your doctor for guidance.

Habit-Forming Potential: None; however, a withdrawal syndrome characterized by dizziness, confusion, sweating, and tremor has been described.

Effects of Overdosage: Confusion, heart rhythm changes, seizures.

Possible Effects of Long-Term Use: Not defined.

Suggested Periodic Examinations While Taking This Drug (at physician's discretion)
Liver function tests.

▷ **While Taking This Drug, Observe the Following**

Foods: No restrictions.
Beverages: No restrictions.
▷   *Alcohol:* The manufacturer recommends avoiding alcohol while taking this medicine.
Tobacco Smoking: No interactions expected, but I advise everyone to quit smoking.
Marijuana Smoking: Additive sedation.
▷   *Other Drugs*
Paroxetine may *increase* the effects of
• benzodiazepines (see Drug Classes).
• desipramine (and potentially other tricyclic antidepressants; see Drug Classes).
• haloperidol (Haldol), because paroxetine blocks an enzyme system needed to remove haloperidol.
• labetalol (Normodyne) and perhaps other beta-blockers (see Drug Classes), because paroxetine inhibits an enzyme system needed to remove labetalol.
• minimally sedating antihistamines astemizole and terfenadine, because paroxetine may inhibit some liver systems that usually remove them from the body. This effect has not been documented, but is theoretically possible.
Paroxetine *taken concurrently* with
• activated charcoal will reduce absorption of paroxetine.
• MAO inhibitors (see Drug Classes) may result in a fatal serotonin syndrome. **Do not** combine these medicines.
• phenytoin (Dilantin) may result in decreased paroxetine blood levels and lessening of therapeutic benefits. Dose increases may be needed.
• quinidine (Quinaglute, others) may result in increased paroxetine levels and toxicity. Decreased paroxetine doses may be needed.
• tramadol (Ultram) may lead to increased risk of seizures. DO NOT combine.
• tryptophan may result in sweating, nausea, and dizziness.

- warfarin (Coumadin) may result in bleeding. More frequent INR (pro-thrombin time or protime) testing is recommended. Warfarin doses should be adjusted based on laboratory results.

The following drug may *increase* the effects of paroxetine
- cimetidine (Tagamet).

▷ *Driving, Hazardous Activities:* This drug may frequently cause sedation. Restrict activities as necessary.

Aviation Note: The use of this drug *is a disqualification* for piloting. Consult a designated Aviation Medical Examiner.

Exposure to Sun: No specific restrictions.

Exposure to Heat: This medicine can cause excessive sweating. If you work or are frequently in a hot environment, be careful to replace enough fluids to avoid dehydration.

Heavy Exercise or Exertion: Since this medicine may cause excessive sweating, be careful to replace lost fluids.

Occurrence of Unrelated Illness: Illnesses that cause fevers may be worsened in their ability to cause dehydration.

Discontinuation: Do not stop this medicine without first talking with your doctor.

PENBUTOLOL (pen BYU toh lohl)

Introduced: 1976   **Class:** Antihypertensive, beta-adrenergic blocker
Prescription: USA: Yes   **Controlled Drug:** USA: No; Canada: No   **Available as Generic:** No

Brand Name: Levatol

BENEFITS versus RISKS	
Possible Benefits	*Possible Risks*
EFFECTIVE, WELL-TOLERATED ANTIHYPERTENSIVE in mild to moderate high blood pressure	CONGESTIVE HEART FAILURE in advanced heart disease
	Worsening of angina in coronary heart disease (abrupt withdrawal)
	Masking of low blood sugar (hypoglycemia) in drug-treated diabetes
	Provocation of asthma (in asthmatics)

▷ **Principal Uses**

As a Single Drug Product: Uses currently included in FDA-approved labeling: Treatment of mild to moderate high blood pressure. May be used alone or concurrently with other antihypertensive drugs, such as diuretics.

Other (unlabeled) generally accepted uses: (1) May help curb aggressive behavior; (2) can help decrease the frequency and severity of angina attacks; (3) may help decrease death from heart attack (myocardial infarction); (4) can have a supportive role in panic attacks; (5) a small amount of data support penbutolol use in glaucoma, but large trials have not been performed as yet.

How This Drug Works: By blocking certain actions of the sympathetic nervous system, this drug
- reduces heart rate and contraction force, lowering the pressure of the blood leaving the heart.
- reduces the degree of blood vessel wall contraction, resulting in lower blood pressure.

Available Dosage Forms and Strengths
Tablets — 20 mg

▷ **Usual Adult Dosage Range:** Initially 20 mg once daily. The dose may be increased gradually by 10 mg/day at intervals of 2 weeks as needed and tolerated, up to 80 mg/day. Although higher doses have been well tolerated, they have not shown greater efficacy. For maintenance, 20 to 40 mg once daily is usually adequate. The total daily dose should not exceed 80 mg. **Note: Actual dosage and administration schedule must be determined for each patient individually.**

Conditions Requiring Dosing Adjustments
Liver Function: Dosage adjustments should be considered in mild to moderate liver disease; however, specific guidelines are not available.
Kidney Function: No dosing changes are thought to be needed.

▷ **Dosing Instructions:** The tablet may be crushed and taken without regard to eating. Do not stop this drug abruptly.

Usual Duration of Use: Use on a regular schedule for up to 2 weeks determines the full effect in lowering blood pressure. Long-term use of this drug (months to years) will determine your blood pressure over time and response to an overall treatment program (weight reduction, salt restriction, smoking cessation, etc.).

Possible Advantages of This Drug
Adequate control of blood pressure with a single daily dose.
Causes less slowing of the heart rate than most other beta-blocker drugs.

▷ **This Drug Should Not Be Taken If**
- you have had an allergic reaction to it previously.
- you have heart failure (overt).
- you have an abnormally slow heart rate or a serious form of heart block.
- you have abnormal growth of the left side of the heart (left ventricular hypertrophy).
- you have bronchial asthma.

▷ **Inform Your Physician Before Taking This Drug If**
- you have had an adverse reaction to any beta-blocker (see Drug Classes).
- you have a history of serious heart disease.
- you have a history of hay fever (allergic rhinitis), asthma, chronic bronchitis, or emphysema.
- you have a history of overactive thyroid function (hyperthyroidism).
- you have a history of low blood sugar (hypoglycemia).
- you have impaired liver or kidney function.
- you have diabetes or myasthenia gravis.
- you have congestive heart failure.
- you have impaired circulation in the extremities (Raynaud's phenomenon, claudication pains in legs).

- you take any form of digitalis, quinidine, or reserpine, or any calcium-channel-blocker drug (see Drug Classes).
- you plan to have surgery under general anesthesia in the near future.

Possible Side Effects (natural, expected, and unavoidable drug actions)

Lethargy and fatigability, cold extremities, slow heart rate, light-headedness in upright position (see Orthostatic Hypotension in Glossary).

▷ **Possible Adverse Effects** (unusual, unexpected, and infrequent reactions)

If any of the following develop, consult your physician promptly for guidance.

Mild Adverse Effects

Allergic Reactions: Skin rash, itching, reversible hair loss.

Headache, dizziness, blurred vision, insomnia, abnormal dreams—infrequent.

Indigestion, nausea, vomiting, constipation, diarrhea—infrequent.

Joint and muscle discomfort—infrequent.

Serious Adverse Effects

Allergic Reactions: Anaphylactic reaction (see Glossary).

Mental depression, anxiety, disorientation, short-term memory loss, hallucinations—possible.

Carpal tunnel syndrome or aggravation of myasthenia gravis—case reports.

High blood sugar or low blood sugar in diabetics—possible.

Worsening of circulatory problems (with preexisting conditions—Raynaud's phenomenon)—possible.

Bronchospasm—rare.

Chest pain, shortness of breath, precipitation of congestive heart failure—possible.

Rebound hypertension—if abruptly stopped.

Induction of bronchial asthma—possible in asthmatics.

▷ **Possible Effects on Sexual Function:**   Decreased libido and impotence—rare but dose related; Peyronie's disease (see Glossary)—rare.

▷ **Adverse Effects That May Mimic Natural Diseases or Disorders**

Reduced blood flow to extremities may resemble Raynaud's phenomenon (see Glossary).

Natural Diseases or Disorders That May Be Activated by This Drug

Raynaud's disease, intermittent claudication, myasthenia gravis.

Possible Effects on Laboratory Tests

Uric acid, potassium, or blood sugar: increased.

CAUTION

1. ***Do not stop this drug suddenly*** without the knowledge and help of your doctor. Carry a notation that states you are taking this drug.
2. Consult your physician or pharmacist **before** using nasal decongestants in over-the-counter cold preparations and nose drops. These can cause sudden increases in blood pressure when taken with beta-blockers.
3. Report the development of any tendency to emotional depression.

Precautions for Use

By Infants and Children: Safety and effectiveness in infants or children are not established.

By Those Over 60 Years of Age: Unacceptably high blood pressure should be reduced without creating the risks associated with excessively low blood pressure. Small starting doses and frequent blood pressure checks are needed. Sudden, rapid, and excessive reduction of blood pressure can predispose to stroke or heart attack. Observe for dizziness, unsteadiness, tendency to fall, confusion, hallucinations, depression, or urinary frequency.

▷ **Advisability of Use During Pregnancy**
Pregnancy Category: C. See Pregnancy Risk Categories at the back of this book.
Animal studies: No birth defects due to this drug found in rat or rabbit studies.
Human studies: Adequate studies of pregnant women are not available.
Use this drug only if clearly needed. Ask your physician for guidance.

Advisability of Use If Breast-Feeding
Presence of this drug in breast milk: Unknown.
Avoid drug or refrain from nursing.

Habit-Forming Potential: None.

Effects of Overdosage: Weakness, slow pulse, low blood pressure, fainting, cold and sweaty skin, congestive heart failure, possible coma, and convulsions.

Possible Effects of Long-Term Use: Reduced heart reserve and eventual heart failure in susceptible individuals with advanced heart disease.

Suggested Periodic Examinations While Taking This Drug (at physician's discretion)
Measurements of blood pressure, evaluation of heart function.
Complete blood cell counts.

▷ **While Taking This Drug, Observe the Following**
Foods: No restrictions. Avoid excessive salt intake.
Beverages: No restrictions. May be taken with milk.
▷ *Alcohol:* Alcohol may exaggerate this drug's ability to lower blood pressure and may increase its mild sedative effect.
Tobacco Smoking: Nicotine may reduce this drug's benefit in treating high blood pressure. I advise everyone to quit smoking.
Other Drugs
Penbutolol may *increase* the effects of
• other antihypertensive drugs, and cause excessive lowering of blood pressure. Dosage adjustments may be necessary.
• reserpine (Ser-Ap-Es, etc.), and cause sedation, depression, slowing of the heart rate, and lowering of blood pressure. This combination is best avoided.
• verapamil (Calan, Isoptin), and cause excessive depression of heart function; monitor this combination closely.
Penbutolol may *decrease* the effects of
• epinephrine, resulting in decreased benefits when used to correct allergic reactions. Slow heartbeat and elevated blood pressure may also occur.
Penbutolol *taken concurrently* with
• amiodarone (Cordarone) may result in sinus arrest or symptomatic bradycardia. DO NOT combine these medicines.
• clonidine (Catapres) requires close monitoring for rebound high blood pressure if clonidine is withdrawn while penbutolol is still being taken.

- fluoxetine (Prozac) may cause very slow heartbeat (bradycardia) and excessive lowering of blood pressure.
- fluvoxamine (Luvox) may cause very slow heartbeat (bradycardia) and excessive lowering of blood pressure.
- insulin or oral hypoglycemic agents requires close monitoring to avoid undetected hypoglycemia (see Glossary).
- venlafaxine (Effexor) may result in increased risk of toxicity from penbutolol.

The following drugs may *increase* the effects of penbutolol
- birth control pills (oral contraceptives).
- methimazole (Tapazole).
- propylthiouracil (Propacil).
- ritonavir (Norvir) and perhaps other protease inhibitors (see Drug Classes).

The following drugs may *decrease* the effects of penbutolol
- barbiturates (phenobarbital, etc.).
- indomethacin (Indocin) and possibly other "aspirin substitutes," or NSAIDs—may impair penbutolol's antihypertensive effect.
- rifampin (Rifadin, Rimactane).

▷ *Driving, Hazardous Activities:* Use caution until the full extent of fatigue, dizziness, and blood pressure change have been determined.

Aviation Note: The use of this drug *is a disqualification* for piloting. Consult a designated Aviation Medical Examiner.

Exposure to Sun: No restrictions.

Exposure to Heat: Hot environments can lower blood pressure and exaggerate the effects of this drug.

Exposure to Cold: Cold environments can worsen the circulatory deficiency in the extremities that may occur with this drug. The elderly should take precautions to prevent hypothermia (see Glossary).

Heavy Exercise or Exertion: Avoid exertion that produces light-headedness, excessive fatigue, or muscle cramping. The use of this drug may intensify the hypertensive response to isometric exercise.

Occurrence of Unrelated Illness: Fever can lower blood pressure and require adjustment of dosage. Nausea or vomiting may interrupt the regular dosage schedule. Ask your physician for guidance.

Discontinuation: It is advisable to avoid sudden discontinuation of this drug in all situations. If possible, gradual reduction of dose over a period of 2 to 3 weeks is recommended. Ask your physician for specific guidance.

PENCICLOVIR (pen i SIL a meen)

Introduced: 1996   **Class:** Antiviral, anti-herpetic   **Prescription:** USA: Yes   **Controlled Drug:** USA: No; Canada: No   **Available as Generic:** USA: No; Canada: No

Brand Name: Denavir
   Author's Note: This profile will be expanded as more information becomes available.

PENICILLAMINE (pen i SIL a meen)

Introduced: 1963   **Class:** Antiarthritic   **Prescription:** USA: Yes
Controlled Drug: USA: No; Canada: No   **Available as Generic:** USA: No;
Canada: No
Brand Names: Cuprimine, Depen

BENEFITS versus RISKS	
Possible Benefits	*Possible Risks*
EFFECTIVE TREATMENT OF WILSON'S DISEASE (COPPER TOXICITY)	SEVERE ALLERGIC REACTIONS BONE MARROW DEPRESSION
Effective treatment of cystinuria and cystine kidney stones	Drug-induced damage of lungs, liver, pancreas, and kidneys
Partially effective treatment of rheumatoid arthritis and poisoning due to heavy metals: iron, lead, mercury, and zinc	

▷ **Principal Uses**

As a Single Drug Product: Uses currently included in FDA-approved labeling: Treatment of (1) Wilson's disease (copper toxicity of brain, cornea, liver, and kidneys); (2) severe rheumatoid arthritis that has failed to respond to less hazardous conventional treatment; also helps rheumatoid arthritis that presents with interstitial lung disease; (3) cystinuria and cystine stone formation (excessive amounts of cystine in the urine).

Other (unlabeled) generally accepted uses: (1) Treatment of heavy metal poisoning, especially that due to lead and mercury; (2) may help increase survival in scleroderma; (3) eases progression of systemic sclerosis.

Author's Note: Due to proliferation of new medicines, this profile has been abbreviated in order to make room for more widely used medicines.

PENICILLINS

Amoxicillin (a mox i SIL in)   **Amoxicillin/Clavulanate** (a mox i SIL in/KLAV yu lan ayt)   **Ampicillin** (am pi SIL in)   **Bacampicillin** (bak am pi SIL in)   **Cloxacillin** (klox a SIL in)   **Penicillin VK** (pen i SIL in VEE KAY)

Introduced: 1969, 1982, 1961, 1979, 1962, 1953, respectively   **Class:** Antibiotics, penicillins   **Prescription:** USA: Yes   **Controlled Drug:** USA: No; Canada: No   **Available as Generic:** USA: Yes (all but amoxicillin/clavulanate); Canada: Yes

Brand Names: Amoxicillin: Amoxil, ✚Apo-Amoxi, ✚Clavulin, Larotid, ✚Novamoxin, ✚Nu-Amoxi, Polymox, Trimox, Wymox; Amoxicillin/clavulanate: Augmentin, ✚Clavulin; Ampicillin; Amcill, ✚Ampicin, ✚Ampicin PRB [CD], ✚Ampilean, ✚Apo-Ampi, D-Amp, Faspak Ampicillin, 500 Kit [CD], Nu-Ampi, ✚Novo-Ampicillin, Omnipen, Omnipen Pediatric Drops, Pardec Capsules [CD], ✚Penbritin, Polycillin, Polycillin Pediatric Drops, Polycillin-

PRB [CD], ♣Pondocillin, Principen, SK-Ampicillin, Totacillin; Bacampicillin: ♣Penglobe, Spectrobid; Cloxacillin: ♣Apo-Cloxi, ♣Bactopen, Cloxapen, ♣Novo-Cloxin, ♣Nu-Cloxi, ♣Orbenin, Tegopen; Penicillin VK: ♣Apo-Pen-VK, Beepen VK, Betapen-VK, Ledercillin VK, ♣Nadopen-V, ♣Novopen-VK, ♣Nu-Pen-VK, Penapar VK, Pen-V, ♣Pen-Vee, Pen-Vee K, Pfizerpen VK, ♣PVF, ♣PVF K, Robicillin VK, SK-Penicillin VK, Uticillin VK, V-Cillin K, ♣VC-K 500, Veetids

---

BENEFITS versus RISKS

Possible Benefits	*Possible Risks*
EFFECTIVE TREATMENT OF INFECTIONS due to susceptible microorganisms	ALLERGIC REACTIONS, mild to severe Superinfections (yeast) Drug-induced colitis—possible Lowering of white blood cells (amoxicillin/clavulanate, ampicillin, cloxacillin) Decreased kidney function

---

▷ **Principal Uses**

As a Single Drug Product: Uses currently included in FDA-approved labeling: (1) Used to treat responsive infections of the upper and lower respiratory tract, the middle ear (acute otitis media) (amoxicillin is a drug of choice), and the skin; (2) helps prevent rheumatic fever and bacterial endocarditis in people with valvular heart disease; (3) some *Haemophilus influenzae* infections (amoxicillin); (4) some genitourinary tract infections (amoxicillin/clavulanate, ampicillin, penicillin VK); (5) treats some cases of sinusitis; (6) ampicillin is used in combination to treat some kinds of septicemia and meningitis.

Other (unlabeled) generally accepted uses: (1) Combination therapy of animal bite wounds; (2) treatment of stage one Lyme disease in children (amoxicillin or penicillin VK); (3) therapy of Lyme disease involving the central nervous system (penicillin VK); (4) can have a role in treating dental abscesses (penicillin VK); (5) typhoid fever (amoxicillin); (6) combination antibiotic therapy of ulcers caused by *Helicobacter pylori* (amoxicillin); prevention of bacterial endocarditis (amoxicillin); (7) biliary tract infections or chancroid (amoxicillin/clavulanate); (8) cloxacillin may have a role in bone infections where intravenous (IV) medicines are not tolerated.

As a Combination Drug Product [CD]: Amoxicillin and clavulanate are combined (Augmentin) to give the benefits of amoxicillin combined with the ability to treat more resistant bacteria (clavulanate).

How These Drugs Work: These drugs destroy susceptible infecting bacteria by interfering with their ability to produce new protective cell walls as they multiply and grow. Amoxicillin/clavulanate uses the ability of clavulanate to block bacterial enzymes to enable the combination to treat resistant bacteria. Bacampicillin is converted to ampicillin and gives peak blood levels that are three times higher than ampicillin. This allows bacampicillin to be taken every 12 hours.

Available Dosage Forms and Strengths

Amoxicillin:

Capsules — 250 mg, 500 mg
Tablets, chewable — 125 mg, 250 mg
Oral liquid — 3 g
Oral suspension — 50 mg/ml, 125 mg/ml, 250 mg/5 ml
Pediatric drops — 50 mg/ml

Amoxicillin/clavulanate:

Oral suspension — 125 mg (amoxicillin) and 31.25 mg (clavulanate) per 5 ml—250 mg (amoxicillin) and 62.5 mg (clavulanate) per 5 ml—250 mg (amoxicillin) and 125 mg (clavulanate)—500 mg (amoxicillin) and 125 mg (clavulanate)

Pediatric formulation, twice daily — 200 mg (amoxicillin) and 28.6 mg (clavulanate) per 5 ml—400 mg (amoxicillin) and 57.1 (clavulanate) per 5 ml

Tablets, chewable — 125 mg (amoxicillin) and 31.25 mg (clavulanate)—250 mg (amoxicillin) and 62.5 mg (clavulanate)

Tablets, chewable twice-daily formulation — 200 mg (amoxicillin) and 28.6 mg (clavulanate)—400 mg (amoxicillin) and 57.1 (clavulanate)

Ampicillin:

Capsules — 250 mg, 500 mg
Oral suspension — 100 mg/ml, 125 mg/ml, 250 mg/ml, 500 mg/5 ml
Pediatric drops — 100 mg/ml

Bacampicillin:

Oral suspension — 125 mg/5 ml
Tablets — 400 mg, 800 mg (800 mg in Canada only)

Cloxacillin:

Capsules — 250 mg, 500 mg
Oral suspension — 125 mg/5 ml
Oral liquid — 125 mg/5 ml

Penicillin VK:

Oral solution — 125 mg/5 ml, 250 mg/5 ml
Tablets — 125 mg, 250 mg, 500 mg

▷ **Usual Adult Dosage Range:**   Dosage is based upon sensitivity testing of the bacteria causing the infection, severity of the infection, and response of the patient.
Penicillin VK: Depending upon the specific infection, the dosage range is 125

to 500 mg every 6 to 8 hours. For the prevention of bacterial endocarditis: 2 g (2000 mg) taken 1 hour before the procedure, followed by 1 g 6 hours later. The total daily dosage should not exceed 7 g (7000 mg).

Infants and Children: Amoxicillin: Up to 6 kg of body mass—25 to 50 mg every 8 hours. 6 to 8 kg of body mass—50 to 100 mg every 8 hours. 8 to 20 kg of body mass—6.7 to 13.3 mg per kg of body mass every 8 hours. 20 kg of body mass and over—same as 12 to 60 years of age.

Amoxicillin/clavulanate: Up to 40 kg of body mass—6.7 to 13.3 mg (amoxicillin) per kg of body mass, every 8 hours. 40 kg of body mass and over—same as 12 to 60 years of age. 12-hour formula: For severe infections—45 mg amoxicillin per kg of body mass **per day** (divided into two doses given every 12 hours). For less severe infections (as in skin infections)—25 mg per kg of body mass **per day** (divided into two doses given every 12 hours).

Bacampicillin: 25 mg per kg of body mass per day is given, divided into two equal doses every 12 hours, for respiratory infections.

Cloxacillin: For children weighing less than 44 lb (20 kg)—50 to 100 mg per kg of body mass per day, divided into four doses. Children greater than 20 kg receive the adult dose. The intravenous route may be required for severe infections.

12 to 60 Years of Age: Amoxicillin: Usual dose—250 to 500 mg every 8 hours. The total daily dose should not exceed 4.5 g. For gonorrhea—3 g, together with 1 g of probenecid, taken as a single dose. For Lyme disease—250 to 500 mg, three or four times a day, for 10 to 30 days; dose and duration of treatment depends on severity of infection and response to treatment.

Author's Note: New American Heart Association (AHA) guidelines for prevention of bacterial endocarditis in patients at risk for it suggest amoxicillin in an initial dose of 2 g in oral or dental procedures. There is no recommendation for follow-up doses of antibiotics.

Amoxicillin/clavulanate: Usual dose—250 to 500 mg (amoxicillin) every 8 hours. The total daily dose (of amoxicillin) should not exceed 4.5 g.

Ampicillin: 50 to 100 mg per kg of body mass per day divided into four doses, or 500 to 1000 mg every 6 hours. The usual maximal dose is 6000 mg daily.

Bacampicillin: For those with a body mass of 25 kg or more: 400 to 800 mg every 12 hours.

Cloxacillin: 250 to 500 mg every 6 hours. The maximum dose is 6000 mg (6 g) every 24 hours.

Over 60 Years of Age: Amoxicillin: Same as 12 to 60 years of age.

Amoxicillin/clavulanate: Same as 12 to 60 years of age. Note: The above doses refer to the amoxicillin component of amoxicillin/clavulanate. The 250-mg regular tablet and the 250-mg chewable tablet contain different amounts of clavulanate and are not interchangeable. See "Dosage Forms" above.

Ampicillin: This medicine is removed more slowly by patients in this age group; however, specific dose decreases are not defined.

Bacampicillin: Assessment of kidney function should be undertaken. Doses of 400 mg per day have been used because of moderate declines in kidney function (the age-related decline in kidney function may be moderate).

Cloxacillin: No specific dosing changes are available.

Note: Actual dosage and administration schedule must be determined for each patient individually for all of these medicines.

Conditions Requiring Dosing Adjustments

Liver Function: Dosage adjustments do not appear to be needed (amoxicillin, amoxicillin/clavulanate, ampicillin, and penicillin VK). Caution is advised for bacampicillin use by these patients. The dose must be decreased or the time between doses increased for cloxacillin.

Kidney Function: Amoxicillin, amoxicillin/clavulanate, ampicillin: Dosing interval **must** be adjusted in renal compromise.

Bacampicillin: The dose must be decreased to 400 mg per day in moderate kidney failure. In severe kidney failure a dose of 400 mg every 36 hours is used.

Penicillin VK: For patients with severe kidney compromise, the usual dose is taken every 8 hours.

Cloxacillin: Patients should be watched closely for adverse effects in severe kidney compromise.

▷ **Dosing Instructions:**   The tablet (amoxicillin, bacampicillin, penicillin VK) may be crushed (or amoxicillin and amoxicillin/clavulanate chew-tabs chewed), or the capsule (amoxicillin) opened and taken on an empty stomach or with food or milk (amoxicillin). Absorption may be slightly faster if taken when stomach is empty (penicillin VK). Ampicillin, bacampicillin, and cloxacillin are best taken on an empty stomach. Oral suspension forms should be shaken well before measuring each dose.

Usual Duration of Use: For all streptococcal infections—not less than 10 consecutive days (without interruption) to reduce the possibility of developing rheumatic fever or glomerulonephritis. For all other infections—as long as necessary to eradicate the infection. Talk with your doctor before stopping therapy if you feel you must stop this medicine. Incomplete treatment may lead to serious resistance and aggressive infections requiring combination therapy.

▷ **These Drugs Should Not Be Taken If**
- you have had an allergic reaction to any dosage form of it previously.
- you are certain you are allergic to *any* form of penicillin.

▷ **Inform Your Physician Before Taking This Drug If**
- you suspect you may be allergic to penicillin or have a history of a previous "reaction."
- you are allergic to any cephalosporin antibiotic (Ancef, Ceclor, etc.—see Drug Classes).
- you are allergic by nature (hay fever, asthma, hives, eczema).
- you are unsure of how much medicine to take or how often to take it.
- you have a history of liver or kidney disease.
- you have a history of low blood counts (amoxicillin/clavulanate, ampicillin, cloxacillin).

Possible Side Effects (natural, expected, and unavoidable drug actions)
Superinfections (see Glossary), often due to yeast organisms, or for some penicillins due to *Clostridium difficile*.

▷ **Possible Adverse Effects** (unusual, unexpected, and infrequent reactions)
If any of the following develop, consult your physician promptly for guidance.

Mild Adverse Effects
   Allergic Reactions: Skin rashes, hives, itching.
   Irritations of mouth or tongue, "black tongue," nausea, vomiting, diarrhea, dizziness—rare to infrequent.

Serious Adverse Effects
   Allergic Reactions: Anaphylactic reaction (see Glossary), severe skin reactions, drug fever, swollen painful joints, sore throat, abnormal bleeding or bruising.
   Severe skin reactions (Stevens-Johnson syndrome, bullous pemphigoid)—case reports.
   Drug-induced colitis—rare.
   Hemolytic anemia (penicillin VK)—case reports.
   Drug-induced periarteritis nodosa, meningitis, or porphyria—(penicillin VK)—case reports.
   Abnormal liver or kidney changes—rare.
   Drug-induced abnormal lowering of white blood cells (amoxicillin/clavulanate, ampicillin, cloxacillin, penicillin VK)—rare.

▷ **Possible Effects on Sexual Function:** None reported except for case reports of a small decrease in sperm counts for ampicillin.

Possible Effects on Laboratory Tests
   Complete blood counts: decreased red cells, hemoglobin, white cells (therapeutic effects of each antibiotic), and platelets (penicillin VK); increased eosinophils (allergic reactions).
   INR (prothrombin time): occasionally increased (ampicillin, cloxacillin, and penicillin VK).
   Liver function tests: increased aspartate aminotransferase (AST/GOT) and bilirubin (cloxacillin and penicillin VK).
   Coombs' test: may be positive with ampicillin or penicillin VK therapy.

CAUTION
   1. Take the exact dose and the full course prescribed.
   2. If these drugs must be used concurrently with antibiotics such as erythromycin or tetracycline, take the penicillin first.

Precautions for Use
   By Infants and Children: Watch children with allergies closely for evidence of a developing allergy to penicillin. These drugs (amoxicillin, penicillin VK) may cause diarrhea, which sometimes necessitates discontinuation. Up to 90% of patients with mononucleosis who take amoxicillin, amoxicillin/clavulanate, or ampicillin get a rash.
   By Those Over 60 Years of Age: Natural changes in the skin may predispose to prolonged itching reactions in the genital and anal regions. Report such reactions promptly.

▷ **Advisability of Use During Pregnancy**
   Pregnancy Category: B. See Pregnancy Risk Categories at the back of this book.
   Animal studies: Birth defects of the limbs reported in mice (penicillin VK only). (Not confirmed in other studies.)
   Human studies: Adequate studies of pregnant women indicate no increased risk of birth defects in 3,546 pregnancies exposed to penicillin derivatives.
   Ask your doctor for guidance, but these drugs are generally considered safe for use during any period of pregnancy.

Advisability of Use If Breast-Feeding
Presence of this drug in breast milk: Yes.
The nursing infant may be sensitized to penicillin and be at risk for developing diarrhea or yeast infections.
Avoid drug if possible or refrain from nursing.

Habit-Forming Potential: None.

Effects of Overdosage: Possible nausea, vomiting, and/or diarrhea.

Possible Effects of Long-Term Use: Superinfections, often due to yeast organisms or *Clostridium difficile*.

Suggested Periodic Examinations While Taking This Drug (at physician's discretion)
Complete blood cell counts, kidney function tests.

▷ **While Taking This Drug, Observe the Following**
Foods: No restrictions, except ampicillin, bacampicillin, and cloxacillin, which are best taken on an empty stomach.
Beverages: No restrictions (except as above). May be taken with milk.
▷   *Alcohol:* No interactions expected, but alcohol can blunt the immune response. It is best NOT to drink while you have an infection severe enough to require antibiotics.
Tobacco Smoking: No interactions expected, but I advise everyone to quit smoking.
▷   *Other Drugs*
Penicillins **taken concurrently** with
• disulfiram (Antabuse) can cause a disulfiramlike reaction (see Glossary) (bacampicillin only). Avoid the combination of these drugs.
• probenecid (Benemid) will increase and sustain blood levels. This interaction is often used to therapeutic advantage.
Ampicillin **taken concurrently** with
• allopurinol may increase the risk of rashes.
• atenolol can blunt the therapeutic benefits of atenolol.
Ampicillin, cloxacillin, or penicillin VK **taken concurrently** with
• warfarin (Coumadin) may intensify the anticoagulant effect and increase risk of bleeding. More frequent INR (prothrombin time or protime) testing is needed.
Penicillins may **decrease** the effects of
• birth control pills (oral contraceptives), and impair their effectiveness in preventing pregnancy.
The following drugs may **decrease** the effects of penicillins
• antacids, histamine (H_2) blockers, or proton pump inhibitors (see Drug Classes)—may reduce the absorption of penicillins.
• chloramphenicol (Chloromycetin).
• erythromycin (Erythrocin, E-Mycin, etc.).
• tetracyclines (Achromycin, Declomycin, Minocin, etc.—see Drug Classes).
▷   *Driving, Hazardous Activities:* Usually no restrictions. Be alert to the rare occurrence of dizziness and/or nausea, and restrict activities accordingly.
Aviation Note: The use of these drugs **may be a disqualification** for piloting. Consult a designated Aviation Medical Examiner.
Exposure to Sun: Ampicillin may increase sensitivity to the sun. Use caution.
Special Storage Instructions: Oral solutions and pediatric drops (amoxicillin) should be refrigerated.

Observe the Following Expiration Times: Do not take the oral solution of these drugs if older than 7 days (cloxacillin is good for only 3 days) if kept at room temperature, or 14 days when kept refrigerated.

PENTAZOCINE (pen TAZ oh seen)

Introduced: 1967   **Class:** Analgesic, strong   **Prescription:** USA: Yes
Controlled Drug: USA: C-IV*; Canada: No   **Available as Generic:** USA: No; Canada: No

Brand Names: Talacen [CD], Talwin, Talwin Compound [CD], ✦Talwin Compound-50 [CD], Talwin Nx [CD]

BENEFITS versus RISKS

Possible Benefits	*Possible Risks*
EFFECTIVE RELIEF OF MODERATE TO SEVERE PAIN	POTENTIAL FOR HABIT FORMATION (DEPENDENCE) Respiratory depression Sedative effects Mental and behavioral disturbances Low blood pressure, fainting Nausea, constipation

---

▷ **Principal Uses**

As a Single Drug Product: Uses currently included in FDA-approved labeling: Relieves acute or chronic pain of moderate to severe degree from any cause. Other (unlabeled) generally accepted uses: None.

As a Combination Drug Product [CD]: Pentazocine is available in combinations with acetaminophen and with aspirin. These milder pain relievers are added to enhance the analgesic effect and reduce fever when present. In the United States the tablet form of pentazocine also contains naloxone (Talwin Nx), a narcotic antagonist that renders the drug ineffective if abused.

How This Drug Works: Acting primarily as a depressant of certain brain functions, this drug suppresses the perception of pain and calms the emotional response to pain.

Available Dosage Forms and Strengths

Caplet — 25 mg pentazocine and 650 mg acetaminophen
Injection — 30 mg/ml
Tablets — 50 mg (Canada)
Tablets — 50 mg with 0.5 mg of naloxone (U.S.)

▷ **Usual Adult Dosage Range:** Oral dosing: 50 mg every 3 to 4 hours. May be increased to 100 mg every 4 hours for severe pain. The total daily dosage should not exceed 600 mg. Many clinicians now use timed or scheduled dosing of pain medicines (analgesics), particularly early in acute pain, as this tends to prevent pain rather than treat it. Others revert to as-needed dosing once the acute pain is controlled. **Note: Actual dosage and administration schedule must be determined for each patient individually.**

*See schedules of Controlled Drugs at the back of this book.

Conditions Requiring Dosing Adjustments
Liver Function: Doses should be decreased or the time between doses lengthened, otherwise increased adverse effects may occur.
Kidney Function: For moderate to severe kidney failure, the dose should be reduced by 25–50%.

▷ **Dosing Instructions:** The tablet may be crushed and taken with or following food to reduce stomach irritation or nausea.

Usual Duration of Use: As required to control pain. Continual use should not exceed 5 to 7 days without interruption and reassessment of need.

▷ **This Drug Should Not Be Taken If**
- you have had an allergic reaction to any dosage form of it previously.
- you are having an acute attack of asthma.
- you have increased intracranial pressure or brain damage.

▷ **Inform Your Physician Before Taking This Drug If**
- you have had an unfavorable reaction to any narcotic drug in the past.
- you have a history of drug abuse or alcoholism.
- you have chronic lung disease with impaired breathing.
- you have impaired liver or kidney function.
- you have a history of confusion or hallucinations.
- you have gallbladder disease, a seizure disorder, or an underactive thyroid gland.
- you have difficulty emptying the urinary bladder.
- you are taking any other drugs that have a sedative effect.
- you plan to have surgery under general anesthesia in the near future.

Possible Side Effects (natural, expected, and unavoidable drug actions)
Drowsiness, light-headedness, weakness, urinary retention, constipation.

▷ **Possible Adverse Effects** (unusual, unexpected, and infrequent reactions)
If any of the following develop, consult your physician promptly for guidance.
Mild Adverse Effects
Allergic Reactions: Skin rash, hives, itching, swelling of face.
Headache, dizziness, sensation of drunkenness, blurred or double vision, flushing, sweating—infrequent and can be dose related.
Increased or decreased blood pressure—infrequent.
Drug fever—rare.
Nausea, vomiting, indigestion, diarrhea—infrequent to frequent.
Serious Adverse Effects
Marked drop in blood pressure, possible fainting—case reports and dose related.
Impaired breathing (respiratory depression)—possible and dose related.
Mental and behavioral disturbances, hallucinations, psychosis—case reports.
Drug-induced seizure, porphyria, or toxic epidermal necrolysis—rare.
Fibrous muscle replacement (with injection form)—rare.
Kidney problems—rare.
Fixed positioning of the eyes (oculogyric crisis)—case report.
Bone marrow depression (see Glossary) of a mild and reversible nature—rare.
Aggravation of prostatism (see Glossary)—possible.

▷ **Possible Effects on Sexual Function:**   Blunting of sexual response—possible.

Natural Diseases or Disorders That May Be Activated by This Drug
Porphyria (see Glossary).

Possible Effects on Laboratory Tests
White blood cell count: rarely decreased.
Blood amylase and lipase levels: increased (natural side effects).

CAUTION
1. Use of this drug with atropinelike drugs may increase the risk of urinary retention and reduced intestinal function.
2. Do not take this drug following acute head injury.

Precautions for Use
By Infants and Children: Safety and effectiveness for those under 12 years of age are not established.
By Those Over 60 Years of Age: Use small doses initially and increase dosage as needed and tolerated. Limit use to short-term treatment only. There may be increased susceptibility to development of drowsiness, dizziness, unsteadiness, falling, urinary retention, and constipation.

▷ **Advisability of Use During Pregnancy**
Pregnancy Category: C (B or D in high doses at term or extended use). See Pregnancy Risk Categories at the back of this book.
Animal studies: Significant birth defects reported in hamsters.
Human studies: Adequate studies of pregnant women are not available. Pentazocine taken repeatedly during the final few weeks before delivery may cause withdrawal symptoms in the newborn infant.
Avoid this drug during the first 3 months. Use only if clearly needed and in small, infrequent doses during the final 6 months.

Advisability of Use If Breast-Feeding
Presence of this drug in breast milk: Expected.
Avoid drug or refrain from nursing.

Habit-Forming Potential: Psychological and/or physical dependence can develop.

Effects of Overdosage: Anxiety, disturbed thoughts, hallucinations, progressive drowsiness, stupor, depressed breathing.

Possible Effects of Long-Term Use: Psychological and physical dependence, chronic constipation.

Suggested Periodic Examinations While Taking This Drug (at physician's discretion)
Complete blood cell counts, if used for an extended period of time.

▷ **While Taking This Drug, Observe the Following**
Foods: No restrictions.
Beverages: No restrictions. May be taken with milk.
▷ *Alcohol:* Pentazocine can intensify the intoxicating effects of alcohol, and alcohol can intensify the depressant effects of pentazocine on brain function, breathing, and circulation. It is best to avoid this combination.
Tobacco Smoking: Heavy smoking may reduce the effectiveness. I advise everyone to quit smoking.
Marijuana Smoking: Increase in drowsiness and pain relief; impairment of mental and physical performance.

▷ *Other Drugs*

Pentazocine may *increase* the effects of

- atropinelike drugs, and increase the risk of constipation and urinary retention.
- cyclosporine (Sandimmune) and cause toxicity.
- MAO inhibitors (see Drug Classes)—may result in muscle rigidity.
- other drugs with sedative effects (see Drug Classes on benzodiazepines, phenothiazines, and opioids).

▷ *Driving, Hazardous Activities:* This drug can impair mental alertness, judgment, reaction time, and physical coordination. Avoid hazardous activities accordingly.

Aviation Note: The use of this drug *is a disqualification* for piloting. Consult a designated Aviation Medical Examiner.

Exposure to Sun: No restrictions.

Discontinuation: It is advisable to limit this drug to short-term use. If it is necessary to use it for extended periods of time, discontinuation should be gradual to minimize possible effects of withdrawal.

PENTOXIFYLLINE (pen tox I fi leen)

Other Name: Oxpentifylline

Introduced: 1972   **Class:** Blood flow agent, xanthines   **Prescription:** USA: Yes   **Controlled Drug:** USA: No; Canada: No   **Available as Generic:** No

Brand Name: Trental

BENEFITS versus RISKS	
Possible Benefits	*Possible Risks*
IMPROVED BLOOD FLOW IN PERIPHERAL ARTERIAL DISEASE	Reduced blood pressure, angina, abnormal heart rhythms
REDUCTION OF INTERMITTENT CLAUDICATION PAIN	Rare low blood counts and aplastic anemia
May help in some AIDS-related pain	Indigestion, nausea, vomiting
	Dizziness, flushing

▷ **Principal Uses**

As a Single Drug Product: Uses currently included in FDA-approved labeling: Adjunctive treatment in the management of peripheral obstructive arterial disease to improve arterial blood flow and reduce frequency and severity of muscle pain due to intermittent claudication.

Other (unlabeled) generally accepted uses: (1) Decreases hemodialysis shunt clots (thrombosis); (2) may have a role in treating impotence that is caused by blood vessel problems (vascular impotence); (3) can increase the motility of sperm; (4) helps decrease interleukin and tumor necrosis factor in patients with cerebral malaria; (5) has had variable results in AIDS patients in attempting to halt weight loss that may be caused by tumor necrosis factor; (6) may ease skin tightening in some cases; (7) has been used to relieve symptoms of septic shock; (8) has been used to help heal refractory ulcers in diabetics; (9) may decrease insulin requirements in some diabetics and help retinopathy and neuropathy.

How This Drug Works: Improves blood flow and increases oxygen supply to working muscles by way of three mechanisms: (1) reduction of blood viscosity due to decreased levels of fibrinogen in the blood; (2) increased flexibility of the red blood cells (carrying oxygen) due to an increase in cyclic AMP (enzyme) within red blood cells—this permits easier passage through the small blood vessels of the microcirculation; and (3) prevention of red blood cell and platelet aggregation. Inhibits interleukins and tumor necrosis factor (problems in diabetes, heart attacks, and other conditions).

Available Dosage Forms and Strengths
Tablets, prolonged action — 400 mg

▷ **Usual Adult Dosage Range:** 400 mg three times a day. If adverse nervous system or gastrointestinal effects occur, reduce the dose to 400 mg twice daily. **Note: Actual dosage and administration schedule must be determined for each patient individually.**

Conditions Requiring Dosing Adjustments
Liver Function: Dosing changes do not appear to be needed in liver compromise.
Kidney Function: The dose should be decreased. 400 mg twice daily to start has been suggested.

▷ **Dosing Instructions:** Take with or following food to reduce stomach irritation. Swallow the tablet whole without breaking, crushing, or chewing.

Usual Duration of Use: Use on a regular schedule for 2 to 4 weeks determines effectiveness in preventing or delaying the pains of intermittent claudication associated with walking. Treatment for a minimum of 3 months is recommended to determine full effectiveness. Long-term use (months to years) requires physician supervision and periodic evaluation. Dosing is individualized for other conditions.

Possible Advantages of This Drug
Reduces blood viscosity and thereby improves blood flow through small vessels.
Increases supply of oxygen to working muscles.

▷ **This Drug Should Not Be Taken If**
• you have had an allergic reaction to it previously.

▷ **Inform Your Physician Before Taking This Drug If**
• you are allergic to other xanthine drugs: caffeine, theophylline, theobromine.
• you have impaired kidney function.
• you have low blood pressure, impaired brain circulation, or coronary artery disease.
• you are a diabetic.
• you have an ulcer of the stomach or intestine.
• you smoke tobacco.
• you are taking any antihypertensive drugs.

Possible Side Effects (natural, expected, and unavoidable drug actions)
Lowering of blood pressure (usually mild).

▷ **Possible Adverse Effects** (unusual, unexpected, and infrequent reactions)
If any of the following develop, consult your physician promptly for guidance.

Mild Adverse Effects
  Allergic Reaction: Skin rash.
  Headache, blurred vision and scotoma, dizziness, tremor—rare.
  May worsen glucose control in diabetics—possible.
  Nosebleeds—rare.
  Flu-like syndrome. Indigestion, nausea, vomiting—rare to infrequent.
Serious Adverse Effects
  Development of angina or heart rhythm disorders—rare.
  Liver toxicity—rare.
  Low platelets, white blood cells, or all cells—rare.
  Auditory hallucinations—case report.
  Retinal bleeding—case reports.
  Bleeding from ulcers of stomach or intestine—case reports and questionable
    association.

▷ **Possible Effects on Sexual Function**
  May help reverse impotence caused by circulatory problems.

Possible Effects on Laboratory Tests
  Complete blood cell counts: rarely decreased red cells, hemoglobin, white
    cells, and platelets. Liver enzymes—rare increases.

CAUTION
  Use this drug with caution in the presence of impaired circulation within the
    brain (cerebral arteriosclerosis) or coronary artery disease. If any related
    symptoms develop, consult your physician for prompt evaluation.

Precautions for Use
  By Infants and Children: Safety and effectiveness for those under 18 years of age
    are not established. Use by this age group is not anticipated.
  By Those Over 60 Years of Age: You may be more susceptible to the adverse
    effects listed. Observe closely for any indications of dizziness or chest pain
    and report these promptly.

▷ **Advisability of Use During Pregnancy**
  Pregnancy Category: C. See Pregnancy Risk Categories at the back of this book.
    Animal studies: Increased fetal resorptions reported in rats, but no birth de-
      fects found in rats or rabbits.
    Human studies: Adequate studies of pregnant women are not available.
    Avoid use during the first 3 months. Use otherwise only if clearly needed.

Advisability of Use If Breast-Feeding
  Presence of this drug in breast milk: Yes.
  Avoid drug or refrain from nursing.

Habit-Forming Potential: None.

Effects of Overdosage: Drowsiness, flushing, faintness, excitement, seizures.

Possible Effects of Long-Term Use: None reported.

Suggested Periodic Examinations While Taking This Drug (at physician's dis-
    cretion)
  Blood pressure measurements, evaluation of heart status.

▷ **While Taking This Drug, Observe the Following**
  Foods: No restrictions.
  Beverages: No restrictions. May be taken with milk.
▷ *Alcohol:* Alcohol may increase the blood-pressure-lowering effect of this drug.

Tobacco Smoking: Nicotine constricts arteries and impairs pentoxifylline effectiveness significantly. Avoid tobacco.

▷ *Other Drugs*

Pentoxifylline may ***increase*** the effects of
- antihypertensive drugs, and cause excessive lowering of blood pressure.
- warfarin (Coumadin, etc.), and increase the possibility of unwanted bleeding; monitor INR (prothrombin time or protime) more frequently. Dosing should be adjusted to laboratory values.

Pentoxifylline ***taken concurrently*** with
- cimetidine (Tagamet), nizatidine (Axid), famotidine (Pepcid), or ranitidine (Zantac) may result in pentoxifylline toxicity (increases drug absorption).
- theophylline (Theo-Dur, others) may result in theophylline toxicity.

▷ *Driving, Hazardous Activities:* This drug may cause drowsiness or dizziness. Restrict activities as necessary.

Aviation Note: The use of this drug ***may be a disqualification*** for piloting. Consult a designated Aviation Medical Examiner.

Exposure to Sun: No restrictions.

PERGOLIDE (PER go lide)

Introduced: 1980   **Class:** Anti-parkinsonism, ergot derivative   **Prescription:** USA: Yes   **Controlled Drug:** USA: No; Canada: No   **Available as Generic:** USA: No

Brand Name: Permax

BENEFITS versus RISKS	
Possible Benefits	*Possible Risks*
ADDITIVE RELIEF OF SYMPTOMS OF PARKINSON'S DISEASE when used concurrently with levodopa/carbidopa PERMITS A REDUCTION IN SINEMET DOSAGE	ABNORMAL INVOLUNTARY MOVEMENTS HALLUCINATIONS INITIAL FALL IN BLOOD PRESSURE/ORTHOSTATIC HYPOTENSION Premature heart contractions (ventricular)

▷ **Principal Uses**

As a Single Drug Product: Uses currently included in FDA-approved labeling: As an adjunct to levodopa/carbidopa treatment of Parkinson's disease for people who experience intolerable abnormal movements (dyskinesia) and/or increasing "on–off" episodes due to levodopa. The addition of pergolide (1) permits reduction of the daily dose of levodopa with consequent lessening of dyskinesia and erratic drug response, and (2) provides additional relief of parkinsonian symptoms.

Other (unlabeled) generally accepted uses: (1) May have a role in helping reduce drug craving in cocaine withdrawal; (2) helps in some conditions where excess prolactin is made; (3) may be of use in acromegaly.

How This Drug Works: By directly stimulating part of the brain (dopamine receptor sites in the corpus striatum), this drug helps to compensate for the deficiency of dopamine that is responsible for the rigidity, tremor, and sluggish movement characteristic of Parkinson's disease.

Available Dosage Forms and Strengths

Tablets — 0.05 mg, 0.25 mg, 1 mg

▷ **Usual Adult Dosage Range**

Parkinson's (in conjunction with levodopa plus carbidopa): Initially 0.05 mg daily for the first 2 days; gradually increase the daily dose by 0.1 mg or 0.15 mg every third day over the next 12 days. If needed and tolerated, the daily dose may be increased further by 0.25 mg every third day until an optimal response is achieved. The total daily dosage should be divided into three equal portions and taken at 6- to 8-hour intervals. The usual maintenance dose is 3 mg every 24 hours; do not exceed 5 mg every 24 hours.

During the gradual introduction of pergolide, the concurrent dose of levodopa/carbidopa (Sinemet) may be cautiously decreased in accordance with your physician's instructions. **Note: Actual dosage and administration schedule must be determined for each patient individually.**

Conditions Requiring Dosing Adjustments

Liver Function: Specific guidelines for liver compromise are not available. It should be used with caution.

Kidney Function: Consideration should be given to empirical decreases in dosage.

▷ **Dosing Instructions:**   The tablet may be crushed and taken with food or milk to reduce stomach irritation.

Usual Duration of Use: Use on a regular schedule for 4 to 6 weeks determines effectiveness in controlling the symptoms of Parkinson's disease and permitting reduction of levodopa/carbidopa dosage. Long-term use (months to years) requires periodic physician evaluation of response.

Possible Advantages of This Drug: It may provide a more effective and uniform control of parkinsonian symptoms, and a reduction of some adverse effects of long-term levodopa therapy.

▷ **This Drug Should Not Be Taken If**
- you have had an allergic reaction to it previously.
- you have had a serious adverse effect from any ergot preparation.
- you have severe coronary artery disease or peripheral vascular disease.

▷ **Inform Your Physician Before Taking This Drug If**
- you have constitutionally low blood pressure.
- you are pregnant or breast-feeding your infant.
- you are taking any antihypertensive drugs or antipsychotic drugs (see Drug Classes).
- you have any degree of coronary artery disease, especially angina or a history of heart attack.
- you have any type of heart rhythm disorder.
- you have impaired liver or kidney function.
- you have a seizure disorder.

Possible Side Effects (natural, expected, and unavoidable drug actions)

Weakness; chest pain—possibly anginal; peripheral edema; orthostatic hypotension (see Glossary).

▷ **Possible Adverse Effects** (unusual, unexpected, and infrequent reactions)
If any of the following develop, consult your physician promptly for guidance.

Mild Adverse Effects

Allergic Reactions: Skin rash, facial swelling—rare.

Headache, dizziness, hallucinations, drowsiness, insomnia, anxiety, double vision—rare to infrequent.

Nasal congestion, shortness of breath, palpitation, fainting—rare to infrequent.

Altered taste, dry mouth, indigestion, nausea, vomiting, constipation, diarrhea—infrequent.

Serious Adverse Effects

Allergic Reactions: None reported.

Idiosyncratic Reactions: Flu-like symptoms.

Abnormal involuntary movements (dyskinesia)—frequent; psychotic behavior—case reports.

Hallucinations (accounted for 7.8% of patient withdrawals from therapy; 13.8% occurrence).

Abnormal heartbeat (ventricular arrhythmias)—infrequent to frequent.

Anemia—rare.

▷ **Possible Effects on Sexual Function**

Infrequent reports of altered libido (increased or decreased), impotence, breast pain, priapism (see Glossary).

▷ **Adverse Effects That May Mimic Natural Diseases or Disorders**

Effects on mental function and behavior may resemble psychotic disorders.

Natural Diseases or Disorders That May Be Activated by This Drug

Coronary artery disease with anginal syndrome, heart rhythm disorders, Raynaud's phenomenon (see Glossary), seizure disorders.

Possible Effects on Laboratory Tests

Blood prolactin level: decreased (marked reduction).

CAUTION

1. May cause abnormal movements (dyskinesias), intensify existing dyskinesias. Watch carefully for tremors, twitching, or abnormal, involuntary movements of any kind. Report these promptly.
2. Low starting doses help prevent possibility of excessive drop in blood pressure. See dosage routine outlined above.
3. Inform your physician promptly if you become pregnant or plan pregnancy. This drug has been reported (rarely) to cause abortion and birth defects.

Precautions for Use

By Infants and Children: This drug is not utilized by this age group.

By Those Over 60 Years of Age: Small initial doses are mandatory. Watch closely for any tendency to light-headedness or faintness, especially on arising from a lying or sitting position. You may be more susceptible to the development of impaired thinking, confusion, agitation, nightmares, or hallucinations.

▷ **Advisability of Use During Pregnancy**
  Pregnancy Category: B. See Pregnancy Risk Categories at the back of this book.
    Animal studies: No birth defects due to this drug were found in mouse or rabbit studies.
    Human studies: Adequate studies of pregnant women are not available. However, there are four reports of birth defects associated with the use of this drug and infrequent reports of abortion. Causal relationships have not been established, but prudence advises against the use of this drug during pregnancy. Consult your physician for guidance.

Advisability of Use If Breast-Feeding
  Presence of this drug in breast milk: Unknown.
  Avoid drug or refrain from nursing.

Habit-Forming Potential: None.

Effects of Overdosage: Nausea, vomiting, palpitations, low blood pressure, agitation, severe involuntary movements, hallucinations, seizures.

Possible Effects of Long-Term Use: Increased risk of developing dyskinesias.

Suggested Periodic Examinations While Taking This Drug (at physician's discretion)
  Regular evaluation of drug response, heart function, and blood pressure status.

▷ **While Taking This Drug, Observe the Following**
  Foods: No restrictions.
  Beverages: No restrictions. May be taken with milk.
▷ *Alcohol:* Alcohol can exaggerate the blood-pressure-lowering and sedative effects of this drug.
  Tobacco Smoking: No interactions expected, but I advise everyone to quit smoking.
▷ *Other Drugs*
    Pergolide *taken concurrently* with
    • antihypertensive drugs (and other drugs that can lower blood pressure) requires careful monitoring for excessive drops in pressure. Dosage adjustments may be necessary.
    The following drugs may *decrease* the effects of pergolide and diminish its effectiveness
    • chlorprothixene (Taractan).
    • haloperidol (Haldol).
    • metoclopramide (Reglan).
    • phenothiazines (see Drug Classes).
    • thiothixene (Navane).
▷ *Driving, Hazardous Activities:* This drug may cause dizziness, drowsiness, impaired coordination, or fainting. Restrict activities as necessary.
  Aviation Note: The use of this drug *is a disqualification* for piloting. Consult a designated Aviation Medical Examiner.
  Exposure to Sun: No restrictions.
  Exposure to Heat: Use caution until the combined effects have been determined. Hot environments can cause lowering of blood pressure.
  Discontinuation: Do not stop this drug abruptly. Sudden withdrawal can cause confusion, paranoid thinking, and severe hallucinations. Consult your physician regarding a schedule for gradual withdrawal.

PERPHENAZINE (per FEN a zeen)

Introduced: 1957   **Class:** Tranquilizer, major; phenothiazines   **Prescription:** USA: Yes   **Controlled Drug:** USA: No; Canada: No   **Available as Generic:** USA: Yes; Canada: Yes

Brand Names: ✦Apo-Perphenazine, ✦Elavil Plus [CD], ✦Entrafon, Etrafon [CD], Etrafon-A [CD], Etrafon Forte [CD], ✦Phenazine, ✦PMS-Levazine, ✦PMS-Perphenazine, Triavil [CD], Trilafon

---

BENEFITS versus RISKS

Possible Benefits	*Possible Risks*
EFFECTIVE CONTROL OF ACUTE MENTAL DISORDERS	SERIOUS TOXIC EFFECTS ON BRAIN with long-term use
Beneficial effects on thinking, mood, and behavior	Liver damage with jaundice
Relief of anxiety and tension	Blood cell disorders: hemolytic anemia, abnormally low white
Moderately effective control of nausea and vomiting	blood cell and platelet counts

---

▷ **Principal Uses**

As a Single Drug Product: Uses currently included in FDA-approved labeling: (1) Used to treat acute and chronic psychotic disorders such as agitated depression, schizophrenia, and similar states of mental dysfunction; (2) may be used as a tranquilizer to help agitated and disruptive behavior in the absence of true psychosis; (3) sometimes used to treat severe nausea and vomiting.

Other (unlabeled) generally accepted uses: Can ease tremors caused by tricyclic antidepressants.

As a Combination Drug Product [CD]: Available combined with amitriptyline, an effective antidepressant. In some cases of severe agitated depression, the combination of a specific antipsychotic drug and a specific antidepressant drug will be more effective than either drug used alone.

How This Drug Works: By inhibiting dopamine, this drug acts to correct an imbalance of nerve impulse transmissions thought to be responsible for mental disorders.

Available Dosage Forms and Strengths

Concentrate — 16 mg/5 ml

Injection — 5 mg/ml

Tablets — 2 mg, 4 mg, 8 mg, 16 mg

Tablets, prolonged action — 8 mg

▷ **Usual Adult Dosage Range:** Psychotic symptoms (patients not hospitalized): Initially 4 to 8 mg three times daily. Dose may be increased by 4 mg at 3- to 4-day intervals as needed and tolerated. The total daily dosage should not exceed 64 mg. **Note: Actual dosage and administration schedule must be determined for each patient individually.**

Conditions Requiring Dosing Adjustments

Liver Function: The dose should be empirically decreased for patients with liver compromise. Perphenazine is contraindicated for patients with moderate to severe liver compromise.

Kidney Function: The kidney is minimally involved in the elimination of this drug.

▷ **Dosing Instructions:**   This drug may be taken with or following meals to reduce stomach irritation. The regular tablets may be crushed for administration; the prolonged-action tablets should be taken whole, not broken, crushed, or chewed.

Usual Duration of Use: Use on a regular schedule for several weeks determines this drug's effectiveness in controlling psychotic disorders. If it is not significantly beneficial within 6 weeks, it should be stopped. Long-term use (months to years) requires periodic physician evaluation of response, and consideration of continued need.

▷ **This Drug Should Not Be Taken If**
- you are allergic to any of the drugs bearing the brand names listed.
- you have active liver disease.
- you have brain damage in the subcortical area.
- you have cancer of the breast.
- you have a current blood cell or bone marrow disorder.

▷ **Inform Your Physician Before Taking This Drug If**
- you are allergic or abnormally sensitive to any phenothiazine (see Drug Classes).
- you have impaired liver or kidney function.
- you have any type of seizure disorder.
- you have diabetes, glaucoma, lupus erythematosus, or heart disease.
- you are pregnant or breast-feeding your infant.
- you have an allergy to sulfites.
- you have a history of neuroleptic malignant syndrome.
- you are taking any drug with sedative effects.
- you plan to have surgery under general or spinal anesthesia soon.

Possible Side Effects (natural, expected, and unavoidable drug actions)
Drowsiness (usually during the first 2 weeks), orthostatic hypotension (see Glossary), blurred vision, dry mouth, nasal congestion, constipation, impaired urination.
Pink or purple coloration of urine, of no significance.

▷ **Possible Adverse Effects** (unusual, unexpected, and infrequent reactions)
If any of the following develop, consult your physician promptly for guidance.
Mild Adverse Effects
Allergic Reactions: Skin rash, hives, low-grade fever.
Lowering of body temperature, especially in the elderly (see Hypothermia in Glossary)—possible.
Increased appetite and weight gain—possible.
Dizziness, weakness, agitation, insomnia, impaired day and night vision—frequent.
Chronic constipation, fecal impaction—possible.
Serious Adverse Effects
Allergic Reactions: Hepatitis with jaundice (see Glossary), severe skin reactions (systemic lupus erythematosus, Stevens-Johnson syndrome), anaphylaxis—case reports.

Idiosyncratic Reactions: Neuroleptic malignant syndrome (see Glossary).

Depression; disorientation; seizures; deposits in cornea, lens, and retina—possible to infrequent.

Rapid heart rate, heart rhythm disorders—case reports.

Blood cell disorders: hemolytic anemia, reduced white blood cell or platelet counts—case reports.

Nervous system reactions: Parkinson-like disorders (see Glossary), severe restlessness, muscle spasms involving the face and neck, tardive dyskinesia (see Glossary)—case reports.

▷ **Possible Effects on Sexual Function**

Altered timing and pattern of menstruation.

Female breast enlargement with milk production.

False-positive pregnancy test results.

Male breast enlargement and tenderness (gynecomastia).

Painful and extended duration of erection (priapism) or inhibited ejaculation—case reports.

▷ **Adverse Effects That May Mimic Natural Diseases or Disorders**

Nervous system reactions may suggest true Parkinson's disease.

Liver reactions may suggest viral hepatitis.

Reactions resembling systemic lupus erythematosus can occur.

Natural Diseases or Disorders That May Be Activated by This Drug

Latent epilepsy, glaucoma, diabetes mellitus, prostatism (see Glossary).

Possible Effects on Laboratory Tests

White blood cell counts: decreased.

Blood bilirubin level: increased (jaundice—see Glossary).

Blood glucose level: increased.

Glucose tolerance test (GTT): decreased in 35% of those taking this drug.

CAUTION

1. Many over-the-counter medications (see Glossary) for allergies, colds, and coughs contain drugs that can interact unfavorably with this drug. Ask your physician or pharmacist for help **before** using any such medications.
2. Antacids that contain aluminum and/or magnesium can prevent the absorption of this drug and reduce its effectiveness.
3. Obtain prompt evaluation of any change or disturbance of vision.

Precautions for Use

By Infants and Children: Use of this drug is not recommended in children under 12 years of age. Do not use this drug in the presence of symptoms suggestive of Reye syndrome (see Glossary). Children with acute infectious diseases (flu-like infections, chickenpox, measles, etc.) are more prone to develop spasms of the face, back, and extremities if this drug is used to control nausea or vomiting.

By Those Over 60 Years of Age: Small starting doses are advisable. Increased susceptibility to development of drowsiness, lethargy, constipation, lowering of body temperature (hypothermia), and orthostatic hypotension (see Glossary). This drug can enhance existing prostatism (see Glossary). You may also be more susceptible to the development of Parkinson-like reactions and/or tardive dyskinesia (see Glossary). These reactions must be recognized early, as they may become unresponsive to treatment and irreversible.

▷ **Advisability of Use During Pregnancy**

Pregnancy Category: C. See Pregnancy Risk Categories at the back of this book.
Animal studies: Cleft palate reported in mouse and rat studies.
Human studies: No increase in birth defects reported in 166 exposures. Information from adequate studies of pregnant women is not available.
Avoid drug during the first 3 months; avoid during the final month because of possible effects on the newborn infant.

Advisability of Use If Breast-Feeding

Presence of this drug in breast milk: Yes, in minute amounts.
Monitor nursing infant closely and discontinue drug or nursing if adverse effects develop.

Habit-Forming Potential: None.

Effects of Overdosage: Marked drowsiness, weakness, tremor, agitation, unsteadiness, deep sleep, coma, convulsions.

Possible Effects of Long-Term Use: Opacities in the cornea or lens of the eye, pigmentation of the retina.
Tardive dyskinesia (see Glossary).

Suggested Periodic Examinations While Taking This Drug (at physician's discretion)

Complete blood cell counts, especially between the 4th and 10th weeks of treatment.
Liver function tests, electrocardiograms.
Complete eye examinations—eye structures and vision.
Careful inspection of the tongue for early evidence of fine, involuntary, wavelike movements that could indicate the beginning of tardive dyskinesia.

▷ **While Taking This Drug, Observe the Following**

Foods: No restrictions.
Nutritional Support: A riboflavin (vitamin B_2) supplement should be taken with long-term use.
Beverages: No restrictions. May be taken with milk.

▷ *Alcohol:* Avoid completely. Alcohol can increase the sedative action of phenothiazines and accentuate their depressant effects on brain function and blood pressure. Phenothiazines can increase the intoxicating effects of alcohol.

Tobacco Smoking: Possible reduction of drowsiness from drug. I advise everyone to quit smoking.

Marijuana Smoking: Moderate increase in drowsiness; accentuation of orthostatic hypotension; increased risk of precipitating latent psychoses, confusing the interpretation of mental status and drug responses.

▷ *Other Drugs*

Perphenazine may *increase* the effects of
• all atropinelike drugs, and cause nervous system toxicity.
• all sedative drugs, especially meperidine (Demerol), and cause excessive sedation.

Perphenazine may *decrease* the effects of
• guanethidine (Ismelin, Esimil), and reduce its effectiveness in lowering blood pressure.
• oral antidiabetic drugs (see Drug Classes) and cause loss of glucose control.

Perphenazine *taken concurrently* with
- ascorbic acid may blunt the therapeutic effect of perphenazine.
- lithium (Lithobid, Lithotabs) may impair the effectiveness of lithium and cause nervous system toxicity.
- monoamine oxidase (MAO) inhibitor drugs (see Drug Classes) may result in increased extrapyramidal reactions.
- ritonavir (Norvir) and perhaps other protease inhibitors (see Drug Classes) may lead to toxicity.

The following drugs may *decrease* the effects of perphenazine
- antacids containing aluminum and/or magnesium.
- barbiturates (see Drug Classes).
- benztropine (Cogentin).
- disulfiram (Antabuse).
- trihexyphenidyl (Artane).

▷ *Driving, Hazardous Activities:* This drug can impair mental alertness, judgment, and physical coordination. Avoid hazardous activities.

Aviation Note: The use of this drug *is a disqualification* for piloting. Consult a designated Aviation Medical Examiner.

Exposure to Sun: Use caution—some phenothiazines can cause photosensitivity (see Glossary).

Exposure to Heat: Use caution and avoid excessive heat as much as possible. This drug may impair the regulation of body temperature and increase the risk of heatstroke.

Exposure to Cold: Use caution and dress warmly. This drug can increase the risk of hypothermia in the elderly.

Discontinuation: After a period of long-term use, do not stop this drug suddenly. Gradual withdrawal over 2 to 3 weeks under physician supervision is recommended. Do not discontinue this drug without your physician's knowledge and approval. The relapse rate of schizophrenia after discontinuation is 50–60%.

PHENELZINE (FEN el zeen)

Introduced: 1961   **Class:** Antidepressant, MAO type A inhibitor   **Prescription:** USA: Yes   **Controlled Drug:** USA: No; Canada: No   **Available as Generic:** No

Brand Name: Nardil

BENEFITS versus RISKS	
Possible Benefits	*Possible Risks*
EFFECTIVE RELIEF OF REACTIVE, NEUROTIC, ATYPICAL DEPRESSIONS with associated anxiety or phobia	DANGEROUS INTERACTIONS WITH MANY DRUGS AND FOODS
Beneficial in some depressions that are not responsive to other treatments	CONDUCIVE TO HYPERTENSIVE CRISIS
	DISORDERED HEART RATE AND RHYTHM
	Drug-induced hepatitis—rare
	Mental changes: agitation, confusion, impaired memory, hypomania

▷ **Principal Uses**
   As a Single Drug Product: Uses currently included in FDA-approved labeling:
   Used to treat severe situational (reactive or neurotic) depression, atypical
   depression, and (though less effective) severe endogenous depression. Because of the supervision required during its use and its potential for serious
   adverse effects, this drug is usually reserved to treat depressions that have
   not responded satisfactorily to other antidepressant therapy.
   Other (unlabeled) generally accepted uses: (1) Helps control binge eating in
   bulimia; (2) may be useful in treating chronic headache patients who also
   suffer from depression or anxiety; (3) a long-term study found phenelzine
   beneficial in treating social phobia; (4) rare use in intractable narcolepsy;
   (5) may be of benefit in posttraumatic stress disorder.

▷ **Usual Adult Dosage Range:**   Initially 15 mg three times a day (or 1 mg per kg of
   body mass, divided into three equal doses and taken three times daily);
   increase rapidly up to 60 mg/day, as needed and tolerated, until improvement is apparent. For maintenance, reduce dose gradually over several
   weeks to the smallest dose that will maintain improvement; this may be as
   low as 15 mg daily or every other day. The total daily dosage should not
   exceed 90 mg. **Note: Actual dose and dosing schedule must be individually determined.**

▷ **While Taking This Drug, Observe the Following**
▷   *Other Drugs*
   Phenelzine may *increase* the effects of
   • all drugs with stimulant effects on the nervous system, and cause excessive
     rise in blood pressure.
   • all drugs with sedative effects, and cause excessive sedation.
   • amphetamine and related drugs.
   • appetite suppressants.
   • insulin.
   • sulfonylureas (see Drug Classes) or other oral hypoglycemic agents.
   Phenelzine *taken concurrently* with
   • antihistamines (see Drug Classes) can worsen the anticholinergic side ef-
     fects of antihistamines.
   • buspirone (Buspar) may result in undesirable increases in blood pressure.
   • carbamazepine (Tegretol) may cause severe toxic reactions.
   • dextromethorphan (nonprescription cough medicine with a "DM") can
     cause severe toxic reactions.
   • dopamine (Intropin) may cause severe toxic reactions.
   • fluoxetine (Prozac) has resulted in fatal reactions with another MAO inhibi-
     tor (tranylcypromine). This combination is to be avoided.
   • fluvoxamine (Luvox) or other serotonin reuptake inhibitors may result in
     neuroleptic malignant syndrome and other serious reactions. This combi-
     nation is not recommended.
   • levodopa (Dopar, Sinemet) may cause a dangerous rise in blood pressure.
   • meperidine (Demerol) may cause high fever, seizures, and coma. These
     drugs are NOT to be combined.
   • methyldopa (Aldomet) may cause a dangerous rise in blood pressure.
   • methylphenidate (Ritalin) may cause severe headache, weakness, and
     numbness in the extremities.

- nadolol (Corgard) and metoprolol (Lopressor) or other beta-blockers (see Drug Classes) may result in significant decreases in heart rate.
- nefazodone (Serzone) may result in serious adverse effects. DO NOT combine these drugs.
- paroxetine (Paxil) may result in serious adverse effects. DO NOT combine these drugs.
- phenothiazines (see Drug Classes) or other antipsychotics may cause exaggeration of the central nervous system and depression of breathing effects.
- phenylephrine (various) may result in serious increases in blood pressure. DO NOT combine.
- phenylpropanolamine (various) may result in serious increases in blood pressure. DO NOT combine.
- propoxyphene (Darvon) may result in coma, heart problems, or severe increases in temperature. DO NOT combine.
- pseudoephedrine (various) may result in serious adverse effects. DO NOT combine these drugs.
- sertraline (Zoloft) may result in muscle rigidity, CNS toxicity, and chills. DO NOT combine these medicines.
- tryptophan (L-Tryptophan) can cause toxic reactions.
- tricyclic antidepressants (see Drug Classes) may cause severe toxic reactions including high fever, delirium, tremor, seizures, and coma.
- venlafaxine (Effexor) may result in serious adverse reactions. DO NOT combine these medicines.

Note: Consult your physician before taking *any other drugs* while taking phenelzine.

▷ *Driving, Hazardous Activities:* This drug may cause dizziness, drowsiness, and blurred vision. Restrict activities as necessary.

Aviation Note: The use of this drug *is a disqualification* for piloting. Consult a designated Aviation Medical Examiner.

Occurrence of Unrelated Illness: Because of the very serious and life-threatening interactions that can occur between this drug and many others, you **must** tell each health care provider you consult that you are taking this drug.

Discontinuation: If this drug is not effective after 4 weeks of continual use, it should be stopped. If it is effective, continue to take it in proper dosage until advised to stop. Do not stop it abruptly. If another antidepressant is to be tried, a drug-free waiting period of 14 days must pass between stopping this drug and starting the new one. Avoid tyramine-rich foods and other interacting drugs during this 14-day period.

Author's Note: Since other medicines are more widely used, the information in this profile has been shortened.

PHENOBARBITAL (fee noh BAR bi tawl)

Other Name: Phenobarbitone

Introduced: 1912   **Class:** Sedative, anticonvulsant, barbiturates   **Prescription:** USA: Yes   **Controlled Drug:** USA: C-IV*; Canada: Yes   **Available as Generic:** Yes

*See schedules of Controlled Drugs at the back of this book.

Brand Names: Alubelap [CD], Aminodrox-Forte, Antispasmodic [CD], Azpan, Barbidonna [CD], Barbidonna Elixir [CD], Barbita, Belap, Belladenal [CD], Belladenal-S [CD], ✦Belladenal Spacetabs [CD], ✦Bellergal [CD], Bellergal-S [CD], ✦Bellergal Spacetabs [CD], Bronchotabs [CD], Bronkolixir [CD], ✦Cafergot-PB, Chardonna-2 [CD], Daricon PB, ✦Diclophen [CD], Dilantin w/Phenobarbital [CD], Donphen, Donna-Sed, Donnatal [CD], Ergobel [CD], Eskabarb, Eskaphen B [CD], Floramine, ✦Gardenal, Hybephen [CD], Hypnaldyne [CD], Isuprel Compound [CD], Kinesed [CD], Luminal, Mudrane GG Elixir & Tablets [CD], Mudrane Tablets [CD], Neospect, Novalene, ✦Neuro-Spasex [CD], ✦Neuro-Trasentin [CD], ✦Neuro-Trasentin Forte [CD], Phedral [CD], ✦Phenaphen Capsules [CD], ✦Phenaphen No. 2, 3, 4 [CD], Phenergan w/Codeine [CD], Phyldrox, Quadrinal [CD], Relaxadron, SBP [CD], Scodonnar [CD], Sedacord [CD], SK-Phenobarbital, Solfoton, Spasquid [CD], Spazcaps, Tedral Preparations [CD], T.E.P. [CD], Thalfed [CD], Theocardone, Theocord [CD], Theolixer, Vitaphen

---

BENEFITS versus RISKS

Possible Benefits	*Possible Risks*
EFFECTIVE CONTROL OF TONIC-CLONIC SEIZURES AND ALL TYPES OF PARTIAL SEIZURES	POTENTIAL FOR DEPENDENCE LIFE-THREATENING TOXICITY WITH OVERDOSAGE
EFFECTIVE CONTROL OF FEBRILE SEIZURES OF CHILDHOOD	Drug-induced hepatitis or decreased kidney function
Effective relief of anxiety and nervous tension	Blood cell disorders: abnormally low red cell, white cell, and platelet counts

---

▷ **Principal Uses**

As a Single Drug Product: Uses currently included in FDA-approved labeling: (1) Used as a mild sedative; (2) used as an anticonvulsant to control grand mal epilepsy and all types of partial seizures. It is also used to control febrile seizures of childhood; (3) used as a sedative; however, newer agents carry fewer drug interactions and effects on sleep cycles.

Other (unlabeled) generally accepted uses: (1) May be helpful in detoxification of sedative-hypnotic addiction; (2) can help control seizures found in cerebral malaria; (3) eases neonatal seizures; (4) may have a role in treating pain syndromes.

As a Combination Drug Product [CD]: This drug is available in many combinations with derivatives of belladonna, an antispasmodic commonly used to treat functional disorders of the gastrointestinal tract. It is also available in combination with bronchodilators for the treatment of asthma, and with ergotamine for the treatment of headaches.

How This Drug Works: By impeding the transfer of sodium and potassium across cell membranes, this drug selectively blocks the transmission of nerve impulses. This could serve to produce a sedative effect and suppress the spread of nerve impulses that are responsible for epileptic seizures.

Available Dosage Forms and Strengths

Capsules — 16 mg
Elixir — 15 mg/5 ml, 20 mg/5 ml
Tablets — 8 mg, 16 mg, 32 mg, 65 mg, 100 mg

▷ **Usual Adult Dosage Range:** As sedative: 15 to 30 mg two to three times a day. As hypnotic: 100 to 200 mg at bedtime. As anticonvulsant: 60 to 250 mg taken as a single dose at bedtime. Some clinicians give 2 to 3 mg per kg of body mass in order to achieve and maintain a blood level between 15 to 40 mcg/ml. **Note: Actual dose and dosing schedule must be determined for each patient individually.**

Conditions Requiring Dosing Adjustments

Liver Function: This drug should be used with caution in decreased doses and blood levels obtained more frequently by patients with liver compromise.

Kidney Function: This drug should be used with caution and in decreased doses by patients with compromised kidneys. Blood levels should be obtained at prudent intervals. One researcher suggests that patients with severe kidney failure (creatinine clearance less than 10 ml/min) can take typical doses, but only every 12 to 16 hours.

▷ **Dosing Instructions:** Regular tablets may be crushed, and capsules opened and taken with or after food to reduce stomach irritation. Prolonged-action dosage forms should be swallowed whole without alteration.

Usual Duration of Use: Use on a regular schedule for 3 to 5 days determines effectiveness in relieving anxiety and tension, and for 4 to 6 weeks to determine its ability to control seizures. If used to treat anxiety-tension states, its use should not exceed 4 weeks without reappraisal of continued need. Long-term use for seizure control (months to years) requires physician supervision and periodic evaluation.

▷ **This Drug Should Not Be Taken If**
- you have had an allergic reaction to it previously.
- you have severe liver impairment.
- you are subject to acute intermittent porphyria (see Glossary).
- you have a respiratory disease that makes it difficult to breathe.

▷ **Inform Your Physician Before Taking This Drug If**
- you are allergic or overly sensitive to any barbiturate (see Drug Classes).
- you are pregnant or planning pregnancy.
- you have a history of alcohol or drug abuse.
- you are taking any drugs with sedative effects.
- you have a history of depression.
- you have any type of seizure disorder.
- you have myasthenia gravis.
- you have impaired liver, kidney, or thyroid gland function.
- you plan to have surgery under general anesthesia in the near future.

Possible Side Effects (natural, expected, and unavoidable drug actions)
Drowsiness, impaired concentration, mental and physical sluggishness.

▷ **Possible Adverse Effects** (unusual, unexpected, and infrequent reactions)
If any of the following develop, consult your physician promptly for guidance.

Mild Adverse Effects

Allergic Reactions: Skin rashes, hives, localized swellings of face, drug fever (see Glossary).

Dizziness, unsteadiness, impaired vision, double vision—possible and may be dose related.

Nausea, vomiting, diarrhea—infrequent.

Abnormal growth of the gums—case reports.

Shoulder-hand syndrome: pain and stiffness in the shoulder, pain/swelling in the hand—case reports.

Serious Adverse Effects

Allergic Reactions: Drug-induced hepatitis with jaundice (see Glossary), severe skin disorders (Stevens-Johnson syndrome or toxic epidermal necrolysis)—case reports.

Osteoporosis—possible with long-term use.

Idiosyncratic Reactions: Paradoxical excitement and delirium (instead of sedation).

Drug-induced myasthenia gravis, liver, or kidney disease—case reports.

Respiratory depression—dose related.

Mental depression, abnormal involuntary movements—case reports.

Blood cell disorders: lowering of all blood cells (weakness, fever, sore throat, bleeding/bruising)—rare.

Blood clotting disorders in neonates—case reports.

Optic neuropathy—rare.

Drug-induced seizures—possible.

Low blood calcium—case reports.

▷ **Possible Effects on Sexual Function**

Decreased libido and/or impotence—occasional.

Decreased effectiveness of oral contraceptives taken concurrently—frequent.

▷ **Adverse Effects That May Mimic Natural Diseases or Disorders**

Liver reactions may suggest viral hepatitis.

Natural Diseases or Disorders That May Be Activated by This Drug

Acute intermittent and/or cutaneous porphyria, systemic lupus erythematosus.

Possible Effects on Laboratory Tests

Complete blood cell counts: decreased red cells, hemoglobin, white cells, and platelets.

Blood lupus erythematosus (LE) cells: positive.

INR (prothrombin time): decreased (when taken concurrently with warfarin).

Blood calcium level: decreased (with long-term use).

Blood thyroxine (T_4) level: decreased.

Liver function tests: increased liver enzymes (ALT/GPT, AST/GOT, alkaline phosphatase) and bilirubin.

Urine sugar tests: no effect with Tes-Tape; false low results with Clinistix and Diastix.

Urine screening tests for drug abuse: may be **positive**. (Test results depend upon amount of drug taken and testing method used.)

CAUTION

1. Accurate diagnosis and classification of the seizure pattern are essential for correct selection of the most appropriate drug for therapy.
2. Emotional stress or physical trauma (including surgery) may require increased anticonvulsant dosage to control seizures.
3. Prolonged-action dosage forms of this drug are not appropriate for the treatment of seizures and should not be used.

Precautions for Use

By Infants and Children: This drug should not be given to the hyperkinetic child. Possible paradoxical stimulation/hyperactivity can occur in 10 to 40% of children. Changes associated with puberty slow metabolism of this drug and permit its gradual accumulation. Blood levels of this drug in adolescents should be monitored every 3 months to detect rising concentrations and early toxicity.

By Those Over 60 Years of Age: It is advisable for the elderly to avoid all barbiturates. If use of this drug is attempted, small starting doses are indicated. Watch for confusion, delirium, agitation, and excitement. Do not use this drug concurrently with other drugs for mental disorders. This drug is conducive to the development of hypothermia (see Glossary).

▷ **Advisability of Use During Pregnancy**

Pregnancy Category: D. See Pregnancy Risk Categories at the back of this book.

Animal studies: Conflicting reports of cleft palate and skeletal defects in mouse, rat, and rabbit studies.

Human studies: Information from studies of pregnant women indicates no increase in birth defects in 8,037 exposures to this drug. However, it is reported that barbiturates can cause fetal damage when taken during pregnancy.

Avoid use of drug during entire pregnancy if possible. If it is clearly needed to control seizures, the mother should receive vitamin K prior to delivery and the infant should receive it at birth.

Advisability of Use If Breast-Feeding

Presence of this drug in breast milk: Yes, in small amounts.

Monitor nursing infant closely and discontinue drug or nursing if adverse effects develop.

Habit-Forming Potential: Psychological and physical dependence can occur with prolonged use of excessive doses—300 to 700 mg/day for 1 to 2 months. Dependence is not likely to occur with usual sedative or anticonvulsant doses.

Effects of Overdosage: Behavior similar to alcoholic intoxication—confusion, slurred speech, physical incoordination, staggering gait, drowsiness, stupor leading to coma.

Possible Effects of Long-Term Use: Psychological and/or physical dependence; syndrome of chronic intoxication—headache, depression, impaired vision, dizziness, slurred speech, incoordination. Megaloblastic anemia due to folic acid deficiency. Rickets or osteomalacia due to deficiencies of vitamin D and calcium.

Suggested Periodic Examinations While Taking This Drug (at physician's discretion)

When used to control seizures, blood phenobarbital levels are needed.

Time to sample blood for phenobarbital level: just before next dose.

Recommended therapeutic range—for adults: 15–40 mcg/ml; for children: 15–30 mcg/ml.

Complete blood cell counts, liver function tests.

During long-term use: blood levels of folic acid, vitamin B_{12}, calcium, and phosphorus; densitometry (DEXA) studies for demineralization/osteoporosis of bone.

▷ **While Taking This Drug, Observe the Following**

Foods: No restrictions. Eat liberally of foods rich in folic acid—fortified breakfast cereals, liver, legumes, green leafy vegetables.

Beverages: No restrictions. May be taken with milk or fruit juices.

▷ *Alcohol:* Avoid completely. Alcohol can increase greatly the sedative and depressant actions of this drug on brain functions.

Tobacco Smoking: May enhance the sedative effects of this drug and increase drowsiness. I advise everyone to quit smoking.

Marijuana Smoking: Increased drowsiness, unsteadiness; significantly impaired mental and physical performance.

▷ *Other Drugs*

Phenobarbital may ***increase*** the effects of
- all other drugs with sedative effects, and cause excessive sedation.

Phenobarbital may ***decrease*** the effects of
- anticoagulants (Coumadin, etc.), and require dosage adjustments based on more frequent INR (prothrombin time or protime) testing.
- birth control pills (oral contraceptives), and reduce their effectiveness in preventing pregnancy.
- certain beta-blockers (Inderal, Lopressor), and reduce their effectiveness.
- cortisonelike drugs (see Drug Classes).
- cyclosporine (Sandimmune).
- diltiazem (Cardizem).
- disopyramide (Norpace).
- doxycycline (Vibramycin).
- felodipine (Plendil).
- griseofulvin (Fulvicin, etc.).
- metoprolol (Lopressor, others).
- nimodipine (Nimotop).
- quinidine (Quinaglute, etc.), and reduce its effectiveness.
- propranolol (Inderal).
- theophyllines (Aminophyllin, Theo-Dur, etc.), and reduce their antiasthmatic effectiveness.
- tricyclic antidepressants (see Drug Classes).
- verapamil (Calan) and reduce its effectiveness.
- warfarin (Coumadin) and increase risk of clots.

Phenobarbital ***taken concurrently*** with
- chloramphenicol (Chloromycetin) may result in decreased chloramphenicol benefits and phenobarbital toxicity. These drugs are NOT to be combined.
- colestipol (Colestid) and other cholesterol-lowering resins may bind phenobarbital and limit absorption.
- influenza vaccine may cause phenobarbital toxicity.
- itraconazole (and perhaps other antifungals) may decrease the antifungal effect of itraconazole.
- phenytoin (Dilantin) may alter phenytoin blood levels: a high phenobarbital level will increase the phenytoin level; a low phenobarbital level will decrease the phenytoin level. Periodic determination of blood levels of both drugs is advised.
- primidone (Mysoline) may lead to phenobarbital toxicity.
- ritonavir (Norvir) and perhaps other protease inhibitors (see Drug Classes) may blunt ritonavir's effects.

The following drugs may *increase* the effects of phenobarbital
- ascorbic acid (vitamin C).
- felbamate (Felbatol).
- valproic acid (Depakene).

▷ *Driving, Hazardous Activities:* This drug may cause drowsiness and may impair mental alertness, judgment, physical coordination, and reaction time. Restrict activities as necessary.

Aviation Note: The use of this drug *is a disqualification* for piloting. Consult a designated Aviation Medical Examiner.

Exposure to Sun: Use caution—this drug may cause photosensitivity.

Exposure to Cold: Observe the elderly for possible hypothermia (see Glossary) while taking this drug.

Discontinuation: If used as an anticonvulsant, this drug must not be stopped abruptly. Sudden withdrawal can precipitate status epilepticus (repetitive seizures). Gradual reduction in dosage should be made over a period of 3 months. Total drug withdrawal may be attempted after a period of 3 to 5 years without a seizure. However, seizures are likely to recur in 40% of adults and in 20–30% of children.

PHENYTOIN (FEN i toh in)

Other Name: Diphenylhydantoin

Introduced: 1938   **Class:** Anticonvulsant, hydantoins, pain syndrome modifier   **Prescription:** USA: Yes   **Controlled Drug:** USA: No; Canada: No   **Available as Generic:**   USA: Yes; Canada: Yes

Brand Names: Dilantin, Dilantin Infatabs, Dilantin w/Phenobarbital [CD], Di-Phen, Diphenylan, Ekko JR, Ekko SR, Ekko Three, ✚Mebroin [CD]

BENEFITS versus RISKS	
Possible Benefits	*Possible Risks*
EFFECTIVE CONTROL OF TONIC-CLONIC (GRAND MAL), PSYCHOMOTOR (TEMPORAL LOBE), MYOCLONIC, AND FOCAL SEIZURES	VERY NARROW TREATMENT MARGIN
	POSSIBLE BIRTH DEFECTS
	Overgrowth of gums
	Excessive hair growth
	Blood cell disorders: impaired production of all blood cells
	Drug-induced hepatitis or nephritis

▷ **Principal Uses**

As a Single Drug Product: Uses currently included in FDA-approved labeling: As an antiepileptic drug to control grand mal, psychomotor, myoclonic, and focal seizures. It can also be used to control seizures following brain surgery.

Other (unlabeled) generally accepted uses: (1) Used to initiate treatment of trigeminal neuralgia; it is sometimes effective in relieving the severe facial pain of this disorder; (2) used in chronic pain syndromes; (3) may have a role (as an applied powder) in helping heal wounds.

As a Combination Drug Product [CD]: This drug is available in combination with phenobarbital, another effective anticonvulsant. Some seizure disorders require the combined actions of these two drugs for effective control.

How This Drug Works: By promoting the loss of sodium from nerve fibers, this drug lowers and stabilizes their excitability and thereby inhibits the repetitious spread of electrical impulses along nerve pathways. This action may prevent seizures altogether, or it may reduce their frequency and severity.

Available Dosage Forms and Strengths

> Capsules, extended — 30 mg, 100 mg
> Capsules, prompt — 30 mg, 100 mg
> Injection — 50 mg/ml
> Kapseals — 30 mg, 100 mg
> Oral suspension — 30 mg/5 ml, 125 mg/5 ml
> Tablets, chewable — 50 mg

▷ **Usual Adult Dosage Range:**   Seizures: Initially (prompt or extended form) 100 mg three times a day. Dose may be increased cautiously by 100 mg/week as needed and tolerated. Once the optimal maintenance dose has been identified, the total daily dose may be taken as a single dose every 24 hours if Dilantin capsules are used. No other formulation is approved for once-a-day use. The total daily dosage should not exceed 600 mg. **Note: Actual dosage and administration schedule must be determined for each patient individually.**

Conditions Requiring Dosing Adjustments

Liver Function: The maintenance dose should be decreased based on blood levels.

Kidney Function: The dose or dosing interval must be decreased in moderate kidney failure.

Obesity: The way this medicine is distributed (volume of distribution) changes with increasing body fat. Loading doses must be calculated based on ideal body weight. The product of 1.33 times actual weight divided by the ideal weight is then added to the original number to decide the final loading dose.

▷ **Dosing Instructions:**   May be taken with or after food to reduce stomach irritation. The capsule may be opened and the tablet may be crushed for administration.

Usual Duration of Use: Use on a regular schedule for 2 to 3 weeks usually determines benefit in reducing frequency and severity of seizures. Optimal control will require careful dosage adjustments over a period of several months. Long-term use (months to years) requires ongoing physician supervision.

▷ **This Drug Should Not Be Taken If**
- you have had an allergic reaction to this drug or other hydantoin drugs previously.
- you have sinus bradycardia or serious heart block.

▷ **Inform Your Physician Before Taking This Drug If**
- you are taking any other drugs at this time.
- you have a history of liver disease or impaired liver function.
- you have low blood pressure, diabetes, or any type of heart disease.
- you are pregnant or planning pregnancy.
- you plan to have surgery under general anesthesia in the near future.

Possible Side Effects (natural, expected, and unavoidable drug actions)
Mild fatigue, sluggishness, and drowsiness (in sensitive individuals).
Pink to red to brown coloration of urine (of no significance).

▷ **Possible Adverse Effects** (unusual, unexpected, and infrequent reactions)
If any of the following develop, consult your physician promptly for guidance.
Mild Adverse Effects
Allergic Reactions: Skin rashes, hives, drug fever (see Glossary).
Headache, dizziness, nervousness, insomnia, muscle twitching—infrequent.
Nausea, vomiting, constipation—infrequent.
Bed-wetting—case reports.
Abnormal eye movements—dose related.
Low blood calcium (and potential osteoporosis) and elevated blood sugar—possible.
Overgrowth of gum tissues—most common in children.
Excessive growth of body hair—most common in young girls.
Serious Adverse Effects
Allergic Reactions: Drug-induced hepatitis, with or without jaundice (see Glossary). Drug-induced nephritis, with acute kidney failure. Severe skin reactions (toxic epidermal necrolysis, Stevens-Johnson syndrome, or erythema multiforme). Myocarditis, generalized enlargement of lymph glands (pseudolymphoma)—case reports.
Idiosyncratic Reactions: Hemolytic anemia (see Glossary).
Acute psychotic episodes—case reports.
Mental confusion, unsteadiness, double vision, jerky eye movements, slurred speech—possible.
Drug-induced seizures—possible.
Blood clotting disorders in infants of mothers maintained on phenytoin—rare.
Bone marrow depression (see Glossary): weakness, fever, sore throat, bleeding or bruising—case reports.
Drug-induced periarteritis nodosa, low thyroid function, or myasthenia gravis—case reports.
Tardive dyskinesia or porphyria—case reports.
Abnormal IgA (increased risk of respiratory infections)—possible.
Peripheral nerve damage (neuropathy) or muscle damage (myopathy)—case reports.
Serious heart rhythm problems—with rapid intravenous use.
Elevated blood sugar, due to inhibition of insulin release—possible.

▷ **Possible Effects on Sexual Function**
Decreased libido and/or impotence—infrequent.
Swelling and tenderness of male breast tissue (gynecomastia) or Peyronie's disease (see Glossary)—rare.
Decreased effectiveness of oral contraceptives taken concurrently.

▷ **Adverse Effects That May Mimic Natural Diseases or Disorders**
Drug-induced hepatitis may suggest viral hepatitis. Skin reactions may resemble lupus erythematosus.

Natural Diseases or Disorders That May Be Activated by This Drug
Latent diabetes, porphyria, systemic lupus erythematosus, low bone mineral density predisposing to osteoporosis.

Possible Effects on Laboratory Tests

Complete blood cell counts: decreased red cells, hemoglobin, white cells, and platelets; increased eosinophils (allergic reaction).

Blood lupus erythematosus (LE) cells: positive.

Prothrombin time: increased (when phenytoin is taken concurrently with warfarin).

Blood calcium level: decreased.

Blood total cholesterol, LDL and VLDL cholesterol levels: no effects.

Blood HDL cholesterol level: increased.

Blood triglyceride levels: no effect.

Blood glucose level: increased.

Blood thyroid hormone levels: T_3, T_4, and free T_4 increased.

Liver function tests: increased liver enzymes (ALT/GPT, AST/GOT, alkaline phosphatase) and bilirubin.

CAUTION

1. Some brand-name capsules of this drug have a significantly longer duration of action than generic name capsules of the same strength. To assure a correct dosing schedule, it is necessary to distinguish between "prompt"-action and "extended"-action capsules. Do not substitute one for the other without your physician's knowledge and guidance.

2. When used for the treatment of epilepsy, ***this drug must not be stopped abruptly.***

3. Periodic measurements of blood levels of this drug are essential in determining appropriate dosage (see "Therapeutic Drug Monitoring," chapter 2).

4. Regularity of drug use is essential. Take this drug at the same time each day.

5. Shake the suspension form of this drug thoroughly before measuring the dose. Use a standard measuring device to assure that the dose is accurate.

6. Side effects and mild adverse effects are usually most apparent during the first several days of treatment, and often subside with continued use.

7. It may be necessary to take folic acid to prevent anemia. Talk with your doctor about this.

8. This medicine has an unusual pathway for removal that can fill up (become saturated) and stop working. This means that a small change in dose may give a huge change in blood levels. Make certain you know exactly how much phenytoin your doctor wants you to take.

9. Carry a card of personal identification with a notation that you are taking this drug.

Precautions for Use

By Infants and Children: Elimination of this drug varies widely with age. Periodic measurement of blood levels is essential for all ages. Some children will require more than one dose daily for good control. Observe for early indications of drug toxicity: jerky eye movements, unsteadiness in stance and gait, slurred speech, abnormal involuntary movements of the extremities, and odd behavior.

By Those Over 60 Years of Age: You may be more sensitive to all of the actions of this drug and require smaller doses. Observe closely for any indications of early toxicity: drowsiness, fatigue, confusion, unsteadiness, disturbances of vision, slurred speech, muscle twitching.

▷ **Advisability of Use During Pregnancy**

Pregnancy Category: D. See Pregnancy Risk Categories at the back of this book.

Animal studies: Cleft lip and palate, skeletal and visceral defects in mice and rats.

Human studies: Available information is conflicting. Some studies suggest a small but significant increase in birth defects. The incidence of birth defects in children of epileptics not taking anticonvulsant drugs is 3.2%; incidence increases to 6.4% with anticonvulsant use in pregnancy. The "fetal hydantoin syndrome" in infants exposed to phenytoin during pregnancy shows: birth defects of skull, face, and limbs; deficient growth and development; and subnormal intelligence. Other effects on the infant include reduction in blood clotting factors that predispose it to severe bruising and hemorrhage.

Discuss the benefits and risks of using this drug during pregnancy with your doctor. It is advisable to use the smallest maintenance dose that will control seizures. In addition, you should take vitamin K during the final month of pregnancy to prevent a deficiency of fetal blood clotting factors.

Advisability of Use If Breast-Feeding

Presence of this drug in breast milk: Yes, in trace amounts.

Monitor nursing infant closely and discontinue drug or nursing if adverse effects develop.

Habit-Forming Potential: None.

Effects of Overdosage: Drowsiness, jerky eye movements, hand tremor, unsteadiness, slurred speech, hallucinations, delusions, nausea, vomiting, stupor progressing to coma.

Possible Effects of Long-Term Use: Low blood calcium resulting in rickets or osteomalacia; megaloblastic anemia; peripheral neuropathy (see Glossary); schizophreniclike psychosis. Lymphosarcoma, malignant lymphoma, and leukemia have been associated with long-term use; a cause-and-effect relationship (see Glossary) has not been established.

Suggested Periodic Examinations While Taking This Drug (at physician's discretion)

Monitoring of blood phenytoin levels to guide dosage.

Time to sample blood for phenytoin level: just before next dose.

Recommended therapeutic range: 10 to 20 ng/ml.

Complete blood cell counts, liver function tests.

Measurements of the following blood levels: glucose, calcium, phosphorus, folic acid, vitamin B_{12}.

Bone mineral density testing (DEXA) to check risk for osteoporosis and fracture.

▷ **While Taking This Drug, Observe the Following**

Foods: No restrictions.

Nutritional Support: Supplements of folic acid, calcium, vitamin D, and vitamin K may be necessary.

Beverages: No restrictions. May be taken with milk.

▷   *Alcohol:* Use extreme caution. Alcohol (in large quantities or with continual use) may reduce this drug's effectiveness in preventing seizures.

Tobacco Smoking: No interactions expected, but I advise everyone to quit smoking.

▷   *Other Drugs*

Phenytoin may ***decrease*** the effects of

- acetaminophen (Tylenol, others).
- conjugated estrogens (Premarin).
- cortisonelike drugs (see Drug Classes).
- cyclosporine (Sandimmune).
- disopyramide (Norpace).
- doxycycline (Vibramycin, etc.).
- itraconazole (Sporanox).
- levodopa (Larodopa, Sinemet).
- levothyroxine (Synthroid, others).
- meperidine (Demerol).
- methadone (Dolophine).
- mexiletine (Mexitil).
- miconazole (Monistat, Micatin, others).
- oral antidiabetic drugs (see Drug Classes).
- oral contraceptives (birth control pills).
- paroxetine (Paxil).
- quinidine (Quinaglute, etc.).
- ritonavir (Norvir) and perhaps other protease inhibitors (see Drug Classes).

Phenytoin ***taken concurrently*** with

- carbamazepine (Tegretol) may result in increased or decreased levels of phenytoin.
- chlordiazepoxide (Librium—and perhaps other benzodiazepines) may increase or decrease phenytoin levels. Levels should be obtained more frequently if these drugs are combined.
- ciprofloxacin (Cipro) may increase or decrease phenytoin levels.
- dopamine will result in very low blood pressure.
- ketorolac (Toradol) may result in seizures. DO NOT combine these medicines.
- oral anticoagulants (Coumadin, etc.) can either increase or decrease the anticoagulant effect; monitor this combination very closely with INR (serial prothrombin) testing.
- primidone (Mysoline) may alter primidone actions and enhance its toxicity.
- theophyllines (Aminophyllin, Theo-Dur, etc.) may cause a decrease in the effectiveness of both drugs.
- valproic acid (Depakene) may result in altered phenytoin or valproic acid levels. Increased blood level testing of both medicines is needed if these medicines are to be combined.
- warfarin (Coumadin) may lead to initial increased bleeding risk and subsequent decrease in anticoagulation. More frequent INR (prothrombin time or protime) testing is needed. Warfarin doses should be adjusted to results.

The following drugs may *increase* the effects of phenytoin
- amiodarone (Cordarone).
- chloramphenicol (Chloromycetin).
- chlorpheniramine.
- cimetidine (Tagamet).
- cotrimoxazole (Bactrim).
- diltiazem (Cardizem).
- disulfiram (Antabuse).
- felbamate (Felbatol).
- fluconazole (Diflucan).
- fluoxetine (Prozac).
- fluvoxamine (Luvox).
- ibuprofen, and perhaps other NSAIDs.
- isoniazid (INH, Niconyl, etc.).
- nifedipine (Adalat).
- omeprazole (Prilosec).
- phenacemide (Phenurone).
- sulfonamides (see Drug Classes).
- tricyclic antidepressants (see Drug Classes).
- trimethoprim (Proloprim, Trimpex).
- valproic acid (Depakene).
- venlafaxine (Effexor).

The following drugs may *decrease* the effects of phenytoin
- bleomycin (Blenoxane).
- carmustine (BiCNU).
- cisplatin (Platinol).
- diazoxide (Proglycem, Hyperstat).
- folic acid (various).
- methotrexate (Mexate).
- rifampin (Rifadin).
- vinblastine (Velban).

▷ *Driving, Hazardous Activities:* This drug may impair mental alertness, vision, and coordination. Restrict activities as necessary.

Aviation Note: The use of this drug *is a disqualification* for piloting. Consult a designated Aviation Medical Examiner.

Exposure to Sun: Use caution—this drug may cause photosensitivity (see Glossary).

Occurrence of Unrelated Illness: Intercurrent infections may slow the elimination of this drug and increase the risk of toxicity, due to higher blood levels.

*Discontinuation: **This drug must not be discontinued abruptly.*** Sudden withdrawal can precipitate severe and repeated seizures. If this drug is to be discontinued, gradual reduction in dosage should be made over a period of 3 months. Total drug withdrawal may be attempted after a period of 3 to 4 years without a seizure. However, seizures are likely to recur in 40% of adults and in 20–30% of children.

PILOCARPINE (pi loh KAR peen)

Introduced: 1875   **Class:** Anti-glaucoma   **Prescription:** USA: Yes
Controlled Drug: USA: No; Canada: No   **Available as Generic:** Yes
Brand Names: Adsorbocarpine, Akarpine, Almocarpine, E-Pilo Preparations [CD], I-Pilopine, Isopto Carpine, ✦Minims, ✦Miocarpine, Ocusert Pilo-20, -40, PE Preparations [CD], Pilagan, Pilocar, Pilopine HS, Piloptic-1, -2, Pilosyst 20/40, Salagen, ✦Spersacarpine

BENEFITS versus RISKS	
Possible Benefits	*Possible Risks*
EFFECTIVE REDUCTION OF INTERNAL EYE PRESSURE FOR CONTROL OF ACUTE AND CHRONIC GLAUCOMA	Mild side effects with systemic absorption Minor eye discomfort Altered vision

▷ **Principal Uses**

As a Single Drug Product: Uses currently included in FDA-approved labeling: (1) Used exclusively for the management of all types of glaucoma. Selection of the appropriate dosage form and strength must be carefully individualized; (2) can help in dry mouth (xerostomia).

Other (unlabeled) generally accepted uses: (1) Treatment of Adie syndrome; (2) can help before laser surgery in order to prevent excessive increases in eye (intraocular) pressure after surgery.

As a Combination Drug Product [CD]: This drug is combined with epinephrine (in eyedrop solutions) to utilize the actions of both drugs in lowering internal eye pressure. The opposite effects of these two drugs on the size of the pupil (pilocarpine constricts, epinephrine dilates) provides a balance that prevents excessive constriction or dilation.

How This Drug Works: By directly stimulating constriction of the pupil, this drug enlarges the outflow canal in the anterior chamber of the eye and promotes the drainage of excess fluid (aqueous humor), thus lowering the internal eye pressure.

Available Dosage Forms and Strengths

Eyedrop solutions — 0.25%, 0.5%, 1%, 2%, 3%, 4%, 5%, 6%, 8%, 10%
Gel — 4%
Ocuserts — 20 mcg, 40 mcg
Tablets — 5 mg

▷ **Usual Adult Dosage Range:** For open-angle glaucoma: Eyedrop solutions—one drop of a 1 to 2% solution three to four times daily. Eye gel—apply 0.5-inch strip of gel into the eye once daily at bedtime. Ocusert—insert one into affected eye and replace every 7 days with a new one. **Note: Actual dose and dosing schedule must be determined for each patient individually.**

Conditions Requiring Dosing Adjustments

Liver Function: The specific elimination of this drug is unclear.
Kidney Function: The elimination of this drug has yet to be defined.

▷ **Dosing Instructions:** To avoid excessive absorption into the body, press finger against inner corner of the eye (to close off the tear duct) during and for 2 minutes following instillation of the eyedrop. Place the gel and the Ocusert in the eye at bedtime.

Usual Duration of Use: Use on a regular schedule for 1 to 2 weeks usually determines this drug's effectiveness in controlling internal eye pressure. Long-
term use (months to years) requires physician supervision.

▷ **This Drug Should Not Be Taken If**
  • you have had an allergic reaction to it previously.
  • you have acute iritis.
  • you have active bronchial asthma and are using the tablet form.

▷ **Inform Your Physician Before Taking This Drug If**
  • you have a history of bronchial asthma.
  • you have a history of acute iritis.
  • you have significant heart disease.
  • you have chronic obstructive pulmonary disease.
  • you have gallstones.

Possible Side Effects (natural, expected, and unavoidable drug actions)
Temporary impairment of vision, usually lasting 2 to 3 hours following instillation of drops. Burning of the eyes and trouble seeing at night—frequent.

▷ **Possible Adverse Effects** (unusual, unexpected, and infrequent reactions)
**If any of the following develop, consult your physician promptly for
guidance.**
Mild Adverse Effects
Allergic Reactions: Itching of the eyes, eyelid itching and/or swelling.
Headache, heart palpitation, tremors—infrequent.
Sweating—frequent.
Nausea—case reports.
Serious Adverse Effects
Provocation of acute asthma in susceptible individuals.
Mental status changes—case reports.
Atrioventricular block (abnormal heart conduction)—case reports.
Retinal detachment—possible.

▷ **Possible Effects on Sexual Function**
None reported.

Possible Effects on Laboratory Tests
Red blood cell and white blood cell counts: increased.

Precautions for Use
By Those Over 60 Years of Age: Maintain personal cleanliness to prevent eye
infections. Report promptly any indication of possible infection involving
the eyes.

▷ **Advisability of Use During Pregnancy**
Pregnancy Category: C. See Pregnancy Risk Categories at the back of this book.
Animal studies: Significant birth defects due to this drug reported in rats.
Human studies: Adequate studies of pregnant women are not available.
Limit use to the smallest effective dose. Minimize systemic absorption (see
"Dosing Instructions" above).

Advisability of Use If Breast-Feeding
Presence of this drug in breast milk: May be present in small amounts.
Monitor nursing infant closely and discontinue drug or nursing if adverse
effects develop.

Habit-Forming Potential: None.

Effects of Overdosage: Flushing of face, increased flow of saliva, sweating. If solution is swallowed: nausea, vomiting, diarrhea, profuse sweating, rapid pulse, difficult breathing, loss of consciousness.

Possible Effects of Long-Term Use: Development of tolerance (see Glossary), temporary loss of effectiveness.

Suggested Periodic Examinations While Taking This Drug (at physician's discretion)
　　Measurement of internal eye pressure on a regular basis.
　　Examination of eyes for development of cataracts.

▷ **While Taking This Drug, Observe the Following**
　　Foods: No restrictions.
　　Beverages: No restrictions.
▷　*Alcohol:* Use caution. If this drug is absorbed, it may prolong the effect of alcohol on the brain.
　　Tobacco Smoking: No interactions expected, but I advise everyone to quit smoking.
　　Marijuana Smoking: Sustained additional decrease in internal eye pressure.
▷　*Other Drugs*
　　　The following drugs may ***decrease*** the effects of pilocarpine
　　　　• atropine and drugs with atropinelike actions (see Drug Classes).
　　　Pilocarpine ***taken concurrently*** with
　　　　• epinephrine will result in increased myopia.
　　　　• timolol can produce additive effects in treating glaucoma.
▷　*Driving, Hazardous Activities:* This drug may impair your ability to focus your vision properly. Restrict activities as necessary.
　　Aviation Note: The use of this drug ***may be a disqualification*** for piloting. Consult a designated Aviation Medical Examiner.
　　Exposure to Sun: This medicine may make you very sensitive to the sun. Wear sunglasses.
　　Discontinuation: Do not stop regular use of this drug without consulting your physician. Periodic discontinuation and temporary substitution of another drug may be necessary to preserve its effectiveness in treating glaucoma.

PINDOLOL (PIN doh lohl)

Introduced: 1972   **Class:**   Antihypertensive, beta-adrenergic blocker
Prescription: USA: Yes   **Controlled Drug:**   USA: No; Canada: No   **Available as Generic:**   Yes

Brand Names: ✤Apo-Pindol, ✤Novo-Pindol, ✤Nu-Pindol, ✤Syn-Pindolol, ✤Viskazide [CD], Visken

```
┌─────────────────────────────────────────────────────────────────────┐
│                        BENEFITS versus RISKS                          │
│      Possible Benefits                        Possible Risks          │
│  EFFECTIVE, WELL-TOLERATED          CONGESTIVE HEART FAILURE in        │
│  ANTIHYPERTENSIVE in mild to          advanced heart disease          │
│  moderate high blood pressure       Worsening of angina in coronary   │
│                                       heart disease (abrupt withdrawal)│
│                                     Masking of low blood sugar         │
│                                       (hypoglycemia) in drug-treated   │
│                                       diabetes                         │
│                                     Provocation of asthma (with high   │
│                                       doses)                           │
└─────────────────────────────────────────────────────────────────────┘
```

▷ **Principal Uses**

As a Single Drug Product: Uses currently included in FDA-approved labeling: Treatment of mild to moderate high blood pressure, alone or with other antihypertensive drugs, such as diuretics.

Other (unlabeled) generally accepted uses: (1) May be of benefit in helping control aggressive behavior; (2) can help prevent migraine headaches; (3) combination therapy with digoxin may be effective in limiting some abnormal heart rhythms (atrial fibrillation); (4) can be of benefit in some kinds of anxiety; (5) decreases sympathetic output in hyperthyroidism.

As a Combination Drug Product [CD]: This drug is available in combination with hydrochlorothiazide (in Canada). The addition of a thiazide diuretic to this beta-blocker drug enhances its effectiveness as an antihypertensive.

How This Drug Works: By blocking certain actions of the sympathetic nervous system, this drug reduces the rate and contraction force of the heart, thus lowering the ejection pressure of the blood leaving the heart; reduces the degree of contraction of blood vessel walls, resulting in their relaxation and consequent lowering of blood pressure.

Available Dosage Forms and Strengths

Tablets — 5 mg, 10 mg, 15 mg (Canada)

▷ **Usual Adult Dosage Range:**   Hypertension: Initially 5 mg twice daily (12 hours apart). The dose may be increased gradually by 10 mg/day at intervals of 3 to 4 weeks as needed and tolerated, up to 60 mg/day. For maintenance, 5 to 10 mg two or three times daily is often effective. The total daily dose should not exceed 60 mg. **Note: Actual dosage and administration schedule must be determined for each patient individually.**

Conditions Requiring Dosing Adjustments

Liver Function: The dose should be empirically decreased for patients with severe liver compromise and for those with combined liver and kidney compromise.

Kidney Function: The dose should be decreased if urine output is significantly decreased.

▷ **Dosing Instructions:**   The tablet may be crushed and taken without regard to eating. Do not stop this drug abruptly.

Usual Duration of Use: Use on a regular schedule for 2 to 3 weeks usually determines effectiveness in lowering blood pressure. The long-term use of this drug (months to years) will be determined by the course of your blood pressure over time and your response to an overall treatment program (weight reduction, salt restriction, smoking cessation, etc.). Consult your physician on a regular basis.

Possible Advantages of This Drug: Causes less slowing of the heart rate than most other beta-blocker drugs.

Currently a "Drug of Choice"
for initiating treatment of hypertension with a single drug.

▷ **This Drug Should Not Be Taken If**
- you have bronchial asthma.
- you have had an allergic reaction to it previously.
- you have congestive heart failure.
- you have an abnormally slow heart rate or a serious form of heart block.
- you are taking, or have taken within the past 14 days, any monoamine oxidase (MAO) type A inhibitor drug (see Drug Classes).

▷ **Inform Your Physician Before Taking This Drug If**
- you have had an adverse reaction to any beta-blocker in the past (see Drug Classes).
- you have a history of serious heart disease.
- you have a history of hay fever (allergic rhinitis), asthma, chronic bronchitis, or emphysema.
- you have a history of overactive thyroid function (hyperthyroidism).
- you have a history of low blood sugar (hypoglycemia) or diabetes.
- you have impaired liver or kidney function.
- you have diabetes or myasthenia gravis.
- you take digitalis, quinidine, or reserpine, or any calcium-channel-blocker drug (see Drug Classes).
- you have bad circulation to your legs or arms (peripheral vascular disease).
- you plan to have surgery under general anesthesia in the near future.

Possible Side Effects (natural, expected, and unavoidable drug actions)
Lethargy and fatigability, cold extremities, slow heart rate, light-headedness in upright position (see Orthostatic Hypotension in Glossary).

▷ **Possible Adverse Effects** (unusual, unexpected, and infrequent reactions)
If any of the following develop, consult your physician promptly for guidance.
Mild Adverse Effects
Allergic Reactions: Skin rash, itching.
Headache, dizziness, insomnia, abnormal dreams, fainting—infrequent.
Indigestion, nausea, vomiting, constipation, diarrhea—infrequent.
Joint and muscle discomfort, tremor, fluid retention (edema)—infrequent.
Serious Adverse Effects
Mental depression, anxiety—infrequent.
Chest pain, shortness of breath—possible.
Induction of bronchial asthma—in asthmatic individuals.
Abnormally slow heartbeat or congestive heart failure—possible to infrequent.
Drug-induced systemic lupus erythematosus or myasthenia gravis—case reports.

Worsening of poor circulation to the arms or legs (intermittent claudication)—possible.

Carpal tunnel syndrome—reported with other beta-blockers.

▷ **Possible Effects on Sexual Function**

Decreased libido or impaired erection—infrequent.

Possible Effects on Laboratory Tests

Blood lupus erythematosus (LE) cells: positive (one case of drug-induced LE).

Blood total cholesterol level: decreased (with long-term use).

Blood HDL cholesterol level: increased.

Blood LDL and VLDL cholesterol levels: no effects.

Blood triglyceride levels: no effects.

Glucose tolerance test (GTT): decreased or increased.

Liver function tests: slightly increased liver enzymes (ALT/GPT and AST/GOT) possible.

CAUTION

1. ***Do not stop this drug suddenly*** without the knowledge and help of your doctor. Carry a notation that states you are taking this drug.
2. Ask your doctor or pharmacist before using nasal decongestants, which are usually present in over-the-counter cold preparations and nose drops. These can cause sudden increases in blood pressure when taken concurrently with beta-blocker drugs.
3. Report the development of any tendency to emotional depression.

Precautions for Use

By Infants and Children: Safety and effectiveness for those under 12 years of age are not established. However, if this drug is used, observe for the development of low blood sugar (hypoglycemia) during periods of reduced food intake.

By Those Over 60 Years of Age: Unacceptably high blood pressure should be reduced without creating the risks associated with excessively low blood pressure. Small starting doses and frequent blood pressure checks are indicated. Sudden, rapid, and excessive reduction of blood pressure can predispose to stroke or heart attack. Watch for dizziness, unsteadiness, tendency to fall, confusion, hallucinations, depression, or urinary frequency.

▷ **Advisability of Use During Pregnancy**

Pregnancy Category: B. See Pregnancy Risk Categories at the back of this book.

Animal studies: No significant increase in birth defects due to this drug.

Human studies: Adequate studies of pregnant women are not available.

Use this drug only if clearly needed. Ask your physician for guidance.

Advisability of Use If Breast-Feeding

Presence of this drug in breast milk: Yes.

Avoid drug or refrain from nursing.

Habit-Forming Potential: None.

Effects of Overdosage: Weakness, slow pulse, low blood pressure, fainting, cold and sweaty skin, congestive heart failure, possible coma, and convulsions.

Possible Effects of Long-Term Use: Reduced heart reserve and eventual heart failure in susceptible individuals with advanced heart disease.

Suggested Periodic Examinations While Taking This Drug (at physician's discretion)
Measurements of blood pressure, evaluation of heart function.

▷ **While Taking This Drug, Observe the Following**
Foods: No restrictions. Avoid excessive salt intake.
Beverages: No restrictions. May be taken with milk.
▷ *Alcohol:* Use with caution. Alcohol may exaggerate lowering of blood pressure or increase mild sedative effect.
Tobacco Smoking: Nicotine may reduce this drug's effectiveness. I advise everyone to quit smoking.
▷ *Other Drugs*
Pindolol may *increase* the effects of
- other antihypertensive drugs, and cause excessive lowering of blood pressure. Dosage adjustments may be necessary.
- reserpine (Ser-Ap-Es, etc.), and cause sedation, depression, slowing of the heart rate, and lowering of blood pressure.
- verapamil (Calan, Isoptin), and cause excessive depression of heart function; monitor this combination closely.

Pindolol *taken concurrently* with
- amiodarone (Cordarone) may cause extremely slow heartbeats and risk of sinus arrest.
- clonidine (Catapres) requires close monitoring for rebound high blood pressure if clonidine is withdrawn while pindolol is still being taken.
- epinephrine (various) will result in a large increase in blood pressure and reflex increase in heart rate (tachycardia).
- fluoxetine (Prozac) may result in increased risk of pindolol toxicity.
- fluvoxamine (Luvox) may result in increased risk of pindolol toxicity.
- insulin requires close monitoring to avoid undetected hypoglycemia (see Glossary).
- oral antidiabetic drugs (see Drug Classes) can result in slowed recovery from low blood sugar.
- phenylpropanolamine (various) may result in severe increases in blood pressure. Avoid this combination.
- venlafaxine (Effexor) may result in beta-blocker or venlafaxine toxicity. Avoid this combination if possible, or use decreased doses of both medicines.

The following drugs may *increase* the effects of pindolol
- cimetidine (Tagamet).
- methimazole (Tapazole).
- oral contraceptives.
- propylthiouracil (Propacil).
- ritonavir (Norvir), and perhaps other protease inhibitors (see Drug Classes).

The following drugs may *decrease* the effects of pindolol
- barbiturates (phenobarbital, etc.).
- indomethacin (Indocin), and possibly other NSAIDs—may impair pindolol's antihypertensive effect.
- rifampin (Rifadin, Rimactane).
- theophylline (Theo-Dur, others).

▷ *Driving, Hazardous Activities:* Use caution until the full extent of fatigue, dizziness, and blood pressure change have been determined.

Aviation Note: The use of this drug *is a disqualification* for piloting. Consult a designated Aviation Medical Examiner.

Exposure to Sun: No restrictions.

Exposure to Heat: Caution is advised. Hot environments can lower blood pressure and exaggerate the effects of this drug.

Exposure to Cold: Caution is advised. Cold environments can enhance the circulatory deficiency in the extremities that may occur with this drug. The elderly should take precautions to prevent hypothermia (see Glossary).

Heavy Exercise or Exertion: It is advisable to avoid exertion that produces light-headedness, excessive fatigue, or muscle cramping. The use of this drug may intensify the hypertensive response to isometric exercise.

Occurrence of Unrelated Illness: Fever can lower blood pressure and require adjustment of dosage. Nausea or vomiting may interrupt regular doses. Ask your doctor for help.

Discontinuation: It is advisable to avoid sudden discontinuation of this drug in all situations. If possible, gradual reduction of dose over a period of 2 to 3 weeks is recommended. Ask your physician for specific guidance.

PIRBUTEROL (peer BYU ter ohl)

Introduced: 1983   **Class:** Antiasthmatic, bronchodilator   **Prescription:** USA: Yes   **Controlled Drug:**   USA: No; Canada: No   **Available as Generic:** No

Brand Name: Maxair

BENEFITS versus RISKS	
Possible Benefits	*Possible Risks*
VERY EFFECTIVE RELIEF OF BRONCHOSPASM	Increased blood pressure
	Nervousness
	Fine hand tremor
	Irregular heart rhythm (with excessive use)

▷ **Principal Uses**

As a Single Drug Product: Uses currently included in FDA-approved labeling: (1) Relieves acute attacks of bronchial asthma; (2) reduces the frequency and severity of chronic, recurrent asthmatic attacks (prevention); (3) relieves reversible bronchospasm associated with chronic bronchitis, bronchiectasis, and emphysema.

Other (unlabeled) generally accepted uses: May help congestive heart failure.

How This Drug Works: By increasing the production of cyclic AMP, this drug relaxes constricted bronchial muscles to relieve asthmatic wheezing.

Available Dosage Forms and Strengths

Aerosol — 200 mcg per actuation (in canisters of 300 inhalations)

▷ **Usual Adult Dosage Range:**   Inhaler: Two inhalations (400 mcg) every 4 to 6 hours. **Do not exceed** 12 inhalations (2400 mcg) every 24 hours. Oral dosing: 10 to 15 mg three to four times a day. Maximum dose is 60 mg daily.

Note: Actual dosage and administration schedule must be determined for each patient individually.

Conditions Requiring Dosing Adjustments

Liver Function: This drug should be used with caution by patients with liver compromise who use it frequently. Guidelines for dosage adjustments are not available.

Kidney Function: The kidneys do not appear to play a role in the elimination of this drug.

▷ **Dosing Instructions:**   Carefully follow the "Patient's Instructions for Use" provided with the inhaler. Do not overuse.

Usual Duration of Use: According to individual requirements. Do not use beyond the time necessary to terminate episodes of asthma.

Possible Advantages of This Drug

Has a more rapid onset of action and a longer duration of effect than most other drugs of this class.

▷ **This Drug Should Not Be Taken If**

- you have had an allergic reaction to it previously.
- you currently have an irregular heart rhythm.
- you are taking, or have taken within the past 2 weeks, any monoamine oxidase (MAO) type A inhibitor drug (see Drug Classes).

▷ **Inform Your Physician Before Taking This Drug If**

- you have any type of heart or circulatory disorder, especially high blood pressure, coronary heart disease, or heart rhythm abnormality.
- you have diabetes or an excessively active thyroid gland (hyperthyroidism).
- you have any type of seizure disorder.
- you are taking any form of digitalis or any stimulant drug.

Possible Side Effects (natural, expected, and unavoidable drug actions)

Aerosol—dryness or irritation of mouth or throat, altered taste.

▷ **Possible Adverse Effects** (unusual, unexpected, and infrequent reactions)

If any of the following develop, consult your physician promptly for guidance.

Mild Adverse Effects

Allergic Reactions: Skin rash, itching—rare.

Headache, dizziness, nervousness, fine tremor of hands—infrequent.

Palpitations, rapid heart rate, chest pain, cough—rare to infrequent.

Nausea, diarrhea, taste disorders—rare.

Serious Adverse Effects

Irregular heart rhythm, increased blood pressure-possible.

▷ **Possible Effects on Sexual Function**

None reported.

Natural Diseases or Disorders That May Be Activated By This Drug

Latent coronary artery disease, diabetes, epilepsy, or high blood pressure.

Possible Effects on Laboratory Tests

None reported.

CAUTION

1. Combined use of this drug by inhalation with beclomethasone aerosol (Beclovent, Vanceril) may increase the risk of toxicity due to fluorocarbon propellants. It is advisable to use pirbuterol aerosol 20 to 30 minutes **before** beclomethasone aerosol. This will reduce the risk of toxicity and help beclomethasone reach the lung.

2. Excessive or prolonged use of this drug by inhalation can reduce its effectiveness and cause serious heart rhythm disturbances, including cardiac arrest.

Precautions for Use
By Infants and Children: Safety and effectiveness of use in children under 12 years of age have not been established.

By Those Over 60 Years of Age: Avoid excessive and continual use. If acute asthma is not relieved promptly, other drugs may be needed. Watch for nervousness, palpitations, irregular heart rhythm, and muscle tremors.

▷ **Advisability of Use During Pregnancy**
Pregnancy Category: C. See Pregnancy Risk Categories at the back of this book. Animal studies: High-dose studies in rabbits revealed abortion and increased fetal deaths. Studies in rats and rabbits found no drug-associated birth defects.

Human studies: Adequate studies of pregnant women are not available. Avoid use during first 3 months if possible.

Advisability of Use If Breast-Feeding
Presence of this drug in breast milk: Unknown.
Avoid drug or refrain from nursing.

Habit-Forming Potential: None.

Effects of Overdosage: Nervousness, palpitation, rapid heart rate, sweating, headache, tremor, vomiting, chest pain.

Possible Effects of Long-Term Use: Loss of effectiveness.

Suggested Periodic Examinations While Taking This Drug (at physician's discretion)
Blood pressure measurements, evaluation of heart status.

▷ **While Taking This Drug, Observe the Following**
Foods: No restrictions.
Beverages: Avoid excessive use of caffeine-containing beverages—coffee, tea, cola, chocolate.
▷ *Alcohol:* No interactions expected.
Tobacco Smoking: No interactions expected, but I advise everyone to quit smoking.
▷ *Other Drugs*
Pirbuterol *taken concurrently* with
- albuterol (Proventil, Ventolin) may result in adverse effects on the heart.
- monoamine oxidase (MAO) type A inhibitor drugs may cause excessive increase in blood pressure and undesirable heart stimulation.
- phenothiazines (see Drug Classes) may result in blunting of the therapeutic effects of pirbuterol.
▷ *Driving, Hazardous Activities:* Use caution if excessive nervousness or dizziness occurs.
Aviation Note: The use of this drug *is a disqualification* for piloting. Consult a designated Aviation Medical Examiner.
Exposure to Sun: No restrictions.
Heavy Exercise or Exertion: Use caution—excessive exercise can induce asthma in sensitive individuals.

PIROXICAM (peer OX i kam)

See the oxicams (nonsteroidal anti-inflammatory drugs) profile for further information.

PRAVASTATIN (pra vah STA tin)

Introduced: 1986   **Class:** Cholesterol-lowering agent, HMG-CoA reductase inhibitor   **Prescription:** USA: Yes   **Controlled Drug:** USA: No; Canada: No   **Available as Generic:** USA: No; Canada: No

Brand Name: Pravachol

BENEFITS versus RISKS	
Possible Benefits	*Possible Risks*
EFFECTIVE REDUCTION OF TOTAL BLOOD CHOLESTEROL AND LDL CHOLESTEROL	Drug-induced hepatitis
	Drug-induced myositis (muscle inflammation)
EFFECTIVE REDUCTION IN THE NUMBER OF FIRST-TIME HEART ATTACKS	
REDUCTION IN THE NUMBER OF PATIENT DEATHS	

▷ **Principal Uses**

As a Single Drug Product: Uses currently included in FDA-approved labeling: (1) Treatment of abnormally high total blood cholesterol levels (in individuals with types IIa and IIb hypercholesterolemia) due to increased fractions of low-density lipoprotein (LDL) cholesterol. Used in conjunction with a cholesterol-lowering diet after an adequate trial of nondrug methods for lowering cholesterol has proved to be ineffective; (2) the FDA has cleared this medicine to help prevent a first heart attack and reduce death from cardiovascular disease in people with increased blood cholesterol levels who are at risk of a first heart attack; (3) slows progression and in some cases makes small reversals in coronary artery disease.

Other (unlabeled) generally accepted uses: Reduces temporary blood flow (to the heart) problems (myocardial ischemia) when combined with other therapies.

How This Drug Works: This drug blocks the liver enzyme that starts production of cholesterol. Its principal action is the reduction of low-density lipoproteins (LDL), the fraction of total blood cholesterol that is thought to increase the risk of coronary heart disease. This drug may also increase the level of high-density lipoproteins (HDL), the cholesterol fraction that is thought to reduce the risk of heart disease.

Available Dosage Forms and Strengths

Tablets — 10 mg, 20 mg, 40 mg

▷ **Recommended Dosage Ranges** (Actual dosage and administration schedule must be determined for each patient individually.)

Infants and Children: Under 2 years of age—do not use this drug.
   2 to 18 years of age—dosage not established.
18 to 60 Years of Age: Initially 10 to 20 mg daily, taken at bedtime. Maintenance
   dosage is 10 to 20 mg daily, and is adjusted as needed and tolerated at
   intervals of 4 weeks.
Over 60 Years of Age: Starting dose for those with kidney or liver compromise is
   10 mg daily.

Conditions Requiring Dosing Adjustments

Liver Function: This drug should be used with caution by patients with liver
   compromise, and the starting dose decreased to 10 mg per day. Pravastatin
   is contraindicated in sudden (acute) liver disease.
Kidney Function: Patients with significant renal compromise can take a starting
   dose of 10 mg per day. Pravastatin should be used with caution in renal
   compromise.

▷ **Dosing Instructions:**   The tablet may be crushed and can be taken without regard to eating. It is preferably taken at bedtime. (The highest rates of cholesterol production occur between midnight and 5 A.M.)

Usual Duration of Use: Use on a regular schedule for 4 to 6 weeks usually determines effectiveness in reducing blood levels of total and LDL-C cholesterol.
   Long-term use (months to years) requires periodic physician evaluation.

Possible Advantages of This Drug: Recent studies indicate that drugs of this
   class (HMG-CoA reductase inhibitors) are more effective and better tolerated than other drugs currently available for reducing total and LDL-C cholesterol. Its long-term effects are yet to be determined.

▷ **This Drug Should Not Be Taken If**
   • you have had an allergic reaction to it previously.
   • you have active liver disease.
   • you are pregnant or breast-feeding your infant.

▷ **Inform Your Physician Before Taking This Drug If**
   • you have previously taken any other drugs in this class: lovastatin (Meva-
     cor), simvastatin (Zocor).
   • you have a history of liver disease or impaired liver function.
   • you are not using any method of birth control, or you are planning preg-
     nancy.
   • you regularly consume substantial amounts of alcohol.
   • you have kidney disease.
   • you have cataracts or impaired vision.
   • you develop any kind of unexplained muscle weakness, pain, or tenderness.
   • you have any type of chronic muscular disorder.
   • you plan to have major surgery in the near future.

Possible Side Effects (natural, expected, and unavoidable drug actions)
   Development of abnormal liver function tests without associated symptoms.

▷ **Possible Adverse Effects** (unusual, unexpected, and infrequent reactions)
   **If any of the following develop, consult your physician promptly for
      guidance.**
   Mild Adverse Effects
   Allergic Reactions: Skin rash, itching—rare.
   Headache, dizziness, depression—case reports, rare.

Flu-like syndrome, cough—case reports.

Indigestion, stomach pain, nausea, excessive gas, constipation, diarrhea—rare to infrequent.

Muscle cramps and/or pain—rare.

Serious Adverse Effects

Marked and persistent abnormal liver function tests with focal hepatitis (without jaundice)—rare.

Acute myositis (muscle pain and tenderness) during long-term use—case reports.

Rhabdomyolysis—rare and more likely if combined with fibrates.

Low white blood cells (leukopenia)—rare.

Neuropathy—case report.

▷ **Possible Effects on Sexual Function**

Impotence—questionable causation.

Possible Delayed Adverse Effects: Increased liver enzymes.

Natural Diseases or Disorders That May Be Activated By This Drug

Latent liver disease.

Possible Effects on Laboratory Tests

Blood alanine aminotransferase (ALT) enzyme level: increased (with higher doses of drug).

Blood total cholesterol, LDL cholesterol, and triglyceride levels: decreased.

Blood HDL cholesterol level: increased.

CAUTION

1. If pregnancy occurs while taking this drug, discontinue it immediately and consult your physician.
2. Report promptly any development of muscle pain or tenderness, especially if accompanied by fever or malaise.
3. Report promptly the development of altered or impaired vision so that appropriate evaluation can be made.
4. If CPK levels become markedly elevated, this medicine should be stopped.

Precautions for Use

By Infants and Children: Safety and effectiveness for those under 18 years of age are not established.

By Those Over 60 Years of Age: Inform your physician regarding any personal or family history of cataracts. Comply with all recommendations regarding periodic eye examinations. Report promptly any alterations in vision.

▷ **Advisability of Use During Pregnancy**

Pregnancy Category: X. See Pregnancy Risk Categories at the back of this book.

Animal studies: Mouse and rat studies reveal skeletal birth defects due to a closely related drug of this class.

Human studies: Adequate studies of pregnant women are not available.

This drug should be avoided during entire pregnancy.

Advisability of Use If Breast-Feeding

Presence of this drug in breast milk: Yes, in small amounts.

Avoid drug or refrain from nursing.

Habit-Forming Potential: None.

Effects of Overdosage: Increased indigestion, stomach distress, nausea, diarrhea.

Possible Effects of Long-Term Use: Abnormal liver function with focal hepatitis.

Suggested Periodic Examinations While Taking This Drug (at physician's discretion)

Blood cholesterol studies: total cholesterol, HDL and LDL fractions.

Liver function tests before treatment, at 12 weeks of treatment, and every 6 months if the 12-week tests are normal. **This is new labeling, and pravastatin was the first HMG-CoA reductase inhibitor to receive labeling from the FDA for less-frequent liver testing.** Complete eye examination at beginning of treatment and at any time that significant change in vision occurs. Ask your doctor for guidance.

▷ **While Taking This Drug, Observe the Following**

Foods: Follow a standard low-cholesterol diet.

Beverages: No restrictions. May be taken with milk.

▷ *Alcohol:* No interactions expected. Use sparingly.

Tobacco Smoking: No interactions expected, but I advise everyone to quit smoking.

▷ *Other Drugs*

Pravastatin *taken concurrently* with

- clofibrate (Atromid-S) has been associated with muscle damage (rhabdomyolysis).
- cyclosporine (Sandimmune) increases the risk for myopathy.
- gemfibrozil (Lopid) may alter the absorption and excretion of pravastatin; these drugs should not be taken concurrently.
- ritonavir (Norvir) and perhaps other protease inhibitors (see Drug Classes) increases toxicity risk.
- warfarin (Coumadin) can increase the risk of bleeding. More frequent INR (prothrombin time or protime) testing is indicated. Ongoing warfarin doses should be based on laboratory results.

The following drug may *decrease* the effects of pravastatin

- cholestyramine (Questran)—may reduce absorption of pravastatin; take pravastatin 1 hour before or 4 hours after cholestyramine.

▷ *Driving, Hazardous Activities:* This drug may cause dizziness. Restrict activities as necessary.

Aviation Note: The use of this drug *may be a disqualification* for piloting. Consult a designated Aviation Medical Examiner.

Exposure to Sun: No restrictions.

Discontinuation: Do not stop this drug without your doctor's knowledge and help. There may be a significant increase in blood cholesterol levels following discontinuation of this drug.

PRAZOSIN (PRA zoh sin)

Introduced: 1970   **Class:** Antihypertensive   **Prescription:** USA: Yes
Controlled Drug: USA: No; Canada: No   **Available as Generic:** Yes
Brand Names: ✤Apo-Prazo, Minipres, Minizide [CD], ✤Novo-Prazin, ✤Nu-Prazo

```
┌─────────────────────────────────────────────────────────────────┐
│                      BENEFITS versus RISKS                        │
│      Possible Benefits                    Possible Risks          │
│  EFFECTIVE INITIAL THERAPY FOR    "First-dose" drop in blood      │
│    MILD TO MODERATE                 pressure with fainting        │
│    HYPERTENSION                   May cause increased heart rate   │
│  EFFECTIVE ANTIHYPERTENSIVE         (paroxysmal tachycardia)      │
│    IN MODERATE TO SEVERE                                           │
│    HYPERTENSION                                                    │
│  EFFECTIVE CONTROL OF                                              │
│    HYPERTENSION IN                                                 │
│    PHEOCHROMOCYTOMA                                                │
│  May help urine flow in benign                                    │
│    prostatic hyperplasia                                          │
│  Effective in presence of impaired                                │
│    kidney function                                                │
└─────────────────────────────────────────────────────────────────┘
```

▷ **Principal Uses**

As a Single Drug Product: Uses currently included in FDA-approved labeling: Used to start treatment in mild to moderate hypertension. Also used in conjunction with other drugs, to treat moderate to severe hypertension.

Other (unlabeled) generally accepted uses: (1) Combination therapy of congestive heart failure; (2) helps control high blood pressure with a rare tumor (pheochromocytoma); (3) may have an adjunctive role in controlling urine outflow problems caused by prostatic obstruction; (4) may help relieve the symptoms of Raynaud's phenomenon; (5) can ease symptoms of angina; (6) has a role in reducing benign prostatic hyperplasia.

As a Combination Drug Product [CD]: This drug is available in combination with polythiazide, a diuretic of the thiazide class of drugs. By utilizing two different methods of drug action, this combination product is more effective and more convenient for long-term use.

How This Drug Works: By blocking certain actions of the sympathetic nervous system, this drug causes direct relaxation and expansion of blood vessel walls, thus lowering the pressure of the blood within the vessels.

Available Dosage Forms and Strengths

Capsules — 1 mg, 2 mg, 5 mg

▷ **Usual Adult Dosage Range:** Hypertension: A "test dose" of 1 mg is given to determine the patient's response within the first 2 hours. Patients at risk for first-dose excessive lowering in blood pressure include those with pheochromocytoma and those who have recently suffered a stroke (cerebral vascular accident). If tolerated satisfactorily, dose is increased cautiously up to 15 mg every 24 hours in two or three divided doses. The total daily dosage should not exceed 20 mg.

Benign prostatic hyperplasia (BPH): Starting dose is 0.5 mg to 1 mg twice a day. This dose is increased (titrated) as needed and tolerated to 2 mg twice daily. **Note: Actual dose and dosing schedule must be determined for each patient individually.**

Conditions Requiring Dosing Adjustments

Liver Function: This drug should be used with caution and in lower doses by patients with liver compromise. The drug is 97% protein bound. Dose adjustments and more frequent blood pressure checks are needed.

Kidney Function: Patients with kidney failure may have adequate response to smaller doses.

▷ **Dosing Instructions:**   May be taken without regard to food. The capsule may be opened for administration.

Usual Duration of Use: Use on a regular schedule for 4 to 6 weeks usually determines effectiveness in controlling hypertension. Long-term use (months to years) requires supervision and periodic physician evaluation.

Possible Advantages of This Drug
Effective initial treatment of hypertension.
Does not alter blood cholesterol, potassium, or sugar levels.

▷ **This Drug Should Not Be Taken If**
• you have had an allergic reaction to it previously.
• you are experiencing mental depression.
• you have angina (active coronary artery disease) and are not taking a beta-blocking drug. (Call your physician.)

▷ **Inform Your Physician Before Taking This Drug If**
• you have experienced orthostatic hypotension (see Glossary) when using other antihypertensive drugs.
• you have a history of mental depression.
• you have impaired brain circulation or a history of stroke (you may be more sensitive to this medicine).
• you have coronary artery disease.
• you have active liver disease or impaired liver function.
• you plan to have surgery under general anesthesia in the near future.

Possible Side Effects (natural, expected, and unavoidable drug actions)
Orthostatic hypotension, drowsiness, salt and water retention, dry mouth, nasal congestion, constipation. Increased urination—infrequent.

▷ **Possible Adverse Effects** (unusual, unexpected, and infrequent reactions)
If any of the following develop, consult your physician promptly for guidance.
Mild Adverse Effects
Allergic Reactions: Skin rash, itching.
Headache, dizziness, fatigue, nervousness, sweating, numbness and tingling, blurred vision, reddened eyes, ringing in the ears—rare to infrequent.
Edema and weight gain—rare.
Nosebleeds—infrequent.
Palpitation, rapid heart rate, shortness of breath—infrequent .
Nausea, vomiting, diarrhea, abdominal pain, constipation—rare to infrequent.
Incontinence (bed-wetting or enuresis also)—case reports.
Serious Adverse Effects
Mental depression, sleep disturbance—possible.
Paroxysmal tachycardia (heart rates of 120 to 160 beats per min)—case reports.
Slowing of the heart peak and passing out (syncope)—rare.
Lupus-erythematosus-like disorder—case report.

▷ **Possible Effects on Sexual Function**
Decreased libido—infrequent; impotence, retrograde ejaculation, or priapism (see Glossary)—case reports.

Natural Diseases or Disorders That May Be Activated By This Drug
Latent coronary artery insufficiency.

Possible Effects on Laboratory Tests
Blood total cholesterol level: no effect in some; decreased in others.
Blood HDL cholesterol level: no effect in some; increased in others.
Blood LDL cholesterol level: no effect.
Blood VLDL cholesterol level: no effect in some; decreased in others.
Blood triglyceride levels: no effect in some; decreased in others.
Blood glucose level: increased.
Liver function tests: increased—rarely.
Glucose tolerance test (GTT): decreased.
Blood thyroid-stimulating hormone (TSH) level: increased.
Blood thyroxine (T_4) level: increased.

CAUTION
1. Watch for "first-dose" response of precipitous drop in blood pressure; this usually occurs within 30 to 90 minutes. Limit initial doses to 1 mg taken at bedtime for the first 3 days; keep flat (supine) after taking these trial doses.

Precautions for Use
By Infants and Children: Safety and effectiveness for use by those under 12 years of age have not been established.
By Those Over 60 Years of Age: Therapy starts with no more than 1 mg/day for the first 3 days. Any dose increases must be very gradual and supervised by your doctor. Orthostatic hypotension can cause unexpected falls; sit or lie down if you feel light-headed or dizzy. Report any indications of dizziness or chest pain to your doctor promptly.

▷ **Advisability of Use During Pregnancy**
Pregnancy Category: C. See Pregnancy Risk Categories at the back of this book.
Animal studies: No birth defects found.
Human studies: Adequate studies of pregnant women are not available.
Use this drug only if clearly needed. Ask your physician for guidance.

Advisability of Use If Breast-Feeding
Presence of this drug in breast milk: Yes, in small amounts.
Monitor nursing infant closely and discontinue drug or nursing if adverse effects develop.

Habit-Forming Potential: None.

Effects of Overdosage: Orthostatic hypotension, headache, generalized flushing, rapid heart rate, extreme weakness, irregular heart rhythm, circulatory collapse.

Possible Effects of Long-Term Use: None reported.

Suggested Periodic Examinations While Taking This Drug (at physician's discretion)
Measurements of blood pressure in lying, sitting, and standing positions.
Measurements of body weight to detect fluid retention.

▷ **While Taking This Drug, Observe the Following**

Foods: No restrictions. Avoid excessive salt intake.

Beverages: No restrictions. May be taken with milk.

▷ *Alcohol:* Use with extreme caution. Alcohol can exaggerate the blood-pressure-lowering actions of this drug and cause excessive reduction.

Tobacco Smoking: Nicotine can worsen this drug's ability to intensify coronary insufficiency. All forms of tobacco should be avoided.

▷ *Other Drugs*

The following drugs may *increase* the effects of prazosin

- other antihypertensive medications (this is often used to help patients).
- beta-adrenergic-blocking drugs (see Drug Classes); severity and duration of the "first-dose" hypotensive response may be increased.
- verapamil (Calan) may increase the blood level of prazosin and require dose reduction.

Prazosin *taken concurrently* with

- NSAIDs (see Drug Classes) may result in blunting of the blood-pressure-lowering benefit of prazosin.

▷ *Driving, Hazardous Activities:* This drug may cause dizziness or drowsiness. Restrict activities as necessary.

Aviation Note: The use of this drug *is a disqualification* for piloting. Consult a designated Aviation Medical Examiner.

Exposure to Sun: No restrictions.

Exposure to Cold: Use caution until combined effect has been determined. Cold environments may increase risk of coronary insufficiency (angina) in susceptible people.

Heavy Exercise or Exertion: Excessive exertion can augment this drug's ability to induce angina.

Discontinuation: If you are taking this drug as part of your treatment program for congestive heart failure, do not stop it abruptly. Ask your physician for guidance.

PREDNISOLONE (pred NIS oh lohn)

Introduced: 1955   **Class:** Cortisonelike drugs   **Prescription:** USA: Yes
Controlled Drug: USA: No; Canada: No   **Available as Generic:** USA: Yes;
Canada: Yes

Brand Names: ✤Ak-Cide [CD], A & D with Prednisolone [CD], ✤Ak-Pred, ✤Ak-Tate, Blephamide, Cortalone, Delta-Cortef, Duapred, Econopred Ophthalmic, Fernisolone-P, Hydelta-TBA, Hydeltrasol, ✤Inflamase, ✤Inflamase Forte, Isopto Cetapred [CD], Key-Pred, Meticortelone, Menti-Derm, Metimyd [CD], Metreton, ✤Minims Prednisolone, Mydrapred, Niscort, Nor-Pred, ✤Nova-Pred, ✤Novoprednisolone, Ophtho-Tate, Optimyd [CD], Otobione [CD], Pediapred, Pediaject, Polypred, Predcor, ✤Pred Forte, Pred-G [CD], ✤Pred Mild, Prelone, PSP-IV, Savacort, Sterane, TBA Pred, ✤Vasocidin [CD]

BENEFITS versus RISKS

Possible Benefits	*Possible Risks*
EFFECTIVE RELIEF OF SYMPTOMS IN A WIDE VARIETY OF INFLAMMATORY AND ALLERGIC DISORDERS	Use exceeding 2 weeks is associated with many possible adverse effects:
EFFECTIVE IMMUNOSUPPRESSION in selected benign and malignant disorders	ALTERED MOOD AND PERSONALITY
	CATARACTS, GLAUCOMA
	HYPERTENSION
	OSTEOPOROSIS
Prevention of rejection in organ transplantation	ASEPTIC BONE NECROSIS
	INCREASED SUSCEPTIBILITY TO INFECTIONS

Author's Note: Adverse effects from ophthalmic use are much more limited and more rare than those from systemic use.

▷ **Principal Uses**

As a Single Drug Product: Uses currently included in FDA-approved labeling: (1) Used in the treatment of a wide variety of allergic and inflammatory conditions. It is used most commonly in the management of serious skin disorders, asthma, regional enteritis, ulcerative colitis, and all types of major rheumatic disorders including bursitis, tendonitis, most forms of arthritis, and inflammatory eye conditions; (2) used as part of combination therapy in lymphoma; (3) used in some kinds of adrenal insufficiencies; (4) used to help tuberculosis patients who also have inflammation around the heart without fluid buildup; (5) eases symptoms in ulcerative colitis.

Other (unlabeled) generally accepted uses: (1) Used as part of combination therapy in acute leukemias (lymphoblastic, lymphocytic, and myelogenous); (2) may have a role in combination therapy of breast cancer; (3) can help relieve the muscle pain of familial Mediterranean fever; (4) part of a combination therapy in treating abnormal liver tumors (hemangiomas); (5) can help subfertile men decrease seminal antibodies and become fertile; (6) helps people who have drug-induced lowering of white blood cells recover; (7) treats anaphylactic reactions of unknown cause; (8) treats thrombocytopenic purpura of unknown cause; (9) eases symptoms in myasthenia gravis; (10) can help reflex sympathetic dystrophy.

How This Drug Works: Not fully established. It is thought that this drug's anti-inflammatory effect is due to its ability to inhibit the normal defensive functions of certain white blood cells. Its immunosuppressant effect is attributed to a reduced production of lymphocytes and antibodies.

Available Dosage Forms and Strengths

Eye ointment — 0.6%
Eye suspension — 0.5%, 1%
Oral liquid — 6.7 mg/5 ml
Syrup — 15 mg/5 ml
Tablets — 5 mg

▷ **Usual Adult Dosage Range:** 5 to 60 mg daily as a single dose or in divided doses (some patients are put on alternate-day schedules). Once an adequate response is achieved, the dose should be decreased to the lowest effective dose. Ophthalmic drops: One to two drops is instilled into the eye sac (conjunctival sac) every 3 to 12 hours. Dosing may be increased to every hour in severe cases. **Note: Actual dosage and administration schedule must be determined for each patient individually.**

Conditions Requiring Dosing Adjustments

Liver Function: Dosing adjustments do not appear to be needed in liver compromise.

Kidney Function: Dosing adjustments in renal compromise do not appear to be needed. This drug can cause proteinuria. It is a benefit-to-risk decision for kidney compromise (nephropathy) patients who tend to lose protein.

▷ **Dosing Instructions:** The tablet may be crushed and taken with or following food to prevent stomach irritation, preferably in the morning. Suspensions should be gently mixed before using.

Usual Duration of Use: For acute disorders: 4 to 10 days. For chronic disorders: according to individual requirements. Use only for time needed to relieve symptoms in acute self-limiting conditions, or the time required to stabilize a chronic condition and permit gradual withdrawal. Because of its intermediate duration of action, this drug is appropriate for alternate-day administration for many forms. See your doctor regularly.

Author's Note: The information categories provided in this profile are appropriate for prednisolone. For specific information that is normally found in those categories that have been omitted from this profile, the reader is referred to the profile of prednisone, which follows. Prednisolone is a derivative of prednisone; all significant actions and effects are shared by both drugs.

PREDNISONE (PRED ni sohn)

Introduced: 1955   **Class:** Cortisonelike drugs   **Prescription:** USA: Yes
Controlled Drug: USA: No; Canada: No   **Available as Generic:** USA: Yes; Canada: Yes

Brand Names: ✦Apo-Prednisone, Aspred-C [CD], Deltasone, Liquid Pred, Meticorten, ✦Metreton [CD], ✦Novoprednisone, Orasone, Panasol-S, Paracort, Prednicen-M, Prednisone Intensol, SK-Prednisone, Sterapred, Sterapred-DS, ✦Winpred

BENEFITS versus RISKS	
Possible Benefits	*Possible Risks*
EFFECTIVE RELIEF OF SYMPTOMS IN A WIDE VARIETY OF INFLAMMATORY AND ALLERGIC DISORDERS	Use exceeding 2 weeks is associated with many possible adverse effects:
EFFECTIVE IMMUNOSUPPRESSION in selected benign and malignant disorders	ALTERED MOOD AND PERSONALITY
	CATARACTS, GLAUCOMA
	HYPERTENSION
	OSTEOPOROSIS
	ASEPTIC BONE NECROSIS
Prevention of rejection in organ transplantation	INCREASED SUSCEPTIBILITY TO INFECTIONS

▷ **Principal Uses**

As a Single Drug Product: Uses currently included in FDA-approved labeling: (1) Treats a wide variety of allergic and inflammatory conditions. It is used most commonly in the management of serious skin disorders, asthma, gout, lupus erythematosus, regional enteritis, ulcerative colitis, nephrotic syndrome, and all types of major rheumatic disorders including bursitis, tendonitis, and most forms of arthritis; (2) used as part of combination therapy of lymphoma; (3) helps address adrenal insufficiency; (4) used as part of combination therapy of several kinds of leukemia; (5) used in kidney transplant patients; (6) helps patients recover from symptoms of multiple sclerosis.

Other (unlabeled) generally accepted uses: (1) Used in combination therapy of acute (lymphoblastic, lymphocytic, and myelogenous) leukemias; (2) combination therapy of breast cancer; (3) may be helpful in therapy of familial Mediterranean fever; (4) used with other medications to treat liver tumors (hemangiomas); (5) may help subfertile men decrease seminal antibodies and become fertile; (6) helps prevent early lung deterioration in children with AIDS; (7) eases symptoms in alcoholics who have hepatitis and encephalopathy; (8) used in some chronic pain syndromes.

How This Drug Works: It is thought that this drug's anti-inflammatory effect is due to its ability to inhibit the normal defensive functions of certain white blood cells. Its immunosuppressant effect is attributed to a reduced production of lymphocytes and antibodies.

Available Dosage Forms and Strengths

Oral solution — 5 mg/5 ml
Syrup — 5 mg/5 ml (5% alcohol)
Tablets — 1 mg, 2.5 mg, 5 mg, 10 mg, 20 mg, 25 mg, 50 mg

▷ **Usual Adult Dosage Range:**   5 to 60 mg daily as a single dose or in divided doses. With myasthenia gravis, patients not responding to 100 mg will not respond to higher doses. Once the initial inflammation has been overcome, the dose should be gradually lowered to the lowest dose that is effective for the condition being treated. **Note: Actual dosage and administration schedule must be determined for each patient individually.**

Conditions Requiring Dosing Adjustments

Liver Function: Dosing adjustments do not appear to be needed in liver compromise.

Kidney Function: Dosing adjustments in kidney disease do not appear to be needed. The drug itself may cause proteinuria. Its use is a benefit-to-risk decision for patients with protein-losing renal compromise (nephropathy).

▷ **Dosing Instructions:**   The tablet may be crushed and taken with or following food to prevent stomach irritation, preferably in the morning.

Usual Duration of Use: For acute disorders: 4 to 10 days. For chronic disorders: according to individual requirements. Use should not exceed time necessary to get adequate symptomatic relief in acute self-limiting conditions, or the time required to stabilize a chronic condition and permit gradual withdrawal. Intermediate duration of action allows alternate-day administration. See your physician regularly.

▷ **This Drug Should Not Be Taken If**
- you have had an allergic reaction to any dosage form of it previously.
- you have active peptic ulcer disease.
- you have an active herpes simplex virus eye infection.
- you have active tuberculosis.
- you have a fungal infection in a large area inside your body (systemic fungal infection).

▷ **Inform Your Physician Before Taking This Drug If**
- you have had an adverse reaction to any cortisonelike drug.
- you have a history of peptic ulcer disease, thrombophlebitis, or tuberculosis.
- you have diabetes, kidney failure, glaucoma, high blood pressure, deficient thyroid function, or myasthenia gravis.
- you have osteoporosis.
- you have been exposed to any viral illness such as measles or chickenpox. (Cases may be severe if you are taking this medicine.)
- you are prone to depression.
- you have diverticulitis.
- you plan to have surgery of any kind in the near future.

Possible Side Effects (natural, expected, and unavoidable drug actions)

Increased appetite, weight gain, retention of salt and water leading to increased blood pressure, excretion of potassium, increased susceptibility to infection. Mild euphoria.

▷ **Possible Adverse Effects** (unusual, unexpected, and infrequent reactions)
If any of the following develop, consult your physician promptly for guidance.

Mild Adverse Effects

Allergic Reaction: Skin rash.

Headache, dizziness, insomnia—infrequent.

Acid indigestion, abdominal distention—infrequent.

Patchy blue areas on the great toe (blue toe syndrome)—case reports.

Muscle cramping and weakness—possible.

Elevated intracranial pressure (pseudotumor cerebri)—infrequent.

Acne, excessive growth of facial hair—frequent.

Serious Adverse Effects

Mental and emotional disturbances of serious magnitude—case reports.

Reactivation of latent tuberculosis—possible in those with past tuberculosis.

Development of peptic ulcer—possible and more likely in those with previous ulcers.

Development of inflammation of the pancreas—rare.

Thrombophlebitis (inflammation of a vein with the formation of blood clot): pain or tenderness in thigh or leg, with or without swelling of the foot, ankle, or leg—rare.

Increased intraocular (inner eye) pressure, glaucoma, or cataracts—infrequent.

Kaposi's sarcoma—case reports.

Growth retardation—possible in children with long-term use.

Cushing's syndrome—possible with long-term use.

Necrosis of bone—case reports.

Osteoporosis—possible with long-term use.

Superinfections—possible.

Inflammation or wasting of muscle (myositis or myopathy)—infrequent.

Increased blood sugar—possible and may be dose related.

Drug-induced porphyria or seizures—case reports.

Pulmonary embolism (movement of a blood clot to the lung)—sudden shortness of breath, pain in the chest, coughing, bloody sputum—increased risk.

▷ **Possible Effects on Sexual Function**

Altered timing and pattern of menstruation.

Correction of male infertility when due to autoantibodies that suppress sperm activity.

▷ **Adverse Effects That May Mimic Natural Diseases or Disorders**

Pattern of symptoms and signs resembling Cushing's syndrome.

Natural Diseases or Disorders That May Be Activated By This Drug

Latent diabetes, glaucoma, peptic ulcer disease, tuberculosis.

Possible Effects on Laboratory Tests

Complete blood cell counts: decreased eosinophils, lymphocytes, and platelets.

Blood amylase level: increased (possible pancreatitis).

Blood total cholesterol and HDL cholesterol levels: increased.

Blood LDL cholesterol level: no effect.

Blood triglyceride levels: no significant effect.

Blood glucose level: increased.

Glucose tolerance test (GTT): decreased.

Blood potassium or testosterone level: decreased.

Blood thyroid hormone (T_3): decreased.

Blood uric acid level: increased.

Urine sugar tests: no effect with Tes-Tape; false low result with Clinistix and Diastix.

Fecal occult blood test: positive (if gastrointestinal bleeding).

CAUTION

1. If therapy exceeds 1 week, carry an identification card noting that you are taking this drug.

2. Do not stop this drug abruptly after long-term use.

3. If vaccination against measles, rabies, smallpox, or yellow fever is required, discontinue this drug 72 hours before vaccination and do not resume it for at least 14 days after vaccination.

Precautions for Use

By Infants and Children: Avoid prolonged use if possible. During long-term use, observe for suppression of normal growth and the possibility of increased intracranial pressure. Following long-term use, the child may be at risk for adrenal gland deficiency during stress for as long as 18 months after cessation of this drug.

By Those Over 60 Years of Age: Cortisonelike drugs should only be used when the disorder under treatment is unresponsive to adequate trials of unrelated drugs. Avoid the prolonged use of this drug. Continual use (even in small doses) can increase severity of diabetes, enhance fluid retention, raise blood pressure, weaken resistance to infection, induce stomach ulcer, and accelerate development of cataract and osteoporosis.

▷ **Advisability of Use During Pregnancy**

Pregnancy Category: B or C. See Pregnancy Risk Categories at the back of this book.

Animal studies: Birth defects reported in mice, rats, and rabbits.

Human studies: Adequate studies of pregnant women are not available.

Avoid completely during the first 3 months. Limit use during the final 6 months as much as possible. If used, examine infant for possible deficiency of adrenal gland function.

Advisability of Use If Breast-Feeding

Presence of this drug in breast milk: Yes.

Avoid drug or refrain from nursing.

Habit-Forming Potential: Long-term use of this drug may produce a state of functional dependence (see Glossary). In therapy of asthma and rheumatoid arthritis, it is advisable to keep the dose as small as possible and attempt drug withdrawal after periods of reasonable improvement. Such procedures may reduce the degree of "steroid rebound"—the return of symptoms as the drug is withdrawn.

Effects of Overdosage: Fatigue, muscle weakness, stomach irritation, acid indigestion, excessive sweating, facial flushing, fluid retention, swelling of extremities, increased blood pressure.

Possible Effects of Long-Term Use: Increased blood sugar (possible diabetes), increased fat deposits on the trunk of the body ("buffalo hump"), rounding of the face ("moon face"), thinning and fragility of skin, loss of texture and strength of bones (osteoporosis, aseptic necrosis), cataracts, glaucoma, retarded growth and development in children.

Suggested Periodic Examinations While Taking This Drug (at physician's discretion)

Measurements of blood pressure, blood sugar and potassium levels.

Complete eye examinations at regular intervals.

Chest X ray if history of tuberculosis.

Bone mineral density testing (DEXA) to check for osteoporosis.

Determination of the rate of development of the growing child to detect retardation of normal growth.

▷ **While Taking This Drug, Observe the Following**

Foods: No interactions expected. Ask your physician regarding need to restrict salt intake or eat potassium-rich foods. During long-term use of this drug, it is advisable to eat a high-protein diet.

Nutritional Support: During long-term use, take a vitamin D supplement. During wound repair, take a zinc supplement. Potassium loss may need to be replaced.

Beverages: No restrictions. Drink all forms of milk liberally.

▷ *Alcohol:* No interactions expected. Use caution if you are prone to peptic ulcers.

Tobacco Smoking: Nicotine increases the blood levels of naturally produced cortisone. I advise everyone to quit smoking.

Marijuana Smoking: May cause additional impairment of immunity.

▷ *Other Drugs*

Prednisone may ***decrease*** the effects of

- isoniazid (INH, Niconyl, etc.).
- salicylates (aspirin, sodium salicylate, etc.).

Prednisone *taken concurrently* with
- amphotericin B (Abelcet, Fungizone) may result in additive potassium loss.
- birth control pills (oral contraceptives) will prolong the prednisone effect.
- cyclosporine (Sandimmune) can cause increased cyclosporine levels and increased prednisone levels. Dose decreases may be needed for both drugs.
- foscarnet (Foscavir) may result in additive potassium loss.
- ketoconazole (Nizoral) will lessen the therapeutic benefits of ketoconazole.
- loop diuretics (furosemide (Lasix); bumetanide (Bumex)) may have blunt their effects.
- macrolide antibiotics (erythromycin, troleandomycin, and perhaps others) can lead to prednisone toxicity.
- NSAIDs may result in additive stomach and intestinal irritation.
- oral anticoagulants may either increase or decrease their effectiveness; consult your physician regarding the need for prothrombin time testing and dosage adjustment.
- oral antidiabetic drugs (see Drug Classes) or insulin may result in loss of glucose control.
- ritonavir (Norvir) and perhaps other protease inhibitors (see Drug Classes) may lead to toxicity.
- theophylline (Theo-Dur, others) may result in variable responses to this medicine. Increased frequency of theophylline levels are recommended.
- thiazide diuretics (see Drug Classes) or loop diuretics may result in additive potassium loss.
- vaccines (flu, pneumococcal, varicella, and others) may result in blunted response to the vaccine and decreased preventive benefits.

The following drugs may *decrease* the effects of prednisone
- antacids—may reduce its absorption.
- barbiturates (Amytal, Butisol, phenobarbital, etc.).
- carbamazepine (Tegretol).
- phenytoin (Dilantin, etc.).
- primidone (Mysoline).
- rifampin (Rifadin, Rimactane, etc.).

▷ *Driving, Hazardous Activities:* Usually no restrictions. Be alert to the rare occurrence of dizziness.

Aviation Note: The use of this drug *may be a disqualification* for piloting. Consult a designated Aviation Medical Examiner.

Exposure to Sun: No restrictions.

Occurrence of Unrelated Illness: This drug may decrease natural resistance to infection. Tell your doctor if you develop an infection of any kind. It may also reduce your body's ability to respond to the stress of acute illness, injury, or surgery. Keep your doctor informed of any significant changes in your state of health.

Discontinuation: After long-term use, do not stop prednisone abruptly. Ask your physician for guidance regarding gradual withdrawal. For a period of 2 years after discontinuing this drug, it is essential in the event of illness, injury, or surgery that you tell attending medical personnel that you have used this drug in the past. The period of impaired response to stress following the use of cortisonelike drugs may last for 1 to 2 years.

PRIMIDONE (PRI mi dohn)

Introduced: 1953   **Class:** Anticonvulsant   **Prescription:** USA: Yes
Controlled Drug: USA: No; Canada: No   **Available as Generic:** USA: Yes;
Canada: Yes
Brand Names: ✦Apo-Primidone, Myidone, Mysoline✦PMS-Primidone

BENEFITS versus RISKS	
Possible Benefits	*Possible Risks*
EFFECTIVE CONTROL OF TONIC-CLONIC (GRAND MAL) AND ALL TYPES OF PARTIAL SEIZURES	Allergic skin reactions Rare blood cell disorders: megaloblastic anemia, deficient white blood cells and platelets

▷ **Principal Uses**
　　As a Single Drug Product: Uses currently included in FDA-approved labeling:
　　　　This drug is used exclusively to control generalized grand mal seizures and
　　　　all types of partial seizures. It can be used to supplement the anticonvulsant
　　　　action of phenytoin.
　　　　Other (unlabeled) generally accepted uses: (1) May have a minor role in help-
　　　　ing in therapy of orthostatic tremor; (2) can help ringing in the ears.

How This Drug Works: Reduces and stabilizes the excitability of nerve fibers
　　　　and inhibits the repetitious spread of electrical impulses along nerve path-
　　　　ways. This action may prevent seizures altogether, or it may reduce their
　　　　frequency and severity. (Part of this drug's action is attributable to pheno-
　　　　barbital, one of its conversion products in the body.)

Available Dosage Forms and Strengths
　　　　Oral suspensions — 250 mg/5 ml
　　　　　　　　Tablets — 50 mg, 125 mg, 250 mg
　　　　Tablets, chewable — 125 mg

▷ **Usual Adult Dosage Range:**   Initially 100 mg every 24 hours as a single dose at
　　　　bedtime for 3 days; 100 to 125 mg twice a day for days 4–6, 100 to 125 mg
　　　　three times a day for days 7–9, and an ongoing (maintenance) dose of 250
　　　　mg three or four times a day, 6 to 8 hours apart. Total daily dosage should
　　　　not exceed 2000 mg. **Note: Actual dosage and administration schedule
　　　　must be determined for each patient individually.**

Conditions Requiring Dosing Adjustments
　　　　Liver Function: The dose **must** be decreased and blood levels obtained more
　　　　frequently for patients with liver compromise.
　　　　Kidney Function: For patients with mild to moderate kidney failure, the usual
　　　　dose can be taken every 8 hours. Patients with moderate to severe kidney
　　　　failure can take the usual dose every 8–12 hours. Patients with severe kid-
　　　　ney failure should take the usual dose every 12–24 hours. Primidone should
　　　　be used with caution in renal compromise, as it can be a cause of crystallu-
　　　　ria.

▷ **Dosing Instructions:**   The tablet may be crushed and taken with or following
　　　　food to reduce stomach irritation. Shake the suspension well before mea-
　　　　suring the dose.

Usual Duration of Use: Use on a regular schedule for 2 to 4 weeks usually determines effectiveness in reducing the frequency and severity of seizures. Long-term use (months to years) requires physician supervision.

▷ **This Drug Should Not Be Taken If**
- you have had an allergic reaction to it previously.
- you are allergic to phenobarbital.
- you have a history of porphyria.

▷ **Inform Your Physician Before Taking This Drug If**
- you have had an allergic or idiosyncratic reaction to any barbiturate drug in the past.
- you have a family history of intermittent porphyria.
- you have impaired liver, kidney, or thyroid gland function.
- you have asthma, emphysema, or myasthenia gravis.
- you are pregnant or planning pregnancy.
- you plan to have surgery under general anesthesia in the near future.

Possible Side Effects (natural, expected, and unavoidable drug actions)
Drowsiness, impaired concentration, mental and physical sluggishness.

▷ **Possible Adverse Effects** (unusual, unexpected, and infrequent reactions)
If any of the following develop, consult your physician promptly for guidance.

Mild Adverse Effects
Allergic Reactions: Skin rashes, hives, localized swellings. "Hangover" effect, dizziness, unsteadiness, impaired vision, double vision, fatigue, emotional disturbances—more likely during first 3 months, may ease with time.
Low blood pressure, faintness—possible.
Shoulder pain, joint pain—possible with longer-term therapy.
Nausea, vomiting, thirst, increased urine volume—rare to infrequent.

Serious Adverse Effects
Allergic Reactions: Swelling of lymph glands.
Idiosyncratic Reactions: Paradoxical anxiety, seizures, agitation, restlessness, rage.
Visual or auditory hallucinations—rare.
Drug-induced porphyria, systemic lupus erythematosus, or low thyroid gland function (hypothyroidism)—case reports.
Blood cell disorders: megaloblastic anemia; low white blood cells or platelets—case reports.
Drug-induced kidney problems (crystalluria)—case reports.

▷ **Possible Effects on Sexual Function**
Decreased libido and/or impotence—case reports.
Decreased effectiveness of oral contraceptives taken concurrently.

▷ **Adverse Effects That May Mimic Natural Diseases or Disorders**
Allergic swelling of lymph glands may suggest a naturally occurring lymphoma.

Natural Diseases or Disorders That May Be Activated By This Drug
Acute intermittent and/or cutaneous porphyria (see Glossary).
Systemic lupus erythematosus.

Possible Effects on Laboratory Tests
Complete blood cell counts: decreased red cells, hemoglobin, white cells, and platelets; increased eosinophils.

Blood lupus erythematosus (LE) cells: positive.

Prothrombin time: decreased (when taken concurrently with warfarin).

Urine screening tests for drug abuse: may be **positive** for phenobarbital (a normal derivative of this drug). (Test results depend upon amount of drug taken and testing method used.)

CAUTION

1. This drug must not be stopped abruptly.
2. A wide variation of drug action from person to person requires careful individualization of dosage.
3. Regularity of drug use is essential for the successful management of seizure disorders. Take your medication at the same time each day.
4. Side effects and mild adverse effects are usually most apparent during the first several weeks of treatment, and often subside with continued use.
5. It may be necessary to take folic acid to prevent anemia while taking this drug. Consult your physician.
6. It is advisable to carry a card of personal identification with a notation that you are taking this drug.

Precautions for Use

By Infants and Children: This drug should be used with caution in the hyperkinetic (overactive) child. Paradoxical hyperactivity is possible. Puberty changes characteristically slow phenobarbital metabolism, permitting gradual accumulation. Measurements of blood levels in young adolescents can detect rising concentrations of this drug that could lead to toxicity (see "Therapeutic Drug Monitoring," chapter 2).

By Those Over 60 Years of Age: It is advisable for the elderly to avoid all barbiturates. If use of this drug is attempted, small starting doses are indicated. Watch for confusion, delirium, agitation, or paradoxical excitement. This drug may be conducive to hypothermia (see Glossary).

▷ Advisability of Use During Pregnancy

Pregnancy Category: D. See Pregnancy Risk Categories at the back of this book.

Animal studies: Birth defects due to this drug reported in mice.

Human studies: Adequate studies of pregnant women are not available. However, recent reports suggest a possible association between the use of this drug during the first 3 months of pregnancy and the development of birth defects in the fetus. Discuss with your physician the advantages and possible disadvantages of using this drug during pregnancy. If it is used, determine the smallest maintenance dose that will prevent seizures.

The newborn infants of mothers who take this drug during pregnancy may develop abnormal bleeding or bruising due to the deficiency of certain blood clotting factors in the blood. Consult your physician regarding the need to take vitamin K during the final month of pregnancy.

Advisability of Use If Breast-Feeding

Presence of this drug in breast milk: Yes.

Monitor nursing infant closely and discontinue drug or nursing if adverse effects develop.

Habit-Forming Potential: None.

Effects of Overdosage: Drowsiness, jerky eye movements, blurred vision, staggering gait, incoordination, slurred speech, stupor progressing to coma.

Possible Effects of Long-Term Use: Enlargement of lymph glands; enlargement of thyroid gland. Megaloblastic anemia due to folic acid deficiency. Reduced blood levels of calcium and phosphorus, leading to rickets in children and loss of bone texture (osteomalacia) in adults.

Suggested Periodic Examinations While Taking This Drug (at physician's discretion)

Complete blood cell counts. Measurements of blood levels of calcium and phosphorus. Evaluation of lymph and thyroid glands. Skeletal X-ray examinations for bone demineralization during long-term use.

▷ **While Taking This Drug, Observe the Following**

Foods: No restrictions.

Nutritional Support: Talk with your doctor about calcium, vitamin D and K, and folic acid supplements.

Beverages: No restrictions. May be taken with milk or fruit juice.

▷   *Alcohol:* Avoid completely. Alcohol can increase greatly the sedative and depressant effects of this drug on brain function.

Tobacco Smoking: May enhance the sedative effects of this drug. I advise everyone to quit smoking.

▷   *Other Drugs*

Note: 15% of primidone is converted to phenobarbital in the body. See the profile of phenobarbital for possible interactions with other drugs.

▷   *Driving, Hazardous Activities:* This drug may cause drowsiness and dizziness; it can also impair mental alertness, vision, and physical coordination. Restrict activities as necessary.

Aviation Note: The use of this drug *is a disqualification* for piloting. Consult a designated Aviation Medical Examiner.

Exposure to Sun: No restrictions.

Occurrence of Unrelated Illness: Notify your physician of any illness or injury that prevents the use of this drug according to your regular dosage schedule.

Discontinuation: Do not stop this drug without your physician's knowledge and approval. Sudden withdrawal of any anticonvulsant drug can cause severe and repeated seizures.

PROBENECID (proh BEN e sid)

Introduced: 1951   **Class:** Anti-gout   **Prescription:** USA: Yes   **Controlled Drug:** USA: No; Canada: No   **Available as Generic:** USA: Yes; Canada: No

Brand Names: ✦Ampicin PRB [CD], Benemid, ✦Benuryl, Colabid [CD], Col-Benemid [CD], Polycillin-PRB [CD], Probalan, Probampacin [CD], Proben-C [CD], ✦Pro-Biosan 500 Kit [CD], SK-Probenecid

BENEFITS versus RISKS	
Possible Benefits	*Possible Risks*
EFFECTIVE LONG-TERM PREVENTION OF ACUTE ATTACKS OF GOUT	Formation of uric acid kidney stones
	Bone marrow depression (aplastic anemia)
Useful adjunct to penicillin therapy (to achieve high blood and tissue levels of penicillin)	Drug-induced liver and kidney damage

▷ **Principal Uses**

As a Single Drug Product: Uses currently included in FDA-approved labeling: (1) Used in helping maintain penicillin levels in therapy of gonorrhea; (2) helps decrease elevated uric acid levels caused by thiazide diuretics; (3) helps prevent gout.

Other (unlabeled) generally accepted uses: (1) May have a role in preventing kidney toxicity in cisplatin chemotherapy; (2) adjunctive use in maintaining effective antibiotic levels in treatment of syphilis; (3) helps decrease uric acid in gout patients.

As a Combination Drug Product [CD]: This drug is available in combination with colchicine, a drug often used for the treatment of acute gout. Each drug works in a different way; when used in combination they provide both relief of the acute gout and some measure of protection from recurrence of acute attacks.

How This Drug Works: Works in the kidney (tubular systems) to increase uric acid excretion in the urine; this drug reduces the levels of uric acid in the blood and body tissues. It also works in the kidney to decrease the amount of penicillin excreted in the urine, and prolongs the presence of penicillin in the blood and helps achieve higher concentrations in body tissues.

Available Dosage Forms and Strengths

Tablets — 500 mg

▷ **Usual Adult Dosage Range:**   Anti-gout: Initially 250 mg twice a day for 1 week; then 500 mg twice a day. Adjunct to penicillin therapy: 500 mg four times a day. **Note: Actual dosage and administration schedule must be determined for each patient individually.**

Conditions Requiring Dosing Adjustments

Liver Function: Specific guidelines for dosage adjustment in liver compromise are not available. This drug should be used with caution.

Kidney Function: Patients with kidney failure (creatinine clearance less than 30 ml/min) should **not** use this drug, as the effectiveness is questionable. Those with moderate kidney failure may still benefit from this medicine, and dose increases (as needed and tolerated) in 500-mg steps up to 2000 mg a day in equally divided doses may be required.

▷ **Dosing Instructions:**   The tablet may be crushed and taken with or following food to reduce stomach irritation. Drink 2.5 to 3 quarts of liquids daily.

Usual Duration of Use: Use on a regular schedule for several months usually determines effectiveness in preventing acute attacks of gout. Long-term use (months to years) requires supervision and periodic evaluation by your physician.

▷ **This Drug Should Not Be Taken If**
- you have had an allergic reaction to it previously.
- you have active liver disease.
- you have acute kidney failure or kidney stones made of uric acid.
- you have an active blood cell or bone marrow disorder.
- you are experiencing an attack of acute gout at the present time.

▷ **Inform Your Physician Before Taking This Drug If**
- you have a history of kidney disease or kidney stones.
- you have a history of liver disease or impaired liver function.
- you have a history of peptic ulcer disease.
- you have a history of a blood cell or bone marrow disorder.
- you are taking any drug product that contains aspirin or aspirinlike drugs.

Possible Side Effects (natural, expected, and unavoidable drug actions)
Development of kidney stones (composed of uric acid); this is preventable. Consult your physician regarding the use of sodium bicarbonate (or other urine alkalizer) to prevent stone formation.

▷ **Possible Adverse Effects** (unusual, unexpected, and infrequent reactions)
If any of the following develop, consult your physician promptly for guidance.
Mild Adverse Effects
Allergic Reactions: Skin rash, itching, drug fever (see Glossary).
Headache, dizziness, flushing of face—infrequent.
Reduced appetite, sore gums, nausea, vomiting—possible to infrequent.
Serious Adverse Effects
Allergic Reactions: Anaphylactic reaction (see Glossary).
Idiosyncratic Reactions: Hemolytic anemia (see Glossary).
Bone marrow depression (see Glossary): fatigue, sore throat, bleeding/bruising—case reports.
Drug-induced liver damage with jaundice (see Glossary) or porphyria—case reports.
Fluid in the retina (retinal edema)—case reports.
Drug-induced kidney damage: marked fluid retention, reduced urine formation—case reports.

▷ **Possible Effects on Sexual Function**
None reported.

▷ **Adverse Effects That May Mimic Natural Diseases or Disorders**
Liver reactions may suggest viral hepatitis. Kidney reactions may suggest nephrosis.

Possible Effects on Laboratory Tests
Complete blood cell counts: decreased red cells, hemoglobin, white cells, and platelets.
INR (prothrombin time): increased (when taken concurrently with warfarin).
Blood glucose level and uric acid level: decreased.
Blood urea nitrogen (BUN) level: increased (kidney damage).
Liver function tests: increased enzymes (ALT/GPT, AST/GOT, alkaline phosphatase), or bilirubin.
Urine sugar tests: false positive with Benedict's solution and Clinitest.

CAUTION
1. This drug should not be started until 2 to 3 weeks after an acute attack of gout has subsided.
2. This drug may increase the frequency of acute attacks of gout during the first few months of treatment. Concurrent use of colchicine is advised to prevent acute attacks.
3. Aspirin (and aspirin-containing drug products) can reduce the effectiveness of this drug. Use acetaminophen or a nonaspirin analgesic for pain relief as needed.

Precautions for Use

By Infants and Children: Safety and effectiveness for those under 2 years of age are not established.

By Those Over 60 Years of Age: The natural decline in kidney function that occurs after 60 may require adjustment of your dosage. You may be more susceptible to the serious adverse effects of this drug. Report any unusual symptoms promptly for evaluation.

▷ **Advisability of Use During Pregnancy**

Pregnancy Category: B. See Pregnancy Risk Categories at the back of this book.
Animal studies: No information available.
Human studies: Adequate studies of pregnant women are not available.
This drug has been used during pregnancy with no reports of birth defects or adverse effects on the fetus. Ask your physician for guidance.

Advisability of Use If Breast-Feeding

Presence of this drug in breast milk: Unknown.
Avoid drug or refrain from nursing.

Habit-Forming Potential: None.

Effects of Overdosage: Stomach irritation, nausea, vomiting, nervous agitation, delirium, seizures, coma.

Possible Effects of Long-Term Use: Formation of kidney stones. Kidney damage in sensitive individuals.

Suggested Periodic Examinations While Taking This Drug (at physician's discretion)

Complete blood cell counts, blood uric acid, liver and kidney function tests.

▷ **While Taking This Drug, Observe the Following**

Foods: Follow your physician's advice regarding the need for a low-purine diet.

Beverages: A large intake of coffee, tea, or cola beverages may reduce the effectiveness of treatment.

▷ *Alcohol:* No interactions expected. However, large amounts of alcohol can raise the blood uric acid level and reduce the effectiveness of treatment.

Tobacco Smoking: No interactions expected, but I advise everyone to quit smoking.

▷ *Other Drugs*

Probenecid may *increase* the effects of
- acyclovir (Zovirax) and result in toxicity unless doses are reduced.
- clofibrate (Atromid-S).
- dyphylline (Neothylline).
- ketoprofen and perhaps other NSAIDs (see Drug Classes).
- methotrexate (Mexate), and increase its toxicity.

- midazolam (Versed) and increase CNS depression.
- oral antidiabetic agents (see Drug Classes).
- thiopental (Pentothal), and prolong its anesthetic effect.
- valacyclovir (Valtrex) and result in toxicity unless doses are reduced.
- zalcitabine (Hivid).
- zidovudine (Retrovir) and increase toxicity risk.

Probenecid *taken concurrently* with
- allopurinol (Zyloprim) may result in extended allopurinol half-life.
- cephalosporins (see Drug Classes) may cause a doubling of antibiotic levels. Caution must be used to avoid toxicity.
- dapsone may cause up to a 50% increased dapsone level and result in toxicity unless dapsone doses are decreased.
- penicillins (see Drug Classes) may cause a threefold to fivefold increase in penicillin blood levels, greatly increasing the effectiveness of each penicillin dose.
- rifampin (Rifadin, others) may result in increased blood levels of rifampin.
- ritonavir (Norvir) may lead to changes in probenecid blood levels.

The following drugs may *decrease* the effects of probenecid
- aspirin and other salicylates—may reduce its effectiveness in promoting the excretion of uric acid.
- bismuth subsalicylate (Pepto-Bismol, others).

▷ *Driving, Hazardous Activities:* This drug may cause dizziness. Restrict activities as necessary.

Aviation Note: The use of this drug *may be a disqualification* for piloting. Consult a designated Aviation Medical Examiner.

Exposure to Sun: No restrictions.

Discontinuation: Do not stop this drug without consulting your physician.

PROCAINAMIDE (proh KAYN a mide)

Introduced: 1950   **Class:** Antiarrhythmic   **Prescription:** USA: Yes
Controlled Drug: USA: No; Canada: No   **Available as Generic:** USA: Yes; Canada: No

Brand Names: ✦Apo-Procainamide, Procamide SR, Procanbid, Procan SR, Promine, Pronestyl, Pronestyl-SR, Rhythmin

BENEFITS versus RISKS	
Possible Benefits	*Possible Risks*
EFFECTIVE TREATMENT OF SELECTED HEART RHYTHM DISORDERS	NARROW TREATMENT RANGE INDUCTION OF SYSTEMIC LUPUS ERYTHEMATOSUS SYNDROME Provocation of abnormal heart rhythms Blood cell disorders: insufficient white blood cells and platelets

▷ **Principal Uses**

As a Single Drug Product: Uses currently included in FDA-approved labeling: Used to abolish and prevent the recurrence of premature beats arising in the ventricles (lower chambers) of the heart.

Other (unlabeled) generally accepted uses: (1) Used to treat and prevent atrial fibrillation, atrial flutter, and abnormally rapid heart rates (tachycardia) that originate in the atria or the ventricles; (2) helps treat myotonia and improve breathing in myotonic dystrophy.

How This Drug Works: By slowing the activity of the pacemaker and delaying the transmission of electrical impulses through the conduction system and muscle of the heart, this drug assists in restoring normal heart rate and rhythm.

Available Dosage Forms and Strengths

Capsules — 250 mg, 375 mg, 500 mg
Injections — 100 mg/ml, 500 mg/ml
Tablets — 250 mg, 375 mg, 500 mg
Tablets, prolonged action — 250 mg, 500 mg, 750 mg, 1000 mg

▷ **Usual Adult Dosage Range:** Dose varies according to indication: Starting dose is up to 50 mg per kg of body mass per day of the immediate-release form. This calculated dose is then divided into equal doses and is taken every 3, 4, or 6 hours. The ongoing daily dose should be adjusted to individual patient response and blood levels. People over 50 years old may get an acceptable clinical response and blood level from a lower dose. The sustained-release form is usually started in younger patients who do not have kidney problems at 50 mg per kg of body mass per day. This calculated dose is divided into equal doses and is taken every 6 to 12 hours, depending on patient response and blood levels. **Note: Actual dosage and administration schedule must be determined for each patient individually.**

Conditions Requiring Dosing Adjustments

Liver Function: This drug should be used with caution by patients with liver compromise, and blood levels appropriately obtained. Lower ongoing doses are generally used. Procainamide should be a benefit-to-risk decision for patients with compromised livers, as it may be more likely to cause liver problems in this patient population.

Kidney Function: Patients with moderate to severe kidney failure can be given the usual doses every 6–12 hours. Patients with severe kidney failure can be given the usual dose every 8–24 hours. The drug should be used with caution in renal compromise, and appropriate blood levels obtained.

▷ **Dosing Instructions:** Preferably taken on an empty stomach, 1 hour before or 2 hours after eating. However, it may be taken with or following food to reduce stomach irritation. The regular capsules may be opened and the regular tablets may be crushed for administration; however, the prolonged-action tablets should be swallowed whole without alteration.

Usual Duration of Use: Use on a regular schedule for 24 to 48 hours usually determines effectiveness in correcting or preventing responsive rhythm disorders. Long-term use requires supervision and periodic evaluation by your physician.

▷ **This Drug Should Not Be Taken If**
- you have had an allergic reaction to it previously.
- you have systemic lupus erythematosus.
- you have second- or third-degree heart block (determined by electrocardiogram).
- you have myasthenia gravis.

▷ **Inform Your Physician Before Taking This Drug If**
  • you are allergic to procaine (Novocain) or other local anesthetics of the "-cain" drug class, such as those commonly used for glaucoma testing and dental procedures.
  • you have had any adverse reactions to other antiarrhythmic drugs.
  • you have a history of heart disease of any kind, especially "heart block."
  • you have a history of low blood pressure.
  • you have a history of lupus erythematosus or myasthenia gravis.
  • you have a history of abnormally low blood platelet counts.
  • you have impaired liver or kidney function.
  • you have an enlarged prostate gland.
  • you are taking any form of digitalis or any diuretic drug that can cause excessive loss of body potassium (ask your physician).
  • you plan to have surgery under general anesthesia in the near future.

Possible Side Effects (natural, expected, and unavoidable drug actions)
  Drop in blood pressure in susceptible individuals.

▷ **Possible Adverse Effects** (unusual, unexpected, and infrequent reactions)
  If any of the following develop, consult your physician promptly for guidance.
  Mild Adverse Effects
  Allergic Reactions: Skin rash, hives, itching, drug fever (see Glossary).
  Weakness, light-headedness—case reports.
  Loss of appetite, bitter taste, indigestion, nausea, vomiting, diarrhea—infrequent.
  Serious Adverse Effects
  Allergic Reactions: Systemic lupus-erythematosus-like syndrome: fever, skin eruptions, joint and muscle pains, pleurisy. **This is reported to occur in up to 20% of users.**
  Idiosyncratic Reactions: Mental depression, hallucinations, psychotic behavior, hemolytic anemia (see Glossary).
  Severe drop in blood pressure, fainting—possible.
  Drug-induced pancreatitis, liver toxicity, or myopathy—case reports.
  Drug-induced myasthenia gravis, pancreatitis, or peripheral neuropathy—case reports.
  Pericardial effusions—rare.
  Asthmalike breathing difficulties—case reports.
  Induction of new heart rhythm disturbances—possible.
  Inability to empty urinary bladder, prostatism (see Glossary).
  Anticholinergic syndrome—rare.
  Blood cell disorders: abnormally low white blood cell or platelet count—case reports.

▷ **Possible Effects on Sexual Function**
  None reported.

▷ **Adverse Effects That May Mimic Natural Diseases or Disorders**
  Rare liver reaction may suggest viral hepatitis.

Natural Diseases or Disorders That May Be Activated By This Drug
  Systemic lupus erythematosus, myasthenia gravis.

Possible Effects on Laboratory Tests

Complete blood cell counts: decreased red cells, hemoglobin, white cells, and platelets; increased eosinophils.

Blood lupus erythematosus (LE) cells: positive.

Blood antinuclear antibodies (ANA): positive (in 50–80% of those using drug after 3 to 6 months).

Liver function tests: increased liver enzymes (ALT/GPT, AST/GOT, alkaline phosphatase) and bilirubin.

Urine screening tests for drug abuse: **initial** test result may be falsely **positive**; **confirmatory** test result will be **negative**. (Test results depend upon amount of drug taken and testing method used.)

CAUTION

1. Thorough evaluation of your heart function (including electrocardiograms) is necessary prior to using this drug.
2. Periodic evaluation of your heart function is necessary to determine your response to this drug. Some individuals may experience worsening of their heart rhythm disorder and/or deterioration of heart function. Close monitoring of heart rate, rhythm, and overall performance is essential.
3. Dosage must be adjusted carefully for each individual. Do not change your dosage without the knowledge and supervision of your physician.
4. Do not combine any antiarrhythmic drugs unless directed to do so by your doctor.
5. Call your doctor IMMEDIATELY if you develop aching joints, muscle pain, or unexplained fever.

Precautions for Use

By Infants and Children: Blood cell counts should be monitored for loss of white blood cells.

By Those Over 60 Years of Age: Reduced kidney function may require reduction in dosage. Observe carefully for light-headedness, dizziness, unsteadiness, and tendency to fall.

▷ **Advisability of Use During Pregnancy**

Pregnancy Category: C. See Pregnancy Risk Categories at the back of this book.
Animal studies: No information available.
Human studies: Adequate studies of pregnant women are not available.
Use this drug only if clearly needed.

Advisability of Use If Breast-Feeding

Presence of this drug in breast milk: Yes.
Avoid drug or refrain from nursing.

Habit-Forming Potential: None.

Effects of Overdosage: Loss of appetite, nausea, vomiting, weakness, faintness, irregular heart rhythm, stupor, circulatory collapse, heart arrest.

Possible Effects of Long-Term Use: Lupus-erythematosus-like syndrome (see above).

Suggested Periodic Examinations While Taking This Drug (at physician's discretion)

Complete blood cell counts.
Blood tests for the development of lupus erythematosus (LE) cells and antinuclear antibodies.

Electrocardiograms to monitor drug effect on mechanisms that influence heart rate and rhythm.

▷ **While Taking This Drug, Observe the Following**

Foods: No restrictions.

Beverages: Avoid excessive intake of coffee, tea, and cola beverages. Avoid iced drinks. May be taken with milk.

▷ *Alcohol:* Use caution—alcohol can increase the blood-pressure-lowering effects of this drug.

Tobacco Smoking: Nicotine can cause heart irritability and reduce the effectiveness. I advise everyone to quit smoking.

▷ *Other Drugs*

Procainamide may *increase* the effects of
- antihypertensive drugs, and cause excessive lowering of blood pressure.
- metformin (Glucophage).

The following drugs may *increase* the effects of procainamide
- amiodarone (Cordarone).
- cimetidine (Tagamet).
- propranolol (Inderal).
- quinidine (Quinaglute).
- ranitidine (Zantac).
- trimethoprim (Proloprim, Bactrim).

▷ *Driving, Hazardous Activities:* This drug may cause dizziness or weakness. Restrict activities as necessary.

Aviation Note: The use of this drug *may be a disqualification* for piloting. Consult a designated Aviation Medical Examiner.

Exposure to Sun: No restrictions.

Exposure to Heat: Use caution—hot environments are conducive to lowering blood pressure.

Occurrence of Unrelated Illness: Vomiting, diarrhea, or dehydration can affect this drug's action. Report such developments promptly.

Discontinuation: This drug should not be stopped abruptly after long-term use. Ask your physician for guidance regarding gradual dose reduction.

PROCHLORPERAZINE (proh klor PER a zeen)

Introduced: 1956   **Class:** Antipsychotic, antiemetic, phenothiazines
Prescription: USA: Yes   **Controlled Drug:** USA: No; Canada: No   **Available as Generic:** USA: Yes; Canada: Yes

Brand Names: ✦Combid [CD], Compazine, Eskatrol, ✦PMS-Prochlorperazine, Pro-Iso, ✦Stemetil, Ultrazine [CD]

BENEFITS versus RISKS	
Possible Benefits	*Possible Risks*
EFFECTIVE CONTROL OF ACUTE MENTAL DISORDERS, NAUSEA, AND VOMITING	SERIOUS TOXIC EFFECTS ON BRAIN with long-term use
	Liver damage with jaundice
Relief of anxiety and nervous tension	Blood cell disorders: abnormally low white cell and platelet counts

▷ **Principal Uses**

As a Single Drug Product: Uses currently included in FDA-approved labeling: (1) Relieves severe nausea and vomiting; (2) may be used to treat schizophrenia; (3) helps prevent motion sickness.

Other (unlabeled) generally accepted uses: (1) Sometimes used to increase the effects of anesthesia; (2) may be of use in treating Ménière's disease (for nausea and vomiting).

How This Drug Works: By inhibiting the action of dopamine, this drug acts to correct an imbalance of nerve impulse transmissions that is thought to be responsible for certain mental disorders. By blocking dopamine in the brain's chemoreceptor trigger zone, this drug prevents stimulation of the vomiting center.

Available Dosage Forms and Strengths

Capsules, prolonged action — 10 mg, 15 mg, 30 mg
Injection — 5 mg/ml
Suppositories — 2.5 mg, 5 mg, 25 mg
Syrup — 5 mg/5 ml
Tablets — 5 mg, 10 mg, 25 mg

▷ **Usual Adult Dosage Range:** Initially 5 mg of the immediate-release form every 6 to 8 hours. If needed and tolerated, dose may be increased by 5 mg at intervals of 3 to 4 days. Usual range is 50 to 75 mg daily. The total daily dosage should not exceed 150 mg.

Nausea and vomiting: 5 to 10 mg three or four times daily. The sustained-release form can be taken as 15 mg when you wake up in the morning, or 10 mg of the sustained-release form every 12 hours. **Note: Actual dose and dosing schedule must be determined for each patient individually.**

Conditions Requiring Dosing Adjustments

Liver Function: This drug should be used with caution by patients with liver compromise. Specific guidelines for dosage adjustment are not available.

Kidney Function: Specific guidelines for adjustment of dosages are not available.

▷ **Dosing Instructions:** The tablets may be crushed and taken with or following food to reduce stomach irritation. Prolonged-action capsules should be swallowed whole without alteration.

Duration of Use: Use on a regular schedule for 12 to 24 hours usually determines effectiveness in controlling nausea and vomiting. If used for severe anxiety-tension states or acute psychotic behavior, a trial of several weeks is usually necessary to determine effectiveness. If not significantly beneficial within 6 weeks, it should be stopped. Consult your physician on a regular basis.

▷ **This Drug Should Not Be Taken If**
- you have had an allergic reaction to it previously.
- you have active liver disease.
- you have signs that are indicative of Reye syndrome.
- you have extremely low blood pressure.
- you have cancer of the breast.

- this drug was prescribed for a child who is less than 2 years old or who weighs less than 20 lb.
- you have a current blood cell or bone marrow disorder.

▷ **Inform Your Physician Before Taking This Drug If**
- you are allergic or abnormally sensitive to any phenothiazine drug (see Drug Classes).
- you have impaired liver or kidney function.
- you have any type of seizure disorder.
- you have bone marrow depression or a history of blood diseases.
- you have diabetes, glaucoma, or heart disease.
- you have prostate trouble (prostatic hypertrophy).
- you are pregnant.
- you have had neuroleptic malignant syndrome or lupus erythematosus.
- you are taking any drug with sedative effects.
- you plan to have surgery under general or spinal anesthesia in the near future.

Possible Side Effects (natural, expected, and unavoidable drug actions)
Drowsiness (usually during the first 2 weeks), orthostatic hypotension (see Glossary), blurred vision, dry mouth, nasal congestion, constipation, impaired urination.
Pink or purple coloration of urine, of no significance.

▷ **Possible Adverse Effects** (unusual, unexpected, and infrequent reactions)
If any of the following develop, consult your physician promptly for guidance.
Mild Adverse Effects
Allergic Reactions: Skin rash, hives, low-grade fever.
Lowering of body temperature, especially in the elderly (see Hypothermia in Glossary)—possible.
Increased appetite and weight gain—possible.
Increased blood pressure—infrequent.
Dizziness, weakness—frequent; agitation, insomnia, impaired day and night vision—infrequent.
Chronic constipation, fecal impaction, incontinence—infrequent.
Serious Adverse Effects
Allergic Reactions: Hepatitis with jaundice (see Glossary), usually between second and fourth week; high fever; asthma; anaphylactic reaction (see Glossary).
Idiosyncratic Reactions: Toxic dermatitis, Stevens-Johnson syndrome. Neuroleptic malignant syndrome (see Glossary).
Liver toxicity or porphyria—case reports.
Abnormal eye positioning (oculogyric crisis)—case reports.
Depression, disorientation, seizures—case reports.
Abnormally high blood pressure—rare.
Disturbances of heart rhythm, rapid heart rate—rare.
Bone marrow depression (see Glossary)—case reports.
Parkinson-like disorders (see Glossary); muscle spasms of face, jaw, neck, back, extremities; slowed movements, muscle rigidity, tremors; tardive dyskinesias (see Glossary)—case reports.

▷ **Possible Effects on Sexual Function**

Altered timing and pattern of menstruation.

Female breast enlargement with milk production—case reports. Causes false-positive pregnancy test result.

Male breast enlargement and tenderness (gynecomastia), inhibited ejaculation or priapism (see Glossary)—case reports.

▷ **Adverse Effects That May Mimic Natural Diseases or Disorders**

Nervous system reactions may suggest Parkinson's disease.

Liver reactions may suggest viral hepatitis.

Reactions resembling systemic lupus erythematosus can occur.

Natural Diseases or Disorders That May Be Activated By This Drug

Latent epilepsy, glaucoma, diabetes mellitus, prostatism (see Glossary).

Possible Effects on Laboratory Tests

White blood cell count: decreased.

Liver function tests: increased enzymes (ALT/GPT, AST/GOT, alkaline phosphatase), or bilirubin.

CAUTION

1. Many over-the-counter medications (see Glossary) for allergies, colds, and coughs contain drugs that can interact unfavorably with this drug. Ask your doctor or pharmacist for help before using any such medications.

2. Aluminum or magnesium containing antacids can limit absorption of this drug and reduce its effectiveness.

3. Obtain prompt evaluation of any change or disturbance of vision.

Precautions for Use

By Infants and Children: Do not use this drug in infants under 2 years of age, or in children of any age with symptoms suggestive of Reye syndrome (see Glossary). Children with acute illnesses ("flu-like" infections, measles, chickenpox, etc.) are very susceptible to adverse effects when this drug is given to control nausea and vomiting.

By Those Over 60 Years of Age: Small starting doses are advisable. You may be more susceptible to drowsiness, lethargy, constipation, lowering of body temperature (hypothermia), and orthostatic hypotension (see Glossary). This drug can worsen existing prostatism (see Glossary). You may also be more susceptible to the development of Parkinson-like reactions and/or tardive dyskinesia (see discussion of these terms in Glossary). These reactions must be recognized early since they may become unresponsive to treatment and irreversible.

▷ **Advisability of Use During Pregnancy**

Pregnancy Category: C. See Pregnancy Risk Categories at the back of this book.

Animal studies: Cleft palate reported in mouse and rat studies.

Human studies: No increase in birth defects reported in 2,023 exposures. Information from adequate studies of pregnant women is not available.

Limit use to small and infrequent doses. Avoid drug during the final month because of possible effects on the newborn infant.

Advisability of Use If Breast-Feeding

Presence of this drug in breast milk: Yes, in small amounts.

Monitor nursing infant closely and discontinue drug or nursing if adverse effects develop.

Habit-Forming Potential: None, but it has been used in combination with pentazocine as a heroin substitute by drug abusers.

Effects of Overdosage: Marked drowsiness, weakness, tremor, agitation, unsteadiness, deep sleep, coma, convulsions.

Possible Effects of Long-Term Use: Tardive dyskinesias. Eye changes: opacities in cornea or lens, retinal pigmentation.

Suggested Periodic Examinations While Taking This Drug (at physician's discretion)

Complete blood cell counts, especially between the 4th and 10th weeks of treatment.

Liver function tests, electrocardiograms.

Complete eye examinations—eye structures and vision.

Careful inspection of the tongue for early evidence of fine, involuntary, wave-like movements that could indicate the beginning of tardive dyskinesia.

▷ **While Taking This Drug, Observe the Following**

Foods: No restrictions. Vitamin C in high doses may lower therapeutic benefits.

Nutritional Support: A riboflavin (vitamin B$_2$) supplement should be taken with long-term use.

Beverages: No restrictions. May be taken with milk.

▷ *Alcohol:* Avoid completely. Alcohol can increase phenothiazine sedation and accentuate depressant effects on brain function and blood pressure. Phenothiazines can increase intoxicating effects of alcohol.

Tobacco Smoking: Possible reduction of drowsiness from drug. I advise everyone to quit smoking.

Marijuana Smoking: Moderate increase in drowsiness; accentuation of orthostatic hypotension; increased risk of precipitating latent psychoses, confusing the interpretation of mental status and drug responses.

▷ *Other Drugs*

Prochlorperazine may ***increase*** the effects of

• all atropinelike drugs, and cause nervous system toxicity.

• all sedative drugs, especially meperidine (Demerol), and cause excessive sedation.

Prochlorperazine may ***decrease*** the effects of

• guanethidine (Ismelin, Esimil), and reduce its effectiveness in lowering blood pressure.

Prochlorperazine ***taken concurrently*** with

• MAO inhibitors (see Drug Classes) may result in increased risk of abnormal body movements (extrapyramidal reactions).

• oral antidiabetic drugs (see Drug Classes) agents may blunt their therapeutic benefits.

• propranolol (Inderal) may cause increased effects of both drugs; monitor drug effects closely and adjust dosages as necessary.

The following drugs may ***decrease*** the effects of prochlorperazine

• antacids containing aluminum and/or magnesium.

• benztropine (Cogentin).

• trihexyphenidyl (Artane).

▷ *Driving, Hazardous Activities:* This drug can impair mental alertness, judgment, and physical coordination. Avoid hazardous activities.

Aviation Note: The use of this drug *is a disqualification* for piloting. Consult a designated Aviation Medical Examiner.

Exposure to Sun: Use caution until sensitivity has been determined. Some phenothiazines can cause photosensitivity (see Glossary).

Exposure to Heat: Use caution and avoid excessive heat as much as possible. This drug may impair the regulation of body temperature and increase the risk of heatstroke.

Exposure to Cold: Use caution and dress warmly. This drug can increase the risk of hypothermia in the elderly.

Discontinuation: After long-term use, do not stop this drug suddenly. Gradual withdrawal over 2 to 3 weeks under physician supervision is recommended.

PROPIONIC ACIDS
(Nonsteroidal Anti-Inflammatory Drugs)

Ibuprofen (i BYU proh fen)   **Fenoprofen** (FEN oh proh fen)   **Flurbiprofen** (flur BI proh fen)   **Ketoprofen** (kee toh PROH fen)   **Naproxen** (na PROX in) **Oxaprozin** (OX a proh zin)

Introduced: 1974, 1976, 1977, 1973, 1974, 1992, respectively   **Class:** Analgesic, mild; NSAIDs   **Prescription:** USA: Varies   **Controlled Drug:** USA: No; Canada: No   **Available as Generic:** Yes: ibuprofen, fenoprofen, flurbiprofen, ketoprofen, and naproxen

Brand Names: Ibuprofen: Aches-N-Pain, Actiprofen, Advil, ✦Amersol, ✦Apo-Ibuprofen, Arthritis Foundation Pain Reliever/Fever Reducer, Bayer Select, Children's Advil, Children's Motrin, Children's Motrin Drops (nonprescription), Children's Motrin Suspension (nonprescription), CoAdvil [CD], Dimetapp Sinus [CD], Dologesic, Dristan Sinus, Excedrin IB, Genpril, Guildprofen, Haltran, Ibuprohm, Ibu, Junior Strength Motrin Caplets (nonprescription), Medipren, Medi-Profen, Midol IB, Motrin, Motrin IB, ✦Novo-Profen, Nuprin, PediaProfen, Profen-IB, Rufen, Superior Pain Medicine, Supreme Pain Medicine, Tab-Profen, Fenoprofen: Nalfon; Flurbiprofen: Ansaid, ✦Apo-Flurbiprofen, ✦Froben, ✦Froben-SR, Ocufen; Ketoprofen: Actron (12.5-mg nonprescription), ✦Apo-Keto, ✦Apo-Keto E, Orudis, Orudis E-50, Orudis E-100, Orudis KT (nonprescription), Orudis SR, Oruvail, Oruvail ER, ✦Oruvail SR, ✦Rhodis, ✦Rhodis EC, ✦Rhodis EC Suppository; Naproxen: Aleve (nonprescription), Anaprox, Anaprox DS, ✦Apo-Naproxen, Naprelan, Naprelan Once Daily, Naprosyn, ✦Naxen, Neo-Prox, ✦Novo-Naprox, ✦Nu-Naprox, ✦Synflex; Oxaprozin: Daypro

---

BENEFITS versus RISKS

Possible Benefits	*Possible Risks*
EFFECTIVE RELIEF OF MILD TO MODERATE PAIN AND INFLAMMATION	Gastrointestinal pain, ulceration, bleeding
EFFECTIVE RELIEF OF FEVER	Kidney damage
	Fluid retention
	Bone marrow depression (except oxaprozin)
	Liver toxicity (naproxen, ketoprofen, and flurbiprofen)
	(All rare)

▷ **Principal Uses**

As a Single Drug Product: Uses currently included in FDA-approved labeling: (1) All of the six agents in this class treat rheumatoid and osteoarthritis; (2) naproxen is useful in treating bursitis, gout, dysmenorrhea (ketoprofen and ibuprofen are also approved for use in primary dysmenorrhea), pain, juvenile rheumatoid arthritis, and tendonitis; (3) fenoprofen is the only agent approved to treat tennis elbow.

Other (unlabeled) generally accepted uses: (1) Naproxen has been used to treat migraine and colds caused by rhinoviruses; (2) oxaprozin is useful in gout and tendonitis; (3) ketoprofen may have a role in temporal arteritis; (4) flurbiprofen has some support for therapy of periodontal disease and miosis inhibition; (5) fenoprofen has been used successfully in therapy of migraine; (6) ibuprofen treats interleukin-2 toxicity, and chronic urticaria, and can decrease IUD-associated bleeding. All of the agents have been used for a variety of pains and fever.

How These Drugs Work: It is thought that these drugs reduces the tissue concentrations of prostaglandins (and related compounds), chemicals involved in the production of inflammation and pain.

Available Dosage Forms and Strengths

Ibuprofen:

Caplets —	200 mg
Tablets, chewable —	50 mg, 100 mg
Oral suspension —	100 mg/5 ml
Tablets —	40 mg, 200 mg, 300 mg, 400 mg, 600 mg, 800 mg

Fenoprofen:

Capsules —	200 mg, 300 mg, 600 mg
Tablets —	600 mg

Flurbiprofen:

Ophthalmic drops —	0.03%
Tablets —	50 mg, 100 mg

Ketoprofen:

Capsules —	50 mg, 75 mg, 100 mg, 150 mg
Suppositories —	100 mg (in Canada)
Tablets (nonprescription) —	12.5 mg
Tablets, enteric —	50 mg (in Canada)

Naproxen:

Caplets — 220 mg
Oral suspension — 125 mg/5 ml
Rectal suppository — 500 mg (Canada)
Tablets — 125 mg, 250 mg, 275 mg, 375 mg, 500 mg,
550 mg
Tablets, controlled release — 375 mg, 500 mg
Naprelan Once Daily — 375 mg, 500 mg
Oxaprozin:

Caplets — 600 mg

▷ **Usual Adult Dosage Range:**   Ibuprofen: 200 to 800 mg three or four times daily.
Total daily dosage should not exceed 3200 mg.

Fenoprofen: 300 to 600 mg three or four times daily. Daily maximum is 3200
mg.

Flurbiprofen: 100 to 300 mg daily in two to four divided doses. The lowest
effective dose should be used. Daily maximum is 300 mg.

Ketoprofen: 75 mg three times daily or 50 mg four times daily. Usual daily
dose is 100 to 300 mg, divided into three or four doses. Daily maximum is
300 mg.

Naproxen: Gout—750 mg initially, then 250 mg every 8 hours until attack is
relieved. Arthritis—250 mg, 375 mg, or 500 mg twice daily, 12 hours apart.

The new sustained-release form (Naprelan) offers an intestinal-protective
drug absorption system (IPDAS) and once-daily (two tablets once a day)
dosing. Menstrual pain—500 mg initially, then 250 mg every 6 to 8 hours as
needed. Maximum dose for pain is 1375 mg.

Oxaprozin: 1200 mg as a single daily dose in the morning. Daily maximum is
1800 mg (or 26 mg per kg of body mass for patients with normal liver and
kidney function).

**Author's Note: Medicines in this class with available nonprescription
forms usually have lower daily maximum doses. For example: Children's Motrin—approved for nonprescription use as temporary relief
of minor aches and pains or reduction of fever in children 2 years of
age and older. Adverse effects are also less common and fewer in number. Less than 11 kg of body mass and under 2 years old: consult your
doctor; 2 to 3 years old and 11–15.9 kg of body mass: 100 mg every 6 to
8 hours. Up to four doses may be given a day. Use should NOT go on for
longer than 3 days. Please consult individual package labels or ask
your pharmacist or doctor for dosing advice.**

**Note: Actual dose and dosing schedule must be determined for each
patient individually.**

Conditions Requiring Dosing Adjustments

Liver Function: All of these drugs are metabolized in the liver and therefore
should be used with caution, and consideration given to lower doses, by
patients with liver compromise.

Kidney Function: These drugs share the risks common to most nonsteroidal
anti-inflammatory drugs (NSAIDs). Some patients with kidney compromise are dependent on prostaglandins for kidney function. A benefit-to-risk
decision must be made regarding the use of NSAIDs by these patients.

▷ **Dosing Instructions:** Take either on an empty stomach or with food or milk to prevent stomach irritation. Take with a full glass of water and remain upright (do not lie down) for 30 minutes. The tablets may be crushed and the capsules opened for administration, except for ketoprofen tablets (should not be crushed or altered).

Usual Duration of Use: Use on a regular schedule for 1 to 2 weeks usually determines effectiveness. Peak oxaprozin effect may take 6 weeks. Long-term use requires supervision and periodic physician evaluation.

▷ **These Drugs Should Not Be Taken If**
- you have had an allergic reaction to them previously.
- you are subject to asthma or nasal polyps caused by aspirin.
- you have a bleeding disorder or a blood cell disorder.
- flurbiprofen ophthalmic drops should NOT be used by people with herpes simplex keratitis.
- you have severe impairment of kidney function (some cases).

▷ **Inform Your Physician Before Taking These Drugs If**
- you are allergic to aspirin or other aspirin substitutes.
- you have active peptic ulcer disease or any form of gastrointestinal bleeding.
- you have a history of peptic ulcer disease or any type of bleeding disorder.
- you have impaired liver or kidney function.
- you have high blood pressure or a history of heart failure.
- you are taking acetaminophen, aspirin, or other aspirin substitutes or anticoagulants.

Possible Side Effects (natural, expected, and unavoidable drug actions)
Fluid retention (weight gain); pink, red, purple, or rust coloration of urine (ibuprofen only). Ringing in the ears.

▷ **Possible Adverse Effects** (unusual, unexpected, and infrequent reactions)
If any of the following develop, consult your physician promptly for guidance.
Mild Adverse Effects
Allergic Reactions: Skin rash, hives, itching.
Headache, dizziness, altered or blurred vision, ringing in the ears, depression—infrequent.
Stinging or burning of the eyes with ophthalmic flurbiprofen drops—possible.
Sleep disturbances (oxaprozin)—infrequent.
Mouth sores, indigestion, nausea, vomiting, constipation, diarrhea—infrequent.
Palpitations (fenoprofen)—rare.
Serious Adverse Effects
Allergic Reactions: Anaphylactic reaction (see Glossary), severe skin reactions—rare; lung inflammation (naproxen—pneumonitis)—rare.
Idiosyncratic Reactions: Drug-induced meningitis with fever and coma (ibuprofen and naproxen)—rare.
Active peptic ulcer, with or without bleeding—rare with 6 months use, infrequent after 1 year of use.
Inflammation of the colon—rare.
Porphyria (some drugs in this class)—case reports.
Pancreatitis or lupus erythematosus—two case reports with naproxen.

Some medicines in this class may cause Parkinson-like symptoms in susceptible patients—case reports.

Inflammation of the esophagus—probable if patients lie down soon after taking these medicines.

Liver damage with jaundice (see Glossary)—case reports.

Kidney damage with painful urination, bloody urine, reduced urine formation—possible.

Bone marrow depression (see Glossary)—fatigue, sore throat, abnormal
bleeding/bruising—case reports.

▷ **Possible Effects on Sexual Function**

Altered timing and pattern of menstruation (ibuprofen, ketoprofen, and naproxen), and excessive menstrual bleeding (ibuprofen and ketoprofen)—
case reports.

Male breast enlargement and tenderness (ibuprofen)—rare.

Naproxen may rarely inhibit ejaculation.

Ketoprofen may rarely decrease libido.

Possible Delayed Adverse Effects: Mild anemia due to "silent" blood loss from
the stomach (less than that caused by aspirin).

▷ **Adverse Effects That May Mimic Natural Diseases or Disorders**

Liver reaction may suggest viral hepatitis.

Natural Diseases or Disorders That May Be Activated by These Drugs

Peptic ulcer disease, ulcerative colitis.

Possible Effects on Laboratory Tests

Complete blood cell counts: decreased red cells, hemoglobin, white cells, and
platelets.

Blood cholesterol or uric acid levels: increased.

Blood lithium level: increased.

Liver function tests: increased enzymes (ALT/GPT, AST/GOT, alkaline phosphatase) or bilirubin.

Kidney function tests: increased blood creatinine and urea nitrogen (BUN)
levels.

Fecal occult blood test: positive.

CAUTION

1. Dosage should always be limited to the smallest amount that produces
reasonable improvement.

2. These drugs may mask early indications of infection. Inform your physician if you think you are developing an infection of any kind.

Precautions for Use

By Infants and Children: Safety and effectiveness for those under 12 years of age
are not established.

By Those Over 60 Years of Age: Small doses are advisable until tolerance is determined. Watch for signs of liver or kidney toxicity, fluid retention, dizziness,
confusion, impaired memory, stomach bleeding, or constipation.

▷ **Advisability of Use During Pregnancy**

Pregnancy Category: B for ibuprofen, fenoprofen, flurbiprofen, ketoprofen, and
naproxen. C for oxaprozin. Ibuprofen and fenoprofen are FDA category D if
used in the final 3 months (trimester) of pregnancy. The manufacturers of
ketoprofen and flurbiprofen say that both medicines should be avoided in
late pregnancy. See Pregnancy Risk Categories at the back of this book.

Animal studies: No birth defects reported in rats or rabbits.

Human studies: Adequate studies of pregnant women are not available.

Avoid these drugs during the final 3 months. Use during the first 6 months only if clearly needed. Ask your physician for guidance.

Advisability of Use If Breast-Feeding

Presence of these drugs in breast milk: Yes, or expected.

Avoid drugs or refrain from nursing.

Habit-Forming Potential: None.

Effects of Overdosage: Drowsiness, dizziness, ringing in the ears, nausea, vomiting, diarrhea, confusion, unsteadiness, stupor progressing to coma.

Possible Effects of Long-Term Use: Fluid retention.

Suggested Periodic Examinations While Taking These Drugs (at physician's discretion)

Complete blood cell counts, liver and kidney function tests, complete eye examinations if vision is altered in any way.

▷ **While Taking These Drugs, Observe the Following**

Foods: No restrictions.

Beverages: No restrictions. May be taken with milk.

▷ *Alcohol:* Use with caution. The irritant action of alcohol on the stomach lining, added to the irritant action of these drugs, can increase the risk of stomach ulceration and/or bleeding.

Tobacco Smoking: No interactions expected, but I advise everyone to quit smoking.

▷ *Other Drugs*

These medicines may *increase* the effects of

- acetaminophen (Tylenol, etc.), and increase the risk of kidney damage; avoid prolonged use of this combination.
- anticoagulants (Coumadin, etc.), and increase the risk of bleeding. More frequent INR (prothrombin time or protime) tests are needed, and ongoing doses should be adjusted to the laboratory test results.
- enoxaparin (Lovenox) if NSAIDs are used before hip replacement surgery, and enoxaparin is used after surgery.
- lithium (Lithobid, others) by causing toxic lithium levels.
- methotrexate (Mexate, others) and result in major methotrexate toxicity with possible anemia, hemorrhage, and blood infections.

These medicines may *decrease* the effects of

- beta-blockers (see Drug Classes) such as carteolol (Cartrol).
- diuretics (see Drug Classes) such as hydrochlorothiazide (Esidrix) and furosemide (Lasix).

These medicines *taken concurrently* with the following drugs may increase the risk of bleeding; avoid these combinations:

- ACE inhibitors (see Drug Classes)—can worsen kidney diseases.
- aspirin.
- dipyridamole (Persantine).
- enoxaparin (Lovenox).
- histamine (H_2) blockers (see Drug Classes)—may increase toxicity from NSAIDs.
- indomethacin (Indocin).

- sulfinpyrazone (Anturane).
- valproic acid (Depakene).
- warfarin (Coumadin).

▷ *Driving, Hazardous Activities:* These drugs may cause drowsiness or dizziness. Restrict activities as necessary.

Aviation Note: The use of these drugs *may be a disqualification* for piloting. Consult a designated Aviation Medical Examiner.

Exposure to Sun: Use caution until sensitivity is determined. Ibuprofen, keto-profen, flurbiprofen, and naproxen cause photosensitivity (see Glossary).

PROPRANOLOL (proh PRAN oh lohl)

Introduced: 1966 **Class:** Anti-anginal, antiarrhythmic, antihypertensive, anti-migraine drug, beta-blocker **Prescription:** USA: Yes **Controlled Drug:** USA: No; Canada: No **Available as Generic:** Yes

Brand Names: ✦Apo-Propranolol, ✦Detensol, Inderal, Inderal-LA, Inderide [CD], Inderide LA [CD], Ipran, ✦Novo-Pranol, ✦PMS Propranolol

---

BENEFITS versus RISKS

Possible Benefits	*Possible Risks*
EFFECTIVE, WELL-TOLERATED AS: ANTI-ANGINAL DRUG in effort-induced angina; ANTIARRHYTHMIC DRUG in certain heart rhythm disorders; ANTIHYPERTENSIVE DRUG in mild to moderate hypertension EFFECTIVE PREVENTION OF MIGRAINE HEADACHES Effective adjunct in the prevention of recurrent heart attack and the management of pheochromocytoma	CONGESTIVE HEART FAILURE in advanced heart disease Worsening of angina in coronary heart disease (if drug is abruptly withdrawn) Masking of low blood sugar (hypoglycemia) in drug-treated diabetes Provocation of asthma Depression Blood cell disorders: low white cell and platelet counts

---

▷ **Principal Uses**

As a Single Drug Product: Uses currently included in FDA-approved labeling: (1) Used to treat several serious cardiovascular disorders: classical effort-induced angina, certain types of heart rhythm disturbance, and high blood pressure. It is also beneficial in preventing the recurrence of heart attacks (myocardial infarction); (2) used to reduce the frequency and severity of migraine headaches; (3) helps decrease tremors in those afflicted with essential tremor.

Other (unlabeled) generally accepted uses: (1) Control of physical signs of anxiety and nervous tension (as in stage fright); (2) helps control familial tremors and symptoms seen with markedly overactive thyroid function (thyrotoxicosis); (3) decreases abnormal abdominal fluid accumulation (ascites) in people with cirrhosis of the liver; (4) may have a role in combination therapy with metronidazole in resistant *Giardia* infections; (5) helps control headaches caused by cyclosporine (Sandimmune); (6) may be useful in certain kinds of pain, especially after amputations; (7) can help control panic attacks; (8) useful in helping decrease bleeding in patients with esophageal varices and liver cirrhosis; (9) helps fight symptoms in narcotic withdrawal cases.

As a Combination Drug Product [CD]: This drug is available in combination with hydrochlorothiazide for the treatment of hypertension. This combination product includes two drugs with different mechanisms of action; it is intended to provide greater effectiveness and convenience for long-term use.

How This Drug Works: By blocking certain actions of the sympathetic nervous system, this drug

- reduces rate and contraction force of the heart, lowering the ejection pressure of the blood leaving the heart and reducing the oxygen requirement for heart function.
- reduces the degree of contraction of blood vessel walls, resulting in their expansion and consequent lowering of blood pressure.
- prolongs the conduction time of nerve impulses through the heart, of benefit in the management of certain heart rhythm disorders.

Available Dosage Forms and Strengths

Capsules, prolonged action — 60 mg, 80 mg, 120 mg, 160 mg

Concentrate — 80 mg/ml

Injection — 1 mg/ml

Oral solution — 4 mg/ml, 8 mg/ml

Tablets — 10 mg, 20 mg, 40 mg, 60 mg, 80 mg, 90 mg, 120 mg

▷ **Usual Adult Dosage Range:**   Anti-anginal: Initially 10 mg three or four times a day; increase dose gradually every 3 to 7 days as needed and tolerated. The total daily dosage should not exceed 400 mg.

Antiarrhythmic: 10 to 30 mg three or four times a day as needed and tolerated.

Antihypertensive: Initially 40 mg twice a day; increase dose gradually as needed and tolerated. The total daily dosage should not exceed 640 mg.

Migraine headache prevention: Initially 20 mg four times a day; increase dose gradually as needed and tolerated. The total daily dosage should not exceed 480 mg. Long-acting formulations offer the advantage of once-daily dosing for many patients. **Note: Actual dosage and administration schedule must be determined for each patient individually.**

Conditions Requiring Dosing Adjustments

Liver Function: This drug should be used with caution by patients with liver compromise. In general, lower starting doses and slower increases as needed and tolerated are indicated.

Kidney Function: This drug should be used with caution by people with combined kidney and liver compromise. Dose adjustments are not needed for people with compromised kidneys.

▷ **Dosing Instructions:**   This drug is preferably taken 1 hour before eating to maximize absorption. The tablet may be crushed for administration; to prevent harmless possible numbing effect, mix with soft food and swallow promptly. The prolonged-action capsules should be swallowed whole. Do not stop this drug abruptly.

Usual Duration of Use: Use on a regular schedule for 10 to 14 days usually determines effectiveness in preventing angina, controlling heart rhythm disorders, and lowering blood pressure. Maximal effectiveness may require continual use for 6 to 8 weeks. The long-term use of this drug (months to years) will be determined by the course of your symptoms over time and your response to the overall treatment program (weight reduction, salt restriction, smoking cessation, etc.). Consult your physician on a regular basis.

▷ **This Drug Should Not Be Taken If**
- you have bronchial asthma.
- you have had an allergic reaction to it previously.
- you have Prinzmetal's variant angina (coronary artery spasm).
- you have heart failure (overt).
- you have Raynaud's disease.
- you have an abnormally slow heart rate or a serious form of heart block.
- you are taking, or have taken within the past 14 days, any monoamine oxidase (MAO) type A inhibitor drug (see Drug Classes).

▷ **Inform Your Physician Before Taking This Drug If**
- you have had an adverse reaction to any beta-blocker drug in the past (see Drug Classes).
- you have a history of serious heart disease.
- you have a history of hay fever (allergic rhinitis), asthma, chronic bronchitis, or emphysema.
- you have a history of overactive thyroid function (hyperthyroidism).
- you have a history of low blood sugar (hypoglycemia).
- you have impaired liver or kidney function.
- you are allergic to bee stings.
- you have diabetes or myasthenia gravis.
- you take digitalis, quinidine, or reserpine, or any calcium-channel-blocker drug (see Drug Classes).
- you plan to have surgery under general anesthesia in the near future.

Possible Side Effects (natural, expected, and unavoidable drug actions)
Lethargy and fatigability, cold extremities, slow heart rate, light-headedness in upright position (see Orthostatic Hypotension in Glossary). Increased bowel movements.

▷ **Possible Adverse Effects** (unusual, unexpected, and infrequent reactions)
If any of the following develop, consult your physician promptly for guidance.
Mild Adverse Effects
Allergic Reactions: Skin rash, temporary loss of hair, drug fever (see Glossary).
Joint pain—case reports.
Headache, dizziness, insomnia, vivid dreams—infrequent.
Indigestion, taste disorder, nausea, vomiting, diarrhea—infrequent.
Weight gain—possible.
Serious Adverse Effects
Allergic Reactions: Anaphylaxis.
Idiosyncratic Reactions: Acute behavioral disturbances: disorientation, confusion, hallucinations, amnesia.

Paradoxical hypertension—case reports.

Mental depression, anxiety—case reports and dose related.

Chest pain, shortness of breath, precipitation of congestive heart failure—possible.

Peripheral neuropathy or hyperthyroidism—rare.

Drug-induced systemic lupus erythematosus, myasthenia gravis, or porphyria—case reports.

Kidney problems (interstitial nephritis)—rare.

Induction of bronchial asthma—in asthmatics.

May precipitate problems walking (intermittent claudication)—possible.

Blood cell disorders: abnormally low white blood cell or platelet counts—case reports.

Carpal tunnel syndrome—case reports.

▷ **Possible Effects on Sexual Function**

Decreased libido; impaired erection; impotence—infrequent. Has the highest incidence of libido reduction and erectile impairment of all beta-blocker drugs.

Male infertility (inhibited sperm motility); Peyronie's disease (see Glossary)—possible.

▷ **Adverse Effects That May Mimic Natural Diseases or Disorders**

Reduced blood flow to extremities may resemble Raynaud's phenomenon (see Glossary).

Natural Diseases or Disorders That May Be Activated By This Drug

Prinzmetal's variant angina, Raynaud's disease, intermittent claudication, myasthenia gravis (questionable).

Possible Effects on Laboratory Tests

White blood cell count: occasionally decreased.

Blood platelet count: increased or decreased.

Bleeding time: increased.

Blood total cholesterol level: no effect in some; increased in others.

Blood HDL cholesterol level: no effect in some; decreased in others.

Blood LDL cholesterol level: no effect in some; increased and decreased in others.

Blood VLDL cholesterol level: no effect in some; increased in others.

Blood triglyceride levels: no effect in some; increased in others.

Blood glucose level: no effect in some; increased or decreased in others.

Glucose tolerance test (GTT): decreased.

Blood thyroid hormone levels: T_3—no effect in some, decreased in others; T_4—increased; free T_4—increased.

Blood uric acid level: no effect in some; increased in others.

Liver function tests: increased liver enzymes (ALT/GPT, AST/GOT, and alkaline phosphatase); effects probably not due to liver damage.

CAUTION

1. ***Do not stop this drug suddenly*** without the knowledge and help of your doctor. Carry a notation that states you are taking this drug.
2. Ask your physician or pharmacist before using nasal decongestants, which are usually present in over-the-counter cold preparations and nose drops. These can cause sudden increases in blood pressure when taken concurrently with beta-blocker drugs.
3. Report the development of any tendency to emotional depression.

Precautions for Use

By Infants and Children: Safety and effectiveness for those under 12 years of age are not established. However, if this drug is used, observe for the development of low blood sugar (hypoglycemia) during periods of reduced food intake.

By Those Over 60 Years of Age: Unacceptably high blood pressure should be reduced without creating the risks associated with excessively low blood pressure. Therapy is started with small doses, and blood pressure checked frequently. Sudden, rapid, and excessive reduction of blood pressure can predispose to stroke or heart attack. Observe for dizziness, unsteadiness, tendency to fall, confusion, hallucinations, depression, or urinary frequency.

▷ **Advisability of Use During Pregnancy**

Pregnancy Category: C. See Pregnancy Risk Categories at the back of this book.

Animal studies: No significant increase in birth defects due to this drug. Some toxic effects on embryo reported.

Human studies: Adequate studies of pregnant women are not available.

Avoid use of drug during the first 3 months if possible. Use this drug only if clearly needed. Ask your physician for guidance.

Advisability of Use If Breast-Feeding

Presence of this drug in breast milk: Yes.

Monitor nursing infant closely and discontinue drug or nursing if adverse effects develop.

Habit-Forming Potential: None.

Effects of Overdosage: Weakness, slow pulse, low blood pressure, fainting, cold and sweaty skin, congestive heart failure, possible coma, and convulsions.

Possible Effects of Long-Term Use: Reduced heart reserve and eventual heart failure in susceptible patients with advanced heart disease.

Suggested Periodic Examinations While Taking This Drug (at physician's discretion)

Complete blood cell counts.

Measurements of blood pressure, evaluation of heart function.

Liver function tests.

▷ **While Taking This Drug, Observe the Following**

Foods: No restrictions. Avoid excessive salt intake.

Beverages: No restrictions. May be taken with milk.

▷ *Alcohol:* Use with caution. Alcohol may exaggerate this drug's ability to lower blood pressure and may increase its mild sedative effect.

Tobacco Smoking: Nicotine may reduce this drug's effectiveness in treating angina, heart rhythm disorders, and high blood pressure. Smoking increases the rate of elimination of this drug. I advise everyone to quit smoking.

▷ *Other Drugs*

Propranolol may *increase* the effects of

- other antihypertensive drugs, and cause excessive lowering of blood pressure. Dosage adjustments may be necessary.
- lidocaine (Xylocaine, etc.).
- reserpine (Ser-Ap-Es, etc.), and cause sedation, depression, slowing of the heart rate, and lowering of blood pressure.

- verapamil (Calan, Isoptin), and cause excessive depression of heart function; monitor this combination closely.
- warfarin (Coumadin) and increase bleeding risk. More frequent INR (prothrombin time or protime) testing are needed. Warfarin dosing should be adjusted to laboratory results.

Propranolol may *decrease* the effects of
- albuterol (Proventil).
- theophyllines (Aminophyllin, Theo-Dur, etc.), and reduce their antiasthmatic effectiveness.

Propranolol *taken concurrently* with
- amiodarone (Cordarone) may result in abnormal heart rhythms and low pulse. These agents should not be combined.
- clonidine (Catapres) requires close monitoring for rebound high blood pressure if clonidine is withdrawn while propranolol is still being taken.
- digoxin can result in severe slowing of the heart (bradycardia).
- epinephrine (Adrenalin, etc.) may cause marked rise in blood pressure and slowing of the heart rate.
- fluoxetine (Prozac) may increase the risk of slow heartbeat and sedation.
- fluvoxamine (Luvox) may increase the risk of slow heartbeat and sedation.
- insulin requires close monitoring to avoid undetected hypoglycemia (see Glossary).
- oral antidiabetic drugs (see Drug Classes) and cause slow recovery from any low blood sugar that may occur.
- quinidine (Quinaglute) can increase adverse effects without increased therapeutic benefits.
- venlafaxine (Effexor) may result in increased risk of propranolol toxicity.
- X-ray contrast media such as diatrizoate results in up to an eightfold increase in risk of severe allergic (anaphylactic) drug reactions.

The following drugs may *increase* the effects of propranolol
- chlorpromazine (Thorazine, etc.).
- cimetidine (Tagamet).
- diltiazem (Cardizem).
- disopyramide (Norpace).
- furosemide or other diuretics.
- methimazole (Tapazole).
- nicardipine (Cardene).
- propylthiouracil (Propacil).
- ritonavir (Norvir) and perhaps other protease inhibitors (see Drug Classes).

The following drugs may *decrease* the effects of propranolol
- antacids.
- barbiturates (phenobarbital, etc.).
- indomethacin (Indocin) and possibly other "aspirin substitutes," or NSAIDs—may impair propranolol's antihypertensive effect.
- rifampin (Rifadin, Rimactane).

▷ *Driving, Hazardous Activities:* Use caution until the full extent of drowsiness, lethargy, and blood pressure change have been determined.

Aviation Note: The use of this drug *may be a disqualification* for piloting. Consult a designated Aviation Medical Examiner.

Exposure to Sun: No restrictions.

Exposure to Heat: Caution is advised. Hot environments can lower blood pressure and exaggerate the effects of this drug.

Exposure to Cold: Caution is advised. Cold environments can enhance the circulatory deficiency in the extremities that may occur with this drug. The elderly should take precautions to prevent hypothermia (see Glossary).

Heavy Exercise or Exertion: It is advisable to avoid exertion that produces lightheadedness, excessive fatigue, or muscle cramping. The use of this drug may intensify the hypertensive response to isometric exercise.

Occurrence of Unrelated Illness: Fever can lower blood pressure and require adjustment of dosage. Nausea or vomiting may interrupt the regular dosage schedule. Ask your physician for guidance.

Discontinuation: It is advisable to avoid sudden discontinuation of this drug in all situations; this is especially true in the presence of coronary artery disease. If possible, a gradual reduction of dose over a period of 2 to 3 weeks is recommended. Ask your physician for specific guidance.

PROTEASE INHIBITORS

Indinavir (in DIN a veer)   **Nelfinavir** (nel FIN a veer)   **Ritonavir** (ri TOHN a veer)   **Saquinavir** (sa KWIN a veer)

Introduced: 1996, 1997, 1996, 1995, respectively   **Class:** Protease inhibitor, antiviral, anti-AIDS drug   **Prescription:** USA: Yes   **Controlled Drug:** USA: No; Canada: Yes   **Available as Generic:** USA: No; Canada: No

Brand Names: Indinavir: Crixivan; Nelfinavir: Viracept; Ritonavir: Norvir; Saquinavir: Invirase
> **Author's Note: This profile will be a combination profile next year when more data are available about protease inhibitors. For this edition, the focus is on indinavir.**

BENEFITS versus RISKS	
Possible Benefits	*Possible Risks*
INCREASED CD4 COUNTS	SERIOUS CHANGES IN INSULIN
DECREASED OPPORTUNISTIC	LEVELS TO KETOACIDOSIS
INFECTIONS	Increased liver function tests
EFFECTIVE COMBINATION	Kidney stones
THERAPY OF HIV	Skin rash
MAY HAVE A ROLE IN	
ERADICATION OF HIV WITH	
EARLY THERAPY	

▷ **Principal Uses**
> *As a Single Drug Product:* Uses currently included in FDA-approved labeling: Treatment of HIV infection when antiretroviral therapy is indicated.
>> **Author's Note: *The Panel on Clinical Practices for Treatment of HIV Infection Report* says that the preferred regimen is: Two nucleoside analogs and one potent protease inhibitor. Single-agent therapy (with the exception of AZT use in preventing HIV transmission from mother to fetus) was rejected by the panel.**
>
> Other (unlabeled) generally accepted uses: (1) Combination therapy of HIV infection; (2) possible use in eradicating HIV infection.

How This Drug Works: This drug inhibits HIV reproduction (replication) by inhibiting an HIV enzyme (protease), which blocks the ability of the virus to make mature, infectious virus particles.

Available Dosage Forms and Strengths
Capsules — 200 mg, 400 mg

▷ **Recommended Dosage Ranges** (Actual dosage and administration schedule must be determined for each patient individually.)
Infants and Children: Safety and efficacy are not established.
18 to 60 Years of Age: 800 mg by mouth every 8 hours.
Over 65 Years of Age: This drug has **not** been studied in those over 65.

Conditions Requiring Dosing Adjustments
Liver Function: The dose should be decreased to 600 mg by mouth every 8 hours in mild to moderate liver failure.
Kidney Function: Less than 20 % of a given dose is removed by the kidneys. Dose changes are not needed.

▷ **Dosing Instructions:**   This drug is best taken on an empty stomach, but may be taken with a light meal, such as dry toast with jelly, apple juice, or coffee. IT IS CRITICAL THAT INDINAVIR DOSES NOT BE MISSED, as resistance may develop. Since case reports of altered blood sugar have been made, knowledge of signs and symptoms of high blood sugar or ketoacidosis and periodic checks of blood sugar appear prudent.

Usual Duration of Use: Use on a regular schedule for several months usually determines effectiveness in lowering the viral burden to nondetectable levels. The lowest level of viral burden, the 12-week level of viral burden, and compliance are key factors in long-term results. Long-term use (months to years) requires periodic physician evaluation of response (viral burden and CD4).

Possible Advantages of This Drug
May have a role in eradicating HIV.
Part of a combination regimen (AZT, lamivudine, and indinavir) that lowered viral burden to nondetectable levels in many patients in one study.
Favorable profile for combination therapy.

▷ **This Drug Should Not Be Taken If**
• you have had an allergic reaction to any dosage form of it previously.

▷ **Inform Your Physician Before Taking This Drug If**
• you have diabetes or a history of blood sugar regulation problems.
• you have had kidney stones previously.
• you have kidney or liver compromise.
• you have had adverse reactions to other protease inhibitors.
• you are uncertain of how much indinavir to take or how often to take it.

Possible Side Effects (natural, expected, and unavoidable drug actions)
Rare kidney stones. Increased liver function tests.

▷ **Possible Adverse Effects** (unusual, unexpected, and infrequent reactions)
If any of the following develop, consult your physician promptly for guidance.
Mild Adverse Effects
Allergic Reactions: Skin rash.
Headache or dizziness—rare.

Blurred vision—rare.

Chills, fever, or sweating—rare.

Nausea and vomiting or abdominal pain—infrequent to frequent.

Palpitations—rare.

Joint pain—rare.

Serious Adverse Effects

Allergic Reactions: Not reported.

Anemia or spleen disorder—rare.

Kidney stones—infrequent.

Changes in insulin levels (increased blood sugar (hyperglycemia) or ketoacidosis)—84 case reports for the protease inhibitors.

▷ **Possible Effects on Sexual Function**

Rare reports of premenstrual syndrome in some early studies.

Possible Delayed Adverse Effects: Kidney stones. Blood sugar problems (low blood sugar or ketoacidosis).

▷ **Adverse Effects That May Mimic Natural Diseases or Disorders**

Increased liver function tests may mimic hepatitis. Changes in insulin levels may mimic diabetes.

Possible Effects on Laboratory Tests

Liver function tests: increased.

Complete blood counts: decreased red blood cells and hematocrit.

Insulin levels: lowered.

Blood sugar (glucose): increased.

CAUTION

1. Serious increases in blood sugar has been reported in 84 case reports to date for protease inhibitors. This effect has been seen on average after 76 days of therapy, but has also been reported after as little as 4 days of treatment with protease inhibitors.

2. Make certain you know high blood sugar (hyperglycemia) and ketoacidosis signs and symptoms if you are taking this medicine. Blood sugar problems have been reported for protease inhibitors.

3. Indinavir has **not** been shown to decrease the risk of giving (transmission) HIV to others through sexual contact or blood contamination.

4. Promptly report flank pain or blood in the urine; this could indicate a kidney stone.

5. Periodic measures of viral load and CD4 are critical to make certain therapy is still working.

6. IT IS CRITICAL to take this medicine exactly as directed to get the best results.

Precautions for Use

By Infants and Children: Safety and effectiveness for those under 18 years of age are not established.

By Those Over 65 Years of Age: This drug has not been studied in this age group.

▷ **Advisability of Use During Pregnancy**

Pregnancy Category: C. See Pregnancy Risk Categories at the back of this book.

Animal studies: Clinical doses in rats and rabbits have not revealed teratogenicity.

Human studies: Adequate studies of pregnant women are not available.

Ask your doctor for guidance.

Advisability of Use If Breast-Feeding

Presence of this drug in breast milk: Yes in rats.

Refrain from nursing if you are HIV-positive or are taking this drug. Breast milk may also transfer the AIDS virus from mother to infant.

Habit-Forming Potential: None.

Effects of Overdosage: No human data are available. Doses of 20 times the human dose in rats and 10 times the human dose in mice were not lethal.

Possible Effects of Long-Term Use: Resistance may develop.

Suggested Periodic Examinations While Taking This Drug (at physician's discretion)

Liver function tests, complete blood counts.

CD4 or viral load measurement.

Measurement of blood sugar (glucose), especially for those with prior blood sugar problems or patients who show signs or symptoms of hyperglycemia or ketoacidosis.

▷ **While Taking This Drug, Observe the Following**

Foods: If indinavir is taken with a meal high in fat, calories, or protein, a 77 to 91% decrease in the total amount of drug absorbed has been reported.

Beverages: No restrictions.

▷ *Alcohol:* No interactions expected.

Tobacco Smoking: No interactions expected, but I advise everyone to quit smoking.

▷ *Other Drugs*

Indinavir ***taken concurrently*** with

- astemizole (Hismanal) may cause serious toxicity. DO NOT COMBINE.
- cisapride (Propulsid) may cause serious toxicity. DO NOT COMBINE.
- didanosine (Videx) may blunt therapeutic benefits. Separate doses by 1 hour.
- ketoconazole (Nizoral) may cause toxicity. Doses of indinavir may need to be reduced.
- midazolam (Versed) may cause serious toxicity. DO NOT COMBINE.
- nevirapine (Viramune) may blunt therapeutic effects. DO NOT COMBINE.
- other antiretrovirals may reduce viral load to nondetectable levels.
- other drugs that are toxic to the liver may result in additive toxicity.
- other drugs that can lead to kidney stones may result in additive risk.
- rifabutin (Mycobutin) may increase rifabutin and decrease indinavir levels. Half the usual dose of rifabutin is used if these drugs are combined.
- rifampin (Rifater, others) may cause loss of indinavir's benefits. DO NOT COMBINE.
- terfenadine (Seldane) may cause serious toxicity. DO NOT COMBINE.
- triazolam (Halcion) and perhaps other benzodiazepines may cause serious toxicity.

▷ *Driving, Hazardous Activities:* This drug may rarely cause sleepiness. Restrict activities as necessary.

Aviation Note: The use of this drug ***may be a disqualification*** for piloting. Consult a designated Aviation Medical Examiner.

Exposure to Sun: No restrictions.

Discontinuation: Do not stop this drug without your doctor's knowledge and guidance.

PROTRIPTYLINE (proh TRIP ti leen)

Introduced: 1966   **Class:** Antidepressant   **Prescription:** USA: Yes
Controlled Drug: USA: No; Canada: No   **Available as Generic:** USA: Yes;
Canada: No
Brand Names: ✦Triptil, Vivactil

BENEFITS versus RISKS	
Possible Benefits	*Possible Risks*
EFFECTIVE RELIEF OF MAJOR ENDOGENOUS DEPRESSIONS	ADVERSE BEHAVIORAL EFFECTS: confusion, disorientation, hallucinations, delusions
HELPS MANAGE OTHER DEPRESSIVE DISORDERS	CONVERSION OF DEPRESSION TO MANIA in manic-depressive (bipolar) disorders
Possibly beneficial in the management of attention deficit disorder and of narcolepsy/cataplexy syndrome	Aggravation of schizophrenia Irregular heart rhythms Blood cell abnormalities

▷ **Principal Uses**

As a Single Drug Product: Uses currently included in FDA-approved labeling: Relieves symptoms associated with major spontaneous (endogenous) depression, depressed bipolar disorder, and mixed bipolar disorder.

Other (unlabeled) generally accepted uses: (1) Treatment of sleep disorders such as apnea, hypersomnia, and impaired morning arousal; (2) may have a role in treating glaucoma; (3) used in combination with methylphenidate or amphetamines in treating narcolepsy.

How This Drug Works: It is thought that this drug relieves depression by slowly restoring to normal levels certain constituents of brain tissue (norepinephrine and serotonin) that transmit nerve impulses.

Available Dosage Forms and Strengths

Tablets — 5 mg, 10 mg

▷ **Recommended Dosage Ranges** (Actual dosage and administration schedule must be determined for each patient individually.)

Infants and Children: Dosage not established.

12 to 60 Years of Age: For depression: Initially 5 to 10 mg, three or four times daily. The dose is increased cautiously as needed and tolerated by 5 mg daily at intervals of 1 week. The usual maintenance dose is 15 to 40 mg a day, divided into three or four doses. The total daily dose should not exceed 60 mg.

Over 60 Years of Age: Initially 5 mg, two or three times daily to evaluate tolerance. Increase dose cautiously as needed and tolerated by 5 mg daily at intervals of 1 week. Doses above 20 mg daily require careful monitoring of heart function and blood pressure. The total daily dose should not exceed 40 mg.

Conditions Requiring Dosing Adjustments

Liver Function: The dose should be empirically decreased, and blood levels obtained at appropriate intervals. Protriptyline is a rare cause of hepatotoxicity.

Kidney Function: The kidney plays a minor role in the elimination of this drug.

▷ **Dosing Instructions:** The tablet may be crushed and taken without regard to meals. If a stimulating effect occurs: (1) necessary dosage increases should be made in the morning; (2) the last daily dose should be taken in the afternoon (3 to 4 P.M.) to avoid insomnia and disturbed dreaming.

Usual Duration of Use: Some benefit may be apparent within 1 to 2 weeks, but adequate response may require continual use for 3 months or longer. Long-term use should not exceed 6 months without evaluation regarding the need for continuation of the drug. Consult your physician on a regular basis.

Possible Advantages of This Drug

Causes less daytime sedation than some other agents.

Causes orthostatic hypotension less frequently (see Glossary).

▷ **This Drug Should Not Be Taken If**
- you have had an allergic reaction to it previously.
- you are taking, or have taken within the past 14 days, any monoamine oxidase (MAO) type A inhibitor drug (see Drug Classes).
- you are recovering from a recent heart attack.
- you have narrow-angle glaucoma.

▷ **Inform Your Physician Before Taking This Drug If**
- you are allergic or sensitive to any other tricyclic antidepressant (see Drug Classes).
- you have a history of any of the following: diabetes, epilepsy, glaucoma, heart disease, prostate gland enlargement, or overactive thyroid function.
- you have a history of psychosis.
- you work outside, particularly in hot weather.
- you plan to have surgery under general anesthesia in the near future.

Possible Side Effects (natural, expected, and unavoidable drug actions)

Severe lowering of blood pressure on standing (orthostatic hypotension), blurred vision, dry mouth, constipation, impaired urination (see Prostatism in Glossary).

▷ **Possible Adverse Effects** (unusual, unexpected, and infrequent reactions)

If any of the following develop, consult your physician promptly for guidance.

Mild Adverse Effects

Allergic Reactions: Skin rash, hives, swelling of face or tongue, drug fever (see Glossary).

Cavities (dental caries) or ringing in the ears— case reports.

Headache, dizziness, weakness, fainting, unsteady gait, tremors—rare to infrequent.

Peculiar taste, irritation of tongue or mouth, nausea, indigestion—infrequent.

Fluctuation of blood sugar levels—case reports.

Serious Adverse Effects

Allergic Reactions: Hepatitis, with or without jaundice (see Glossary).

Confusion, disorientation, hallucinations, delusions—case reports.

Aggravation of paranoid psychoses and schizophrenia; seizures—possible.

Heart palpitation and irregular rhythm—case reports.

Bone marrow depression (see Glossary): fatigue, abnormal bleeding or bruising—case reports.

Peripheral neuritis (see Glossary): numbness, tingling—case reports.

Parkinson-like disorders (see Glossary)—usually mild and infrequent; more likely to occur in the elderly.

▷ **Possible Effects on Sexual Function**

Decreased libido, increased libido (antidepressant effect), male impotence, inhibited female orgasm, male and female breast enlargement, milk production, swelling of testicles—case reports.

▷ **Adverse Effects That May Mimic Natural Diseases or Disorders**

Liver toxicity may suggest viral hepatitis.

Natural Diseases or Disorders That May Be Activated by This Drug

Latent diabetes, epilepsy, glaucoma, prostatism.

Possible Effects on Laboratory Tests

White blood cell and platelet counts: decreased.

Blood glucose levels: increased and decreased (fluctuations).

Liver function tests: increased liver enzymes (ALT/GPT, AST/GOT, and alkaline phosphatase), increased bilirubin.

CAUTION

1. Dosage must be adjusted for each person individually. Report for follow-up evaluation and laboratory tests as directed by your physician.
2. It is advisable to withhold this drug if electroconvulsive therapy (ECT, "shock" treatment) is to be used to treat your depression.

Precautions for Use

By Infants and Children: Safety and effectiveness for those under 6 years of age are not established. This drug may be used to relieve symptoms of attention deficit disorder, with or without hyperactivity, in selected children over 6 years of age.

By Those Over 60 Years of Age: Usual dosage is 15 to 30 mg daily in divided doses. During the first 2 weeks of treatment, observe for the development of confusion, agitation, forgetfulness, disorientation, delusions, and hallucinations. Reduction of dosage or discontinuation may be necessary. Unsteadiness may predispose to falling and injury. This drug can increase the degree of impaired urination associated with prostate gland enlargement (prostatism).

▷ **Advisability of Use During Pregnancy**

Pregnancy Category: C. See Pregnancy Risk Categories at the back of this book.

Animal studies: No birth defects found in mouse, rat, and rabbit studies.

Human studies: No defects reported in 21 exposures to amitriptyline, a closely related drug. Adequate studies of pregnant women are not available.

Avoid use of drug during first 3 months. Use during final 6 months only if clearly needed. Ask your physician for guidance.

Advisability of Use If Breast-Feeding

Presence of this drug in breast milk: Yes, in small amounts.

Monitor nursing infant closely and discontinue drug or nursing if adverse effects develop: excessive drowsiness and failure to feed.

Habit-Forming Potential: Psychological or physical dependence is rare and unexpected.

Effects of Overdosage: Confusion, hallucinations, marked drowsiness, heart palpitations, dilated pupils, tremors, stupor, deep sleep, coma, convulsions.

Suggested Periodic Examinations While Taking This Drug (at physician's discretion)

Complete blood cell counts, liver function tests, serial blood pressure readings, and electrocardiograms.

▷ **While Taking This Drug, Observe the Following**

Foods: No restrictions. This drug may increase the appetite and cause excessive weight gain.

Beverages: No restrictions. May be taken with milk.

▷ *Alcohol:* Avoid completely. This drug can markedly increase the intoxicating effects of alcohol and accentuate its depressant action on brain function.

Tobacco Smoking: May hasten the elimination of this drug. I advise everyone to quit smoking.

Marijuana Smoking: Increased heart rate greater than either drug alone. DO NOT COMBINE.

▷ *Other Drugs*

Protriptyline may *increase* the effects of

- atropinelike drugs (see Drug Classes).
- dicumarol, and increase the risk of bleeding.
- epinephrine (Adrenalin).
- norepinephrine.
- phenytoin (Dilantin) and lead to toxicity.
- pseudoephedrine and cause high blood pressure and arrhythmias.

Protriptyline may *decrease* the effects of

- clonidine (Catapres), and cause loss of blood pressure control; do not use these drugs concurrently.
- guanethidine (Ismelin).

Protriptyline *taken concurrently* with

- carbamazepine (Tegretol) may result in increased carbamazepine levels (toxicity risk) and decreased protriptyline levels (loss of therapeutic benefits).
- disulfiram (Antabuse) may cause acute dementia: confusion, disorientation, hallucinations.
- monoamine oxidase (MAO) inhibitor drugs (see Drug Classes) may cause high fever, delirium, and convulsions.
- thyroid preparations (see Drug Classes) may impair heart rhythm and function. Ask your physician for guidance regarding adjustment of thyroid dose.
- tramadol (Ultram) may increase seizure risk. DO NOT COMBINE.
- venlafaxine (Effexor) may result in increased protriptyline levels and toxicity.
- warfarin (Coumadin) may result in prolonged anticoagulation. Increased INR (prothrombin time or protime) testing is needed.

The following drugs may *increase* the effects of protriptyline

- cimetidine (Tagamet).
- conjugated estrogens (Premarin).

- fluoxetine (Prozac).
- lithium (Lithobid, etc.).
- methylphenidate (Ritalin).
- oral contraceptives (birth control pills).
- quinidine (Quinaglute, others).
- ranitidine (Zantac).
- sertraline (Zoloft).

The following drugs may *decrease* the effects of protriptyline
- barbiturates (see Drug Classes), and reduce its effectiveness.

▷ *Driving, Hazardous Activities:* This drug may impair mental alertness, judgment, physical coordination, and reaction time. Avoid hazardous activities.

Aviation Note: The use of this drug *is a disqualification* for piloting. Consult a designated Aviation Medical Examiner.

Exposure to Sun: Use caution—this drug may cause photosensitivity (see Glossary).

Exposure to Heat: This drug can inhibit sweating and impair the body's adaptation to hot environments, increasing the risk of heatstroke. Avoid saunas.

Exposure to Cold: The elderly should use caution and avoid conditions conducive to hypothermia (see Glossary).

Discontinuation: It is advisable to discontinue this drug gradually. Abrupt withdrawal after long-term use can cause headache, malaise, and nausea.

PYRAZINAMIDE (peer a ZIN a mide)

Introduced: 1968   **Class:** Anti-infective, antituberculosis drug   **Prescription:** USA: Yes   **Controlled Drug:** USA: No; Canada: No   **Available as Generic:** USA: Yes; Canada: No

Brand Names: ✦PMS Pyrazinamide, Rifater, ✦Tebrazid

BENEFITS versus RISKS	
Possible Benefits	*Possible Risks*
EFFECTIVE ADJUNCTIVE TREATMENT OF TUBERCULOSIS	DRUG-INDUCED HEPATITIS—rare Activation of gouty arthritis and porphyria Decreased platelets and hemoglobin

▷ **Principal Uses**

As a Single Drug Product: Uses currently included in FDA-approved labeling: Treatment of active tuberculosis, in combination with other antitubercular drugs.

Other (unlabeled) generally accepted uses: (1) Combination therapy of *Mycobacterium xenopi* infections; (2) combination therapy of resistant tuberculosis; (3) combination therapy of tuberculosis in AIDS.

As a Combination Drug Product [CD]: This medicine is combined with two other antituberculosis (isoniazid and rifampin) medicines in order to attack tuberculosis with combination treatment with a single dosage form.

How This Drug Works: This drug is ideal for killing tuberculosis organisms that are in acid environments, such as in some kinds of white blood (macrophages) cells.

Available Dosage Forms and Strengths
Tablets — 500 mg

▷ **Recommended Dosage Ranges** (Actual dosage and administration schedule must be determined for each patient individually.)

Infants and Children: 7.5 to 15 mg per kg of body mass, twice daily; or 15 to 30 mg per kg of body mass, once daily. Total daily dosage should not exceed 1.5 g.

12 to 60 Years of Age: For tuberculosis—15 to 30 mg per kg of body mass (up to a maximum of 2000 mg) daily. Some patients do better with twice-weekly dosing: 50 to 70 mg per kg of body mass (up to 4000 mg).

> **Author's Note: Because of the current resistant tuberculosis problem, most clinicians start all patients on a four-antituberculosis-medicine regimen until laboratory culture results are available.**

Over 60 Years of Age: Same as 12 to 60 years of age.

Conditions Requiring Dosing Adjustments

Liver Function: This drug should be used with caution and in decreased doses by patients with liver compromise. Contraindicated in patients with severe liver dysfunction.

Kidney Function: For patients with endstage renal failure, the dose **must** be adjusted. One researcher recommends: 60 mg per kg of body mass, twice weekly. The dose of pyrazinamide should be given at least 24 hours before any given dialysis session. Patients should be closely monitored.

▷ **Dosing Instructions:**   The tablet may be crushed and taken with or following food to reduce stomach irritation. Take the full course prescribed. This drug should be taken concurrently with other antitubercular drugs to prevent the development of drug-resistant strains of tuberculosis bacteria.

Usual Duration of Use: Use on a regular schedule for 2 months usually determines effectiveness in controlling active tuberculosis. Long-term use of antitubercular drugs (6 months) requires periodic physician evaluation.

Possible Advantages of This Drug
May reduce the period of drug treatment from 9 to 6 months in responsive infections.

▷ **This Drug Should Not Be Taken If**
- you have had an allergic reaction to it previously.
- you have permanent liver damage with impaired function.
- you have active gout.
- you have active peptic ulcer disease.

▷ **Inform Your Physician Before Taking This Drug If**
- you have had an allergic reaction to ethionamide, isoniazid, niacin (nicotinic acid).
- you have a history of liver disease.
- you have a history of peptic ulcer or porphyria.
- you tried to take medicines for tuberculosis before, but did not complete the prescribed therapy.
- you have gout or diabetes.
- you have impaired kidney function.

Possible Side Effects (natural, expected, and unavoidable drug actions)
Increased blood uric acid levels. Fever.

▷ **Possible Adverse Effects** (unusual, unexpected, and infrequent reactions)
   If any of the following develop, consult your physician promptly for guidance.
   Mild Adverse Effects
   Allergic Reactions: Skin rash, itching, fever.
   Loss of appetite, mild nausea, vomiting—frequent.
   Joint pain—frequent.
   Acne—rare.
   Serious Adverse Effects
   Idiosyncratic Reactions: Rare sideroblastic anemia.
   Decreased blood platelets—rare.
   Seizures—rare.
   Drug-induced porphyria or pellagra—case reports.
   Kidney problems (interstitial nephritis)—case reports.
   Drug-induced hepatitis, with and without jaundice (see Glossary)—case reports.
   Gouty arthritis, due to increased blood uric acid levels—possible.

▷ **Possible Effects on Sexual Function**
   None reported.

▷ **Adverse Effects That May Mimic Natural Diseases or Disorders**
   Drug-induced hepatitis may suggest viral hepatitis.

Natural Diseases or Disorders That May Be Activated by This Drug
   Gout, peptic ulcer, porphyria.

Possible Effects on Laboratory Tests
   Complete blood cell counts: decreased red cells, hemoglobin, and platelets.
   INR (prothrombin time): increased.
   Blood uric acid level: increased.
   Liver function tests: increased enzymes (ALT/GPT, AST/GOT, alkaline phosphatase), or bilirubin.
   Urine ketone tests: false-positive test result with Acetest and Ketostix.

CAUTION
   1. When this drug is used alone, tuberculosis bacteria rapidly develop resistance to it. To be effective, this drug must be used in combination with other effective antitubercular drugs, such as isoniazid and rifampin.
   2. This drug may interfere with control of diabetes.

Precautions for Use
   By Infants and Children: Safety and effectiveness for those under 12 years of age are not established. The rare occurrence of drug-related seizure has been reported in a 2-year-old child.
   By Those Over 60 Years of Age: No specific information available.

▷ **Advisability of Use During Pregnancy**
   Pregnancy Category: C. See Pregnancy Risk Categories at the back of this book.
   Animal studies: No information available.
   Human studies: Adequate studies of pregnant women are not available.
   Use this drug only if clearly needed. Ask your physician for guidance.

Advisability of Use If Breast-Feeding
   Presence of this drug in breast milk: Yes.
   Avoid drug or refrain from nursing.

Habit-Forming Potential: None.

Effects of Overdosage: Nausea, vomiting, malaise.

Possible Effects of Long-Term Use: Liver damage.

Suggested Periodic Examinations While Taking This Drug (at physician's discretion)
> Complete blood cell counts.
> Liver function tests.
> Uric acid blood levels.

▷ **While Taking This Drug, Observe the Following**
> *Foods:* No restrictions.
> *Beverages:* No restrictions. May be taken with milk.
▷ *Alcohol:* Use sparingly to minimize liver toxicity.
> *Tobacco Smoking:* No interactions expected, but I advise everyone to quit smoking.
▷ *Other Drugs*
> Pyrazinamide may *decrease* the effects of
> • allopurinol (Zyloprim).
> • BCG vaccine.
> • cyclosporine (Sandimmune).
> • probenecid (Benemid).
> • sulfinpyrazone (Anturane).
> Pyrazinamide *taken concurrently* with
> • phenytoin (Dilantin) may lead to phenytoin toxicity.
▷ *Driving, Hazardous Activities:* No restrictions.
> *Aviation Note:* The use of this drug is probably *not a disqualification* for piloting. Consult a designated Aviation Medical Examiner.
> *Exposure to Sun:* Use caution—this drug may cause photosensitivity (see Glossary).
> *Discontinuation:* If tolerated, this drug is usually taken for a minimum of 2 months. Do not stop it without your physician's knowledge and guidance.

PYRIDOSTIGMINE (peer id oh STIG meen)

Introduced: 1962   **Class:** Antimyasthenic   **Prescription:** USA: Yes
Controlled Drug: USA: No; Canada: No   **Available as Generic:** USA: No;
Canada: No

Brand Names: ✤Anaplex SR, Mestinon, Mestinon-SR, Mestinon Timespan, Regonol

BENEFITS versus RISKS	
Possible Benefits	*Possible Risks*
MODERATELY EFFECTIVE TREATMENT OF OCULAR AND MILD FORMS OF MYASTHENIA GRAVIS (symptomatic relief of muscle weakness)	Cholinergic crisis (overdose): excessive salivation, nausea, vomiting, stomach cramps, diarrhea, shortness of breath (asthmalike wheezing), excessive weakness

▷ **Principal Uses**

As a Single Drug Product: Uses currently included in FDA-approved labeling: (1) Used to treat the ocular and milder forms of myasthenia gravis by providing temporary relief of muscle weakness and fatigability. Most useful in long-term treatment when there is little or no swallowing difficulty; (2) used to reverse muscle relaxants.

Other (unlabeled) generally accepted uses: (1) Combination therapy in chronic pain; (2) may help in combination therapy of Huntington's chorea and Lambert-Eaton syndrome; (3) adjunctive use with scopolamine to prevent side effects of scopolamine in treating motion sickness; (4) used in war zones to treat the effects of nerve gas; (5) may have a role in treating nonepidemic parotitis.

How This Drug Works: This drug inhibits cholinesterase, the enzyme that destroys acetylcholine. This results in higher levels of acetylcholine, the nerve transmitter that facilitates the stimulation of muscular activity. The net effects are increased muscle strength and endurance.

Available Dosage Forms and Strengths

Syrup — 60 mg/5 ml (5% alcohol)

Tablets — 30 mg, 60 mg

Tablets, prolonged action — 180 mg

▷ **Usual Adult Dosage Range:**   Myasthenia gravis: Initially one to six normal-release tablets, spaced throughout the day when maximum strength is needed. Maintenance varies with the severity of the disease: one to three extended-release tablets taken every 6 hours. Some patients may need to supplement the extended-release tablets with the 30-mg, immediate-release tablets or the syrup in order to best control symptoms.

Nerve gas or agent protection: 30 mg every 8 hours when the threat of a nerve agent attack is present. **Note: Actual dosage and administration schedule must be determined for each patient individually.**

Conditions Requiring Dosing Adjustments

Liver Function: No dosing changes are defined in liver compromise.

Kidney Function: This drug is primarily eliminated in the urine; however, specific guidelines for dosage adjustments in renal compromise are not available.

▷ **Dosing Instructions:**   Take with food or milk to reduce the intensity of side effects. Larger portions of the daily maintenance dosage should be timed according to the pattern of fatigue and weakness. The syrup will permit a finer adjustment of dosage. The regular tablet may be crushed for administration. The prolonged-action tablet should be taken whole (not altered).

Usual Duration of Use: Use on a regular schedule (with dosage adjustment) for 10 to 14 days usually determines effectiveness in relieving myasthenia symptoms. Long-term use (months to years) requires periodic physician evaluation.

▷ **This Drug Should Not Be Taken If**
- you are known to be allergic to bromide compounds.
- you have a urinary obstruction or mechanical intestinal obstruction.

▷ **Inform Your Physician Before Taking This Drug If**
- you are subject to heart rhythm disorders or bronchial asthma.
- you are sensitive to bromides.

- you have recurrent urinary tract infections.
- you have prostatism (see Glossary).
- you plan to have surgery under general anesthesia in the near future.

Possible Side Effects (natural, expected, and unavoidable drug actions)

Small pupils (miosis), watering of eyes, slow pulse, excessive salivation, nausea, vomiting, stomach cramps, diarrhea, urge to urinate, increased sweating, increased bronchial secretions.

▷ **Possible Adverse Effects** (unusual, unexpected, and infrequent reactions)

If any of the following develop, consult your physician promptly for guidance.

Mild Adverse Effects

Allergic Reactions: Skin rash.

Nervousness, anxiety, unsteadiness, muscle cramps or twitching—infrequent.

Loss of scalp hair (alopecia)—case report.

Serious Adverse Effects

Confusion, slurred speech, seizures, difficult breathing (asthmatic wheezing).

Increased muscle weakness or paralysis—case report.

Psychosis—rare.

Excessive vomiting or diarrhea may induce abnormally low blood potassium levels (hypokalemia). This will accentuate muscle weakness.

▷ **Possible Effects on Sexual Function**

None reported.

▷ **Adverse Effects That May Mimic Natural Diseases or Disorders**

Seizures may suggest the possibility of epilepsy.

Natural Diseases or Disorders That May Be Activated by This Drug

Latent bronchial asthma.

Possible Effects on Laboratory Tests

None reported.

CAUTION

1. Some drugs block this drug, reducing effectiveness in treating myasthenia gravis (see "Other Drugs" below). Ask your doctor before starting any prescription or over-the-counter drug.
2. Variations in response may occur from time to time. Because generalized muscle weakness is a major symptom of both myasthenia crisis (underdosage) and cholinergic crisis (overdosage), it may be difficult to recognize the correct cause. As a rule, weakness that starts an hour after taking this drug probably represents overdosage; weakness that begins 3 or more hours after taking this drug is probably due to underdosage. Observe these time relationships and tell your doctor.
3. During long-term use, watch for development of resistance to the therapeutic action (loss of effect). Ask your doctor if the drug should be stopped for a few days to see if response can be restored.

Precautions for Use

By Infants and Children: The syrup form of this drug permits greater precision of dosage adjustment and ease of administration in this age group. Neonates have received 5 mg every 4 to 6 hours. Since this is often self-limiting in neonates, the medicine can frequently be tapered and stopped.

By Those Over 60 Years of Age: The natural decline of kidney function with aging may require smaller doses to prevent accumulation of this drug to toxic levels.

▷ **Advisability of Use During Pregnancy**

Pregnancy Category: C. See Pregnancy Risk Categories at the back of this book.

Animal studies: No information available.

Human studies: Adequate studies of pregnant women are not available.

There are no reports of birth defects due to the use of this drug during pregnancy. However, there are reports of significant muscular weakness in newborn infants whose mothers had taken this drug during pregnancy. Ask your physician for guidance.

Advisability of Use If Breast-Feeding

Presence of this drug in breast milk: Yes, as roughly 0.01% of the mother's dose.

Monitor nursing infant closely and discontinue drug or nursing if adverse effects develop.

Habit-Forming Potential: None.

Effects of Overdosage: Generalized muscular weakness, blurred vision, very small pupils, slow heart rate, difficult breathing (wheezing), excessive salivation, nausea, vomiting, stomach cramps, diarrhea, muscle cramps or twitching. This syndrome constitutes the cholinergic crisis.

Possible Effects of Long-Term Use: Development of tolerance (see Glossary) with loss of therapeutic effectiveness.

Suggested Periodic Examinations While Taking This Drug (at physician's discretion)

Assessment of drug effectiveness and dosage schedule for optimal therapeutic results.

▷ **While Taking This Drug, Observe the Following**

Foods: No restrictions.

Beverages: No restrictions. May be taken with milk.

▷ *Alcohol:* Use caution until the combined effects are determined. Weakness and unsteadiness may be accentuated.

Tobacco Smoking: No interactions expected, but I advise everyone to quit smoking.

▷ *Other Drugs*

Pyridostigmine ***taken concurrently*** with
- disopyramide (Norpace) may help the decreased sweating, difficulty urinating, and other anticholinergic effects.

The following drugs may ***decrease*** the effects of pyridostigmine
- adrenocortical steroids (see Drug Classes).
- atropine (belladonna).
- clindamycin (Cleocin).
- guanadrel (Hylorel).
- guanethidine (Esimil, Ismelin).
- procainamide (Procan SR, Pronestyl).
- quinidine (Cardioquin, Duraquin, etc.).
- quinine (Quinamm).

▷ *Driving, Hazardous Activities:* This drug may cause blurred vision, confusion, or generalized weakness. Restrict activities as necessary.

Aviation Note: The use of this drug *is a disqualification* for piloting. Consult a designated Aviation Medical Examiner.

Exposure to Sun: No restrictions.

Exposure to Heat: Use caution—this drug may cause excessive sweating and increased weakness.

Exposure to Environmental Chemicals: Avoid excessive exposure (inhalation, skin contamination) to the insecticides Baygon, Diazinon, and Sevin. These can worsen potential drug toxicity.

Discontinuation: Do not stop this drug abruptly without your doctor's knowledge and guidance.

QUAZEPAM (KWAH zee pam)

Introduced: 1982   **Class:** Hypnotic, benzodiazepines   **Prescription:** USA: Yes   **Controlled Drug:** USA: C-IV*   **Available as Generic:** USA: No
Brand Names: Doral, Dormalin

Author's Note: The information in this profile has been abbreviated to make room for more widely used medicines.

QUINACRINE (KWIN a kreen)

Other Name: Mepacrine

Author's Note: This medicine is derived from a natural source that is no longer available.

QUINAPRIL (KWIN a pril)

Introduced: 1984   **Class:** Antihypertensive, ACE inhibitor   **Prescription:** USA: Yes   **Controlled Drug:** USA: No; Canada: No   **Available as Generic:** No
Brand Name: Accupril

BENEFITS versus RISKS	
Possible Benefits	*Possible Risks*
EFFECTIVE CONTROL OF MILD TO MODERATE HIGH BLOOD PRESSURE	Low blood pressure Low white blood cell counts Allergic swelling of face, tongue, throat, vocal cords

*See schedules of Controlled Drugs at the back of this book.

▷ **Principal Uses**

As a Single Drug Product: Uses currently included in FDA-approved labeling: (1) Treats mild to moderate high blood pressure, either alone or combined with a thiazide diuretic; (2) treats symptoms of congestive heart failure.

Other (unlabeled) generally accepted uses: (1) Improves survival in patients with congestive heart failure; (2) may improve survival in patients with atherosclerosis; (3) other medicines from this class have helped decrease the number of deaths and the severity of ongoing heart compromise.

How This Drug Works: By blocking certain enzyme systems (angiotensin-converting enzyme, ACE) that influence arterial function, this drug helps relax arterial walls and lowers resistance to blood flow that causes high blood pressure. This, in turn, reduces the workload of the heart and improves its performance.

Available Dosage Forms and Strengths

Tablets — 5 mg, 10 mg, 20 mg, 40 mg

▷ **Recommended Dosage Ranges** (Actual dosage and administration schedule must be determined for each patient individually.)

Infants and Children: Dosage not established.

12 to 60 Years of Age: Initially 10 mg once daily for those not taking a diuretic; 5 mg once daily for those taking a diuretic. Usual maintenance dose is 20 to 40 mg daily, taken in a single dose. If once-a-day dosing does not give stable control of blood pressure over a 24-hour period, divide the dose equally into morning and evening doses. The total daily dosage should not exceed 80 mg.

Over 60 Years of Age: Same as 12 to 60 years of age, if kidney function is normal. If kidney function is significantly impaired, reduce dose by 50%. The total daily dose should not exceed 40 mg.

Conditions Requiring Dosing Adjustments

Liver Function: Decreases in dose are not needed.

Kidney Function: Patients with mild kidney failure can take 10 mg daily. Those with moderate kidney failure should take 5 mg daily. In severe kidney failure, 2.5 mg per day may be taken. If needed and tolerated, dose increases should only be made every 2 weeks.

▷ **Dosing Instructions:** The tablet may be crushed and taken on an empty stomach or with food, at same time each day.

Usual Duration of Use: Use on a regular schedule for 2 to 3 weeks usually determines effectiveness in controlling high blood pressure. The proper treatment of high blood pressure usually requires the long-term use of effective medications. Consult your physician on a regular basis.

Possible Advantages of This Drug

Usually controls blood pressure effectively with one daily dose.

Relatively low incidence of adverse effects.

No adverse influence on asthma, cholesterol blood levels, or diabetes.

Sudden withdrawal does not result in a rapid increase in blood pressure.

▷ **This Drug Should Not Be Taken If**

- you have had an allergic reaction to it previously.
- you are pregnant (final 6 months).

- you have experienced swelling of the face (angioedema) from this or other ACE inhibitors.
- you have an abnormally high level of blood potassium.

▷ **Inform Your Physician Before Taking This Drug If**
- you have had an allergic reaction (or other adverse effect) on using any other ACE inhibitor drug (see Drug Classes).
- you currently have a blood cell or bone marrow disorder.
- you are planning pregnancy or are breast-feeding your infant.
- you have a history of kidney disease or impaired kidney function.
- you have severe liver disease.
- you are immunosuppressed or taking an immunosuppressant medicine.
- you are taking potassium supplements or have an elevated blood potassium.
- you have a low white blood cell count.
- you have scleroderma or systemic lupus erythematosus.
- you have cerebral artery disease.
- you have any form of heart disease.
- you are taking other antihypertensives, diuretics, nitrates, or potassium supplements.
- you plan to have surgery under general anesthesia in the near future.

Possible Side Effects (natural, expected, and unavoidable drug actions)
Dizziness, orthostatic hypotension (see Glossary), fainting, increased blood potassium level—all rare.

▷ **Possible Adverse Effects** (unusual, unexpected, and infrequent reactions)
If any of the following develop, consult your physician promptly for guidance.
Mild Adverse Effects
Allergic Reactions: Skin rash, itching—rare.
Headache, fatigue, drowsiness, numbness and tingling, weakness—infrequent.
Taste disorders—rare.
Cough, chest pain, muscle pain, palpitation—rare to infrequent.
Indigestion, nausea/vomiting, constipation—infrequent.
Serious Adverse Effects
Allergic Reactions: Swelling (angioedema) of face, tongue, and/or vocal cords—rare; can be life-threatening—case reports.
Impairment of kidney function—rare.
Blood cell problems (reported with other ACE inhibitors). Caution is advised.
Increased blood potassium—infrequent.

▷ **Possible Effects on Sexual Function:**   Swelling and tenderness of male breast tissue (gynecomastia), impotence—ACE case reports.

Possible Effects on Laboratory Tests
Complete blood cell counts: decreased white cells and platelets.
Blood potassium level: increased.
LDL: decreased.
HDL: increased.
Liver function tests: increased liver enzymes (ALT/GPT, AST/GOT, and alkaline phosphatase).
Kidney function tests: increased blood urea nitrogen (BUN) and creatinine.

CAUTION
1. Ask your doctor if other antihypertensive drugs (especially diuretics) should be stopped for 1 week before starting this drug.
2. **Inform your physician immediately if you become pregnant.** This drug should not be taken beyond the first 3 months of pregnancy.
3. **Report promptly** any indications of infection (fever, sore throat), and any indications of water retention (weight gain, puffiness, swollen feet or ankles).
4. Do not use a salt substitute without your physician's knowledge and approval. (Many salt substitutes contain potassium.)
5. Blood cell counts and urine analyses should be checked **before** starting this drug.

Precautions for Use
By Infants and Children: Safety and effectiveness for those in this age group not established.

By Those Over 60 Years of Age: Small starting doses are indicated. Sudden and excessive lowering of blood pressure can predispose to stroke or heart attack in those with impaired brain circulation or coronary artery heart disease.

▷ **Advisability of Use During Pregnancy**
Pregnancy Category: C during the first 3 months (trimester). D in the final 6 months of pregnancy. See Pregnancy Risk Categories at the back of this book.

Animal studies: No information available.

Human studies: The use of ACE inhibitor drugs during the final 6 months of pregnancy is known to possibly cause very serious injury and possible death to the fetus; skull and limb malformations, lung defects, and kidney failure have been reported in over 50 cases worldwide.

Avoid this drug completely during the final 6 months. During the first 3 months of pregnancy, use this drug only if clearly needed. Ask your physician for guidance.

Advisability of Use If Breast-Feeding
Presence of this drug in breast milk: Unknown.

Avoid drug or refrain from nursing.

Habit-Forming Potential: None.

Effects of Overdosage: Excessive drop in blood pressure, light-headedness, dizziness, fainting.

Possible Effects of Long-Term Use: Gradual increase in blood potassium level.

Suggested Periodic Examinations While Taking This Drug (at physician's discretion)
Before starting drug: Complete blood cell counts; urine analysis with measurement of protein content; blood potassium level.

During use of drug: Blood cell counts; measurements of blood potassium.

▷ **While Taking This Drug, Observe the Following**
Foods: Consult your physician regarding salt intake.

Nutritional Support: **Do not** take potassium supplements unless directed by your physician.

Beverages: No restrictions. May be taken with milk.

▷ *Alcohol:* Use caution until combined effect has been determined. Alcohol may enhance the blood-pressure-lowering effect of this drug.

Tobacco Smoking: No interactions expected, but I advise everyone to quit smoking.

▷ *Other Drugs*

Quinapril *taken concurrently* with

- aspirin or other NSAIDs (see Drug Classes) may block prostaglandin synthesis and blunt the therapeutic benefits of quinapril.
- cyclosporine (Sandimmune) may cause increased kidney toxicity.
- furosemide (Lasix) or bumetanide (Bumex) may cause decreased blood pressure on standing (postural hypotension).
- interferon alfa or beta may increase risk of blood (hematological) toxicity.
- lithium (Lithobid, others) can cause increased lithium blood levels and toxicity; monitor lithium blood levels and adjust dosage as necessary.
- potassium preparations (K-Lyte, Slow-K, etc.) may cause increased blood levels of potassium with risk of serious heart rhythm disturbances.
- potassium-sparing diuretics such as amiloride (Moduretic), spironolactone (Aldactazide), or triamterene (Dyazide) may cause increased blood levels of potassium with risk of serious heart rhythm disturbances.

▷ *Driving, Hazardous Activities:* Usually no restrictions. Be aware of possible drops in blood pressure with resultant dizziness or faintness.

Aviation Note: The use of this drug *may be a disqualification* for piloting. Consult a designated Aviation Medical Examiner.

Exposure to Sun: Caution is advised. A similar drug of this class can cause photosensitivity.

Exposure to Heat: Caution is advised. Avoid excessive perspiring with resultant loss of body water and drop in blood pressure.

Occurrence of Unrelated Illness: Report promptly any disorder that causes nausea, vomiting, or diarrhea. Fluid and chemical imbalances must be corrected as soon as possible.

Discontinuation: This drug may be stopped abruptly without causing a sudden increase in blood pressure. However, you should consult your physician regarding withdrawal of this drug for any reason.

QUINIDINE (KWIN i deen)

Introduced: 1918   **Class:** Antiarrhythmic   **Prescription:** USA: Yes
Controlled Drug: USA: No; Canada: No   **Available as Generic:** Yes

Brand Names: ✦Apo-Quinidine, ✦Biquin Durules, Cardioquin, Cin-Quin, Duraquin, ✦Natisedine, ✦Novoquinidine, Quinaglute Dura-Tabs, ✦Quinate, Quinatime, Quinidex Extentabs, ✦Quinobarb [CD]*, Quinora, Quin-Release, SK-Quinidine sulfate

*Quinobarb contains phenylethylbarbiturate, a sedative of the barbiturate class.

BENEFITS versus RISKS

Possible Benefits	*Possible Risks*
EFFECTIVE TREATMENT OF SELECTED HEART RHYTHM DISORDERS	NARROW TREATMENT RANGE FREQUENT ADVERSE EFFECTS NUMEROUS ALLERGIC AND IDIOSYNCRATIC REACTIONS Dose-related toxicity Provocation of abnormal heart rhythms Abnormally low blood platelet count Hemolytic anemia Kidney or liver toxicity

---

▷ **Principal Uses**

As a Single Drug Product: Uses currently included in FDA-approved labeling: (1) Helps control the following types of abnormal heart rhythm: atrial fibrillation and flutter, paroxysmal atrial tachycardia, paroxysmal ventricular tachycardia, premature atrial and ventricular contractions; (2) intravenous treatment of malaria in people who can not take medicine by mouth.

Other (unlabeled) generally accepted uses: None.

As a Combination Drug Product [CD]: This drug is available (in Canada) in combination with a barbiturate, a mild sedative that is added to allay the anxiety and nervous tension that often accompany heart rhythm disorders.

How This Drug Works: By slowing the activity of the pacemaker and delaying transmission of electrical impulses through the conduction system and muscle of the heart, this drug assists in restoring normal heart rate and rhythm.

Available Dosage Forms and Strengths

Capsules — 200 mg, 300 mg

Injections—80 mg/ml, 200 mg/ml

Tablets—100 mg, 200 mg, 275 mg, 300 mg

Tablets, prolonged action—250 mg, 300 mg, 324 mg, 330 mg

▷ **Usual Adult Dosage Range:**   Premature atrial or ventricular contractions: 200 to 400 mg every 4 to 6 hours.

Paroxysmal atrial tachycardia: 400 to 600 mg every 2 to 3 hours until paroxysm is terminated.

Atrial flutter: Digitalize first; then individualize dosage schedule as appropriate.

Atrial fibrillation: Digitalize first; then try 200 mg every 2 to 3 hours for five to eight doses; increase dose daily until normal rhythm is restored or toxic effects develop.

Maintenance schedule: 200 to 300 mg three or four times daily. Total daily dosage should not exceed 4000 mg.

Note: Actual dosage and administration schedule must be determined for each patient individually.

Conditions Requiring Dosing Adjustments

Liver Function: This drug is extensively metabolized in the liver. Blood levels should be obtained to guide dosing. A larger loading dose and a 50% decreased maintenance dose may be indicated.

Kidney Function: Blood levels should be obtained, and used to guide dosing. Quinidine should be used with caution in renal compromise.

▷ **Dosing Instructions:**   This drug is preferably taken on an empty stomach to achieve high blood levels rapidly. However, it may be taken with or following food to reduce stomach irritation. The regular tablets may be crushed and the capsules opened for administration. The prolonged-action forms should be swallowed whole without alteration.

Usual Duration of Use: Use on a regular schedule for 2 to 4 days usually determines effectiveness in correcting or preventing responsive abnormal rhythms. Long-term use (months to years) requires physician supervision and periodic evaluation.

▷ **This Drug Should Not Be Taken If**
- you have had an allergic or idiosyncratic reaction to it previously.
- you currently have an acute infection of any kind.
- you have taken too much digoxin (digoxin toxicity).
- you have myasthenia gravis.
- you have abnormal heart rhythms caused by an escape mechanism (ask your specialist).

▷ **Inform Your Physician Before Taking This Drug If**
- you have coronary artery disease or myasthenia gravis.
- you have a history of excessive thyroid function (hyperthyroidism).
- you usually have very low blood pressure.
- you have had a deficiency of blood platelets in the past from any cause.
- you are now taking, or have taken recently, any digitalis preparation (digitoxin, digoxin, etc.).
- you plan to have surgery under general anesthesia in the near future.
- you have acute rheumatic fever or subacute bacterial endocarditis (SBE).

Possible Side Effects (natural, expected, and unavoidable drug actions)

Drop in blood pressure, may be marked in some patients and cause passing out (syncope).

▷ **Possible Adverse Effects** (unusual, unexpected, and infrequent reactions)

If any of the following develop, consult your physician promptly for guidance.

Mild Adverse Effects

Allergic Reactions: Skin rash, hives, itching, drug fever—rare.

Irritation of the esophagus (esophagitis)—possible.

Nausea, vomiting, diarrhea—infrequent.

Serious Adverse Effects

Allergic Reactions: Severe skin reactions, hemolytic anemia (see Glossary), joint and muscle pains, anaphylactic reaction (see Glossary), reduced blood platelet count, drug-induced hepatitis (see Glossary).

Idiosyncratic Reactions: Skin rash, fast heart rate, delirium, difficult breathing.

Dose-related toxicity (cinchonism): blurred vision, ringing ears, hearing loss, heart arrest.

Drug-induced myasthenia gravis, systemic lupus erythematosus (SLE), or carpal tunnel syndrome—case reports.

Swelling of the lymph glands in the inguinal area (lymphadenopathy)—case report.

Kidney toxicity—case reports.

Heart conduction abnormalities—case reports.

Optic neuritis, impaired vision—case report.

Abnormally low white blood cell count: fever, sore throat, infections—case reports.

▷ **Possible Effects on Sexual Function:** None reported.

▷ **Adverse Effects That May Mimic Natural Diseases or Disorders**

Drug-induced hepatitis may suggest viral hepatitis.

Natural Diseases or Disorders That May Be Activated by This Drug

Systemic lupus erythematosus, myasthenia gravis, psoriasis (in sensitive individuals).

Possible Effects on Laboratory Tests

Complete blood cell counts: decreased red cells, hemoglobin, white cells, and platelets; increased eosinophils (allergic reaction); marked increase of white blood cells in association with "quinidine fever"—very rare.

Antinuclear antibodies (ANA): positive.

INR (protime): increased (when taken concurrently with warfarin).

Liver function tests: increased enzymes (ALT/GPT, AST/GOT, alkaline phosphatase) or bilirubin.

CAUTION

1. There is a wide variation in response from person to person. Dosage adjustments must be based upon individual reaction. Notify your physician of any events that you suspect may be drug related.

2. It is advisable to carry a card of personal identification which notes that you are taking this drug.

Precautions for Use

By Infants and Children: A test for drug idiosyncrasy should be made before starting treatment with this drug. If there is no beneficial response after 3 days of adequate dosage, this drug should be discontinued.

By Those Over 60 Years of Age: Small doses are mandatory until your individual response has been determined. Observe for the development of light-headedness, dizziness, weakness, or sense of impending faint. Use caution to prevent falls.

▷ **Advisability of Use During Pregnancy**

Pregnancy Category: C. See Pregnancy Risk Categories at the back of this book.

Animal studies: No information available.

Human studies: Adequate studies of pregnant women are not available. No birth defects have been reported following use of this drug during pregnancy.

Use this drug only if clearly needed.

Advisability of Use If Breast-Feeding

Presence of this drug in breast milk: Yes.

Avoid drug or refrain from nursing.

Habit-Forming Potential: None.

Effects of Overdosage: Nausea, vomiting, ringing in the ears, headache, jerky eye movements, double vision, altered color vision, confusion, delirium, hot skin, seizures, coma.

Possible Effects of Long-Term Use: None reported.

Suggested Periodic Examinations While Taking This Drug (at physician's discretion)

Complete blood cell counts, electrocardiograms, blood levels.

▷ **While Taking This Drug, Observe the Following**

Foods: No restrictions.

Beverages: No restrictions. May be taken with milk.

▷ *Alcohol:* Use caution—alcohol may enhance the blood-pressure-lowering effects of this drug.

Tobacco Smoking: Nicotine can increase irritability of the heart and aggravate rhythm disorders. Avoid all forms of tobacco.

▷ *Other Drugs*

Quinapril *taken concurrently* with

- aspirin may prolong the bleeding time.
- beta-blockers may result in additive and undesirable beta-blockade. Lower starting doses may be needed for both medicines.
- codeine may blunt the effectiveness of codeine.
- tricyclic antidepressants (see Drug Classes) may result in antidepressant toxicity.
- venlafaxine (Effexor) may result in venlafaxine toxicity.

Quinidine may *increase* the effects of

- anticoagulants (Coumadin, etc.), and increase the risk of bleeding. More frequent INR (prothrombin time or protime) testing is needed.
- digitoxin and digoxin (Lanoxin), and cause digitalis toxicity.
- disopyramide (Norpace).
- tricyclic antidepressants (doxepin).

The following drugs may *increase* the effects of quinidine

- amiodarone (Cordarone).
- cimetidine (Tagamet).
- ketoconazole (Nizoral).
- ritonavir (Norvir) and perhaps other protease inhibitors (see Drug Classes). Do not combine.
- verapamil (Verelan).

The following drugs may *decrease* the effects of quinidine

- barbiturates (phenobarbital, etc.).
- phenytoin (Dilantin).
- rifampin (Rifadin, Rimactane).
- sucralfate (Carafate).

▷ *Driving, Hazardous Activities:* This drug may cause dizziness and alter vision. Restrict activities as necessary.

Aviation Note: The use of this drug *may be a disqualification* for piloting. Consult a designated Aviation Medical Examiner.

Exposure to Sun: Use caution—this drug may cause photosensitivity (see Glossary).

RAMIPRIL (ra MI pril)

Introduced: 1985   **Class:** Antihypertensive, ACE inhibitor   **Prescription:** USA: Yes   **Controlled Drug:** USA: No; Canada: No   **Available as Generic:** No

Brand Name: Altace

BENEFITS versus RISKS	
Possible Benefits	*Possible Risks*
EFFECTIVE CONTROL OF MILD TO SEVERE HIGH BLOOD PRESSURE	Low blood pressure Allergic swelling of face, tongue, or vocal cords

▷ **Principal Uses**

As a Single Drug Product

Uses currently included in FDA-approved labeling: (1) Treats all degrees of high blood pressure, alone or concurrently with thiazide-type diuretics. Mild to moderate high blood pressure usually responds to low doses; severe high blood pressure may require higher doses, with greater risk of serious adverse effects; (2) helps decrease the size of the left ventricle and control blood pressure in people with left ventricular hypertrophy; (3) helps control blood pressure caused by abnormalities (stenosis) in the renal artery; (4) used in patients with atherosclerosis to help prevent heart attacks, angina, and need for surgery; (5) used after heart attacks to help prevent death, a second heart attack, and undesirable compromises from the first heart attack.

Other (unlabeled) generally accepted uses: Helps improve survival in patients with congestive heart failure.

How This Drug Works: By blocking enzyme systems that influence arterial function, this drug helps relax arterial walls and lower resistance to blood flow that causes high blood pressure. This, in turn, reduces the workload of the heart and improves its performance.

Available Dosage Forms and Strengths

Capsules — 1.25 mg, 2.5 mg, 5 mg, 10 mg

▷ **Usual Adult Dosage Range:** Initially 2.5 mg once daily for 2 to 4 weeks. Usual maintenance dose is 2.5 to 20 mg daily in a single dose or two divided doses.

If taking diuretics: Either discontinue the diuretic for 3 days before initiating this drug, or begin treatment with 1.25 mg of this drug. Total daily dose should not exceed 5 mg if kidney function is significantly impaired.**Note: Actual dosage and dosing schedule must be determined for each patient individually.**

Conditions Requiring Dosing Adjustments

Liver Function: Patients should be followed closely if they have compromised livers. No specific dosage recommendations are available.

Kidney Function: For patients with moderate kidney failure or creatinine values of greater than 2.5 mg/dl, 1.25 mg of ramipril can be taken daily.

▷ **Dosing Instructions:** Take on an empty stomach or with food, at same time each day. The capsule may be opened.

Usual Duration of Use: Use on a regular schedule for 2 to 4 weeks usually determines effectiveness in controlling high blood pressure. The proper treatment of high blood pressure usually requires the long-term use of effective medications. Consult your physician on a regular basis.

▷ **This Drug Should Not Be Taken If**
- you have had an allergic reaction to it previously.
- you are pregnant (final 6 months).
- you have a history of angioedema (a serious allergic reaction) from any cause.
- you have active liver disease.
- you have an abnormally high level of blood potassium.

▷ **Inform Your Physician Before Taking This Drug If**
- you have had an unfavorable reaction to angiotensin-converting enzyme (ACE) inhibitor drugs previously: captopril (Capoten), enalapril (Vasotec), lisinopril (Prinivil, Zestril), others (see Drug Classes).
- you are pregnant (first 3 months), planning pregnancy, or breast-feeding.
- you have impaired liver or kidney function.
- you have scleroderma or systemic lupus erythematosus.
- you have any form of heart disease or diabetes.
- you take other antihypertensives, diuretics, nitrates, or potassium supplements.
- you have abnormal kidney circulation (ask your doctor).
- you take immunosuppressant therapy or have an autoimmune disease.
- you have an abnormally elevated blood potassium level or take a potassium-sparing diuretic.
- you have a condition that causes increased temperature.
- you have had low white blood cell counts.
- you plan to have surgery under general anesthesia in the near future.

Possible Side Effects (natural, expected, and unavoidable drug actions)
Dizziness, light-headedness. Profound lowering of the blood pressure—rare.

▷ **Possible Adverse Effects** (unusual, unexpected, and infrequent reactions)
If any of the following develop, consult your physician promptly for guidance.
Mild Adverse Effects
Allergic Reactions: Skin rash, itching.
Headache, fatigue, drowsiness, nervousness, numbness and tingling, insomnia—infrequent.
Palpitation, drug-induced cough—infrequent.
Indigestion, stomach pain, nausea, vomiting, diarrhea—rare to infrequent.
Excessive sweating, joint and muscle aches—possible.
Serious Adverse Effects
Allergic Reactions: Swelling (angioedema) of face, tongue, and/or vocal cords; can be life-threatening—rare.
Liver toxicity or pancreatitis—case reports.
Chest pain (angina) when used after a heart attack—infrequent to frequent.
Increased blood potassium—infrequent.
Pancreatitis—reported with other ACE inhibitors.

▷ **Possible Effects on Sexual Function:**   Impotence or swelling and tenderness of male breast tissue (gynecomastia)—rare.

Possible Effects on Laboratory Tests

Complete blood cell counts: decreased red cells and hemoglobin (0.4% using this drug alone; 1.5% using this drug and a diuretic); decreased white cells, increased eosinophils—both rare.

Blood potassium level: increased (1%).

Liver function tests: increased enzymes (ALT/GPT, AST/GOT, alkaline phosphatase), or bilirubin.

Kidney function tests: increased blood urea nitrogen (BUN) (0.5% using this drug alone; 3% using this drug and a diuretic); increased creatinine (1.2% using this drug alone; 1.5% using this drug and a diuretic).

Erythrocyte sedimentation rate or uric acid: increased.

Blood sodium level: decreased.

CAUTION

1. Ask your doctor if other antihypertensive drugs (especially diuretics) should be stopped for 1 week before starting this drug.
2. **Report promptly** any indications of infection (fever, sore throat), and any indications of water retention (weight gain, puffiness, swollen feet or ankles).
3. Do not use a salt substitute without your physician's knowledge and approval. (Many salt substitutes contain potassium.)
4. It is advisable to obtain blood cell counts and urine analyses **before** starting this drug.
5. **Notify your physician immediately if pregnancy occurs.** This drug should not be taken beyond the first 3 months of pregnancy.

Precautions for Use

By Infants and Children: Safety and effectiveness for use by those in this age group have not been established.

By Those Over 60 Years of Age: Small doses are advisable until tolerance has been determined. Sudden and excessive lowering of blood pressure can predispose to stroke or heart attack in those with impaired brain circulation or coronary artery heart disease.

▷ Advisability of Use During Pregnancy

Pregnancy Category: C during the first 3 months. D during the final 6 months. See Pregnancy Risk Categories at the back of this book.

Animal studies: Fetal kidney defects found in rat studies; retarded growth found in mouse studies.

Human studies: Adequate studies of pregnant women are not available. However, drugs of this class taken during the final 6 months of pregnancy have been reported to cause serious fetal defects: skull and facial malformations, limb deformities, lung defects, and kidney failure (over 50 cases reported worldwide).

Avoid this drug completely during the final 6 months. During the first 3 months of pregnancy, use this drug only if clearly needed. Ask your physician for guidance.

Advisability of Use If Breast-Feeding

Presence of this drug in breast milk: Yes.

Avoid drug or refrain from nursing.

Habit-Forming Potential: None.

Effects of Overdosage: Excessive drop in blood pressure—light-headedness, dizziness, fainting.

Possible Effects of Long-Term Use: Gradual increase in blood potassium level.

Suggested Periodic Examinations While Taking This Drug (at physician's discretion)

Before starting drug: Complete blood cell counts; urine analysis with measurement of protein content; blood potassium level.

During use of drug: Blood cell counts; measurements of blood potassium.

▷ **While Taking This Drug, Observe the Following**

Foods: Consult your physician regarding salt intake.

Nutritional Support: **Do not** take potassium supplements unless directed by your physician.

Beverages: No restrictions. May be taken with milk.

▷ *Alcohol:* Use caution until combined effect has been determined. Alcohol may enhance the blood-pressure-lowering effect of this drug.

Tobacco Smoking: No interactions expected, but I advise everyone to quit smoking.

▷ *Other Drugs*

Ramipril *taken concurrently* with

- aspirin or other NSAIDs (see Drug Classes) may blunt the blood-pressure-lowering response.
- cyclosporine (Sandimmune) may pose increased risk of kidney toxicity.
- interferon alfa or beta may lead to increased blood (hematological) toxicity.
- lithium (Lithane, Lithotab, etc.) may cause increased blood lithium levels and symptoms of lithium toxicity. Monitor lithium levels closely.
- loop diuretics such as furosemide (Lasix) or bumetanide (Bumex) may cause severe postural hypotension (see Glossary).
- phenothiazines (see Drug Classes) has been reported to cause hypotension with other ACE inhibitors. Caution is advised.
- potassium preparations (K-Lyte, Slow-K, etc.) may cause increased blood levels of potassium with risk of serious heart rhythm disturbances.
- potassium-sparing diuretics such as amiloride (Moduretic), spironolactone (Aldactazide), or triamterene (Dyazide) may cause increased blood levels of potassium with risk of serious heart rhythm disturbances.

▷ *Driving, Hazardous Activities:* Usually no restrictions. Be aware of possible drops in blood pressure with resultant dizziness or faintness.

Aviation Note: The use of this drug *may be a disqualification* for piloting. Consult a designated Aviation Medical Examiner.

Exposure to Sun: Caution is advised. A similar drug of this class can cause photosensitivity.

Exposure to Heat: Caution is advised. Avoid excessive perspiring with resultant loss of body water and drop in blood pressure.

Occurrence of Unrelated Illness: Nausea, vomiting, or diarrhea may cause fluid and chemical imbalances that must be corrected as soon as possible.

RANITIDINE (ra NI te deen)

Author's Note: ALL of the four available histamine (H_2) receptor blocking drugs are now available without prescription. See the new histamine (H_2) blocking drugs profile for further information.

RIFABUTIN (RIF a byu tin)

Introduced: 1993   **Class:** Anti-mycobacterial agent (antitubercular)
Prescription: USA: Yes   **Controlled Drug:** USA: No; Canada: No   **Available as Generic:** USA: No; Canada: No
Brand Name: Mycobutin
Warning: Rifabutin prophylaxis must not be taken by people with active tuberculosis.

```
┌─────────────────────────────────────────────────────────────┐
│                    BENEFITS versus RISKS                     │
│     Possible Benefits              Possible Risks            │
│ PREVENTION OF DISSEMINATED     NEUTROPENIA                   │
│   MYCOBACTERIUM                 Low platelet counts          │
│   AVIUM-INTRACELLULARE                                       │
│ COMPLEX IN PEOPLE WITH                                       │
│   ADVANCED HIV INFECTION                                     │
└─────────────────────────────────────────────────────────────┘
```

▷ **Principal Uses**
As a Single Drug Product: Uses currently included in FDA-approved labeling: (1) Prevention of disseminated *Mycobacterium avium-intracellulare complex* in patients with advanced HIV infection; (2) combination treatment of *Mycobacterium avium-intracellulare complex* infection.
Other (unlabeled) generally accepted uses: None.

How This Drug Works: Rifabutin inhibits DNA-dependent RNA polymerase (an enzyme critical to cells that are dividing) in *E. coli*. The exact mechanism of action of rifabutin in *Mycobacterium avium* or *Mycobacterium avium-intracellulare complex* is not known.

Available Dosage Forms and Strengths
Rifabutin (Mycobutin) capsules—150 mg

How to Store
Keep at room temperature and avoid exposure to excessive humidity.

▷ **Recommended Dosage Ranges** (Actual dosage and administration schedule must be determined for each patient individually.)
Infants and Children: Safety and effectiveness of rifabutin in *Mycobacterium avium-intracellulare complex* prophylaxis has not clearly been established. Safety data comes from a trial of 22 children who were HIV positive:
Infants 1 year of age—18.5 mg per kg of body mass per day.
Children 2–10 years—8.6 mg per kg of body mass per day.
Adolescents up to 14 years—4.0 mg per kg of body mass per day.
14 to 60 Years of Age: 300 mg once a day. Those prone to nausea and vomiting may take 150 mg two times a day with food.
Over 60 Years of Age: Same as 12 to 60 years of age.

Conditions Requiring Dosing Adjustments

Liver Function: At present, clear adjustments of dose in hepatic compromise are not defined, but the drug should be used with caution.

Kidney Function: Elimination of rifabutin may actually be increased in people with compromised kidneys, yet the clinical effect is as yet unknown.

▷ **Dosing Instructions:**   May be taken with food if you are prone to nausea and vomiting. May be mixed with foods such as applesauce for use in children.

Usual Duration of Use: Use on a regular schedule indefinitely is usually needed to assure this drug's effectiveness in prophylaxis of disseminated *Mycobacterium avium-intracellulare complex*. Long-term use (months to years) requires periodic physician evaluation of response.

If rifabutin is being used as a part of combination therapy of a *Mycobacterium avium-intracellulare* infection, the ideal duration of treatment has not been identified, but treatment is usually ongoing.

Possible Advantages of This Drug

Oral treatment of very resistant organisms.

Currently a "Drug of Choice"

for prophylaxis (prevention) of disseminated *Mycobacterium avium-intracellulare complex*.

▷ **This Drug Should Not Be Taken If**

- you have had an allergic reaction to any dosage form of it previously.
- you have active tuberculosis (combination therapy with several medications is indicated).

▷ **Inform Your Physician Before Taking This Drug If**

- you are pregnant or plan to become pregnant.
- you are taking an oral contraceptive (a nonhormonal alternative method is advised).
- you have a history of blood disorders.
- you are taking an anticoagulant such as warfarin (Coumadin).
- you take other prescription or nonprescription medicines that were not discussed with your doctor when this medicine was prescribed.
- you are uncertain of how much to take or how often to take rifabutin.

Possible Side Effects (natural, expected, and unavoidable drug actions)

This medication may color saliva, urine, feces, sputum, perspiration, tears, and skin a brown-orange color. Soft contact lenses may become permanently stained by rifabutin or its metabolites.

Emergence of resistant *Mycobacterium tuberculosis*.

▷ **Possible Adverse Effects** (unusual, unexpected, and infrequent reactions)

If any of the following develop, consult your physician promptly for guidance.

Mild Adverse Effects

Allergic Reactions: Skin rash, fever.

Change in taste perceptions; headache—infrequent.

Loss of appetite; nausea, vomiting, and diarrhea; muscle aches, and a flu-like syndrome—infrequent.

Taste disturbances—possible.

Increased liver enzymes—infrequent.

Serious Adverse Effects
Neutropenia—infrequent.
Anemia and lowered blood platelets (thrombocytopenia)—case reports.

▷ **Possible Effects on Sexual Function:**   Potential alteration of pattern and timing of menstruation.
Decreased effectiveness of oral contraceptives taken together with this drug.

▷ **Adverse Effects That May Mimic Natural Diseases or Disorders**
Liver reactions similar to viral hepatitis.

Possible Effects on Laboratory Tests
Complete blood cell counts: neutropenia (decreases in a specific kind of white blood cells), thrombocytopenia (decreased platelets), anemia, leukopenia (decreased white blood cells).
Coagulation (clotting tests), decreased prothrombin time (when taken at the same time as warfarin).
Liver enzymes (alkaline phosphatase, SGOT, and SGPT) can be increased.

CAUTION
1. The effectiveness of oral contraceptives may be decreased.
2. This drug may hasten the development of resistant *Mycobacterium tuberculosis* if used as monotherapy (as a single drug).
3. Urine, feces, saliva, sputum, sweat, tears, and skin may be colored brown-orange by rifabutin and some of its metabolites. Soft contact lenses may be permanently stained.

Precautions for Use
By Infants and Children: Safety and effectiveness for use in children has not been established.
By Those Over 60 Years of Age: Specific precautions have not yet been developed; however, since the drug is similar to rifampin, those over 60 may be more sensitive to the adverse effects of rifabutin.

▷ **Advisability of Use During Pregnancy**
Pregnancy Category: B. See Pregnancy Risk Categories at the back of this book.
Animal studies: At doses equal to eight times the usual human dose, rifabutin caused an increase in skeletal variants in rats. Doses of 16 times the usual human dose caused maternotoxicity and fetal skeletal anomalies in rabbits.
Human studies: Adequate studies of pregnant women are not available.
Ask your physician for guidance.

Advisability of Use If Breast-Feeding
Presence of this drug in breast milk: It is not known whether rifabutin is excreted in breast milk.
A decision should be made to avoid drug or refrain from nursing.

Habit-Forming Potential: None.

Effects of Overdosage: No information is currently available on overdosage in humans.

Suggested Periodic Examinations While Taking This Drug (at physician's discretion)
This medication may cause neutropenia and thrombocytopenia, therefore white blood cell counts and platelet counts should be checked. Liver function tests should also be obtained periodically.

▷ **While Taking This Drug, Observe the Following**

Foods: No restrictions.

Beverages: No restrictions.

▷ *Alcohol:* The potential exists for additive liver toxicity. It is best to avoid alcohol.

Tobacco Smoking: No interactions expected, but I advise everyone to quit smoking.

Marijuana Smoking: May be an additive cause of rashes and seizures in people with existing seizure disorders. Avoid marijuana completely.

▷ *Other Drugs*

Rifabutin may *decrease* the effects of

- antianxiety agents such as diazepam and perhaps other benzodiazepines (see Drug Classes).
- anticoagulants such as warfarin (Coumadin).
- anticonvulsant drugs such as phenytoin (Dilantin).
- barbiturates (see Drug Classes).
- BCG live-attenuated vaccine.
- beta-blockers such as metoprolol or propranolol (see Drug Classes).
- birth control pills (oral contraceptives).
- chloramphenicol (Chloromycetin).
- clofibrate (Atromid-S).
- cortisonelike drugs (see Drug Classes).
- cyclosporine (Sandimmune).
- dapsone.
- digitalis preparations (Lanoxin, others).
- disopyramide (Norpace).
- ketoconazole (Nizoral).
- mexiletine (Mexitil).
- narcotics such as methadone (see Opioids in Drug Classes).
- oral hypoglycemic agents (sulfonylureas such as tolbutamide—see Sulfonylureas and Oral Antidiabetic Drugs in Drug Classes).
- quinidine (Quinaglute, others).
- theophylline (Theo-Dur, others).
- verapamil (Verelan).
- zidovudine (AZT) (the therapeutic effect will be lessened by a decreased drug level).

Rifabutin *taken concurrently* with

- anticoagulants such as warfarin (Coumadin) will result in a decreased anticoagulant effect (the INR [protime] will decrease). More frequent INR testing is needed. Warfarin dosing should then be adjusted to INR results.
- fluconazole (Diflucan) may result in increased rifabutin concentrations.
- macrolide antibiotics (see Drug Classes) may lower therapeutic antibiotic benefits.
- ritonavir (Norvir) and perhaps other protease inhibitors (see Drug Classes) may lead to loss of protease inhibitor benefits and rifabutin toxicity as well.
- trimetrexate (Neutrexin) may result in lowered trimetrexate levels and decreased therapeutic benefits from trimetrexate.

▷ *Driving, Hazardous Activities:* This drug may rarely be associated with confusion and seizures. Restrict activities as necessary.

Aviation Note: The use of this drug *may be a disqualification* for piloting. Consult a designated Aviation Medical Examiner.

Exposure to Sun: No restrictions.

Discontinuation: Do not stop or interrupt taking this medication without asking your doctor.

Special Storage Instructions: Keep at room temperature and avoid exposure to excessive humidity.

RIFAMPIN (ri FAM pin)

Other Name: Rifampicin

Introduced: 1967   **Class:** Antibiotic, rifamycins   **Prescription:** USA: Yes   **Controlled Drug:** USA: No; Canada: No   **Available as Generic:** Yes

Brand Names: Rifadin, Rifadin IV, Rifamate [CD], Rifater [CD], Rimactane, Rimactane/INH Dual Pack [CD], ✦Rofact

BENEFITS versus RISKS	
Possible Benefits	*Possible Risks*
EFFECTIVE TREATMENT OF TUBERCULOSIS in combination with other drugs	DRUG-INDUCED HEPATITIS
	DRUG-INDUCED NEPHRITIS
	Blood cell or coagulation disorders
EFFECTIVE PREVENTION OF MENINGITIS by the elimination of meningococcus from the throat of carriers	Colitis (pseudomembranous)

▷ **Principal Uses**

As a Single Drug Product: Uses currently included in FDA-approved labeling: (1) Treats active tuberculosis. It is usually given concurrently with other antitubercular drugs to enhance its effectiveness. It is also used to eliminate the meningitis germ (meningococcus) from the throats of healthy carriers so it cannot be spread to others; (2) treats tuberculosis in coal workers with good outcomes when combined with other antitubercular drugs; (3) used to prevent tuberculosis in people exposed to patients with active disease.

Other (unlabeled) generally accepted uses: (1) Second-line agent in combination with doxycycline in treatment of brucellosis; (2) has a place in preventing *Haemophilus influenzae* infections in people exposed to patients with active disease; (3) combination therapy of lepromatous leprosy; (4) used in combination with cotrimoxazole to eliminate methicillin-resistant *Staphylococcus aureus* (MRSA) from people who carry the bacteria.

As a Combination Drug Product [CD]: This drug is available in combination with isoniazid, another antitubercular drug that delays the development of drug-resistant strains of the tuberculosis germ.

How This Drug Works: This drug prevents the growth and multiplication of susceptible tuberculosis organisms by blocking specific enzyme systems that are involved in the formation of essential proteins.

Available Dosage Forms and Strengths

Capsules — 150 mg, 300 mg

▷ **Usual Adult Dosage Range:**   For tuberculosis: 10 mg per kg of body mass per day, up to 600 mg once daily.

For meningococcus carriers: 600 mg once daily for 4 days. The total daily dosage should not exceed 600 mg. **Note: Actual dosage and administration schedule must be determined for each patient individually.**

Conditions Requiring Dosing Adjustments

Liver Function: This drug can cause liver damage, and patients should be followed closely. In severe failure, the dose should be limited to 6 to 8 mg per kg of body mass twice a week.

Kidney Function: For patients with a creatinine clearance (see Glossary) of 10 to 50 ml/min, one researcher suggests that 50 to 100% of the usual dose should be given.

▷ **Dosing Instructions:**   This drug is preferably taken with 8 ounces of water on an empty stomach (1 hour before or 2 hours after eating). However, it may be taken with food if necessary to reduce stomach irritation. The capsule may be opened and the contents mixed with applesauce or jelly for administration.

Usual Duration of Use: Use on a regular schedule for several months usually determines effectiveness in promoting recovery from tuberculosis. Long-term use (possibly 1 to 2 years) requires ongoing physician supervision and periodic evaluation.

▷ **This Drug Should Not Be Taken If**
  • you have had an allergic reaction to it previously.

▷ **Inform Your Physician Before Taking This Drug If**
  • you are pregnant.
  • you have a history of liver disease or impaired liver function.
  • you have active liver disease.
  • you consume alcohol daily.
  • you are taking an oral contraceptive. (An alternate method of contraception is advised.)
  • you are taking an anticoagulant.

Possible Side Effects (natural, expected, and unavoidable drug actions)

Red, orange, or brown discoloration of tears, sweat, saliva, sputum, urine, or stool. Yellow discoloration of the skin (not jaundice). Note: In the absence of symptoms indicating illness, any discoloration is a harmless drug effect and does not indicate toxicity. Possible fungal superinfections (see Glossary).

▷ **Possible Adverse Effects** (unusual, unexpected, and infrequent reactions)

If any of the following develop, consult your physician promptly for guidance.

Mild Adverse Effects

Allergic Reactions: Skin rash, hives, itching, drug fever (see Glossary).

Headache, dizziness, blurred vision, impaired hearing, vague numbness and tingling—infrequent.

Joint and muscle pain—infrequent and often subsides after a few weeks.

Loss of appetite, heartburn, nausea, vomiting, abdominal cramps, diarrhea—infrequent.

Serious Adverse Effects
Skin problems (Stevens-Johnson syndrome or toxic epidermal necrolysis)—case reports.
Flu-like syndrome: fever, headache, dizziness, musculoskeletal pain, difficult breathing—case reports.
Drug-induced liver damage, with or without jaundice—frequent.
Kidney damage—infrequent.
Drug-induced porphyria, pancreatitis, gallstones, or pseudomembranous colitis—case reports.
Excessively low blood platelet count: abnormal bleeding or bruising—rare.
Blood clotting problems (disseminated intravascular coagulopathy)—case report.
Hemolytic anemia—case reports.
Suppression of the adrenal gland—possible.

▷ **Possible Effects on Sexual Function**
Altered timing and pattern of menstruation—case reports.
Decreased effectiveness of oral contraceptives taken concurrently.

▷ **Adverse Effects That May Mimic Natural Diseases or Disorders**
Liver reactions may suggest viral hepatitis.
Kidney reactions may suggest an infectious nephritis.

Possible Effects on Laboratory Tests
Complete blood cell counts: decreased red cells, hemoglobin, white cells, and platelets; increased eosinophils (allergic reaction).
INR (protime): increased (when taken concurrently with warfarin).
Liver function tests: increased liver enzymes (ALT/GPT, AST/GOT, and alkaline phosphatase), increased bilirubin.

CAUTION
1. This drug may permanently discolor soft contact lenses.
2. This drug may reduce the effectiveness of oral contraceptives—unplanned pregnancy could occur. An alternate method of contraception is advised.
3. When this drug is used alone in the treatment of tuberculosis, resistance can develop rapidly. This drug should only be used in conjunction with other antitubercular drugs.
4. To ensure the best possible response to treatment, take the full course of medication prescribed; this may be for several months or years.

Precautions for Use
By Infants and Children: Monitor closely for possible liver toxicity or deficiency of blood platelets.
By Those Over 60 Years of Age: Natural changes in body composition and function make you more susceptible to the adverse effects of this drug. Report promptly any indications of possible drug toxicity.

▷ **Advisability of Use During Pregnancy**
Pregnancy Category: C. See Pregnancy Risk Categories at the back of this book.
Animal studies: Cleft palate and spinal defects reported in rodent studies.
Human studies: Adequate studies of pregnant women are not available.
If possible, avoid use of drug during the first 3 months.

Advisability of Use If Breast-Feeding
Presence of this drug in breast milk: Yes.
Avoid drug or refrain from nursing.

Habit-Forming Potential: None.

Effects of Overdosage: Nausea, vomiting, drowsiness, unconsciousness, severe liver damage, jaundice.

Possible Effects of Long-Term Use: Superinfections, fungal overgrowth of mouth or tongue.

Suggested Periodic Examinations While Taking This Drug (at physician's discretion)
Complete blood cell counts, liver and kidney function tests.
Hearing acuity tests if hearing loss is suspected.

▷ **While Taking This Drug, Observe the Following**
Foods: No restrictions.
Beverages: No restrictions.
▷ *Alcohol:* It is best to avoid alcohol completely to reduce the risk of liver toxicity.
Tobacco Smoking: No interactions expected, but I advise everyone to quit smoking.
▷ *Other Drugs*
Rifampin **taken concurrently** with
• halothane anesthesia may result in serious liver damage.
Rifampin may **decrease** the effects of
• antianxiety agents such as diazepam and perhaps other benzodiazepines (see Drug Classes).
• anticoagulants such as warfarin (Coumadin).
• anticonvulsant drugs such as phenytoin (Dilantin).
• barbiturates (see Drug Classes).
• BCG live-attenuated vaccine.
• beta-blockers such as metoprolol or propranolol (see Drug Classes).
• birth control pills (oral contraceptives).
• some calcium channel blockers (see Drug Classes).
• chloramphenicol (Chloromycetin).
• clofibrate (Atromid-S).
• cortisonelike drugs (see Drug Classes).
• cyclosporine (Sandimmune).
• dapsone.
• digitalis preparations (Lanoxin, others).
• disopyramide (Norpace).
• enalapril (Vasotec).
• fluconazole (Diflucan).
• indinavir (Crixivan).
• itraconazole (Sporanox).
• ketoconazole (Nizoral).
• methadone (Dolophine).
• mexiletine (Mexitil).
• narcotics such as methadone (see Opioids in Drug Classes).
• nifedipine (Adalat).
• oral hypoglycemic agents (sulfonylureas such as tolbutamide—see Drug Classes).

- phenytoin (Dilantin).
- progestins.
- quinidine (Quinaglute, others).
- ritonavir (Norvir)—this combination may also lead to rifampin toxicity.
- theophylline (Theo-Dur, others).
- tricyclic antidepressants (see Drug Classes).
- verapamil (Verelan).
- warfarin (Coumadin). Increased INR testing is needed.
- zidovudine (AZT) (the therapeutic effect will be lessened by a decreased drug level).

The following drug may *decrease* the effects of rifampin

- *para*-aminosalicylic acid (PAS), and reduce its antitubercular effectiveness.

▷ *Driving, Hazardous Activities:* This drug may cause dizziness, drowsiness, impaired vision, and impaired hearing. Restrict activities as necessary.

Aviation Note: The use of this drug *may be a disqualification* for piloting. Consult a designated Aviation Medical Examiner.

Exposure to Sun: No restrictions.

Discontinuation: It is advisable not to interrupt or stop this drug without consulting your physician. Intermittent administration can increase the possibility of developing allergic reactions.

RISPERIDONE (RIS peer i dohn)

Introduced: 1993   **Class:** Antipsychotic agent   **Prescription:** USA: Yes
Controlled Drug: USA: No; Canada: No   **Available as Generic:** USA: No; Canada: No

Brand Name: Risperdal

BENEFITS versus RISKS	
Possible Benefits	*Possible Risks*
TREATMENT OF SCHIZOPHRENIA REFRACTORY TO OTHER AGENTS	Change in heart function
	Involuntary movement disorder
	Neuroleptic malignant syndrome
DECREASED SIDE EFFECTS COMPARED TO OTHER AVAILABLE DRUGS	
EFFECTIVE TREATMENT OF CERTAIN PSYCHOTIC DISORDERS	

▷ **Principal Uses**

As a Single Drug Product: Uses currently included in FDA-approved labeling: Management of the effects (manifestations) of psychotic disorders such as chronic schizophrenia.

Other (unlabeled) generally accepted uses: (1) Treatment of acute schizophrenia; (2) treatment of aggression; (3) treatment of Tourette syndrome; (4) can have a role in helping behavioral problems in people with mental retardation.

How This Drug Works: This medication acts to balance two nerve transmitters (dopamine and serotonin) and, by doing so, helps restore more normal thinking and mood.

Available Dosage Forms and Strengths

Oral solution — 1 mg/ml
Tablets — 1 mg, 2 mg, 3 mg, 4 mg

▷ **Recommended Dosage Ranges** (Actual dosage and administration schedule must be determined for each patient individually.)

Infants and Children: Safety and efficacy for those less than 18 years of age are not established.

18 to 60 Years of Age: Usual starting dose is 1 mg taken twice daily. Dosage may be increased as needed and tolerated by 1 mg on the second and third day, for a total of 3 mg twice daily by the third day. If further dose changes are needed, they should be made at 1-week intervals. Doses greater than 6 mg per day are not recommended.

Over 60 Years of Age: Therapy is started with 0.5 mg twice daily. The dose is increased if needed and tolerated by 0.5 mg twice daily. Doses greater than 1.5 mg daily are achieved by small increases made at 1-week intervals. Careful attention must be paid to blood pressure and development of adverse effects.

Conditions Requiring Dosing Adjustments

Liver Function: The starting dose must be decreased and adjusted as for those over 60 years old. Additionally, there may be an increased amount of the active drug that results from each dose (increased free fraction), and as such a greater than expected effect may be seen.

Kidney Function: The starting dose must be decreased and adjusted as for those over 60 years old.

▷ **Dosing Instructions:**   The tablet may be crushed, and the medication's effect is not changed by food.

Usual Duration of Use: Use on a regular schedule for 1 to 2 weeks usually determines effectiveness in helping control chronic schizophrenia. If long-term use is attempted, the lowest effective dose should be used. Periodic physician evaluation of response and dose is required.

Possible Advantages of This Drug

Treatment of schizophrenia refractory to other therapy.

▷ **This Drug Should Not Be Taken If**

- you have had an allergic reaction to any dosage form of it previously.
- you have had neuroleptic malignant syndrome (ask your doctor).

▷ **Inform Your Physician Before Taking This Drug If**

- you have a history of breast cancer.
- you have liver or kidney compromise.
- you are pregnant or plan to become pregnant or are breast-feeding your infant.
- you have had tardive dyskinesia in the past.
- you have a history of Parkinson's disease or seizures.
- you have a history of heart rhythm disturbances.
- you are uncertain of your risperidone dose or how often to take it.

Possible Side Effects (natural, expected, and unavoidable drug actions)

Increased prolactin levels may result in male and female breast tenderness and swelling. Sleepiness. Orthostatic hypotension (see Glossary)—rare. Weight gain—infrequent.

▷ **Possible Adverse Effects** (unusual, unexpected, and infrequent reactions)

If any of the following develop, consult your physician promptly for guidance.

Mild Adverse Effects

Allergic Reactions: Skin rash.

Difficulty in concentrating—rare.

Headache or increased dreaming—rare to infrequent.

Constipation, diarrhea, or nausea—infrequent.

Palpitations—rare.

Increased urination—rare.

Serious Adverse Effects

Allergic Reactions: Anaphylactic reactions.

Abnormal heart function (prolonged QT interval)—rare.

Tardive dyskinesia (see Glossary) or neuroleptic malignant syndrome—case reports.

Low sodium—rare.

Seizures—rare.

Lowered white blood cells or platelets—case reports.

Abnormal liver function—rare.

▷ **Possible Effects on Sexual Function:** Diminished sexual desire; delayed or absent orgasm; erectile dysfunction including priapism; male or female breast tenderness or swelling; dry vagina or menstrual changes (hypermenorrhea)—rare. Ejaculation failure—case reports.

Possible Delayed Adverse Effects: Swelling and tenderness of male and female breast tissue.

Natural Diseases or Disorders That May Be Activated by This Drug

Some human cancers depend on prolactin for growth, and since risperidone increases prolactin, it should be used with caution by people with previously diagnosed breast cancer.

Possible Effects on Laboratory Tests

Liver function tests: increased SGPT, SGOT, and LDH.

Complete blood counts: decreased platelets, white blood cells, and hemoglobin.

Prolactin: increased.

CAUTION

1. This drug should be used with great caution, if at all, by patients with cancer.
2. Call your doctor promptly if you have an increased tendency to infection or abnormal bleeding or bruising while taking this drug.
3. This drug should be used with great caution, if at all, by patients with a history of seizures.

Precautions for Use

By Infants and Children: Safety and effectiveness for those under 18 years of age are not established.

By Those Over 60 Years of Age: The starting dose of 0.5 mg twice daily is used for patients who are elderly or debilitated, and slower increases in dose as needed and tolerated are indicated. Great care should be taken by those with heart disease. You may be more likely to experience postural hypotension (see Glossary) and problems with motor skills. Those with prostate problems may have increased risk of urine retention.

▷ **Advisability of Use During Pregnancy**
Pregnancy Category: C. See Pregnancy Risk Categories at the back of this book. Animal studies: Increased rat pup death during the first few days of lactation. Human studies: Adequate studies of pregnant women are not available. One case report of lack of formation of the corpus callosum of the brain in a fetus exposed to this drug while in the uterus.
Ask your doctor for guidance.

Advisability of Use If Breast-Feeding
Presence of this drug in breast milk: Yes.
Avoid drug or refrain from nursing.

Habit-Forming Potential: None.

Effects of Overdosage: Drowsiness, hypotension, tachycardia, low sodium and potassium, ECG changes (prolonged QT interval), and seizure.

Suggested Periodic Examinations While Taking This Drug (at physician's discretion)
Liver function tests.
Electrolytes (sodium and potassium).
ECG.
Prolactin levels.

▷ **While Taking This Drug, Observe the Following**
Foods: No restrictions.
Beverages: No restrictions.
▷ *Alcohol:* Patients should avoid alcohol while taking risperidone.
Tobacco Smoking: No interactions expected, but I advise everyone to quit smoking.
Marijuana Smoking: Increased somnolence.
▷ *Other Drugs*
Risperidone may *decrease* the effects of
• levodopa (Sinemet, others).
Risperidone *taken concurrently* with
• carbamazepine (Tegretol) will decrease the drug level and perhaps the therapeutic effects of risperidone.
• clozapine (Clozaril) may decrease the therapeutic effects of risperidone.
• other centrally acting medicines may result in increased central effects.
• ritonavir (Norvir) and perhaps other protease inhibitors (see Drug Classes) may lead to toxicity.
▷ *Driving, Hazardous Activities:* This drug may cause drowsiness and difficulty in concentrating. Restrict activities as necessary.
Aviation Note: The use of this drug *is a disqualification* for piloting. Consult a designated Aviation Medical Examiner.
Exposure to Sun: Use caution— this drug may cause photosensitivity.
Discontinuation: Consult your doctor before stopping this medication.

SALMETEROL (sal ME ter ohl)

Introduced: 1994   **Class:** Bronchodilator   **Prescription:** USA: Yes
Controlled Drug: USA: No; Canada: Not available in Canada   **Available as**
Generic: USA: No
Brand Names: Serevent, Aeromax

BENEFITS versus RISKS	
Possible Benefits	*Possible Risks*
LONG-ACTING RELIEF OF BRONCHIAL ASTHMA PREVENTION OF NOCTURNAL ASTHMA SYMPTOMS	Rapid heart rate (tachycardia)

▷ **Principal Uses**
As a Single Drug Product: Uses currently included in FDA-approved labeling: (1) Treatment and prevention of bronchospasm in asthma; (2) prevention of nocturnal asthma; (3) prevention of exercise-induced bronchospasm.
Other (unlabeled) generally accepted uses: May have a role in treating chronic obstructive pulmonary disease (COPD).

How This Drug Works: This drug acts at specific sites (beta-2) in the lung and results in opening of the airways (bronchodilation), decreased airway reactivity, and increased movement of mucus. It also appears to block release of chemicals from certain (mast) cells that worsen asthma.

Available Dosage Forms and Strengths
Inhaler — 13-g canister that gives 21 mcg of salmeterol per use

▷ **Recommended Dosage Ranges** (Actual dosage and administration schedule must be determined for each patient individually.)
Infants and Children: Safety and efficacy in those less than 12 years of age are not established.
12 to 60 Years of Age: For prevention of asthma: Two inhalations (42 mcg) twice daily in the morning and evening. Doses should be taken 12 hours apart.
For prevention of exercised-induced asthma: Two inhalations at least 30 to 60 minutes **before** exercise. Additional doses of salmeterol should **not** be taken for 12 hours.
Over 60 Years of Age: Same as 12 to 60 years of age.

Conditions Requiring Dosing Adjustments
Liver Function: Use with caution, as the drug may accumulate in liver failure.
Kidney Function: Salmeterol has not been studied in kidney failure patients.

▷ **Dosing Instructions:**   Follow written instructions on the inhaler closely. This drug has not been studied for use with a spacer or similar device. Shake well before using.

Usual Duration of Use: Use on a regular schedule for 4 to 6 weeks usually determines effectiveness in preventing asthma attacks. Long-term use (months to years) requires periodic physician evaluation of response and dosage adjustment.

Possible Advantages of This Drug
Longer-acting beta-2 agent than medications previously available.

▷ **This Drug Should Not Be Taken If**
- you have had an allergic reaction to any dosage form of it previously.
- you currently have an irregular heart rhythm.
- you are taking, or have taken within the past 2 weeks, any monoamine oxidase (MAO) type A inhibitor.
- you are having sudden (acute) symptoms or worsening (exacerbation) of your asthma.

▷ **Inform Your Physician Before Taking This Drug If**
- your breathing does not improve after administration of this drug.
- you have an overactive thyroid (hyperthyroidism).
- you have diabetes.
- you have a history of heart problems.
- you have abnormally high blood pressure.
- you are uncertain of how much salmeterol to take or how often to take it.

Possible Side Effects (natural, expected, and unavoidable drug actions)
  Dryness or irritation of the mouth or throat, altered taste. Nervousness, tremor, or palpitations.

▷ **Possible Adverse Effects** (unusual, unexpected, and infrequent reactions)
  If any of the following develop, consult your physician promptly for guidance.
  Mild Adverse Effects
  Allergic Reactions: Skin rash and urticaria.
  Rhinitis and laryngitis—possible.
  Rapid heart rate (tachycardia)—case reports.
  Headache, tremor, dizziness, and nervousness—infrequent.
  Serious Adverse Effects
  Allergic Reactions: Not defined.
  Paradoxical bronchospasm.
  Respiratory arrest—case reports.

▷ **Possible Effects on Sexual Function:**   Not defined.

Possible Delayed Adverse Effects: None defined at present.

▷ **Adverse Effects That May Mimic Natural Diseases or Disorders**
  Rapid heart rate may mimic heart disease. Bronchospasm may mimic asthma.

Natural Diseases or Disorders That May Be Activated by This Drug
  Latent coronary artery disease. Diabetes or high blood pressure.

Possible Effects on Laboratory Tests
  Blood cholesterol profile: may be increased.
  Blood glucose level: increased.

CAUTION
  1. Use of this drug by inhalation with beclomethasone aerosol (Beclovent, Vanceril) may increase the risk of fluorocarbon propellant toxicity. Use salmeterol aerosol 20 to 30 minutes **before** beclomethasone aerosol to reduce toxicity and enhance penetration of beclomethasone into the lungs.
  2. Serious heart rhythm problems or cardiac arrest can result from excessive and prolonged use.
  3. Call your doctor if you begin to have symptoms more frequently than

usual, or if you begin to increase your use of the immediate bronchodilator that was prescribed for you.
4. The recent *Guidelines for the Diagnosis and Management of Asthma* from
the National Institutes of Health state that salmeterol should NOT be
used for treatment of acute symptoms or exacerbations of asthma.

Precautions for Use

By Infants and Children: Safety and effectiveness for those under 12 years of age
are not established.

By Those Over 60 Years of Age: Avoid increased use. If asthma is not controlled as
it has been in the past, call your doctor.

▷ **Advisability of Use During Pregnancy**

Pregnancy Category: C. See Pregnancy Risk Categories at the back of this book.
Animal studies: Rabbit studies have revealed cleft palate, limb and paw flex-
ures, and delayed bone formation.
Human studies: Adequate studies of pregnant women are not available.
Ask your doctor for guidance.

Advisability of Use If Breast-Feeding

Presence of this drug in breast milk: Yes, but extent not defined.
Avoid drug or refrain from nursing.

Habit-Forming Potential: None.

Effects of Overdosage: Exaggeration of pharmacological effects: tachycardia
and/or arrhythmia, muscle cramps, cardiac arrest, and death.

Suggested Periodic Examinations While Taking This Drug (at physician's discretion)
Blood pressure checks, evaluations of heart (cardiac) status.

▷ **While Taking This Drug, Observe the Following**

Foods: No restrictions.
Beverages: Avoid excessive caffeine as in coffee, tea, cola, and chocolate.
▷ *Alcohol:* No interactions expected.
Tobacco Smoking: No interactions expected, but I advise everyone to quit smok-
ing.
▷ *Other Drugs*
Salmeterol *taken concurrently* with
• monoamine oxidase (MAO) type A inhibitor drugs can cause extreme in-
creases in blood pressure and heart stimulation.
The following drugs may *increase* the effects of salmeterol
• methylxanthines such as caffeine or theophylline.
• tricyclic antidepressants.
▷ *Driving, Hazardous Activities:* This drug may cause nervousness or dizziness.
Restrict activities as necessary.
Aviation Note: The use of this drug *is a disqualification* for piloting. Consult a
designated Aviation Medical Examiner.
Exposure to Sun: No restrictions.
Heavy Exercise or Exertion: Use caution—this may stress protective effects of
this drug.

SELEGILINE (se LEDGE i leen)

Other Name: Deprenyl

Introduced: 1981   **Class:** Anti-parkinsonism, monoamine oxidase (MAO) type B inhibitor   **Prescription:** USA: Yes   **Controlled Drug:** USA: No; Canada: No   **Available as Generic:** USA: No

Brand Name: Eldepryl

BENEFITS versus RISKS	
Possible Benefits	*Possible Risks*
EFFECTIVE INITIAL TREATMENT OF PARKINSON'S DISEASE when started at the onset of symptoms ADDITIVE RELIEF OF SYMPTOMS OF PARKINSON'S DISEASE when used concurrently with levodopa/carbidopa PERMITS REDUCTION IN SINEMET DOSAGE May have a role in Alzheimer's disease	ABNORMAL INVOLUNTARY MOVEMENTS HALLUCINATIONS INITIAL FALL IN BLOOD PRESSURE/ORTHOSTATIC HYPOTENSION

▷ **Principal Uses**

As a Single Drug Product: Uses currently included in FDA-approved labeling: (1) Used to start drug treatment of very early Parkinson's disease (soon after onset of symptoms), thus delaying the use of levodopa/carbidopa; (2) also used as an adjunct to levodopa/carbidopa treatment of Parkinson's disease if intolerable abnormal movements (dyskinesia) and/or increasing "on–off" episodes occur. Addition of selegiline (1) permits reduction of the daily dose of levodopa with consequent lessening of dyskinesia and erratic drug response, and (2) provides additional relief of parkinsonian symptoms.

Other (unlabeled) generally accepted uses: Some improvement achieved in Alzheimer's disease (some trials also used high-dose vitamin E) in patients treated with this drug.

How This Drug Works: By (1) inhibiting monoamine oxidase type B, the enzyme that inactivates dopamine in the brain, and by (2) slowing the restorage of released dopamine at nerve terminals, this drug helps correct dopamine deficiency responsible for rigidity, tremor, and sluggish movement characteristic of Parkinson's disease.

Available Dosage Forms and Strengths

Capsules — 5 mg

Tablets — 5 mg

Author's Note: The capsule form of this medicine will eventually replace the tablet form, and is an astute attempt by the company to help avoid confusion with other white tablets or counterfeit copies of Eldepryl.

▷ **Usual Adult Dosage Range**

Parkinsonism: 5 mg once or twice daily. The usual maintenance dose is 5 mg after breakfast and 5 mg after lunch. A total daily dose of 10 mg is adequate to achieve optimal benefit from this drug. Higher doses do not result in further improvement and are not advised. During gradual introduction of selegiline, concurrent dose of levodopa/carbidopa (Sinemet) may be cautiously decreased. Concurrent Sinemet dosage should be reduced by 10 to 20% when selegiline is started. **Note: Actual dosage and administration schedule must be determined for each patient individually.**

Conditions Requiring Dosing Adjustments

Liver Function: This drug is extensively metabolized in the liver. Patients with liver compromise should be followed closely.

Kidney Function: The kidney does not have a major role in the elimination of this medication. It can cause prostatic hypertrophy, and should be used with caution by patients with urine outflow problems.

▷ **Dosing Instructions:** The tablet may be crushed and taken with food or milk to reduce stomach irritation.

Usual Duration of Use: Use on a regular schedule for 4 to 6 weeks usually determines effectiveness in controlling the symptoms of Parkinson's disease and permitting reduction of levodopa/carbidopa dosage. Long-term use (months to years) requires periodic physician evaluation of response and dosage adjustment.

Possible Advantages of This Drug

It may provide a more effective and uniform control of parkinsonian symptoms and a significant reduction of some adverse effects associated with long-term levodopa therapy. It does not lose its effectiveness with long-term use, and does not require avoidance of foods containing tyramine, as is necessary with monoamine oxidase (MAO) type A inhibitors.

▷ **This Drug Should Not Be Taken If**

- you have had an allergic reaction to it previously.
- you have Huntington's disease, hereditary (essential) tremor, or tardive dyskinesia (see Glossary).
- you are pregnant or breast-feeding.
- you take meperidine (Demerol).

▷ **Inform Your Physician Before Taking This Drug If**

- you have constitutionally low blood pressure.
- you have peptic ulcer disease.
- you are taking levodopa.
- you have a history of heart rhythm disorder.
- you are taking any antihypertensive drugs or antipsychotic drugs (see Drug Classes).

Possible Side Effects (natural, expected, and unavoidable drug actions)

Weakness, orthostatic hypotension (see Glossary), dry mouth, insomnia—all rare.

▷ **Possible Adverse Effects** (unusual, unexpected, and infrequent reactions)

If any of the following develop, consult your physician promptly for guidance.

Mild Adverse Effects

Headache, dizziness, blurred vision, agitation—rare.

Palpitations, fainting—rare.

Altered taste—rare, nausea and vomiting, stomach pain, anorexia—common.

Serious Adverse Effects

Dyskinesias: abnormal involuntary movements—infrequent.

Confusion and hallucinations, depression, psychosis, vivid dreams—rare.

Aggravation of peptic ulcer, gastrointestinal bleeding—rare.
Growth of the prostate—rare.

▷ **Possible Effects on Sexual Function:**   Transient decreases in penile sensation and anorgasmia have rarely been reported if doses exceed 10 mg per day. Increased libido may occur.

▷ **Adverse Effects That May Mimic Natural Diseases or Disorders**
Effects on mental function and behavior may resemble psychotic disorders.

Natural Diseases or Disorders That May Be Activated by This Drug
Peptic ulcer disease.

Possible Effects on Laboratory Tests
None reported.

CAUTION
1. This drug can initiate dyskinesias and intensify existing dyskinesias. Watch carefully for the development of tremors, twitching, or abnormal, involuntary movements of any kind. Report these promptly.
2. This drug potentiates the effects of levodopa. When this drug is added to current levodopa treatment, adverse effects of levodopa may develop or be intensified. The dose of levodopa must be reduced by 10 to 20% when treatment with selegiline begins.
3. Tell your doctor promptly if you become pregnant or plan pregnancy. The manufacturer does not recommend the use of this drug during pregnancy.

Precautions for Use
By Infants and Children: This drug is not utilized by this age group.
By Those Over 60 Years of Age: This drug is well tolerated by the elderly. Observe closely for any tendency to light-headedness or faintness, especially on arising from a lying or sitting position.

▷ **Advisability of Use During Pregnancy**
Pregnancy Category: C. See Pregnancy Risk Categories at the back of this book.
Animal studies: No birth defects due to this drug were found in rat studies.
Human studies: Adequate studies of pregnant women are not available. The manufacturer advises that this drug should not be taken during pregnancy.

Advisability of Use If Breast-Feeding
Presence of this drug in breast milk: Unknown.
Avoid drug or refrain from nursing.

Habit-Forming Potential: None.

Effects of Overdosage: Nausea, vomiting, palpitations, low blood pressure, agitation, severe involuntary movements, hallucinations.

Possible Effects of Long-Term Use: None reported.

Suggested Periodic Examinations While Taking This Drug (at physician's discretion)
Regular evaluation of drug response, heart function, and blood pressure status.

▷ **While Taking This Drug, Observe the Following**
Foods: Caution should be used regarding foods containing tyramine (see Glossary for a list), although the reaction with this drug may not be as severe as that seen with other MAO inhibitors.

Beverages: No restrictions. May be taken with milk.

▷ *Alcohol:* Use caution until the combined effects have been determined. Alcohol may exaggerate the blood-pressure-lowering and sedative effects of this drug.

Tobacco Smoking: No interactions expected, but I advise everyone to quit smoking.

Marijuana Smoking: Additive drowsiness may occur.

▷ *Other Drugs*

Selegiline *taken concurrently* with

- albuterol (Ventolin, others) may result in increased adverse vascular effects.
- amphetamine (Dexedrine) can cause a severe increase in blood pressure.
- antidepressants (see Drug Classes) such as amitriptyline (Elavil) may cause neurotoxic reactions such as seizures.
- antihypertensive drugs (and other drugs that can lower blood pressure) require careful monitoring for excessive drops in pressure. Dosage adjustments may be necessary.
- benzodiazepines (see Drug Classes) may result in increased central nervous system depression.
- buspirone (Buspar) may result in increases in blood pressure.
- dextromethorphan (various), a cough suppressant used in many nonprescription cough medicines, has been reported to cause toxicity with low blood pressure, spasms, high fevers, and some deaths. These medicines should not be combined.
- ephedrine (various) can result in severe increases in temperature.
- fluoxetine (Prozac) may cause serotonin toxicity syndrome.
- fluvoxamine (Luvox) may result in extreme agitation, rigidity, excessive temperatures, and coma. DO NOT combine these medicines.
- lithium (Lithobid) may increase risk of the serotonin toxicity syndrome.
- meperidine (Demerol) may cause a life-threatening reaction of unknown cause; avoid this combination.
- oral hypoglycemic agents (see Oral Antidiabetic Drugs in Drug Classes) may cause very low blood sugars.
- paroxetine (Paxil) may result in central nervous system toxicity.
- phenothiazines (see Drug Classes) may result in increased occurrence of movement disorders.
- phenylpropanolamine (various) can cause severe increases in temperature and blood pressure. DO NOT combine.
- pseudoephedrine (various) can cause severe increases in temperature and blood pressure. DO NOT combine.
- sertraline (Zoloft) may result in central nervous system toxicity.
- tryptophan may cause a fatal serotonin syndrome.
- venlafaxine (Effexor) can result in central and autonomic nervous system toxicity.

The following drugs may *decrease* the effects of selegiline and diminish its effectiveness

- chlorprothixene (Taractan).
- haloperidol (Haldol).
- metoclopramide (Reglan).
- phenothiazines (see Drug Classes).

- reserpine (Ser-Ap-Es, etc.), in high doses.
- thiothixene (Navane).

▷ *Driving, Hazardous Activities:* This drug may cause dizziness, drowsiness, impaired coordination, or fainting. Restrict activities as necessary.

Aviation Note: The use of this drug *is a disqualification* for piloting. Consult a designated Aviation Medical Examiner.

Exposure to Sun: Use caution—photosensitivity has been reported.

Exposure to Heat: Use caution until the combined effects have been determined. Hot environments can cause lowering of blood pressure.

Discontinuation: Do not stop this drug abruptly. Sudden withdrawal can cause prompt increase in parkinsonian symptoms and deterioration of control. Consult your physician regarding a schedule for gradual withdrawal and concurrent adjustment of Sinemet or other appropriate drugs.

SERTRALINE (SER tra leen)

Introduced: 1986   **Class:** Antidepressant   **Prescription:** USA: Yes
Controlled Drug: USA: No; Canada: No   **Available as Generic:** USA: No
Brand Name: Zoloft

BENEFITS versus RISKS	
Possible Benefits	*Possible Risks*
EFFECTIVE TREATMENT OF MAJOR DEPRESSIVE DISORDERS	Male sexual dysfunction Seizures
Possibly effective in relieving the symptoms of obsessive-compulsive disorder	

▷ **Principal Uses**

As a Single Drug Product: Uses currently included in FDA-approved labeling: Treats major forms of depression that have not responded well to other therapies. This drug should be used only when a diagnosis of a true, primary depression of significant degree has been established.

Other (unlabeled) generally accepted uses: (1) May have a role in treating obesity. Rat studies have shown a decrease in eating that depends on the dose that is taken. Studies in humans are being conducted; (2) treatment of obsessive-compulsive disorder.

How This Drug Works: This drug relieves depression by slowly restoring to normal levels a specific constituent of brain tissue (serotonin) that transmits nerve impulses.

Available Dosage Forms and Strengths

Tablets — 50 mg, 100 mg

▷ **Recommended Dosage Ranges** (Actual dosage and administration schedule must be determined for each patient individually.)

Infants and Children: Dosage not established.

12 to 60 Years of Age: Initially 50 mg once daily, taken in the morning or evening. The dose is then gradually increased, as needed and tolerated, in increments of 50 mg at intervals of 1 week. The total daily dosage should not exceed 200 mg.

Over 60 Years of Age: Same as 12 to 60 years of age. Adjust dosage as appropriate for impaired liver or kidney function.

Conditions Requiring Dosing Adjustments

Liver Function: This drug is a rare cause of liver damage. Patients should be followed closely, and less frequent or lower doses should be used.

Kidney Function: The role of the kidneys in the elimination of this drug is unknown.

▷ **Dosing Instructions:**   The tablet may be crushed and is best taken with food to enhance absorption, but may be taken at any time with or without food.

Usual Duration of Use: Use on a regular schedule for 4 to 8 weeks usually determines (1) this drug's effectiveness in relieving depression; (2) the pattern of both favorable and unfavorable drug effects. Long-term use (months to years) requires periodic physician evaluation of response and dosage adjustment.

Possible Advantages of This Drug

Does not cause weight gain, a common side effect of tricyclic antidepressants.

Less likely to cause dry mouth, constipation, urinary retention, orthostatic hypotension (see Glossary), and heart rhythm disturbances than tricyclic antidepressants.

Does not cause Parkinson-like reactions.

▷ **This Drug Should Not Be Taken If**

- you have had an allergic reaction to it previously.
- you are currently taking, or have taken within the past 14 days, any monoamine oxidase (MAO) type A inhibitor drug (see Drug Classes).

▷ **Inform Your Physician Before Taking This Drug If**

- you have experienced any adverse effects from antidepressant drugs.
- you have impaired liver or kidney function.
- you have Parkinson's disease.
- you have had a recent heart attack.
- you have a seizure disorder.
- you are pregnant or plan pregnancy while taking this drug.

Possible Side Effects (natural, expected, and unavoidable drug actions)

Decreased appetite, weight loss (average 1 to 2 lb).

▷ **Possible Adverse Effects** (unusual, unexpected, and infrequent reactions)

If any of the following develop, consult your physician promptly for guidance.

Mild Adverse Effects

Allergic Reactions: Skin rash, itching—rare.

Headache, nervousness, insomnia, fatigue, tremor, dizziness, impaired concentration—rare; abnormal vision, numbness, and tingling—rare; confusion—rare; hallucinations—rare to infrequent.

Chest pain and increased blood pressure—rare.

Paresthesias—rare.

Dry mouth, altered taste, nausea, vomiting, diarrhea, tongue ulceration—rare to infrequent.

Serious Adverse Effects
Allergic Reactions: Dermatitis (various forms)—rare.
Drug-induced seizures—rare.
Hemorrhage into the anterior chamber of the eye or anemia—rare.
Increased blood cholesterol (hypercholesterolemia)—infrequent.
Low blood sugar—case reports.
Bronchospasm—infrequent.
Low blood sodium—rare; case reports of SIADH (may also occur with other selective serotonin reuptake inhibitors).

▷ **Possible Effects on Sexual Function:**   Male sexual dysfunction: Delayed ejaculation—may be frequent; female sexual dysfunction: inhibited orgasm—rare.
Swelling and tenderness of male and female breast tissue—case reports.
Infrequent dysmenorrhea, intermenstrual bleeding, or atrophic vaginitis.

Natural Diseases or Disorders That May Be Activated by This Drug
Latent epilepsy.

Possible Effects on Laboratory Tests
Blood total cholesterol and triglyceride levels: increased—infrequent.
Blood uric acid levels: decreased.
Hemoglobin or hematocrit: decreased—rare.
Liver function tests: increased liver enzymes (ALT/GPT, AST/GOT, and alkaline phosphatase).
Blood sodium: decreased (with rare SIADH).

CAUTION
1. If any type of skin reaction develops (rash, hives, etc.), discontinue this drug and inform your physician promptly.
2. If dryness of the mouth develops and persists for more than 2 weeks, consult your dentist for guidance.
3. Ask your doctor or pharmacist before taking any other prescription or over-the-counter drug while taking sertraline.
4. If you are advised to take any monoamine oxidase (MAO) type A inhibitor drug (see Drug Classes), allow an interval of 5 weeks after discontinuing this drug before starting the MAO inhibitor.
5. It is advisable to withhold this drug if electroconvulsive therapy (ECT, "shock" treatment) is to be used to treat your depression.

Precautions for Use
By Infants and Children: Safety and effectiveness for those under 12 years of age are not established.
By Those Over 60 Years of Age: The lowest effective dose should be used for maintenance treatment and adjusted as needed for reduced kidney function.

▷ **Advisability of Use During Pregnancy**
Pregnancy Category: B. See Pregnancy Risk Categories at the back of this book.
Animal studies: Delayed bone development due to this drug found in rat and rabbit studies.
Human studies: Adequate studies of pregnant women are not available.
Use this drug only if clearly needed. Ask your physician for guidance.

Advisability of Use If Breast-Feeding
>   Presence of this drug in breast milk: Unknown.
>   Avoid drug or refrain from nursing.

Habit-Forming Potential: None.

Effects of Overdosage: Agitation, restlessness, excitement, nausea, vomiting, seizures.

Possible Effects of Long-Term Use: None reported.

Suggested Periodic Examinations While Taking This Drug (at physician's discretion)
>   None.

▷ **While Taking This Drug, Observe the Following**
>   *Foods:* May increase peak blood level.
>   *Beverages:* No restrictions. May be taken with milk.

▷   *Alcohol:* Avoid completely.
>   *Tobacco Smoking:* No interactions expected, but I advise everyone to quit smoking.

▷   *Other Drugs*
>   Sertraline may ***increase*** the effects of
>   • diazepam (Valium) and perhaps other benzodiazepines (see Drug Classes).
>   • tolbutamide (Orinase).
>   • warfarin (Coumadin) and related oral anticoagulants. More frequent INR (prothrombin time or protime) testing is needed. Ongoing warfarin doses should be based on INR results.
>
>   Sertraline ***taken concurrently*** with
>   • antidiabetic drugs (insulin, oral hypoglycemics—see Oral Antidiabetic Drugs in Drug Classes) may increase the risk of hypoglycemic reactions; monitor blood and urine sugar levels carefully.
>   • cimetidine (Tagamet, Tagamet HB 200) may lead to sertraline toxicity.
>   • flecainide (Tambocor) may lead to flecainide toxicity.
>   • monoamine oxidase (MAO) type A inhibitor drugs may cause confusion, agitation, high fever, seizures, and dangerous elevations of blood pressure. Avoid the concurrent use of these drugs.
>   • ritonavir (Norvir) and perhaps other protease inhibitors (see Drug Classes) may lead to toxicity.

▷   *Driving, Hazardous Activities:* This drug may cause drowsiness, dizziness, impaired judgment, and altered vision. Restrict activities as necessary.
>   *Aviation Note:* The use of this drug ***is a disqualification*** for piloting. Consult a designated Aviation Medical Examiner.
>   *Exposure to Sun:* Use caution—this drug may (rarely) cause photosensitivity (see Glossary).
>   *Discontinuation:* The slow elimination of this drug from the body makes it unlikely that any withdrawal effects will result from abrupt discontinuation. However, call your doctor if you plan to stop this drug for any reason.

SIMVASTATIN (sim vah STA tin)

Introduced: 1986   **Class:** Anticholesterol   **Prescription:** USA: Yes
Controlled Drug: USA: No; Canada: No   **Available as Generic:** USA: No;
Canada: No

Brand Name: Zocor

BENEFITS versus RISKS

Possible Benefits	*Possible Risks*
EFFECTIVE REDUCTION OF TOTAL BLOOD CHOLESTEROL AND LDL CHOLESTEROL	Drug-induced hepatitis
	Drug-induced myositis
REDUCES RISK FROM CORONARY DISEASE	
REDUCES DEATH FROM CORONARY REVASCULARIZATION	
REDUCES NONFATAL MYOCARDIAL INFARCTIONS	

▷ **Principal Uses**

As a Single Drug Product: Uses currently included in FDA-approved labeling: (1) Used by patients with elevated cholesterol to reduce death from heart disease (42% in one study) and decrease the number of nonfatal heart attacks; (2) treatment of abnormally high total blood cholesterol levels (in people with types IIa and IIb hypercholesterolemia) due to increased fractions of low-density lipoprotein (LDL) cholesterol. It is used in conjunction with a cholesterol-lowering diet. It should not be used until an adequate trial of nondrug methods for lowering cholesterol has proved to be ineffective; (3) stops the progression and decreases the number of deaths of patients with coronary artery disease.

Author's Note: This drug was found to be the second drug of choice in treating patients with high blood cholesterol in a recent *Clinical Therapeutics* study.

Other (unlabeled) generally accepted uses: (1) may help reduce lipid disorders that occur in kidney (nephrotic syndrome) problems; (2) can have a role as part of combination therapy in preventing gallstones.

How This Drug Works: This drug blocks the liver enzyme that starts production of cholesterol. It reduces low-density lipoproteins (LDL), the fraction of total blood cholesterol that is thought to increase the risk of coronary heart disease. This drug may also increase the level of high-density lipoproteins (HDL), the cholesterol fraction that reduces the risk of heart disease.

Available Dosage Forms and Strengths

Tablets — 5 mg, 10 mg, 20 mg, 40 mg

Author's Note: The maker of this medicine is planning a double-strength version of simvastatin.

▷ **Recommended Dosage Ranges** (Actual dosage and administration schedule must be determined for each patient individually.)

Infants and Children: Under 2 years of age—do not use this drug.
2 to 20 years of age—dosage not established.

20 to 60 Years of Age: Initially 5 to 10 mg daily, taken at bedtime. Dose is increased as needed to reach desired goals (such as decreased LDL-C percent). More aggressive goals may require the 10-mg starting dose. The drug is then increased as needed and tolerated by increments of 5 to 10 mg at intervals of 4 weeks. The total daily dose should not exceed 40 mg.

Over 60 Years of Age: Initially 5 mg daily. Increase dose as needed and tolerated by increments of 5 mg at intervals of 4 weeks. The total daily dose should not exceed 20 mg.

Conditions Requiring Dosing Adjustments

Liver Function: This drug achieves a high concentration in the liver, and is subsequently eliminated in the bile. It can be a rare cause of liver damage, and patients should be followed closely.

Kidney Function: In severe kidney failure, the dose should be started at 5 mg, and the patient closely followed.

▷ **Dosing Instructions:** The tablet may be crushed and taken without regard to eating, preferably taken at bedtime (the highest rates of cholesterol production occur between midnight and 5 A.M.).

Usual Duration of Use: Use on a regular schedule for 4 to 6 weeks usually determines effectiveness in reducing blood levels of total and LDL cholesterol. Long-term use (months to years) requires periodic physician evaluation of response and dosage adjustment. Consult your physician on a regular basis.

Possible Advantages of This Drug: Recent studies indicate that drugs of this class (HMG-CoA reductase inhibitors) are more effective and better tolerated than other drugs currently available for reducing total and LDL cholesterol. Its long-term effects are yet to be determined.

▷ **This Drug Should Not Be Taken If**
- you have had an allergic reaction to it previously.
- you have active liver disease.
- you are pregnant or breast-feeding your infant.

▷ **Inform Your Physician Before Taking This Drug If**
- you have previously taken any other drugs in this class: lovastatin (Mevacor) or pravastatin (Pravachol).
- you have a history of liver disease or impaired liver function.
- you are not using any method of birth control, or you are planning pregnancy.
- you regularly consume substantial amounts of alcohol.
- you have cataracts or impaired vision.
- you have any type of chronic muscular disorder.
- you develop muscle pain, weakness, or soreness that is unexplained while taking this medicine.
- you plan to have major surgery in the near future.

Possible Side Effects (natural, expected, and unavoidable drug actions)
Development of abnormal liver function tests without associated symptoms.

▷ **Possible Adverse Effects** (unusual, unexpected, and infrequent reactions)
If any of the following develop, consult your physician promptly for guidance.

Mild Adverse Effects
    Allergic Reactions: Rash.
    Headache—infrequent.
    Nausea, excessive gas, constipation, diarrhea—rare to infrequent.
    Lowering of blood pressure—possible.
Serious Adverse Effects
    Marked and persistent abnormal liver function tests with focal hepatitis—
        rare.
    Acute myositis (muscle pain and tenderness)—infrequent.
    Rhabdomyolysis—rare.
    Potential for cataracts—based on animal data, not reported in humans.
    Depression—rare.
    Protein in the urine—rare.
    Lichen planus skin rash—rare.

▷ **Possible Effects on Sexual Function:**   None reported.

Possible Delayed Adverse Effects: None reported to date. Doses 15 to 33 times
    the human dose given to rats caused an increase in liver cancers.

Natural Diseases or Disorders That May Be Activated by This Drug
    Latent liver disease.

Possible Effects on Laboratory Tests
    Blood alanine aminotransferase (ALT) enzyme level: increased (with higher
        doses of drug).
    Blood total cholesterol, LDL cholesterol, and triglyceride levels: decreased.
    Blood HDL cholesterol level: increased.

CAUTION
    1. If pregnancy occurs while taking this drug, stop it immediately and con-
       sult your physician.
    2. Report promptly any development of muscle pain or tenderness, espe-
       cially if accompanied by fever or weakness (malaise).
    3. Promptly report altered or impaired vision so that appropriate evaluation
       can be made.

Precautions for Use
    By Infants and Children: Safety and effectiveness for those under 20 years of age
        are not established.
    By Those Over 60 Years of Age: Inform your physician regarding any personal or
        family history of cataracts. Comply with all recommendations regarding
        periodic eye examinations. Report promptly any alterations in vision.

▷ **Advisability of Use During Pregnancy**
    Pregnancy Category: X. See Pregnancy Risk Categories at the back of this book.
        Animal studies: Mouse and rat studies reveal skeletal birth defects due to a
        closely related drug of this class.
    Human studies: Adequate studies of pregnant women are not available.
    This drug should be avoided during entire pregnancy.

Advisability of Use If Breast-Feeding
    Presence of this drug in breast milk: Unknown.
    Avoid drug or refrain from nursing.

Habit-Forming Potential: None.

Effects of Overdosage: Increased indigestion, stomach distress, nausea, diarrhea.

Possible Effects of Long-Term Use: Abnormal liver function with focal hepatitis.

Suggested Periodic Examinations While Taking This Drug (at physician's discretion)

Blood cholesterol studies: total cholesterol, HDL, and LDL fractions.

Liver function tests before treatment, and at 6-month intervals for 1 year. In patients who have had an increase in liver enzymes, testing should continue at 6-month intervals until 1 year after the last liver function test elevation.

Complete eye examination at beginning of treatment and at any time that significant change in vision occurs. Ask your doctor for help.

▷ **While Taking This Drug, Observe the Following**

Foods: Follow a standard low-cholesterol diet.

Beverages: No restrictions. May be taken with milk.

▷ *Alcohol:* No interactions expected. Use sparingly.

Tobacco Smoking: No interactions expected, but I advise everyone to quit smoking.

▷ *Other Drugs*

Simvastatin may *increase* the effects of

- digoxin (Lanoxin).
- warfarin (Coumadin); more frequent testing of INR (prothrombin time or protime) will be needed.

Simvastatin *taken concurrently* with

- clofibrate (Atromid-S) or other fibrates may result in increased risk of serious muscle toxicity.
- cyclosporine (Sandimmune) can result in kidney failure and myopathy.
- gemfibrozil (Lopid) may alter absorption and excretion of simvastatin. DO NOT COMBINE.
- niacin may cause an increased frequency of muscle problems (myopathy) when combined with a related medicine (lovastatin). Caution is advised.

The following drug may *decrease* the effects of simvastatin

- cholestyramine (Questran) may reduce absorption of simvastatin; take simvastatin 1 hour before or 4 hours after cholestyramine.

▷ *Driving, Hazardous Activities:* No restrictions.

Aviation Note: No restrictions.

Exposure to Sun: No restrictions.

Discontinuation: Do not stop this drug without your physician's knowledge and guidance. There may be significant increase in blood cholesterol levels following discontinuation of this drug.

SPIRONOLACTONE (speer on oh LAK tohn)

Introduced: 1959   **Class:** Diuretic   **Prescription:** USA: Yes   **Controlled Drug:** USA: No; Canada: No   **Available as Generic:** USA: Yes

Brand Names: Alatone, Aldactazide [CD], Aldactone, ✦Apo-Spirozide, ✦Novospiroton, ✦Novospirozine [CD], ✦Sincomen, Spironazide

```
┌─────────────────────────────────────────────────────────────────┐
│                    BENEFITS versus RISKS                          │
│      Possible Benefits              Possible Risks                │
│   EFFECTIVE PREVENTION OF       ABNORMALLY HIGH BLOOD             │
│     POTASSIUM LOSS when used      POTASSIUM LEVEL with excessive  │
│     adjunctively with other diuretics  use                       │
│   EFFECTIVE DIURETIC IN          Enlargement of male breast tissue│
│     REFRACTORY CASES OF FLUID    Masculinization effects in women:│
│     RETENTION when used            excessive hair growth, deepening of│
│     adjunctively with other diuretics  the voice                 │
│                                  Hepatitis                        │
└─────────────────────────────────────────────────────────────────┘
```

▷ **Principal Uses**

As a Single Drug Product: Uses currently included in FDA-approved labeling: (1) Manages congestive heart failure and disorders of the liver and kidney that are accompanied by excessive fluid retention (edema); (2) also used with other measures to treat high blood pressure where prevention of potassium loss is needed; (3) used to decrease fluid in patients who have failed glucocorticoid treatment and have nephrotic syndrome.

Other (unlabeled) generally accepted uses: (1) May have an adjunctive role in treating acne; (2) can help treat lung problems (bronchopulmonary dysplasia) and slow the disease process; (3) can help precocious puberty in females; (4) eases fluid buildup in premenstrual syndrome; (5) may help women with excessive facial hair growth (hirsutism).

As a Combination Drug Product [CD]: This drug is available in combination with hydrochlorothiazide, a different kind of diuretic that promotes the loss of potassium from the body. Spironolactone is used in this combination to counteract the potassium-wasting effect of the thiazide diuretic.

How This Drug Works: By inhibiting the action of aldosterone (an adrenal gland hormone), this drug prevents the reabsorption of sodium and the excretion of potassium by the kidney. Thus the drug promotes the excretion of sodium (and water with it) and the retention of potassium.

Available Dosage Forms and Strengths

Tablets — 25 mg, 50 mg, 100 mg

▷ **Usual Adult Dosage Range:**   For edema: Initially 100 mg per day in one dose or divided into several doses. The dose is then adjusted according to individual response. The usual maintenance dose is 50 to 200 mg daily, divided into two to four doses. If response is not adequate after 5 days, a second fluid medicine (diuretic) is added. **Note: Actual dosage and administration schedule must be determined for each patient individually.**

Conditions Requiring Dosing Adjustments

Liver Function: This drug can be a rare cause of liver damage, and patients should be followed closely.

Kidney Function: For patients with mild kidney failure, the drug can be taken every 12 hours in the usual dose. In moderate kidney failure, spironolactone can be taken every 12 to 24 hours in the usual dose. In severe kidney failure, this drug should **not** be taken. Spironolactone is contraindicated in acute renal failure and severe chronic renal compromise.

▷ **Dosing Instructions:**   The tablet may be crushed and taken with or following meals to promote absorption of the drug and reduce stomach irritation.

Usual Duration of Use: Use on a regular schedule for 5 to 10 days usually determines effectiveness in clearing edema, and for 2 to 3 weeks to determine its effect on hypertension. Long-term use (months to years) requires physician supervision and periodic evaluation.

▷ **This Drug Should Not Be Taken If**
- you have had an allergic reaction to it previously.
- you have severely impaired liver or kidney function.
- your kidneys are not making any urine.
- your blood potassium is excessively high (hyperkalemia).
- your creatinine is greater than 2.5 mg/dl.

▷ **Inform Your Physician Before Taking This Drug If**
- you have a history of liver or kidney disease.
- you have diabetes.
- you take an anticoagulant, antihypertensives, a digitalis preparation, another diuretic, lithium, or a potassium preparation.
- you plan to have surgery under general anesthesia in the near future.

Possible Side Effects (natural, expected, and unavoidable drug actions)
Abnormally high blood potassium levels—frequent; abnormally low blood sodium levels or dehydration—infrequent.

▷ **Possible Adverse Effects** (unusual, unexpected, and infrequent reactions)
If any of the following develop, consult your physician promptly for guidance.
Mild Adverse Effects
Allergic Reactions: Skin rash, hives, itching, drug fever (see Glossary).
Headache, dizziness, unsteadiness, weakness, drowsiness, lethargy, confusion—infrequent.
Dry mouth, nausea, vomiting, diarrhea—infrequent.
Taste disturbances—possible.
Serious Adverse Effects
Allergic Reactions: Abnormally low blood platelet count—rare.
Symptomatic potassium excess: confusion, numbness and tingling in lips and extremities, fatigue, weakness, shortness of breath, slow heart rate, low blood pressure—possible.
Masculine pattern of hair growth and deepening of the voice in women—case reports.
Stomach ulceration with bleeding—case reports.
Possible association with decreased white blood cell counts.
Disruption in the acid–base balance of body (hyperchloremic or hyperkalemic acidosis)—possible.
Liver toxicity (hepatitis)—rare.
Porphyria or systemic-lupus-erythematosus-like syndrome—case reports.
Decreased platelet counts—rare.
Thinning of the bones—case reports.

▷ **Possible Effects on Sexual Function**
Decreased libido or impaired erection or impotence—frequent.
Male breast enlargement and tenderness (gynecomastia) (increases with higher doses).

Female breast enlargement (100% with high doses); altered timing and pattern of menstruation; postmenopausal bleeding. Decreased vaginal secretion—case reports.

Possible Effects on Laboratory Tests

White blood cell count: decreased (one report only).
Blood platelet count or INR (protime): decreased.
Blood potassium level: increased.
Blood uric acid level: no effect in some; increased and decreased in others.

CAUTION

1. Do not take potassium supplements or increase intake of potassium-rich foods while taking this drug.
2. Do not stop this drug abruptly unless abnormally high blood levels of potassium develop.
3. Ordinary doses of aspirin (600 mg) may reverse the diuretic effect of this drug. Observe your response to this drug combination.
4. Avoid excessive use of salt substitutes containing potassium; these are potential causes of potassium excess.

Precautions for Use

By Infants and Children: Limit the continual use of this drug in children to 1 month. Observe closely for indications of potassium accumulation.

By Those Over 60 Years of Age: The natural decline in kidney function may predispose to potassium retention in the body. Watch for indications of potassium excess: slow heart rate, irregular heart rhythms, low blood pressure, confusion, drowsiness. The excessive use of diuretics can cause harmful loss of body water (dehydration), increased viscosity of the blood, and an increased tendency of the blood to clot, predisposing to stroke, heart attack, or thrombophlebitis.

▷ Advisability of Use During Pregnancy

Pregnancy Category: B. See Pregnancy Risk Categories at the back of this book.
Animal studies: This drug causes feminization of male rat fetuses.
Human studies: Adequate studies of pregnant women are not available.
This drug should not be used during pregnancy unless a very serious complication of pregnancy occurs for which this drug is significantly beneficial.

Advisability of Use If Breast-Feeding

Presence of this drug in breast milk: A metabolic end product (canrenone) is present.
Avoid drug or refrain from nursing.

Habit-Forming Potential: None.

Effects of Overdosage: Thirst, drowsiness, fatigue, weakness, nausea, vomiting, confusion, irregular heart rhythm, low blood pressure.

Possible Effects of Long-Term Use: Potassium accumulation to abnormally high blood levels. Male breast enlargement.

Suggested Periodic Examinations While Taking This Drug (at physician's discretion)

Measurements of blood sodium, potassium, and chloride levels.
Kidney function tests.

▷ **While Taking This Drug, Observe the Following**

Foods: No restrictions. Avoid excessive restriction of salt.

Beverages: No restrictions. May be taken with milk.

▷ *Alcohol:* Use with caution. Alcohol may enhance the drowsiness and the blood-pressure-lowering effect of this drug.

Tobacco Smoking: No interactions expected, but I advise everyone to quit smoking.

▷ *Other Drugs*

Spironolactone may *increase* the effects of
- digoxin (Lanoxin).

Spironolactone may *decrease* the effects of
- anticoagulants (Coumadin, etc.). Increased frequency of INR (prothrombin time or protime) testing is needed.

Spironolactone *taken concurrently* with
- captopril (Capoten) or other ACE inhibitors (see Drug Classes) may cause excessively high blood potassium levels.
- cyclosporine (Sandimmune) may result in very elevated potassium levels.
- digitoxin (Crystodigin) may cause either increased or decreased digitoxin effects (unpredictable).
- lithium (Lithobid, others) may cause accumulation of lithium to toxic levels.
- potassium preparations may cause excessively high blood potassium levels.

The following drugs may *decrease* the effects of spironolactone
- aspirin or other NSAIDs (see Drug Classes)—may reduce its diuretic effectiveness.

▷ *Driving, Hazardous Activities:* This drug may cause dizziness and drowsiness. Restrict activities as necessary.

Aviation Note: The use of this drug *may be a disqualification* for piloting. Consult a designated Aviation Medical Examiner.

Exposure to Sun: No restrictions.

Discontinuation: With high dosage or prolonged use, it is advisable to withdraw this drug gradually. Ask your physician for guidance.

STAVUDINE (STAV u dine)

Other Names: D4T

Introduced: 1994   **Class:** Anti-AIDS drug   **Prescription:** USA: Yes
Controlled Drug: USA: No; Canada: No   **Available as Generic:** USA: No; Canada: No

Brand Name: Zerit

```
┌─────────────────────────────────────────────────────────────┐
│                   BENEFITS versus RISKS                      │
│      Possible Benefits              Possible Risks           │
│  INCREASED CD4 COUNTS IN       PERIPHERAL NEUROPATHY         │
│    ADULTS WITH ADVANCED HIV    Pancreatitis                  │
│  THERAPEUTIC OPTION VERSUS                                   │
│    AZT OR OTHER NUCLEOSIDE                                   │
│    ANALOGS                                                   │
│  LESS LIKELY THAN OTHER                                      │
│    AGENTS TO DEVELOP                                         │
│    RESISTANCE                                               │
│  EFFECTIVE COMBINATION                                       │
│    THERAPY OF HIV                                           │
└─────────────────────────────────────────────────────────────┘
```

▷ **Principal Uses**

As a Single Drug Product: Uses currently included in FDA-approved labeling: Treatment of HIV in adults who have received prior AZT (zidovudine) therapy. **Author's Note: *The Panel on Clinical Practices for Treatment of HIV Infection Report* says that the preferred regimen is: Two nucleoside analogs and one potent protease inhibitor. Single-agent therapy (with the exception of AZT use in preventing HIV transmission from mother to fetus) was rejected by the panel.**

Other (unlabeled) generally accepted uses: (1) This drug has been used in a small number of children; (2) approval is pending for initial use in HIV-positive patients; (3) combination therapy may offer a durable increase in CD4 count and decrease in viral load.

How This Drug Works: This drug inhibits HIV reproduction (replication) by: (1) Inhibiting an HIV enzyme (reverse transcriptase), which blocks the ability of the virus to make nuclear material; (2) inhibiting an enzyme (DNA polymerase-gamma and -beta), which blocks the ability to make DNA in the mitochondria.

Available Dosage Forms and Strengths

Capsules — 15 mg, 20 mg, 30 mg, 40 mg

▷ **Recommended Dosage Ranges** (Actual dosage and administration schedule must be determined for each patient individually.)

Infants and Children: Safety and efficacy are not established.

18 to 60 Years of Age: Patients with a body mass of 60 kg (132 lb) or more should take 40 mg twice daily. Patients with a body mass of less than 60 kg should take 30 mg twice daily.

For those who have had to stop because of peripheral neuropathy (after complete resolution of symptoms): 20 mg twice daily for patients with a body mass of 60 kg or more; 15 mg twice daily for those with a body mass less than 60 kg.

Over 65 Years of Age: This drug has **not** been studied in those over 65.

Conditions Requiring Dosing Adjustments

Liver Function: Liver involvement in elimination has not been studied in humans.

Kidney Function: Patients with mild kidney compromise (creatinine clearance greater than 50 ml/min) failure may take the usual weight-adjusted dose for adults. Those with mild to moderate kidney failure (creatinine clearance 26 to 50 ml/min) should take one-half of the usual weight-adjusted dose every 12 hours. In severe kidney compromise (creatinine clearance 10 to 25 ml/min) one-half the usual weight-adjusted dose should be taken every 24 hours.

▷ **Dosing Instructions:**   This drug may be taken without regard to food.

Usual Duration of Use: Use on a regular schedule for several months usually determines effectiveness in slowing AIDS progression and increasing CD4 counts. Long-term use (months to years) requires periodic physician evaluation of response (viral burden and CD4).

Possible Advantages of This Drug
More favorable side-effect profile than other nucleoside analogs.
Favorable profile for combination therapy.

▷ **This Drug Should Not Be Taken If**
• you have had an allergic reaction to any dosage form of it previously.

▷ **Inform Your Physician Before Taking This Drug If**
• you have had peripheral neuropathy caused by other drugs before.
• you have kidney or liver compromise.
• you have had pancreatitis.
• your bone marrow is depressed.
• you have vitamin B_{12} deficiency or folic acid deficiency.
• you are uncertain of how much stavudine to take or how often to take it.

Possible Side Effects (natural, expected, and unavoidable drug actions)
Chills or fever—infrequent. Peripheral neuropathy—infrequent to frequent. Pancreatitis—infrequent.

▷ **Possible Adverse Effects** (unusual, unexpected, and infrequent reactions)
If any of the following develop, consult your physician promptly for guidance.
Mild Adverse Effects
Allergic Reactions: Skin rash.
Nausea and vomiting or abdominal pain—infrequent.
Increased liver enzymes—frequent.
Serious Adverse Effects
Allergic Reactions: Anaphylactic reactions—rare.
Anemia—case reports.
Low white blood cell or platelet counts—rare to infrequent in phase three data, not found in later data.

▷ **Possible Effects on Sexual Function:**   Impotence—rare in phase three data.

Possible Delayed Adverse Effects: Peripheral neuropathy.

▷ **Adverse Effects That May Mimic Natural Diseases or Disorders**
Increased liver function tests may mimic hepatitis.

Possible Effects on Laboratory Tests
Liver function tests: increased.
Amylase: increased.
Complete blood counts: decreased platelets and white blood cells.

CAUTION
1. Stavudine has **not** been shown to decrease the risk of giving (transmission) HIV to others through sexual contact or blood contamination.

2. Promptly report the development of stomach pain and vomiting; this could indicate pancreatitis.
3. Report development of pain, numbness, tingling or burning in the hands or feet, as this may be peripheral neuropathy.

Precautions for Use

By Infants and Children: Safety and effectiveness for those under 18 years of age are not established.

By Those Over 65 Years of Age: The drug has not been studied in this age group.

▷ **Advisability of Use During Pregnancy**

Pregnancy Category: C. See Pregnancy Risk Categories at the back of this book.

Animal studies: Clinical doses in rats have not revealed teratogenicity; however, doses of 399 times those used in humans have resulted in skeletal problems. Increased early rat death has also occurred at 399 times the human dose.

Human studies: Adequate studies of pregnant women are not available.

Ask your doctor for guidance.

Advisability of Use If Breast-Feeding

Presence of this drug in breast milk: Yes.

Refrain from nursing if you are HIV positive or are taking this drug.

Habit-Forming Potential: None.

Effects of Overdosage: Adults treated with 12 to 24 times the recommended daily dose revealed no acute toxicity.

Possible Effects of Long-Term Use: Peripheral neuropathy and hepatic toxicity.

Suggested Periodic Examinations While Taking This Drug (at physician's discretion)

Liver function tests, amylase and complete blood counts.

CD4 or viral load measurement.

▷ **While Taking This Drug, Observe the Following**

Foods: No restrictions.

Beverages: No restrictions.

▷   *Alcohol:* No interactions expected.

Tobacco Smoking: No interactions expected, but I advise everyone to quit smoking.

▷   *Other Drugs*

Stavudine **taken concurrently** with
• other drugs such as metronidazole (Flagyl) that can cause peripheral neuropathy should be avoided if possible.

Stavudine may **increase** the effects of
• didanosine (Videx) at specific drug concentration ratios.
• zidovudine (AZT) at specific drug concentration ratios.

Stavudine may **decrease** the effects of
• didanosine (Videx) at specific drug concentration ratios.
• zidovudine (AZT) at specific drug concentration ratios.

▷   *Driving, Hazardous Activities:* This drug may cause dizziness. Restrict activities as necessary.

Aviation Note: The use of this drug **may be a disqualification** for piloting. Consult a designated Aviation Medical Examiner.

Exposure to Sun: No restrictions.

Discontinuation: Do not stop this drug without your doctor's knowledge and guidance.

STRONTIUM-89 (STRON tee um)

Introduced: 1993   **Class:** Systemic radionuclide, pain syndrome modifier
Prescription: USA: Yes   **Controlled Drug:** USA: No; Canada: No   **Available as Generic:** USA: No; Canada: No

Brand Name: Metastron

BENEFITS versus RISKS	
Possible Benefits	*Possible Risks*
EFFECTIVE RELIEF OF PRIMARY OR METASTATIC BONE CANCER PAIN	BONE MARROW TOXICITY (decreased white blood cells and platelets)
	Transient increase in bone pain

▷ **Principal Uses**

As a Single Drug Product: Uses currently included in FDA-approved labeling: Used to treat metastatic bone cancer pain.

Other (unlabeled) generally accepted uses: None at present.

How This Drug Works: This radiopharmaceutical is selectively taken up by areas of bone cancer. Once it accumulates in cancerous areas, it emits radiation directly at the site of the cancer.

Available Dosage Forms and Strengths

Injection — 10.9 to 22.6 mg of strontium in a total of 1 ml of water

▷ **Recommended Dosage Ranges** (Actual dosage and administration schedule must be determined for each patient individually.)

Infants and Children: Safety and efficacy for those less than 18 years old are not established.

18 to 60 Years of Age: A dose of 4 mCi (148 MBq) is given intravenously over 1 to 2 min. The dose may also be calculated using 40 to 60 mcCI/kg. The dose may be repeated at 90-day intervals, if needed.

Over 60 Years of Age: Same as 18 to 60 years of age.

Conditions Requiring Dosing Adjustments

Liver Function: Dosing changes in liver compromise do not appear to be needed.

Kidney Function: This agent is primarily removed by the kidneys; however, decreases in doses are not presently defined.

▷ **Dosing Instructions:** You may eat and drink as you normally would. During the first week after injection, strontium-89 will be present in the blood and the urine. A normal toilet should be used in preference to a urinal.

Usual Duration of Use: Use of previously prescribed pain medicine will be expected for 7 to 20 days after the injection. A maximum of 20 days after injection has been needed to determine peak effectiveness in controlling bone cancer pain. The dose may be repeated (if blood tests are acceptable) 90 days after the prior dose was given. Consult your physician on a regular basis.

Possible Advantages of This Drug
> Effective control of bone cancer pain without the risks or compromise of narcotics.

▷ **This Drug Should Not Be Taken If**
- you have had an allergic reaction to any dosage form of it previously.
- you have cancer that does **not** involve the bone.

▷ **Inform Your Physician Before Taking This Drug If**
- you have a history of low platelets or white blood cell counts.
- you take other drugs that may lower white cells or platelets.
- you do not understand how to appropriately dispose of your urine or vomit.

Possible Side Effects (natural, expected, and unavoidable drug actions)
> May cause a calciumlike flushing when injected. May cause transient (up to 72 hours) increase in bone pain.

▷ **Possible Adverse Effects** (unusual, unexpected, and infrequent reactions)
> **If any of the following develop, consult your physician promptly for guidance.**
> *Mild Adverse Effects*
> Allergic Reactions: Chills and fever.
> *Serious Adverse Effects*
> Allergic Reactions: None defined.
> Bone marrow toxicity: 20–30% decrease in white cell or platelet counts—may be dose related.
> Bacterial infection of blood (septicemia) following drug-induced decreases in white blood cells—possible.

▷ **Possible Effects on Sexual Function:**   None reported.

Possible Delayed Adverse Effects: Lowering of white blood cells (recovery in up to 6 months) and blood platelets (lowest count 12 to 16 weeks after therapy).

Natural Diseases or Disorders That May Be Activated by This Drug
> Aplastic anemia.

Possible Effects on Laboratory Tests
> White blood cell counts: decreased.
> Platelet counts: decreased.

CAUTION
1. Promptly report any signs of infection (lethargy, temperature, sore throat).
2. It may take up to 20 days for this agent to work. Narcotics will need to be continued.
3. Your blood and urine will contain radioactive strontium for 7 days after injection. Ask you doctor for help on appropriate disposal.
4. This drug is a potential carcinogen.
5. Promptly report any abnormal bleeding or bruising.

Precautions for Use
> *By Infants and Children:* Safety and effectiveness for those under 18 years of age are not established.
> *By Those Over 60 Years of Age:* Specific changes are not presently needed.

▷ **Advisability of Use During Pregnancy**
> *Pregnancy Category:* D. See Pregnancy Risk Categories at the back of this book.
> Animal studies: Adequate studies evaluating potential to cause birth defects have not been performed.

Human studies: Adequate studies of pregnant women are not available. This drug may cause fetal harm. Ask your doctor for advice.

Advisability of Use If Breast-Feeding
Presence of this drug in breast milk: This drug acts like calcium and is expected to be present in breast milk.
Avoid drug or refrain from nursing.

Habit-Forming Potential: None.

Effects of Overdosage: May result in acute radiation syndrome with initial nausea and vomiting followed by depressed white cells and platelets, and tendency to infections. Careful dosage calculations are indicated, as this drug emits beta-radiation.

Possible Effects of Long-Term Use: Not indicated for long-term use.

Suggested Periodic Examinations While Taking This Drug (at physician's discretion)
Complete blood counts should be tested once every other week during therapy.

▷ **While Taking This Drug, Observe the Following**
Foods: No restrictions.
Beverages: No restrictions.
▷ *Alcohol:* No interactions expected.
Tobacco Smoking: No interactions expected, but I advise everyone to quit smoking.
Marijuana Smoking: No interactions expected.
▷ *Other Drugs*
Strontium-89 *taken concurrently* with
• medications that lower white blood cells or platelets may result in severe decreases.
▷ *Driving, Hazardous Activities:* This drug may cause a transient increase in bone pain. Restrict activities as necessary.
Aviation Note: The use of this drug *may be a disqualification* for piloting. Consult a designated Aviation Medical Examiner.
Exposure to Sun: No restrictions.
Discontinuation: Dosing may be repeated if blood counts are acceptable.

SUCRALFATE (soo KRAL fayt)

Introduced: 1978 **Class:** Antiulcer, gastrointestinal drug **Prescription:** USA: Yes **Controlled Drug:** USA: No; Canada: No **Available as Generic:** Yes

Brand Names: Carafate, ✦Sulcrate

BENEFITS versus RISKS	
Possible Benefits	*Possible Risks*
EFFECTIVE TREATMENT IN DUODENAL ULCER DISEASE	Constipation
No serious adverse effects	Skin rash, hives, itching
	Aluminum toxicity in kidney compromise

▷ **Principal Uses**

As a Single Drug Product: Uses currently included in FDA-approved labeling: Treats and prevents recurrence of duodenal ulcer disease in adults and children. Effective when used alone, but may be used in with antacids for pain relief.

Other (unlabeled) generally accepted uses: (1) May be useful in treating gastric ulcers in people who cannot tolerate other treatment; (2) can reduce the frequency of diarrhea caused by radiation therapy; (3) may have a role as a douche in promoting healing of vaginal ulcerations that are resistant to other measures; (4) can ease the pain and spasms associated with tonsillectomy.

How This Drug Works: This drug promotes ulcer healing in several ways: (1) formation of a protective coating over the ulcer and ulcer margins, preventing further damage; (2) inhibition of the digestive action of pepsin; (3) the stimulation of active healing (tissue repair).

Available Dosage Forms and Strengths
    Tablets — 1 g
    Suspension — 1 g/10 ml

▷ **Usual Adult Dosage Range:**   1 g four times daily. **Note: Actual dosage and administration schedule must be determined for each patient individually.**

Conditions Requiring Dosing Adjustments
Liver Function: Sucralfate is not absorbed.
Kidney Function: Sucralfate is not absorbed.

▷ **Dosing Instructions:**   Take with water on an empty stomach at least 1 hour before or 2 hours after each meal and at bedtime. Swallow the tablets whole; do not alter or chew. Take the full course prescribed.

Usual Duration of Use: Use on a regular schedule for 6 to 8 weeks is usually needed for peak effect in promoting the healing of ulcers. Use beyond 8 weeks must be determined by your physician.

▷ **This Drug Should Not Be Taken If**
    • you have had an allergic reaction to it previously.

▷ **Inform Your Physician Before Taking This Drug If**
    • you have chronic constipation.
    • you have chronic kidney failure.
    • you are taking any other drugs at this time.

Possible Side Effects (natural, expected, and unavoidable drug actions)
    Constipation.

▷ **Possible Adverse Effects** (unusual, unexpected, and infrequent reactions)
    If any of the following develop, consult your physician promptly for guidance.
Mild Adverse Effects
    Allergic Reactions: Skin rash, hives, itching.
    Dizziness, light-headedness, drowsiness—infrequent.
    Dry mouth, indigestion, nausea, cramping, diarrhea—infrequent.
Serious Adverse Effects
    Increased risk of aluminum toxicity (seizures, jerks, and encephalopathy) with patients in end-stage kidney failure.

Bezoar (a clumping of food) formation in the esophagus or proximal stomach—possible.

▷ **Possible Effects on Sexual Function:**   None reported.

Possible Effects on Laboratory Tests
None reported.

CAUTION
1. If antacids are needed to relieve ulcer pain, do not take them within half an hour before or 2 hours after the dose of sucralfate.
2. This drug may impair the absorption of other drugs if they are taken close together. It is advisable to avoid taking any other drugs within 2 hours of taking sucralfate. This applies especially to cimetidine (Tagamet), phenytoin (Dilantin), and tetracyclines.

Precautions for Use
By Infants and Children: This drug has been used to treat reflux esophagitis or long-standing (chronic) duodenal ulcers in those 3 months to 13 years. In esophagitis, 500 mg was used four times daily in those less than 6 years old. The adult dose and interval was used for those 6 or older. Duodenal ulcer treatment used the adult regimen.

By Those Over 60 Years of Age: Specific changes not presently needed.

▷ **Advisability of Use During Pregnancy**
Pregnancy Category: B. See Pregnancy Risk Categories at the back of this book.
Animal studies: No birth defects reported in mouse, rat, and rabbit studies.
Human studies: Adequate studies of pregnant women are not available.
This drug should be used only if clearly needed. Ask your physician for guidance.

Advisability of Use If Breast-Feeding
Presence of this drug in breast milk: Unknown.
Watch nursing infant closely and stop drug or nursing if adverse effects develop.

Habit-Forming Potential: None.

Effects of Overdosage: Nausea, stomach cramping, possible diarrhea.

Possible Effects of Long-Term Use: Deficiencies of vitamins A, D, E, and K due to impaired absorption from the intestine.

Suggested Periodic Examinations While Taking This Drug (at physician's discretion)
None required.

▷ **While Taking This Drug, Observe the Following**
Foods: No restrictions. Follow diet prescribed by your physician.
Beverages: No restrictions. This drug is preferably taken with water.

▷ *Alcohol:* No interactions with drug expected. However, alcohol is best avoided because of its irritant effect on the stomach.
Tobacco Smoking: Nicotine can delay ulcer healing and reduce the effectiveness of this drug. Avoid all forms of tobacco.

▷ *Other Drugs*
Sucralfate may ***decrease*** the effects of
• cimetidine (Tagamet).
• ciprofloxacin (Cipro).
• digoxin (Lanoxin).

- enoxacin (Penetrex).
- fleroxacin (Megalone).
- ketoconazole (Nizoral).
- lomefloxacin (Maxaquin).
- norfloxacin (Noroxin).
- ofloxacin (Floxin) or temafloxacin (Omniflox).
- phenytoin (Dilantin, etc.).
- quinidine (Quinaglute).
- tetracycline (Achromycin, Tetracyn, etc.).
- warfarin (Coumadin, etc.), and reduce its anticoagulant effect. Increased frequency of INR testing (prothrombin time or protime) is needed.

▷ *Driving, Hazardous Activities:* This drug may cause dizziness or drowsiness. Restrict activities as necessary.

Aviation Note: The use of this drug *may be a disqualification* for piloting. Consult a designated Aviation Medical Examiner.

Exposure to Sun: No restrictions.

SULFAMETHOXAZOLE (sul fa meth OX a zohl)

See the new sulfonamide antibiotics profile for more information.

SULFASALAZINE (sul fa SAL a zeen)

Introduced: 1949   **Class:** Bowel anti-inflammatory, sulfonamides   **Prescription:** USA: Yes   **Controlled Drug:** USA: No; Canada: No   **Available as Generic:** USA: Yes; Canada: No

Brand Names: Azaline, Azulfidine, Azulfidine EN-Tabs, ✦PMS Sulfasalazine, ✦PMS Sulfasalazine E.C., ✦Salazopyrin, ✦Salazopyrin EN, ✦SAS-Enema, ✦SAS Enteric-500, SAS-500

BENEFITS versus RISKS	
Possible Benefits	*Possible Risks*
EFFECTIVE SUPPRESSION OF INFLAMMATORY BOWEL DISEASE	Allergic reactions: Mild to severe skin reactions
SYMPTOMATIC RELIEF OF REGIONAL ENTERITIS AND ULCERATIVE COLITIS	Blood cell disorders: Aplastic anemia, hemolytic anemia, abnormally low white cell or platelet counts
HELPFUL IN REFRACTORY RHEUMATOID ARTHRITIS	Drug-induced liver damage
	Drug-induced kidney damage
	Seizures

▷ **Principal Uses**

As a Single Drug Product: Uses currently included in FDA-approved labeling: (1) Treats inflammatory disease of the lower intestinal tract: regional enteritis (Crohn's disease) and ulcerative colitis. It is usually taken by mouth, but may also be used in retention enemas; (2) helps rheumatoid arthritis (second-line agent).

Other (unlabeled) generally accepted uses: (1) Short-term use in therapy of ankylosing spondylitis; (2) treatment of mild to moderate psoriasis.

How This Drug Works: Suppresses the formation of prostaglandins (and related compounds), tissue substances that induce inflammation, tissue destruction, and diarrhea.

Available Dosage Forms and Strengths

> Oral suspension — 250 mg/5-ml
> Tablets — 500 mg
> Tablets, enteric coated — 500 mg

▷ **Usual Adult Dosage Range:** Ulcerative colitis: Initially 1 to 2 g every 6 to 8 hours until symptoms are adequately controlled. For maintenance, 500 mg every 6 hours. The total daily dosage should not exceed 12 g. If diarrhea occurs, the dose is often decreased to the earlier dose that worked and did not cause diarrhea.

Rheumatoid arthritis (when salicylates or NSAIDs have not worked): 2 g daily is taken in equally divided doses. If the delayed-release form (Azulfidine EN-Tabs) is used, 500 mg is taken for 1 week in the evening, then 500 mg twice daily for a week, then 500 mg in the morning and 1 g in the evening for a week, and continuing with 1 g twice a day. **Note: Actual dosage and administration schedule must be determined for each patient individually.**

Conditions Requiring Dosing Adjustments

Liver Function: This drug can be a cause of liver damage, and patients should be followed closely.

Kidney Function: Empiric decreases in doses should be considered. This drug should be used with caution in kidney compromise.

▷ **Dosing Instructions:** This drug is preferably taken with 8 ounces of water on an empty stomach, 1 hour before or 2 hours after eating. However, it may be taken with or following food to reduce stomach irritation. Intervals between doses (day and night) should be no longer than 8 hours. The regular tablet may be crushed for administration; the enteric-coated tablet should be swallowed whole without alteration.

Usual Duration of Use: Use on a regular schedule for 1 to 3 weeks usually determines effectiveness in controlling the symptoms of regional enteritis or ulcerative colitis. Benefits in rheumatoid arthritis may be seen in 4 to 12 weeks. Long-term use (months to years) requires physician supervision.

▷ **This Drug Should Not Be Taken If**
  • you are allergic to *any* sulfonamide drug (see Drug Classes), or aspirin (or other salicylates).
  • you are in the final month of pregnancy.
  • it has been prescribed for an infant less than 2 years old.
  • you have a urinary or intestinal obstruction or porphyria.
  • you are breast-feeding.

▷ **Inform Your Physician Before Taking This Drug If**
  • you are allergic to any sulfonamide: acetazolamide, thiazide diuretics, or sulfonylurea antidiabetics (see Drug Classes).
  • you are allergic by nature: history of hay fever, asthma, hives, eczema.
  • you have asthma.

- you have impaired liver or kidney function.
- you have a glucose-6-phosphate dehydrogenase (G6PD) deficiency.
- you have a personal or family history of porphyria.
- you have had a drug-induced blood cell or bone marrow disorder.
- you currently take any oral anticoagulant, antidiabetic drug, or phenytoin.
- you plan to have surgery under pentothal anesthesia soon.

Possible Side Effects (natural, expected, and unavoidable drug actions)

Brownish coloration of the urine, of no significance. Skin pigmentation. Superinfections, bacterial or fungal (see Glossary).

▷ **Possible Adverse Effects** (unusual, unexpected, and infrequent reactions)

If any of the following develop, consult your physician promptly for guidance.

Mild Adverse Effects

Allergic Reactions: Skin rashes, hives, itching.

Headache—frequent; dizziness—infrequent.

Discoloration of contact lenses—possible.

Ringing in the ears—case reports.

Loss of appetite, irritation of mouth or tongue, nausea, vomiting, diarrhea—infrequent to frequent.

Taste disorders—rare.

Serious Adverse Effects

Allergic Reactions: Drug fever (see Glossary), swollen glands, painful joints, anaphylaxis (see Glossary). Allergic pneumonitis, allergic hepatitis. Severe skin reactions (Stevens-Johnson syndrome or toxic epidermal necrolysis).

Idiosyncratic Reactions: Hemolytic anemia (see Glossary).

Bone marrow depression (see Glossary): fever, sore throat, abnormal bleeding/bruising—rare to infrequent.

Pancreatitis, myopathy, or drug-induced lupus erythematosus—case reports.

Folic acid deficiency—possible.

Kidney damage—case reports.

Peripheral neuropathy (see Glossary)—case reports.

Inflammation of the tissue around the heart (pericarditis)—case reports.

▷ **Possible Effects on Sexual Function:**   Decreased production of sperm, reversible infertility—case reports.

▷ **Adverse Effects That May Mimic Natural Diseases or Disorders**

Liver reactions may suggest viral hepatitis. Lung reactions may suggest an infectious pneumonia.

Natural Diseases or Disorders That May Be Activated by This Drug

Goiter, acute intermittent porphyria.

Possible Effects on Laboratory Tests

Complete blood cell counts: decreased red cells, hemoglobin, white cells, and platelets; increased eosinophils (allergic reaction).

Liver function tests: increased enzymes (ALT/GPT, AST/GOT, alkaline phosphatase) or bilirubin.

Sperm count: decreased; abnormal sperm common; effects reversible on discontinuation of drug.

CAUTION

1. A large intake of water (up to 2 quarts daily) is necessary to ensure an adequate volume of urine.
2. Shake liquid dosage forms thoroughly before measuring each dose.

Precautions for Use

By Infants and Children: Safety and effectiveness for those under 2 years of age are not established.

By Those Over 60 Years of Age: Observe for the development of reduced urine volume, fever, sore throat, abnormal bleeding or bruising, or skin irritation with itching, particularly in the anal or genital regions.

▷ **Advisability of Use During Pregnancy**

Pregnancy Category: B; however, this drug should **not** be used near the time of the birth of the baby. See Pregnancy Risk Categories at the back of this book.

Animal studies: Cleft palate and skeletal birth defects due to sulfonamides reported in mice and rats.

Human studies: No increase in birth defects reported in 4,584 exposures to various sulfonamides during pregnancy.

Avoid use of drug during the final month of pregnancy because of possible adverse effects on the newborn infant.

Advisability of Use If Breast-Feeding

Presence of this drug in breast milk: Yes.

Avoid drug or refrain from nursing.

Habit-Forming Potential: None.

Effects of Overdosage: Headache, dizziness, nausea, vomiting, abdominal cramping, toxic fever, coma, jaundice, kidney failure.

Possible Effects of Long-Term Use: Development of goiter, with or without hypothyroidism. An orange-yellow discoloration of the skin has been reported. This is not jaundice.

Suggested Periodic Examinations While Taking This Drug (at physician's discretion)

Complete blood cell counts, weekly for the first 8 weeks.

Urine analysis weekly.

Liver and kidney function tests.

▷ **While Taking This Drug, Observe the Following**

Foods: No restrictions. Follow prescribed diet.

Beverages: No restrictions. May be taken with milk.

▷ *Alcohol:* Use caution. Sulfonamide drugs can increase the intoxicating effects of alcohol.

Tobacco Smoking: No interactions expected, but I advise everyone to quit smoking.

▷ *Other Drugs*

Sulfasalazine may *increase* the effects of
- anticoagulants (Coumadin, etc.), and increase bleeding risk. More frequent INR (prothrombin time or protime) testing is needed.
- sulfonylureas or other oral hypoglycemic agents (see Sulfonylureas and Oral Antidiabetic Drugs in Drug Classes), and increase the risk of hypoglycemia.

Sulfasalazine may *decrease* the effects of
- digoxin (Lanoxin).

Sulfasalazine *taken concurrently* with
- ampicillin and perhaps other penicillins may lower therapeutic benefits from sulfasalazine.

- calcium supplements (Calcium Gluconate) may result in decreased therapeutic benefits from sulfasalazine.
- iron salts or calcium may decrease sulfasalazine's benefits.
- some barbiturates (see Drug Classes) may result in decreased sulfasalazine therapeutic benefits.

▷ *Driving, Hazardous Activities:* This drug may cause dizziness. Restrict activities as necessary.

Aviation Note: The use of this drug **may be a disqualification** for piloting. Consult a designated Aviation Medical Examiner.

Exposure to Sun: Use caution—some sulfonamide drugs can cause photosensitivity (see Glossary).

SULFONAMIDE ANTIBIOTICS

Sulfamethoxazole (sul fa meth OX a zohl)   **Sulfisoxazole** (sul fi SOX a zohl)

Introduced: 1961, 1949, respectively   **Class:** Anti-infective, sulfonamides
Prescription: USA: Yes   **Controlled Drug:** USA: No; Canada: No   **Available as Generic:** Yes

Brand Names: Sulfamethoxazole: ✦Apo-Sulfamethoxazole, ✦Apo-Sulfatrim [CD], ✦Apo-Sulfatrim DS [CD], Azo Gantanol [CD], Bactrim [CD], Bactrim DS [CD], Bethaprim [CD], Comoxol [CD], Cotrim [CD], Gantanol, ✦Novo-Trimel [CD], ✦Novo-Trimel DS [CD], ✦Nu-Cotrimox, ✦Protrin [CD], ✦Protrin DF [CD], ✦Roubac [CD], Septra [CD], Septra DS [CD], Sulfatrim [CD], ✦Uro Gantanol [CD], Uroplus DS [CD], Uroplus SS [CD], Vagitrol; Sulfisoxazole: Azo Gantrisin [CD], Azo-Sulfisoxazole, Eryzole [CD], Gantrisin, Gulfasin, Lipo Gantrisin, ✦Novosoxazole, Pediazole [CD], SK-Soxazole, Sulfalar

BENEFITS versus RISKS	
Possible Benefits	*Possible Risks*
EFFECTIVE ANTIMICROBIAL ACTION against susceptible bacteria and protozoa	Allergic reactions: Mild to severe skin reactions, anaphylaxis, myocarditis
Effective adjunctive prevention and treatment of *Pneumocystis carinii* pneumonia (AIDS-related—sulfamethoxazole)	Blood cell disorders: Aplastic anemia, hemolytic anemia, abnormally low white cell or platelet counts
	Drug-induced liver or kidney damage

▷ **Principal Uses**

As a Single Drug Product: Uses currently included in FDA-approved labeling: (1) Used to treat a variety of bacterial and protozoan infections: chancroid, cystitis, and other infections of the urinary tract. **Sulfamethoxasole should not be used to treat group A streptococcal infections;** (2) Sulfisoxazole is used in treating ear infections and toxoplasmosis.

Other (unlabeled) generally accepted uses: (1) *Chlamydia* infections; (2) combination therapy of resistant *Mycobacterium kansasii* infections; (3) sulfisoxazole may work in long-term prevention of ear infections.

As a Combination Drug Product [CD]: These medicines are available in combination with phenazopyridine, an analgesic to ease discomfort associated with acute urethral infections. Sulfamethoxazole is also available in combination with another antibacterial drug, trimethoprim; in some countries this combination is given the generic name cotrimoxazole. This combination is quite effective in the treatment of certain types of middle ear infection, bronchitis, pneumonia, and certain infections of the intestinal tract and urinary tract. It is now used as primary prevention and treatment for *Pneumocystis carinii* pneumonia associated with AIDS.

How These Drugs Work: Prevents the growth and multiplication of susceptible bacteria or protozoa by interfering with their formation of folic acid, an essential nutrient.

Available Dosage Forms and Strengths

Sulfamethoxazole:

Oral suspension —	500 mg/5 ml
Tablets —	500 mg, 1 g

Sulfisoxazole:

Emulsion, prolonged action —	1 g/5 ml
Eyedrops —	4%
Eye ointment —	4%
Injection —	400 mg/ml
Pediatric suspension —	500 mg/5 ml
Syrup —	500 mg/5 ml
Tablets —	500 mg

▷ **Usual Adult Dosage Range:**   Sulfamethoxazole: Children over 2 months—50 to 60 mg per kg of body mass to start, then 25 to 30 mg per kg of body mass every 12 hours, up to a maximum of 75 mg per kg of body mass daily. Adults—Initially 2 g, then 1 g every 8 to 12 hours, depending upon the severity of the infection. The total daily dosage should not exceed 3 g.

Sulfisoxazole: Children over 2 months—50 mg per kg of body mass to start, then 100 mg per kg of body mass per day, divided into equal doses given two to four times daily. Adults—Initially 2 to 4 g, then 750 to 1500 mg (1.5 g) every 4 hours, or 1 to 2 g every 6 hours, depending upon the severity of the infection. The total daily dosage should not exceed 8 g. **Note: Actual dosage and administration schedule must be determined for each patient individually.**

Conditions Requiring Dosing Adjustments

Liver Function: Patients with compromised livers should be followed closely; however, specific guidelines for decreasing doses are not defined. Sulfisoxazole may cause liver damage.

Kidney Function: Doses should be decreased for patients with compromised kidneys. For patients with mild to moderate kidney failure, sulfisoxazole can be taken every 6 hours in the usual dose. In moderate to severe kidney failure, it can be taken every 12 to 24 hours in the usual dose. In severe kidney failure, it can be taken once a day. Increased elimination of this drug may be seen in patients with alkaline urine. It should be used with caution in renal compromise.

▷ **Dosing Instructions:**   The tablet may be crushed and is preferably taken on an empty stomach, 1 hour before or 2 hours after eating. However, both drugs may be taken with or following food to reduce stomach irritation. Be certain to drink liberal amounts of water while taking this medicine if you are not restricted from doing so.

Usual Duration of Use: Use on a regular schedule for 4 to 7 days usually determines effectiveness in controlling responsive infections. Treatment should be continued until the patient is free of symptoms for 48 hours. Limit treatment to no more than 14 days if possible. Preventive use of trimethoprim/sulfamethoxazole will be ongoing.

Currently a "Drug of Choice"

Sulfamethoxazole (when combined with trimethoprim) for preventing pneumonia (due to *Pneumocystis carinii*) in patients with AIDS.

▷ **These Drugs Should Not Be Taken If**
- you are allergic to **any** sulfonamide drug (see Drug Classes).
- you are in the final month of pregnancy.
- you are breast-feeding your infant.
- it has been prescribed for an infant less than 2 months old (unless congenital toxoplasmosis is being treated—sulfisoxazole).

▷ **Inform Your Physician Before Taking These Drugs If**
- you are allergic to any sulfonamide derivative: acetazolamide, thiazide diuretics, sulfonylurea antidiabetics (see Drug Classes).
- you are allergic by nature: history of hay fever, asthma, hives, eczema.
- you have impaired liver or kidney function.
- you have a personal or family history of porphyria.
- you have had a drug-induced blood cell or bone marrow disorder.
- you have a glucose-6-phosphate dehydrogenase (G6PD) deficiency in your red blood cells (ask your doctor).
- you currently take any oral anticoagulant, antidiabetic drug, or phenytoin.
- you plan to have surgery under pentothal anesthesia while taking this drug.

Possible Side Effects (natural, expected, and unavoidable drug actions)

Brownish coloration of the urine, of no significance. Superinfections, bacterial or fungal (see Glossary).

▷ **Possible Adverse Effects** (unusual, unexpected, and infrequent reactions)

If any of the following develop, consult your physician promptly for guidance.

Mild Adverse Effects

Allergic Reactions: Skin rashes, hives, itching, localized swellings, reddened eyes.

Myopia—infrequent.

Headache, dizziness, unsteadiness, ringing in the ears—possible.

Loss of appetite, irritation of mouth or tongue, nausea, vomiting, abdominal pain, diarrhea—infrequent.

Serious Adverse Effects

Allergic Reactions: Drug fever (see Glossary), swollen glands, painful joints, anaphylaxis (see Glossary). Allergic reaction in the heart muscle (myocarditis), allergic pneumonitis, allergic hepatitis. Severe skin reactions—rare.

Idiosyncratic Reactions: Hemolytic anemia (see Glossary)—possible.

Bone marrow depression (see Glossary): fatigue, weakness, fever, sore throat, abnormal bleeding or bruising—case reports.

Liver damage—rare.

Pancreatitis—case reports.

Kidney damage: bloody or cloudy urine, reduced urine volume—possible.

Psychotic reactions, hallucinations, seizures, hearing changes (loss or vestibular symptoms), peripheral neuropathy (see Glossary)—case reports.

Severe hypoglycemia—case report (sulfamethoxazole).

Methemoglobinemia—rare.

Drug-induced lupus erythematosus or blood clotting problems (hypoprothrombinemia)—rare.

Drug-induced disulfiramlike reaction (sulfisoxazole)—possible.

▷ **Possible Effects on Sexual Function:** None reported.

▷ **Adverse Effects That May Mimic Natural Diseases or Disorders**

Liver reactions may suggest viral hepatitis. Lung reactions may suggest an infectious pneumonia.

Natural Diseases or Disorders That May Be Activated by These Drugs

Goiter, acute intermittent porphyria, polyarteritis nodosa, systemic lupus erythematosus (questionable).

Possible Effects on Laboratory Tests

Complete blood cell counts: decreased red cells, hemoglobin, white cells, and platelets; increased eosinophils (allergic reaction).

INR (prothrombin time): increased (when taken concurrently with warfarin).

Liver function tests: increased enzymes (ALT/GPT, AST/GOT, alkaline phosphatase), or bilirubin.

CAUTION

1. A large intake of water (up to 2 quarts daily) is necessary to ensure an adequate volume of urine.
2. Shake liquid dosage forms thoroughly before measuring each dose.

Precautions for Use

By Infants and Children: These drugs should not be used in infants under 2 months of age.

By Those Over 60 Years of Age: Small doses taken at longer intervals often achieve adequate blood and tissue drug levels. Observe for the development of reduced urine volume, fever, sore throat, abnormal bleeding or bruising, or skin irritation with itching, particularly in the anal or genital regions.

▷ **Advisability of Use During Pregnancy**

Pregnancy Category: C; however, these drugs **SHOULD NOT BE TAKEN** (is contraindicated) near the time of the birth of the baby. See Pregnancy Risk Categories at the back of this book.

Animal studies: Cleft palate and skeletal birth defects reported in mice and rats.

Human studies: No increase in birth defects reported in 4,584 exposures to various sulfonamides during pregnancy.

Avoid use of drug during the final 3 months of pregnancy because of possible adverse effects on the newborn infant.

Advisability of Use If Breast-Feeding

Presence of this drug in breast milk: Yes.

Avoid drug or refrain from nursing.

Habit-Forming Potential: None.

Effects of Overdosage: Headache, dizziness, nausea, vomiting, abdominal cramping, toxic fever, coma, jaundice, kidney failure.

Possible Effects of Long-Term Use: Superinfections, bacterial or fungal. Development of goiter, with or without hypothyroidism. Excessive loss of vitamin C via urine.

Suggested Periodic Examinations While Taking This Drug (at physician's discretion)

Complete blood cell counts, weekly for the first 8 weeks.

Urine analysis weekly.

Liver and kidney function tests.

▷ **While Taking This Drug, Observe the Following**

Foods: No restrictions.

Beverages: No restrictions. May be taken with milk. Note recommendations for increased fluid intake.

▷ *Alcohol:* Use caution. Sulfonamide drugs can increase the intoxicating effects of alcohol.

Tobacco Smoking: No interactions expected, but I advise everyone to quit smoking.

▷ *Other Drugs*

These medicines may ***increase*** the effects of

- amantadine (Symmetrel) and cause abnormal heart rhythms and CNS stimulation (confusion, disorientation).
- anticoagulants (Coumadin, etc.), and increase the risk of bleeding. More frequent INR testing (prothrombin time or protime) is needed. Ongoing warfarin doses should be decided based on laboratory results.
- methotrexate (Mexate) and cause severe blood toxicity.
- sulfonylureas (see Drug Classes) or other oral hypoglycemic agents, and increase the risk of excessively low blood sugar (hypoglycemia).
- warfarin (Coumadin) and result in bleeding. More frequent INR testing is needed.
- zidovudine (AZT) and result in zidovudine toxicity.

These medicines may ***decrease*** the effects of

- birth control pills (oral contraceptives).
- cyclosporine (Sandimmune), and reduce its immunosuppressive effect.
- penicillins (see Drug Classes).

▷ *Driving, Hazardous Activities:* This drug may cause dizziness. Restrict activities as necessary.

Aviation Note: The use of this drug ***may be a disqualification*** for piloting. Consult a designated Aviation Medical Examiner.

Exposure to Sun: Use caution. Some sulfonamide drugs can cause photosensitivity (see Glossary).

SULINDAC (sul IN dak)

See the acetic acids (nonsteroidal anti-inflammatory drugs) profile for further information.

SUMATRIPTAN (soo ma TRIP tan)

Introduced: 1993   **Class:** Anti-migraine drug, serotonin-1-receptor agonist
Prescription: USA: Yes   **Controlled Drug:** USA: No; Canada: No   **Available as Generic:** USA: No; Canada: No
Brand Name: Imitrex

```
┌─────────────────────────────────────────────────────────────┐
│                    BENEFITS versus RISKS                     │
│        Possible Benefits              Possible Risks         │
│  RAPID AND EFFECTIVE RELIEF OR  Fainting                     │
│    PREVENTION OF MIGRAINE       Myocardial infarction (probably │
│  GENERALLY WELL TOLERATED         secondary to coronary vasospasm) │
│  NEWLY AVAILABLE IN A NASAL     Serious atrial and ventricular │
│    SPRAY FORM                     arrhythmias                │
│  Relieves photophobia (light                                 │
│    sensitivity)                                              │
│  Relieves phonophobia (sound                                 │
│    sensitivity)                                              │
│  Relieves nausea and vomiting                                │
└─────────────────────────────────────────────────────────────┘
```

▷ **Principal Uses**

As a Single Drug Product: Uses currently included in FDA-approved labeling: Acute treatment of migraine with or without aura in adults.

Other (unlabeled) generally accepted uses: (1) Treatment of cluster headache; (2) may have a role in treating posttraumatic headaches.

How This Drug Works: Sumatriptan acts on blood vessels to cause vasoconstriction (shrinking of the blood vessels). This relieves swelling, thought to be the cause of migraine. The drug binds to receptor arteries such as the basilar artery and in vasculature (blood vessels) associated with the dura mater (part of the lining of the brain).

Available Dosage Forms and Strengths

Nasal spray (newly approved)—20 mg per spray (final dosage form is pending)

Sumatriptan succinate (Imitrex) injection

SELFdose system kit, which has two syringes with 6 mg in 0.5 ml of liquid in a 1-ml size syringe, a dosing device, and instructions.

Unit-of-use syringes with 6 mg in 0.5 ml of liquid in a 1-ml syringe in a carton of two syringes.

6 mg single-dose vials with 0.5 ml of liquid in a 2-ml vial. These vials are packaged in cartons of five vials.

All of the liquid in these products should be a colorless to pale yellow clear solution. Particles or precipitates should never be present.

Tablets — 25 mg, 50 mg

How To Store

Keep out of reach of children. Store at room temperature in a room where the temperature will not exceed 86 degrees F (30 degress C). Keep away from heat and light.

▷ **Recommended Dosage Ranges** (Actual dosage and administration schedule must be determined for each patient individually.)

Infants and Children: The safety and effectiveness in pediatrics have **not** been determined.

18 to 60 Years of Age: Subcutaneous: Maximum adult dose is 6 mg. The dose should be taken as soon as possible after the symptoms of acute migraine are recognized. Controlled clinical trials have failed to demonstrate a benefit of repeated injections if the initial injection is unsuccessful. If symptoms return, a second 6-mg injection may be taken 12 hours after the first injection. If side effects occur, use the lowest dose in the approved dosage range that is effective for you.

Oral: 25 mg taken as soon as headache pain starts. If the symptoms do not improve after 2 hours, a second 25 to 100 mg may be taken. Maximum single oral dose is 100 mg, but there is presently no evidence that doses this large provide greater relief of symptoms.

Nasal: 20 mg as a one-time dose. If symptoms return, a second spray may be taken 12 hours after the first spray.

Over 65 Years of Age: Safety and effectiveness have **not** been evaluated in this age group. Since declines in renal and hepatic function and coronary artery disease are more common in those over 65, the possibility of an increase in side effects would be expected.

Conditions Requiring Dosing Adjustments

Liver Function: The effect of liver impairment on sumatriptan has not been specifically studied, and dosage or interval adjustments have not been established.

Kidney Function: Presently there are no determined requirements for dosage adjustment in renal compromise.

▷ **Dosing Instructions:**   The injection form must be given subcutaneously, **not intravenously**. Intravenous injection must be avoided because of potential to cause coronary vasospasm (constriction of the blood vessels that supply the heart). This medicine should be colorless to pale yellow and clear. Particles should never be present. There is extensive information on self-injection available from your doctor or pharmacist. The first dose is usually given in the doctor's office. The tablet form may take more than an hour to work. The tablet form may be taken with food. Follow directions for the nasal form closely.

Usual Duration of Use: The maximum dose is two 6-mg doses (injections) in 24 hours. This medication relieves existing migraines, and will not change the frequency or number of attacks. Recurring use of this medicine will be needed. If your migraines increase in frequency or severity, consult your doctor. If this medicine is not effective in helping your migraine, call your doctor.

Possible Advantages of This Drug

Effective subcutaneous treatment of acute nonbasilar, nonhemiplegic migraine. Better side-effect profile and treatment of migraine-associated nausea and vomiting, phonophobia, and photophobia than other currently available agents.

Currently a "Drug of Choice"

for nonbasilar, nonhemiplegic migraine.

▷ **This Drug Should Not Be Taken If**
- you have had an allergic reaction to any dosage form of it previously.
- you are unfamiliar with the subcutaneous route. Particular care must be taken to avoid intravenous use because this may lead to coronary vasospasm (constriction of the blood vessels that supply the heart).
- you have ischemic heart disease with symptoms such as angina pectoris or silent ischemia, or history of MI (myocardial infarction).
- you have Prinzmetal's angina (a specific kind of chest pain).

- you have uncontrolled hypertension (high blood pressure).
- you have basilar or hemiplegic migraine.
- you have taken a MAO inhibitor within the last 2 weeks.
- you have (within 24 hours) taken an ergotamine preparation.

▷ **Inform Your Physician Before Taking This Drug If**
- you are pregnant or plan to become pregnant.
- you are breast-feeding your infant.
- you have high blood pressure.
- you have chest pain, heart disease, or irregular heartbeats.
- you have had a heart attack.
- you have taken or have prescriptions for other migraine medications.
- you have allergies or trouble taking other medications, whether prescription or over the counter.
- you have liver or kidney disease.
- you are uncertain of how much to take or when to take this medicine.
- you do not understand the subcutaneous injection technique.
- you have Raynaud's phenomenon.

Possible Side Effects (natural, expected, and unavoidable drug actions)
Excessive thirst and frequent urination. Transient rises in blood pressure. Vision changes—rare.

▷ **Possible Adverse Effects** (unusual, unexpected, and infrequent reactions)
If any of the following develop, consult your physician promptly for guidance.
Mild Adverse Effects
Allergic Reactions: Red, itching skin; skin rash and tenderness.
Atypical sensations such as tingling (rare with injection, infrequent with tablet form).
Confusion and other mental changes or dizziness—rare.
Flushing—rare; tightness in the chest or jaw—infrequent.
Gastroesophageal reflux and diarrhea—case report.
Pain at the injection site; joint pain, weakness, and stiffness—rare.
Serious Adverse Effects
Allergic Reactions: Anaphylactic reactions.
Syncope (fainting), CVA, dysphasia, seizure—rare.
Serious changes in heart rate and rhythm—rare.
Raynaud's phenomenon, dyspnea (difficulty breathing)—rare.
Kidney stones (renal calculi)—rare.
Prinzmetal's angina—rare.
Heart attack (myocardial infarction)—rare.

▷ **Possible Effects on Sexual Function:** Dysmenorrhea, erection problems—case reports.

Possible Delayed Adverse Effects: None identified.

▷ **Adverse Effects That May Mimic Natural Diseases or Disorders**
Changes in heart rate and rhythm may mimic a number of cardiac conditions. Drug-induced acute renal failure (ARF) may mimic non-drug-induced ARF. Drug-induced hypertension may mimic hypertension from other causes. Urological symptoms may mimic benign prostatic hypertrophy. Sumatriptan can mimic Raynaud's phenomenon.

Natural Diseases or Disorders That May Be Activated by This Drug
Hypertension.

Possible Effects on Laboratory Tests
Liver function tests: rare increases in SGOT and SGPT.

CAUTION
1. Do not use sumatriptan if you are pregnant.
2. Call your doctor if you have any pain or tightness in the chest or throat when you use this medicine.
3. Do not use sumatriptan if you have used an ergotamine preparation within the last 24 hours.
4. This medication is **not** to be used intravenously.
5. If you are diagnosed as having ischemic heart disease after sumatriptan has been prescribed for you, do not use the medicine again.

Precautions for Use
By Infants and Children: Safety and effectiveness for those under 18 years of age are not established.
By Those Over 65 Years of Age: Not established.

▷ **Advisability of Use During Pregnancy**
Pregnancy Category: C. See Pregnancy Risk Categories at the back of this book.
Animal studies: Sumatriptan has been lethal to rabbit embryos when given in doses that were threefold higher than those produced by a 6-mg dose. Term fetuses from rabbits treated with sumatriptan exhibited an increase in cervicothoracic vascular defects and minor skeletal abnormalities.
Human studies: Adequate studies of pregnant women are not available.
Ask your physician for guidance.

Advisability of Use If Breast-Feeding
Presence of this drug in breast milk: Yes.
Use of this medication by nursing mothers is a benefit-to-risk decision to be made by a physician.

Habit-Forming Potential: Not clearly defined.

Effects of Overdosage: Patients have received doses of 8 to 12 mg without adverse effects. Healthy volunteers have taken up to 16 mg subcutaneously without serious adverse events. Coronary vasospasm has resulted from intravenous administration of normal doses. Animal data presents convulsions, tremor, flushing, decreased breathing and activity, cyanosis, ataxia, and paralysis.

Possible Effects of Long-Term Use: Not defined.

Suggested Periodic Examinations While Taking This Drug (at physician's discretion)
Liver function tests, electrocardiogram.

▷ **While Taking This Drug, Observe the Following**
Foods: No restrictions; however, some foods or additives such as monosodium glutamate or chocolate may be a risk factor for migraines. Skipping meals can also be a risk factor for migraines.
Beverages: No restrictions.
▷   *Alcohol:* May cause additive sedation. Alcohol may also be a precipitating factor for migraine.

Tobacco Smoking: No interactions expected, but I advise everyone to quit smoking.

Marijuana Smoking: May cause additive dizziness, drowsiness, and lethargy; may cause additive increases in blood pressure.

▷ *Other Drugs*

Sumatriptan *taken concurrently* with

- dexfenfluramine (Redux) may cause serotonin syndrome. DO NOT combine.
- ergotamine-containing preparations (see Drug Classes) may result in additive vasospasm (prolonged constriction of the blood vessels). These medicines should not be taken within 24 hours of any sumatriptan dose.
- monoamine oxidase (MAO) inhibitors (see Drug Classes) may result in toxic levels of sumatriptan. MAO inhibitors and sumatriptan should never be combined. It is important that 14 days go by after your last dose of an MAO inhibitor before you take any form of sumatriptan.

▷ *Driving, Hazardous Activities:* This drug may cause dizziness and drowsiness. Restrict activities as necessary.

Aviation Note: The use of this drug *may be a disqualification* for piloting. Consult a designated Aviation Medical Examiner.

Exposure to Sun: No restrictions.

Exposure to Cold: Use caution until tolerance is determined. Cold may enhance sumatriptan vasoconstriction.

Heavy Exercise or Exertion: Strenuous exercise can be a risk factor for migraines in some patients.

Special Storage Instructions: Keep this medicine out of reach of children. Store at room temperature in a room where the temperature will not exceed 86 degrees F (30 degress C). Keep away from heat and light.

Observe the Following Expiration Times: There is an expiration date printed on the treatment package. Throw the medication away if it has expired. The autoinjector may be used again.

TACRINE (TA kreen)

See the new anti-Alzheimer's drugs profile for more information.

TAMOXIFEN (ta MOX i fen)

Introduced: 1973   **Class:** Antiestrogen, anticancer   **Prescription:** USA: Yes   **Controlled Drug:** USA: No; Canada: No   **Available as Generic:** No

Brand Names: ✦Alpha-Tamoxifen, ✦Apo-Tamox, Nolvadex, ✦Nolvadex-D, ✦Novo-Tamoxifen, ✦Tamofen, ✦Tamone

BENEFITS versus RISKS	
Possible Benefits	*Possible Risks*
EFFECTIVE ADJUNCTIVE TREATMENT IN ADVANCED BREAST CANCER	UTERINE CANCER Severe increase in tumor or bone pain, transient Thrombophlebitis, pulmonary embolism Abnormally high blood calcium levels Eye changes: corneal opacities, retinal injury

▷ **Principal Uses**

As a Single Drug Product: Uses currently included in FDA-approved labeling: (1) An alternative to estrogens and androgens (male sex hormones) to treat advanced breast cancer in postmenopausal women; (2) treats advanced breast cancer in men that has spread (metastasized) from a prior site; (3) used to delay the recurrence of breast cancer in women.

Other (unlabeled) generally accepted uses: (1) May have a role in treating cancer of the liver or lung; (2) used to stimulate ovulation in premenopausal women with infertility; (3) used to treat rare desmoid tumors; (4) helps prevent osteoporosis in women in whom the drug is being used to prevent the recurrence of cancer; (5) can help retroperitoneal fibrosis; (6) could have a role in treating tenderness and swelling of male breast tissue (gynecomastia) of unknown cause (idiopathic); (7) helps lipid (cholesterol) levels.

How This Drug Works: It is thought that by blocking the uptake of estradiol (estrogen), this drug removes or reduces a stimulus to breast cancer cells.

Available Dosage Forms and Strengths

Tablets — 10 mg, 15.2 mg (in Canada), 20 mg (in Canada), 30.4 mg (in Canada)

▷ **Usual Adult Dosage Range:**   Breast cancer: 10 to 20 mg two to three times a day for 2 to 5 years. **Note: Actual dosage and administration schedule must be determined for each patient individually.**

Conditions Requiring Dosing Adjustments

Liver Function: Dose decreases are not defined for patients with compromised livers.

Kidney Function: The kidney plays a minor role in the elimination of this drug; however, tamoxifen should be used with caution in renal compromise.

▷ **Dosing Instructions:**   The tablet may be crushed and taken either on an empty stomach or with food.

Usual Duration of Use: Use on a regular schedule for 4 to 10 weeks usually determines effectiveness in controlling growth and spread of advanced breast cancer. In the presence of bone involvement, treatment for several months may be required to evaluate effectiveness. Long-term use (months to years) requires physician supervision and periodic evaluation.

▷ **This Drug Should Not Be Taken If**

• you have had a serious allergic or adverse reaction to it previously.
• you have active phlebitis.

- you have a significant deficiency of white blood cells or blood platelets.
- you are pregnant.

▷ **Inform Your Physician Before Taking This Drug If**
- you have a history of thrombophlebitis or pulmonary embolism.
- you have a history of abnormally high blood calcium levels.
- you have a history of any type of blood cell or bone marrow disorder.
- you have cataracts or other visual impairment.
- you have impaired liver function.
- you plan to have surgery in the near future.

Possible Side Effects (natural, expected, and unavoidable drug actions)
Hot flashes—frequent, fluid retention, weight gain.

▷ **Possible Adverse Effects** (unusual, unexpected, and infrequent reactions)
If any of the following develop, consult your physician promptly for guidance.
Mild Adverse Effects
Allergic Reactions: Skin rash.
Visual impairment—infrequent.
Increased calcium—infrequent.
Headache, dizziness, drowsiness, depression, fatigue, confusion—infrequent.
Nausea, vomiting—frequent; itching in genital area, loss of hair—infrequent.
Serious Adverse Effects
Initial "flare" of severe pain in tumor or involved bone—possible.
Development of thrombophlebitis, risk of pulmonary embolism—increased risk.
Eye changes: corneal opacities, retinal injury—case reports.
Delusions—rare.
Increased uterine cancer risk (increased karyopyknotic index of vaginal epithelium)—questionable.
Development of abnormally high blood calcium levels—possible.
Transient decreases in white blood cells and blood platelets—frequent.
Neutropenia or decrease in all blood cells (pancytopenia)—case reports.
Liver toxicity—rare.

▷ **Possible Effects on Sexual Function**
Premenopausal: Altered timing and pattern of menstruation. Postmenopausal: Vaginal bleeding.
Decreased libido.
Abnormal and painful erections (priapism)—case reports.
This drug may be effective in treating the following conditions:
- male infertility due to abnormally low sperm counts.
- male breast enlargement and tenderness.
- chronic female breast pain (mastodynia).

Possible Effects on Laboratory Tests
Complete blood cell counts: decreased red cells, hemoglobin, white cells, and platelets.
Blood calcium level: increased.
Blood thyroid hormone levels: T_3, T_4, and free T_4 increased.
Liver function tests: increased liver enzyme (AST/GOT), increased bilirubin (one case report).
Sperm count: increased or decreased.

CAUTION

1. If this drug is used prior to your menopause, it may induce ovulation and predispose to pregnancy. Since this drug should not be used during pregnancy, some method of contraception (other than oral contraceptives) is advised.

2. Do not take any form of estrogen while taking this drug; estrogens can inhibit tamoxifen's effectiveness.

3. Tamoxifen has recently been shown to cause an increased incidence of uterine cancer. Women who have received or are receiving this drug should have regular gynecological examinations. Report menstrual irregularity, abnormal vaginal bleeding or vaginal discharge, pelvic pain or pressure promptly to your doctor.

▷ **Advisability of Use During Pregnancy**

Pregnancy Category: D. See Pregnancy Risk Categories at the back of this book.

Animal studies: No birth defects due to this drug reported.

Human studies: Adequate studies of pregnant women are not available.

This drug can have estrogenic effects. It should not be used during pregnancy.

Advisability of Use If Breast-Feeding

Presence of this drug in breast milk: Unknown.

Avoid drug or refrain from nursing.

Habit-Forming Potential: None.

Effects of Overdosage: Severe extension of the pharmacological effects.

Possible Effects of Long-Term Use: Development of abnormally high blood calcium levels.

Suggested Periodic Examinations While Taking This Drug (at physician's discretion)

Complete blood cell counts, measurements of blood calcium levels.

Complete eye examinations if impaired vision occurs.

Women who have been given or are now receiving tamoxifen **must** have regular gynecological examinations.

▷ **While Taking This Drug, Observe the Following**

Foods: No restrictions.

Beverages: No restrictions. May be taken with milk.

▷ *Alcohol:* No interactions expected.

Tobacco Smoking: No interactions expected, but I advise everyone to quit smoking.

Marijuana Smoking: Animal studies show an increased suppression of the immune system; significance in humans is not known.

▷ *Other Drugs*

The following drugs may *decrease* the effects of tamoxifen

- estrogens.
- oral contraceptives (those that contain estrogens).

Tamoxifen *taken concurrently* with

- allopurinol (Zyloprim) may worsen allopurinol toxicity to the liver.
- cyclosporine (Sandimmune) may increase cyclosporine levels and cause toxicity.
- mitomycin will cause increased risk of hemolytic uremic syndrome.

- pneumococcal and perhaps other vaccines will blunt the vaccine's immune response (benefit).
- ritonavir (Norvir) and perhaps other protease inhibitors (see Drug Classes) may lead to toxicity.
- warfarin (Coumadin) presents an increased risk of bleeding. Increased frequency of INR (prothrombin time or protime) testing is needed.

▷ *Driving, Hazardous Activities:* This drug may cause dizziness or drowsiness. Restrict activities as necessary.

Aviation Note: The use of this drug *may be a disqualification* for piloting. Consult a designated Aviation Medical Examiner.

Exposure to Sun: No restrictions.

TERAZOSIN (ter AY zoh sin)

Introduced: 1987   **Class:** Antihypertensive   **Prescription:** USA: Yes
Controlled Drug: USA: No   **Available as Generic:** No
Brand Name: Hytrin

BENEFITS versus RISKS	
Possible Benefits	*Possible Risks*
EFFECTIVE TREATMENT OF MILD TO MODERATE HYPERTENSION	"First-dose" drop in blood pressure with fainting
LOWERED LOW-DENSITY LIPOPROTEINS AND TOTAL CHOLESTEROL	Fluid retention
LOWERED TRIGLYCERIDE LEVELS	
TREATS BENIGN PROSTATIC HYPERPLASIA	

▷ **Principal Uses**

As a Single Drug Product: Uses currently included in FDA-approved labeling: (1) Used to treat mild to moderate hypertension. Also used in combination with other drugs to treat moderate to severe hypertension; (2) treats symptomatic benign prostatic hyperplasia (BPH).

Other (unlabeled) generally accepted uses: (1) Used to help correct symptoms in congestive heart failure; (2) may have a beneficial effect in lowering cholesterol levels.

How This Drug Works: Terazosin blocks some actions of the sympathetic nervous system, causing direct opening of blood vessel walls and lowering blood pressure. In BPH it relaxes the smooth muscle around the bladder neck and prostate, allowing opening of the urethra and increased urine flow.

Available Dosage Forms and Strengths

Tablets — 1 mg, 2 mg, 5 mg, 10 mg

▷ **Usual Adult Dosage Range:** Treatment is started with a test dose of 1 mg; the patient's response is observed for 2 hours (some physicians have the patient take the medicine at bedtime). If terazosin is tolerated, dose can be slowly (as needed and tolerated) increased up to 5 mg daily. Maximum daily dosage should not exceed 20 mg.

Benign prostatic hyperplasia: 1 mg is taken at bedtime. This dose is gradually increased as needed and tolerated to the desired response. Many patients need 10 mg for 4 to 6 weeks in order to get symptom relief. **Note: Actual dosage and administration schedule must be determined for each patient individually.**

Conditions Requiring Dosing Adjustments

Liver Function: Dose should be decreased for patients with severe liver problems.

Kidney Function: Dose changes are not needed for patients with severe kidney failure.

▷ **Dosing Instructions:**   The tablet may be crushed and taken without regard to food. It is best taken at bedtime to avoid orthostatic hypotension (see Glossary).

Usual Duration of Use: Use on a regular schedule for 6 to 8 weeks usually determines effectiveness in hypertension; 4 to 6 weeks of scheduled use are needed in benign prostatic hyperplasia (BPH). See your doctor regularly.

Possible Advantages of This Drug

May be used to initiate treatment.

Usually effective with once-a-day dosage.

Rarely causes depression or impotence.

Does not alter blood cholesterol, potassium, or sugar.

▷ **This Drug Should Not Be Taken If**

- you have had an allergic reaction to it previously.
- you are experiencing mental depression.
- you have angina (active coronary artery disease) and are not taking a beta-blocking drug. (See your physician.)

▷ **Inform Your Physician Before Taking This Drug If**

- you have experienced orthostatic hypotension (see Glossary).
- you have a history of mental depression.
- you have impaired circulation to the brain or a history of stroke.
- your job requires alertness or dexterity in operating heavy machinery (this medicine may cause somnolence or drowsiness).
- you have coronary artery disease.
- you have impaired liver or kidney function.
- you plan to have surgery under general anesthesia soon.

Possible Side Effects (natural, expected, and unavoidable drug actions)

Orthostatic hypotension—rare; drowsiness, salt and water retention, dry mouth, nasal congestion, constipation.

▷ **Possible Adverse Effects** (unusual, unexpected, and infrequent reactions)

If any of the following develop, consult your physician promptly for guidance.

Mild Adverse Effects

Allergic Reactions: Skin rash.

Headache, dizziness, fatigue, nervousness, sweating, numbness/tingling, blurred vision—rare to infrequent.

Weight gain—case reports.

Palpitation, rapid heart rate, shortness of breath—infrequent.

Nausea, vomiting, diarrhea—infrequent.

Serious Adverse Effects

Mental depression—rare.

▷ **Possible Effects on Sexual Function:** Impotence—rare.

Natural Diseases or Disorders That May Be Activated by This Drug

Latent coronary artery insufficiency.

Possible Effects on Laboratory Tests

Blood total cholesterol, LDL and VLDL cholesterol levels: decreased.

Blood HDL cholesterol level or blood triglyceride levels: increased or no effect.

CAUTION

1. A "first-dose" precipitous drop in blood pressure, with or without fainting, can occur (usually within 30 to 90 minutes). Limit initial doses to 1 mg taken at bedtime (for first 3 days); lie down and remain prone after taking trial doses.

2. Call your doctor if you plan to use over-the-counter remedies for allergic rhinitis or head colds. Serious drug interactions are possible.

Precautions for Use

By Infants and Children: Safety and effectiveness for those under 12 years of age are not established.

By Those Over 60 Years of Age: Therapy is started with no more than 1 mg/day for the first 3 days. Any dose increases must be very gradual and closely supervised by your physician. Orthostatic hypotension can cause falls and injury. Sit or lie down promptly if you feel light-headed or dizzy. Report dizziness or chest pain promptly.

▷ **Advisability of Use During Pregnancy**

Pregnancy Category: C. See Pregnancy Risk Categories at the back of this book.

Animal studies: No birth defects found in rat or rabbit studies.

Human studies: Adequate studies of pregnant women are not available.

Use this drug only if clearly needed. Ask your physician for guidance.

Advisability of Use If Breast-Feeding

Presence of this drug in breast milk: Unknown.

Watch infant closely and stop drug or nursing if adverse effects start.

Habit-Forming Potential: None.

Effects of Overdosage: Orthostatic hypotension, headache, flushing, fast heart rate, extreme weakness, irregular heart rhythm, circulatory collapse.

Possible Effects of Long-Term Use: None reported.

Suggested Periodic Examinations While Taking This Drug (at physician's discretion)

Measurements of blood pressure in lying, sitting, and standing positions.

Measurements of body weight to detect fluid retention.

▷ **While Taking This Drug, Observe the Following**

Foods: No restrictions. Avoid excessive salt intake.

Beverages: No restrictions. May be taken with milk.

▷ *Alcohol:* Alcohol can exaggerate the blood-pressure-lowering actions of this drug and cause excessive reduction. Use with extreme caution.

Tobacco Smoking: Nicotine can intensify this drug's ability to worsen coronary insufficiency. Avoid all forms of tobacco.

▷ *Other Drugs*

The following drugs may ***increase*** the effects of terazosin
- beta-adrenergic-blocking drugs (see Drug Classes); severity and duration of the "first-dose" response may be increased.
- verapamil (Verelan, Calan, others) and cause excessive lowering of blood pressure.

The following drugs may ***decrease*** the effects of terazosin
- estrogens (see Drug Classes).
- indomethacin (Indocin) and other NSAIDs (see Drug Classes).

▷ *Driving, Hazardous Activities:* This drug may cause dizziness or drowsiness. Restrict activities as necessary.

Aviation Note: The use of this drug ***is a disqualification*** for piloting. Consult a designated Aviation Medical Examiner.

Exposure to Sun: No restrictions.

Exposure to Cold: Cold environments may increase this drug's ability to cause coronary insufficiency (angina) and hypothermia (see Glossary). Use caution.

Heavy Exercise or Exertion: Excessive exertion can increase likelihood of chest pain. See Hypothermia in Section Two.

Discontinuation: Do not stop this medicine abruptly if it is being used to treat congestive heart failure. Ask your physician for guidance.

TERBUTALINE (ter BYU ta leen)

Introduced: 1974   **Class:** Antiasthmatic, bronchodilator   **Prescription:** USA: Yes   **Controlled Drug:** USA: No; Canada: No   **Available as Generic:** No

Brand Names: Brethaire, Brethine, Bricanyl, ✦Bricanyl Spacer

BENEFITS versus RISKS	
Possible Benefits	*Possible Risks*
VERY EFFECTIVE RELIEF OF BRONCHOSPASM	Increased blood pressure
	Fine hand tremor
	Irregular heart rhythm (with excessive use)

▷ **Principal Uses**

As a Single Drug Product: Uses currently included in FDA-approved labeling: (1) Relieves acute bronchial asthma and reduces frequency and severity of chronic, recurrent asthmatic attacks; (2) also used to relieve reversible bronchospasm associated with chronic bronchitis and emphysema.

Other (unlabeled) generally accepted uses: (1) May have a role in helping ease fetal distress in some patients; (2) used to help stop premature labor; (3) an alternative to intravenous isoproterenol in therapy of status asthmaticus; (4) has a role in easing sustained and painful erections (priapism); (5) used in combination therapy in patients who have wheals/itching of unknown cause (idiopathic urticaria).

How This Drug Works: By stimulating certain sympathetic nerve terminals, this drug acts to dilate those bronchial tubes that are in sustained constriction, thereby increasing the size of the airway and improving the ability to breathe.

Available Dosage Forms and Strengths

Aerosol—0.2 mg per actuation, 0.25 mg per actuation (Canada)

Injection—1 mg/ml

Tablets—2.5 mg, 5 mg

▷ **Usual Adult Dosage Range:** Aerosol: 0.4 mg taken in two separate inhalations 1 minute apart; repeat every 4 to 6 hours as needed.

Tablets: 2.5 to 5 mg taken every 6 hours. The total daily dosage **should not exceed 15 mg. Note: Actual dosage and administration schedule must be determined for each patient individually.**

Conditions Requiring Dosing Adjustments

Liver Function: This drug is extensively metabolized in the liver; however, guidelines for dosing changes for patients with compromised livers are not available.

Kidney Function: For patients with moderate to severe kidney failure, 50% of the usual dose can be taken at the usual time. In severe failure, the drug should not be used.

▷ **Dosing Instructions:** Tablets may be crushed and taken on an empty stomach or with food or milk. For aerosol, follow the written instructions carefully. Do not overuse.

Usual Duration of Use: Individualized. Do not use beyond the time necessary to terminate episodes of asthma.

Possible Advantages of This Drug

Rapid onset of action.

Long duration of action.

Highly effective relief of asthma.

▷ **This Drug Should Not Be Taken If**

• you have had an allergic reaction to any dosage form of it previously.

• you currently have an irregular heart rhythm.

• you are taking, or have taken within the past 2 weeks, any monoamine oxidase (MAO) type A inhibitor drug (see Drug Classes).

▷ **Inform Your Physician Before Taking This Drug If**

• you are overly sensitive to other drugs that stimulate the sympathetic nervous system.

• you are currently using epinephrine (Adrenalin, Primatene Mist, etc.) to relieve asthmatic breathing.

• you have a seizure disorder.

• you have liver or kidney failure.

• you have any type of heart or circulatory disorder, especially high blood pressure or coronary heart disease.

• you have diabetes or an overactive thyroid gland (hyperthyroidism).

• you are taking any form of digitalis or any stimulant drug.

Possible Side Effects (natural, expected, and unavoidable drug actions)

Aerosol: dryness or irritation of mouth or throat, altered taste. Tablet: nervousness, tremor, palpitation.

▷ **Possible Adverse Effects** (unusual, unexpected, and infrequent reactions)
If any of the following develop, consult your physician promptly for guidance.

Mild Adverse Effects

Headache, dizziness, drowsiness, restlessness, insomnia—infrequent.

Rapid, pounding heartbeat; increased sweating; muscle cramps in arms and legs—infrequent to frequent.

Nausea, heartburn, vomiting—rare with oral form, frequent with IV.

Increased blood sugar—frequent (40% abnormal one-hour glucose).

Serious Adverse Effects

Rapid or irregular heart rhythm, intensification of angina, increased blood pressure—infrequent.

Lowered blood calcium or potassium (especially with intravenous use)—possible.

Liver toxicity—case reports.

Severe lowering of blood pressure (hypotension)—case reports.

Increased blood sugar—infrequent.

▷ **Possible Effects on Sexual Function:**   None reported.

Natural Diseases or Disorders That May Be Activated by This Drug

Latent coronary artery disease, diabetes, or high blood pressure.

Possible Effects on Laboratory Tests

Blood total cholesterol and LDL cholesterol levels: no effect.

Blood HDL cholesterol level: increased.

Blood triglyceride levels: no effect.

Blood thyroid hormone levels: T_3 increased; T_4 decreased; free T_4 no effect.

Glucose tolerance test: abnormal test.

Liver function tests: may be elevated.

CAUTION

1. Combination of this drug by aerosol with beclomethasone aerosol (Beclovent, Vanceril) may increase the risk of toxicity due to fluorocarbon propellants. It is best to use this aerosol 20 to 30 minutes **before** beclomethasone aerosol. This reduces toxicity risk and will help beclomethasone get into the lungs.

2. **Avoid excessive use of aerosol inhalation.** Excessive or prolonged use by inhalation can reduce its effectiveness and cause serious heart rhythm disturbances, including cardiac arrest.

3. Do not use this drug concurrently with epinephrine. These two drugs may be used alternately if an interval of 4 hours is allowed between doses.

4. If you do not respond to your usually effective dose, ask your physician for guidance. Do not increase the size or frequency of the dose without your physician's approval.

Precautions for Use

By Infants and Children: Safety and effectiveness for those under 12 years of age are not established.

By Those Over 60 Years of Age: Avoid excessive and continual use. If acute asthma is not relieved promptly, other drugs will be needed. Watch for nervousness, palpitations, irregular heart rhythm, and muscle tremors. Use with extreme caution if you have hardening of the arteries, heart disease, or high blood pressure.

▷ **Advisability of Use During Pregnancy**
  Pregnancy Category: B. See Pregnancy Risk Categories at the back of this book.
    Animal studies: No significant birth defects reported in mouse and rat studies.
    Human studies: Adequate studies of pregnant women are not available.
    Use only if clearly needed. Ask your physician for guidance.

Advisability of Use If Breast-Feeding
  Presence of this drug in breast milk: Yes.
  Monitor nursing infant closely and discontinue drug or nursing if adverse effects develop.

Habit-Forming Potential: None.

Effects of Overdosage: Nervousness, palpitation, rapid heart rate, sweating, headache, tremor, vomiting, chest pain.

Possible Effects of Long-Term Use: Loss of effectiveness. See "CAUTION" above.

Suggested Periodic Examinations While Taking This Drug (at physician's discretion)
  Blood pressure measurements, evaluation of heart status.

▷ **While Taking This Drug, Observe the Following**
  Foods: No restrictions.
  Beverages: Avoid excessive use of caffeine-containing beverages: coffee, tea, cola, chocolate.
▷ *Alcohol:* No interactions expected.
  Tobacco Smoking: No interactions expected, but I advise everyone to quit smoking.
▷ *Other Drugs*
    Terbutaline *taken concurrently* with
    • monoamine oxidase (MAO) type A inhibitor drugs may cause excessive increase in blood pressure and undesirable heart stimulation (see Drug Classes).
    • theophylline (Theo-Dur, others) may cause decreased theophylline effectiveness.
    The following drugs may *decrease* the effects of terbutaline
    • beta-blocker drugs—may impair terbutaline's effectiveness (see Drug Classes).
▷ *Driving, Hazardous Activities:* Usually no restrictions. Use caution if excessive nervousness or dizziness occurs.
  Aviation Note: The use of this drug *is a disqualification* for piloting. Consult a designated Aviation Medical Examiner.
  Exposure to Sun: No restrictions.
  Heavy Exercise or Exertion: Use caution—excessive exercise can induce asthma in some patients.

TERFENADINE (ter FEN a deen)

See the new minimally sedating antihistamines profile for further information.

TETRACYCLINE (te trah SI kleen)

Introduced: 1953   **Class:** Antibiotic, tetracyclines   **Prescription:** USA: Yes   **Controlled Drug:** USA: No; Canada: No   **Available as Generic:** Yes

Brand Names: Achromycin, Achromycin V, ✦Acrocidin, ✦Apo-Tetra, Actisite, Aureomycin, Contimycin, Cyclinex, Cyclopar, Lemtrex, ✦Medicycline, Mysteclin-F [CD], ✦Neo-Tetrine, ✦Nor-Tet, ✦Novo-Tetra, ✦Nu-Tetra, Panmycin, Retet, Robitet, SK-Tetracycline, Sumycin, Teline, Tetra-C, Tetracap, Tetra-Con, Tetracyn, Tetralan, Tetram, Tropicycline

---

BENEFITS versus RISKS

Possible Benefits	*Possible Risks*
EFFECTIVE TREATMENT OF INFECTIONS due to susceptible bacteria and protozoa	ALLERGIC REACTIONS, mild to severe: ANAPHYLAXIS, DRUG-INDUCED HEPATITIS Drug-induced colitis Superinfections (bacterial or fungal) Blood cell disorders: hemolytic anemia, abnormally low white cell and platelet counts

---

▷ **Principal Uses**

As a Single Drug Product: Uses currently included in FDA-approved labeling: (1) Treats a broad range of infections caused by susceptible bacteria and protozoa (short-term use); (2) treats severe, resistant pustular acne (long-term use); (3) used in a sustained-release form (Actisite) to treat gum disease (periodontitis) in adults.

Other (unlabeled) generally accepted uses: (1) Combination antibiotic treatment of duodenal ulcers caused by *Helicobacter pylori*; (2) used in vaginal and vulval cysts (Gartner's) and in vaginal hydrocele; (3) topical tetracycline is useful in chronic eye problems (blepharitis); (4) treats cancer (malignant) fluid (pericardial effusion) buildup around the heart; (5) used to treat stage one Lyme disease; (6) has a role in acne rosacea in decreasing the number of papules or nodules.

As a Combination Drug Product [CD]: This drug is available in combination with amphotericin B, an antifungal antibiotic that is provided to reduce the risk of developing an overgrowth of yeast organisms (superinfection) of the gastrointestinal tract.

How This Drug Works: This drug prevents the growth and multiplication of susceptible bacteria by interfering with their formation of essential proteins.

Available Dosage Forms and Strengths

Capsules — 100 mg, 250 mg, 500 mg
Ointment — 3%
Ointment, ophthalmic — 10 mg/g
Periodontal fiber — 12.7 mg per fiber
Solution, topical — 2.2 mg/ml
Suspension, ophthalmic — 10 mg/ml
Suspension, oral — 125 mg/5 ml
Tablets — 250 mg, 500 mg

▷ **Usual Adult Dosage Range:**   250 to 500 mg every 6 hours, or 500 to 1000 mg every 12 hours. The total daily dosage should not exceed 4000 mg (4 g). **Note: Actual dosage and administration schedule must be determined for each patient individually.**

Conditions Requiring Dosing Adjustments

Liver Function: Tetracycline is a cause of hepatoxicity. A benefit-to-risk decision should be made for patients with compromised livers to use this drug. The maximum daily dose in liver disease is 1 g a day.

Kidney Function: Patients with mild to moderate kidney failure can take the usual dose every 8 to 12 hours. Patients with moderate to severe kidney failure can take the usual dose every 12 to 24 hours. In severe kidney failure (creatinine clearance less than 10 ml/min), tetracycline should be avoided.

▷ **Dosing Instructions:**   The tablet may be crushed and the capsule opened and preferably taken on an empty stomach, 1 hour before or 2 hours after eating. However, to reduce stomach irritation it may be taken with crackers that contain insignificant amounts of iron, calcium, magnesium, or zinc. Avoid all dairy products for 2 hours before and after taking this drug. Take at the same time each day, with a full glass of water. Take the full course prescribed.

Usual Duration of Use: The time required to control the acute infection and be free of fever and symptoms for 48 hours. This varies with the nature of the infection. Long-term use (months to years, as for treatment of acne) requires supervision and periodic evaluation. Treatment of stage one Lyme disease requires 3 to 4 weeks in adults.

▷ **This Drug Should Not Be Taken If**
- you are allergic to any tetracycline (see Drug Classes).
- you are pregnant or breast-feeding.
- you have severe liver compromise.

▷ **Inform Your Physician Before Taking This Drug If**
- it is prescribed for a child under 8 years of age.
- you have a history of liver or kidney disease.
- you have systemic lupus erythematosus.
- you are taking any penicillin drug.
- you are taking any anticoagulant drug.
- you plan to have surgery under general anesthesia in the near future.

Possible Side Effects (natural, expected, and unavoidable drug actions)

Superinfections (see Glossary), often due to yeast organisms. These can occur in the mouth, intestinal tract, rectum, and/or vagina, resulting in rectal and vaginal itching. Tooth discoloration (when used in children less than 8 years old). Metallic taste.

▷ **Possible Adverse Effects** (unusual, unexpected, and infrequent reactions)
If any of the following develop, consult your physician promptly for guidance.

Mild Adverse Effects

Allergic Reactions: Skin rash, hives, itching of hands and feet, swelling of face or extremities.

Loss of appetite, stomach irritation, taste disorders, nausea, vomiting, diarrhea—infrequent.

Warts—very rare and of questionable causality.

Irritation of mouth or tongue, "black tongue," sore throat, abdominal cramping or pain—infrequent.

Serious Adverse Effects

Allergic Reactions: Anaphylactic reaction (see Glossary), asthma, fever, swollen joints and lymph glands.

Serious skin problems (Stevens-Johnson syndrome, Jarisch-Herxheimer reaction)—case reports.

Drug-induced hepatitis with jaundice—case reports.

Permanent discoloration and/or malformation of teeth when taken by children under 8 years of age, including unborn child and infant.

Drug-induced colitis, myasthenia gravis, or pancreatitis—case reports.

Worsening of existing systemic lupus erythematosus—case reports.

Rare blood cell disorders: hemolytic anemia (see Glossary); abnormally low white blood cell count, causing fever and infections; abnormally low blood platelet count—case reports.

Impairment of blood clotting—case reports.

Increased intracranial pressure (pseudotumor cerebri) or kidney problems—rare.

Drug-induced porphyria, esophageal ulcers, or low blood potassium—case reports.

▷ **Possible Effects on Sexual Function:** Decreased effectiveness of oral contraceptives taken concurrently (several case reports of pregnancy).
Decreased male fertility—case reports.

▷ **Adverse Effects That May Mimic Natural Diseases or Disorders**
Drug-induced hepatitis may suggest viral hepatitis.

Natural Diseases or Disorders That May Be Activated by This Drug
Systemic lupus erythematosus.

Possible Effects on Laboratory Tests
Complete blood cell counts: decreased red cells, hemoglobin, white cells, and platelets; increased eosinophils (allergic reaction).

Blood lupus erythematosus (LE) cells: positive.

Blood amylase level: increased (toxic effect in pregnant women).

Liver function tests: increased enzymes (ALT/GPT, AST/GOT, alkaline phosphatase) or bilirubin.

Kidney function tests: increased blood creatinine and urea nitrogen (BUN) levels (kidney damage).

Urine sugar tests: false-positive results with Benedict's solution and Clinitest.

CAUTION

1. Antacids, dairy products, and preparations containing aluminum, bismuth, calcium, iron, magnesium, or zinc can prevent adequate absorption of this drug and reduce its effectiveness significantly.
2. Troublesome and persistent diarrhea can develop. If diarrhea persists for more than 24 hours, stop this drug and call your doctor.
3. If general anesthesia is required while taking this drug, the choice of anesthetic agent must be selected carefully to prevent kidney damage.

Precautions for Use

By Infants and Children: If possible, tetracyclines should not be given to children under 8 years of age because of the risk of permanent discoloration and deformity of the teeth. Rarely, infants may develop increased intracranial pressure within the first 4 days of receiving this drug. Tetracyclines may inhibit normal bone growth and development.

By Those Over 60 Years of Age: Dosage must be carefully individualized based on kidney function. Natural skin changes may predispose to severe and prolonged itching reactions in the genital and anal regions.

▷ **Advisability of Use During Pregnancy**

Pregnancy Category: D. See Pregnancy Risk Categories at the back of this book. Animal studies: Tetracycline causes limb defects in rats, rabbits, and chickens.

Human studies: Information from studies of pregnant women indicates that this drug can cause impaired development and discoloration of teeth and other developmental defects.

It is advisable to avoid this drug completely during entire pregnancy.

Advisability of Use If Breast-Feeding

Presence of this drug in breast milk: Yes.

Avoid drug or refrain from nursing.

Habit-Forming Potential: None.

Effects of Overdosage: Stomach burning, nausea, vomiting, diarrhea.

Possible Effects of Long-Term Use: Superinfections; rarely impairment of bone marrow, liver, or kidney function.

Suggested Periodic Examinations While Taking This Drug (at physician's discretion)

Complete blood cell counts, liver and kidney function tests.

During extended use, sputum and stool examinations may detect early superinfection due to yeast organisms.

▷ **While Taking This Drug, Observe the Following**

Foods: Avoid cheeses, yogurt, ice cream, iron-fortified cereals and supplements, and meats for 2 hours before and after taking this drug. Calcium and iron can combine with this drug and reduce its absorption significantly.

Beverages: Avoid all forms of milk for 2 hours before and after taking this drug.

▷ *Alcohol:* Reduces doxycycline blood levels. Alcohol should be avoided with doxycycline, and perhaps another tetracycline substituted, particularly for those who have drinking problems. Alcohol is also best avoided if you have active liver disease.

Tobacco Smoking: No interactions expected, but I advise everyone to quit smoking.

▷ *Other Drugs*

Tetracyclines may ***increase*** the effects of

- digoxin (Lanoxin), and cause digitalis toxicity.
- lithium (Eskalith, Lithane, etc.), and increase the risk of lithium toxicity.
- oral anticoagulants such as warfarin (Coumadin), and make it necessary to reduce their dosage. Increased INR (prothrombin time or protime) testing is needed.

Tetracyclines may *decrease* the effects of
- birth control pills (oral contraceptives), and impair their effectiveness in preventing pregnancy.
- penicillins (see Drug Classes) and impair their effectiveness in treating infections.

Tetracyclines *taken concurrently* with
- furosemide (Lasix) will tend to increase blood urea nitrogen (BUN).
- isotretinoin (Accutane) may worsen tetracycline-caused increased intracranial pressure and cause additive toxicity.
- methoxyflurane anesthesia may impair kidney function.
- theophylline (Theo-Dur) may result in variable changes in drug levels. More frequent theophylline blood levels are needed if these medicines are to be combined.
- warfarin (Coumadin) poses an increased risk of bleeding. INR (prothrombin time or protime) testing should be checked more frequently, and doses adjusted if needed.

The following drugs may *decrease* the effects of tetracyclines
- antacids (aluminum or magnesium preparations, sodium bicarbonate, etc.)—may reduce drug absorption.
- bismuth subsalicylate (Pepto-Bismol, others).
- calcium supplements (various brands).
- cholestyramine (Questran) and other cholesterol-lowering resins.
- colestipol (Colestid).
- iron, zinc, magnesium, and mineral preparations—may reduce drug absorption.
- sucralfate (Carafate).

▷ *Driving, Hazardous Activities:* Usually no restrictions. However, this drug may cause nausea or diarrhea. Restrict activities as necessary.

Aviation Note: The use of this drug *may be a disqualification* for piloting. Consult a designated Aviation Medical Examiner.

Exposure to Sun: Use caution—some tetracyclines can cause photosensitivity (see Glossary).

THEOPHYLLINE (thee OFF i lin)

Introduced: 1900   **Class:** Antiasthmatic, bronchodilator, xanthines
Prescription: USA: Yes   **Controlled Drug:** USA: No; Canada: No   **Available as Generic:** Yes

Brand Names: Accurbron, ✦Acet-Am, A.E.A., Aerolate, Aminodrox-Forte, ✦Apo-Oxtriphylline, ✦Aquaphyllim, ✦Asbron [CD], Asmalix, Azpan, Brocomar, Bronchial Gelatin Capsule, Broncomar, Bronkotabs, Bronkaid Tablets [CD], Bronkodyl, Bronkolixir [CD], Bronkotabs [CD], Constant-T, Duraphyl, Elixicon, Elixomin, Elixophyllin, For-Az-Ma [CD], Isuprel Compound [CD], Labid, Lanophyllin, Lixolin, Lodrane, Lodrane CR, Marax [CD], Marax DF [CD], Mudrane GG Elixir [CD], Phedral [CD], Phyllocontin, Physpan, ✦PMS Theophylline, Primatene, ✦Pulmophylline, Quadrinal [CD], Quibron [CD], Quibron-300 [CD], Quibron Plus [CD], Quibron-T Dividose, Quibron-T/SR, Respbid, Slo-bid, Slo-bid Gyrocaps, Slo-Phyllin, Slo-Phyllin GG [CD], Slo-Phyllin Gyrocaps, Somophyllin, Sompphyllin-12,

Sustaire, Tedral [CD], Tedral SA [CD], T.E.H. [CD], T.E.P., Thalfed, Theobid Duracaps, ♣Theo-Bronc, Theochron, Theoclear, Theoclear L.A., Theocord, Theo-Dur, Theo-Dur Sprinkle, Theolair, Theolair-SR, Theolate [CD], Theolixir, Theomar [CD], Theomax DF, Theon, Theophyl-SR, Theo-24, Theospan-SR, Theo-SR, Theo-Time, Theovent, Theox, Theozine, Therex [CD], Uni-Dur, ♣Uniphyl, Vitaphen [CD]

BENEFITS versus RISKS

Possible Benefits	*Possible Risks*
EFFECTIVE PREVENTION AND RELIEF OF ACUTE BRONCHIAL ASTHMA	NARROW TREATMENT RANGE FREQUENT STOMACH DISTRESS
MODERATELY EFFECTIVE CONTROL OF CHRONIC, RECURRENT BRONCHIAL ASTHMA	Gastrointestinal bleeding
	Central nervous system toxicity, seizures
Moderately effective symptomatic relief in chronic bronchitis and emphysema	Heart rhythm disturbances

---

▷ **Principal Uses**

As a Single Drug Product: Uses currently included in FDA-approved labeling: (1) Used to relieve shortness of breath and wheezing of acute bronchial asthma, and to prevent the recurrence of asthmatic episodes; (2) useful in relieving asthmaticlike symptoms associated with some types of chronic bronchitis, chronic obstructive pulmonary disease, and emphysema.

Other (unlabeled) generally accepted uses: (1) May have a role in combination therapy of cystic fibrosis; (2) can help decrease excessive production of red blood cells in kidney transplant patients; (3) may have a role in helping decrease the risk of sudden infant death syndrome (SIDS); (4) may have a supportive role with steroids and other agents in helping prevent rejection of transplanted kidneys; (5) can help ease essential tremor; (6) decreases risk of breathing cessation in neonatal apnea; (7) helps in treating SIDS children; (8) may have a role in treating sleep apnea.

As a Combination Drug Product [CD]: Available in combination with several other drugs that help in overall management of bronchial asthma and related conditions. Ephedrine is added to enhance the bronchodilator's effects; guaifenesin is added to provide an expectorant effect that thins mucus in the bronchial tubes; mild sedatives such as phenobarbital are added to allay the anxiety that often accompanies acute attacks of asthma.

How This Drug Works: By inhibiting the enzyme phosphodiesterase, this drug produces an increase in the tissue chemical cyclic AMP. This causes relaxation of the muscles in the bronchial tubes and blood vessels of the lung, resulting in relief of bronchospasm, expanded lung capacity, and improved lung circulation.

Available Dosage Forms and Strengths

Capsules — 100 mg, 200 mg, 250 mg, 260 mg

Capsules, prolonged action — 50 mg, 60 mg, 65 mg, 75 mg, 100 mg, 125 mg, 130 mg, 200 mg, 250 mg, 260 mg, 300 mg

$$\begin{aligned}
\text{Elixir} &— \text{27 mg/5 ml, 50 mg/5 ml} \\
\text{Oral solution} &— \text{27 mg/5 ml, 53.3 mg/5 ml} \\
\text{Oral suspension} &— \text{100 mg/5 ml} \\
\text{Syrup} &— \text{27 mg/5 ml, 50 mg/5 ml} \\
\text{Tablets} &— \text{100 mg, 125 mg, 200 mg, 250 mg, 300 mg} \\
\text{Tablets, prolonged action} &— \text{50 mg, 60 mg, 65 mg, 75 mg, 100 mg, 125} \\
&\quad\ \text{mg, 130 mg, 200 mg, 225 mg, 250 mg, 260} \\
&\quad\ \text{mg, 300 mg, 350 mg, 400 mg, 450 mg, 500} \\
&\quad\ \text{mg, 600 mg}
\end{aligned}$$

▷ **Recommended Dosage Ranges** (Actual dosage and administration schedule must be determined for each patient individually.)

Infants and Children: For acute attack of asthma (not currently taking theophylline)—loading dose of 5 mg per kg of body mass.

For acute attack while currently taking theophylline—a single dose of 2.5 mg per kg of body mass, if no indications of theophylline toxicity. Monitor blood levels of theophylline.

For maintenance during acute attack—dosage is based on age:

Up to 6 months of age—0.07 for each week of age + 1.7 = the mg per kg of body mass, given every 8 hours.

6 months to 1 year of age—0.05 for each week of age + 1.25 = the mg per kg of body mass, given every 6 hours.

1 to 9 years of age—5 mg per kg of body mass, every 6 hours.

9 to 12 years of age—4 mg per kg of body mass, every 6 hours.

12 to 16 years of age—3 mg per kg of body mass, every 6 hours.

For chronic treatment to prevent recurrence of asthma—dosage is based on age: once slow increase in dosing is accomplished, daily doses should be adjusted to reach blood levels of 10 to 15 mcg/ml.

Note: It is advisable to measure blood levels of theophylline periodically during chronic therapy.

16 to 60 Years of Age: For acute attack of asthma (not currently taking theophylline)—loading dose of 5 mg per kg of body mass.

For acute attack while currently taking theophylline—a single dose of 2.5 mg per kg of body mass, if no indications of theophylline toxicity. Monitor blood levels of theophylline.

For maintenance during acute attack—for nonsmokers: 3 mg per kg of body mass, every 8 hours; for smokers: 4 mg per kg of body mass, every 6 hours.

For chronic treatment to prevent recurrence of asthma—initially 6 to 8 mg per kg of body mass, in three or four divided doses at 6- to 8-hour intervals, up to a maximum of 400 mg daily. Increase dose as needed and tolerated by increments of 25% every 2 to 3 days. The total daily dosage should not exceed 13 mg per kg of body mass or 900 mg, whichever is less.

Prolonged-action formulations may allow twice-daily dosing with good results.

Over 60 Years of Age: Theophylline is removed some 30% more slowly than in younger patients. Decreased doses and more frequent blood levels are prudent.

Conditions Requiring Dosing Adjustments

Liver Function: The dose **must** be lowered, and blood levels obtained frequently. Doses may need to be decreased by 50% in some cases.

Kidney Function: Lower doses and more frequent blood levels are indicated.

▷ **Dosing Instructions:**   May be taken with or following food to reduce stomach irritation. The regular capsules may be opened and the regular tablets may be crushed for administration. The prolonged-action dosage forms should be swallowed whole and not altered. Shake the oral suspension well before measuring each dose. Do not refrigerate any liquid dosage forms of this drug.

Usual Duration of Use: Use on a regular schedule for 48 to 72 hours usually determines effectiveness in controlling the breathing impairment associated with bronchial asthma and chronic lung disease. Long-term use (months to years) requires supervision and periodic physician evaluation.

▷ **This Drug Should Not Be Taken If**
- you have had an allergic reaction to it, or to aminophylline, dyphylline, or oxtriphylline.
- you have active peptic ulcer disease.
- you have an uncontrolled seizure disorder.
- you have had a blood level drawn and it is in the "toxic" range.

▷ **Inform Your Physician Before Taking This Drug If**
- you have had an unfavorable reaction to any xanthine (see Drug Classes).
- you have a seizure disorder of any kind.
- you have a history of peptic ulcer disease.
- you have a history of underactive thyroid (hypothyroidism).
- you have impaired liver or kidney function.
- you take any of the drugs listed in the "Other Drugs" section below.
- you have hypertension, heart disease, or any type of heart rhythm disorder.

Possible Side Effects (natural, expected, and unavoidable drug actions)
Nervousness, insomnia, rapid heart rate, increased urine volume.

▷ **Possible Adverse Effects** (unusual, unexpected, and infrequent reactions)
If any of the following develop, consult your physician promptly for guidance.
Mild Adverse Effects
Allergic Reactions: Skin rash, hives.
Headache, dizziness, irritability, tremor, fatigue, weakness—infrequent.
Loss of appetite, nausea, vomiting (may be an early warning of toxicity), abdominal pain, diarrhea, excessive thirst—infrequent.
Flushing of face—case reports.
Serious Adverse Effects
Allergic Reactions: Severe skin rash (Stevens-Johnson syndrome)—case reports.
Idiosyncratic Reactions: Marked anxiety, confusion, behavioral disturbances.
Central nervous system toxicity: muscle twitching, seizures—dose related.
Heart rhythm abnormalities, rapid breathing, low blood pressure—variable and dose related.
Gastrointestinal bleeding—rare.
Defects in clotting (coagulation)—case reports.
Drug-induced abnormal urine production (SIADH) or porphyria—case reports.
Worsening of ulcers—possible.
Liver toxicity—case reports.

▷ **Possible Effects on Sexual Function:**   None reported.

Natural Diseases or Disorders That May Be Activated by This Drug
Latent peptic ulcer disease.

Possible Effects on Laboratory Tests
Blood uric acid level: increased.
Fecal occult blood test: positive (large doses may cause stomach bleeding).

CAUTION
1. This drug should not be taken at the same time as other antiasthmatic drugs unless your doctor prescribes the combination. Serious overdose could result.
2. Influenza vaccine may delay the elimination of this drug and cause accumulation to toxic levels.

Precautions for Use
By Infants and Children: Do not exceed recommended doses. Watch for toxicity: irritability, agitation, tremors, lethargy, fever, vomiting, rapid heart rate and breathing, seizures. Blood levels are needed during long-term use.
By Those Over 60 Years of Age: Small starting doses are indicated. You may be at increased risk for stomach irritation, nausea, vomiting, or diarrhea. When used concurrently with coffee (caffeine) or nasal decongestants, this drug may cause excessive stimulation and a hyperactivity syndrome.

▷ **Advisability of Use During Pregnancy**
Pregnancy Category: C. See Pregnancy Risk Categories at the back of this book.
Animal studies: Significant birth defects due to this drug reported in mice.
Human studies: Adequate studies of pregnant women are not available. No increase in birth defects reported in 394 exposures to this drug.
Avoid this drug during the first 3 months. Use it otherwise only if clearly needed. Ask your physician for guidance.

Advisability of Use If Breast-Feeding
Presence of this drug in breast milk: Yes.
Avoid drug or refrain from nursing.

Habit-Forming Potential: None.

Effects of Overdosage: Nausea, vomiting, restlessness, irritability, confusion, delirium, seizures, high fever, weak pulse, coma.

Possible Effects of Long-Term Use: Gastrointestinal irritation.

Suggested Periodic Examinations While Taking This Drug (at physician's discretion)
Periodic testing of blood theophylline levels (see "Therapeutic Drug Monitoring," chapter 2). Time to sample blood for theophylline level: 2 hours after regular (standard) dosage forms; 5 hours after sustained-release dosage forms. Recommended therapeutic range: 10 to 20 mcg/ml.

▷ **While Taking This Drug, Observe the Following**
Foods: No restrictions.
Beverages: Avoid excessive use of caffeine-containing beverages: coffee, tea, cola, or chocolate; this combination could cause nervousness and insomnia.
▷ *Alcohol:* No interactions expected. May have additive effect on stomach irritation.
Tobacco Smoking: May hasten the elimination of this drug and reduce its effectiveness. I advise everyone to quit smoking.

Marijuana Smoking: May hasten the elimination of this drug and reduce its effectiveness. Higher doses may be necessary to maintain a therapeutic blood level.

▷   *Other Drugs*

Theophylline may ***decrease*** the effects of
- lithium (Lithane, Lithobid, etc.), and reduce its effectiveness.

Theophylline ***taken concurrently*** with
- halothane (anesthesia) may cause heart rhythm abnormalities.
- phenytoin (Dilantin) may cause decreased effects of both drugs. Monitor blood levels and adjust dosages as appropriate.

The following drugs may ***increase*** the effects of theophylline
- allopurinol (Lopurin, Zyloprim).
- amiodarone (Cordarone).
- birth control pills (oral contraceptives).
- cimetidine (Tagamet).
- ciprofloxacin (Cipro).
- clarithromycin (Biaxin).
- disulfiram (Antabuse).
- doxycycline and other tetracyclines.
- enoxacin (Penetrex).
- ephedrine.
- erythromycin (E-Mycin, Erythrocin, etc.).
- famotidine (Pepcid).
- flu vaccine (influenza vaccine).
- fluvoxamine (Luvox).
- furosemide (Lasix).
- imipenem/cilastatin (Primaxin).
- interferon alfa.
- isoniazid (INH).
- methotrexate (Mexate)
- mexiletine (Mexitil).
- nicotine (Nicorette, Pro-Step, others).
- norfloxacin (Noroxin).
- pentoxifylline (Trental).
- ranitidine (Zantac).
- tacrine (Cognex).
- thiabendazole.
- ticlopidine (Ticlid).
- troleandomycin (TAO).
- verapamil (Calan, Verelan).
- viloxazine.

The following drugs may ***decrease*** the effects of theophylline
- barbiturates (phenobarbital, etc.).
- beta-blocker drugs (see Drug Classes).
- carbamazepine (Tegretol).
- isoproterenol.
- primidone (Mysoline).
- rifampin (Rifadin, Rimactane, etc.).
- ritonavir (Norvir) and perhaps other protease inhibitors (see Drug Classes).
- sulfinpyrazone (Anturane).

▷ *Driving, Hazardous Activities:* This drug may cause dizziness. Restrict activities as necessary.

Aviation Note: The use of this drug *may be a disqualification* for piloting. Consult a designated Aviation Medical Examiner.

Exposure to Sun: No restrictions.

Occurrence of Unrelated Illness: Acute viral respiratory infections may decrease drug elimination. Watch for signs of toxicity. Dosing **must** be changed if this occurs. Fever can decrease the rate of removal (clearance) of this medicine. Increased frequency of blood levels are suggested. Seizure disorders may be worsened by this medicine. This drug should be used with extreme caution by seizure patients. Theophylline should also be used with extreme caution in active peptic ulcer disease or heart arrhythmias (cardiac, not including slow or bradyarrhythmias).

Discontinuation: Avoid prolonged or unnecessary use of this drug. When your asthma resolves, withdraw this drug gradually over several days.

THIAZIDE DIURETICS

Bendroflumethiazide (ben droh meh THI a zide)   **Hydrochlorothiazide** (hi droh klor oh THI a zide)   **Hydroflumethiazide** (hi droh flu meh THI a zide) **Chlorothiazide** (klor oh THI a zide)   **Methyclothiazide** (METH i klo THI a zide) **Trichlormethiazide** (tri klor me THI a zide)   **Chlorthalidone** (KLOR thal i dohn)   **Metolazone** (me TOHL a zohn)

Introduced: 1960, 1959, 1961, 1957, 1959, 1962, 1960, 1974, respectively **Class:**   Antihypertensive, diuretic, thiazides   **Prescription:**   USA: Yes **Controlled Drug:**   USA: No; Canada: No   **Available as Generic:**   USA: Yes; Canada: Yes

Brand Names: Bendroflumethiazide: Naturetin; Hydrochlorothiazide: Aldactazide [CD], Aldoril-15/25 [CD], Aldoril D30/D50 [CD], ♣Apo-Amilzide, ♣Apo-Hydro, ♣Apo-Methazide [CD], ♣Apo-Triazide [CD], Apresazide [CD], Apresoline-Esidrix [CD], Capozide [CD], ♣Co-Betaloc [CD], Diaqua, ♣Diuchlor H, Dyazide [CD], Esidrix, Ezide, H-H-R, H.H.R., HydroDiuril, Hydromal, Hydro-Par, Hydropres [CD], Hydroserpine [CD], Hydroserpine Plus [CD], Hydro-T, Hydro-Z-50, Inderide [CD], Inderide LA [CD], ♣Ismelin-Esidrix [CD], Lopressor HCT [CD], Maxzide [CD], Maxzide-25 [CD], M Dopazide [CD], Microzide, Mictrin, ♣Moduret [CD], Moduretic [CD], ♣Natrimax, ♣Neo-Codema, Normozide [CD], ♣Novo-Doparil [CD], ♣Novo-Hydrazide, ♣Novo-Spirozine [CD], ♣Novo-Triamzide [CD], Oretic, Oreticyl [CD], ♣PMS Dopazide [CD], Prinzide [CD], Ser-Ap-Es [CD], Serpasil-Esidrix [CD], SK-Hydrochlorothiazide, Thiuretic, Timolide [CD], Trandate HCT [CD], Unipres [CD], ♣Urozide, Vaseretic [CD], ♣Viskazide [CD], Zestoretic [CD], Ziac, Zide; Chlorothiazide: Aldochlor [CD], Diachlor, Diupres [CD], Diurigen, Diuril, SK-Chlorothiazide, ♣Supres [CD]; Hydroflumethiazide: Diucardin, Saluron; Methyclothiazide: Aquatensen, ♣Duretic, Enduron; Trichlormethiazide:Diurese, Marazide II, Metahydrin, Naqua, Naquival [CD]; Chlorthalidone: ♣Apo-Chlorthalidone, Combipress [CD], Demi-Regroton [CD], Hygroton, ♣Hygroton-Resperpine [CD], Hylidone, ♣Novothalidone, Regroton [CD], Thalitone, ♣Uridon, Tenoretic; Metolazone: Diulo, Microx, Mykrox, Zaroxolyn

BENEFITS versus RISKS	
Possible Benefits	*Possible Risks*
EFFECTIVE, WELL-TOLERATED DIURETICS	Loss of body potassium and magnesium (especially with higher doses)
POSSIBLY EFFECTIVE IN MILD HYPERTENSION	
ENHANCES EFFECTIVENESS OF OTHER ANTIHYPERTENSIVES	Cardiac arrhythmias caused by decreased electrolytes (studied in chlorthalidone and hydrochlorothiazide)
Beneficial in treatment of diabetes insipidus	
	Increased blood sugar, uric acid, or calcium
	Rare blood cell disorders
	Rare liver toxicity (chlorothiazide or hydrochlorothiazide)

▷ **Principal Uses**

As a Single Drug Product: Uses currently included in FDA-approved labeling: (1) Increases the volume of urine (diuresis) to correct fluid retention (edema) seen in congestive heart failure, corticosteroid or estrogen use, and certain types of liver and kidney disease; and (2) starting therapy for high blood pressure (hypertension).

Author's Note: Recent data show that hydrochlorothiazide achieves benefits (outcomes) in decreasing left ventricular size equal to more expensive agents such as ACE inhibitors.

Other (unlabeled) generally accepted uses: (1) Prevention of kidney stones that contain calcium; (2) may help decrease the frequency of hip fractures in the elderly; (3) methyclothiazide has been used to help maintain blood calcium levels in Paget's disease; (4) may have a role in helping prevent osteoporosis (by correcting abnormally high elimination of calcium in the urine or hypercalciuria); (5) of use in diabetes insipidus (nephrogenic) in decreasing the urine volume.

As Combination Drug Products [CD]: Used to treat blood pressure that has not responded to single-drug therapy.

How These Drugs Work: By increasing the elimination of salt and water in the urine, these drugs reduce fluid volume and body sodium. They also relax the walls of smaller arteries and the combined effect of these two actions (reduced blood volume in expanded space) results in lowering of the blood pressure.

Available Dosage Forms and Strengths

Bendroflumethiazide:
        Tablets — 5 mg, 10 mg
Hydrochlorothiazide:
        Solution — 50 mg/5 ml
     Solution, intensol — 100 mg/ml
        Tablets — 12.5 mg, 25 mg, 50 mg, 100 mg
Chlorothiazide:
        Injection — 500 mg/20 ml

         Oral suspension — 250 mg/5 ml
                Tablets — 250 mg, 500 mg
Methyclothiazide:
                Tablets — 2.5 mg, 5 mg
Trichlormethiazide:
                Tablets — 2 mg, 4 mg
Chlorthalidone:
                Tablets — 25 mg, 50 mg, 100 mg
Metolazone:
                Tablets — 0.5 mg, 2.5 mg, 5 mg, 10 mg

▷ **Usual Adult Dosage Range:**   Bendroflumethiazide: As antihypertensive—12.5 to 5 mg daily, in a single dose.

Hydrochlorothiazide: As antihypertensive—12.5 to 100 mg daily initially; 12.5 to 200 mg daily for maintenance. As diuretic—variable; 12.5 to 200 mg daily. Many patients require 100–200 mg; the smallest effective dose should be determined (see "CAUTION" below). The total daily dose should not exceed 200 mg. Microzide is a new once-daily formulation (12.5 mg) of this medicine.

Author's Note: Many patients with mild to moderate high blood pressure get acceptable blood-pressure-lowering results from 12.5 mg of hydrochlorothiazide. If results are obtained with this dose, it can minimize loss of potassium and magnesium as well!

Chlorothiazide: As antihypertensive—500 to 1000 mg per day to start and 500 to 2000 mg daily as a maintenance dose. As a diuretic—500 to 2000 mg per day, using the smallest effective dose. Daily maximum is 2000 mg.

Methyclothiazide: As antihypertensive or diuretic—2.5 to 5 mg daily. Maximum daily diuretic dose is 10 mg. Pediatric dose—0.05 to 0.2 mg per kg of body mass daily.

Trichlormethiazide: As antihypertensive or diuretic—Therapy may be started with 1 to 4 mg twice daily. Usual maintenance dose is 1 to 4 mg once daily.

Chlorthalidone: As antihypertensive—25 to 50 mg daily to start therapy, then 50 to 100 mg for maintenance. As a diuretic—50 to 100 mg daily, then maintenance with the smallest effective dose (see "CAUTION" below). Daily maximum is 200 mg; however, this may change with recently published data.

Note: Actual dosage and administration schedule must be determined for each patient individually.

Conditions Requiring Dosing Adjustments

Liver Function: Electrolyte balance is critical in liver failure. These drugs may precipitate encephalopathy. Hydrochlorothiazide and chlorothiazide are also a rare cause of cholestatic jaundice and should be used with caution in liver failure.

Kidney Function: These drugs can be used with caution by patients with mild kidney failure, and are not effective for patients with moderate failure. They should not be used in severe kidney failure; they can be a rare cause of kidney damage.

▷ **Dosing Instructions:**   The tablets may be crushed and taken with or following meals to reduce stomach irritation. They are best taken in the morning to avoid nighttime urination.

Usual Duration of Use: Use on a regular schedule for 2 to 3 weeks determines effectiveness in lowering high blood pressure. Long-term use (months to years) requires periodic physician evaluation.

Possible Advantages of This Drug
> Hydrochlorothiazide was studied in more than 1,100 Veterans Administration patients with mild to moderate high blood pressure. It was found to have met blood pressure reduction goals while offering decreased left ventricular mass. These outcomes or results were accomplished using low-dose therapy, avoiding many of the undesirable changes in blood chemistry that can be seen with higher doses. This was also accomplished at a fraction of the cost of ACE inhibitors or calcium channel blockers.

▷ **These Drugs Should Not Be Taken If**
  • you have had an allergic reaction to any dosage form of it previously.
  • your kidneys are not making urine.

▷ **Inform Your Physician Before Taking These Drugs If**
  • you are allergic to any form of "sulfa" drug.
  • you are pregnant or planning pregnancy.
  • you have a history of kidney or liver disease.
  • you have a history of pancreatitis.
  • you have asthma or allergies to other medicines.
  • you have had testing of electrolytes ordered by another physician, which your doctor has not seen.
  • you develop muscle cramps, weakness, or abnormal heartbeats while taking one of these medicines.
  • you have diabetes, gout, or lupus erythematosus.
  • you are allergic to the dye tartrazine, as some of these medicines contain it.
  • you take any form of cortisone, digitalis, oral antidiabetic drug, or insulin.
  • you plan to have surgery under general anesthesia in the near future.

Possible Side Effects (natural, expected, and unavoidable drug actions)
Light-headedness on arising from sitting or lying position (see Orthostatic Hypotension in Glossary).
Increased blood sugar or uric acid level; decreased blood potassium or magnesium level. Decreased blood magnesium, combined with loss of potassium, may lead to increased risk of sudden cardiac death, especially if high doses are used for extended periods.

▷ **Possible Adverse Effects** (unusual, unexpected, and infrequent reactions)
If any of the following develop, consult your physician promptly for guidance.
Mild Adverse Effects
Allergic Reactions: Skin rashes, hives, drug fever (see Glossary).
Headache, dizziness, blurred or yellow vision—infrequent.
Reduced appetite, indigestion, nausea, vomiting, diarrhea—infrequent.
Serious Adverse Effects
Allergic Reactions: Hepatitis with jaundice (see Glossary), anaphylactic reaction (see Glossary), severe skin reactions.
Inflammation of the pancreas—case reports.
Bone marrow depression (see Glossary): fever, sore throat, abnormal bleeding/bruising—case reports.
Data from studies of hydrochlorothiazide and chlorthalidone suggest that po-

tassium and magnesium loss associated with higher-dose therapy increases the risk of sudden cardiac death.

Acute gout in some patients (because these medicines decrease uric acid removal).

Loss of blood glucose control—possible.

Short-term (less than 1 year) increase in serum lipids (returns to pretreatment levels in about 1 year).

▷ **Possible Effects on Sexual Function:**   Decreased libido (hydrochlorothiazide, chlorthalidone); impotence (bendroflumethiazide, chlorothiazide, hydrochlorothiazide)—case reports.

▷ **Adverse Effects That May Mimic Natural Diseases or Disorders**

Liver reaction may suggest viral hepatitis.

Natural Diseases or Disorders That May Be Activated by These Drugs

Diabetes, gout, systemic lupus erythematosus. People with asthma or other drug allergies may be more likely to have allergic reactions.

Possible Effects on Laboratory Tests

Complete blood counts: decreased red cells, hemoglobin, white cells, and platelets.

Blood amylase level: increased (possible pancreatitis).

Blood calcium or uric acid level: increased.

Blood sodium and chloride levels: decreased.

Blood cholesterol and triglyceride levels: increased, short term.

Blood glucose level: increased.

Glucose tolerance test (GTT): decreased.

Blood lithium level: increased.

Blood potassium and magnesium level: decreased.

Blood urea nitrogen (BUN) level: increased with long-term use.

Liver function tests (hydrochlorothiazide and chlorothiazide): increased liver enzymes (ALT/GPT, AST/GOT, and alkaline phosphatase), increased bilirubin.

CAUTION

1. One study found a strong association between higher doses of hydrochlorothiazide and chlorthalidone and combination drugs containing these diuretics and electrolyte loss and sudden cardiac death. This appeared to be a result of magnesium and potassium loss, and may be circumvented by close following of those electrolytes.

2. Take these exactly as prescribed. Excessive loss of sodium and potassium can lead to loss of appetite, nausea, fatigue, weakness, confusion, and tingling in the extremities.

3. If you take digitalis (digitoxin, digoxin), adequate potassium is critical. Periodic testing and high-potassium foods may be needed to prevent potassium deficiency—a potential cause of digitalis toxicity (see Table 13, "High Potassium Foods," Section Six).

Precautions for Use

By Infants and Children: Overdose could cause serious dehydration. Significant potassium loss can occur within the first 2 weeks of drug use.

By Those Over 60 Years of Age: Starting doses may be as low as 12.5 mg. Increased risk of impaired thinking, orthostatic hypotension, potassium loss, and blood sugar increase. Overdose or extended use can cause excessive loss of body water, thickening (increased viscosity) of blood, and increased tendency for the blood to clot—predisposing to stroke, heart attack, or thrombophlebitis (vein inflammation with blood clot).

▷ **Advisability of Use During Pregnancy**
Pregnancy Category: Metolazone: B by manufacturer, D by other independent researchers. All other thiazides in this class are D. See Pregnancy Risk Categories at the back of this book.
Animal studies: No birth defects found in rat studies.
Human studies: Reports are conflicting and inconclusive. Use of thiazides can cause a variety of maternal complications that may cause adverse fetal effects, including death. They should not be used during pregnancy unless a very serious complication occurs for which this drug is significantly beneficial. Ask your physician for guidance.

Advisability of Use If Breast-Feeding
Presence of these drugs in breast milk: Yes.
Avoid drugs or refrain from nursing.

Habit-Forming Potential: None.

Effects of Overdosage: Dry mouth, thirst, lethargy, weakness, muscle cramping, nausea, vomiting, drowsiness progressing to stupor or coma.

Possible Effects of Long-Term Use: Impaired balance of water, salt, magnesium, and potassium in blood and body tissues. Impaired tolerance of glucose. Pathological changes in parathyroid glands with increased blood calcium levels and decreased blood phosphate levels.

Suggested Periodic Examinations While Taking These Drugs (at physician's discretion)
Complete blood cell counts; measurements of blood levels of sodium, potassium, chloride, magnesium, sugar, and uric acid.
Kidney and liver function tests.

▷ **While Taking These Drugs, Observe the Following**
Foods: Ask your doctor if you need to eat foods rich in potassium. See Table 13, "High Potassium Foods," Section Six, if needed. Follow your physician's advice regarding the use of salt. Magnesium should be routinely checked and supplemented if these medicines have lowered blood levels.
Beverages: No restrictions. This drug may be taken with milk.
▷ *Alcohol:* Use with caution—alcohol may exaggerate the blood-pressure-lowering effects of these drugs and cause orthostatic hypotension.
Tobacco Smoking: No interactions expected, but I advise everyone to quit smoking.
▷ *Other Drugs*
These drugs may ***increase*** the effects of
• lithium (Lithobid, others), and cause lithium toxicity.
• other antihypertensive drugs; dosage adjustments may be necessary to prevent excessive lowering of blood pressure.
These drugs may ***decrease*** the effects of
• oral anticoagulants such as warfarin (Coumadin). Increased frequency of INR (prothrombin time or protime) testing is needed.
• oral antidiabetic drugs (sulfonylureas—see Drug Classes); dosage adjustments may be necessary for proper control of blood sugar.

These drugs *taken concurrently* with

- allopurinol (Zyloprim) may decrease kidney function.
- amphotericin B (Fungizone) may result in additive potassium loss. Increased frequency of laboratory testing is needed.
- calcium may result in the milk-alkali syndrome with increased calcium, alkalosis, and kidney failure.
- carbamazepine (Tegretol) may result in low sodium levels and symptomatic hyponatremia.
- cortisone or other corticosteroid medicines may result in excessive potassium loss with resultant heart rhythm changes and lethargy.
- digitalis preparations (digitoxin, digoxin) requires careful monitoring and dose changes to prevent low potassium levels and serious disturbances of heart rhythm.
- nonsteroidal anti-inflammatory drugs (see Drug Classes) such as sulindac (Clinoril) and naproxen (Naprosyn, Aleve, Anaprox, others) may result in decreased thiazide effectiveness.

The following drugs may *decrease* the effects of these thiazides

- cholestyramine (Cuemid, Questran)—may interfere with its absorption.
- colestipol (Colestid)—may interfere with its absorption.

Take cholestyramine and colestipol 1 hour before any oral diuretic.

▷ *Driving, Hazardous Activities:* Use caution until the possible occurrence of orthostatic hypotension, dizziness, or impaired vision has been determined.

Aviation Note: The use of these drugs *may be a disqualification* for piloting. Consult a designated Aviation Medical Examiner.

Exposure to Sun: Use caution until sensitivity has been determined. These drugs can cause photosensitivity (see Glossary).

Exposure to Heat: Caution—excessive perspiring could cause additional loss of salt and water from the body.

Heavy Exercise or Exertion: Avoid exertion that produces light-headedness, excessive fatigue, or muscle cramping. Isometric exercises can raise blood pressure significantly. Ask your doctor for help regarding participation in this form of exercise.

Occurrence of Unrelated Illness: Vomiting or diarrhea can produce a serious imbalance of important body chemistry. Consult your physician for guidance.

Discontinuation: These drugs should not be stopped abruptly following long-term use; sudden discontinuation can cause serious thiazide-withdrawal fluid retention (edema). The dose should be reduced gradually. It may be advisable to discontinue this drug 5 to 7 days before major surgery. Ask your physician, surgeon, and/or anesthesiologist for guidance.

THIORIDAZINE (thi oh RID a zeen)

Introduced: 1959   **Class:** Antipsychotic; tranquilizer, major; phenothiazines   **Prescription:** USA: Yes   **Controlled Drug:** USA: No; Canada: No
Available as Generic: USA: Yes; Canada: Yes

Brand Names: ✦Apo-Thioridazine, Mellaril, Mellaril-S, Millazine, ✦Novoridazine, ✦PMS-Thioridazine, SK-Thioridazine

```
┌─────────────────────────────────────────────────────────────────┐
│                    BENEFITS versus RISKS                          │
│        Possible Benefits              Possible Risks              │
│  EFFECTIVE CONTROL OF ACUTE      TARDIVE DYSKINESIA (SERIOUS      │
│    MENTAL DISORDERS                TOXIC BRAIN EFFECT with        │
│  Relief of anxiety, agitation, and  long-term use)               │
│    tension                       NEUROLEPTIC MALIGNANT           │
│  Possibly effective in the management  SYNDROME                   │
│    of the hyperactivity syndrome in  Liver damage with jaundice   │
│    children                        (infrequent)                  │
│                                  Blood cell disorder: abnormally low │
│                                    white blood cell count        │
└─────────────────────────────────────────────────────────────────┘
```

▷ **Principal Uses**

> *As a Single Drug Product:* Uses currently included in FDA-approved labeling: (1) Helps manage symptoms of psychotic disorders as well as: moderate to marked depression with significant anxiety and nervous tension; agitation, anxiety, depression, and exaggerated fears in the elderly; (2) used in severe behavioral problems in children characterized by hyperexcitability, short attention span and rapid swings in mood (temper tantrums).

> Other (unlabeled) generally accepted uses: (1) May have a role in treating alcohol withdrawal in patients who cannot tolerate benzodiazepines; (2) can be used to treat unexplained infertility; (3) may help control premature ejaculation and nocturnal emissions in men; (4) can help borderline personality disorder; (5) of use in some chronic pain syndromes; (6) may be of use in hypersexuality.

How This Drug Works: By inhibiting the action of dopamine in certain brain centers, this drug acts to correct an imbalance of nerve impulse transmissions that is thought to be responsible for certain mental disorders. May help control premature ejaculation by inhibiting the muscle (longitudinal) that controls the vas deferens.

Available Dosage Forms and Strengths

> Concentrate — 30 mg/ml, 100 mg/ml
> Oral suspension — 25 mg/5 ml, 100 mg/5 ml
> Tablets — 10 mg, 15 mg, 25 mg, 50 mg, 100 mg, 150 mg, 200 mg

▷ **Usual Adult Dosage Range:** Initially 25 to 100 mg three times daily. Dose may be increased by 25 to 50 mg at 3- to 4-day intervals as needed and tolerated. Usual dosage range (psychosis) is 200 to 800 mg daily, divided into two to four doses. The total daily dosage should not exceed 800 mg. **Note: Actual dosage and administration schedule must be determined for each patient individually.**

Conditions Requiring Dosing Adjustments

> *Liver Function:* This drug is extensively metabolized in the liver and should be used with caution in liver compromise, and the patient closely monitored.
> *Kidney Function:* Patients with compromised kidneys should be closely followed.

▷ **Dosing Instructions:** The tablets may be crushed and taken with or following meals to reduce stomach irritation.

Usual Duration of Use: Use on a regular schedule for 3 to 4 weeks usually determines effectiveness in controlling psychotic disorders. If not significantly beneficial within 6 weeks, it should be stopped. Long-term use (months to years) requires periodic physician evaluation of response, appropriate dosage adjustment, and consideration of continued need.

▷ **This Drug Should Not Be Taken If**
   - you are allergic to any of the drugs bearing the brand names listed above.
   - you have active liver disease.
   - you have cancer of the breast.
   - you have a constitutionally low blood pressure.
   - you have a current blood cell or bone marrow disorder.

▷ **Inform Your Physician Before Taking This Drug If**
   - you are allergic or abnormally sensitive to any phenothiazine (see Drug Classes).
   - you have impaired liver or kidney function.
   - you have any type of seizure disorder.
   - you have diabetes, glaucoma, or heart disease.
   - you have a history of lupus erythematosus.
   - you are taking any drug with sedative effects.
   - you plan to have surgery under general or spinal anesthesia in the near future.

Possible Side Effects (natural, expected, and unavoidable drug actions)
   Drowsiness (usually during the first 2 weeks), orthostatic hypotension (see Glossary), blurred vision, dry mouth, nasal congestion, constipation, impaired urination. Pink or purple coloration of urine, of no significance.

▷ **Possible Adverse Effects** (unusual, unexpected, and infrequent reactions)
   If any of the following develop, consult your physician promptly for guidance.

   Mild Adverse Effects
   Allergic Reactions: Skin rash, hives, low-grade fever.
   Lowering of body temperature, especially in the elderly (see Hypothermia in Glossary)—possible.
   Abnormal body hair growth (hirsutism)—case reports.
   Urinary incontinence—possible.
   Increased appetite and weight gain—case reports.
   Inflammation of the parotid gland—case reports.
   Weakness, agitation, insomnia, impaired day and night vision—infrequent.
   Chronic constipation, fecal impaction—infrequent.

   Serious Adverse Effects
   Allergic Reactions: Hepatitis with jaundice (see Glossary), severe skin reactions (Stevens-Johnson syndrome or erythema multiforme).
   Idiosyncratic Reactions: Neuroleptic malignant syndrome (see Glossary).
   Depression, disorientation, seizures, loss of peripheral vision—case reports.
   Rapid heart rate, heart rhythm disorders—case reports.
   Blood cell disorders: reduced white blood cell count—more common in the elderly.
   Excessive production of urine (SIADH) or pituitary tumors—case reports.
   Nervous system reactions: Parkinson-like disorders (see Glossary), severe restlessness, muscle spasms involving the face and neck, tardive dyskinesia (see Glossary)—case reports.

Retinopathy—case reports.

Liver toxicity (cholestatic jaundice)—infrequent.

Abnormally low blood pressure—possible.

▷ **Possible Effects on Sexual Function**

Decreased male and female libido; inhibited ejaculation; impotence—frequent; impaired female orgasm; priapism (see Glossary)—infrequent.

Male breast enlargement and tenderness (gynecomastia), female breast enlargement with milk production.

Altered timing and pattern of menstruation. False positive pregnancy test results—case reports.

May help control premature ejaculation and nocturnal emissions.

▷ **Adverse Effects That May Mimic Natural Diseases or Disorders**

Nervous system reactions may suggest true Parkinson's disease.

Liver reactions may suggest viral hepatitis.

Reactions resembling systemic lupus erythematosus can occur.

Natural Diseases or Disorders That May Be Activated by This Drug

Latent epilepsy, glaucoma, diabetes mellitus, prostatism (see Glossary).

Possible Effects on Laboratory Tests

Complete blood cell counts: decreased red cells, hemoglobin, white cells, and platelets.

Liver function tests: increased enzymes (ALT/GPT, AST/GOT, alkaline phosphatase) or bilirubin.

Urine pregnancy tests: false-positive result with Prognosticon.

CAUTION

1. Many over-the-counter medications (see Glossary) for allergies, colds, and coughs contain drugs that can interact unfavorably with this drug. Ask your doctor or pharmacist for help **before** using any such medications.

2. Antacids that contain aluminum and/or magnesium can limit drug absorption and benefits.

3. Obtain prompt evaluation of any change or disturbance of vision.

Precautions for Use

By Infants and Children: NOT recommended for children under 2 years of age. Do not use this drug in the presence of symptoms suggestive of Reye syndrome (see Glossary). Children with acute infectious diseases (flu-like infections, chickenpox, measles, etc.) are more prone to develop muscular spasms of the face, back, and extremities when this drug is given for any reason.

By Those Over 60 Years of Age: Small starting doses are advisable. You may be more susceptible to drowsiness, lethargy, constipation, lowering of body temperature (hypothermia), and orthostatic hypotension (see Glossary). This drug can worsen existing prostatism (see Glossary). You may also be more susceptible to Parkinson-like reactions and/or tardive dyskinesia (see discussion of these terms in Glossary). These reactions must be recognized early since they may become unresponsive to treatment and permanent.

▷ **Advisability of Use During Pregnancy**

Pregnancy Category: C. See Pregnancy Risk Categories at the back of this book.

Animal studies: The results of rodent studies are conflicting.

Human studies: No increase in birth defects reported in 23 exposures. Adequate studies of pregnant women are not available.

Avoid drug during the first 3 months. Use it otherwise only if clearly needed. Ask your physician for guidance.

Advisability of Use If Breast-Feeding

Presence of this drug in breast milk: Yes, in minute amounts.

Monitor nursing infant closely and discontinue drug or nursing if adverse effects develop.

Habit-Forming Potential: None.

Effects of Overdosage: Marked drowsiness, weakness, tremor, agitation, unsteadiness, deep sleep, coma, convulsions.

Possible Effects of Long-Term Use: Opacities in the cornea or lens of the eye, pigmentation of the retina. Tardive dyskinesia (see Glossary).

Suggested Periodic Examinations While Taking This Drug (at physician's discretion)

Complete blood cell counts, especially between the 4th and 10th weeks of treatment.

Liver function tests, electrocardiograms.

Complete eye examinations—eye structures and vision.

Careful inspection of the tongue for early evidence of fine, involuntary, wavelike movements that could be the beginning of tardive dyskinesia.

▷ **While Taking This Drug, Observe the Following**

Foods: No restrictions.

Nutritional Support: A riboflavin (vitamin B_2) supplement should be taken with long-term use.

Beverages: No restrictions. May be taken with milk.

▷ *Alcohol:* Avoid completely. Alcohol can increase the sedative action of phenothiazines and accentuate their depressant effects on brain function and blood pressure. Phenothiazines can increase the intoxicating effects of alcohol.

Tobacco Smoking: There may be a reduction of drowsiness from this drug if you smoke, but I advise everyone to quit smoking.

Marijuana Smoking: Moderate increase in drowsiness; accentuation of orthostatic hypotension; increased risk of precipitating latent psychoses, confusing the interpretation of mental status and drug responses.

▷ *Other Drugs*

Thioridazine may *increase* the effects of
- all atropinelike drugs, and cause nervous system toxicity.
- all sedative drugs, especially meperidine (Demerol), and cause excessive sedation.

Thioridazine may *decrease* the effects of
- amphetamines.
- bromocriptine (Parlodel).
- guanethidine (Ismelin, Esimil), and reduce its effectiveness in lowering blood pressure.
- oral hypoglycemic agents (see Oral Antidiabetic Drugs in Drug Classes).

Thioridazine *taken concurrently* with
- ascorbic acid (vitamin C) may result in decreased thioridazine therapeutic benefits.
- lithium (Lithobid, Lithotabs) may impair the effectiveness of lithium and cause nervous system toxicity.
- monoamine oxidase (MAO) inhibitors may lead to prolonged thioridazine effects.
- phenytoin (Dilantin) may increase or decrease blood levels.
- ritonavir (Norvir) and perhaps other protease inhibitors (see Drug Classes) may lead to toxicity.
- tramadol (Ultram) may increase seizure risk.

The following drugs may *decrease* the effects of thioridazine
- antacids containing aluminum and/or magnesium.
- barbiturates (see Drug Classes).
- benztropine (Cogentin).
- disulfiram (Antabuse).
- trihexyphenidyl (Artane).

▷ *Driving, Hazardous Activities:* This drug can impair mental alertness, judgment, and physical coordination. Avoid hazardous activities.

Aviation Note: The use of this drug *is a disqualification* for piloting. Consult a designated Aviation Medical Examiner.

Exposure to Sun: Use caution—some phenothiazines can cause photosensitivity (see Glossary).

Exposure to Heat: Use caution and avoid excessive heat as much as possible. This drug may impair the regulation of body temperature and increase the risk of heatstroke.

Exposure to Cold: Use caution and dress warmly. This drug can increase the risk of hypothermia in the elderly.

Discontinuation: After long-term use, do not stop this drug suddenly. Gradual withdrawal over 2 to 3 weeks under physician supervision is recommended. Do not discontinue this drug without your physician's knowledge and approval.

THIOTHIXENE (thi oh THIX een)

Introduced: 1967   **Class:** Tranquilizer, major; thioxanthenes   **Prescription:** USA: Yes   **Controlled Drug:** USA: No; Canada: No   **Available as Generic:** USA: Yes; Canada: No

Brand Name: Navane

BENEFITS versus RISKS	
Possible Benefits	*Possible Risks*
EFFECTIVE CONTROL OF ACUTE MENTAL DISORDERS	SERIOUS TOXIC EFFECTS ON BRAIN with long-term use
	Liver damage with jaundice
	Blood cell disorder: abnormally low white blood cell count

▷ **Principal Uses**

As a Single Drug Product: Uses currently included in FDA-approved labeling: Relieves psychotic thinking and behavior associated with acute psychoses, episodes of mania and paranoia, and acute schizophrenia.

Other (unlabeled) generally accepted uses: Can be of use in significant borderline personality disorder.

How This Drug Works: By inhibiting dopamine, this drug corrects an imbalance of nerve impulse transmissions (at both D1 and D2 receptors) that is thought to be responsible for certain mental disorders.

Available Dosage Forms and Strengths

Capsules — 1 mg, 2 mg, 5 mg, 10 mg, 20 mg

Concentrate — 5 mg/ml

Injections — 2 mg/ml, 5 mg/ml

▷ **Usual Adult Dosage Range:**   Initially 2 to 5 mg two or three times daily. Dose may be increased by 2 mg at 3- to 4-day intervals as needed and tolerated. Usual dosage range is 20 to 30 mg daily. The total daily dosage should not exceed 60 mg. **Note: Actual dosage and administration schedule must be determined for each patient individually.**

Conditions Requiring Dosing Adjustments

Liver Function: This drug should be used with caution in liver compromise.

Kidney Function: Patients with compromised kidneys should be closely followed.

▷ **Dosing Instructions:**   The capsules may be opened and taken with or following meals to reduce stomach irritation. The liquid concentrate must be diluted just before administration by adding it to 8 ounces of water, milk, fruit juice, or carbonated beverage.

Usual Duration of Use: Use on a regular schedule for several weeks usually determines control of psychotic disorders. If not beneficial within 6 weeks, it should be stopped. Long-term use (months to years) requires periodic physician evaluation of response, appropriate dosage adjustment, and consideration of continued need.

▷ **This Drug Should Not Be Taken If**

- you have had an allergic reaction to it previously.
- you have active liver disease.
- you have cancer of the breast.
- you have a current blood cell or bone marrow disorder.

▷ **Inform Your Physician Before Taking This Drug If**

- you are allergic or abnormally sensitive to other thioxanthene drugs or any phenothiazine drug (see Drug Classes).
- you have impaired liver or kidney function.
- you have any type of seizure disorder.
- you have diabetes, glaucoma, or heart disease.
- you have a history of lupus erythematosus.
- you have Parkinson's disease.
- you have had neuroleptic malignant syndrome.
- you are taking any drug with sedative effects.
- you drink alcohol daily.
- you plan to have surgery under general or spinal anesthesia in the near future.

Possible Side Effects (natural, expected, and unavoidable drug actions)
> Mild drowsiness (usually during the first 2 weeks), orthostatic hypotension (see Glossary), blurred vision, dry mouth, nasal congestion, constipation, impaired urination.

▷ **Possible Adverse Effects** (unusual, unexpected, and infrequent reactions)
> **If any of the following develop, consult your physician promptly for guidance.**

Mild Adverse Effects
> Allergic Reactions: Skin rash, hives, itching.
> Lowering of body temperature, especially in the elderly (see Hypothermia in Glossary).
> Fluid retention, weight gain—possible.
> Dizziness, weakness, agitation, insomnia, impaired vision—infrequent to frequent.
> Nausea, vomiting—infrequent.

Serious Adverse Effects
> Allergic Reactions: Rare hepatitis with jaundice (see Glossary), anaphylactic reaction (see Glossary).
> Idiosyncratic Reactions: Paradoxical worsening of psychotic symptoms. Development of the neuroleptic malignant syndrome (see Glossary).
> Abnormal production of urine and loss of blood sodium (SIADH)—case reports.
> Depression, disorientation, seizures—case reports.
> Deposits in cornea and lens of the eye—infrequent.
> Abnormal fixed eye positioning (oculogyric crisis)—frequent extrapyramidal effect.
> Rapid heart rate, heart rhythm disorders—possible.
> Systemic lupus erythematosus or blood cell disorders: reduced white blood count—case reports.
> Nervous system reactions: Parkinson-like disorders (see Glossary), severe restlessness, muscle spasms involving the face and neck, tardive dyskinesia (see Glossary)—infrequent.
> Severe reduction in blood pressure—rare.

▷ **Possible Effects on Sexual Function**
> Altered timing and pattern of menstruation.
> Impotence, priapism, and retrograde ejaculation—rare.
> Male breast enlargement and tenderness (gynecomastia)—case reports.
> Female breast enlargement with milk production—rare.

▷ **Adverse Effects That May Mimic Natural Diseases or Disorders**
> Nervous system reactions may suggest true Parkinson's disease or Reye syndrome (see Glossary). Liver reactions may suggest viral hepatitis.

Natural Diseases or Disorders That May Be Activated by This Drug
> Latent epilepsy, glaucoma, prostatism (see Glossary).

Possible Effects on Laboratory Tests
> Complete blood cell counts: decreased red cells, hemoglobin, white cells, and platelets; increased eosinophils.
> Blood glucose level: increased and decreased (fluctuations).
> Liver function tests: increased enzymes (ALT/GPT, AST/GOT, alkaline phosphatase) or bilirubin.
> Urine pregnancy tests: false-positive result with some tests.

CAUTION
1. Many over-the-counter medications (see Glossary) for allergies, colds, and coughs contain drugs that can interact unfavorably with this drug. Ask your doctor or pharmacist for help **before** using any such medications.
2. Antacids that contain aluminum and/or magnesium may limit drug absorption and effectiveness.
3. Obtain prompt evaluation of any change or disturbance of vision.

Precautions for Use

By Infants and Children: Use of this drug is not recommended for children under 12 years of age. Do not use this drug in the presence of symptoms suggestive of Reye syndrome (see Glossary). Children with acute infectious diseases (flu-like infections, chickenpox, measles, etc.) are more prone to develop muscular spasms of the face, back, and extremities when this drug is given.

By Those Over 60 Years of Age: Small starting doses are advisable. Increased risk of drowsiness, lethargy, constipation, lowering of body temperature (hypothermia), and orthostatic hypotension (see Glossary). This drug can worsen existing prostatism (see Glossary). You may also be more susceptible to the development of Parkinson-like reactions and/or tardive dyskinesia (see discussion of these terms in Glossary). These reactions must be recognized early since they may become unresponsive to treatment and irreversible.

▷ **Advisability of Use During Pregnancy**
Pregnancy Category: C. See Pregnancy Risk Categories at the back of this book.
Animal studies: No birth defects reported in rats, rabbits, or monkeys.
Human studies: Adequate studies of pregnant women are not available.
Avoid drug during the first 3 months if possible. Avoid during the final month because of possible effects on the newborn infant.

Advisability of Use If Breast-Feeding
Presence of this drug in breast milk: Expected in small amounts, but no data are available.
Avoid drug or refrain from nursing.

Habit-Forming Potential: None.

Effects of Overdosage: Marked drowsiness, weakness, tremor, agitation, unsteadiness, deep sleep, coma, convulsions.

Possible Effects of Long-Term Use: Opacities in the cornea or lens of the eye, pigmentation of the retina. Tardive dyskinesia (see Glossary).

Suggested Periodic Examinations While Taking This Drug (at physician's discretion)
Complete blood cell counts, especially between the 4th and 10th weeks of treatment.
Liver function tests, electrocardiograms.
Complete eye examinations—eye structures and vision.
Careful inspection of the tongue for early evidence of fine, involuntary, wave-like movements that could indicate the beginning of tardive dyskinesia.

▷ **While Taking This Drug, Observe the Following**
Foods: No restrictions.
Beverages: No restrictions. May be taken with milk.

▷   *Alcohol:* Avoid completely. Alcohol can increase the sedative action of thiothixene and accentuate its depressant effects on brain function and blood pressure. Thiothixene can increase the intoxicating effects of alcohol.

Tobacco Smoking: No interactions expected, but I advise everyone to quit smoking.

Marijuana Smoking: Moderate increase in drowsiness; accentuation of orthostatic hypotension; increased risk of precipitating latent psychoses, confusing the interpretation of mental status and drug responses.

▷   *Other Drugs*

Thiothixene may ***increase*** the effects of
- all atropinelike drugs, and cause nervous system toxicity.
- all sedative drugs, especially barbiturates and narcotic analgesics, and
cause excessive sedation.

Thiothixene may ***decrease*** the effects of
- guanethidine (Ismelin, Esimil), and reduce its effectiveness in lowering
blood pressure.

Thiothixene ***taken concurrently*** with
- ketorolac (Toradol) may result in hallucinations.
- lithium (Lithobid, others) may result in exaggerated neurotoxicity (rigidity
and tremor).
- monoamine oxidase (MAO) inhibitors (see Drug Classes) may result in
worsening of the depressive effects of thiothixene on the central nervous
system and breathing.
- tramadol (Ultram) may increase seizure risk.

The following drugs may ***decrease*** the effects of thiothixene
- antacids containing aluminum and/or magnesium.
- barbiturates (see Drug Classes).
- benztropine (Cogentin).
- trihexyphenidyl (Artane).

▷   *Driving, Hazardous Activities:* This drug can impair mental alertness, judgment,
and physical coordination. Avoid hazardous activities.

Aviation Note: The use of this drug ***is a disqualification*** for piloting. Consult a
designated Aviation Medical Examiner.

Exposure to Sun: Use caution until sensitivity has been determined. This drug
can cause photosensitivity (see Glossary).

Exposure to Heat: Use caution and avoid excessive heat as much as possible.
This drug may impair the regulation of body temperature and increase the
risk of heatstroke.

Exposure to Cold: Use caution and dress warmly. This drug can increase the risk
of hypothermia in the elderly.

Discontinuation: After a period of long-term use, do not stop this drug suddenly.
Gradual withdrawal over 2 to 3 weeks under physician supervision is recommended. Do not discontinue this drug without your physician's knowledge and approval. The relapse rate of schizophrenia after discontinuation
is 50 to 60%.

TICLOPIDINE (ti KLOH pi deen)

Introduced: 1985   **Class:** Antiplatelet   **Prescription:** USA: Yes
Controlled Drug: USA: No; Canada: No   **Available as Generic:** USA: No
Brand Name: Ticlid

BENEFITS versus RISKS	
Possible Benefits	*Possible Risks*
SIGNIFICANT REDUCTION IN THE RISK OF STROKE FOR THOSE WITH TRANSIENT ISCHEMIC ATTACK (TIA) OR PREVIOUS STROKE	SIGNIFICANT REDUCTION IN WHITE BLOOD CELL COUNTS (uncommon) Increase of 8–10% in total blood cholesterol level Drug-induced hepatitis with jaundice

▷ **Principal Uses**

As a Single Drug Product: Uses currently included in FDA-approved labeling: Used in selected individuals (who are intolerant to aspirin) to prevent recurrent stroke following initial thrombotic stroke.

Other (unlabeled) generally accepted uses: (1) Used in some patients with peripheral vascular disease and intermittent claudication to prevent blood clots (thrombosis); (2) used by people who have had bypass surgery to help prevent clot formation and keep the graft working; may have a role in slowing the progression of eye problems (retinopathy) in diabetics; (3) combined with other agents to keep patients with angina from having heart attacks; (4) used in combination therapy to help lessen the symptoms of rheumatoid arthritis; (5) may help prevent strokes in patients who have experienced transient ischemic attacks (TIAs); (6) can help patients with kidney failure keep from building up phosphate, urea, and creatinine.

How this Drug Works: By inhibiting clumping of blood platelets, this drug prevents the beginning of processes that lead to blood clot formation within atherosclerotic vessels (arterial thrombosis).

Available Dosage Forms and Strengths

Tablets — 250 mg

▷ **Recommended Dosage Ranges** (Actual dosage and administration schedule must be determined for each patient individually.)

Infants and Children: Dosage not established.

18 to 60 Years of Age: 250 mg twice daily, 12 hours apart, taken with food.

Over 60 Years of Age: Same as 18 to 60 years of age.

Conditions Requiring Dosing Adjustments

Liver Function: This drug is contraindicated in patients with severe liver impairment. Doses may need to be decreased for people with compromised livers.

Kidney Function: Changes in dosing for kidney compromise patients do not appear to be needed.

▷ **Dosing Instructions:**   The tablet may be crushed and is best taken with meals to enhance absorption and reduce stomach irritation.

Usual Duration of Use: Use on a regular schedule for 6 to 12 months usually determines effectiveness in preventing stroke. Long-term use (months to years) requires periodic physician evaluation of response and dosage adjustment.

Possible Advantages of This Drug

A reduction in risk of initial stroke during first year following TIA (in contrast to aspirin).

A reduction in risk of recurrent stroke during the first year following initial stroke.

Effective in both men and women.

▷ **This Drug Should Not Be Taken If**
- you have had an allergic reaction to it previously.
- you currently have a bone marrow, blood cell, or bleeding disorder.
- you have active peptic ulcer disease, Crohn's disease, or ulcerative colitis.
- you have severely impaired liver function.
- you are taking aspirin, anticoagulants, or cortisonelike drugs.

▷ **Inform Your Physician Before Taking This Drug If**
- you have a history of a drug-induced bone marrow depression or blood cell disorder.
- you have gastric or duodenal ulcers.
- you have impaired liver or kidney function.
- you plan to have surgery in the near future; this drug should be discontinued 10 to 14 days prior to surgery.

Possible Side Effects (natural, expected, and unavoidable drug actions)

Spontaneous bruising (purpura)—rare.

▷ **Possible Adverse Effects** (unusual, unexpected, and infrequent reactions)

If any of the following develop, consult your physician promptly for guidance.

Mild Adverse Effects

Allergic Reactions: Rash, itching—rare.

Dizziness, ringing in the ears—rare.

Loss of appetite, indigestion, nausea, vomiting, stomach pain, diarrhea—rare to infrequent.

Serious Adverse Effects

Allergic Reactions: Drug-induced hepatitis with jaundice—rare. This usually occurs during the first 4 months of treatment (see Jaundice in Glossary).

Idiosyncratic Reactions: Decreased production of white blood cells (neutrophils and granulocytes): fever, sore throat, susceptibility to infection.

Liver damage—infrequent.

Aplastic anemia (see Glossary) or lupus erythematosus—case reports.

▷ **Possible Effects on Sexual Function:**   None reported.

▷ **Adverse Effects That May Mimic Natural Diseases or Disorders**

Drug-induced hepatitis may suggest viral hepatitis.

Possible Effects on Laboratory Tests

Complete blood cell counts: decreased red cells, hemoglobin, white cells, and platelets.

Bleeding time: increased.

Total cholesterol and triglyceride levels: increased.

Liver function tests: increased liver enzymes (ALT/GPT, AST/GOT, and alkaline phosphatase), increased bilirubin.

CAUTION

1. If significantly low white blood cell counts occur, they usually begin between 3 weeks and 3 months after treatment starts. White blood cell counts **must** be obtained every 2 weeks from the second week to the end of the third month of drug administration.
2. Report promptly any indications of infection: fever, chills, sore throat, cough, etc.
3. Report promptly any abnormal or unusual bleeding or bruising.
4. While taking this drug, do not take any type of aspirin or anticoagulant drug without your physician's approval.
5. Inform all health care professionals who prescribe medicines for you that you are taking this drug.

Precautions for Use

By Infants and Children: Safety and effectiveness for those under 18 years of age are not established.

By Those Over 60 Years of Age: You may be more susceptible to bone marrow depression and blood cell decreases. Observe carefully for any tendency to infections or unusual bleeding or bruising. Report such developments promptly.

▷ **Advisability of Use During Pregnancy**

Pregnancy Category: B. See Pregnancy Risk Categories at the back of this book.
Animal studies: No drug-induced birth defects found in mouse, rat, or rabbit studies.
Human studies: Adequate studies of pregnant women are not available.
Use this drug only if clearly needed. Ask your physician for guidance.

Advisability of Use If Breast-Feeding

Presence of this drug in breast milk: Unknown.
Avoid drug or refrain from nursing.

Habit-Forming Potential: None.

Effects of Overdosage: Abnormal bleeding or bruising, dizziness, nausea, diarrhea.

Possible Effects of Long-Term Use: None reported.

Suggested Periodic Examinations While Taking This Drug (at physician's discretion)

Complete blood cell counts. See "CAUTION" above.
Liver function tests.

▷ **While Taking This Drug, Observe the Following**

Foods: High-fat meals may increase absorption by 20%.
Beverages: No restrictions. May be taken with milk.
▷ *Alcohol:* No interactions expected. Avoid if you have active peptic ulcer disease.
Tobacco Smoking: No interactions expected, but I advise everyone to quit smoking.
▷ *Other Drugs*

Ticlopidine may *increase* the effects of
• aspirin.
• theophylline (Theo-Dur, others).
• warfarin (Coumadin), and also increase the risk of hepatitis. This combination is **not** recommended.

Ticlopidine may **decrease** the effects of
- cyclosporine (Sandimmune) and decrease its effectiveness.
- digoxin (Lanoxin).

The following drug may **increase** the effects of ticlopidine
- cimetidine (Tagamet).

The following drugs may **decrease** the effects of ticlopidine
- antacids—decreases absorption of ticlopidine.

▷ *Driving, Hazardous Activities:* This drug may cause dizziness. Restrict activities as necessary.

Aviation Note: The use of this drug **may be a disqualification** for piloting. Consult a designated Aviation Medical Examiner.

Exposure to Sun: No restrictions.

Discontinuation: To be determined and guided by your physician.

TIMOLOL (TI moh lohl)

Introduced: 1972   **Class:** Anti-anginal, anti-glaucoma, antihypertensive, beta-blocker   **Prescription:** USA: Yes   **Controlled Drug:** USA: No; Canada: No   **Available as Generic:** USA: Yes; Canada: No

Brand Names: ✦Apo-Timolol, ✦Apo-Timop, Betimol, Blocadren, ✦Timolide [CD], Timoptic, Timoptic Ocudose, Timoptic-XE

BENEFITS versus RISKS	
Possible Benefits	*Possible Risks*
EFFECTIVE, WELL-TOLERATED ANTI-ANGINAL DRUG	CONGESTIVE HEART FAILURE in advanced heart disease
ANTI-GLAUCOMA DRUG	Worsening of angina in coronary
ANTIHYPERTENSIVE DRUG in mild to moderate hypertension	heart disease (if drug is abruptly withdrawn)
EFFECTIVE PREVENTION OF MIGRAINE HEADACHES	Masking of low blood sugar (hypoglycemia) in drug-treated
Effective adjunct in the prevention of recurrent heart attack (myocardial infarction)	diabetes
	Provocation of asthma

▷ **Principal Uses**

As a Single Drug Product: Uses currently included in FDA-approved labeling: (1) Treats classical effort-induced angina, certain types of heart rhythm disturbance, and high blood pressure; (2) helps lower increased internal eye pressure in chronic open-angle glaucoma; (3) beneficial when taken within 24 hours and for 28 days thereafter in decreasing the size of the heart damage, decreasing arrhythmias, and preventing repeat heart attacks (myocardial infarction); (4) used to reduce the frequency and severity of migraine headaches.

Other (unlabeled) generally accepted uses: (1) Has been used by people who are afraid to fly on airplanes (air travel phobia); (2) may be helpful in decreasing the incidence of abnormal heart rhythms that arise in the atria of the heart (atrial fibrillation and flutter); (3) helps prevent abnormally increased intraocular pressure following cataract surgery; (4) of use in patients with detached retinas that have not torn.

As a Combination Drug Product [CD]: This drug is available in combination with hydrochlorothiazide for the treatment of hypertension. This combination product includes two drugs with different mechanisms of action; it is intended to provide greater effectiveness and convenience for long-term use.

How This Drug Works: By blocking certain actions of the sympathetic nervous system, this drug
- reduces rate and contraction force of the heart, lowering the ejection pressure of blood and reducing the amount of oxygen the heart needs to work.
- reduces the degree of contraction of blood vessel walls, resulting in their expansion and consequent lowering of blood pressure.
- prolongs the conduction time of nerve impulses through the heart, of benefit in the management of certain heart rhythm disorders.
- slows formation of fluid (aqueous humor) in the anterior chamber of the eye and improves its drainage from the eye, lowering the internal eye pressure.

Available Dosage Forms and Strengths
>   Eye solutions — 0.25%, 0.5%
>   Tablets — 5 mg, 10 mg, 20 mg

▷ **Usual Adult Dosage Range:**   Varies with indication.
>   Anti-anginal and antihypertensive: Initially 10 mg two times daily; increase dose gradually every 7 days as needed and tolerated. Usual maintenance dose is 10 to 20 mg once a day or divided into two equal doses and taken twice daily. The total daily dosage should not exceed 60 mg.
>   Migraine headache prevention: Initially 10 mg two times daily; increase dose as needed to 10 mg in the morning and 20 mg at night.
>   Preventing repeat heart attack: 10 mg twice daily.
>   Anti-glaucoma: one drop in affected eye twice daily. **Note: Timoptic-XE form is a clear gel and may be used once daily.**
>   **Note: Actual dosage and administration schedule must be determined for each patient individually.**

Conditions Requiring Dosing Adjustments
>   *Liver Function:* Consideration must be given to empirically decreasing the dose for patients with compromised livers.
>   *Kidney Function:* Patients with kidney compromise should be followed closely, and the dose decreased if the medication appears to be accumulating.

▷ **Dosing Instructions:**   Preferably taken 1 hour before eating to maximize absorption. The tablet may be crushed for administration. Do not stop this drug abruptly.

Usual Duration of Use: Use on a regular schedule for 10 to 14 days usually determines effectiveness in preventing angina, controlling heart rhythm disorders, and lowering blood pressure. Peak benefit may require continual use for 6 to 8 weeks. The long-term use of this drug (months to years) will be determined by the course of your symptoms over time and your response to an overall treatment program (weight reduction, salt restriction, smoking cessation, etc.). Consult your physician on a regular basis.

▷ **This Drug Should Not Be Taken If**
- you have bronchial asthma or severe obstructive lung disease.
- you have had an allergic reaction to it previously.

- you have Prinzmetal's variant angina (coronary artery spasm).
- you have congestive heart failure.
- you have an abnormally slow heart rate or a serious form of heart block.
- you are taking, or have taken within the past 14 days, any monoamine oxidase (MAO) type A inhibitor drug (see Drug Classes).

▷ **Inform Your Physician Before Taking This Drug If**
- you have had an adverse reaction to any beta-blocker (see Drug Classes).
- you have a history of serious heart disease.
- you have a history of hay fever (allergic rhinitis), asthma, chronic bronchitis, or emphysema.
- you have a history of overactive thyroid function (hyperthyroidism).
- you have a history of low blood sugar (hypoglycemia).
- you have impaired liver or kidney function.
- you have Raynaud's phenomenon.
- you have diabetes or myasthenia gravis.
- you currently take digitalis, quinidine, or reserpine, or any calcium-channel-blocker drug (see Drug Classes).
- you plan to have surgery under general anesthesia in the near future.

Possible Side Effects (natural, expected, and unavoidable drug actions)
Lethargy and fatigability, cold extremities, slow heart rate, light-headedness in upright position (see Orthostatic Hypotension in Glossary).

▷ **Possible Adverse Effects** (unusual, unexpected, and infrequent reactions)
If any of the following develop, consult your physician promptly for guidance.
Mild Adverse Effects
Allergic Reactions: Skin rash, itching.
Loss of hair involving the scalp, eyebrows, and/or eyelashes. This effect can occur with use of the oral tablets or the eyedrops (used to treat glaucoma). Regrowth occurs with discontinuation of this drug.
Headache, dizziness, visual disturbances, vivid dreams—infrequent.
Indigestion, nausea, vomiting, diarrhea—infrequent.
Numbness and tingling in extremities, joint pain—case reports.
Serious Adverse Effects
Allergic Reactions: Laryngospasm, severe dermatitis.
Idiosyncratic Reactions: Acute behavioral disturbances—depression, hallucinations.
Chest pain, shortness of breath, precipitation of congestive heart failure—case reports.
Induction of bronchial asthma (in asthmatic individuals)—possible.
May mask warning signs of impending low blood sugar (hypoglycemia) in drug-treated diabetes.
Drug-induced myasthenia gravis—case reports.
Periodic cramping of the leg (intermittent claudication)—possible.
Stopping of breathing (respiratory arrest)—case report.

▷ **Possible Effects on Sexual Function**
Decreased libido, impaired erection, impotence. **Note: All of these effects can occur with the use of timolol eyedrops at recommended dosage, albeit less often.**

▷ **Adverse Effects That May Mimic Natural Diseases or Disorders**

Reduced blood flow to extremities may resemble Raynaud's phenomenon (see Glossary).

Natural Diseases or Disorders That May Be Activated by This Drug

Prinzmetal's variant angina, Raynaud's disease, intermittent claudication, myasthenia gravis (questionable).

Possible Effects on Laboratory Tests

None reported.

CAUTION

1. ***Do not stop this drug suddenly*** without the knowledge and guidance of your doctor. Carry a notation which states that you take this drug.
2. Ask your doctor or pharmacist before using nasal decongestants usually present in over-the-counter cold preparations and nose drops. These can cause sudden increases in blood pressure when taken concurrently with beta-blocker drugs.
3. Report the development of any tendency to emotional depression (rare with this drug).

Precautions for Use

By Infants and Children: Safety and effectiveness for those under 12 years of age are not established. However, if this drug is used, watch for low blood sugar (hypoglycemia) during periods of reduced food intake.

By Those Over 60 Years of Age: Unacceptably high blood pressure should be reduced without creating the risks associated with excessively low blood pressure. Small starting doses and frequent blood pressure checks are needed. Sudden, rapid, and excessive reduction of blood pressure can predispose to stroke or heart attack. Observe for dizziness, unsteadiness, tendency to fall, confusion, hallucinations, depression, or urinary frequency.

▷ **Advisability of Use During Pregnancy**

Pregnancy Category: C. See Pregnancy Risk Categories at the back of this book.

Animal studies: No significant increase in birth defects due to this drug.

Human studies: Adequate studies of pregnant women are not available.

Avoid use of drug during the first 3 months if possible. Use this drug only if clearly needed. Ask your physician for guidance.

Advisability of Use If Breast-Feeding

Presence of this drug in breast milk: Yes.

Monitor nursing infant closely and discontinue drug or nursing if adverse effects develop.

Habit-Forming Potential: None.

Effects of Overdosage: Weakness, slow pulse, low blood pressure, fainting, cold and sweaty skin, congestive heart failure, possible coma and convulsions.

Possible Effects of Long-Term Use: Reduced heart reserve and eventual heart failure in susceptible individuals with advanced heart disease.

Suggested Periodic Examinations While Taking This Drug (at physician's discretion)

Complete blood cell counts (because of adverse effects of other drugs of this class).

Measurements of blood pressure, evaluation of heart function.

▷ **While Taking This Drug, Observe the Following**
  Foods: No restrictions. Avoid excessive salt intake.
  Beverages: No restrictions. May be taken with milk.
▷ *Alcohol:* Use with caution. Alcohol may exaggerate this drug's ability to lower the blood pressure and may increase its mild sedative effect.
  Tobacco Smoking: Nicotine may reduce this drug's effectiveness. I advise everyone to quit smoking.
▷ *Other Drugs*
  Timolol may *increase* the effects of
  • amiodarone (Cordarone) and cause cardiac arrest and bradycardia.
  • lidocaine (Xylocaine, etc.).
  • other antihypertensive drugs, and cause excessive lowering of blood pressure. Dosage adjustments may be necessary.
  • reserpine (Ser-Ap-Es, etc.), and cause sedation, depression, slowing of the heart rate, and lowering of blood pressure.
  • verapamil (Calan, Isoptin), and cause excessive depression of heart function; monitor this combination closely.
  Timolol may *decrease* the effects of
  • theophyllines (Aminophyllin, Theo-Dur, etc.), and reduce their antiasthmatic effectiveness.
  Timolol *taken concurrently* with
  • clonidine (Catapres) requires close monitoring for rebound high blood pressure if clonidine is withdrawn while timolol is still being taken.
  • epinephrine (Adrenalin, etc.) may cause marked rise in blood pressure and slowing of the heart rate.
  • insulin may hide the symptoms of hypoglycemia (see Glossary).
  • oral hypoglycemic agents (see Oral Antidiabetic Drugs in Drug Classes) such as acetohexamide (Dymelor) and glipizide (Glucotrol) may result in prolonged low blood sugar.
  • venlafaxine (Effexor) may result in increased risk of timolol toxicity.
  The following drugs may *increase* the effects of timolol
  • chlorpromazine (Thorazine, etc.).
  • cimetidine (Tagamet).
  • fluoxetine (Prozac).
  • fluvoxamine (Luvox).
  • methimazole (Tapazole).
  • propylthiouracil (Propacil).
  • ritonavir (Norvir) and perhaps other protease inhibitors (see Drug Classes).
  The following drugs may *decrease* the effects of timolol
  • antacids (when taken at the same time).
  • barbiturates (phenobarbital, etc.).
  • indomethacin (Indocin) and possibly other "aspirin substitutes," or NSAIDs—may impair timolol's antihypertensive effect.
  • rifampin (Rifadin, Rimactane).
▷ *Driving, Hazardous Activities:* Use caution until the full extent of dizziness, lethargy, and blood pressure change have been determined.
  Aviation Note: The use of this drug *may be a disqualification* for piloting. Consult a designated Aviation Medical Examiner.
  Exposure to Sun: No restrictions.

Exposure to Heat: Caution is advised. Hot environments can exaggerate the effects of this drug.

Exposure to Cold: Caution is advised. Cold environments can worsen circulatory deficiency in the extremities that may occur with this drug. The elderly should take precautions to prevent hypothermia (see Glossary).

Heavy Exercise or Exertion: It is advisable to avoid exertion that produces lightheadedness, excessive fatigue, or muscle cramping. The use of this drug may intensify the hypertensive response to isometric exercise.

Occurrence of Unrelated Illness: Fever can lower blood pressure and require adjustment of dosage. Nausea or vomiting may interrupt the dosing schedule. Ask your doctor for help.

Discontinuation: It is advisable to avoid sudden discontinuation of this drug in all situations; this is especially true in the presence of coronary artery disease. If possible, gradual reduction of dose over a period of 2 to 3 weeks is recommended. Ask your physician for specific guidance.

TOLBUTAMIDE (tohl BYU ta mide)

Introduced: 1956   **Class:** Antidiabetic, sulfonylureas   **Prescription:** USA: Yes   **Controlled Drug:** USA: No; Canada: No   **Available as Generic:** Yes

Brand Names: ✦Apo-Tolbutamide, ✦Mobenol, ✦Novobutamide, Oramide, Orinase, SK-Tolbutamide

Warning: The brand names Orinase, Ornade, and Ornex are similar and can be mistaken for each other; this can lead to serious medication errors. These names represent very different drugs. Orinase is the generic drug tolbutamide; it is used to treat diabetes. Ornade is a combination of chlorpheniramine and phenylpropanolamine, and is used to treat nasal and sinus congestion. Ornex is a combination of acetaminophen and phenylpropanolamine, used to treat head colds and sinus pain. Verify that you are taking the correct drug.

BENEFITS versus RISKS	
Possible Benefits	*Possible Risks*
Assistance in regulating blood sugar in noninsulin-dependent diabetes (adjunctive to appropriate diet and weight control)	HYPOGLYCEMIA, severe and prolonged Drug-induced liver damage Bone marrow depression Hemolytic anemia

▷ **Principal Uses**

As a Single Drug Product: Uses currently included in FDA-approved labeling: Helps control mild to moderately severe type II diabetes mellitus (adult, maturity-onset) that does not require insulin, but that cannot be adequately controlled by diet alone.

Other (unlabeled) generally accepted uses: Has been used intravenously to help diagnose tumors that secrete insulin.

How This Drug Works: It is thought that this drug (1) stimulates the release of insulin (by a pancreas that is capable of responding to stimulation), and (2) enhances the utilization of insulin by appropriate tissues.

Available Dosage Forms and Strengths
Tablets — 250 mg, 500 mg

▷ **Usual Adult Dosage Range:** Initially 500 mg twice a day. The dose may be increased or decreased every 48 to 72 hours until the minimal amount required for satisfactory control is determined. The usual range is 500 to 2000 mg a day. 3 g (3000 mg) is the maximum daily dose. **Note: Actual dosage and administration schedule must be determined for each patient individually.**

Conditions Requiring Dosing Adjustments
Liver Function: Consideration should be given to decreasing the dose for patients with compromised livers. Tolbutamide can be a rare cause of liver damage, and patients should be followed closely.
Kidney Function: Dosing decreases are not needed in kidney compromise.

▷ **Dosing Instructions:** May be taken with food (morning and evening meals) to reduce stomach irritation. The tablet may be crushed for administration.

Usual Duration of Use: Use on a regular schedule for 5 to 7 days weeks usually determines effectiveness in controlling diabetes. Failure to respond to maximal doses within 1 month constitutes a primary failure. Up to 15% of those who respond initially may develop secondary failure of the drug within the first year. Ongoing blood sugar testing is required. See your physician on a regular basis.

▷ **This Drug Should Not Be Taken If**
- you have had an allergic reaction to it previously.
- you have severe impairment of liver or kidney function.
- you are undergoing major surgery.
- you have a severe infection.
- you have diabetes complicated by formation of excess acid (acidosis).
- you are pregnant.

▷ **Inform Your Physician Before Taking This Drug If**
- you are allergic to other sulfonylurea drugs or "sulfa" drugs (see Drug Classes).
- your diabetes has been unstable or "brittle" in the past.
- you do not know how to recognize or treat hypoglycemia (see Glossary).
- you have an infection and a fever.
- you have a deficiency of glucose-6-phosphate dehydrogenase (G6PD) in your red blood cells (ask your doctor).
- you have a history of congestive heart failure, peptic ulcer disease, cirrhosis of the liver, hypothyroidism, or porphyria.

Possible Side Effects (natural, expected, and unavoidable drug actions)
If drug dose is excessive or food intake is delayed or inadequate, abnormally low blood sugar (hypoglycemia) will occur.

▷ **Possible Adverse Effects** (unusual, unexpected, and infrequent reactions)
If any of the following develop, consult your physician promptly for guidance.
Mild Adverse Effects
Allergic Reactions: Skin rash, hives, itching, drug fever (see Glossary).
Headache, ringing in the ears, weakness—infrequent.
Indigestion, heartburn, nausea, vomiting—infrequent.

Serious Adverse Effects

Allergic Reactions: Hepatitis with jaundice (see Glossary).

Idiosyncratic Reactions: Hemolytic anemia (see Glossary); disulfiramlike reaction with concurrent use of alcohol (see Glossary)—infrequent with this drug.

Seizures—case reports.

Low blood sodium (SIADH), porphyria, or urinary tract stones (urolithiasis)—case reports.

Disulfiramlike reaction—possible if taken with alcohol.

Bone marrow depression (see Glossary): fatigue, fever, abnormal bleeding or bruising—case reports.

Abnormally low thyroid gland function (hypothyroidism)—case reports.

Increased risk of cardiovascular death versus management by diet or insulin (based on a single study).

▷ **Possible Effects on Sexual Function**

None reported.

▷ **Adverse Effects That May Mimic Natural Diseases or Disorders**

Liver reactions may suggest viral hepatitis.

Natural Diseases or Disorders That May Be Activated by This Drug

Acute intermittent porphyria (see Glossary).

Possible Effects on Laboratory Tests

Complete blood cell counts: decreased red cells, hemoglobin, white cells, and platelets.

Blood glucose level: decreased.

Liver function tests: increased enzymes (ALT/GPT, AST/GOT, alkaline phosphatase) or bilirubin.

CAUTION

1. This drug is only one part of the total program for the management of your diabetes. It is not a substitute for a properly prescribed diet and regular exercise.

2. Over a period of time (usually several months), this drug may lose its effectiveness in controlling blood sugar levels. Periodic follow-up examinations are needed to monitor response to drug treatment.

Precautions for Use

By Infants and Children: This drug is not effective in type I (juvenile, growth-onset) insulin-dependent diabetes.

By Those Over 60 Years of Age: This drug should be used with caution in this age group. Start treatment with 500 mg/day; increase dosage cautiously and monitor closely to prevent hypoglycemic reactions. Repeated episodes of hypoglycemia in the elderly can cause brain damage.

▷ **Advisability of Use During Pregnancy**

Pregnancy Category: C. See Pregnancy Risk Categories at the back of this book.

Animal studies: Ocular and bone birth defects reported in rat studies.

Human studies: Adequate studies of pregnant women are not available.

Because uncontrolled blood sugar levels during pregnancy are associated with a higher incidence of birth defects, many experts recommend that insulin (instead of an oral agent) be used as necessary to control diabetes during the entire pregnancy.

Use of this drug during pregnancy is not recommended by the manufacturer.

Advisability of Use If Breast-Feeding
Presence of this drug in breast milk: Yes.
Avoid drug or refrain from nursing.

Habit-Forming Potential: None.

Effects of Overdosage: Symptoms of mild to severe hypoglycemia: headache, light-headedness, faintness, nervousness, confusion, tremor, sweating, heart palpitation, weakness, hunger, nausea, vomiting, stupor progressing to coma.

Possible Effects of Long-Term Use: Reduced function of the thyroid gland (hypothyroidism). Reports of increased frequency and severity of heart and blood vessel diseases associated with long-term use of this class of drugs are highly controversial and inconclusive. A direct cause-and-effect relationship (see Glossary) is tenuous. Ask your physician for guidance.

Suggested Periodic Examinations While Taking This Drug (at physician's discretion)
Complete blood cell counts, liver function tests, thyroid function tests, periodic evaluation of heart and circulatory system.

▷ **While Taking This Drug, Observe the Following**
Foods: Follow the diabetic diet prescribed by your physician.
Beverages: As directed in the diabetic diet. May be taken with milk.
▷ *Alcohol:* Use with extreme caution. Alcohol can exaggerate this drug's hypoglycemic effect. This drug infrequently causes a marked intolerance of alcohol resulting in a disulfiramlike reaction (see Glossary): facial flushing, sweating, palpitation.
Tobacco Smoking: Decreased tolbutamide blood levels are found in smokers. I advise everyone to quit smoking.
▷ *Other Drugs*
The following drugs may *increase* the effects of tolbutamide
• acarbose (Precose).
• aspirin and other salicylates.
• chloramphenicol (Chloromycetin).
• cimetidine (Tagamet).
• cisapride (Propulsid).
• clofibrate (Atromid-S).
• cotrimoxazole (Bactrim, others).
• fenfluramine (Pondimin).
• fluconazole (Diflucan).
• itraconazole (Sporanox).
• ketoconazole (Nizoral).
• monoamine oxidase (MAO) type A inhibitors (see Drug Classes).
• phenylbutazone (Butazolidin).
• ranitidine (Zantac).
• sulfonamide drugs (see Drug Classes).
• valproic acid (Depakene).
The following drugs may *decrease* the effects of tolbutamide
• beta-blocker drugs (see Drug Classes).
• bumetanide (Bumex).
• corticosteroids (see Adrenocortical Steroids in Drug Classes).
• diazoxide (Proglycem).
• ethacrynic acid (Edecrin).

- furosemide (Lasix).
- phenytoin (Dilantin).
- rifampin (Rifadin, Rimactane).
- thiazide diuretics (see Drug Classes).
- thyroid hormones (see Drug Classes).

Tolbutamide *taken concurrently* with

- colestipol (Colestid) can result in decreased colestipol response.
- digoxin may result in increased risk of digoxin toxicity.
- insulin will result in additive lowering of the blood sugar.
- sulfonamides (see Drug Classes) may result in a greater than expected effect of tolbutamide. Caution against hypoglycemia is advised, along with consideration for lower tolbutamide doses while the medicines are combined.

▷ *Driving, Hazardous Activities:* Regulate your dosage schedule, eating schedule, and physical activities very carefully to prevent hypoglycemia. Be able to recognize the early symptoms of hypoglycemia so you can avoid hazardous activities and take corrective measures.

Aviation Note: Diabetes *is a disqualification* for piloting. Consult a designated Aviation Medical Examiner.

Exposure to Sun: Use caution—some drugs of this class can cause photosensitivity (see Glossary).

Occurrence of Unrelated Illness: Acute infections, illnesses causing vomiting or diarrhea, serious injuries, and surgical procedures can interfere with diabetic control and may require insulin. If any of these conditions occur, call your doctor promptly.

Discontinuation: Because of the possibility of secondary failure, it is advisable to evaluate the continued benefit of this drug every 6 months.

TOLMETIN (TOHL met in)

See the new acetic acids (nonsteroidal anti-inflammatory drugs) profile for further information.

TRAMADOL (TRAM ah doll

Introduced: 1996   **Class:** Analgesic   **Prescription:** USA: Yes   **Controlled Drug:** USA: Yes; Canada: No   **Available as Generic:** USA: No; Canada: No

Brand Name: Ultram

BENEFITS versus RISKS	
Possible Benefits	*Possible Risks*
EFFECTIVE TREATMENT OF PAIN	DROWSINESS
MINIMAL SIDE EFFECTS VERSUS	May decrease the seizure threshold
MORPHINE	Constipation

▷ **Principal Uses**

As a Single Drug Product: Uses currently included in FDA-approved labeling: Used to provide symptomatic relief in all types of pain.

Other (unlabeled) generally accepted uses: May have a role in pain where depression is also a therapeutic problem.

How This Drug Works: It is thought that this drug increases the availability of the nerve impulse transmitter serotonin within certain brain centers and thereby relieves the symptoms of emotional depression.

Available Dosage Forms and Strengths

Tablets — 50 mg

▷ **Usual Adult Dosage Range:**   50 to 100 mg every 4 to 6 hours. Most patients respond to 150 to 300 mg daily.

The total daily dosage should not exceed 400 mg. German data uses 5.6 mg per kg of body mass per day as a maximum for those over 18 years of age. **Note: Actual dosage and administration schedule must be determined for each patient individually.**

Conditions Requiring Dosing Adjustments

Liver Function: Patients with cirrhosis should be closely watched for adverse effects and may take only 50 mg every 12 hours.

Kidney Function: In patients with creatinine clearances less than 30 ml/min, the usual dose is taken every 12 hours and the daily maximum is 200 mg.

▷ **Dosing Instructions:**   May be taken without regard to meals. The tablet may be crushed for administration. If excessive drowsiness or dizziness occurs, call your doctor.

Usual Duration of Use: Peak effect usually happens in half an hour. Use on a regular schedule depends on the condition being treated. Many chronic pain syndromes are treated with combinations of medicines. Long-term use requires supervision and periodic evaluation by your physician.

▷ **This Drug Should Not Be Taken If**
- you have had an allergic reaction to it previously.
- you are allergic to codeine or similar compounds.
- you are intoxicated by morphinelike drugs or alcohol.
- you are taking, or have taken within the last 14 days, a monoamine oxidase (MAO) inhibitor.

▷ **Inform Your Physician Before Taking This Drug If**
- you have a history of seizures or take medicines that may make seizures more likely.
- you have a history of alcoholism, epilepsy, narcotic addiction, or thyroid gland problems.
- you are prone to constipation.
- you have impaired liver or kidney function.
- you are pregnant or breast-feeding your infant.
- you plan to have surgery under general anesthesia in the near future.

Possible Side Effects (natural, expected, and unavoidable drug actions)

Drowsiness, light-headedness, blurred vision, dry mouth, constipation—infrequent to frequent.

▷ **Possible Adverse Effects** (unusual, unexpected, and infrequent reactions)

If any of the following develop, consult your physician promptly for guidance.

Mild Adverse Effects

Allergic Reactions: Skin rash.

Rapid heart rate, palpitations—case reports.

Nausea, vomiting, diarrhea—infrequent to frequent.

Urinary retention—possible.

Serious Adverse Effects

Allergic Reactions: Anaphylaxis—case reports.

Behavioral effects: confusion, hallucinations—case reports.

Seizures—increased risk, especially in those with seizure disorders.

Lowered blood pressure or breathing rate (respiration)—possible and dose related.

▷ **Possible Effects on Sexual Function**

Decreased male or female libido—possible.

Possible Effects on Laboratory Tests

Liver enzymes: increased.

CAUTION

1. If you experience a significant degree of mouth dryness while using this drug, consult your dentist regarding the risk of gum erosion or tooth decay. Ask for guidance in ways to keep the mouth comfortably moist.

2. If you have breathing problems (such as chronic obstructive pulmonary disease [COPD]), you may be at greater risk for respiratory depression.

3. DO NOT take this medicine if you are allergic to codeine (more likely to have a serious reaction).

Precautions for Use

By Infants and Children: Safety and effectiveness for use by those under 16 years of age have not been established.

By Those Over 60 Years of Age: During the first 2 weeks of treatment, observe for the confusion or disorientation. Be aware of possible unsteadiness and in-coordination that may predispose to falling. This drug may enhance prostatism (see Glossary).

▷ **Advisability of Use During Pregnancy**

Pregnancy Category: C. See Pregnancy Risk Categories at the back of this book.

Animal studies: Fetal deaths and birth defects reported at doses 3 to 15 times the human dose.

Human studies: Adequate studies of pregnant women are not available.

Avoid this drug completely during the first 3 months. Use otherwise only if clearly needed. Ask your physician for guidance.

Advisability of Use If Breast-Feeding

Presence of this drug in breast milk: Yes.

Avoid drug or refrain from nursing.

Habit-Forming Potential: May cause psychological or physical dependence.

Effects of Overdosage: Marked drowsiness, weakness, confusion, tremors, stupor, coma, possible seizures.

Possible Effects of Long-Term Use: May increase likelihood of dependence.

Suggested Periodic Examinations While Taking This Drug (at physician's discretion)

Heart rate and blood pressure, bowel and bladder status, evaluation for tremor or hallucination. Liver function tests.

▷ **While Taking This Drug, Observe the Following**

Foods: No restrictions.

Beverages: No restrictions. May be taken with milk.

▷ *Alcohol:* Avoid completely. This drug can increase markedly the intoxicating effects of alcohol and accentuate its depressant action on brain functions.

Tobacco Smoking: No interactions expected, but I advise everyone to quit smoking.

▷ *Other Drugs*

Tramadol may *increase* the effects of

- antihypertensive drugs and cause excessive lowering of blood pressure; dosage adjustments may be necessary.
- drugs with sedative effects and cause excessive sedation (see Antihistamines, Opioids, Antianxiety drugs, etc., in Drug Classes).
- tricyclic antidepressants (see Drug Classes) in leading to seizures.

Tramadol *taken concurrently* with

- clonidine will lessen clonidine's therapeutic effect.
- digoxin (Lanoxin) may lead to digoxin toxicity. DO NOT combine.
- fluoxetine (Prozac) may result in an increased seizure risk.
- fluvoxamine (Luvox) may result in an increased seizure risk.
- monoamine oxidase (MAO) inhibitors (see Drug Classes) may result in undesirable side effects.
- other drugs that cause central nervous system depression (see Benzodiazepines, Opioids, and Tranquilizers in Drug Classes) may have additive effects.
- other drugs that increase seizure risks may have additive effects.
- some phenothiazines (see Drug Classes) may result in excessively lowered blood pressure.
- ritonavir (Norvir) and perhaps other protease inhibitors (see Drug Classes) may lead to toxicity.

▷ *Driving, Hazardous Activities:* This drug may cause dizziness or drowsiness. Restrict activities as necessary.

Aviation Note: The use of this drug *is a disqualification* for piloting. Consult a designated Aviation Medical Examiner.

Exposure to Sun: No restrictions.

Discontinuation: It is advisable to discontinue this drug gradually. Ask your physician for guidance in dosage reduction over an appropriate period of time.

TRAZODONE (TRAZ oh dohn)

Introduced: 1967   **Class:** Antidepressants   **Prescription:** USA: Yes
Controlled Drug: USA: No; Canada: No   **Available as Generic:** USA: Yes; Canada: No

Brand Names: Desyrel, ✦Desyrel Dividose, Trialodine

BENEFITS versus RISKS	
Possible Benefits	*Possible Risks*
EFFECTIVE TREATMENT IN ALL TYPES OF DEPRESSIVE ILLNESS	Adverse behavioral effects Potential for causing heart rhythm disorders in people with heart disease

▷ **Principal Uses**

    As a Single Drug Product: Uses currently included in FDA-approved labeling: Used to provide symptomatic relief in all types of depression, with or without anxiety or agitation.

        Other (unlabeled) generally accepted uses: (1) May have a role in reducing the symptoms of agoraphobia; (2) may help drug-induced (such as MAO inhibitors) insomnia; (3) can have a role in combination therapy of some pain syndromes; (4) may be of help in essential tremor; (5) can ease bouts of repetitive screaming.

How This Drug Works: It is thought that this drug increases the availability of the nerve impulse transmitter serotonin within certain brain centers and thereby relieves the symptoms of emotional depression.

Available Dosage Forms and Strengths

    Tablets — 50 mg, 100 mg, 150 mg, 300 mg

▷ **Usual Adult Dosage Range:**   Initially 50 mg three times daily. The dose may be increased by 50 mg daily at intervals of 3 or 4 days, as needed and tolerated. The total daily dosage should not exceed 400 mg. **Note: Actual dosage and administration schedule must be determined for each patient individually.**

Conditions Requiring Dosing Adjustments

    Liver Function: Blood levels should be obtained to guide dosing. This drug can be a rare cause of liver damage, and patients should be followed closely.

    Kidney Function: Metabolites are removed by the kidneys; however, dosage adjustment in renal compromise is not defined.

▷ **Dosing Instructions:**   This drug is best taken with food to improve absorption. The tablet may be crushed for administration. If excessive drowsiness or dizziness occurs, it is advisable to take a larger portion of the total daily dose at bedtime and divide the remaining amount into two or three smaller doses to be taken during the day.

Usual Duration of Use: Use on a regular schedule for 2 to 4 weeks usually determines effectiveness in relieving the symptoms of depression. Long-term use (weeks to months) requires supervision and periodic evaluation by your physician.

▷ **This Drug Should Not Be Taken If**

- you have had an allergic reaction to it previously.
- you are recovering from a recent heart attack (myocardial infarction).
- you have carcinoid syndrome.
- you are taking, or have taken within the past 14 days, any monoamine oxidase (MAO) type A inhibitor (see Drug Classes).

▷ **Inform Your Physician Before Taking This Drug If**

- you have a history of alcoholism, epilepsy, or heart disease (especially heart rhythm disorders).
- you have impaired liver or kidney function.
- you are pregnant or breast-feeding your infant.
- you are taking any antihypertensive drugs.
- you plan to have surgery under general anesthesia in the near future.

Possible Side Effects (natural, expected, and unavoidable drug actions)

    Drowsiness, light-headedness, blurred vision, weight gain, dry mouth, constipation.

▷ **Possible Adverse Effects** (unusual, unexpected, and infrequent reactions)
  If any of the following develop, consult your physician promptly for guidance.
  Mild Adverse Effects
    Allergic Reactions: Skin rash.
    Headache, dizziness, fatigue, impaired concentration, nervousness, tremors—infrequent.
    Rapid heart rate, palpitations—rare.
    Peculiar taste, stomach discomfort, nausea, vomiting, diarrhea—infrequent.
    Urinary retention—possible.
    Cavities (dental caries)—case reports.
    Muscular aches and pains—infrequent.
  Serious Adverse Effects
    Allergic Reactions: Serious skin rashes (erythema multiforme).
    Behavioral effects: confusion, anger, hostility, delusions, hallucinations, nightmares—case reports.
    Irregular heart rhythms, low blood pressure, fainting—case reports.
    Erythema multiforme—case reports.
    Seizures—rare.
    Liver toxicity—possible.

▷ **Possible Effects on Sexual Function**
    Decreased male libido; increased female libido.
    Inhibited ejaculation, impotence, priapism (see Glossary), or altered timing and pattern of menstruation—case reports.

Possible Effects on Laboratory Tests
    Liver enzymes: increased.

CAUTION
    1. If you experience a significant degree of mouth dryness while using this drug, consult your dentist regarding the risk of gum erosion or tooth decay. Ask for guidance in ways to keep the mouth comfortably moist.
    2. It is advisable to withhold this drug if electroconvulsive therapy (ECT) is to be used to treat your depression.

Precautions for Use
    By Infants and Children: Safety and effectiveness for use by those under 18 years of age have not been established.
    By Those Over 60 Years of Age: During the first 2 weeks of treatment, observe for the development of restlessness, agitation, excitement, forgetfulness, confusion, or disorientation. Be aware of possible unsteadiness and incoordination that may predispose to falling. This drug may enhance prostatism (see Glossary).

▷ **Advisability of Use During Pregnancy**
    Pregnancy Category: C. See Pregnancy Risk Categories at the back of this book.
    Animal studies: Fetal deaths and birth defects reported.
    Human studies: Adequate studies of pregnant women are not available.
    Avoid this drug completely during the first 3 months. Use otherwise only if clearly needed. Ask your physician for guidance.

Advisability of Use If Breast-Feeding
    Presence of this drug in breast milk: Yes.
    Avoid drug or refrain from nursing.

Habit-Forming Potential: None.

Effects of Overdosage: Marked drowsiness, confusion, tremors, low blood pressure, rapid heart rate, stupor, coma, or seizures.

Possible Effects of Long-Term Use: None reported.

Suggested Periodic Examinations While Taking This Drug (at physician's discretion)
   Complete blood cell counts. (This drug may cause slight reductions in white blood cell counts. This should be monitored closely if infection, sore throat, or fever develops.)
   Serial blood pressure readings and electrocardiograms.

▷ **While Taking This Drug, Observe the Following**
   Foods: No restrictions.
   Beverages: No restrictions. May be taken with milk.
▷   *Alcohol:* Avoid completely. This drug can increase markedly the intoxicating effects of alcohol and accentuate its depressant action on brain functions.
   Tobacco Smoking: No interactions expected, but I advise everyone to quit smoking.
▷   *Other Drugs*
      Trazodone may ***increase*** the effects of
      • antihypertensive drugs, and cause excessive lowering of blood pressure; dosage adjustments may be necessary.
      • drugs with sedative effects, and cause excessive sedation.
      • phenytoin (Dilantin), by raising its blood level; observe for phenytoin toxicity.
      Trazodone ***taken concurrently*** with
      • clonidine (Catapres) will lessen the therapeutic effect of clonidine.
      • fluoxetine (Prozac) may result in an increased trazodone level and toxicity.
      • monoamine oxidase (MAO) inhibitors (see Drug Classes) may result in undesirable side effects in some patients, and beneficial therapeutic effects in others.
      • other drugs that cause central nervous system depression (see Benzodiazepines, Opioids, and Tranquilizers in Drug Classes) may have additive effects.
      • ritonavir (Norvir) and perhaps other protease inhibitors (see Drug Classes) may lead to toxicity.
      • some phenothiazines (see Drug Classes) may result in excessively lowered blood pressure.
      • warfarin (Coumadin) may result in decreased therapeutic benefits of warfarin. INR (prothrombin time or protime) should be checked three times a week while combined warfarin and trazodone therapy are undertaken.
▷   *Driving, Hazardous Activities:* This drug may cause dizziness or drowsiness. Restrict activities as necessary.
   Aviation Note: The use of this drug ***is a disqualification*** for piloting. Consult a designated Aviation Medical Examiner.
   Exposure to Sun: No restrictions.
   Discontinuation: It is advisable to discontinue this drug gradually. Ask your physician for guidance in dosage reduction over an appropriate period of time.

TRIAMCINOLONE (tri am SIN oh lohn)

Introduced: 1985 **Class:** Antiasthmatic, cortisonelike drugs **Prescription:** USA: Yes **Controlled Drug:** USA: No; Canada: No **Available as Generic:** Yes

Brand Name: Amcort, Aristocort, Aristocort R, Aristoform D, ✦Aristospan, Articulose LA, ✦Aureocort, Azmacort, Cenocort, Cenocort Forte, Flutex, ✦Kenacomb, Kenacort, Kenaject, Kenalog, Kenalog H, Kenalog IN, Kenalone, Mycogen II, Mycomar, Mytrex [CD], Nasacort, Nasacort AQ, SK-Triamcinolone, TAC-40, TAC-D, Triacet, ✦Triaderm Mild, ✦Triaderm Regular, Triam-A, Triam-Forte, Triamolone 40, Triderm, Tri-Kort, Trilog, Tristoject, ✦Viaderm-K.C.

BENEFITS versus RISKS

Possible Benefits	*Possible Risks*
EFFECTIVE CONTROL OF SEVERE, CHRONIC BRONCHIAL ASTHMA	Yeast infections of mouth and throat
EFFECTIVE SUPPRESSION OF A VARIETY OF INFLAMMATORY DISORDERS	Suppression of normal cortisone production
POSSIBLE REDUCTION IN SYSTEMIC STEROID USE	Euphoria and psychotic episodes
EFFECTIVE TREATMENT OF SEASONAL OR PERENNIAL ALLERGIC RHINITIS IN ADULTS AND CHILDREN	Cushing's syndrome ("moon face," obesity, and "buffalo hump")
	Muscle wasting (with long-term use)
	Osteoporosis (with long-term use)

▷ **Principal Uses**

As a Single Drug Product: Uses currently included in FDA-approved labeling: (1) Inhaler form is used to treat chronic bronchial asthma in people who require cortisonelike drugs for asthma control. This is better than cortisone taken by mouth (swallowed) or injection because it works more locally on the respiratory tract, not requiring systemic distribution. This helps prevent some serious adverse effects that usually result from the long-term use of cortisone taken for systemic effects; (2) tablet form can be used in a variety of inflammatory disorders; (3) tablet form is used to ease drug reactions; (4) used as part of combination treatment of acute lymphocytic leukemia in children; (5) used in autoimmune hemolytic anemia; (6) nasal inhaler form helps adults and children with symptoms of seasonal or perennial allergic rhinitis.

Other (unlabeled) generally accepted uses: (1) May have a role in postherpetic nerve pain (neuralgia); (2) corticosteroids may be of use with *Pneumocystis carinii* pneumonia in extreme cases where conventional therapy has not worked; (3) may help Guillain-Barre syndrome; (4) can help myasthenia gravis; (5) short-term therapy of psoriasis.

How This Drug Works: By increasing the amount of cyclic AMP in appropriate tissues, this drug may thereby increase the concentration of epinephrine, which is an effective bronchodilator and antiasthmatic. Additional benefit is due to the drug's ability to reduce local allergic reaction and inflammation in the lining tissues of the respiratory tract.

Available Dosage Forms and Strengths

Inhalation aerosol — 0.1 mg per metered spray

Tablets — 1 mg, 2 mg, 4 mg, 8 mg

Topical cream — 0.1%, 0.25%, 0.5%

Topical ointment — 0.25%, 0.5%

▷ **Recommended Dosage Ranges** (Actual dosage and administration schedule must be determined for each patient individually.)

Infants and Children: Up to 6 years of age: Dosage not established.

6 to 12 years of age: 0.1 to 0.2 mg (one or two metered sprays) three or four times a day. Adjust dosage as needed and tolerated. Limit total daily dosage to 1.2 mg (12 metered sprays).

12 to 60 Years of Age: Initially 0.2 mg (two metered sprays) three or four times a day.

For severe asthma: 1.2 to 1.6 mg (12 to 16 metered sprays) per day, in divided doses. Adjust dosage as needed and tolerated. It is usually used as two inhalations three to four times a day. Results are better when used in this fashion versus on an as-needed basis. Limit total daily dose to 1.6 mg (16 metered sprays).

Nasacort AQ and Nasacort may prove effective with a starting dose of 220 mcg per day.

Tablets: 4 to 48 mg daily for inflammatory conditions.

Cream: 0.025% is usually applied to the affected area two to four times a day.

Over 60 Years of Age: Same as 12 to 60 years of age.

Conditions Requiring Dosing Adjustments

Liver Function: This drug is metabolized in the liver. Dosing changes in liver compromise are not defined.

Kidney Function: Dosing adjustments do not appear warranted for patients with compromised kidneys.

▷ **Dosing Instructions:** Inhalation form: May be used as needed without regard to eating. Shake the container well before using. Carefully follow the printed patient instructions provided with the unit. Rinse the mouth and throat (gargle) with water thoroughly after each inhalation; do not swallow the rinse water. The Nasacort AQ form is water based for treatment of allergic rhinitis and does not contain chlorofluorocarbon propellants.

Oral tablets: May cause stomach upset, and can be taken with meals or snacks.

Usual Duration of Use: Use on a regular schedule for 1 to 2 weeks usually determines effectiveness in controlling severe, chronic asthma. Long-term use requires the supervision and guidance of the physician.

▷ **This Drug Should Not Be Taken If**

- you have had an allergic reaction to it previously.
- you are having severe acute asthma or status asthmaticus that requires immediate relief.
- you have a form of nonallergic bronchitis with asthmatic features.
- you have a systemic fungal infection.

▷ **Inform Your Physician Before Taking This Drug If**

- you are now taking, or have recently taken, any cortisone-related drug (including ACTH by injection) for any reason (see Drug Classes).

- you have a history of tuberculosis of the lungs.
- you have chronic bronchitis or bronchiectasis.
- you have diabetes, glaucoma, myasthenia gravis, or peptic ulcer disease.
- you have had unexpected surgery (may delay wound healing).
- you have an underactive thyroid (hypothyroidism).
- you think you may have an active infection of any kind, especially a respiratory infection.
- you are taking any of the following drugs: warfarin, oral antidiabetic drugs, insulin, or digoxin.

Possible Side Effects (natural, expected, and unavoidable drug actions)
Yeast infections (thrush) of the mouth and throat. Irritation of mouth, tongue, or throat. May cause euphoria, manic-depressive illness, or paranoid states with long-term oral use. Can cause a syndrome (Cushing's) characterized by "moon face," obesity, and poorly controlled high blood pressure.

▷ **Possible Adverse Effects** (unusual, unexpected, and infrequent reactions)
If any of the following develop, consult your physician promptly for guidance.
Mild Adverse Effects
Allergic Reactions: Skin rash.
Easy bruising (ecchymosis)—infrequent.
Swelling of face, hoarseness, voice change, cough—possible to infrequent.
Serious Adverse Effects
Allergic Reactions—rare.
Bronchospasm, asthmatic wheezing—rare.
Can be a cause of high blood pressure with long-term use.
Edema or swelling, especially with kidney or heart vessel disease—infrequent.
Decrease of circulating T lymphocytes—possible.
Drug-induced seizures, ulcer development, pancreatitis, or osteoporosis—possible to infrequent.
Electrolyte disturbances (decreased blood potassium)—infrequent..
Excessive thyroid activity (hyperthyroidism).
Cataract formation or muscle wasting has occurred with long-term use.
Elevated blood sugar—possible.
Toxic megacolon—rare.
Toxic psychosis has occurred with other steroids.
Author's Note: The inhalation form and topical forms do not have many of the systemic side effects of the oral form.

▷ **Possible Effects on Sexual Function:**   None reported.

Natural Diseases or Disorders That May Be Activated by This Drug
Latent amebiasis, congestive heart failure, diabetes, glaucoma, hypertension, myasthenia gravis, peptic ulcer.
Cortisone-related drugs (used by inhalation) that produce systemic effects can impair immunity and lead to reactivation of "healed" or quiescent tuberculosis of the lungs. Individuals with a history of tuberculosis should be observed closely during use of cortisonelike drugs by inhalation.

Possible Effects on Laboratory Tests

Blood calcium levels: decreased.

Blood total cholesterol levels: increased.

Blood glucose or sodium levels: increased.

Blood potassium levels: decreased.

CAUTION

1. This drug should not be relied upon for the immediate relief of acute asthma.
2. If you were using any cortisone-related drugs for treatment of your asthma *before* transferring to this inhaler drug, it may be necessary to resume the former cortisone-related drug if you experience injury or infection of any kind, or if you require surgery. Tell your doctor about prior use of cortisone-related drugs taken either by mouth or injection.
3. If you experience a return of severe asthma while using this drug, call your doctor immediately so that additional supportive treatment with cortisone-related drugs by mouth or injection can be provided.
4. Carry a card noting (if applicable) that you have used cortisone-related drugs within the past year. During periods of stress resumption of cortisone treatment may be required.
5. Approximately 5 to 10 minutes should separate the inhalation of bronchodilators such as albuterol, epinephrine, pirbuterol, etc. (which should be used first), and the inhalation of this drug. This sequence will permit greater penetration of triamcinolone into the bronchial tubes. This will also reduce the possibility of adverse effects from the propellants used in the two inhalers.

Precautions for Use

By Infants and Children: Safety and effectiveness for use of the oral inhaler by those under 6 years of age have not been established. To ensure adequate penetration of the drug and obtain maximal benefit, the use of a spacer device is recommended for inhalation therapy in children.

By Those Over 60 Years of Age: Individuals with chronic bronchitis or bronchiectasis should be observed closely for the development of lung infections.

▷ **Advisability of Use During Pregnancy**

Pregnancy Category: C. See Pregnancy Risk Categories at the back of this book.

Animal studies: Rat and rabbit studies reveal significant toxic effects on the embryo and fetus and multiple birth defects due to this drug.

Human studies: Adequate studies of pregnant women are not available.

Limit use to very serious illness for which no satisfactory treatment alternatives are available.

Advisability of Use If Breast-Feeding

Presence of this drug in breast milk: Unknown.

Ask your doctor for guidance.

Habit-Forming Potential: With recommended dosage, a state of functional dependence (see Glossary) is not likely to develop.

Effects of Overdosage: Indications of cortisone excess (due to systemic absorption)—fluid retention, flushing of the face, stomach irritation, nervousness.

Possible Effects of Long-Term Use: Significant suppression of normal cortisone production.

Suggested Periodic Examinations While Taking This Drug (at physician's discretion)

Inspection of mouth and throat for evidence of yeast infection.

Assessment of the status of adrenal gland function (cortisone production).

X-ray examination of the lungs of individuals with a prior history of tuberculosis.

Bone mineral density tests to assess osteoporosis.

▷ **While Taking This Drug, Observe the Following**

Foods: No specific restrictions beyond those advised by your physician.

Beverages: No specific restrictions.

▷ *Alcohol:* No interactions expected.

Tobacco Smoking: No interactions expected, but I advise everyone to quit smoking.

▷ *Other Drugs*

The following drugs may *increase* the effects of triamcinolone

- inhalant bronchodilators—albuterol, bitolterol, epinephrine, pirbuterol, etc.
- oral bronchodilators—aminophylline, ephedrine, terbutaline, theophylline, etc.

The following drugs may *decrease* the effects of triamcinolone

- carbamazepine (Tegretol)—increases triamcinolone metabolism and may result in decreased effectiveness.
- phenytoin (Dilantin)—increases triamcinolone metabolism and may result in decreased effectiveness.
- primidone (Mysoline)—increases steroid metabolism and may result in decreased triamcinolone metabolism.
- rifampin (Rifadin).

Triamcinolone *taken concurrently* with

- amphotericin B (Abelcet) may lead to additive potassium loss.
- aspirin may result in blunting of the therapeutic benefits of aspirin.
- cyclosporine (Sandimmune) may result in changes in the blood levels of both medicines.
- oral hypoglycemic agents (see Oral Antidiabetic Drugs in Drug Classes) may result in loss of glucose control.
- thiazide diuretics (see Drug Classes) can result in loss of glucose control.
- vaccines (flu, rabies, others) may result in a less than optimal vaccine response.
- warfarin (Coumadin) can result in variation in the degree of anticoagulation. Increased INR (prothrombin time or protime) testing is indicated.

▷ *Driving, Hazardous Activities:* No restrictions.

Aviation Note: The use of this drug and the disorder for which this drug is prescribed *may be disqualifications* for piloting. Consult a designated Aviation Medical Examiner.

Exposure to Sun: No restrictions.

Occurrence of Unrelated Illness: Acute infections, serious injuries, and surgical procedures can create an urgent need for the administration of additional supportive cortisone-related drugs given by mouth and/or injection. Notify your physician immediately in the event of new illness or injury of any kind.

Discontinuation: If the regular use of this drug has made it possible to reduce or stop doses of cortisonelike drugs by mouth, *do not* discontinue this drug abruptly. Call your doctor if you must stop this drug for any reason. Restarting cortisone preparations may be required.

Special Storage Instructions: Store at room temperature. Avoid exposure to temperatures above 120 degrees F (49 degrees C). Do not store or use this inhaler near heat or open flame.

TRIAMTERENE (tri AM ter een)

Introduced: 1964   **Class:** Diuretic   **Prescription:** USA: Yes   **Controlled Drug:** USA: No; Canada: No   **Available as Generic:** Yes

Brand Names: ✦Apo-Triazide [CD], Dyazide [CD], Dyrenium, Maxzide [CD], Maxzide-25 [CD], ✦Novo-Triamzide [CD], ✦Nu-Triazide

BENEFITS versus RISKS	
Possible Benefits	*Possible Risks*
EFFECTIVE PREVENTION OF POTASSIUM LOSS when used adjunctively with other diuretics	ABNORMALLY HIGH BLOOD POTASSIUM LEVEL with excessive use
EFFECTIVE DIURETIC IN REFRACTORY CASES OF FLUID RETENTION when used adjunctively with other diuretics	Possible blood cell disorders: megaloblastic anemia, abnormally low white blood cell and platelet counts
	Possible kidney stone formation

▷ **Principal Uses**

As a Single Drug Product: Uses currently included in FDA-approved labeling: (1) Used as part of combination therapy of congestive heart failure or liver and kidney disorders accompanied by excessive fluid retention (edema); (2) used in conjunction with other measures to treat high blood pressure. It is used primarily in situations where it is advisable to prevent loss of potassium from the body.

Other (unlabeled) generally accepted uses: None.

As a Combination Drug Product [CD]: This drug is available in combination with hydrochlorothiazide, a different kind of diuretic that promotes the loss of potassium from the body. Triamterene is used in this combination to counteract the potassium-wasting effect of the thiazide diuretic.

How This Drug Works: By inhibiting the enzyme system that initiates the sodium–potassium exchange process, this drug prevents the reabsorption of sodium and the excretion of potassium by the kidney. Thus the drug promotes the excretion of sodium (and water with it) and the retention of potassium.

Available Dosage Forms and Strengths

Capsules — 50 mg, 100 mg

▷ **Usual Adult Dosage Range:** Hypertension: Initially 50 to 100 mg twice daily. The dose is then adjusted according to individual response. The usual maintenance dose is 100 to 200 mg daily, divided into two doses. The total daily dosage should not exceed 300 mg. **Note: Actual dosage and administration schedule must be determined for each patient individually.**

Conditions Requiring Dosing Adjustments

Liver Function: The dose should be reduced and used with extreme caution by patients with severe liver disease.

Kidney Function: Patients with mild to moderate kidney failure may take the usual dose every 12 hours. In severe or progressive kidney failure, this medication should **not** be used.

▷ **Dosing Instructions:**   May be taken with or following meals to promote absorption of the drug and reduce stomach irritation. The capsule may be opened for administration. Intermittent or alternate-day use is recommended to minimize the possibility of sodium and potassium imbalance.

Usual Duration of Use: Use on a regular schedule for 3 to 5 days usually determines effectiveness in clearing edema, and for 2 to 3 weeks to determine its effect on hypertension. Long-term use (months to years) requires physician supervision and periodic evaluation.

▷ **This Drug Should Not Be Taken If**
- you have had an allergic reaction to it previously.
- you have severely impaired liver or kidney function.
- your kidney disease is progressive or you have a creatinine clearance greater than 2.5 mg/dl (ask your doctor).
- your blood potassium level is significantly elevated (ask your doctor).

▷ **Inform Your Physician Before Taking This Drug If**
- you have a history of liver or kidney disease.
- you have diabetes or gout.
- you are taking any of the following: antihypertensives, a digitalis preparation, another diuretic, lithium, or a potassium preparation.
- you have a history of glucose-6-phosphate dehydrogenase (G6PD) deficiency (ask your doctor).
- you have a history of blood cell disorders.
- you plan to have surgery under general anesthesia in the near future.

Possible Side Effects (natural, expected, and unavoidable drug actions)

With excessive use: abnormally high blood potassium levels, abnormally low blood sodium levels, dehydration.

Blue coloration of the urine (of no significance).

▷ **Possible Adverse Effects** (unusual, unexpected, and infrequent reactions)

If any of the following develop, consult your physician promptly for guidance.

Mild Adverse Effects

Allergic Reactions: Skin rash, itching.

Headache, dizziness, unsteadiness, weakness, drowsiness, lethargy—infrequent.

Dry mouth, nausea, vomiting, diarrhea—infrequent.

Serious Adverse Effects

Allergic Reaction: Anaphylactic reaction (see Glossary).

Symptomatic potassium excess: confusion, numbness and tingling in lips and extremities, fatigue, weakness, shortness of breath, slow heart rate, low blood pressure—possible.

Blood cell disorders: megaloblastic anemia, abnormally low white blood cell count, or abnormally low blood platelet count—case reports.

Hemolytic anemia—in those with deficiency of G6PD in red cells.

Abnormal urine production (SIADH)—case reports.

Formation of kidney stones and kidney toxicity—rare.

Liver toxicity—rare.

▷ **Possible Effects on Sexual Function:**   None reported.

Possible Effects on Laboratory Tests

Complete blood cell counts: decreased red cells, hemoglobin, white cells, and platelets; increased eosinophils (allergic reaction).

Blood glucose level: increased in diabetics.

Blood lithium, potassium, or uric acid level: increased.

Kidney function tests: increased blood creatinine and urea nitrogen (BUN) levels (kidney damage).

CAUTION

1. Do not take potassium supplements or increase your intake of potassium-rich foods while taking this drug.
2. Patients who take quinidine (Quinaglute, others) may have falsely increased laboratory test results if fluorescent measurement techniques are used.
3. Do not stop this drug abruptly unless abnormally high blood levels of potassium develop.
4. Avoid liberal use of salt substitutes with potassium in them (potential causes of potassium excess).

Precautions for Use

By Infants and Children: This drug is not recommended for use in children.

By Those Over 60 Years of Age: Natural decline in kidney function may predispose to potassium retention. Watch for potassium excess: slow heart rate, irregular heart rhythms, low blood pressure, confusion, drowsiness. Excessive use of diuretics can cause harmful loss of body water (dehydration), increased viscosity of the blood and an increased tendency of the blood to clot, predisposing to stroke, heart attack, or thrombophlebitis.

▷ **Advisability of Use During Pregnancy**

Pregnancy Category: B by the manufacturer, D by one researcher. See Pregnancy Risk Categories at the back of this book.

Animal studies: No birth defects due to this drug reported.

Human studies: Adequate studies of pregnant women are not available.

This drug should not be used during pregnancy unless a very serious complication of pregnancy occurs for which this drug is significantly beneficial.

Advisability of Use If Breast-Feeding

Presence of this drug in breast milk: Yes.

Avoid drug or refrain from nursing.

Habit-Forming Potential: None.

Effects of Overdosage: Thirst, drowsiness, fatigue, nausea, vomiting, confusion, irregular heart rhythm, low blood pressure.

Possible Effects of Long-Term Use: Potassium accumulation to abnormally high blood levels.

Suggested Periodic Examinations While Taking This Drug (at physician's discretion)

Complete blood cell counts.

Measurements of blood sodium, potassium, and chloride levels.
Kidney function tests.

▷ **While Taking This Drug, Observe the Following**

Foods: Diets high in high-potassium foods (see Table 13, Section Six) may cause problems. Avoid excessive restriction of salt.

Beverages: No restrictions. May be taken with milk.

▷ *Alcohol:* Use with caution. Alcohol may enhance the drowsiness and the blood-pressure-lowering effect of this drug.

Tobacco Smoking: No interactions expected, but I advise everyone to quit smoking.

▷ *Other Drugs*

Triamterene may *increase* the effects of

• amantadine (Symmetrel).
• digoxin (Lanoxin).

Triamterene *taken concurrently* with

• captopril (Capoten) or other ACE inhibitors may cause excessively high blood potassium levels.
• histamine (H_2) blockers (see Drug Classes) may decrease triamterene absorption and its therapeutic effects.
• indomethacin (Indocin) may increase the risk of kidney damage.
• lithium may cause accumulation of lithium to toxic levels.
• NSAIDs (see Drug Classes) may blunt the blood-pressure-lowering effect of triamterene.
• potassium preparations may cause excessively high blood potassium levels.

▷ *Driving, Hazardous Activities:* This drug may cause dizziness and drowsiness. Restrict activities as necessary.

Aviation Note: The use of this drug *may be a disqualification* for piloting. Consult a designated Aviation Medical Examiner.

Exposure to Sun: Use caution—this drug may cause photosensitivity (see Glossary).

Discontinuation: With high dosage or prolonged use, it is best to slowly withdraw this drug. Sudden discontinuation may cause rebound potassium excretion and potassium deficiency. Ask your physician for guidance.

TRICHLORMETHIAZIDE (tri KLOR meth i a zide)

See the thiazide diuretics profile for further information.

TRIFLUOPERAZINE (tri flu oh PER a zeen)

Introduced: 1958   **Class:** Tranquilizer, major; phenothiazines   **Prescription:** USA: Yes   **Controlled Drug:** USA: No; Canada: No   **Available as Generic:** USA: Yes; Canada: No

Brand Names: ✚Apo-Trifluoperazine, ✚Novo-Flurazine, ✚Solazine, Stelabid [CD], Stelazine, Suprazine, ✚Terfluzine

```
┌──────────────────────────────────────────────────────────────┐
│                    BENEFITS versus RISKS                       │
│      Possible Benefits              Possible Risks             │
│  EFFECTIVE CONTROL OF ACUTE    SERIOUS TOXIC EFFECTS ON        │
│    MENTAL DISORDERS: beneficial   BRAIN with long-term use     │
│    effects on thinking, mood, and Liver damage with jaundice   │
│    behavior                         (infrequent)               │
│                                   Rare blood cell disorders: Abnormally │
│                                     low red and white blood cell and    │
│                                     platelet counts            │
└──────────────────────────────────────────────────────────────┘
```

▷ **Principal Uses**

As a Single Drug Product: Uses currently included in FDA-approved labeling: (1) Treats psychotic thinking and behavior associated with acute psychoses of unknown nature, mania, paranoid states, and acute schizophrenia. It is most effective in those who are withdrawn and apathetic and those with agitation, delusions, and hallucinations; (2) approved for treatment of anxiety disorders, but is not a drug of first choice.

Other (unlabeled) generally accepted uses: (1) May have a role in combination therapy of some kinds of chronic pain; (2) may help in combination therapy of chemotherapy-induced nausea or vomiting.

How This Drug Works: Present theory is that by inhibiting the action of dopamine, this drug acts to correct an imbalance of nerve impulse transmissions that is thought to be responsible for certain mental disorders.

Available Dosage Forms and Strengths

Concentrate — 10 mg/ml
Injection — 2 mg/ml
Tablets — 1 mg, 2 mg, 5 mg, 10 mg

▷ **Usual Adult Dosage Range:**   Nonpsychotic anxiety: Initially 1 or 2 mg twice daily. The dose may be increased by 1 or 2 mg at 3- to 4-day intervals to a maximum dose of 4 mg for patients who are not in the hospital.

For psychosis: 2 to 5 mg twice a day. The dose is then increased every 3 or 4 days as needed and tolerated. Usual dosage range is 15 to 20 mg daily. The total daily dosage should not exceed 40 mg. Some rare cases have required 100 mg per day. **Note: Actual dosage and administration schedule must be determined for each patient individually.**

Conditions Requiring Dosing Adjustments

Liver Function: This drug should be used with caution in liver compromise.
Kidney Function: Patients with compromised kidneys should be closely followed.

▷ **Dosing Instructions:**   The tablets may be crushed and taken with or following meals to reduce stomach irritation.

Usual Duration of Use: Use on a regular schedule for several weeks usually determines effectiveness in psychotic disorders. If not significantly beneficial within 6 weeks, it should be stopped. Long-term use (months to years) requires periodic physician evaluation of response, dosage adjustment, and consideration of continued need.

▷ **This Drug Should Not Be Taken If**

• you are allergic to any of the drugs bearing the brand names listed above.
• you have active liver disease.

- you have cancer of the breast.
- you have a current blood cell or bone marrow disorder.

▷ **Inform Your Physician Before Taking This Drug If**
- you are allergic or abnormally sensitive to any phenothiazine drug (see Drug Classes).
- you have impaired liver or kidney function.
- you have a history of anginal pain (this drug may worsen it).
- you have any type of seizure disorder.
- you have diabetes, glaucoma, or heart disease.
- you have a history of lupus erythematosus.
- you are taking any drug with sedative effects.
- you have had neuroleptic malignant syndrome (ask your doctor).
- you plan to have surgery under general or spinal anesthesia in the near future.

Possible Side Effects (natural, expected, and unavoidable drug actions)
> Drowsiness (usually during the first 2 weeks), orthostatic hypotension (see Glossary), blurred vision, dry mouth, nasal congestion, constipation, impaired urination.
> Pink or purple coloration of urine, of no significance.

▷ **Possible Adverse Effects** (unusual, unexpected, and infrequent reactions)
> **If any of the following develop, consult your physician promptly for guidance.**

Mild Adverse Effects
> Allergic Reactions: Skin rash, hives, low-grade fever.
> Lowering of body temperature, especially in the elderly (see Hypothermia in Glossary).
> Increased appetite and weight gain—possible.
> Dizziness, weakness, agitation, insomnia, impaired day and night vision—infrequent.

Serious Adverse Effects
> Allergic Reactions: Hepatitis with jaundice (see Glossary), severe skin reactions, anaphylactic reaction (see Glossary).
> Idiosyncratic Reactions: Neuroleptic malignant syndrome (see Glossary).
> Depression, disorientation, loss of peripheral vision—case reports.
> Serious skin disorders (Stevens-Johnson syndrome)—rare.
> Drug-induced glaucoma or abnormal eye positioning (oculogyric crisis)—case reports.
> Drug-induced porphyrias, pituitary tumors, or seizures—case reports.
> Rapid heart rate, heart rhythm disorders—possible.
> Blood cell disorders: reduction in all cellular elements of the blood (see Bone Marrow Depression in Glossary)—case reports.
> Phenothiazine-induced sudden death syndrome—case reports.
> Nervous system reactions: Parkinson-like disorders (see Glossary), severe restlessness, muscle spasms involving the face and neck, tardive dyskinesia (see Glossary)—rare to infrequent.

▷ **Possible Effects on Sexual Function**
> Altered timing and pattern of menstruation.
> Male breast enlargement and tenderness (gynecomastia).
> Female breast enlargement with milk production.
> Spontaneous male orgasm, paradoxical—one case reported. Inhibited ejacu-

lation, painful ejaculation, painful and extended erections (priapism) (see Glossary).

Delayed female orgasm—case reports.

▷ **Adverse Effects That May Mimic Natural Diseases or Disorders**

Nervous system reactions may suggest true Parkinson's disease. Liver reactions may suggest viral hepatitis.

Reactions resembling systemic lupus erythematosus may occur.

Natural Diseases or Disorders That May Be Activated by This Drug

Latent epilepsy, glaucoma, diabetes mellitus, prostatism (see Glossary).

Possible Effects on Laboratory Tests

Complete blood cell counts: decreased red cells, hemoglobin, white cells, and platelets.

Liver function tests: increased enzymes (ALT/GPT, AST/GOT, alkaline phosphatase) or bilirubin.

Urine pregnancy tests: falsely positive result with some tests.

CAUTION

1. Many over-the-counter medications (see Glossary) for allergies, colds, and coughs contain drugs that can interact unfavorably with this drug. Ask your doctor or pharmacist for help before using any such medications.
2. Antacids that contain aluminum and/or magnesium may prevent the absorption of this drug and reduce its effectiveness.
3. Obtain prompt evaluation of any change or disturbance of vision.

Precautions for Use

By Infants and Children: Use of this drug is not recommended in children under 6 years of age. Do not use this drug in the presence of symptoms suggestive of Reye syndrome (see Glossary). Children with acute infectious diseases (flu-like infections, chickenpox, measles, etc.) are more prone to develop muscular spasms of the face, back, and extremities when this drug is given.

By Those Over 60 Years of Age: Small starting doses are prudent to try to decrease risk of drowsiness, lethargy, constipation, lowering of body temperature (hypothermia), and orthostatic hypotension (see Glossary). This drug may enhance existing prostatism (see Glossary). You may also be more susceptible to Parkinson-like reactions and/or tardive dyskinesia (see discussion of these terms in Glossary). These reactions must be recognized early since they may become unresponsive to treatment and irreversible.

▷ **Advisability of Use During Pregnancy**

Pregnancy Category: C. See Pregnancy Risk Categories at the back of this book.

Animal studies: Significant birth defects reported in mouse and rat studies.

Human studies: No increase in birth defects reported in 700 exposures. Adequate studies of pregnant women are not available.

Avoid drug during the first 3 months; avoid during the final month because of possible adverse effects on the newborn infant.

Advisability of Use If Breast-Feeding

Presence of this drug in breast milk: Yes, in minute amounts.

Monitor nursing infant closely and discontinue drug or nursing if adverse effects develop.

Habit-Forming Potential: None.

Effects of Overdosage: Marked drowsiness, weakness, tremor, agitation, unsteadiness, deep sleep, coma, convulsions.

Possible Effects of Long-Term Use: Tardive dyskinesia (see Glossary).

Suggested Periodic Examinations While Taking This Drug (at physician's discretion)
> Complete blood cell counts, especially between the 4th and 10th weeks of treatment.
> Liver function tests, electrocardiograms.
> Complete eye examinations of eye structures and vision.
> Careful inspection of the tongue for early evidence of fine, involuntary, wavelike movements that could indicate the beginning of tardive dyskinesia.

▷ **While Taking This Drug, Observe the Following**
Foods: No restrictions.
Nutritional Support: A riboflavin (vitamin B_2) supplement should be taken with long-term use.
Beverages: Caffeine may slightly blunt the calming effect of this medicine. May be taken with milk.
▷ *Alcohol:* Avoid completely. Alcohol can increase the sedative action of phenothiazines and accentuate their depressant effects on brain function and blood pressure. Phenothiazines can increase the intoxicating effects of alcohol.
Tobacco Smoking: Possible reduction of drowsiness from drug, but I advise everyone to quit smoking.
Marijuana Smoking: Moderate increase in drowsiness; accentuation of orthostatic hypotension; increased risk of precipitating latent psychoses, confusing the interpretation of mental status and drug responses.
▷ *Other Drugs*
Trifluoperazine may *increase* the effects of
- all atropinelike drugs, and cause nervous system toxicity.
- all sedative drugs, especially narcotic analgesics (also see Drug Classes for Opioids and Benzodiazepines), and cause excessive sedation.

Trifluoperazine may *decrease* the effects of
- guanethidine (Ismelin, Esimil), and reduce its effectiveness in lowering blood pressure.

Trifluoperazine *taken concurrently* with
- ascorbic acid (vitamin C) may result in decreased therapeutic benefits from trifluoperazine.
- lithium (Lithobid, Lithotabs) may impair the effectiveness of lithium and cause nervous system toxicity.
- monoamine oxidase (MAO) inhibitors (see Drug Classes) may result in an increased risk of Parkinson-like disorders (see Glossary) reactions.
- oral hypoglycemic agents (see Oral Antidiabetic Drugs in Drug Classes) will blunt the beneficial effects of the oral hypoglycemic agents.
- tramadol (Ultram) may increase risk of seizures.

The following drugs may *decrease* the effects of trifluoperazine
- antacids containing aluminum and/or magnesium.
- barbiturates (see Drug Classes).
- benztropine (Cogentin).

- disulfiram (Antabuse).
- trihexyphenidyl (Artane).

▷ *Driving, Hazardous Activities:* This drug can impair mental alertness, judgment, and physical coordination. Avoid hazardous activities.

Aviation Note: The use of this drug *is a disqualification* for piloting. Consult a designated Aviation Medical Examiner.

Exposure to Sun: Use caution—some phenothiazines can cause photosensitivity (see Glossary).

Exposure to Heat: Use caution and avoid excessive heat as much as possible. This drug may impair the regulation of body temperature and increase the risk of heatstroke.

Exposure to Cold: Use caution and dress warmly. This drug can increase the risk of hypothermia in the elderly.

Discontinuation: After a period of long-term use, do not stop this drug suddenly. Gradual withdrawal over 2 to 3 weeks under physician supervision is recommended. Do not discontinue this drug without your physician's knowledge and approval. The relapse rate of schizophrenia after discontinuation is 50–60%.

TRIMETHOPRIM (tri METH oh prim)

Introduced: 1966   **Class:** Anti-infective   **Prescription:** USA: Yes
Controlled Drug: USA: No; Canada: No   **Available as Generic:** USA: Yes; Canada: No

Brand Names: ✦Apo-Sulfatrim [CD], ✦Apo-Sulfatrim DS [CD], Bactrim [CD], Bactrim DS [CD], Bethaprim [CD], Comoxol [CD], ✦Coptin [CD], Cotrim [CD], ✦Novo-Trimel [CD], ✦Novo-Trimel DS [CD], ✦Nu-Cotrimox, Polytrim, Proloprim, ✦Protrin [CD], ✦Protrin DF [CD], ✦Roubac [CD], Septra [CD], Septra DS [CD], SMZ-TMP [CD], Sulfatrim D/S, Trimpex, Uroplus DS [CD], Uroplus SS [CD]

BENEFITS versus RISKS	
Possible Benefits	*Possible Risks*
EFFECTIVE TREATMENT OF INFECTIONS due to susceptible microorganisms	Blood cell disorders: megaloblastic anemia, methemoglobinemia, abnormally low white cells or platelets
Effective adjunctive prevention and treatment of *Pneumocystis carinii* pneumonia (AIDS related)	

▷ **Principal Uses**

As a Single Drug Product: Uses currently included in FDA-approved labeling: (1) Treats or prevents certain infections of the urinary tract not complicated by the presence of kidney stones or obstructions to the normal flow of urine; (2) treats eye infections caused by sensitive organisms.

Other (unlabeled) generally accepted uses: (1) Used in combination with dapsone to treat *Pneumocystis carinii* pneumonia in AIDS patients; (2) may have a role in combination therapy of resistant acne; (3) prevention (prophylaxis) of urinary tract infections.

As a Combination Drug Product [CD]: This drug is available in combination with sulfamethoxazole; the generic name cotrimoxazole is used in some countries to identify this combination. It is very effective in the treatment of certain urinary tract infections, middle ear infections, chronic bronchitis, acute enteritis, and certain types of pneumonia. It is now used as primary prevention and treatment of *Pneumocystis carinii* pneumonia associated with AIDS.

How This Drug Works: This drug prevents the growth and multiplication of susceptible infecting organisms by inactivating the enzyme systems that are necessary for the formation of essential nuclear elements and cell proteins.

Available Dosage Forms and Strengths

>   Tablets — 100 mg, 200 mg
>   Tablets — 80 mg combined with 400 mg of sulfamethoxazole
>   Tablets — 160 mg combined with 800 mg of sulfamethoxazole
>   Ophthalmic — 1 mg/ml
> Oral suspension — 40 mg combined with 200 mg of sulfamethoxazole per
>   , 5 ml

▷ **Usual Adult Dosage Range:**   Orally for infections: 100 mg every 12 hours for 10 days. For certain pneumonias, the same dose is taken every 6 hours. The total daily dosage should not exceed 640 mg.

Ophthalmic: one drop in the affected eye every 3 hours (up to six doses a day) for 7 to 10 days. **Note: Actual dosage and administration schedule must be determined for each patient individually.**

Conditions Requiring Dosing Adjustments

Liver Function: This drug should be used with caution by patients with both liver and kidney compromise.

Kidney Function: Patients with mild kidney compromise can take the usual dose every 12 hours. Patients with moderate to severe kidney failure (creatinine clearances of 15 to 50 ml/min) can take the usual dose every 18 hours. This drug is contraindicated in patients with severe and worsening kidney failure.

▷ **Dosing Instructions:**   The tablet may be crushed and taken without regard to meals. However, it may also be taken with or following food if necessary to reduce stomach irritation.

Usual Duration of Use: Use on a regular schedule for 7 to 14 days usually determines effectiveness in controlling responsive infections. The actual duration of use will depend upon the nature of the infection.

Currently a "Drug of Choice"

(when combined with sulfamethoxazole) for preventing pneumonia (due to *Pneumocystis carinii*) in patients with AIDS.

▷ **This Drug Should Not Be Taken If**
- you have had an allergic reaction to it previously.
- you have an anemia due to folic acid deficiency (megaloblastic anemia).

▷ **Inform Your Physician Before Taking This Drug If**
- you have a history of folic acid deficiency.
- you have impaired liver or kidney function.
- you are pregnant or breast-feeding.

Possible Side Effects (natural, expected, and unavoidable drug actions)
None with short-term use.

▷ **Possible Adverse Effects** (unusual, unexpected, and infrequent reactions)
If any of the following develop, consult your physician promptly for guidance.
Mild Adverse Effects
Allergic Reactions: Skin rash, itching, drug fever (see Glossary).
Headache, abnormal taste, sore mouth or tongue, nausea, vomiting, cramping, diarrhea—infrequent.
Serious Adverse Effects
Allergic Reactions: Severe dermatitis with peeling of skin (toxic epidermal necrolysis).
Blood cell disorders: megaloblastic anemia, methemoglobinemia, abnormally low white blood cell and platelet counts—rare.
Worsening of hyperkalemia (increased blood potassium)—possible.
Kidney or liver toxicity—rare.
Aseptic meningitis (of questionable causal relationship)—case reports.

▷ **Possible Effects on Sexual Function:**   None reported.

Possible Effects on Laboratory Tests
Complete blood cell counts: decreased red cells, hemoglobin, white cells, and platelets.
INR (prothrombin time): increased (when taken concurrently with warfarin).

CAUTION
1. Certain strains of bacteria that cause urinary tract infections can develop resistance to this drug. If you do not show significant improvement within 2 days, call your physician.
2. Comply with your physician's request for periodic blood counts during long-term therapy.

Precautions for Use
By Infants and Children: Safety and effectiveness for those under 2 months of age are not established.
By Those Over 60 Years of Age: The natural decline in liver and kidney function may require smaller doses. If you develop itching reactions in the genital or anal areas, report this promptly.

▷ **Advisability of Use During Pregnancy**
Pregnancy Category: C. See Pregnancy Risk Categories at the back of this book.
Animal studies: Birth defects due to this drug reported in rat and rabbit studies.
Human studies: Adequate studies of pregnant women are not available.
Avoid use of drug during the first 3 months and during the final 2 weeks of pregnancy. Use this drug otherwise only if clearly needed. Ask your physician for guidance.

Advisability of Use If Breast-Feeding
Presence of this drug in breast milk: Yes.
Avoid drug or refrain from nursing.

Habit-Forming Potential: None.

Effects of Overdosage: Headache, dizziness, confusion, depression, nausea, vomiting, bone marrow depression, possible liver toxicity with jaundice.

Possible Effects of Long-Term Use: Impaired production of red and white blood cells and blood platelets.

Suggested Periodic Examinations While Taking This Drug (at physician's discretion)
Complete blood cell counts.

▷ **While Taking This Drug, Observe the Following**
Foods: No restrictions.
Beverages: No restrictions. May be taken with milk.
▷ *Alcohol:* No interactions expected.
Tobacco Smoking: No interactions expected, but I advise everyone to quit smoking.
▷ *Other Drugs*
Trimethoprim may *increase* the effects of
- amantadine (Symmetrel) and also result in increased levels of trimethoprim, resulting in toxicity.
- cyclosporine (Sandimmune) and result in increased kidney toxicity.
- dapsone and result in dapsone or trimethoprim toxicity.
- metformin (Glucophage) and other cationic drugs.
- phenytoin (Dilantin), and cause phenytoin toxicity.
- procainamide (Procan SR) and result in procainamide toxicity.
The following drugs may *decrease* the effects of trimethoprim
- cholestyramine (Questran) and perhaps other cholesterol-lowering medicines (see Drug Classes) of the same class—these will bind trimethoprim and blunt its beneficial effects by inhibiting absorption.
- rifampin (Rifadin, Rimactane).
▷ *Driving, Hazardous Activities:* No restrictions.
Aviation Note: The use of this drug is *probably not a disqualification* for piloting. Consult a designated Aviation Medical Examiner.
Exposure to Sun: No restrictions.

TROGLITAZONE (troh GLIT a zoan)

Introduced: 1996   **Class:** Antidiabetic, thiazolidinedione   **Prescription:** USA: Yes   **Controlled Drug:** USA: No; Canada: No   **Available as Generic:** No

Brand Name: Rezulin

BENEFITS versus RISKS	
Possible Benefits	*Possible Risks*
DECREASED INSULIN RESISTANCE	HYPOGLYCEMIA
EFFECTIVE CONTROL OF BLOOD SUGAR (GLUCOSE)	
POSSIBLE AVOIDANCE OF LONG-TERM EFFECTS (BLOOD VESSEL, NERVE, KIDNEY, HIGH BLOOD PRESSURE, AND HEART ADVERSE EFFECTS) FROM DIABETES	
Assistance in regulating blood sugar in insulin-dependent diabetes (adjunctive to appropriate diet and weight control)	

▷ **Principal Uses**

As a Single Drug Product: Uses currently included in FDA-approved labeling: Helps control mild to moderately severe type II diabetes mellitus (adult, maturity-onset) that requires 30 (or more) units of insulin daily as multiple injections, and still cannot be adequately controlled.

Other (unlabeled) generally accepted uses: None at present.

How This Drug Works: It is thought that this drug (1) improves how cells (target cells) respond to insulin; (2) decreases liver (hepatic) sugar (glucose) output, and (3) enhances the utilization of insulin (insulin-dependent functions) by appropriate tissues (skeletal muscle glucose disposal).

Available Dosage Forms and Strengths

Tablets — 200 mg, 400 mg

▷ **Usual Adult Dosage Range:**   Initially 200 mg once daily. The dose may be increased, if needed and tolerated, to 400 mg once daily after 2 to 4 weeks. Insulin doses should be decreased by 10–25% when fasting plasma glucose decreases to less than 120 mg/dl. 600 mg is the maximum daily troglitazone dose. **Note: Actual dosage and schedule must be determined for each patient individually.**

Conditions Requiring Dosing Adjustments

Liver Function: This drug should be used with caution by patients with liver damage.

Kidney Function: Dosing decreases are not needed in kidney compromise.

▷ **Dosing Instructions:**   Should be taken with a meal. The tablet may be crushed for administration.

Usual Duration of Use: Use on a regular schedule for 2 to 4 weeks usually determines peak effectiveness in controlling diabetes. Failure to respond after this period requires a dosage increase. Insulin doses should be decreased by 10 to 25% when the fasting glucose decreases to less than 120 mg/dl. Effective use can only be determined by periodic measurement of the blood sugar. See your physician on a regular basis.

▷ **This Drug Should Not Be Taken If**
- you have had an allergic reaction to it previously.
- you have diabetes complicated by formation of excess acid (acidosis).

▷ **Inform Your Physician Before Taking This Drug If**
- you are over 60 years old.
- your diabetes has been unstable or "brittle" in the past.
- you are pregnant.
- you do not know how to recognize or treat hypoglycemia (see Glossary).
- you have an infection and a fever.
- you have a deficiency of red blood cells (anemia)—ask your doctor.
- you take an oral hypoglycemic agent (not studied).
- you have NYHA class lll or IV heart failure (not studied).

Possible Side Effects (natural, expected, and unavoidable drug actions)
> If drug dose is excessive or food intake is delayed or inadequate, abnormally low blood sugar (hypoglycemia) may occur.

▷ **Possible Adverse Effects** (unusual, unexpected, and infrequent reactions)
> **If any of the following develop, consult your physician promptly for guidance.**
>
> *Mild Adverse Effects*
> Allergic Reactions: Skin rash—rare.
> Hypoglycemia (more likely with use of insulin at the same time)—infrequent.
> Decreased hemoglobin (mild and limited)—infrequent.
> Increased liver enzymes—rare.
> Increased blood urea nitrogen (BUN)—rare and not present in all studies.
> Nausea, vomiting, or diarrhea—infrequent.
> *Serious Adverse Effects*
> Allergic Reactions: Not reported.
> Idiosyncratic Reactions: Not reported.
> Hypoglycemia—more likely with insulin use at the same time.

▷ **Possible Effects on Sexual Function**
> None reported.

▷ **Adverse Effects That May Mimic Natural Diseases or Disorders**
> Liver reactions may suggest viral hepatitis.

Natural Diseases or Disorders That May Be Activated by This Drug
> None reported.

Possible Effects on Laboratory Tests
> Complete blood cell counts: decreased red cells, hemoglobin, and hematocrit—mild and stabilizes after 4–8 weeks.
> Blood glucose or glycosylated hemoglobin level: decreased.
> Liver function tests: increased liver enzymes (ALT/GPT, AST/GOT, and alkaline phosphatase).
> Blood urea nitrogen (BUN): rarely increased in some clinical studies.

CAUTION
1. This drug must be regarded as only one part of the total program for the management of your diabetes. It is not a substitute for a properly prescribed diet, insulin, and regular exercise.
2. This medicine may reduce the effectiveness of birth control pills. Talk

about alternative contraception options with your doctor. Periodic follow-up examinations are necessary.

Precautions for Use

By Infants and Children: This drug is approved for type II insulin-dependent diabetes.

By Those Over 65 Years of Age: This drug should be used with caution in this age group and monitored closely to prevent hypoglycemic reactions. Repeated episodes of hypoglycemia in the elderly can cause brain damage. Clinical trials did not reveal differences in safety or effectiveness in those over 65.

▷ **Advisability of Use During Pregnancy**

Pregnancy Category: B. See Pregnancy Risk Categories at the back of this book. Animal studies: No effects were seen in rats given 10 or 20 mg per kg of body mass.

Human studies: Adequate studies of pregnant women are not available.

Because uncontrolled blood sugar levels during pregnancy are associated with a higher incidence of birth defects, many experts recommend that insulin (instead of an oral agent) be used as necessary to control diabetes during the entire pregnancy.

Use of this drug during pregnancy is not recommended by the manufacturer.

Advisability of Use If Breast-Feeding

Presence of this drug in breast milk: Yes in rats; unknown in women.

Avoid drug or refrain from nursing.

Habit-Forming Potential: None.

Effects of Overdosage: Symptoms of mild to severe hypoglycemia: headache, light-headedness, faintness, nervousness, confusion, tremor, sweating, heart palpitation, weakness, hunger, nausea, vomiting, stupor progressing to coma.

Possible Effects of Long-Term Use: Not defined at present.

Suggested Periodic Examinations While Taking This Drug (at physician's discretion)

Complete blood cell counts, liver function tests, follow-up tests (such as fingerstick testing) of blood sugar. Glycosylated hemoglobin.

▷ **While Taking This Drug, Observe the Following**

Foods: Follow the diabetic diet prescribed by your physician.

Beverages: As directed in the diabetic diet. May be taken with milk.

▷ *Alcohol:* Use with caution. Single doses of moderate amounts of alcohol did not increase risk of hypoglycemia.

Tobacco Smoking: No interaction expected, but I advise everyone to quit smoking.

▷ *Other Drugs*

The following drugs may *decrease* the effects of troglitazone
- cholestyramine (Questran).
- thiazide diuretics (see Drug Classes).
- thyroid hormones (see Drug Classes).

Troglitazone *taken concurrently* with
- birth control pills (oral contraceptives) may decrease their effectiveness resulting in unwanted pregnancy.
- insulin will result in additive lowering of the blood sugar.

- oral hypoglycemic agents such as sulfonylureas (see Drug Classes) may further decrease fasting blood sugar. Caution is advised, as this combination was not well studied.
- terfenadine (Seldane) may decrease terfenadine concentrations and lessen its therapeutic effect.

▷ *Driving, Hazardous Activities:* Regulate your dosage schedule, eating schedule, and physical activities very carefully to prevent hypoglycemia. Be able to recognize the early symptoms of hypoglycemia so you can avoid hazardous activities and take corrective measures.

Aviation Note: Diabetes *is a disqualification* for piloting. Consult a designated Aviation Medical Examiner.

Exposure to Sun: Not defined.

Occurrence of Unrelated Illness: Acute infections, illnesses causing vomiting or diarrhea, serious injuries, and surgical procedures can interfere with diabetic control and may require insulin. If any of these conditions occur, call your doctor promptly.

Discontinuation: Talk with your doctor before changing the dosing schedule of this medicine or considering stopping troglitazone.

VALACYCLOVIR (VALA si klo veer)

Introduced: 1996   **Class:** Antiviral   **Prescription:** USA: Yes   **Controlled Drug:** USA: No; Canada: No   **Available as Generic:** USA: No; Canada: No

Brand Name: Valtrex

BENEFITS versus RISKS	
Possible Benefits	*Possible Risks*
EFFECTIVE TREATMENT OF HERPES ZOSTER (SHINGLES) EFFECTIVE EPISODIC TREATMENT OF GENITAL HERPES	Rare reports of thrombotic thrombocytopenic purpura (TTP) in HIV and bone marrow or kidney transplant patients Nausea

▷ **Principal Uses**

As a Single Drug Product: Uses currently included in FDA-approved labeling: (1) To treat herpes zoster (shingles); (2) used in recurrent genital herpes in patients with intact immune systems.

Other (unlabeled) generally accepted uses: None at present; since this medicine is rapidly converted to acyclovir, see the acyclovir profile for some possible unlabeled uses.

How This Drug Works: This medicine is rapidly converted to acyclovir, and moves into the body to a much greater extent (dose to dose) than acyclovir. It is thought that by blocking the formation of genetic material by the virus, this medicine stops the ability of the virus to multiply and spread.

Available Dosage Forms and Strengths

Caplets — 500 mg

▷ **Usual Adult Dosage Range** (Actual dosage and administration schedule must be determined for each patient individually.)

Herpes zoster (shingles): Best started within 48 hours of the zoster rash. Dose: 1 g (1000 mg) three times a day for 7 days.

Genital herpes simplex: This medicine is best started within 24 hours of the onset of symptoms, and is taken as 500 mg twice daily for 5 days.

Conditions Requiring Dosing Adjustments

Liver Function: In moderate to severe cases of liver compromise dose changes are not needed.

Kidney Function: Dosing changes **MUST** be made for patients with compromised kidneys, including the typical age-related decline in kidney function (ask your doctor about this if you are over 60 years old).

▷ **Dosing Instructions:**   May be taken without regard to meals.

Usual Duration of Use: Treatment is best started within 48 hours of onset of the zoster rash. Use on a regular schedule for 7 days for herpes zoster has been effective. Treatment is best started within 24 hours of signs of genital herpes; regular use for 5 days has been effective for genital herpes. Take the full course as prescribed.

Possible Advantages of This Drug: Generally well-tolerated antiviral that decreases the length of time patients are in pain from genital herpes and herpes zoster. Achieves blood levels similar to INTRAVENOUS acyclovir with a medicine taken by mouth (the oral route). Patients do not have to take it as many times a day as with acyclovir.

▷ **This Drug Should Not Be Taken If**
• you have had an allergic reaction to it previously.
• you have advanced HIV disease or have had a bone marrow or kidney transplant (increased risk of thrombotic thrombocytopenic purpura).

▷ **Inform Your Physician Before Taking This Drug If**
• you have impaired liver or kidney function.
• you are taking any other drugs at this time.
• you think you are dehydrated.
• you are unsure of how much or how often to take valacyclovir.

Possible Side Effects (natural, expected, and unavoidable drug actions)
With use of caplets—none.

▷ **Possible Adverse Effects** (unusual, unexpected, and infrequent reactions)
If any of the following develop, consult your physician promptly for guidance.

Mild Adverse Effects

Allergic Reactions: Skin rash.

Headache, dizziness, nervousness, insomnia, depression, fatigue—infrequent.

Nausea, vomiting, diarrhea—infrequent.

Serious Adverse Effects

Thrombotic thrombocytopenic purpura—rare and in immunocompromised patients.

Kidney problems—reported with high doses of acyclovir and rare.

▷ **Possible Effects on Sexual Function:**   Altered timing and pattern of menstruation reported with acyclovir, not with valacyclovir.

Possible Effects on Laboratory Tests
>Complete blood cell counts: decreased red cells and hemoglobin.
>Blood urea nitrogen (BUN) or creatinine: increased.

CAUTION
>1. This drug does **not** eliminate all herpes virus and **is not a cure**. Recurrence is possible (with genital herpes use). Resume treatment at the earliest sign of infection.
>2. Avoid sexual intercourse if herpes blisters and swelling are present.
>3. Do not exceed the prescribed dosage.
>4. Tell your doctor if frequency (genital herpes) or severity (herpes zoster) doesn't improve.

Precautions for Use
>*By Infants and Children:* Safety and effectiveness for use in pediatrics have not been established.
>*By Those Over 60 Years of Age:* Avoid dehydration. Drink 2 to 3 quarts of liquids daily. Lower doses are required if you are over 60 years old and your kidneys have undergone the usual age-related decline in how well they work.

▷ **Advisability of Use During Pregnancy**
>*Pregnancy Category:* B. See Pregnancy Risk Categories at the back of this book.
>Animal studies: NOT teratogenic in rabbits or rats (up to 10 times the human dose).
>Human studies: Adequate studies of pregnant women are not available.
>Physicians should call 1–800–722–9292, extension 58465, to register their patients.

Advisability of Use If Breast-Feeding
>Presence of this drug in breast milk: Yes (documented in two women; 0.6 to 4.1 times the plasma levels). Given to breast-feeding mothers with caution or not at all. Discuss the benefits versus risks with your doctor.

Habit-Forming Potential: None.

Effects of Overdosage: Possible kidney damage (based on formation of crystals in the kidney with excessive doses).

Possible Effects of Long-Term Use: Development of acyclovir-resistant strains of genital herpes virus. Treatment will fail if this occurs.

▷ **While Taking This Drug, Observe the Following**
>*Foods:* No restrictions.
>*Beverages:* No restrictions. May be taken with milk. **Drink 2 to 3 quarts of liquids** (if not contraindicated for you) **daily.**
▷ *Alcohol:* Use caution; dizziness or fatigue may be accentuated.
>*Tobacco Smoking:* No interactions expected, but I advise everyone to quit smoking.
▷ *Other Drugs*
>The following drugs may *increase* the effects of valacyclovir
>• cyclosporine use may result in increased risk of kidney toxicity.
>• probenecid (Benemid) may delay acyclovir elimination.
>Valacyclovir *taken concurrently* with
>• cimetidine (Tagamet) may caused decreased elimination by the kidney.
>• meperidine may result in neurological problems (based on acyclovir data).
>• varicella vaccine (Varivax) may blunt the vaccine's effectiveness (acyclovir data).

- zidovudine (AZT) may result in severe fatigue and lethargy with acyclovir, and may result in similar results with valacyclovir. An increased risk of thrombotic thrombocytopenic purpura (TTP) is possible in immunocompromised patients.

▷ *Driving, Hazardous Activities:* Use caution if dizziness or fatigue occurs.

Aviation Note: The use of this drug **may be a disqualification** for piloting. Consult a designated Aviation Medical Examiner.

Exposure to Sun: No restrictions.

Discontinuation: Talk with your doctor or pharmacist about how long and how best to take this medicine.

VALPROIC ACID (val PROH ik a sid)

Introduced: 1967   **Class:** Anticonvulsant   **Prescription:** USA: Yes
Controlled Drug: USA: No; Canada: No   **Available as Generic:** USA: Yes;
Canada: No

Brand Names: Depa, Depakene, Depakote (divalproex sodium), Deproic, ✦Epival

BENEFITS versus RISKS	
Possible Benefits	*Possible Risks*
EFFECTIVE CONTROL OF MULTIPLE SEIZURE TYPES: ABSENCE SEIZURES, TONIC-CLONIC SEIZURES, MYOCLONIC SEIZURES, PSYCHOMOTOR SEIZURES, when used adjunctively with other antiseizure drugs HELPS CONTROL REFRACTORY MIGRAINES DIVALPROEX SODIUM HELPS MANIA	LIVER TOXICITY, infrequent but may be severe Reduction of blood platelets and impaired platelet function with risk of bleeding Possible pancreatitis or liver toxicity

▷ **Principal Uses**

As a Single Drug Product: Uses currently included in FDA-approved labeling: (1) Used to manage the following types of epilepsy: simple and complex absence seizures (petit mal); tonic-clonic seizures (grand mal); myoclonic seizures; complex partial seizures (psychomotor, temporal lobe epilepsy). Sometimes used adjunctively with other anticonvulsants as needed; (2) used for people who do not respond to medicine once they have a migraine or have more than two migraines a month; (3) divalproex sodium (Depakote) is now approved for use in treating mania.

Other (unlabeled) generally accepted uses: (1) Can help relieve the symptoms of trigeminal neuralgia; (2) can have a role in intractable hiccups; (3) some use in patients with epilepsy and hepatic porphyria; (4) may be of help for writer's cramp.

How This Drug Works: It is thought that by increasing the availability of the nerve impulse transmitter gamma-aminobutyric acid (GABA), this drug suppresses the spread of abnormal electrical discharges that cause seizures.

Available Dosage Forms and Strengths
Capsules — 250 mg
Capsules, sprinkle — 125 mg
Syrup — 250 mg/5 ml
Tablets, enteric coated — 125 mg, 250 mg, 500 mg

▷ **Usual Adult Dosage Range:**   Starting dose is 15 mg per kg of body mass per day. The dose is increased cautiously by 5 to 10 mg per kg of body mass daily, every 7 days as needed and tolerated. *The usual daily dose is from 1000 mg to 1600 mg in divided doses.* The total daily dosage should not exceed 60 mg per kg of body mass. Blood levels are used to guide ongoing dosing.
For migraines: Starting dose is 250 mg, which is then slowly increased, as needed and tolerated, to 500 to 750 mg daily in divided doses. **Note: Actual dosage and administration schedule must be determined for each patient individually.**

Conditions Requiring Dosing Adjustments
Liver Function: This medicine SHOULD NOT be taken by patients with significant liver compromise or liver disease.
Kidney Function: No dosing changes are anticipated for patients with compromised kidneys.

▷ **Dosing Instructions:**   Preferably taken 1 hour before meals. However, it may be taken with or following food if necessary to prevent stomach irritation. The regular capsule should not be opened and the tablet should not be crushed for administration. The sprinkle capsule may be opened and the contents sprinkled on soft food for administration. Do not administer the syrup in carbonated beverages; it may be diluted in water or milk.

Usual Duration of Use: Use on a regular schedule for 2 weeks usually determines effectiveness in reducing the frequency and severity of seizures. Long-term use (months to years) requires physician supervision and periodic evaluation.

▷ **This Drug Should Not Be Taken If**
- you have had an allergic reaction to it previously.
- you have active liver disease.
- you are pregnant.
- you have an active bleeding disorder.

▷ **Inform Your Physician Before Taking This Drug If**
- you have a history of liver disease or impaired liver function.
- you have a history of any type of bleeding disorder.
- you are pregnant or planning pregnancy.
- you have myasthenia gravis.
- you are taking anticoagulants; other anticonvulsants; antidepressants, either the tricyclic type or monoamine oxidase (MAO) type A inhibitors (see Drug Classes).
- you plan to have surgery or dental extraction in the near future.

Possible Side Effects (natural, expected, and unavoidable drug actions)
   Drowsiness and lethargy.

▷ **Possible Adverse Effects** (unusual, unexpected, and infrequent reactions)
   If any of the following develop, consult your physician promptly for guidance.

   Mild Adverse Effects

   Allergic Reactions: Skin rash—rare.
   Headache, dizziness, confusion, unsteadiness, tremor—dose related; slurred speech—infrequent.
   Nausea, indigestion, stomach cramps, diarrhea—infrequent.
   Weight gain—case reports.
   Bed-wetting at night—case reports.
   Temporary loss of scalp hair—case reports.

   Serious Adverse Effects

   Idiosyncratic Reactions: Bizarre behavior, psychosis, hallucinations.
   Drug-induced hepatitis with jaundice (see Glossary). **Children less than 2 years old have considerably increased risk of fatal hepatotoxicity.**
   Blood ammonia level or blood glucose—increased.
   Drug-induced pancreatitis, porphyria, lowered thyroid gland function (hypothyroidism)—case reports.
   Selenium levels—decreased.
   Reduced formation of blood platelets, impaired platelet function, and anemia—case reports.
   Increased pressure in the head (pseudotumor cerebri)—case reports.
   Can cause a Reye-like syndrome.

▷ **Possible Effects on Sexual Function**
   Altered timing and pattern of menstruation.
   Female breast enlargement with milk production.
   Decreased libido—case reports.
   Decreased effectiveness of oral contraceptives taken concurrently (6%).

▷ **Adverse Effects That May Mimic Natural Diseases or Disorders**
   Liver reactions may suggest viral hepatitis.

Possible Effects on Laboratory Tests
   Complete blood cell counts: decreased white cells and platelets.
   Bleeding time or INR (prothrombin time): increased.
   Blood amylase level: increased (possible pancreatitis).
   Liver function tests: increased enzymes (ALT/GPT, AST/GOT, alkaline phosphatase) or bilirubin.

CAUTION
   1. The capsules and tablets should be swallowed whole to avoid irritation of the mouth and throat.
   2. This drug can impair normal blood clotting mechanisms. In the event of injury, dental extraction, or need for surgery, inform your physician or dentist that you are taking this drug.
   3. Because this drug can impair the normal function of blood platelets, it is best to avoid aspirin (which has the same effect).
   4. Over-the-counter drug products that contain antihistamines (allergy and cold remedies, sleep aids) can enhance sedative effects.

Precautions for Use

By Infants and Children: The concurrent use of aspirin with this drug can cause abnormal bleeding or bruising. Children with mental retardation, organic brain disease, or severe seizure disorders may be at increased risk for severe liver toxicity while taking this drug. Observe closely for the development of fever that could indicate the onset of a drug-induced Reye syndrome (see Glossary). Avoid concurrent use of clonazepam (Klonopin); the combined use could result in continuous petit mal episodes.

By Those Over 60 Years of Age: Start treatment with small doses and increase dosage cautiously. Observe closely for excessive sedation, confusion, or unsteadiness that could predispose to falling and injury.

▷ **Advisability of Use During Pregnancy**

Pregnancy Category: D. See Pregnancy Risk Categories at the back of this book.

Animal studies: Palate and skeletal birth defects reported in mouse, rat, and rabbit studies.

Human studies: Adequate studies of pregnant women are not available. There have been several reports of birth defects attributed to the use of this drug during early pregnancy.

Consult your physician regarding the advantages and disadvantages of using this drug. If it is used, it is advisable to keep the dose as low as possible.

Advisability of Use If Breast-Feeding

Presence of this drug in breast milk: Yes.

Monitor nursing infant closely and discontinue drug or nursing if adverse effects develop.

Habit-Forming Potential: None.

Effects of Overdosage: Increased drowsiness, weakness, unsteadiness, confusion, stupor progressing to coma.

Possible Effects of Long-Term Use: None reported.

Suggested Periodic Examinations While Taking This Drug (at physician's discretion)

Complete blood cell counts and baseline liver function tests should be done before treatment is started. During treatment, blood counts should be repeated every month and liver function tests repeated every 2 months.

▷ **While Taking This Drug, Observe the Following**

Foods: No restrictions.

Beverages: Do not administer the syrup in carbonated beverages; this could liberate the valproic acid and irritate the mouth and throat. This drug may be taken with milk.

▷ *Alcohol:* Alcohol can increase the sedative effect of this drug. Also, this drug can increase the depressant effects of alcohol on brain function.

Tobacco Smoking: No interactions expected, but I advise everyone to quit smoking.

▷ *Other Drugs*

Valproic acid may ***increase*** the effects of

- anticoagulants (Coumadin, etc.), and increase the risk of bleeding. Increased frequency of INR (prothrombin time or protime) testing is needed.
- antidepressants, both monoamine oxidase (MAO) type A inhibitors and tricyclics, and cause toxicity.

- nimodipine (Nimotop) and cause nimodipine toxicity.
- phenobarbital, and cause barbiturate intoxication.
- phenytoin (Dilantin), and cause phenytoin toxicity.

Valproic acid *taken concurrently* with

- antacids (Maalox) will decrease absorption and their therapeutic benefits.
- antiplatelet drugs—aspirin, dipyridamole (Persantine), sulfinpyrazone (Anturane)—may enhance the inhibition of platelet function and increase the risk of bleeding.
- aspirin can lead to valproic acid toxicity.
- carbamazepine (Tegretol) may have a variable effect on blood levels. More frequent blood level testing is advised.
- clonazepam (Klonopin) may result in repeated episodes of absence seizures (absence status).
- cyclosporine (Sandimmune) may increase risk of liver toxicity.
- erythromycin (Ery-Tab, others) may increase the level of valproic acid and result in toxicity. The newer macrolides (azithromycin or clarithromycin) may also cause problems.
- felbamate (Felbatol) can lead to increased valproic acid levels.
- isoniazid (INH) can cause valproic acid or isoniazid toxicity.

▷ *Driving, Hazardous Activities:* This drug may cause drowsiness, dizziness, or confusion. Restrict activities as necessary.

Aviation Note: The use of this drug *is a disqualification* for piloting. Consult a designated Aviation Medical Examiner.

Exposure to Sun: Caution: this drug has caused photosensitivity.

Discontinuation: Do not stop this drug suddenly. Abrupt withdrawal can cause repetitive seizures that are difficult to control.

VANCOMYCIN (van koh MI sin)

Introduced: 1974   **Class:** Anti-infective   **Prescription:** USA: Yes
Controlled Drug: USA: No; Canada: No   **Available as Generic:** USA: Yes; Canada: No

Brand Names: Vancocin, Vancoled, Vancor

Note: Vancomycin is used to treat a variety of serious infections. It is given intravenously to treat some infections and orally to treat others. In the past, the information provided in this profile was limited to the use of vancomycin taken by mouth. Since resistant organisms have increased use of this medicine by vein (intravenously), this profile has been expanded to help patients understand vancomycin's broadened role in infectious disease.

BENEFITS versus RISKS	
Possible Benefits	*Possible Risks*
TREATS SERIOUS INFECTIONS CAUSED BY RESISTANT GRAM-POSITIVE ORGANISMS SUCH AS "STAPH" AND "STREP" TREATS ANTIBIOTIC-ASSOCIATED PSEUDOMEMBRANOUS COLITIS	Ringing in ears (tinnitus) Loss of hearing

▷ **Principal Uses**

As a Single Drug Product: Uses currently included in FDA-approved labeling: (1) Oral form is used in antibiotic-associated pseudomembranous colitis caused by *Clostridium difficile*; (2) the oral form is also used in enterocolitis caused by staphylococcal organisms; (3) the intravenous form is used to treat a variety of serious infections such those in heart valves, bones (osteo-myelitis), endocarditis, and meningitis, including those caused by methicil-lin-resistant *Staphylococcus aureus* (MRSA).

Other (unlabeled) generally accepted uses: None.

How This Drug Works: By inhibiting the formation of bacterial cell walls and the production of RNA, this drug destroys susceptible strains of infecting bacteria.

Available Dosage Forms and Strengths

Capsules — 125 mg, 250 mg

Intravenous — 500 mg/15 ml, 1 g/15 ml

Oral solution — 250 mg/5 ml teaspoonful and 500 mg/5 ml

▷ **Recommended Dosage Ranges** (Actual dosage and administration schedule must be determined for each patient individually.)

Infants and Children: 10 mg per kg of body mass every 6 hours, for 5 to 10 days. The total daily dose should not exceed 2000 mg (2 g). Repeat course as necessary.

12 to 60 Years of Age: Many clinicians use a 15-mg-per-kg-of-body-mass loading dose and then calculate ongoing doses based on individual patient height, weight, kidney function, and suspected bacteria (bacterial pathogen). Cal-culations are made in order to attain a peak blood level of 30–40 mcg/ml and a lowest blood level (trough) of 5–10 mcg/ml.

Oral dosing for pseudomembranous colitis caused by *Clostridium difficile*: 125 mg by mouth every 6 hours for 10 days.

Over 60 Years of Age: Intravenous dosing: The loading dose is the same as for younger patients. Ongoing doses may be much smaller and may need to be taken much less often than in younger patients (such as once a day or once every 2 days).

For oral dosing: Same as 12 to 60 years of age (vancomycin in pseudomem-branous colitis is not absorbed).

Conditions Requiring Dosing Adjustments

Liver Function: The liver is not involved in the elimination of vancomycin.

Kidney Function: Oral vancomycin is minimally absorbed. Intravenous vanco-mycin MUST be taken in decreased dose or increased interval in kidney failure. This drug is also a potential cause of kidney failure, and should only be taken if other alternatives are not available. Daily measures of kidney function and more frequent blood levels are indicated if this medicine is used by patients with compromised kidneys.

▷ **Dosing Instructions:**   Oral form may be taken with or following food to reduce stomach irritation. Because of this drug's unpleasant taste, it is preferable to swallow the capsule whole without alteration. Use a measuring device to ensure accuracy of dose when taking the oral solution. Observe the expira-tion date.

Usual Duration of Use: Oral use: use on a regular schedule for 48 to 72 hours usually determines effectiveness in controlling infection in the colon. If response is prompt, limit treatment to 10 days. If symptoms warrant, continue treatment for 14 to 21 days. Consult your physician on a regular basis. For intravenous use, the length of treatment depends on the severity and site of the infection (for example, bone infections may take 6 weeks to cure).

Currently a "Drug of Choice"
for treating metronidazole-treatment failures in antibiotic-associated pseudomembranous colitis caused by *Clostridium difficile*. Used in methicillin-resistant *Staphylococcus aureus* (MRSA).

▷ **This Drug Should Not Be Taken If**
- you have had an allergic reaction to it previously.

▷ **Inform Your Physician Before Taking This Drug If**
- you have a history of Crohn's disease or ulcerative colitis.
- you have impaired kidney function.
- you are pregnant.
- you have any degree of hearing loss.
- you are taking cholestyramine (Questran) or colestipol (Colestid).

Possible Side Effects (natural, expected, and unavoidable drug actions)
Bitter, unpleasant taste for the oral form. Kidney damage with long-term, high-dose use of the intravenous form. Red-man syndrome (lowering of blood pressure; sudden rash of neck, chest, face, and extremities).

▷ **Possible Adverse Effects** (unusual, unexpected, and infrequent reactions)
If any of the following develop, consult your physician promptly for guidance.
Mild Adverse Effects
Allergic Reactions: Skin rash (with large doses or prolonged use).
Nausea, vomiting—infrequent with oral form and rare with intravenous form.
Chills—infrequent.
Serious Adverse Effects
Allergic Reactions: Anaphylaxis. Serious skin rashes (exfoliative dermatitis or Stevens-Johnson syndrome).
Ringing or buzzing in ears, sensation of ear fullness, loss of hearing—toxicity sign.
Lowering of white blood cells—reversible, and seen with the intravenous form.
Cardiac arrest—rare.
Hearing loss—may be reversible and more likely with high dose or long-term use.
Kidney toxicity—may be dose dependent and more likely with higher doses and long-term use.
Thrombophlebitis—infrequent with the intravenous form.

▷ **Possible Effects on Sexual Function:** None reported.

Natural Diseases or Disorders That May Be Activated by This Drug
Latent hearing loss, kidney failure.

Possible Effects on Laboratory Tests
Serum creatinine: increased (a sign of kidney toxicity).

CAUTION
1. Report promptly the development of fullness, ringing, or buzzing in either ear. This may indicate the onset of nerve damage that could lead to hearing loss.
2. Do not take any medication to stop your diarrhea without calling your doctor. The bacterial toxin that causes colitis is eliminated by diarrhea; stopping the elimination could intensify and prolong your illness.
3. Blood levels MUST be used to guide dosing. Keep all appointments for laboratory work.

Precautions for Use

By Infants and Children: Some cases may require doses up to 50 mg per kg of body mass daily.

By Those Over 60 Years of Age: You may be more susceptible to drug-induced hearing loss. Use the minimum course of treatment required to cure your colitis or other infection.

▷ **Advisability of Use During Pregnancy**

Pregnancy Category: B. See Pregnancy Risk Categories at the back of this book. Animal studies: Rat and rabbit studies reveal no drug-induced birth defects. Human studies: Adequate studies of pregnant women are not available. Use this drug only if clearly needed. Ask your physician for guidance.

Advisability of Use If Breast-Feeding

Presence of this drug in breast milk: Yes.
Avoid drug or refrain from nursing.

Habit-Forming Potential: None.

Effects of Overdosage: Possible nausea, vomiting, ringing in ears.

Possible Effects of Long-Term Use: Hearing loss.

Suggested Periodic Examinations While Taking This Drug (at physician's discretion)

Hearing tests. Measures of kidney function and blood vancomycin levels with intravenous use.

▷ **While Taking This Drug, Observe the Following**

Foods: No restrictions.

Beverages: No restrictions. May be taken with milk.

▷   *Alcohol:* No interactions expected. Use sparingly; alcohol may aggravate colitis.

Tobacco Smoking: No interactions expected, but I advise everyone to quit smoking.

▷   *Other Drugs*

The following drugs may *decrease* the effects of vancomycin
- cholestyramine (Questran).
- colestipol (Colestid).

Vancomycin *taken concurrently* with
- aminoglycoside antibiotics (see Drug Classes) such as gentamicin or tobramycin may cause additive toxicity risk to the ears and kidneys.
- cyclosporine (Sandimmune) may result in increased toxicity risk.
- other medicines that cause kidney toxicity may pose an additive toxicity risk.
- warfarin (Coumadin) may cause increased bleeding risk. Increased INR (prothrombin time or protime) testing is needed.

▷ *Driving, Hazardous Activities:* Usually no restrictions.
Aviation Note: The use of this drug is ***probably not a disqualification*** for pilot-
ing. Consult a designated Aviation Medical Examiner.
Exposure to Sun: No restrictions.
Discontinuation: To be determined by your physician.
Special Storage Instructions: Refrigerate the oral solution. A home IV service
will explain storage of the intravenous form.
Observe the Following Expiration Times: Provided on your prescription label by
your pharmacist.

VARICELLA VIRUS VACCINE (VAIR a sell ah)

Introduced: 1995   **Class:** Vaccine   **Prescription:** USA: Yes   **Controlled Drug:** USA: No; Canada: No   **Available as Generic:** USA: No; Canada: No

Brand Name: Varivax

BENEFITS versus RISKS	
Possible Benefits	*Possible Risks*
PREVENTION OF VARICELLA (chickenpox)	Rash Soreness at the injection site Anaphylactic reaction

▷ **Principal Uses**
As a Single Drug Product: Uses currently included in FDA-approved labeling:
Prevention of chickenpox.
Other (unlabeled) generally accepted uses: None.

How This Drug Works: By stimulating the immune system, the vaccine pre-
pares the body to fight any exposure to the wild-type virus.

Available Dosage Forms and Strengths
Vaccine, multidose vial—a single-dose vial of vaccine (1500 PFU per dose)

How to Store
This product **must** be kept frozen prior to use.
**Author's Note: The Center for Disease Control's (CDC) Immunization
Practices Committee has recommended that all children 12 to 18
months old should be given varicella vaccine if they have not previously contracted chickenpox. The vaccine is also recommended by the
committee for children 19 months to 13 years old. Finally, adults or
adolescents who have not had chickenpox and are at risk for exposure
should also be given the vaccine.**

▷ **Recommended Dosage Ranges** (Actual dosage and administration schedule
must be determined for each patient individually.)
Infants and Children 1 to 12 Years Old: Not indicated in infants. Children 1 year
old or older are given 0.5 ml injected under the skin.
12 to 55 Years of Age: Same as the children's dose, providing the patient has not
had chickenpox.
Over 55 Years of Age: Not studied.

Conditions Requiring Dosing Adjustments
  Liver Function: Not a consideration.
  Kidney Function: Not a consideration.

▷ **Dosing Instructions:**   This vaccine is to be injected under the skin. It may be given with measles, mumps, and rubella vaccine.

Usual Duration of Benefit: Exposure to chickenpox 5 years after vaccination may result in 20% of patients developing mild disease. More experience is needed before the question of repeat vaccination is answered.

Possible Advantages of This Drug
  Prevention of chickenpox.

Currently a "Drug of Choice"
  for prevention of chickenpox.

▷ **This Drug Should Not Be Taken If**
  • you have had an allergic reaction to any dosage form of it previously.
  • you have a history of anaphylactic reaction to neomycin.
  • you have a history of blood diseases or leukemia, or have AIDS.
  • you are taking medicines that suppress the immune system.
  • you have tuberculosis that has not been treated.
  • you are allergic to eggs.
  • you are pregnant.
  • you have an active infection.

▷ **Inform Your Physician Before Taking This Drug If**
  • you are planning pregnancy in the near future.
  • you have a condition that may require steroids.
  • you take salicylates (aspirin, others) on a regular basis. This should NOT be done for 6 weeks following vaccination, as it is a risk for Reye syndrome.
  • you live with someone who has a depressed immune system (such as an AIDS patient). Because this vaccine is a live-virus vaccine, you may be infectious to them.

Possible Side Effects (natural, expected, and unavoidable drug actions)
  Pain at the injection site, fever.

▷ **Possible Adverse Effects** (unusual, unexpected, and infrequent reactions)
  If any of the following develop, consult your physician promptly for guidance.
  Mild Adverse Effects
  Allergic Reactions: Skin rash.
  Varicellalike rash—infrequent.
  Headache, irritability, fatigue, and loss of appetite—rare to infrequent.
  Chills, stiff neck, and joint pain—infrequent.
  Nausea, vomiting—rare.
  Serious Adverse Effects
  Allergic Reactions: Anaphylactic reaction.
  Idiosyncratic Reactions: None reported.
  Febrile seizures—case reports.
  Herpes zoster—possible.
  Pneumonitis—case report and of questionable causation.

▷ **Possible Effects on Sexual Function:**   None reported.

Possible Delayed Adverse Effects: None reported.

▷ **Adverse Effects That May Mimic Natural Diseases or Disorders**
    Rash may resemble chickenpox.

Natural Diseases or Disorders That May Be Activated by This Drug
    None reported.

Possible Effects on Laboratory Tests
    None reported.

CAUTION
    1. **Do not** give aspirin or other salicylates to patients who have recently
    received the vaccine. The risk of Reye syndrome is associated with such
    aspirin use.

Precautions for Use
    By Infants and Children: Safety and effectiveness for use by those under 12
    months of age have not been established.
    By Those Over 60 Years of Age: Not studied.

▷ **Advisability of Use During Pregnancy**
    Pregnancy Category: C. See Pregnancy Risk Categories at the back of this book.
    Animal studies: Have not been conducted with this vaccine.
    Human studies: Information from adequate studies of pregnant women is not
    available. The manufacturer says that the vaccine should not be given to
    pregnant women and pregnancy should be avoided for 3 months following
    vaccination.

Advisability of Use If Breast-Feeding
    Presence of this drug in breast milk: Expected.
    Avoid drug or refrain from nursing.

Habit-Forming Potential: None.

Effects of Overdosage: Not defined.

Possible Effects of Long-Term Use: Not intended for long-term use.

Suggested Periodic Examinations While Taking This Drug (at physician's dis-
    cretion)
    None suggested.

▷ **While Taking This Drug, Observe the Following**
    Foods: No restrictions.
    Beverages: No restrictions.
▷   *Alcohol:* No interactions expected.
    Tobacco Smoking: No interactions expected, but I advise everyone to quit smok-
        ing.
▷   *Other Drugs*
        Varicella vaccine *taken concurrently* with
        • acyclovir (Zovirax) may result in a blunted immune benefit from the vac-
          cine.
        • aspirin or any salicylates (various) may result in Reye syndrome. DO NOT
          take aspirin for 6 weeks after vaccination.
        • corticosteroids (see Drug Classes) may result in extreme reactions.
        • immune globulins may result in decreased beneficial response to the vac-
          cine.

- immunosuppressant medicines (such as cyclosporine—Sandimmune) may result in extreme reactions.
- mesalamine (Asacol) may result in risk of Reye syndrome. DO NOT take salicylates for 6 weeks after vaccination.
- olsalazine (Dipentum) may result in risk of Reye syndrome. DO NOT take salicylates for 6 weeks after vaccination.

▷ *Driving, Hazardous Activities:* This drug may cause soreness at the injection site. Restrict activities as necessary.

Aviation Note: The use of this drug *is probably not a disqualification* for piloting. Consult a designated Aviation Medical Examiner.

Exposure to Sun: No restrictions.

Occurrence of Unrelated Illness: This vaccination should not be given in the presence of any other active infection.

Special Storage Instructions: This vaccine must be stored frozen.

Author's Note: There is now a Vaccine Adverse Event Reporting System (VAERS). The toll-free number is 1–800–822–7967.

VENLAFAXINE (ven la FAX een)

Introduced: 1993   **Class:** Antidepressant   **Prescription:** USA: Yes
Controlled Drug: USA: No; Canada: No   **Available as Generic:** USA: No
Brand Names: Effexor, Effexor XR (approvable)

BENEFITS versus RISKS	
Possible Benefits	*Possible Risks*
EFFECTIVE TREATMENT OF DEPRESSION	INCREASED BLOOD PRESSURE
	Seizures
BETTER SIDE-EFFECT PROFILE THAN TRICYCLIC ANTIDEPRESSANTS	Constipation
	Increased heart rate
RAPID ONSET OF EFFECT	Increased serum lipids

▷ **Principal Uses**

As a Single Drug Product: Uses currently included in FDA-approved labeling: Treatment of depression.

Other (unlabeled) generally accepted uses: May be useful in treatment of obsessive-compulsive disorder.

How This Drug Works: This bicyclic (second-generation) antidepressant inhibits the return (reuptake) of nerve transmitters (serotonin, norepinephrine, and dopamine) and helps return normal mood and thinking.

Available Dosage Forms and Strengths

Tablets — 25 mg, 37.5 mg, 50 mg, 75 mg, 100 mg
Tablets, extended release — pending

▷ **Recommended Dosage Ranges** (Actual dosage and administration schedule must be determined for each patient individually.)

Infants and Children: Safety and efficacy for those under 18 years of age are not established.

18 to 60 Years of Age: For depression: start with 75 mg per day, as 25-mg doses three times daily. If needed and tolerated, the dose may be increased at 4-day intervals up to a maximum of 225 mg per day. Some hospitalized patients have been given a maximum of 375 mg per day.
   The XR form has not yet been fully described.

Over 60 Years of Age: Low starting doses and slow increases are indicated. Natural declines in kidney function may lead to drug accumulation at higher doses. May worsen a constipation problem that you already face.

Conditions Requiring Dosing Adjustments
Liver Function: Total daily dose must be reduced by 50% for patients with moderate liver compromise. Further dose decreases and individualized dosing is indicated in patients with liver cirrhosis. The drug is changed to an active form in the liver.

Kidney Function: Patients with compromised kidneys (creatinine clearance of 10 to 70 ml/min) should take 75% of the usual daily dose.

▷ **Dosing Instructions:**   Food has no clinically significant effect on venlafaxine absorption.

Usual Duration of Use: Use on a regular schedule for 2 weeks usually determines effectiveness in treating depression. Long-term use (months to years) requires periodic physician evaluation of response and dosage adjustment.

Possible Advantages of This Drug
Effective treatment of depression with fewer side effects than other currently available agents.
Starts to have a therapeutic effect more rapidly than other available agents.

▷ **This Drug Should Not Be Taken If**
   • you have had an allergic reaction to any dosage form of it previously.
   • you are taking a monoamine oxidase (MAO) inhibitor (see Drug Classes).

▷ **Inform Your Physician Before Taking This Drug If**
   • you have a history of high blood pressure.
   • you have a history of abnormally increased lipids (hyperlipidemia).
   • you have a history of seizures.
   • you have a history of hypomania or mania.
   • you are uncertain of how much venlafaxine to take or how often to take it.

Possible Side Effects (natural, expected, and unavoidable drug actions)
Constipation and headache. Weight loss, dry mouth. Small increases in cholesterol (2–3 mg/dl).

▷ **Possible Adverse Effects** (unusual, unexpected, and infrequent reactions)
   If any of the following develop, consult your physician promptly for guidance.
Mild Adverse Effects
Allergic Reactions: Not characterized.
Palpitations—rare.
Nausea and vomiting—infrequent.
Dizziness (may disappear without treatment), fatigue, and headache—infrequent.
Anxiety, somnolence or insomnia (may stop on its own).
Blurred vision—possible.
Sweating—possible.

Serious Adverse Effects
Allergic Reactions: None reported.
Idiosyncratic Reactions: None reported.
Increased blood pressure—case reports.
Seizures—very rare during premarketing studies.

▷ **Possible Effects on Sexual Function:**   Delayed orgasm, abnormal ejaculation, impotence, and erectile failure—all rare.

Possible Delayed Adverse Effects: None reported.

▷ **Adverse Effects That May Mimic Natural Diseases or Disorders**
None reported.

Natural Diseases or Disorders That May Be Activated by This Drug
None reported.

Possible Effects on Laboratory Tests
Serum cholesterol: increased slightly.

CAUTION
1. This drug should **not** be taken with MAO inhibitor (see Glossary) drugs. If you have recently stopped an MAO inhibitor, 14 days should pass before venlafaxine is started.

▷ **Advisability of Use During Pregnancy**
Pregnancy Category: C. See Pregnancy Risk Categories at the back of this book.
Animal studies: There was an increase in stillborn rats at 10 times the usual human dose.
Human studies: Adequate studies of pregnant women are not available.
Ask your doctor for guidance.

Advisability of Use If Breast-Feeding
Presence of this drug in breast milk: Unknown.
Monitor nursing infant closely and discontinue drug or nursing if adverse effects develop.

Habit-Forming Potential: None.

Effects of Overdosage: Nausea, vomiting, constipation, seizure potential.

Possible Effects of Long-Term Use: None noted.

Suggested Periodic Examinations While Taking This Drug (at physician's discretion)
Blood pressure checks.

▷ **While Taking This Drug, Observe the Following**
Foods: No restrictions.
Nutritional Support: No special support indicated.
Beverages: Since venlafaxine is metabolized in the liver, and grapefruit juice has been shown to inhibit the removal (metabolism) of some other medications, caution is advised. Water may be the best liquid to take this medicine with.

▷ *Alcohol:* May increase somnolence if combined.
Tobacco Smoking: No interactions expected, but I advise everyone to quit smoking.
Marijuana Smoking: Additive effect on somnolence.

▷ *Other Drugs*
Venlafaxine ***taken concurrently*** with
• beta-blockers (see Drug Classes) may result in larger than expected pharmacological effects from the beta-blockers. Because these agents are me-

tabolized in the liver, and venlafaxine may block this metabolism, caution is advised.

- calcium channel blockers (see Drug Classes) may result in toxicity. Because these agents are metabolized in the liver, and venlafaxine may block this metabolism, caution is advised.
- cimetidine (Tagamet) may lead to venlafaxine toxicity.
- drugs with sedative properties will increase those effects.
- MAO inhibitors may lead to undesirable side effects. Do not combine.
- quinidine (Quinaglute, others) may result in venlafaxine toxicity.
- tricyclic antidepressants (see Drug Classes) may result in toxicity. Because these agents are metabolized in the liver, and venlafaxine may block this metabolism, caution is advised.
- warfarin (Coumadin) may result in bleeding. More frequent INR (prothrombin time or protime) testing is needed. Ongoing warfarin doses should be adjusted to laboratory results.

▷ *Driving, Hazardous Activities:* This drug may cause somnolence. Restrict activities as necessary.

Aviation Note: The use of this drug *is a disqualification* for piloting. Consult a designated Aviation Medical Examiner.

Exposure to Sun: No restrictions.

Exposure to Heat: No restrictions.

Discontinuation: Talk to your doctor before stopping this medication.

VERAPAMIL (ver AP a mil)

Introduced: 1967   **Class:** Anti-anginal, antiarrhythmic, antihypertensive, calcium channel blocker   **Prescription:** USA: Yes   **Controlled Drug:** USA: No; Canada: No   **Available as Generic:** USA: Yes; Canada: No

Brand Names: ✦Apo-Verap, Calan, Calan SR, Isoptin, Isoptin SR, ✦Novo-Veramil, ✦Nu-Verap, Verelan

Controversies in Medicine: Medicines in this class have been subject to much conflicting data. There have also been several FDA hearings held on the calcium-channel-blocker class. **More recent data found the long-acting forms of calcium channel blockers to be safe and effective.**

BENEFITS versus RISKS	
Possible Benefits	*Possible Risks*
EFFECTIVE PREVENTION OF BOTH MAJOR TYPES OF ANGINA	Congestive heart failure
EFFECTIVE CONTROL OF HEART RATE IN CHRONIC ATRIAL FIBRILLATION AND FLUTTER	Low blood pressure (infrequent)
	Heart rhythm disturbance
	Fluid retention
EFFECTIVE PREVENTION OF PAROXYSMAL ATRIAL TACHYCARDIA (PAT)	Liver damage without jaundice
	Swelling of male breast tissue
EFFECTIVE TREATMENT OF HYPERTENSION	

▷ **Principal Uses**

As a Single Drug Product: Uses currently included in FDA-approved labeling: Used to treat (1) angina pectoris due to coronary artery spasm (Prinzmetal's variant angina) that occurs spontaneously and is not associated with exertion; (2) classical angina-of-effort (due to atherosclerotic disease of the coronary arteries) in individuals who have not responded to or cannot tolerate the nitrates and beta-blocker drugs customarily used to treat this disorder; (3) abnormally rapid heart rate due to chronic atrial fibrillation or flutter; (4) recurrent paroxysmal atrial tachycardia; and (5) primary hypertension.

Other (unlabeled) generally accepted uses: (1) May help prevent abnormal heart rhythms that occur after surgery; (2) can help relieve symptoms and may help reverse hypertrophic cardiomyopathy; (3) may help decrease the severity or occurrence of cluster headaches; (4) used to help control the symptoms of panic attacks; (5) can be of use in post-ischemic-acute-kidney failure; (6) may stop the progression of abnormal buildup on the inside of blood vessels (atherosclerosis); (7) may help decrease severity and occurrence of nocturnal leg cramps; (8) could have a place in combination therapy of multiple myeloma; (9) can help stuttering; (10) may have a role in treating Tourette syndrome.

How This Drug Works: By blocking passage of calcium through certain cell walls (which is necessary for the function of nerve and muscle tissue), this drug slows the spread of electrical activity through the heart and inhibits the contraction of coronary arteries and peripheral arterioles. As a result of these combined effects, this drug

- prevents spontaneous coronary artery spasm (Prinzmetal's type of angina).
- reduces heart rate and contraction force during exertion, thus lowering the oxygen requirement of the heart muscle; this reduces the occurrence of effort-induced angina (classical angina pectoris).
- reduces degree of contraction of peripheral arterial walls, resulting in relaxation and lowering of blood pressure. This further reduces the workload of the heart during exertion and contributes to the prevention of angina.
- slows the rate of electrical impulses through the heart and thereby prevents excessively rapid heart action (tachycardia).

Available Dosage Forms and Strengths

Caplets, sustained release — 120 mg, 180 mg, 240 mg
Capsules, sustained release — 360 mg
Injection — 5 mg/2 ml
Tablets — 40 mg, 80 mg, 120 mg
Tablets, sustained release — 120 mg, 180 mg, 240 mg

▷ **Usual Adult Dosage Range:** Hypertension: Initially 80 mg three times daily. The dose may be increased gradually at 1- to 7-day intervals as needed and tolerated. The usual maintenance dose is from 240 to 360 mg daily in three or four divided doses. The prolonged-action (sustained-release) dosage forms permit once-a-day dosing. The total daily dosage should not exceed 360 mg.

Once-a-day treatment may be initiated with one prolonged-action capsule of 120 mg or one tablet of 180 mg.

Note: Actual dosage and administration schedule must be determined for each patient individually.

Conditions Requiring Dosing Adjustments

Liver Function: Blood levels should be obtained and used to guide dosing. For patients with liver compromise, the dose should be decreased to 20–50% of the usual dose and may be taken at the usual interval. Verapamil can be a rare cause of liver damage, and patients should be followed closely. Changes in the electrocardiogram may provide an early indication of increasing blood levels.

Kidney Function: In severe kidney compromise, the dose should be decreased by 50–75%.

▷ **Dosing Instructions:** Preferably taken with meals and with food at bedtime. The regular tablet may be crushed for administration. The prolonged-action dosage forms (capsules and tablets) should be swallowed whole and not altered. Verelan capsules may be taken without regard to food intake.

Usual Duration of Use: Use on a regular schedule for 2 to 4 weeks usually determines effectiveness in reducing the frequency and severity of angina. Reduction of elevated blood pressure may be apparent within the first 1 to 2 weeks. For long-term use (months to years), the smallest effective dose should be used. Periodic physician evaluation is needed.

Possible Advantages of This Drug

No adverse effects on blood levels of glucose, potassium, or uric acid.

Does not increase blood cholesterol or triglyceride levels.

Does not impair capacity for exercise.

The new 360-mg strength of Verelan allows once-daily dosing for those patients who require more than 240 mg daily. The company has noted that there is no increase in side effects when comparing the 240-mg capsules to the new 360-mg ones.

Currently a "Drug of Choice"

for treating hypertension in African-Americans.

▷ **This Drug Should Not Be Taken If**

- you have had an allergic reaction to it previously.
- you have active liver disease.
- you have a "sick sinus" syndrome (and do not have an artificial pacemaker).
- you have a fast heart rate (ventricular tachycardia) arising in the ventricles.
- you have been told that you have a second- or third-degree heart block.
- you have low blood pressure (systolic pressure below 90).
- you have advanced aortic stenosis (ask your doctor).

▷ **Inform Your Physician Before Taking This Drug If**

- you have had an unfavorable response to any calcium channel blocker.
- you are currently taking any other drugs, especially digitalis or a beta-blocker drug (see Drug Classes).
- you have had a recent stroke or heart attack.
- you have a history of congestive heart failure or heart rhythm disorders.
- you have poor circulation to your extremities, or gangrene.
- you have impaired liver or kidney function.
- you have a history of drug-induced liver damage.

Possible Side Effects (natural, expected, and unavoidable drug actions)

Low blood pressure, fluid retention—rare.

▷ **Possible Adverse Effects** (unusual, unexpected, and infrequent reactions)
If any of the following develop, consult your physician promptly for guidance.
Mild Adverse Effects
Allergic Reactions: Skin rash, hives, itching, aching joints.
Headache—frequent; dizziness, fatigue—infrequent.
Nausea, indigestion, constipation—rare.
Abnormal growth of the gums—infrequent.
Sensation of numbness or coldness in the extremities—case reports.
Serious Adverse Effects
Serious disturbances of heart rate and/or rhythm, congestive heart failure—rare.
Drug-induced liver damage without jaundice—case reports.
Antiplatelet effect and extended time to form blood clots—possible.
Excessive lowering of blood pressure—case reports.
Unmasking of parkinsonism—rare.
Low blood sugar—possible.

▷ **Possible Effects on Sexual Function**
Altered timing and pattern of menstruation.
Male breast enlargement and tenderness (gynecomastia)—case reports.
Impotence—frequent.

Possible Effects on Laboratory Tests
Blood total cholesterol and HDL cholesterol levels: no effect in some; decreased in others.
Blood LDL cholesterol or triglyceride level: no effect.
Glucose tolerance test (GTT): decreased.
Liver function tests: increased enzymes (ALT/GPT, AST/GOT), increased bilirubin (one case report).

CAUTION
1. Be sure to inform all physicians and other health care professionals who provide medical care for you that you take this drug. Note the use of this drug on your card of personal identification.
2. You may use nitroglycerin and other nitrate drugs as needed to relieve acute episodes of angina pain. If your angina attacks are becoming more frequent or intense, call your doctor promptly.
3. If this drug is used concurrently with a beta-blocker drug, you may develop excessively low blood pressure.
4. This drug may cause swelling of the feet and ankles. This may not be indicative of either heart or kidney dysfunction.

Precautions for Use
By Infants and Children: Safety and effectiveness for those under 12 years of age are not established.
By Those Over 60 Years of Age: You may be more susceptible to weakness, dizziness, fainting, and falling. Take necessary precautions to prevent injury. Report promptly any changes in your pattern of thirst and urination.

▷ **Advisability of Use During Pregnancy**
Pregnancy Category: C. See Pregnancy Risk Categories at the back of this book.
Animal studies: Toxic effects on the embryo and retarded growth of the fetus (but no birth defects) reported in rat studies.

Human studies: Adequate studies of pregnant women are not available. Avoid this drug during the first 3 months. Use during the final 6 months only if clearly needed. Ask your physician for guidance.

Advisability of Use If Breast-Feeding
Presence of this drug in breast milk: Yes.
Discuss the benefits and risks of nursing your infant. Although levels are present in the infant, most researchers find them to be below clinically significant levels. Monitor infant for adverse effects.

Habit-Forming Potential: None.

Effects of Overdosage: Flushed and warm skin, sweating, light-headedness, irritability, rapid heart rate, low blood pressure, loss of consciousness.

Possible Effects of Long-Term Use: None reported.

Suggested Periodic Examinations While Taking This Drug (at physician's discretion)
Evaluations of heart function, including electrocardiograms; liver and kidney function tests, with long-term use.

▷ **While Taking This Drug, Observe the Following**
Foods: No restrictions. Avoid excessive salt intake.
Beverages: Caffeine levels will be increased if caffeine-containing beverages are consumed while you are on verapamil. May be taken with milk.
▷ *Alcohol:* Use with caution until combined effects have been determined. Alcohol may exaggerate the drop in blood pressure, and change the elimination of alcohol (experienced by some patients).
Tobacco Smoking: Nicotine can reduce the effectiveness of this drug. Avoid all forms of tobacco.
Marijuana Smoking: Possible reduced effectiveness of this drug; mild to moderate increase in angina; possible changes in electrocardiogram, confusing interpretation.
▷ *Other Drugs*
Verapamil may *increase* the effects of
- carbamazepine (Tegretol), and cause carbamazepine toxicity.
- digitoxin and digoxin, and cause digitalis toxicity.
Verapamil *taken concurrently* with
- aspirin may result in bleeding.
- amiodarone (Cordarone) may result in cardiac arrest.
- beta-blocker drugs (see Drug Classes) may affect heart rate and rhythm adversely. Careful monitoring by your physician is necessary if these drugs are taken concurrently.
- calcium supplements (various) may blunt the therapeutic benefits of verapamil. Separate calcium and verapamil dosing by 2 hours.
- cyclosporine (Sandimmune) may result in cyclosporine toxicity and renal compromise.
- dantrolene will cause elevated blood potassium and depression of the heart.
- disopyramide (Norpace) can cause congestive heart failure.
- lithium (Lithobid, others) may result in lithium toxicity and mania.
- NSAIDs (see Drug Classes) may blunt the therapeutic effect of verapamil on blood pressure.

- oral hypoglycemic agents (see Oral Antidiabetic Drugs in Drug Classes) may lead to excessively low blood sugar.
- phenytoin (Dilantin) may result in decreased effectiveness of verapamil.
- quinidine (Quinaglute, others) can result in quinidine toxicity.
- rifampin (Rifadin, others) will decrease the therapeutic benefits of verapamil.
- sulfinpyrazone increases the removal of verapamil and lessens its therapeutic effects.
- terazosin (Hytrin) can lead to excessive decreases in blood pressure.
- theophylline (Theo-Dur, others) can lead to theophylline toxicity.

The following drugs may *increase* the effects of verapamil

- cimetidine (Tagamet) and other histamine (H_2) blocking drugs (see Drug Classes).
- ritonavir (Norvir) and perhaps other protease inhibitors (see Drug Classes).
- tricyclic antidepressants (see Drug Classes).

▷ *Driving, Hazardous Activities:* Usually no restrictions. This drug may cause dizziness. Restrict activities as necessary.

Aviation Note: Coronary artery disease *is a disqualification* for piloting. Consult a designated Aviation Medical Examiner.

Exposure to Sun: Use caution until sensitivity has been determined. This drug may cause photosensitivity (see Glossary).

Exposure to Heat: Caution is advised. Hot environments can exaggerate the blood-pressure-lowering effects of this drug. Observe for light-headedness or weakness.

Heavy Exercise or Exertion: This drug may improve your ability to be more active without resulting angina pain. Use caution and avoid excessive exercise that could impair heart function in the absence of warning pain.

Discontinuation: Do not stop this drug abruptly. Consult your physician regarding gradual withdrawal to prevent the development of rebound angina.

WARFARIN (WAR far in)

Introduced: 1941   **Class:** Anticoagulant, coumarins   **Prescription:** USA: Yes   **Controlled Drug:** USA: No; Canada: No   **Available as Generic:** USA: Yes, a Barr generic was recently approved; Canada: No
Brand Names: Coumadin, Warfarin Sodium

BENEFITS versus RISKS	
Possible Benefits	*Possible Risks*
EFFECTIVE PREVENTION OF BOTH ARTERIAL AND VENOUS THROMBOSIS	NARROW TREATMENT RANGE Dose-related bleeding Skin and soft tissue hemorrhage with tissue death
EFFECTIVE PREVENTION OF EMBOLIZATION IN THROMBOEMBOLIC DISORDERS	
HELPS PREVENT RECURRENCE OF HEART ATTACK	
HELPS PREVENT STROKES IN PATIENTS WITH ATRIAL FIBRILLATION	

▷ **Principal Uses**

As a Single Drug Product: Uses currently included in FDA-approved labeling: Used in: (1) Acute thrombosis (clot) or thrombophlebitis of the deep veins; (2) acute pulmonary embolism, resulting from blood clots that originate anywhere in the body; (3) atrial fibrillation, to prevent clotting of blood inside the heart that could result in embolization of small clots to any part of the body; (4) acute myocardial infarction (heart attack), to prevent clotting and embolization and therefore a recurrence of heart attack; (5) mitral valve replacement; (6) helps prevent blood clots in the lungs (pulmonary embolism) that may start after hip replacement surgery.

Other (unlabeled) generally accepted uses: (1) Helps prevent embolization from the heart in individuals with artificial heart valves; (2) may help patients with low blood platelets caused by heparin.

How This Drug Works: The coumarin anticoagulants interfere with the production of four essential blood clotting factors by blocking the action of vitamin K. This leads to a deficiency of these clotting factors in circulating blood and inhibits blood clotting mechanisms.

Available Dosage Forms and Strengths

Injection — 5 mg

Tablets — 1 mg, 2 mg, 2.5 mg, 5 mg, 7.5 mg, 10 mg

▷ **Usual Adult Dosage Range:**   Initially 2 to 5 mg daily for 2 to 3 days. A large loading dose is inappropriate and may be hazardous. For maintenance, the dose is decided based on INR (prothrombin time or protime) results and the condition being treated. In many conditions an INR of 2 to 3 is considered therapeutic. **Note: Actual dosage and schedule must be determined for each patient individually.**

Conditions Requiring Dosing Adjustments

Liver Function: Blood testing (prothrombin times) should be obtained to guide dosing. This drug is contraindicated in patients with liver disease.

Kidney Function: This drug should be used with caution in renal compromise, as warfarin may cause microscopic kidney stones.

▷ **Dosing Instructions:**   The tablet may be crushed and is preferably taken when the stomach is empty, and at the same time each day to ensure uniform results.

Usual Duration of Use: Use on a regular schedule for 3 to 5 days usually determines effectiveness in providing significant anticoagulation. An additional 10 to 14 days is required to determine the optimal maintenance dose for each individual. Long-term use (months to years) requires physician supervision.

▷ **This Drug Should Not Be Taken If**

• you have had an allergic reaction to it previously.
• you have an active peptic ulcer or active ulcerative colitis.
• you are pregnant.
• you have had recent anesthesia (lumbar block) to the spine.
• you have arterial aneurysm.
• you have low blood platelets.
• you have infective pericarditis.
• you have liver disease.

- you have esophageal varices (ask your doctor).
- you have had a recent stroke.

▷ **Inform Your Physician Before Taking This Drug If**
- you are now taking *any other drugs,* either prescription drugs or over-the-counter drug products.
- you are planning pregnancy.
- you have a history of a bleeding disorder.
- you have high blood pressure.
- you have abnormally heavy or prolonged menstrual bleeding.
- you have diabetes.
- you are using an indwelling catheter.
- you have impaired liver or kidney function.
- you plan to have surgery or dental extraction in the near future.

Possible Side Effects (natural, expected, and unavoidable drug actions)
Minor episodes of bleeding may occur even though dosage and prothrombin times are well within the recommended range.

▷ **Possible Adverse Effects** (unusual, unexpected, and infrequent reactions)
If any of the following develop, consult your physician promptly for guidance.
Mild Adverse Effects
Allergic Reactions: Skin rash, hives.
Loss of scalp hair—case reports.
Loss of appetite, nausea, vomiting, cramping, diarrhea—case reports.
Serious Adverse Effects
Allergic Reactions: Drug fever (see Glossary).
Idiosyncratic Reactions: Bleeding into skin and soft tissues, causing gangrene of breast, toes, and localized areas anywhere—rare.
Hereditary warfarin resistance—rare.
Abnormal bleeding from nose, gastrointestinal tract, lungs, urinary tract, or uterus—possible and dose related.
Pericardial tamponade—case reports.
Hemolytic anemia—rare.
Sudden nerve damage (femoral neuropathy)—case reports.
Kidney problems (tubulointerstitial nephritis)—case reports.

▷ **Possible Effects on Sexual Function:**   None reported.

▷ **Adverse Effects That May Mimic Natural Diseases or Disorders**
Drug-induced fever may suggest infection.

Natural Diseases or Disorders That May Be Activated by This Drug
Bleeding from "silent" peptic ulcer, intestinal or bladder polyp or tumor.

Possible Effects on Laboratory Tests
Complete blood cell counts: decreased red cells, hemoglobin, and white cells.
Bleeding time: increased.
INR (prothrombin time): increased.
Blood uric acid level: increased (in men).
Liver function tests: increased liver enzymes (ALT/GPT, AST/GOT, and alkaline phosphatase).

CAUTION

1. Always carry a personal identification card that includes a statement that *you are taking an anticoagulant drug.*
2. While taking this drug, always consult your physician *before* starting any new drug, changing the dosage schedule of any drug, or stopping any drug.
3. Data from the Agency for Health Care Policy and Research have shown that expanded use of warfarin could cut in half the 80,000 strokes that occur every year in patients who have atrial fibrillation.

Precautions for Use

By Those Over 60 Years of Age: Small starting doses are mandatory. Watch regularly for excessive drug effects: prolonged bleeding from shaving cuts, bleeding gums, bloody urine, rectal bleeding, excessive bruising. Some study data reveal that the beneficial effects of this medicine are not as widely known as needed and it is underprescribed for those over 60.

▷ **Advisability of Use During Pregnancy**

Pregnancy Category: X. See Pregnancy Risk Categories at the back of this book. Animal studies: Fetal hemorrhage and death due to this drug reported in mice.

Human studies: Information from studies of pregnant women indicates fetal defects and fetal hemorrhage due to this drug.

The manufacturers state that this drug is contraindicated during entire pregnancy.

Advisability of Use If Breast-Feeding

Presence of this drug in breast milk: Yes.

Avoid drug or refrain from nursing.

Habit-Forming Potential: None.

Effects of Overdosage: Episodes of bleeding from minor surface bleeding (nose, gums, small lacerations) to major internal bleeding: vomiting blood, bloody urine or stool.

Possible Effects of Long-Term Use: None reported.

Suggested Periodic Examinations While Taking This Drug (at physician's discretion)

Regular determinations of INR (prothrombin time or protime) are essential to safe dosage and proper control. Urine analyses for blood.

▷ **While Taking This Drug, Observe the Following**

Foods: A larger intake than usual of foods rich in vitamin K may reduce the effectiveness of this drug and make larger doses necessary. Foods rich in vitamin K include: asparagus, bacon, beef liver, cabbage, fish, cauliflower, green leafy vegetables. Vitamin E may increase risk of bleeding.

Beverages: No restrictions. May be taken with milk.

▷ *Alcohol:* Limit alcohol to one drink daily. Note: Heavy users of alcohol with liver damage may be very sensitive to anticoagulants and require smaller than usual doses.

Tobacco Smoking: Heavy smokers may require relatively larger doses of this drug. I advise everyone to quit smoking.

▷ *Other Drugs*

Warfarin may *increase* the effects of

- oral hypoglycemic agents (see Oral Antidiabetic Drugs in Drug Classes).
- phenytoin (Dilantin).

The following drugs may *increase* the effects of warfarin
- acetaminophen (high dose).
- allopurinol (Zyloprim).
- amiodarone (Cordarone).
- androgens (see Drug Classes).
- aspirin and some other NSAIDs (see Drug Classes).
- azithromycin (Zithromax).
- bismuth subsalicylate (Pepto-Bismol).
- carbamazepine (Tegretol).
- cephalosporins (see Drug Classes).
- chloral hydrate (Noctec).
- chloramphenicol (Chloromycetin).
- cimetidine (Tagamet).
- ciprofloxacin and other quinolone antibiotics (see Drug Classes).
- cisapride (Propulsid).
- clarithromycin (Biaxin).
- clofibrate (Atromid-S).
- cotrimoxazole (Bactrim).
- dextrothyroxine.
- dirithromycin and other macrolide antibiotics (see Drug Classes).
- disopyramide (Norpace).
- disulfiram (Antabuse).
- erythromycin (various).
- felbamate (Felbatol).
- fluconazole (Diflucan).
- fluoxetine (Prozac).
- fluvoxamine (Luvox).
- gemfibrozil (Lopid).
- glucagon.
- HMG CoA-reductase inhibitors.
- influenza vaccine (various).
- isoniazid (INH).
- itraconazole (Sporanox).
- ketoconazole (Nizoral).
- mesna (Mesnex).
- metronidazole (Flagyl).
- miconazole (Monistat).
- nonsteroidal anti-inflammatory drugs (see Drug Classes).
- omeprazole (Prilosec).
- pravastatin (Pravachol).
- propranolol (Inderal).
- quinidine (Quinaglute).
- ranitidine (Zantac).
- ritonavir (Norvir) and perhaps other protease inhibitors (see Drug Classes).
- salicylates (aspirin, etc.).
- sertraline (Zoloft).
- simvastatin (Zocor).
- streptokinase.
- sulfinpyrazone (Anturane).
- sulfonamides (see Drug Classes).
- tamoxifen (Nolvadex).

- tetracyclines (see Drug Classes).
- thyroid hormones (various).
- tricyclic antidepressants (see Drug Classes).
- vancomycin (Vancoled).
- vitamin E.

The following drugs may *decrease* the effects of warfarin

- azathioprine (Imuran).
- barbiturates (see Drug Classes).
- birth control pills (oral contraceptives).
- carbamazepine (Tegretol).
- cholestyramine (Questran).
- estrogens (unclear, but possible).
- ethchlorvynol (Placidyl).
- glutethimide (Doriden).
- griseofulvin (Gris-PEG).
- phytonadione (vitamin K).
- primidone (Mysoline).
- some penicillins (see Drug Classes).
- spironolactone.
- sucralfate (Carafate).
- rifampin (Rifadin).
- thiazide diuretics (see Drug Classes).
- vitamin K.

▷ *Driving, Hazardous Activities:* No restrictions.

Aviation Note: The use of this drug *is a disqualification* for piloting. Consult a designated Aviation Medical Examiner.

Exposure to Sun: No restrictions.

Discontinuation: Do not stop this drug abruptly unless abnormal bleeding occurs. Ask your physician for guidance regarding gradual reduction in dosage over a period of 3 to 4 weeks.

ZALCITABINE (zal SIT a been)

Other Names: Dideoxycytidine, DDC

Introduced: 1987   **Class:** Antiviral, anti-AIDS drug   **Prescription:** USA: Yes   **Controlled Drug:** USA: No; Canada: No   **Available as Generic:** USA: No

Brand Name: Hivid

BENEFITS versus RISKS	
Possible Benefits	*Possible Risks*
DELAYED PROGRESSION OF DISEASE IN HIV-INFECTED PATIENTS	DRUG-INDUCED PERIPHERAL NEURITIS
PART OF EFFECTIVE COMBINATION REGIMENS	Drug-induced pancreatitis, esophageal ulcers, or arthritis
	Drug-induced cardiomyopathy/congestive heart failure

▷ **Principal Uses**

As a Single Drug Product: Uses currently included in FDA-approved labeling: (1) This drug is approved for advanced (CD4 cell count less than or equal to 300 cells per cubic mm) HIV infection in adults who do not tolerate alternative antiretroviral therapy or have progression of their disease while taking alternative antiretrovirals; (2) used in combination therapy with zidovudine in patients with limited prior treatment with zidovudine (< 3 months). This drug is not a cure for AIDS.

Author's Note: *The Panel on Clinical Practices for Treatment of HIV Infection Report* says that the preferred regimen is: Two nucleoside analogs and one potent protease inhibitor. Single-agent therapy (with the exception of AZT use in preventing HIV transmission from mother to fetus) was rejected by the panel.

Other (unlabeled) generally accepted uses: (1) Combination therapy with saquinavir (Invirase); (2) may have a role in pediatric AIDS.

How This Drug Works: By interfering with essential HIV enzyme systems, this drug is thought to prevent the growth and reproduction of HIV particles within infected cells, thus limiting the severity and extent of HIV infection.

Available Dosage Forms and Strengths

Tablets — 0.375 mg, 0.75 mg

▷ **Recommended Dosage Ranges** (Actual dosage and administration schedule must be determined for each patient individually.)

Infants and Children: Under investigation.

12 to 60 Years of Age: The recommended combination regimen is: one 0.75-mg tablet every 8 hours. In combination therapy: one 0.75-mg tablet orally, to be taken with 200 mg of zidovudine every 8 hours. The total daily dose for both drugs then becomes 2.25 mg of zalcitabine and 600 mg of zidovudine. The initial dose does not need to be reduced unless the patient has a body mass of less than 30 kg (66 lb).

Conditions Requiring Dosing Adjustments

Liver Function: Liver toxicity may be more likely in people with a prior history of alcohol abuse or liver damage. The patient should be monitored closely, and the dosage reduced or the medication interrupted if toxicity occurs. Patients with liver function enzymes that are more than five times the upper limit of the normal range should stop the drug.

Kidney Function: Patients with moderate kidney failure can take 0.75 mg of zalcitabine every 12 hours. In severe kidney failure, the patient can take 0.75 mg every 24 hours.

▷ **Dosing Instructions:**   When combination therapy is being given, dose adjustments must be based on the toxicity profiles for each drug. For example: if peripheral neuropathy or severe oral ulcers occur, the zalcitabine dose should be decreased or interrupted. Second, if the patient experiences anemia or granulocytopenia, the zidovudine dose should be decreased or interrupted. If the zalcitabine is interrupted or stopped, the zidovudine dose should be changed from 200 mg every 8 hours to 100 mg every 4 hours. Zalcitabine is **not** indicated for use as the only therapy. If zalcitabine is stopped, the physician **must** consider alternative antiretroviral therapy.

The largest peak concentration, the time that it takes for the peak to be achieved, and the amount absorbed are all changed if this drug is taken with food. It is better to take this medication on an empty stomach.

Usual Duration of Use: Use on a regular schedule for several months usually determines effectiveness in slowing the progression of AIDS. Long-term use (months to years) requires periodic physician evaluation of response (viral load and CD4) and dosage adjustment.

Possible Advantages of This Drug
Does not cause serious depression of bone marrow function (production of blood cells).

▷ **This Drug Should Not Be Taken If**
- you have had an allergic reaction to it previously.
- you have had pancreatitis recently.
- you have severe myelosuppression (ask your doctor).

▷ **Inform Your Physician Before Taking This Drug If**
- you have had allergic reactions to any drugs in the past.
- you are taking any other drugs currently.
- you have a history of pancreatitis or peripheral neuritis.
- you have a history of severe myelosuppression (ask your doctor).
- you have a history of esophageal ulcers.
- you have congestive heart failure or cardiac muscle damage (cardiac myopathy).
- you have a history of alcoholism.
- you have impaired liver or kidney function.

Possible Side Effects (natural, expected, and unavoidable drug actions)
Mild and infrequent decreases in red blood cell, white blood cell, and platelet counts.

▷ **Possible Adverse Effects** (unusual, unexpected, and infrequent reactions)
If any of the following develop, consult your physician promptly for guidance.
Mild Adverse Effects
Allergic Reactions: Skin rash and itching.
Fever, joint pains—infrequent.
Ringing in the ears—case reports.
Mouth sores, nausea, vomiting, diarrhea, stomach pain—infrequent.
Serious Adverse Effects
Allergic Reactions: Anaphylaxis—rare.
Drug-induced peripheral neuritis (see Glossary), usually occurring after 7 to 18 weeks of treatment. This is more frequent and severe with high doses, and less frequent and mild with low doses.
Drug-induced cardiomyopathy/congestive heart failure—infrequent.
Drug-induced pancreatitis, usually within the first 6 months of treatment—rare.
Electrolyte changes (lowered phosphorous, sodium, magnesium, or calcium)—rare to infrequent.
Ototoxicity and hearing loss—rare.
Lowered white blood cell counts—infrequent.
Worsening of preexisting liver disease or hepatotoxicity—rare.

▷ **Possible Effects on Sexual Function:** None reported.

▷ **Adverse Effects That May Mimic Natural Diseases or Disorders**
None reported to date.

Possible Effects on Laboratory Tests
Complete blood cell counts: decreased red cells, white cells, and platelets (infrequent and mild).
Blood amylase level: increased (infrequent).
Blood glucose level: increased.
Liver function tests: increased (SGOT, SGPT, and LDH).

CAUTION
1. This drug does not cure HIV infection.
2. Call your doctor right away if stomach pain with nausea and vomiting occurs; this could indicate the onset of pancreatitis. It may be necessary to discontinue this drug.
3. MOST clinicians advocate combination therapy for this disease.
4. Pain, numbness, tingling, or burning in the hands or feet should prompt a call to your doctor; this could indicate the onset of peripheral neuritis. It may be necessary to stop this drug.
5. It is advisable to avoid all other drugs that are known to cause pancreatitis or peripheral neuritis; ask your physician for guidance.

Precautions for Use
By Infants and Children: Safety and effectiveness for use by this age group have not been established. Children may also be at risk for developing drug-induced pancreatitis and peripheral neuritis; monitor closely for significant symptoms.
By Those Over 60 Years of Age: Reduced kidney function may require dosage reduction.

▷ **Advisability of Use During Pregnancy**
Pregnancy Category: C. See Pregnancy Risk Categories at the back of this book.
Animal studies: This drug has been shown to be teratogenic in mice at doses of 1,365 and 2,730 times of the maximum recommended human dose (MRHD). Increased embryolethality was observed in mice with doses of 2,730 times the MRHD.
Human studies: Information from adequate studies of pregnant women is not available. The manufacturer recommends that fertile women should not receive zalcitabine unless they are using effective contraception during therapy.
Consult your physician for specific guidance.

Advisability of Use If Breast-Feeding
Presence of this drug in breast milk: Unknown.
Avoid drug or refrain from nursing.
Note: HIV has been found in human breast milk. Breast-feeding may result in transmission of HIV infection to the nursing infant.

Habit-Forming Potential: None.

Effects of Overdosage: Nausea, vomiting, stomach pain, diarrhea, pain in hands and feet.

Possible Effects of Long-Term Use: Peripheral neuritis (see Glossary).

Suggested Periodic Examinations While Taking This Drug (at physician's discretion)

Complete blood cell counts before starting treatment and weekly thereafter until tolerance is established.

Blood amylase levels, fractionated for salivary gland and pancreatic origin.

Triglyceride levels should be tested at baseline (before therapy is started) and periodically during therapy.

Assessment of CD4 counts and viral load. These give the clearest indication of pending failure and reason to change to other agents.

▷ **While Taking This Drug, Observe the Following**

Foods: No restrictions.

Beverages: No restrictions.

▷ *Alcohol:* No interactions expected.

Tobacco Smoking: No interactions expected, but I advise everyone to quit smoking.

▷ *Other Drugs*

Zalcitabine may ***increase*** the effects of

- zidovudine (Retrovir), and enhance its antiviral effect against HIV. Serious patient reactions to either of these medicines should be reported to the FDA.

Zalcitabine ***taken concurrently*** with

- cimetidine (Tagamet) may result in toxic zalcitabine levels.
- didanosine (Videx) may result in additive neurotoxicity.
- metoclopramide (Reglan) may result in lowered blood levels of zalcitabine and reduced therapeutic benefits.
- other drugs that cause neurotoxicity or pancreatitis—this combination is best avoided.
- probenecid (Benemid) may lead to zalcitabine toxicity.

▷ *Driving, Hazardous Activities:* This drug may cause pain and weakness in the extremities. Restrict activities as necessary.

Aviation Note: The use of this drug ***is a disqualification*** for piloting. Consult a designated Aviation Medical Examiner.

Exposure to Sun: No restrictions.

Discontinuation: Do not stop this drug without your physician's knowledge and guidance.

ZIDOVUDINE (zi DOH vyoo deen)

Other Names: AZT, azidothymidine, Compound S, ZDV

Introduced: 1987   **Class:** Antiviral, anti-AIDS drugs   **Prescription:** USA: Yes   **Controlled Drug:** USA: No; Canada: No   **Available as Generic:** USA: No; Canada: No

Brand Name: Retrovir

```
┌─────────────────────────────────────────────────────────────┐
│                    BENEFITS versus RISKS                      │
│      Possible Benefits              Possible Risks            │
│   DELAYED PROGRESSION OF        SERIOUS BONE MARROW           │
│   DISEASE IN HIV-INFECTED         DEPRESSION                  │
│   PATIENTS WHEN COMBINATION     Brain toxicity               │
│   TREATMENT IS USED             Lip, mouth, and tongue sores │
│   REDUCED INCIDENCE OF                                        │
│   INFECTIONS WITH                                             │
│   COMBINATION THERAPY                                         │
└─────────────────────────────────────────────────────────────┘
```

▷ **Principal Uses**

As a Single Drug Product: Uses currently included in FDA-approved labeling: (1) Used to treat selected patients who have acquired immunodeficiency syndrome (AIDS). This drug is not a cure for AIDS, and it does not reduce the risk of transmission of AIDS infection to others through sexual contact or contamination of blood; (2) approved to help prevent transmission of HIV from mother to infant; (3) approved for combination therapy with other agents; (4) approved for children 3 months or older who have laboratory values that indicate HIV infection or HIV immunosuppression; (5) approved for use in HIV-positive patients who are as yet asymptomatic.

Author's Note: *The Panel on Clinical Practices for Treatment of HIV Infection Report* **says that the preferred regimen is: Two nucleoside analogs and one potent protease inhibitor. Single-agent therapy (with the exception of AZT use in preventing HIV transmission from mother to fetus) was rejected by the panel.**

Other (unlabeled) generally accepted uses: (1) Used to treat Kaposi's sarcoma; (2) helps remove hairy leukoplakia in the mouth; (3) used to treat heart dysfunction in people with HIV; (4) may prevent HIV in health care workers exposed to the AIDS virus; (5) appears to increase AIDS-related low platelet counts; (6) may have a role in treating adult T-cell leukemia or lymphoma in combination with interferon alpha.

Author's Note: Although this drug has historically been used as a single drug to treat AIDS, a medical consensus has developed that limits the use of this drug to combination therapy.

How This Drug Works: By interfering with essential enzyme systems, this drug is thought to prevent the growth and reproduction of HIV particles within tissue cells, thus limiting the severity and extent of HIV infection.

Available Dosage Forms and Strengths

Capsules — 100 mg
Injection — 10 mg/ml
Syrup — 50 mg/5 ml

▷ **Usual Adult Dosage Range:** HIV infection: The product information insert for zidovudine recommends 600 mg daily, divided into equal doses in combination with other antiretroviral agents. Further, 500 mg as 100 mg every 4 hours while awake or 600 mg daily divided into equal doses is suggested for monotherapy.

For prevention of maternal fetal transmission in pregnancy: 100 mg by mouth five times per day until the start of labor. During labor, AZT is given intravenously (2 mg per kg of body mass), followed by 1 mg per kg of body mass per hour. This dose is continued until the umbilical cord is clamped. The infant then receives 1.5 mg per kg of body mass every 6 hours.

Note: Actual dosage and administration schedule must be determined for each patient individually. Author's Note: There is controversy as to the ideal time to start antiretroviral therapy. Current recommendations call for combination therapy once the infection is diagnosed.

Conditions Requiring Dosing Adjustments

Liver Function: The dose should be decreased by 50% or the dosing interval should be doubled for patients with significant liver compromise. This drug can be a rare cause of liver damage, and patients should be followed closely.

Kidney Function: Specific guidelines for dosage adjustments in patients with compromised kidneys are not available. This drug should be used with caution in kidney compromise.

▷ **Dosing Instructions:**   Preferably taken on an empty stomach, but may be taken with or following food. Take exactly as prescribed. The capsule may be opened and the contents mixed with food just prior to administration. It is best to take the capsule with at least 120 ml of water.

Usual Duration of Use: Use on a regular schedule for 10 to 12 weeks usually determines effectiveness in improving the course of symptomatic AIDS infection. Long-term use requires periodic physician evaluation of response (viral load and CD4) and dosage adjustment.

▷ **This Drug Should Not Be Taken If**
- you have had a serious allergic reaction to it previously.
- you have a serious degree of uncorrected bone marrow depression.

▷ **Inform Your Physician Before Taking This Drug If**
- you have a history of either folic acid or vitamin B_{12} deficiency.
- you have impaired liver or kidney function.
- you take other drugs that can have a bad effect on the bone marrow (are myelosuppressive).

Possible Side Effects (natural, expected, and unavoidable drug actions)
None reported.

▷ **Possible Adverse Effects** (unusual, unexpected, and infrequent reactions)
If any of the following develop, consult your physician promptly for guidance.

Mild Adverse Effects
Allergic Reactions: Skin rash, hives, itching.
Headache, weakness, drowsiness, dizziness, nervousness, insomnia—infrequent.
Nausea, diarrhea, vomiting, altered taste, lip sores, swollen mouth or tongue—infrequent.
Paresthesias, muscle aches, fever, sweating—infrequent.

Serious Adverse Effects
Confusion, loss of speech, twitching, tremors, seizures (representing brain toxicity)—infrequent.
Eye problems (macular edema)—case reports.
Muscle toxicity (myopathy)—infrequent.
Mania or seizures—rare.
Muscle toxicity of the heart (cardiomyopathy)—case reports.

Bone marrow depression (see Glossary): fatigue, weakness, fever, sore throat, abnormal bleeding or bruising. Anemia occurs most commonly after 4 to 6 weeks of treatment; abnormally low white blood cell counts occur after 6 to 8 weeks of treatment—infrequent.

Esophageal ulcers (patients should take this medicine with at least 120 ml of water and not lie down for an hour)—possible.

Liver toxicity—infrequent.

▷ **Possible Effects on Sexual Function**

None reported.

Possible Delayed Adverse Effects: Significant anemia and deficient white blood cell counts may develop after this drug has been discontinued. Myopathy.

▷ **Adverse Effects That May Mimic Natural Diseases or Disorders**

Seizures may suggest the possibility of epilepsy.

Possible Effects on Laboratory Tests

Complete blood cell counts: decreased red cells, hemoglobin, white cells, and platelets.

CAUTION

1. This drug is not a cure for AIDS, nor does it protect completely against other infections or complications. Follow your physician's instructions and take all medications exactly as prescribed.
2. This drug does not reduce the risk of transmitting AIDS to others through sexual contact or contamination of the blood. The use of an effective condom is mandatory. Needles for drug administration should not be shared.

Precautions for Use

By Infants and Children: Zidovudine syrup is used in HIV-infected pediatric patients who are greater than 3 months old. The usual dose is 180 mg per square meter.

By Those Over 60 Years of Age: Impaired kidney function will require dosage reduction.

▷ **Advisability of Use During Pregnancy**

Pregnancy Category: C. See Pregnancy Risk Categories at the back of this book.

Animal studies: Rat studies reveal no birth defects.

Human studies: Adequate studies of pregnant women are not available.

Consult your physician for specific guidance. This medicine has been shown to dramatically reduce the transference of HIV from mother to infant. If the decision is made to use this medicine in pregnancy, cases should be reported to 1–800–722–9292, extention 8465.

Advisability of Use If Breast-Feeding

Presence of this drug in breast milk: Unknown.

Avoid drug or refrain from nursing.

Habit-Forming Potential: None.

Effects of Overdosage: Nausea, vomiting, diarrhea, bone marrow depression.

Possible Effects of Long-Term Use: Serious anemia and loss of white blood cells. Muscle toxicity (myopathy).

Suggested Periodic Examinations While Taking This Drug (at physician's discretion)

Complete blood cell counts before starting treatment and weekly thereafter until tolerance is established. Continual monitoring for bone marrow depression is necessary during entire course of treatment. Periodic CD4 counts or measurements of viral load are indicators that treatment is failing and demand change of antiretroviral therapy.

▷ **While Taking This Drug, Observe the Following**

Foods: No restrictions.

Beverages: No restrictions. May be taken with milk.

▷ *Alcohol:* No interactions expected.

Tobacco Smoking: No interactions expected, but I advise everyone to quit smoking.

▷ *Other Drugs*

The following drugs may ***increase*** the effects of zidovudine and enhance its toxicity

- acetaminophen (Tylenol, others).
- acyclovir (Zovirax).
- amphotericin B (Fungizone).
- aspirin.
- benzodiazepines (see Drug Classes).
- cimetidine (Tagamet).
- fluconazole (Diflucan).
- ganciclovir (Cytovene).
- indomethacin.
- interferon beta.
- morphine (various).
- probenecid (Benemid).
- sulfonamides (see Drug Classes).

Zidovudine ***taken concurrently*** with

- didanosine may result in increased risk of myelosuppression.
- filgrastim (Neupogen) may help maintain the white blood cell count.
- rifampin (Rifadin) can lead to decreased zidovudine blood levels.
- stavudine (D4T) may lessen effectiveness, as both agents are cell cycle specific.
- trimexate may cause additive hematological toxicity.

▷ *Driving, Hazardous Activities:* This drug may cause dizziness or fainting. Restrict activities as necessary.

Aviation Note: The use of this drug ***is a disqualification*** for piloting. Consult a designated Aviation Medical Examiner.

Exposure to Sun: No restrictions.

Discontinuation: Do not stop this drug without your physician's knowledge and guidance.

ZOLPIDEM (ZOL pi dem)

Introduced: 1993 **Class:** Hypnotic, imidazopyridine **Prescription:**
USA: Yes **Controlled Drug:** USA: C-IV*; Canada: Prescription **Available**
as Generic: USA: No
Brand Name: Ambien

BENEFITS versus RISKS	
Possible Benefits	*Possible Risks*
GIVES SHORT-TERM RELIEF OF INSOMNIA WITH MINIMAL SLEEP DISRUPTION (REM)	Habit-forming potential with prolonged use
	Rebound insomnia upon withdrawal

▷ **Principal Uses**
As a Single Drug Product: Uses currently included in FDA-approved labeling:
Short-term treatment of insomnia in adults.
Other (unlabeled) generally accepted uses: Long-term (more than 1 year)
treatment of insomnia has been accomplished successfully in limited trials.

How This Drug Works: This drug attaches (binds) to a specific receptor
(omega-1) and: reduces the time it takes to fall asleep, and increases total
sleep time while producing a pattern and benefit of sleep that is similar to
normal sleep patterns.

Available Dosage Forms and Strengths
Tablets — 5 mg, 10 mg

▷ **Recommended Dosage Ranges** (Actual dosage and administration schedule
must be determined for each patient individually.)
Infants and Children: Safety and efficacy for those under 18 years of age are not
established.
18 to 60 Years of Age: 10 mg is taken immediately before bedtime. Patients
should be reevaluated after taking this drug for 10 days.
Over 60 Years of Age: Therapy should be started with 5 mg taken at bedtime. The
dose may be cautiously increased to 10 mg at bedtime.

Conditions Requiring Dosing Adjustments
Liver Function: The dose should be reduced by 50% in liver compromise.
Kidney Function: The half-life is doubled in chronic kidney compromise, and
the dose must be decreased.

▷ **Dosing Instructions:** The tablet may be crushed and is best taken on an empty
stomach. Do **not** stop this drug abruptly if taken for more than 7 days.

Usual Duration of Use: Use on a regular schedule for 2 nights usually determines effectiveness in treating insomnia. Your physician should assess the
benefit of this drug after 10 days.

Possible Advantages of This Drug
Low occurrence of adverse effects.
May produce less of an undesirable effect on normal sleep patterns.

Currently a "Drug of Choice"
for short-term management of insomnia in adults.

*See schedules of Controlled Drugs at the back of this book.

▷ **This Drug Should Not Be Taken If**
- you have had an allergic reaction to any dosage form of it previously.

▷ **Inform Your Physician Before Taking This Drug If**
- you have abnormal liver or kidney function.
- you are pregnant or planning pregnancy.
- you have a history of alcoholism or drug abuse.
- you have a serious lung problem (respiratory impairment).
- you have a history of serious depression or mental disorder.
- you are uncertain of how much zolpidem to take or how often to take it.

Possible Side Effects (natural, expected, and unavoidable drug actions)
Drowsiness and blurred vision, "hangover" effects following long-term use.

▷ **Possible Adverse Effects** (unusual, unexpected, and infrequent reactions)
If any of the following develop, consult your physician promptly for guidance.
Mild Adverse Effects
Allergic Reactions: Skin rash.
Drowsiness and dizziness—rare.
Nausea and diarrhea—infrequent.
Elevation of liver function tests—rare.
Muscle tremors—infrequent.
Blurred vision—infrequent.
Serious Adverse Effects
Allergic Reactions: Not defined.
Abnormal thoughts or hallucinations—case reports.
Paradoxical aggression, agitation, or suicidal thoughts—rare.

▷ **Possible Effects on Sexual Function:**   None reported.

Possible Effects on Laboratory Tests
Liver function tests: increased SGOT, SGPT, and CPK.

CAUTION
1. This drug works quickly. It is best to take it just before bedtime.
2. Do **not** drink alcohol while taking this drug.
3. Withdrawal (see Glossary) may occur, even if this drug was only taken for a week or two. Ask your doctor for advice before stopping zolpidem.
4. You may experience trouble going to sleep for 1 or 2 nights after stopping this drug (rebound insomnia). This effect is usually short term.
5. Sleep disturbances may be a symptom of underlying psychological problems. Tell your doctor if unusual behaviors or odd thoughts occur.
6. Drugs that depress the central nervous system may produce additive effects with this drug. Ask your doctor or pharmacist **before** combining other prescription or nonprescription drugs with zolpidem.

Precautions for Use
By Infants and Children: Safety and effectiveness for those under 18 years of age are not established.
By Those Over 60 Years of Age: The starting dose should be decreased to 5 mg. Since this drug works quickly, it is best taken immediately before going to bed. You may be at increased risk for falls if the drug remains in your system in the morning. Watch for lethargy, unsteadiness, nightmares, and paradoxical agitation and anger.

▷ **Advisability of Use During Pregnancy**
    Pregnancy Category: B. See Pregnancy Risk Categories at the back of this book.
    Animal studies: In rats, abnormal skull bone formation was reported. In rabbits, abnormal bone formation was found.
    Human studies: Adequate studies of pregnant women are not available.
    Use during pregnancy is **not** advisable. Ask your doctor for guidance.

Advisability of Use If Breast-Feeding
    Presence of this drug in breast milk: Yes.
    Avoid drug or refrain from nursing.

Habit-Forming Potential: This drug may cause dependence (see Glossary).

Effects of Overdosage: Marked change from lethargy to coma. Cardiovascular and respiratory compromise was also reported. The drug flumazenil may help reverse symptoms.

Possible Effects of Long-Term Use: Psychological and/or physical dependence.

Suggested Periodic Examinations While Taking This Drug (at physician's discretion)
    Liver function tests.

▷ **While Taking This Drug, Observe the Following**
    Foods: This drug should **not** be taken with food.
    Beverages: Avoid caffeine-containing beverages: coffee, tea, cola, chocolate.
▷   *Alcohol:* This drug should **not** be combined with alcohol.
    Tobacco Smoking: Nicotine is a stimulant and should be avoided. I advise everyone to quit smoking.
    Marijuana Smoking: May cause additive drowsiness.
▷   *Other Drugs*
        Zolpidem *taken concurrently* with
- ritonavir (Norvir) and perhaps other protease inhibitors (see Drug Classes) may lead to toxicity.

        Zolpidem may *increase* the effects of
- chlorpromazine (Thorazine).
- narcotics or other CNS-depressant drugs (see Drug Classes for Opioids, Phenothiazines, Antihistamines, and Benzodiazepines).

▷   *Driving, Hazardous Activities:* This drug may cause drowsiness and impair coordination. Restrict activities as necessary.
    Aviation Note: The use of this drug *is a disqualification* for piloting. Consult a designated Aviation Medical Examiner.
    Discontinuation: This drug should **not** be stopped abruptly, even after a week of use. Ask your doctor for help regarding an appropriate withdrawal schedule.

THE LEADING EDGE

This section is designed to help you become more fully aware of medicines that show promise in novel applications or are FDA approvable. "The Leading Edge" is also intended to bring information about new concepts in medication delivery. Also, a few interesting medications or therapeutic products still in early clinical trials are included as "stars on the horizon."

It is impossible to predict which medicines or delivery systems **will** achieve final FDA approval or be used in specific drugs, but many of those successful ones will be covered in subsequent editions. Finally, there will be many potential medicines or delivery systems which could be covered in a given year. The author will choose those which in his opinion offer the most potential benefit to his readers.

AIDS VACCINE (AYDS)

Star on the Horizon

President Clinton has promised 19 million dollars to further the development of an AIDS vaccine. To date, compounds have been elusive. An approach targeting the genetic material (DNA) of the virus has hope, but will take time to develop.

ANTIESTROGENS (ANT eye s troh genz)

Star on the Horizon

These compounds (also known as SERMs or selective estrogen receptor modulators) appear to have many of the desirable properties of estrogens, but do not have the undesirable side effects of estrogens. Several members of this class are in therapeutic trials. A medicine called raloxifene is presently in phase three clinical trials and has been referred to as a "designer estrogen."

ESTROGENS (S troh genz)

Novel Application
In a study of 400 women at Johns Hopkins, these compounds have been shown to possibly prevent Alzheimer's. Further study is needed, however; researchers are having difficulty enrolling patients in a placebo-controlled trial.

HOMOCYSTEINE (HOMO sis teen)

Star on the Horizon
This compound is not a medicine, but was recently confirmed by the European Concerted Action Project as a powerful risk factor for blood vessel disease, and found to be equal in importance to smoking or increased blood lipids. Early data appear to show that folic acid and possibly pyridoxine can reduce homocysteine blood levels and decrease this risk factor for patients in whom it is elevated.

INTEGRASE (IN ta grace)

Star on the Horizon
Integrase, and research into medicines that can interfere with it, has continued with two companies currently having compounds in clinical trials. This drug acts at a different point in the life cycle of the virus than the four nucleoside analogs, the two nonnucleoside analogs, or the new protease inhibitors that are currently available. Still another point of attack may be found in preventing HIV's ability to enter and infect cells. A new drug known as ALX40–4C appears to block viral entry. Recent X-ray crystallography evidence shows that the attachment protein which the HIV virus uses has two parts and appears to require joining to be active. Both of these new approaches used alone or in combination with existing medicines may well turn AIDS into a more survivable, chronic disease.

INTERLEUKINS (inter LEW kenz)

Star on the Horizon
These compounds appear to have a role in many aspects of human physiology: for example, interleukin 1 (IL-1) has a role in causing osteoporosis. Other interleukins may have a role in treating certain problems. Interleukin 11 (IL-11) is in phase three trials for use in preventing lowering of blood platelets in patients who are given cancer chemotherapy.

LAMIVUDINE (lam IV you deen)

Novel Application
This medicine is currently available under the name Epivir for treating AIDS. It is also in clinical trials for use in treating sudden (acute) and long-standing (chronic) hepatitis B infections. Results so far are very promising and appear to offer results where previously little could be done.

LIPOSOMES (LIP oh soams)

Medication Delivery
Once again liposomes, and the ability to place medications in them, appear to offer greatly improved results (outcomes) from medicines. Sequus and Bayer AG are working to enclose an antibiotic called ciprofloxacin into long-circulating liposomes.

LYME DISEASE VACCINE

Star on the Horizon
Progress into a vaccine for this prevalent infection has continued. Presently, two companies (Connaught and SmithKline Beecham) are completing research and plan to seek FDA approval for their respective versions of a Lyme disease vaccine. Once again, **"Rybacki's recommendation number one:"** It is always better to prevent a disease or condition than to have to treat it.

MINOCYCLINE (MIN oh seye clean)

Novel Application
This medicine is an antibiotic that has been in use for many years. In addition to its antibiotic effect, it also has an anti-inflammatory action. Minocycline appears to inhibit proteinases that may be involved in causing rheumatoid arthritis (RA). It has modest benefits in long-standing RA, but shows much promise in early treatment of RA. There may also be a role for this medicine in ankylosing spondylitis.

NSAIDS (EN saydz)

Novel Application
NSAIDs are nonsteroidal anti-inflammatory drugs. Some data have been made public which show that long-term use of some NSAIDs appears to offer protection from Alzheimer's disease. Further research is required to find out how this effect occurs, which of the medicines in this very broad class are best at preventing Alzheimer's, and what are the best doses and risk profiles to consider when using one of these medicines for long-term therapy.

PHYSOSTIGMINE (fi soh STIG mean)

Novel Application
This medicine is an anticholinesterase agent. In the past, it has been used intravenously to reverse toxic effects of anticholinergic drugs, and in some cases as an eyedrop in glaucoma. Recent data show that this medicine helps short-term memory in normal patients, and it appears to have an effect in Alzheimer's patients. It is presently available as the brand name Antilirium (tablets and intravenous injection) and Isopto (eserine ophthalmic drops).

ROTAVIRUS VACCINE (ROW ta vi russ)

Star on the Horizon

Rotavirus is a significant cause of mortality and morbidity in infants and young children because of dehydrating gastroenteritis. New research involving 1,278 healthy infants showed significant results. Future trials are needed to confirm safety and efficacy, but it appears a final vaccine formulation is not far away.

ST.-JOHN'S-WORT (saint jahns wort)

Star on the Horizon

Many herbs and plant extracts have been touted as having significant health benefits. This one (also known as *Hypericum*) appears to have a legitimate role in mild to moderate depression. In Germany, St.-John's-wort or *Hypericum* is the leading antidepressant used to help this condition. Some research also finds that this product has fewer side effects than available prescription agents. Several key points must be made: First, this agent appears to have a role in mild to moderate depression; next, more medicine-to-medicine research needs to be done; and finally, dosing and results or outcomes should be supervised by your doctor.

THALIDOMIDE (tha LID oh myde)

Novel Application

This medicine is NEVER to be used in pregnancy and carries a pregnancy category X labeling. A recently published study reveals its benefits in severe canker sores in AIDS patients. The previous edition of *The Essential Guide to Prescription Drugs* discussed ongoing research into AIDS wasting, rheumatoid arthritis, and systemic lupus erythematosus. These new uses for thalidomide (Synovir) provide new hope for patients using a medicine with a very dark past.

TOLCAPONE (TOLL ka pohn)

Star on the Horizon

This medicine (Tasmar) is the first of a new class of medicines called catechol-*O*-methyltransferase (COMT) inhibitors. It is to be used in addition to levodopa to help improve the quality of life for patients with Parkinson's disease. COMT inhibitors help increase levodopa levels by inhibiting catechol-*O*-methyltransferase.

VITAMIN E (VI da min)

Novel Application

The American Psychiatric Association has developed clinical guidelines on treatment of Alzheimer's. These guidelines recommend vitamin E for delay in progression of symptoms in patients with mild to moderate Alzheimer's disease. The vitamin is recommended both alone or in combination with donepezil (Aricept) as the first-line approach.

DRUG CLASSES

Throughout the drug profiles reference is made to various drug classes. Use this section to protect yourself and your family. Learn which medicines belong to a particular class of drugs. Medicines in the same class often share important characteristics in their chemistry or how they work in the body. *Any* drug (or *all* drugs) in a given class can be expected to behave in a particular way. This knowledge helps you prevent interactions or unanticipated or hazardous adverse effects. Each Drug Class is named, followed by an alphabetic listing of the generic names of the drugs in the class. Following each generic name (and enclosed in parentheses) is the widely recognized brand name(s) of that particular drug. A complete listing is not possible. If your medicine is not present, call your doctor or pharmacist to get the generic name of the drug that concerns you. The generic name listings are sufficiently complete to serve the scope of this book.

ACE (Angiotensin-Converting Enzyme) Inhibitors

benazepril (Lotensin)
captopril (Capoten)
enalapril (Vasotec)
fosinopril (Monopril)
lisinopril (Prinivil, Zestril)

moexipril (Univasc)
quinapril (Accupril)
ramipril (Altace)
spirapril (Renormax)
trandolapril (Mavik)

Adrenocortical Steroids (Cortisonelike Drugs)

amcinonide (Cyclocort)
beclomethasone (Beclovent, Vanceril)
betamethasone (Celestone)
budesonide (Pulmicort)
cortisone (Cortone)
dexamethasone (Decadron)
fludrocortisone (Florinef)
flunisolide (AeroBid, Nasarel)
fluorometholone (FML)
fluticasone (Flonase)
halcinonide (Halog)

halobetasol (Ultravate)
hydrocortisone (Cortef)
medrysone (HMS Ophthalmic
    Suspension)
methylpredisolone (Medrol)
mometasone (Elocon)
paramethasone (Haldrone)
prednisolone (Delta-Cortef)
prednisone (Deltasone)
rimexalone (Vexol)
triamcinolone (Aristocort, Azmacort)

Alpha-Glucosidase Inhibitors

acarbose (Precose)   miglitol (Glyset)

Amebicides (Anti-Infectives)

chloroquine (Aralen)   metronidazole (Flagyl)
emetine   paromomycin (Humatin)
iodoquinol (Yodoxin)

Aminoglycosides (Anti-Infectives)

amikacin (Amikin)   neomycin (Mycifradin, Neobiotic)
gentamicin (Garamycin)   paromomycin (Humatin)
kanamycin (Kantrex)   tobramycin (Tobicin)

Amphetaminelike Drugs

amphetamine   phendimetrazine (Adipost, Anorex, Plegine)
benzphetamine (Didrex)   phenmetrazine (Preludin)
dextroamphetamine (Dexedrine)   phentermine (Adipex-P, Fastin)
diethylpropion (Tenuate, Tepanil)   phentermine resin complex (Ionamin)
methamphetamine (Desoxyn)   phenylpropanolamine (Dexatrim)
methylphenidate (Ritalin)

Analgesics

acetaminophen (Datril, Tylenol)   propoxyphene (Darvon)
acetaminophen/propoxyphene (Darvocet-N tramadol (Ultram)
   100)   See also Nonsteroidal Anti-Inflammatory
aspirin   Drugs (NSAIDs) and Opioid Drugs
lidocaine/prilocaine cream (Emla)

Androgens (Male Sex Hormones)

fluoxymesterone (Halotestin)   testosterone (Androderm, Depotest,
methyltestosterone (Android, Metandren,   Testone)
   Oreton)

Angiotensin-2-Receptor Antagonists

losartan (Cozaar)   valsartan (Diovan)

Anorexiants (Appetite Suppressants)

dexfenfluramine (Redux)   mazindol (Mazanor, Sanorex)
REMOVED FROM THE MARKET   See also Amphetaminelike Drugs

Anti-Acne Drugs

adapalene (Differin)   isotretinoin (Accutane)
azelaic acid (Azelex)   sodium sulfacetamide 10% lotion (Klaron)
benzoyl peroxide (Epi-Clear, others)   tetracycline (Achromycin V)
erythromycin (Eryderm)   tretinoin (Retin-A)

Anti-AIDS Drugs (Anti-Retrovirals)

delavirdine (Rescriptor)
didanosine (DDI, Videx)
indinavir (Crixivan)
integrase (Zintevir)
lamivudine (3TC, Epivir)
nelfinavir (Viracept)

nevirapine (Viramune)
ritonavir (Norvir)
saquinavir (Invirase)
stavudine (D4T, Zerit)
zalcitabine (dideoxycytidine, DDC, Hivid)
zidovudine (AZT, Retrovir)

Antialcoholism Drugs

disulfiram (Antabuse)

naltrexone (Trexan, ReVia)

Anti-Alzheimer's Drugs

donepezil (Aricept)
tacrine (Cognex)

vitamin E (various brands)

Anti-Anginal Drugs

bepridil (Vascor)
diltiazem (Cardizem)
nicardipine (Cardene)
nifedipine (Adalat, Procardia)

nitrates (see class below)
verapamil (Calan, Isoptin)
See also Beta-Blockers

Antianxiety Drugs (Mild Tranquilizers)

buspirone (Buspar)
chlormezanone (Trancopal)
hydroxyzine (Atarax, Vistaril)

lorazepam (Ativan)
meprobamate (Equanil, Miltown)
See also Benzodiazepines

Antiarrhythmic Drugs (Heart Rhythm Regulators)

acebutolol (Sectral)
adenosine (Adenocard)
amiodarone (Cordarone)
atenolol (Tenormin)
digitoxin (Crystodigin)
digoxin (Lanoxin)
disopyramide (Norpace)
flecainide (Tambocor)
ibutilide (Corvert)

lidocaine (Xylocaine)
mexiletine (Mexitil)
procainamide (Procan SR, Pronestyl)
propafenone (Rythmol)
propranolol (Inderal)
quinidine (Quinaglute, Quinidex, Quinora)
sotalol (Betapace)
tocainide (Tonocard)
verapamil (Calan, Isoptin)

Antiarthritics

aspirin
azathioprine (Imuran; rheumatoid only)
chloroquine (Aralen; rheumatoid only)

penicillamine (Cuprimine)
See also Nonsteroidal Anti-Inflammatory
    Drugs (NSAIDs) and Adrenocorticosteroids

Antiasthmatic Drugs

Anti-Inflammatory Agents, Corticosteroids

beclomethasone (Beclovent, Vanceril)
flunisolide (AeroBid)

fluticasone (Flovent)
triamcinolone (Azmacort)

Anti-Leukotrienes

zafirlukast (Accolate)

zileuton (Zyflo)

Bronchodilators

albuterol (Proventil, Ventolin)
aminophylline (Phyllocontin)
bitolterol (Tornalate)
dyphylline (Lufyllin)
ephedrine (Efed II)
epinephrine (Adrenalin, Bronkaid Mist,
    Primatene Mist)
ipratropium
isoetharine (Bronkosol, Dey-Lute)

isoproterenol (Isuprel)
metaproterenol (Alupent, Metaprel)
oxtriphylline (Choledyl)
pirbuterol (Maxair)
salmeterol (Serevent)
terbutaline (Brethaire, Brethine, Bricanyl)
theophylline (Bronkodyl, Elixophyllin,
    Slo-Phyllin, others)

Mast-Cell-Stabilizing Agents

cromolyn sodium (Gastrocrom, Intal)

nedocromil (Tilade)

Preventive Agents

cromolyn (Intal)

nedocromil (Tilade)

Xanthines

theophylline (Slo-bid, Theo-Dur)

Anti-Attention-Deficit-Hyperactivity-Disorder Drugs

clonidine (Catapres)
methylphenidate (Ritalin)

pemoline (Cylert)

Anti-Benign-Prostatic-Hyperplasia Drugs

doxazosin (Cardura)
finasteride (Proscar)
prazosin (Minipres)

tamsulosin (Flomax)
terazosin (Hytrin)

Antibiotics

See specific antibiotic class (Cephalosporins, Penicillins, Tetracyclines, etc.)

Topical, Anti-Infectives

mupirocin (Bactroban)

Anticancer Drugs (Antineoplastics or Chemotherapy)

chlorambucil (Leukeran)
cyclophosphamide (Cytoxan)
flutamide (Eulexin)
hydroxyurea (Hydrea)

mercaptopurine (Purinethol)
methotrexate (Rheumatrex)
tamoxifen (Nolvadex)

Anti-Canker-Sore Drugs

amlexanox (Apthasol)

Anticholesterol Drugs

See Cholesterol-Reducing Drugs

Anticholinergic Drugs (Atropinelike Drugs)

atropine
belladonna
hyoscyamine
scopolamine

See also the specific drug class:
Antidepressant Drugs, Tricyclic
Antihistamines, some
Anti-Parkinsonism Drugs, some
Antispasmodics, Synthetic, some
Muscle Relaxants, some

Anticoagulant Drugs

anisindione (Miradon)
dicumarol

warfarin (Coumadin and generic)

Anticonvulsant Drugs (Antiepileptic Drugs)

acetazolamide (Diamox)
carbamazepine (Tegretol)
clonazepam (Klonopin)
clorazepate (Tranxene)
diazepam (Valium)
ethosuximide (Zarontin)
ethotoin (Peganone)
felbamate (Felbatol)
gabapentin (Neurontin)
lamotrigine (Lamictal)
mephenytoin (Mesantoin)

methsuximide (Celontin)
paramethadione (Paradione)
phenacemide (Phenurone)
phenobarbital (Luminal)
phensuximide (Milontin)
phenytoin (Dilantin)
primidone (Mysoline)
topiramate (Topamax)
trimethadione (Tridione)
valproic acid (Depakene)

Anti-Cystic-Fibrosis Agents (Recombinant DNase)

dornase alfa (Pulmozyme)

Antidepressant Drugs

Bicyclic Antidepressants

fluoxetine (Prozac)

venlafaxine (Effexor)

Tricyclic Antidepressants

amitriptyline (Elavil, Endep)
amoxapine (Asendin)
clomipramine (Anafranil)
desipramine (Norpramin, Pertofrane)
doxepin (Adapin, Sinequan)

imipramine (Tofranil)
nortriptyline (Aventyl, Pamelor)
protriptyline (Vivactil)
trimipramine (Surmontil)

Tetracyclic Antidepressants

maprotiline (Ludiomil)

mirtazapine (Remeron)

Other Antidepressants

bupropion (Wellbutrin, Wellbutrin SR)
fluvoxamine (Luvox)
Hypericum (St.-John's-wort)
nefazodone (Serzone)
paroxetine (Paxil)

sertraline (Zoloft)
trazodone (Desyrel)
See also Monoamine Oxidase (MAO)
    Inhibitors

Antidiabetic Drugs

Oral

See Alpha-Glucosidase Inhibitors, Biguanides, Sulfonylureas, and Thiazolindinediones

Injectable

insulin

Antidiarrheal Drugs

loperamide

Antiemetic Drugs (Anti-Motion-Sickness, Antinausea Drugs)

chlorpromazine (Thorazine)
cyclizine (Marezine)
dimenhydrinate (Dramamine)
diphenhydramine (Benadryl)
granisetron (Kytril)
hydroxyzine (Atarax, Vistaril)

meclizine (Antivert, Bonine)
ondansetron (Zofran)
prochlorperazine (Compazine)
promethazine (Phenergan)
scopolamine (Transderm Scop)
trimethobenzamide (Tigan)

Antiepileptic Drugs

See Anticonvulsant Drugs

Antifungal Drugs (Anti-Infectives)

amphotericin B (Fungizone)
butenafine (Mentax)
fluconazole (Diflucan)
flucytosine (Ancobon)
griseofulvin (Fulvicin, Grifulvin, Grisactin)
itraconazole (Sporanox)

ketoconazole (Nizoral)
lipid-associated amphotericin B (Abelcet)
miconazole (Monistat)
nystatin (Mycostatin)
terbinafine (Lamisil)
tioconazole (Vagistat-1)

Anti-Glaucoma Drugs

acetazolamide (Diamox)
betaxolol (Betoptic)
brimonidine (Alphagan)
dipivefrin (Propine)
dorzolamide (Trusopt)
epinephrine (Glaucon)

lanoprost (Xalatan)
levobunolol (Betagan)
metipranolol (Optipranolol)
pilocarpine (Pilocar)
timolol (Betimol, Timoptic, Timoptic-XE)

Anti-Gout Drugs

allopurinol (Zyloprim)
colchicine
diclofenac (Cataflam, Voltaren)
fenoprofen (Nalfon)
ibuprofen (Advil, Motrin, Nuprin, Rufin)
indomethacin (Indocin)
ketoprofen (Orudis)

mefenamic acid (Ponstel)
naproxen (Anaprox, Naprosyn)
oxaprozin (Daypro)
piroxicam (Feldene)
probenecid (Benemid)
sulfinpyrazone (Anturane)
sulindac (Clinoril)

Antihistamines

astemizole (Hismanal)
azatadine (Optimine)
azelastine (Astelin)
brompheniramine (Dimetane, others)
carbinoxamine (Clistin, Rondec)
cetirizine (Zyrtec)
chlorpheniramine (Chlor-Trimeton, Teldrin)
clemastine (Tavist)
cyclizine (Marezine)
cyproheptadine (Periactin)
dimenhydrinate (Dramamine)
diphenhydramine (Benadryl)

doxylamine (Unisom)
hydroxyzine (Atarax)
loratadine (Claritin, Claritin Extra)
meclizine (Antivert, Bonine)
orphenadrine (Norflex)
pheniramine (component of Triaminic)
promethazine (Phenergan, others)
pyrilamine (component of Triaminic)
terfenadine (Seldane)
tripelennamine (Pyribenzamine, PBZ)
triprolidine (component of Actifed and
    Sudahist)

Nonsedating or Minimally Sedating

astemizole (Hismanal)
cetirizine (Zyrtec)
fexofenadine (Allegra)

loratadine (Claritin)
terfenadine (Seldane)

Antihypertensive Drugs

amlodipine/benazepril (Lotrel)
bisoprolol/hydrochlorothiazide (Ziac)
clonidine (Catapres)
doxazosin (Cardura)
enalapril/felodipine (Lexxel)
guanabenz (Wytensin)
guanadrel (Hylorel)
guanethidine (Ismelin)
See also ACE Inhibitors,
Angiotensin-2-Receptor Antagonists,
Beta-Blockers, Calcium Blockers, and
Diuretics

guanfacine (Tenex)
hydralazine (Apresoline)
hydrochlorothiazide/benazepril (Lotensin)
methyldopa (Aldomet)
minoxidil (Loniten)
prazosin (Minipres)
reserpine (Serpasil)
terazosin (Hytrin)

Anti-Infective Drugs

See the specific anti-infective drug class:
Amebicides
Aminoglycosides
Antifungal Drugs
Antileprosy Drugs
Antimalarial Drugs
Antituberculosis Drugs

Antiviral Drugs
Cephalosporins
Fluoroquinolones
Macrolide Antibiotics
Penicillins
Sulfonamides
Tetracyclines

Miscellaneous Anti-Infective Drugs

atovaquone (Mepron)
chloramphenicol (Chloromycetin)
clindamycin (Cleocin)
colistin (Coly-Mycin S)
furazolidone (Furoxone)
lincomycin (Lincocin)

nalidixic acid (NegGram)
nitrofurantoin (Furadantin, Macrodantin)
novobiocin (Albamycin)
pentamidine (Pentam-300)
trimethoprim (Proloprim, Trimpex)
vancomycin (Vancocin)

Antileprosy Drugs (Anti-Infectives)

clofazimine (Lamprene)

dapsone

Antimalarial Drugs (Anti-Infectives)

chloroquine (Aralen)
doxycycline (Vibramycin)
hydroxychloroquine (Plaquenil)
mefloquine (Lariam)
primaquine

pyrimethamine (Daraprim)
quinacrine (Atabrine)
quinine
sulfadoxine/pyrimethamine (Fansidar)

Anti-Migraine Drugs

atenolol (Tenormin)
ergotamine (Ergostat)
methysergide (Sansert)
metoprolol (Lopressor)
nadolol (Corgard)

nifedipine (Procardia)
propranolol (Inderal)
sumatriptan (Imitrex)
timolol (Blocadren)
verapamil (Calan, Isoptin)

Anti-Motion-Sickness/Antinausea Drugs

See Antiemetic Drugs

Anti-Myasthenics

neostigmine

Anti-Mycobacterial Agents

rifabutin (Mycobutin)

Anti-Osteoporotics

alendronate (Fosamax)
antiestrogens (SERM)
calcitonin (Miacalcin)

calcium
estrogen (various brands)
tiludronate (Skelid)

Anti-Parkinsonism Drugs

amantadine (Symmetrel)
benztropine (Cogentin)
bromocriptine (Parlodel)
diphenhydramine (Benadryl)
levodopa (Dopar, Larodopa)
levodopa/bensarazide (Prolopa)

levodopa/carbidopa (Sinemet, Sinemet CR)
pergolide (Permax)
selegiline (Eldepryl)
tolcapone (Tasmar)
trihexyphenidyl (Artane)

Antiplatelet Drugs (Platelet Aggregation Inhibitors)

aspirin
dipyridamole (Persantine)

sulfinpyrazone (Anturane)
ticlopidine (Ticlid)

Anti-Psoriatic Drugs

etretinate

methotrexate

Antipsychotic Drugs (Neuroleptics, Major Tranquilizers)

chlorprothixene (Taractan)
clozapine (Clozaril)

haloperidol (Haldol)
loxapine (Loxitane)

molindone (Moban)
olanzapine (Zyprexa)
pimozide (Orap)
risperidone (Risperdal)

thiothixene (Navane)
See also Phenothiazines and
    Thienobenzodiazepines

Antipyretic Drugs (Fever-Reducing Drugs)

acetaminophen
aspirin

See also Nonsteroidal Anti-Inflammatory
    Drugs (NSAIDs)

Anti-Sickle-Cell-Anemia Drugs

hydroxyurea (Hydrea)

Antispasmodics, Synthetic

anisotropine (Valpin)
clidinium (Quarzan)
glycopyrrolate (Robinul)
hexocyclium (Tral)
isopropamide (Darbid)

mepenzolate (Cantil)
methantheline (Banthine)
methscopolamine (Pamine)
propantheline (Pro-Banthine)
tridihexethyl (Pathilon)

Antituberculosis Drugs

aminosalicylate sodium (Sodium P.A.S.)
capreomycin (Capastat)
cycloserine (Seromycin)
ethambutol (Myambutol)
ethionamide (Trecator-SC)

isoniazid (Laniazid, Nydrazid)
pyrazinamide
rifampin (Rifadin, Rimactane)
rifabutin (Mycobutin)
streptomycin

Antitussive Drugs (Cough Suppressants)

benzonatate (Tessalon)
codeine (various brands)
dextromethorphan (Hold DM, Suppress)
diphenhydramine (Benylin)

hydrocodone (Hycodan)
hydromorphone (Dilaudid)
promethazine (Phenergan)

Antiulcer Drugs

Antacids

various brands

Antibiotics

amoxicillin
clarithromycin
metronidazole

tetracycline
See Histamine (H_2) Blockers
See Proton Pump Inhibitors

Miscellaneous Antiulcer Drugs

bismuth subsalicylate (Pepto-Bismol, others)
misoprostol (Cytotec)

ranitidine bismuth citrate (Tritec)
sucralfate (Carafate)

Antiviral Drugs (Anti-Infectives)

acyclovir (Zovirax)
amantadine (Symmetrel)

cidofovir (Vistide)
didanosine (Videx)

famciclovir (Famvir)
foscarnet (Foscavir)
ganciclovir (Cytovene)
indinavir (Crixivan)
lamivudine (Epivir)
nelfinavir (Viracept)
nevirapine (Viramune)
penciclovir (Denavir)
ribavirin (Virazole)

rimantadine (Flumadine)
ritonavir (Norvir)
saquinavir (Invirase)
stavudine (Zerit)
valacyclovir (Valtrex)
vidarabine (Vira A)
zalcitabine (Hivid)
zidovudine (Retrovir)

Appetite Suppressants

See Anorexiants

Atropinelike Drugs

See Anticholinergic Drugs

Barbiturates

amobarbital (Amytal)
aprobarbital (Alurate)
butabarbital (Butisol)
mephobarbital (Mebaral)
metharbital (Gemonil)

pentobarbital (Nembutal)
phenobarbital (Luminal, Solfoton)
secobarbital (Seconal)
talbutal (Lotusate)

Benzodiazepines

alprazolam (Xanax)
bromazepam (Lectopam)
chlordiazepoxide (Libritabs, Librium)
clonazepam (Klonopin)
clorazepate (Tranxene)
diazepam (Valium, Vazepam)
flurazepam (Dalmane)
halazepam (Paxipam)
ketazolam (Loftran)

lorazepam (Ativan)
midazolam (Versed)
nitrazepam (Mogadon)
oxazepam (Serax)
prazepam (Centrax)
quazepam (Doral)
temazepam (Restoril)
triazolam (Halcion)

Beta-Blockers (Beta-Adrenergic-Blocking Drugs)

acebutolol (Sectral)
atenolol (Tenormin)
betaxolol (Kerlone)
bisoprolol (Zebeta)
bisoprolol/hydrochlorothiazide (Ziac)
carteolol (Cartrol)
carvedilol (Coreg)

labetalol (Normodyne, Trandate)
metoprolol (Lopressor)
nadolol (Corgard)
penbutolol (Levatol)
pindolol (Visken)
propranolol (Inderal)
timolol (Blocadren)

Biguanides (Oral Antidiabetic Drugs)

metformin (Glucophage)

Blood Flow Agents

pentoxifylline (Trental)

Bowel Anti-Inflammatory Drugs (Inflammatory Bowel Disease Suppressants)

azathioprine (Imuran)
mesalamine (Rowasa, Asacol)
metronidazole (Flagyl)

olsalazine (Dipentum)
sulfasalazine (Azulfidine)

Bronchodilators

See Antiasthmatic Drugs

Calcium Blockers (Calcium-Channel-Blocking Drugs)

amlodipine (Norvasc)
bepridil (Vascor)
diltiazem (Cardizem, Tiazac)
felodipine (Plendil)
isradipine (DynaCirc)
mibefradil (Posicor)

nicardipine (Cardene, Cardene SR)
nifedipine (Adalat CC, Procardia XL)
nimodipine (Nimotop)
nisoldipine (Sular)
verapamil (Calan, Isoptin, Verelan)

Cephalosporins (Anti-Infectives)

cefaclor (Ceclor)
cefadroxil (Duricef, Ultracef)
cefamandole (Mandol)
cefazolin (Ancef, Kefzol, Zolicef)
cefepime (Maxipime)
cefixime (Suprax)
cefmetazole (Zefazone)
cefonicid (Monocid)
cefoperazone (Cefobid)
ceforanide (Precef)
cefotaxime (Claforan)
cefotetan (Cefotan)
cefoxitin (Mefoxin)

cefpodoxime (Vantin)
cefprozil (Cefzil)
ceftazidime (Fortaz, Tazidime, Tazicef)
ceftibuten (Cedax)
ceftizoxime (Cefizox)
ceftriaxone (Rocephin)
cefuroxime (Ceftin, Kefurox, Zinacef)
cephalexin (Keflex, Keftab)
cephalothin (Keflin)
cephapirin (Cefadyl)
cephradine (Anspor, Velosef)
moxalactam (Moxam)

Cholesterol-Reducing Drugs

atorvastatin (Lipitor)
cerivastatin (Baycol)
cholestyramine (Questran, Prevalite)
clofibrate (Atromid-S)
colestipol (Colestid)
dextrothyroxine (Choloxin)
fenofibrate (Lipidil)

fluvastatin (Lescol)
gemfibrozil (Lopid)
lovastatin (Mevacor)
niacin (Nicobid, Slo-Niacin, others)
pravastatin (Pravachol)
probucol (Lorelco)
simvastatin (Zocor)

Cortisonelike Drugs

See Adrenocortical Steroids

Cough Suppressants

See Antitussive Drugs

Decongestants

ephedrine (Efedron, Ephedrol)
naphazoline (Naphcon, Vasocon)
oxymetazoline (Afrin, Duration, others)
phenylephrine (Neo-Synephrine, others)
phenylpropanolamine (Propadrine,

Propagest, others)
pseudoephedrine (Afrinol, Sudafed, others)
tetrahydrozoline (Tyzine, Visine, others)
xylometazoline (Otrivin)

Digitalis Preparations

deslanoside (Cedilanid-D)
digitoxin (Crystodigin)

digoxin (Lanoxicaps, Lanoxin)

Diuretics

acetazolamide (Diamox)
amiloride (Midamor)
bumetanide (Bumex)
chlorthalidone (Hygroton)
ethacrynic acid (Edecrin)
furosemide (Lasix)

indapamide (Lozol)
metolazone (Diulo, Zaroxolyn)
spironolactone (Aldactone)
triamterene (Dyrenium)
See also Thiazide Diuretics

Ergot Derivatives

bromocriptine (Parlodel)
ergotamine (Bellergal)

methysergide (Sansert)
pergolide (Permax)

Estrogens (Female Sex Hormones)

chlorotrianisene (Tace)
diethylstilbestrol (DES, Stilphostrol)
estradiol (Estrace, Estraderm, others)
estrogens, conjugated (Premarin)
estrogens, esterified (Estratab, Menest)

estrone (Theelin, others)
estropipate (Ogen)
ethinyl estradiol (Estinyl)
quinestrol (Estrovis)

Female Sex Hormones

See Estrogens and Progestins

Fever-Reducing Drugs

See Antipyretic Drugs

5-Alpha-Reductase Inhibitors

finasteride (Proscar)

Fluoroquinolones (Anti-Infectives)

ciprofloxacin (Cipro)
levofloxacin (Levaquin)
lomefloxacin (Maxaquin)

norfloxacin (Noroxin)
ofloxacin (Floxin)
sparfloxacin (Zagam)

Gastrointestinal Drugs

Miscellaneous

cisapride (Propulsid)

metoclopramide (Reglan)

Ulcer Preventatives

misoprostol (Cytotec)

H$_2$-Blockers (Histamine [H$_2$] Blocking Drugs)

cimetidine (Tagamet, Tagamet HB 200)
famotidine (Pepcid, Pepcid AC)

nizatidine (Axid, Axid AR)
ranitidine (Zantac, Zantac 75)

Hair Growth Stimulants

finasteride (Proscar, Propecia)

minoxidil (Rogaine)

Heart Rhythm Regulators

See Antiarrhythmic Drugs

Hematopoietic Agents

filgrastim (Neupogen)

Hormones

Miscellaneous

nafarelin (Synarel)
See also Androgens for male sex hormones,

Estrogens and Progestins for female sex
hormones

Hypnotic Drugs (Sedatives/Sleep Inducers)

acetylcarbromal (Paxarel)
chloral hydrate (Aquachloral, Noctec)
estazolam (ProSom)
ethchlorvynol (Placidyl)
ethinamate (Valmid)
flurazepam (Dalmane)
glutethimide (Doriden)
methyprylon (Noludar)

paraldehyde (Paral)
propiomazine (Largon)
quazepam (Doral)
temazepam (Restoril)
triazolam (Halcion)
zolpidem (Ambien)
See also Barbiturates

Immunosuppressants

azathioprine (Imuran)
chlorambucil (Leukeran)
cyclophosphamide (Cytoxan)

cyclosporine (Sandimmune)
hydroxychloroquine (Plaquenil)

Macrolide Antibiotics (Anti-Infectives)

azithromycin (Zithromax)
clarithromycin (Biaxin)
dirithromycin (Dynabac)

erythromycin (E-Mycin, Ilosone, Erythrocin,
    E.E.S.)
troleandomycin (TAO)

Male Sex Hormones

See Androgens

Mast-Cell-Stabilizing Agents

See Antiasthmatic Drugs

Monoamine Oxidase (MAO) Inhibitor Drugs (Type A: Antidepressants)

isocarboxazid (Marplan)
phenelzine (Nardil)

tranylcypromine (Parnate)

Muscle Relaxants (Skeletal Muscle Relaxants)

baclofen (Lioresal)
carisoprodol (Rela, Soma, others)
chlorphenesin carbamate (Maolate)
chlorzoxazone (Paraflex, Parafon Forte)
cyclobenzaprine (Flexeril)
dantrolene (Dantrium)

diazepam (Valium)
meprobamate (Equanil, Miltown, others)
metaxalone (Skelaxin)
methocarbamol (Robaxin, others)
orphenadrine (Norflex, others)

Nitrates

amyl nitrate (Amyl Nitrate Vaporole, others)
erythrityl tetranitrate (Cardilate)
isosorbide dinitrate (Isordil, Sorbitrate, others)
isosorbide mononitrate (Ismo, Imdur)

nitroglycerin (Nitrostat, Nitrolingual, Nitrogard, Nitrong, others)
pentaerythritol tetranitrate (Duotrate, Peritrate)

Nonnucleoside Reverse Transcriptase Inhibitors

delavirdine (Rescriptor)

nevirapine (Viramune)

Nonsteroidal Anti-Inflammatory Drugs (NSAIDs) (Aspirin Substitutes)

Acetic Acids

bromfenac sodium (Duract)
diclofenac potassium (Cataflam)
diclofenac sodium (Voltaren)
etodolac (Lodine)
indomethacin (Indochron E-R, Indocin,

Indocin SR)
ketorolac (Toradol)
nabumetone (Relafen)
sulindac (Clinoril)
tolmetin (Tolectin, Tolectin DS)

Fenamates

meclofenamate (Meclomen)

mefenamic acid (Ponstel)

Oxicams

piroxicam (Feldene)

Propionic Acids

diflunisal (Dolobid)
fenoprofen (Nalfon)
flurbiprofen (Ansaid)

ibuprofen
ketoprofen (Orudis, Oruvail)
naproxen (Naprosyn)

naproxen sodium (Aleve, Anaprox, Anaprox DS)
oxaprozin (Daypro)

oxyphenbutazone (Oxalid)
suprofen (Profenal)

Opioid Antagonists

naltrexone (ReVia)

Opioid Drugs (Narcotics)

alfentanil (Alfenta)
codeine
fentanyl (Sublimaze, Duragesic)
hydrocodone (Hycodan)
hydromorphone (Dilaudid)
levorphanol (Levo-Dromoran)
meperidine (Demerol)

methadone (Dolophine)
morphine (Astramorph, Duramorph, MS Contin, Roxanol)
oxycodone (OxyContin, Roxicodone)
oxymorphone (Numorphan)
propoxyphene (Darvon)
sufentanil (Sufenta)

Pain Syndrome Modifiers (also adjuvants)

carbamazepine (Tegretol)
gabapentin (Neurontin)

phenytoin (Dilantin)
strontium-89 (Metastron)

Penicillins (Anti-Infectives)

amoxicillin (Amoxil, Larotid, Polymox, Trimox, others)
amoxicillin/clavulanate (Augmentin)
ampicillin (Omnipen, Polycillin, Principen, Totacillin)
ampicillin/sulbactam (Unasyn)
bacampicillin (Spectrobid)
carbenicillin (Geocillin, Geopen, Pyopen)
cloxacillin (Cloxapen, Tegopen)
dicloxacillin (Dynapen, Pathocil, Veracillin)

methicillin (Staphcillin)
mezlocillin (Mezlin)
nafcillin (Nafcil, Unipen)
oxacillin (Prostaphlin)
penicillin G (Pentids, others)
penicillin V (Pen Vee K, V-Cillin K, Veetids, others)
piperacillin (Pipracil)
ticarcillin (Ticar)
ticarcillin/clavulanate (Timentin)

Phenothiazines (Antipsychotic Drugs)

acetophenazine (Tindal)
chlorpromazine (Thorazine)
fluphenazine (Permitil, Prolixin)
mesoridazine (Serentil)
perphenazine (Trilafon)

prochlorperazine (Compazine)
promazine (Sparine)
thioridazine (Mellaril)
trifluoperazine (Stelazine)
triflupromazine (Vesprin)

Progestins (Female Sex Hormones)

ethynodiol
hydroxyprogesterone (Duralutin, Gesterol L.A., others)
medroxyprogesterone (Amen, Curretab, Prempro, Premphase, Provera)

megestrol (Megace)
norethindrone (Micronor, Norlutate, Norlutin)
norgestrel (Ovrette)
progesterone (Gesterol 50, Progestaject)

Protease Inhibitors

indinavir (Crixivan)
nelfinavir (Viracept)

ritonavir (Norvir)
saquinavir (Invirase)

Proton Pump Inhibitors (H/K ATPase Inhibitors)

lansoprazole (Prevacid)

omeprazole (Prilosec)

Radiopharmaceuticals

samarium-EDTMP (Quadramet)

strontium-89 (Metastron)

Salicylates

aspirin
choline salicylate (Arthropan)
magnesium salicylate (Doan's, Magan,
    Mobidin)

salsalate (Amigesic, Disalcid, Salsitab)
sodium salicylate
sodium thiosalicylate (Rexolate, Tusal)

Sedatives/Sleep Inducers

See Hypnotic Drugs

SERMs (Selective Estrogen Receptor Modulators)

raloxifene (name is pending, as the drug is in
    phase three trials)

Smoking Cessation Adjuncts

bupropion (Zyban)
nicotine (Nicorette, various patch brands
    such as Nicotrol)

Sulfonamides (Anti-Infectives)

multiple sulfonamides (Triple Sulfa No. 2)
sulfacytine (Renoquid)
sulfadiazine
sulfamethizole (Thiosulfil)

sulfamethoxazole (Gantanol)
sulfasalazine (Azulfidine)
sulfisoxazole (Gantrisin)

Sulfonylureas (Oral Antidiabetic Drugs)

acetohexamide (Dymelor)
chlorpropamide (Diabinese)
glimepiride (Amaryl)
glipizide (Glucotrol)

glyburide (DiaBeta, Micronase)
tolazamide (Ronase, Tolamide, Tolinase)
tolbutamide (Orinase)

Tetracyclines (Anti-Infectives)

demeclocycline (Declomycin)
doxycycline (Doryx, Doxychel, Vibramycin)
methacycline (Rondomycin)
minocycline (Minocin)

oxytetracycline (Terramycin)
tetracycline (Achromycin V, Panmycin,
    Sumycin)

Thiazide Diuretics

bendroflumethiazide (Naturetin)
benzthiazide (Aquatag, Exna, Marazide)
chlorothiazide (Diuril)
cyclothiazide (Anhydron)
hydrochlorothiazide (Esidrix, Hydrodiuril,
    Oretic)

hydroflumethiazide (Diucardin, Saluron)
methyclothiazide (Enduron, Aquatensen)
polythiazide (Renese)
trichlormethiazide (Metahydrin, Naqua)

Thiazolidinediones

troglitazone (Rezulin)

Thienobenzodiazepines

olanzapine (Zyprexa)

Thyroid Hormones

levothyroxine (Synthroid)   liothyronine (Cytomel)

Tranquilizers, Major

See Antipsychotic Drugs

Tranquilizers, Minor

See Antianxiety Drugs

Vaccines (Immune Modulators)

influenza vaccine (Fluogen, Flu-Shield,   varicella virus vaccine (Varivax)
   Fluzone)

Vasodilators (Peripheral Vasodilators)

cyclandelate (Cyclospasmol)   nylidrin (Arlidin)
ethaverine (Ethaquin, Isovex)   papaverine (Cerespan, Pavabid)
isoxsuprine (Vasodilan)

Xanthines (Bronchodilators)

aminophylline (Phyllocontin, Truphylline)   theophylline (Bronkodyl, Slo-Phyllin,
dyphylline (Dilor, Lufyllin)   Theolair, others)
oxtriphylline (Choledyl)

A GLOSSARY
OF
DRUG-RELATED TERMS

Glossary

addiction Although there is disagreement about how inclusive this definition should be, addiction is generally recognized as a state of intense dependence (upon a drug), characterized by uncontrollable drug-seeking behavior, *tolerance* for the drug's pleasure-giving effects, and *withdrawal* manifestations when the drug is withheld. These features constitute *physical dependence*—a state where the drug is incorporated into the fundamental biochemistry of specific brain activities. (See the terms DEPENDENCE and TOLERANCE for accounts of physical and psychological dependence.)

adverse effect or reaction An abnormal, unexpected, infrequent, and usually unpredictable injurious response to a drug. Used in this restrictive sense, the term *adverse reaction* does *not* include effects of a drug that are a part of its pharmacological action, even though such effects may be undesirable and unintended. (See SIDE EFFECT.) Adverse reactions are of three basic types: those due to drug *allergy*, those caused by individual *idiosyncrasy,* and those representing *toxic* effects of drugs on tissue structure and function (see ALLERGY [DRUG], IDIOSYNCRASY, and TOXICITY).

allergy (drug) An abnormal drug response that occurs in people who make injurious antibodies* that react with foreign substances—in this instance, a drug. People who are allergic by nature and have a history of hay fever, asthma, hives, or eczema are more likely to develop drug allergies. Allergic reactions to drugs take many forms: skin eruptions of various kinds, fever, swollen glands, painful joints, jaundice, interference with breathing, acute collapse of circulation, etc. Drug allergies can develop gradually, or they can appear suddenly and require life-saving intervention.

alternative delivery system (ADS) A term coined to describe a variety of health care forms other than the traditional fee-for-service model such as HMOs, PPOs, and others.

analgesic A drug that is used to relieve pain. Analgesics are of three types: (1) Simple, nonnarcotic agents relieve pain by suppressing production of prostaglandins and related substances—examples are acetaminophen, aspirin, and nonsteroidal anti-

---

*Antibodies are special proteins that combine with foreign substances. Protective antibodies destroy bacteria and neutralize toxins. Injurious antibodies, reacting with foreign substances, cause release of histamine, a chemical responsible for allergic reactions.

inflammatory drugs or aspirin substitutes (Motrin, Advil, Naprosyn, etc.); (2) narcotic analgesics or opioids ("like-opium" derivatives) that relieve pain by blunting pain perception in the brain—examples are morphine, codeine, and hydrocodone (natural derivatives of opium), and meperidine or pentazocine (synthetic drug products); (3) local anesthetics that prevent or relieve pain by making sensory nerve endings insensitive to pain—such as the urinary tract analgesic phenazopyridine (Pyridium).

anaphylactic (anaphylactoid) reaction A group of symptoms which represent (or resemble) an extreme hypersensitivity to a drug. Anaphylactic reactions, whether mild, moderate, or severe, often involve several body systems. Mild symptoms include itching, hives, nasal congestion, nausea, abdominal cramping, or diarrhea. Sometimes these precede severe symptoms such as choking, shortness of breath, and sudden loss of consciousness (usually referred to as anaphylactic shock). Anaphylactic reactions can result from a very small dose of drug; may develop suddenly, usually within a few minutes after taking the drug; and can be rapidly fatal. A developing anaphylactic reaction is a true medical emergency. Any adverse effect that appears within 20 minutes after taking a drug should be considered an early sign of a possible anaphylactic reaction. Get medical attention immediately! (See ALLERGY [DRUG], and HYPERSENSITIVITY.)

antihypertensive A drug used to lower excessively high blood pressure. The term *hypertension* denotes blood pressure above the normal range. It does not refer to excessive nervous or emotional tension. Today there are more than 80 drug products in use for treating hypertension. Those most frequently prescribed for long-term use fall into three major groups:

1. drugs that increase urine production (the diuretics)
2. drugs that relax blood vessel walls
3. drugs that reduce sympathetic nervous system activity

Regardless of how they work, all these drugs can lower blood pressure. Remember that many other drugs can interact with antihypertensive drugs: some add to their effect, causing excessive reduction in blood pressure; others blunt their action, reducing their effectiveness. If you are taking medicines for high blood pressure, talk with your doctor if other drugs are prescribed to treat other conditions.

antipyretic A drug that treats fever by lowering body temperature. They accomplish this by working on the temperature-regulating center in the hypothalamus of the brain, causing dilation of blood vessels (capillary beds) in the skin and bringing overheated blood to the skin surface for cooling. Sweat glands are also stimulated to help cool the body further through evaporation. An antipyretic drug may also be a pain reliever (analgesic) (acetaminophen), or analgesic and anti-inflammatory (aspirin).

aplastic anemia A form of bone marrow failure (also known as pancytopenia) where production of the three types of blood cells is seriously impaired. Aplastic anemia can occur suddenly from unknown causes, but about half of reported cases are caused by drugs or chemicals. A delay of 1 to 6 months may occur between the use of a causative drug and the detection of anemia. Symptoms reflect consequences of inadequate supplies of all three blood cell types: lower red blood cells (anemia) results in fatigue, weakness, and pallor; deficiency of white blood cells (leukopenia) predisposes to infections; while lowered blood platelets (thrombocytopenia) can cause spontaneous bruising or hemorrhage. Treatment is difficult and the outcome unpredictable. Even with the best of care, half the cases may be fatal. Aplastic anemia is a rare consequence of drug treatment, but anyone taking a drug that can cause it should have periodic complete blood cell counts if the drug is to be used over an extended period of time. For a listing of causative drugs, see Table 5, Section Six.

bioavailability How fast and how much of the active drug is absorbed into the bloodstream. Two types of measurements—(1) blood levels of the drug at certain times after it was taken, and (2) how long the drug stays in the blood—shows how much of the drug is available for biological activity and for how long. This can also be measured by checking (1) the cumulative amount of the drug (or any breakdown product) excreted in the urine, and (2) how much drug accumulates in the urine. The two major factors that govern bioavailability are the chemical and physical characteristics of the dosage form, and the functional state of the digestive system of the person taking it. A drug that falls apart quickly in a normally functioning stomach or small intestine produces blood levels quite promptly. Such a drug product has good bioavailability.

bioequivalence The ability of a drug product to cause its intended therapeutic effect is related to its bioavailability. When a particular drug is marketed by several manufacturers, it is critical that the drug chosen is one that has the bioavailability needed to work. Substantial variations may occur among manufacturers. While the drug ingredient in medicines from different firms may the same chemical, don't assume that they are equally available and are therapeutically equal.

The bioavailability of any drug depends mostly on the physical characteristics of how it is made; these in turn determine how rapidly and how completely the drug disintegrates and releases its active drug component(s). Drug products that contain the same drug but are combined with different inert additives, coated with different substances, or enclosed in different capsules may or may not have the same bioavailability. Those that do are termed bioequivalent, and can be relied upon to give the same therapeutic result.

If you consider having your prescription filled with a generic form, ask your physician *and* pharmacist for help. This decision requires professional judgment in each case. In many cases, reasonable differences in the bioavailability patterns among drug products are acceptable. In some serious illnesses, or because blood levels of the drug must be kept in a narrowly defined range, it is essential to use the drug product that has been shown to have reliable bioavailability.

blood platelets The smallest of the three types of blood cells made by the bone marrow. Platelets are normally present in very large numbers. They form the basis of normal blood clotting and prevent excessive bruising or bleeding in the event of injury. When present in proper numbers and functioning normally, platelets preserve the retaining power of smaller blood vessel walls. By starting clotting processes in the blood, platelets seal small points of leakage in the vessel walls.

Certain drugs and chemicals may lower the number of platelets. Some of these drugs act by suppressing platelet formation; other drugs hasten their destruction. When the number of functioning platelets falls below a critical level, blood begins to leak through the thin walls of smaller vessels. This shows as scattered bruises in the skin of the thighs or legs and is called purpura. Bleeding may occur anywhere in the body, internally as well as superficially into the tissues immediately beneath the skin. For a listing of causative drugs, see Table 5, Section Six.

bone marrow depression A reduction in the ability of bone marrow to make blood cells. This can happen as an adverse reaction to some drugs or chemicals on the bone marrow. When it works normally, bone marrow makes most of the body's blood cells: the red blood cells (erythrocytes), the white blood cells (leukocytes), and the blood platelets (thrombocytes). Each type of cell has one or more functions, all of which are critical to life and health.

Drugs that can depress bone marrow activity may impair production of all types of blood cells at once or only one type selectively. Periodic examinations of the blood can show changes in structure or number of blood cells as a possible drug effect on bone marrow. If fewer red blood cells are made, anemia results. This causes weakness, loss of energy and stamina, cold intolerance, and shortness of breath. Lowered white blood cells can impair immunity and lower resistance to infection. Some symptoms of this can be fever, sore throat, or pneumonia. If blood platelets fall to abnormally low levels, the blood loses its ability to quickly clot. This may lead to abnormal spontaneous bruising or prolonged bleeding of injuries. Any of these symptoms require immediate studies of blood and bone marrow. For a listing of causative drugs, see Table 5, Section Six.

brand name The registered trade name given to a drug by its manufacturer. Each company adopts a distinctive trade name to distinguish its brand of the generic drug from that of its competitors. A brand name designates a proprietary drug— one that is protected by patent or copyright. Generally, brand names are shorter, easier to pronounce, and more readily remembered than their generic counterparts.

capitation A system where a set amount of money is used to cover the cost of health care for a given person. For instance, a health plan or hospital is paid monthly on a negotiated per-person rate and the plan or hospital provides all health services for the people in the plan.

cause-and-effect relationship An association between a drug and a biological event—most commonly a side effect or an adverse effect. Knowledge of a drug's full spectrum of effects (wanted and unwanted) is highly desirable when weighing its benefits and risks. However, it is often impossible to show that a particular drug is the primary cause of an adverse effect. Consideration must be given to factors such as when the drug was given and the possible reaction, use of multiple drugs and possible interactions among these drugs, the effects of the disease being treated, the physiological and psychological characteristics of the patient, and influences of unrecognized disorders or malfunctions.

The majority of adverse drug reactions occur sporadically, unpredictably, and infrequently in the general population. A *definite* cause-and-effect relationship between drug and reaction is shown when (1) the adverse effect immediately follows administration of the drug; or (2) the adverse effect disappears after the drug is discontinued (dechallenge) and promptly reappears when the drug is used again (rechallenge); or (3) the adverse effects are clearly the expected and predictable toxic consequences of drug overdosage.

There is also a large gray area of "probable," "possible," and "coincidental" associations associated with varying degrees of uncertainty. Clarification of cause-and-effect relationships here requires carefully designed observation over a long period of time, followed by sophisticated statistical analysis. Some news stories are based on suggestive but incomplete data. Though early warning is in the public interest, such announcements should make clear whether the presumed relationship is based upon definitive criteria or is simply inferred. It is critical to avoid losing valuable medicine use because of poorly designed or reported studies that find their way to the newspaper or television.

The most competent techniques for evaluating cause-and-effect relationships of adverse drug reactions have been devised by the Division of Tissue Reactions to Drugs, a research unit of the Armed Forces Institute of Pathology. Based upon a highly critical examination of all available evidence, the Division's study of 2,800 drug-related deaths yielded the following levels of certainty:

No association	5.0%
Coincidental	14.5%
Possible	33.0%
Probable	30.0%
Causative	17.5%

It is significant that expert evaluation of 2,800 drug-related cases concluded that only 47.5% could be substantiated as definitely or probably causative.

contraindication A condition or disease that precludes the use of a particular drug. Some contraindications are *absolute,* meaning that the use of the drug would expose the patient to extreme hazard and therefore cannot be justified. Other contraindications are *relative,* meaning that the condition or disease does not entirely bar the use of the drug, but requires that special consideration be given to factors that could aggravate existing disease, interfere with current treatment, or produce new injury.

covered lives A term used by health maintenance organizations to indicate how many people have enrolled in their plan. From the HMO's point of view, a minimum number of covered lives is necessary to support a certain number of family practice physicians, subspecialists, and so on. Understanding their logic helps explain why some HMOs have one urologist while others have several.

creatinine clearance A measure of how well the kidneys are eliminating waste, toxins, and impurities from the body. A low creatinine clearance (such as 20 ml per minute or ml/min) means poorer kidney function; a high creatinine clearance (such as 120 ml/min) means better kidney function. People who have low creatinine clearances often receive lower initial doses and smaller increases of medicines that are removed by the kidneys.

critical or clinical pathway An assortment of coordinated measures taken by a hospital or clinic to organize the care of their patients with specific diseases or conditions. All diagnostic tests, treatments, discharge planning, and other measures are the result of careful study and practice aimed at providing the maximum benefit to all patients in the most cost-effective manner.

dependence A term used to identify the drug-dependent states of *psychological dependence* (or *habituation*) and *physical dependence* (or *addiction*). In addition, a third kind of drug dependence can be included under this term. This might be called *functional dependence*—the need to use a drug continuously in order to sustain a particular body function, the impairment of which causes annoying symptoms of varying degree and significance.

    Psychological dependence is a form of neurotic behavior—an "emotional" dependence. It is an obsession to satisfy a particular desire. Psychological dependence is a very human trait seen often in many socially acceptable patterns and practices such as entertainment, gambling, sports, and collecting. A common form in today's culture is an increasing reliance on drugs to help cope with everyday problems of living: pills for frustration, disappointment, nervous stomach, tension headache, and insomnia. This compulsive drug abuse shows little or no tendency to increase the dose (see TOLERANCE) and no or only minor physical symptoms on withdrawal. Some authorities choose to broaden the definition of addiction to include psychological dependence.

    Physical dependence, which is true addiction, includes two elements: *tolerance* and *withdrawal* manifestations. Addicting drugs provide relief from anguish and pain, but can also cause a physiological tolerance that requires increased doses or repeated use to remain effective. These two features foster continued need for the drug and lead to its becoming a functioning component in the biochemistry of the brain. As this occurs, the drug assumes an "essential" role in ongoing chemical processes. (Thus some authorities prefer the term *chemical dependence*.) Sudden removal of the drug from the system causes a major upheaval in body chemistry and provokes a withdrawal syndrome—the intense mental and physical pain experienced by the addict when intake of the drug is stopped abruptly—that is the hallmark of addiction. It must be noted that true addiction is rare, and fear of addiction, even with potent narcotics, should never stand in the way of effective pain control.

Functional dependence differs significantly from both psychological and physical dependence. It occurs when a drug relieves a distressing condition and the body function involved needs the action of the drug to provide a sense of well-being. Drugs that cause functional dependence are used primarily for the relief of symptoms. They do not act on the brain to produce alteration of mood or consciousness as do those drugs with potential for either psychological or physical dependence. The most familiar example of functional dependence is the "laxative habit." Some types of constipation are made worse by the wrong choice of laxative, and natural bowel function fades as the colon becomes more and more dependent upon the laxative drug.

disease management An approach to the prevention and treatment of a specific condition which attempts to identify the frequency of its occurrence in the population, organize available resources, and allocate money to reach the best balance of dollars spent and results achieved.

disulfiramlike (Antabuse-like) reaction Symptoms that result from the interaction of alcohol and any drug that is capable of provoking the pattern of response typical of the "Antabuse effect." When sufficient levels of both alcohol and drug are present in the blood, the reaction occurs. It consists of intense flushing and warming of the face, a severe throbbing headache, shortness of breath, chest pains, nausea, repeated vomiting, sweating, and weakness. If the amount of alcohol ingested has been large enough, the reaction may progress to blurred vision, vertigo, marked drop in blood pressure, and loss of consciousness. Severe reactions may lead to convulsions and death. The reaction can last from 30 minutes to several hours, depending upon the amount of alcohol in the body. As the symptoms subside, the individual is exhausted and usually sleeps for several hours.

diuretic A drug that alters kidney function to increase the volume of urine. Diuretics use several mechanisms to increase urine volume, and these have different effects on body chemistry. Diuretics are used to (1) remove excess water from the body (as in congestive heart failure and some types of liver and kidney disease) and (2) treat hypertension by promoting the excretion of sodium from the body.

divided doses The total daily dose of a medicine is split into smaller individual doses over the course of a day.

dosage forms and strengths This information category in the individual Drug Profiles (Section Two) uses several abbreviations to designate measurements of weight and volume. These are:

mcg	=	microgram	=	1,000,000th of a gram (weight)
mg	=	milligram	=	1000th of a gram (weight)
ml	=	milliliter	=	1000th of a liter (volume)
gm	=	gram	=	1000 milligrams (weight)

There are approximately 65 mg in 1 grain.
There are approximately 5 ml in 1 teaspoon.
There are approximately 15 ml in 1 tablespoon.
There are approximately 30 ml in 1 ounce.

1 milliliter of water weighs 1 g.
There are approximately 454 g in 1 pound.

drug, drug product Terms often used interchangeably to designate a medicine (in any of its dosage forms) used in medical practice. Strictly speaking, the term *drug* refers to the single chemical entity that provokes a specific response when placed within a biological system—the "active" ingredient. A *drug product* is the manufactured dosage form—tablet, capsule, elixir, etc.—that contains the active drug intermixed with inactive ingredients to provide for convenient administration. Drug products that contain only one active ingredient are referred to as single-entity drugs. Drug products with two or more active ingredients are called combination drugs (designated [CD] in the lists of brand names in the Drug Profiles, Section Two).

drug class A group of drugs that are similar in chemistry, method of action, and use. Because of their common characteristics, many drugs in a class will cause the same side effects and have similar potential for related adverse reactions and interactions. Significant variations among members within a drug class can occur. This can let choices be made if certain beneficial actions are desired or particular side effects are to be minimized. Examples: Antihistamines and phenothiazines (see Drug Classes, Section Four).

drug fever Increased body temperature that occurs as an unwanted drug action. Drugs can cause fever by several mechanisms, such as allergic reactions, drug-induced tissue damage, acceleration of tissue metabolism, constriction of blood vessels in the skin with resulting decrease in loss of body heat, and direct action on the temperature-regulating center in the brain.

The most common form of drug fever is associated with allergic reactions. It may be the only allergic manifestation apparent, or it may be part of a complex of allergic symptoms that can include skin rash, hives, joint swelling and pain, enlarged lymph glands, hemolytic anemia, or hepatitis. The fever usually appears about 7 to 10 days after starting the drug and may vary from low-grade to alarmingly high levels. It may be sustained or intermittent, but it usually persists for as long as the drug is taken. In previously sensitized individuals drug fever may occur within 1 or 2 hours after taking the first dose of medication.

Although many drugs are capable of producing fever, the following are more commonly responsible:

allopurinol	novobiocin
antihistamines	*para*-aminosalicylic acid
atropinelike drugs	penicillin
barbiturates	pentazocine
coumarin anticoagulants	phenytoin
hydralazine	procainamide
iodides	propylthiouracil
isoniazid	quinidine
methyldopa	rifampin
nadolol	sulfonamides

extension effect An unwanted but predictable drug response that is a result of mild to moderate overdose. An extension effect is an exaggeration of the drug's normal pharmacological action; it can be thought of as a mild form of dose-related toxicity (see OVERDOSAGE and TOXICITY).

Example: The continued "hangover" of mental sluggishness that persists after arising in the morning is a common extension effect of a long-acting sleep-inducing drug (hypnotic) taken the night before.

Example: The persistent intestinal cramping and diarrhea that result from too generous a dose of laxative are extension effects of the drug's anticipated action.

FDA approvable A stage in the Food and Drug Administration's review and approval process. A medicine is considered FDA approvable once the panel which reviewed the supporting data submitted to the FDA finds that data acceptable. In general, at this point only final details need to be resolved before the drug becomes FDA approved and is made available for general use.

generic name The official, common, or public name used to designate an active drug, whether in pure form or in dosage form. Generic names are coined by committees of officially appointed drug experts and are approved by governmental agencies for national and international use, thus they are nonproprietary. Many drug products are marketed only under the generic name of the principal active ingredient. Prescriptions for generic medicines account for an increased number of all new prescriptions written in the United States. The drugs most commonly prescribed by generic name are listed below, ranked in descending order of the number of new prescriptions issued.

amoxicillin	erythromycin
penicillin VK	hydrochlorothiazide
ampicillin	acetaminophen/codeine
tetracycline	doxycycline
prednisone	phenobarbital

genetic therapy Perhaps the most promising area of therapy in medicine today. Healthy genetic material is isolated and inserted into appropriate but diseased cells. For example, normal lung genes are given to a person with cystic fibrosis. Still very experimental, it may someday allow people suffering with genetically-based diseases or conditions to receive therapy that changes the affected genes and actually *cure* those conditions.

habituation A form of drug dependence based upon strong psychological gratification. Habitual use of drugs that alter mood or relieve minor discomforts results from a compulsive need to feel pleasure and satisfaction or to escape emotional distress. The abrupt cessation of habituating drugs does not produce the withdrawal syndrome seen in addiction, thus habituation is a *psychological dependence.* (See DEPENDENCE for a further account of psychological and physical dependence.)

hemolytic anemia Lowered red blood cells and hemoglobin resulting from premature destruction (hemolysis) of red blood cells. One way that this happens is from a genetic lowering of glucose-6-phosphate dehydrogenase (G6PD), a needed enzyme. If patients with this condition are given certain antimalarial drugs, sulfa drugs, or other drugs, some of their red cells will disintegrate. Another type of drug-induced hemolytic anemia is a form of drug allergy. Many drugs in wide use (such as quinidine and levodopa) are known to cause hemolytic destruction of red cells as a hypersensitivity (allergic) reaction.

Hemolytic anemia can occur abruptly or silently. The acute form lasts about 7 days and shows as fever, pallor, weakness, dark-colored urine, and varying degrees of jaundice (yellow coloration of eyes and skin). If drug-induced hemolytic anemia is mild, there may be no symptoms. Such episodes are detected only by means of laboratory studies (see IDIOSYNCRASY and ALLERGY [DRUG]). For listings of causative drugs, see Table 5, Section Six.

hepatitislike reaction Some medicines may cause changes in the liver that resemble viral hepatitis. The symptoms of drug-induced hepatitis and virus-induced hepatitis are often so similar that the correct cause cannot be established without precise laboratory studies. Hepatitis due to drugs may be a form of allergy, or it may be a toxic adverse effect. Liver reactions of significance usually result in jaundice and represent serious adverse effects (see JAUNDICE). For listings of causative drugs, see Table 8, Section Six.

HMO Abbreviation for Health Maintenance Organization: A health care delivery system that provides a broad spectrum of medical therapies and services by a collective group of practitioners within a common organization.

hypersensitivity One common use of this term is for over responsiveness to drugs. Used in this sense, the term means that the nature of the response is appropriate but the degree of response is exaggerated. The term is more widely used today to identify a state of allergy. To have a *hypersensitivity* to a drug is to be *allergic* to it (see ALLERGY [DRUG]). Some people develop cross-hypersensitivity. This means that once a person has developed an allergy to one drug, that person will experience an allergic reaction to other drugs that are closely related.

> *Example:* The patient was known to be *hypersensitive* by nature, having a history of seasonal hay fever and asthma since childhood. His *allergy* to penicillin developed after his third course of treatment. This drug *hypersensitivity* manifested itself as a diffuse, measleslike rash.

hypnotic A drug that is used to cause sleep. Classes include: antihistamines, barbiturates, benzodiazepines, and several unrelated compounds. Within the past 15 years, benzodiazepines have largely replaced the barbiturates as the most commonly used hypnotics. In general, they are safer and have lower dependence potential. Since tolerance to the hypnotic effect can happen after several weeks of continual use, hypnotics should be used intermittently for short periods of time.

hypoglycemia A condition where the amount sugar (glucose) in the blood is below the normal range. Since the brain is only able to run on sugar, if blood sugar falls below a critical point, the brain will be seriously impaired. Early warnings include headache, a sensation resembling mild drunkenness, hunger, and an inability to think clearly. If blood sugar levels continue to fall, nervousness and confusion develop. Varying degrees of weakness, numbness, trembling, sweating, and rapid heart action follow. If blood sugar drops further, impaired speech, incoordination, and unconsciousness, with or without convulsions, will follow. Prompt recognition and treatment for any low blood sugar (hypoglycemia) is important. Because of potential for injury to the brain, the mechanisms and management of hypoglycemia should be understood by all who use drugs capable of producing it.

hypothermia A situation where the internal body temperature falls to levels below the norm of 98.6 degrees F or 37 degrees C. By definition, hypothermia means a body temperature of less than 95 degrees F or 35 degrees C. The elderly and debilitated are more prone to develop hypothermia if clothed inadequately and exposed to cool environments. Most episodes are initiated by room temperatures below 65 degrees F or 18.3 degrees C. The condition often develops suddenly, can mimic a stroke, and has a mortality rate of 50%. Some drugs, such as phenothiazines, barbiturates, and benzodiazepines, are conducive to causing hypothermia.

idiosyncrasy An abnormal drug response that occurs in people who have a defect in body chemistry (often hereditary) which produces an effect totally unrelated to the drug's normal action. Idiosyncrasy is not a form of allergy. The actual chemical defects responsible for certain idiosyncratic drug reactions are well understood; others are not.

> *Example:* Approximately 100 million people in the world (including 10% of African-Americans) have an enzyme deficiency of glucose-6-phosphate dehydrogenase (G6PD) in their red blood cells that causes these cells to disintegrate when exposed to drugs such as sulfonamides (Gantrisin, Kynex), nitrofurantoin (Fura-

dantin, Macrodantin), probenecid (Benemid), quinine, and quinidine. As a result of this reaction, these drugs (and others) can cause a significant anemia.

immunosuppressive A drug that significantly suppresses the immune system. In some cases, immunosuppression is an intended drug effect (cyclosporine to prevent rejection of a transplanted kidney). In other instances, it is an unwanted side effect, as in the long-term use of cortisonelike drugs (to control asthma) suppressing the immune system. Immunosuppressant drugs are used to treat several chronic disorders that are thought to be autoimmune diseases, notably advanced rheumatoid arthritis, ulcerative colitis, and systemic lupus erythematosus.

interaction An unwanted change in the body's response to a drug that results when a second drug which can alter the action of the first is administered at the same time. Some drug interactions can enhance the effect of either drug, producing an over response similar to overdose. Other interactions may reduce drug effectiveness and cause inadequate response. A third type of interaction can produce a seemingly unrelated toxic response with no increase or decrease in the actions of the interacting drugs. Many interactions can be anticipated, and appropriate adjustments in dose can be made to prevent or minimize unintended fluctuations in drug response.

jaundice A yellow coloration of the skin (and the white portion of the eyes) that occurs when bile pigments accumulate in the blood as a result of impaired liver function. Jaundice can be produced in several ways: it may be caused by a wide variety of diseases, or it may represent an adverse reaction to a particular drug. At times it is difficult to distinguish between disease-induced jaundice and drug-induced jaundice.

Jaundice due to a drug is always a serious adverse effect. If you take a medicine that can cause jaundice, watch closely for any change in the color of urine or feces. Dark discoloration of the urine and paleness (lack of color) of the stool may be early indications of a developing jaundice. If either of these symptoms occur, it is best to stop the drug and call your doctor promptly. Diagnostic tests are available to clarify the nature of the jaundice. For a listing of causative drugs, see Table 8, Section Six.

lupus erythematosus (LE) A serious disease that occurs in two forms, one limited to the skin (discoid LE) and the other involving several body systems (systemic LE). Both forms occur mostly in young women. About 5% of cases of the discoid form convert to the systemic form. Systemic LE is a disorder of the immune system which may result in chronic, progressive inflammation and destruction of the connective tissue of the skin, blood vessels, joints, brain, heart muscle, lungs, and kidneys. Altered proteins in the blood lead to antibody formation that reacts with certain organ tissues. A reduction in the number of white blood cells and blood platelets often occurs. The course of systemic LE is usually quite protracted and unpredictable. While no cure is known, satisfactory management may be achieved in some cases by the judicious use of cortisonelike drugs.

Several drugs are capable of initiating a form of systemic LE quite similar to that which occurs spontaneously. Symptoms may appear as early as 2 weeks or as late as 8 years after starting the responsible drug. The initial symptoms usually consist of low-grade fever, skin rashes of various kinds, aching muscles, and multiple joint pains. Chest pains (pleurisy) are fairly common. Enlargement of the lymph glands occurs less frequently. Symptoms usually subside if the drug is stopped, but laboratory evidence of the reaction may persist for many months.

medication map (MM) A new concept in medicines pioneered by Dr. Rybacki. One of the flaws in current drug information is that it is provided for individual medicines when patients actually often take medicines during the same day and in combination as well. Patients are not given a schedule that organizes their medicines into a framework which works well with their usual day. The medication map seeks to organize any and all of the medicines a patient takes into a clear schedule using the best possible times, combinations, and results or outcomes data. A medication map helps avoid drug–drug, drug–food, and drug activity interactions, and gives the patient the best possible quality of life.

neuroleptic malignant syndrome (NMS) A rare, serious, sometimes fatal idiosyncratic reaction to the use of neuroleptic (antipsychotic) drugs. Symptoms include hyperthermia (temperatures of 102 to 104 degrees F), marked muscle rigidity, and coma. Other symptoms include rapid heart rate and breathing, profuse sweating, tremors, and seizures. Two-thirds of reported cases occurred in men, one-third in women. The mortality rate is 15 to 20%.

The following drugs may cause this reaction:

amitriptyline + perphenazine (Triavil)	metoclopramide (Reglan, Octamide)
amoxapine (Asendin)	molindone (Moban)
chlorpromazine (Thorazine)	perphenazine (Etrafon, Trilafon)
chlorprothixene (Taractan)	pimozide (Orap)
clomipramine (Anafranil)	prochlorperazine (Compazine)
fluphenazine (Permitil, Prolixin)	thioridazine (Mellaril)
haloperidol (Haldol)	thiothixene (Navane)
imipramine (Tofranil, etc.)	trifluoperazine (Stelazine)
levodopa + carbidopa (Sinemet)	trimeprazine (Temaril)
loxapine (Loxitane)	

orthostatic hypotension A type of low blood pressure that is related to body position or posture (also called postural hypotension). People who get orthostatic hypotension may have a normal blood pressure while lying down, but on sitting upright or standing will experience sudden sensations of light-headedness, dizziness, and a feeling of an impending faint. These symptoms result from inadequate blood flow (oxygen supply) to the brain.

Many drugs may cause orthostatic hypotension. Tell your doctor if you have this effect so that appropriate dosage adjustment can be made. Failure to correct or to compensate for these sudden drops in blood pressure can lead to severe falls and injury. Tendency to orthostatic hypotension can be reduced by avoiding sudden standing, prolonged standing, vigorous exercise, and exposure to hot environments. A new medicine is also available to treat this. Alcoholic beverages should be used cautiously until their combined effect with the drug in use has been determined.

outcomes research A current concept in health care evaluation that considers the comparative benefits (gauged by a variety of measures) of using a particular medication over another. This may lead to the cheapest drug **not** being the drug of choice, because the outcomes from the therapy do not stand up over time or may result in significant treatment failure.

overdosage The meaning of this term should not be limited to the concept of doses that exceed the normal dosage range recommended by the manufacturer. The optimal dose of many drugs varies greatly from person to person. What may be an average dose for most people will be an overdose for some and an underdose for others. Factors such as age, body size, nutritional status, and liver and kidney function have significant impact on dosage requirements. Drugs with narrow safety margins often produce signs of overdosage if something delays the elimination of the daily dose. In this instance, overdosage results from accumulation of prescribed daily doses. Massive overdosage—as occurs with accidental ingestion of drugs by children or with suicidal intention by adults—is referred to as poisoning.

over-the-counter (OTC) drugs Drug products that can be purchased without prescription. Because of the unrestricted availability, many people do not look upon OTC medicines as drugs. They are capable of a wide variety of actions on biological systems. Within the last 30 years, many OTC drugs have assumed greater importance because of their ability to interact unfavorably with widely used prescription drugs. Serious problems in drug management can arise when (1) the patient fails to tell the physician of the OTC drug(s) he or she is taking ("because they really aren't drugs") and (2) the physician fails to specify that his or her question about which medicines are being taken currently *includes all OTC drugs*. During any course of treatment, whether medical or surgical, the patient should consult with the physician regarding any OTC drug that he or she wishes to take.

The major classes of OTC drugs for internal use include:

allergy medicines (antihistamines)	menstrual aids
antacids	motion sickness remedies
anti-worm medicines	pain relievers
aspirin and aspirin combinations	salt substitutes
aspirin substitutes	sedatives and tranquilizers
asthma aids	sleeping pills
cold medicines (decongestants)	smoking cessation products
cough medicines	stimulants (caffeine)
diarrhea remedies	sugar substitutes (saccharin)
digestion aids	tonics
diuretics	vaginal yeast infection medicines
heartburn medicines	vitamins
iron preparations	weight-reducing aids
laxatives	

paradoxical reaction An unexpected drug response not consistent with the known pharmacology of the drug. Such reactions are due to individual sensitivity or variability and can occur in any age group. They are seen more commonly, however, in children and the elderly.

Example: An 80-year-old man was admitted to a nursing home following the death of his wife. He had difficulty adjusting to his new environment and was restless, agitated, and irritable. He was given a trial of the tranquilizer diazepam (Valium) to relax him, starting with small doses. On the second day of medication he became confused and erratic in behavior. The dose of diazepam was increased. On the third day he began to wander, talked incessantly in a loud voice, and displayed anger when attempts were made to help him. Suspecting the possibility of a paradoxical reaction, his health care provider discontinued the diazepam. All behavioral disturbances gradually subsided within 3 days.

Parkinson-like disorders (parkinsonism) A group of symptoms that resembles those caused by Parkinson's disease, a chronic disorder of the nervous system. The characteristic features of parkinsonism include a fixed, emotionless facial expression (masklike in appearance); a prominent trembling of the hands, arms, or legs; and stiffness of the extremities that limits movement and produces a rigid posture and gait. Parkinsonism is a fairly common adverse effect that occurs in about 15% of all patients who take large doses of phenothiazines or use them over an extended period of time. If recognized early, the Parkinson-like features will lessen or disappear with reduced dosage or change in medication. In some instances, however, Parkinson-like changes may become permanent, requiring appropriate medication.

peripheral neuritis (peripheral neuropathy) A group of symptoms that results from injury to nerve tissue in the extremities. A variety of drugs or chemicals can cause this. The characteristic pattern consists of a sensation of numbness and tingling that usually begins in the fingers and toes and is accompanied by an altered sensation to touch and vague discomfort ranging from aching sensations to burning pain. Severe forms of peripheral neuritis may include loss of muscular strength and coordination.

A relatively common form of peripheral neuritis is that seen with the long-term use of isoniazid in the treatment of tuberculosis. If vitamin B_6 (pyridoxine) is not given concurrently with isoniazid, peripheral neuritis may occur in sensitive individuals. Vitamin B_6 can be both preventive and curative in this form of drug-induced peripheral neuritis.

Since peripheral neuritis can also occur as a late complication following many viral infections, care must be taken to avoid assigning a cause-and-effect relationship to a drug that is not responsible for the nerve injury (see CAUSE-AND-EFFECT RELATIONSHIP).

See Table 10, Section Six, for further discussion of drug-induced nerve damage.

Peyronie's disease A permanent deformity of the penis caused by the formation of dense fibrous (scarlike) tissue within the system of penile vessels that become engorged with blood during the process of erection. During sexual arousal, this inelastic fibrous tissue causes a painful downward bowing of the penis that hampers or precludes satisfactory intercourse. This condition has been associated with the use of phenytoin (Dilantin, etc.) and with most members of the beta-blocker class of drugs (see Drug Classes, Section Four). For a listing of causative drugs, see Table 11, Section Six.

pharmacoeconomics The discipline within pharmacology that studies the issues of costs versus benefits, utilizing a variety of measures: material and personnel costs, treatment outcomes, quality of patient life, etc. Study results are used in deciding where and how health care resources should be utilized.

pharmacology The medical science that relates to the development and use of medicinal drugs and their composition and action in animals and man. Used in its broadest sense, pharmacology embraces the related sciences of medicinal chemistry, experimental therapeutics, and toxicology.

photosensitivity A drug-induced change in the skin that results in the development of a rash or exaggerated sunburn on exposure to the sun or ultraviolet lamps. The reaction is confined to uncovered areas of skin, providing a clue to the nature of its cause. For a listing of causative drugs, see Table 2, Section Six.

porphyria A group of hereditary disorders characterized by excessive production of porphins, essential respiratory pigments of the body. (One porphin is a component of hemoglobin, the pigment of red blood cells.) Two forms of porphyria—acute intermittent porphyria and cutaneous porphyria—can be activated by the use of certain drugs. Acute intermittent porphyria involves damage to the nervous system; an acute attack can include fever, rapid heart rate, vomiting, pain in the abdomen and legs, hallucinations, seizures, paralysis, and coma. Some examples include barbiturates, "sulfa" drugs, chlordiazepoxide (Librium), chlorpropamide (Diabinese), methyldopa (Aldomet), and phenytoin (Dilantin). Cutaneous porphyria involves damage to the skin and liver. An episode can include reddening and blistering of the skin, followed by crust formation, scarring, and excessive hair growth; repeated liver damage can lead to cirrhosis. This form of porphyria can be precipitated by chloroquine, estrogen, oral contraceptives, and excessive iron.

priapism Prolonged, painful erection of the penis usually associated with sexual arousal or stimulation. It is caused by obstruction to the outflow (drainage) of blood through the veins at the root of the penis. Erection may persist for 30 minutes to a few hours and then subside spontaneously, or it may persist for up to 30 hours and require surgical drainage of blood from the penis for relief. More than half of the episodes of priapism induced by drugs result in permanent impotence. Sickle cell anemia (or trait) may predispose to priapism; individuals with this disorder should avoid all drugs that may induce priapism.

Drugs reported to induce priapism include the following:

anabolic steroids (male hormonelike
   drugs: Anadrol, Anavar, Android,
   Halotestin, Metandren, Oreton, Testred,
   Winstrol)
chlorpromazine (Thorazine)
cocaine
guanethidine (Ismelin)
haloperidol (Haldol)
heparin
levodopa (Sinemet)
molindone (Moban)
prazosin (Minipres)
prochlorperazine (Compazine)
trazodone (Desyrel)
trifluoperazine (Stelazine)
warfarin (Coumadin)

prostatism This term refers to the difficulties associated with an enlarged prostate. As the prostate enlarges (a natural development in aging men), it constricts the urethra (outflow passage) where it joins the urinary bladder and impedes urination. This causes a reduction in the size and force of the urinary stream, hesitancy in starting the flow of urine, interruption of urination, and incomplete emptying of the bladder. Atropine and drugs with atropinelike effects can impair the bladder's ability to compensate for the obstructing prostate gland, thus intensifying all of the above symptoms.

Raynaud's phenomenon This term refers to intermittent episodes of reduced blood flow into the fingers or toes, with resulting paleness, discomfort, numbness, and tingling. It is due to an exaggerated constriction of the small arteries that supply blood to the digits. Characteristically an attack is precipitated either by emotional stress or exposure to cold. It can occur as part of a systemic disorder (lupus erythematosus, scleroderma), or it can occur without apparent cause (Raynaud's disease). Some widely used drugs, notably beta-adrenergic blockers and products that contain ergotamine, are conducive to the development of Raynaud-like symptoms in predisposed people.

Reye (Reye's) syndrome An acute, often fatal, childhood illness characterized by swelling of the brain and toxic degeneration of the liver. It usually develops during a flu-like infection, measles, or chickenpox. Cases have been reported with some collagen disease such as lupus (SLE). Symptoms include fever, headache, delirium, loss of consciousness, and seizures. It is one of the 10 major causes of death in children ages 1 to 10 years. Those younger than 18 may be affected. Evidence to date suggests that the syndrome may be due to combined effects of viral infection and chemical toxins (possibly drugs) in a genetically predisposed child. Drugs that have been used just prior to the onset of symptoms include salicylates (aspirin) and drugs to control nausea and vomiting. Current recommendations are to avoid the use of salicylates (aspirin and aspirinlike medicines) in children with flu-like infections, chickenpox, or measles. Some clinicians question use of any NSAID. Remember to look for salicylates in combination cold or flu products and inflammatory bowel drugs. Valproic acid (a seizure medicine) has been implicated in a Reye-like syndrome. Acetaminophen appears to the medicine of choice in those less than 18 who have significant fever from a sudden viral illness.

secondary effect A by-product or complication of drug use that does not occur as part of the drug's primary pharmacological activity. Secondary effects are unwanted consequences and may therefore be classified as adverse effects.

Example: The reactivation of dormant tuberculosis can be a *secondary effect* of long-term cortisone administration for arthritis. Cortisone and related drugs (see Cortisonelike Drugs in Drug Classes, Section Four) suppress natural immunity and lower resistance to infection.

Example: The cramping of leg muscles can be a *secondary effect* of diuretic (urine-producing) drug treatment for high blood pressure. Excessive loss of potassium through increased urination renders the muscle vulnerable to painful spasm during exercise.

side effect A normal, expected, and predictable response to a drug that accompanies the principal (intended) response sought in treatment. Side effects are part of a drug's pharmacological activity and thus are unavoidable. Most side effects are undesirable. The majority cause minor annoyance and inconvenience; some may cause serious problems in managing certain diseases; a few can be hazardous.

superinfection (suprainfection) Development of a second infection superimposed on an initial infection currently under treatment. The superinfection is caused by organisms that are not susceptible to the killing action of the drug(s) used to treat the original (primary) infection. Superinfections usually occur during or immediately following treatment with a broad-spectrum antibiotic—one that is capable of altering the customary balance of bacterial populations in various parts of the body. The disturbance of this balance permits the overgrowth of organisms that normally exist in numbers too small to cause disease. The superinfection may also require treatment, using those drugs that are effective against the offending organism.

Example: A woman is given an antibiotic for a sinus infection. This medicine changes the bacteria usually present in her vagina, allowing yeast to grow. The yeast infection must then be treated with a second medicine.

tardive dyskinesia A drug-induced disorder of the nervous system with involuntary bizarre movements of the eyelids, jaws, lips, tongue, neck, and fingers. It can happen after use of more potent drugs used to treat serious mental illness. It may occur in any age group, but is more common in the middle-aged and especially in chronically ill older women. Once it starts, the pattern of uncontrollable chewing, lip puckering, and repetitive tongue protruding (fly-catching movement) may be irreversible. To date, there is no way of identifying which patient may develop this reaction, and there is no known prevention. The abnormal movement (dyskinesia) is not associated with further decline in mental function.

tolerance A situation where the body adapts to a medicine, and reacts to it less vigorously over time. Tolerance can be beneficial or harmful in treatment.

Example: Beneficial tolerance happens when someone with hay fever finds that drowsiness from their antihistamine gradually disappears after 4 or 5 days of continuous use.

Harmful tolerance occurs when the patient with "shingles" (herpes zoster) finds that the usual dose of pain medicine no longer works to relieve pain.

toxicity The capacity of a drug to impair body functions or damage body tissues. Most drug toxicity is related to total dosage: the larger the overdose, the greater the toxic effects. Some drugs can produce toxic reactions when used in normal doses. Toxic effects due to overdosage are generally a harmful extension of the drug's normal pharmacological actions and—to some extent—are predictable and preventable. Toxic reactions that occur with normal dosage are unrelated to the drug's known pharmacology and for the most part are unpredictable and unexplainable.

tyramine A chemical present in many common foods and beverages. The main pharmacological action of tyramine is to raise the blood pressure. Normally, enzymes present in body tissues neutralize this action of tyramine. The principal enzyme that neutralizes tyramine is monoamine oxidase (MAO) type A. If the action of MAO type A is blocked, substances like tyramine function unopposed, and relatively small amounts can cause alarming and dangerous elevations of blood pressure.

Several drugs in use today are capable of blocking the action of monoamine oxidase type A. These drugs are called monoamine oxidase (MAO) type A inhibitors (see Drug Classes, Section Four). If you are taking one of these drugs and your diet includes foods or beverages that have significant tyramine, a sudden increase in blood pressure may happen. Talk with your doctor or pharmacist about an appropriate diet and before combining any other medicine with an MAO inhibitor.

The following foods and beverages have been reported to contain varying amounts of tyramine. Unless their tyramine content is known to be insignificant, they should be avoided altogether while taking an MAO type A inhibitor drug.

FOODS	BEVERAGES
Aged cheeses of all kinds*	Beer (unpasteurized)
Avocado	Chianti wine
Banana skins	Sherry wine
Bean curd	Vermouth
Bologna	
"Bovril" extract	
Broad bean pods	
Chicken liver (unless fresh and used at once)	
Chocolate	
Figs, canned	
Fish, canned	
Fish, dried and salted	
Herring, pickled	
Liver, if not very fresh	
"Marmite" extract	
Meat extracts	
Meat tenderizers	
Pepperoni	
Raisins	
Raspberries	
Salami	
Shrimp paste	
Sour cream	
Soy sauce	
Yeast extracts	

Note: *Any* high-protein food that is aged or has undergone breakdown by putrefaction probably contains tyramine and could produce a hypertensive crisis in anyone taking MAO type A inhibitor drugs.

viral load or viral burden A term used in reference to AIDS patients to describe the amount of HIV virus present in the body at any given time. The amount of virus

*Cottage cheese, cream cheese, and processed cheese are safe to eat.

relates to the effectiveness of the drug therapy that is being used, and can be a reason to change medication if the load increases.

WHO Pain Ladder A therapeutic scheme using increasing strengths and combinations of pain medicines (analgesics) that includes NSAIDs, opiates, and adjuvant drugs to control pain as specified by the World Health Organization. It is *not* an absolute treatment scheme, but should be used to organize the approach to effective analgesia.

TABLES OF DRUG INFORMATION

TABLE 1

Drugs That May Adversely Affect the Fetus and Newborn Infant

In 1961 it was found that thalidomide use during early pregnancy could cause major birth defects. This sparked concern about medicines as possible teratogens. Much research has increased our understanding of how drugs can affect the developing fetus and newborn infant, and which drugs can cause significant harm to the unborn and newborn child. In many instances, it is not possible to clearly separate adverse effects due to the mother's disease or disorder from those that may be caused by medicines. Based on our current knowledge, it is strongly recommended that only those drugs that confer clear and essential benefits should be used during pregnancy.

Drugs that *probably* cause adverse effects when taken during the *first trimester*

aminopterin	fluorouracil	opioid analgesics*
anticonvulsants*	iodides	progestins*
antithyroid drugs	isotretinoin	quinine
cytarabine	kanamycin	streptomycin
danazol	mercaptopurine	testosterone
diethylstilbestrol	methotrexate	warfarin
etretinate	misoprostol	

Drugs that *possibly* cause adverse effects when taken during the *first trimester*

angiotensin-converting enzyme inhibitors*	lithium	piperazine
busulfan	mebendazole	rifampin
chlorambucil	monoamine oxidase inhibitors*	tetracyclines*
estrogens*	oral contraceptives	

Drugs that *probably* cause adverse effects when taken during the *second* and *third trimesters*

amiodarone	iodides	rifampin
androgens*	kanamycin	streptomycin
angiotensin-converting enzyme inhibitors*	lithium	sulfonamides*
antithyroid drugs	nonsteroidal anti-inflammatory drugs*	sulfonylureas*
aspirin		tetracyclines*
benzodiazepines*	opioid analgesics*	thiazide diuretics*
chloramphenicol	phenothiazines*	tricyclic antidepressants*
estrogens*	progestins*	warfarin

Drugs that *possibly* cause adverse effects when taken during the *second* and *third trimesters*

acetazolamide	ethacrynic acid	hydroxyzine
clemastine	fluoroquinolones*	promethazine
diphenhydramine	haloperidol	

*See Drug Class, Section Four.

TABLE 2

Drugs That May Cause Photosensitivity on Exposure to Sun

Some drugs can sensitize skin to ultraviolet light. This can cause the skin to react with a rash or exaggerated burn on exposure to sun or ultraviolet lamps. If you are taking any of the following drugs, ask your doctor for guidance with regard to sun exposure and sunblocks.

acetazolamide
acetohexamide
alprazolam
amantadine
amiloride
aminobenzoic acid
amiodarone
amitriptyline
amoxapine
barbiturates
bendroflumethiazide
benzocaine
benzophenones
benzoyl peroxide
benzthiazide
captopril
carbamazepine
chlordiazepoxide
chloroquine
chlorothiazide
chlorpromazine
chlorpropamide
chlortetracycline
chlorthalidone
ciprofloxacin
clindamycin
clofazimine
clofibrate
clomipramine
cyproheptadine
dacarbazine
dapsone
demeclocycline
desipramine
desoximetasone
diethylstilbestrol
diflunisal
diltiazem
diphenhydramine
disopyramide

doxepin
doxycycline
enoxacin
estrogen
etretinate
flucytosine
fluorescein
fluorouracil
fluphenazine
flutamide
furosemide
glipizide
glyburide
gold preparations
griseofulvin
haloperidol
hexachlorophene
hydrochlorothiazide
hydroflumethiazide
ibuprofen
imipramine
indomethacin
isotretinoin
ketoprofen
lincomycin
lomefloxacin
maprotiline
mesoridazine
methacycline
methotrexate
methyclothiazide
methyldopa
metolazone
minocycline
minoxidil
nabumetone
nalidixic acid
naproxen
nifedipine
norfloxacin

nortriptyline
ofloxacin
oral contraceptives
oxyphenbutazone
oxytetracycline
para-aminobenzoic acid
perphenazine
phenelzine
phenobarbital
phenylbutazone
phenytoin
piroxicam
polythiazide
prochlorperazine
promazine
promethazine
protriptyline
pyrazinamide
quinidine
quinine
sulfonamides
sulindac
tetracycline
thiabendazole
thioridazine
thiothixene
tolazamide
tolbutamide
tranylcypromine
trazodone
tretinoin
triamterene
trichlormethiazide
trifluoperazine
triflupromazine
trimeprazine
trimethoprim
trimipramine
triprolidine
vinblastine

TABLE 3

Drugs That May Adversely Affect Behavior

Medicines can alter mood and disturb emotional stability, and may also cause unpredictable patterns of abnormal thinking and behavior. Such responses are relatively

*See Drug Class, Section Four.

infrequent, but the nature and degree of mental disturbance can be quite alarming and potentially dangerous for both patient and family.

Such paradoxical responses are often of an idiosyncratic nature, and someone with a history of a serious mental or emotional disorder is more likely to experience bizarre reactions. In some cases, it may be difficult to separate the disorder under treatment from an effect of one (or more) drugs the patient may be taking. If in doubt, it is best to talk with your doctor and stop any drug with potential for such side effects and see if thinking changes resolve.

Drugs reported to impair *concentration* and/or *memory*

antihistamines*	isoniazid	primidone
anti-parkinsonism drugs*	monoamine oxidase	scopolamine
barbiturates*	(MAO) inhibitor drugs*	
benzodiazepines*	phenytoin	

Drugs reported to cause *confusion, delirium,* or *disorientation*

acetazolamide	digitalis	metoclopramide
aminophylline	digitoxin	narcotic pain relievers
amphotericin B	digoxin	(analgesics)
antidepressants*	disulfiram	NSAIDs
antihistamines*	diuretics	*para*-aminosalicylic acid
antipsychotics	ethchlorvynol	phenelzine
atropinelike drugs*	ethinamate	phenothiazines*
barbiturates*	fenfluramine	phenytoin
benzodiazepines*	fluoroquinolone antibiotics	piperazine
bromides	glutethimide	primidone
carbamazepine	H_2-receptor antagonists	propranolol
chloroquine	isoniazid	reserpine
cimetidine	levodopa	scopolamine
clonidine	meprobamate	theophylline
cortisonelike drugs*	methyldopa	tricyclic antidepressants
cycloserine		

Drugs reported to cause *paranoid thinking*

bromides	diphenhydramine	isoniazid
cortisonelike drugs*	disulfiram	levodopa

Drugs reported to cause *schizophreniclike behavior*

amphetamines*	fenfluramine	phenylpropanolamine
ephedrine	phenmetrazine	

Drugs reported to cause *maniclike behavior*

antidepressants*	levodopa	(MAO) inhibitor drugs*
cortisonelike drugs*	monoamine oxidase	

Some medicines have mood-altering *side effects*, although they are prescribed for altogether unrelated conditions. Emotional and behavioral secondary effects will be quite unpredictable and vary enormously from person to person. However, the following experiences have been seen with sufficient frequency to establish recognizable patterns.

*See Drug Class, Section Four.

Drugs reported to cause *nervousness* (anxiety and irritability)

amantadine
amphetaminelike drugs*
  (appetite suppressants)
antihistamines*
caffeine
chlorphenesin
cortisonelike drugs*
ephedrine
epinephrine

isoproterenol
levodopa
liothyronine (in excessive
  dosage)
methylphenidate
methysergide
monoamine oxidase
  (MAO) inhibitor drugs*
nylidrin

oral contraceptives
selective serotonin
  reuptake inhibitors
theophylline
thyroid (in excessive
  dosage)
thyroxine (in excessive
  dosage)

Drugs reported to cause *emotional depression*

amantadine
amphetamines* (on
  withdrawal)
benzodiazepines*
beta-adrenergic-blocking
  drugs (some)
carbamazepine
chloramphenicol
cortisonelike drugs*
cycloserine
digitalis
digitoxin
digoxin

diphenoxylate
estrogens
ethionamide
fenfluramine (on
  withdrawal)
fluphenazine
guanethidine
haloperidol
indomethacin
isoniazid
levodopa
methsuximide
methyldopa

methysergide
metoprolol
oral contraceptives
phenylbutazone
procainamide
progesterones
propranolol
reserpine
sulfonamides*
vitamin D (in excessive
  dosage)

Drugs reported to cause *euphoria*

amantadine
aminophylline
amphetamines
antihistamines* (some)
antispasmodics, synthetic*
aspirin
barbiturates*
benzphetamine
chloral hydrate
clorazepate
codeine

cortisonelike drugs*
diethylpropion
diphenoxylate
dronabinol
ethosuximide
flurazepam
haloperidol
levodopa
meprobamate
methysergide

monoamine oxidase
  (MAO) inhibitor drugs*
morphine
opioids
pargyline
pentazocine
phenmetrazine
propoxyphene
scopolamine
tybamate

Drugs reported to cause *excitement*

acetazolamide
amantadine
amphetaminelike drugs*
antidepressants*
antihistamines*
atropinelike drugs*
barbiturates* (paradoxical
  response)
benzodiazepines*
  (paradoxical response)
cortisonelike drugs
cycloserine

diethylpropion
digitalis
ephedrine
epinephrine
ethinamate (paradoxical
  response)
ethionamide
glutethimide (paradoxical
  response)
isoniazid
isoproterenol
levodopa

meperidine and MAO
  inhibitor drugs*
methyldopa and MAO
  inhibitor drugs*
methyprylon (paradoxical
  response)
nalidixic acid
orphenadrine
quinine
scopolamine

*See Drug Class, Section Four.

TABLE 4

Drugs That May Adversely Affect Vision

A significant percentage of all adverse drug effects involve visual changes or eye damage. Some effects, such as blurring of vision or double vision, may occur shortly after starting a drug. More subtle and serious effects, such as cataract development or damage to the retina or optic nerve, may not occur until a drug has been in use for an extended time. Some of these changes are irreversible. If you are taking a drug that can affect the eye, promptly report any eye discomfort or change in vision.

Drugs reported to cause *blurring of vision*

acetazolamide
antiarthritic/anti-inflamm-
   atory drugs
antidepressants*
antihistamines*
atropinelike drugs*

chlorthalidone
ciprofloxacin
cortisonelike drugs*
diethylstilbestrol
etretinate
fenfluramine

norfloxacin
oral contraceptives
phenytoin
sulfonamides*
tetracyclines*
thiazide diuretics*

Drugs reported to cause *double vision*

antidepressants*
antidiabetic drugs*
antihistamines*
aspirin
barbiturates*
benzodiazepines*
bromides
carbamazepine
carisoprodol
chloroquine
chlorprothixene
ciprofloxacin
clomiphene
colchicine
colistin
cortisonelike drugs*

digitalis
digitoxin
digoxin
ethionamide
ethosuximide
etretinate
guanethidine
hydroxychloroquine
indomethacin
isoniazid
levodopa
mephenesin
methocarbamol
methsuximide
morphine
nalidixic acid

nitrofurantoin
norfloxacin
oral contraceptives
orphenadrine
oxyphenbutazone
pentazocine
phenothiazines*
phensuximide
phenylbutazone
phenytoin
primidone
propranolol
quinidine
sedatives/sleep inducers*
thiothixene
tranquilizers*

Drugs reported to cause *farsightedness*

ergot
penicillamine

sulfonamides* (possibly)
tolbutamide (possibly)

Drugs reported to cause *nearsightedness*

acetazolamide
aspirin
carbachol
chlorthalidone
codeine
cortisonelike drugs*

ethosuximide
methsuximide
morphine
oral contraceptives
penicillamine
phenothiazines*

phensuximide
spironolactone
sulfonamides*
tetracyclines*
thiazide diuretics*

Drugs reported to *alter color vision*

acetaminophen
amodiaquine
amyl nitrite
aspirin

atropine
barbiturates*
belladonna
chloramphenicol

chloroquine
chlorpromazine
chlortetracycline
ciprofloxacin

*See Drug Class, Section Four.

Drugs reported to *alter color vision* (cont.)

cortisonelike drugs*
digitalis
digitoxin
digoxin
disulfiram
epinephrine
ergotamine
erythromycin
ethchlorvynol
ethionamide
fluphenazine
furosemide
hydroxychloroquine
indomethacin
isocarboxazid
isoniazid

mefenamic acid
mesoridazine
methysergide
nalidixic acid
norfloxacin
oral contraceptives
oxyphenbutazone
paramethadione
pargyline
penicillamine
pentylenetetrazol
perphenazine
phenacetin
phenylbutazone
primidone
prochlorperazine

promazine
promethazine
quinacrine
quinidine
quinine
reserpine
sodium salicylate
streptomycin
sulfonamides*
thioridazine
tranylcypromine
trifluoperazine
triflupromazine
trimeprazine
trimethadione

Drugs reported to cause *sensitivity to light* (photophobia)

antidiabetic drugs*
atropinelike drugs*
bromides
chloroquine
ciprofloxacin
clomiphene
digitoxin
doxepin
ethambutol

ethionamide
ethosuximide
etretinate
hydroxychloroquine
mephenytoin
methsuximide
monoamine oxidase
    (MAO) inhibitor drugs*
nalidixic acid

norfloxacin
oral contraceptives
paramethadione
phenothiazines*
quinidine
quinine
tetracyclines*
trimethadione

Drugs reported to cause *halos around lights*

amyl nitrite
chloroquine
cortisonelike drugs*
digitalis
digitoxin

digoxin
hydrochloroquine
nitroglycerin
norfloxacin
oral contraceptives

paramethadione
phenothiazines*
quinacrine
trimethadione

Drugs reported to cause *visual hallucinations*

amantadine
amphetaminelike drugs*
amyl nitrite
antihistamines*
aspirin
atropinelike drugs*
barbiturates*
benzodiazepines*
bromides
carbamazepine
cephalexin
cephaloglycin
chloroquine
cycloserine

digitalis
digoxin
disulfiram
ephedrine
furosemide
gabapentin
griseofulvin
haloperidol
hydroxychloroquine
indomethacin
isosorbide
levodopa
nialamide
oxyphenbutazone

pargyline
pentazocine
phenothiazines*
phenylbutazone
phenytoin
primidone
propranolol
quinine
sedatives/sleep inducers*
sulfonamides*
tetracyclines*
tricyclic antidepressants*
tripelennamine

*See Drug Class, Section Four.

Drugs reported to impair the use of *contact lenses*

brompheniramine
carbinoxamine
chlorpheniramine
cyclizine
cyproheptadine

dexbrompheniramine
dexchlorpheniramine
dimethindene
diphenhydramine
furosemide

oral contraceptives
terfenadine
tripelennamine

Drugs reported to cause *cataracts* or *lens deposits*

allopurinol
busulfan
chlorpromazine
chlorprothixene
cortisonelike drugs*
fluphenazine
mesoridazine

methotrimeprazine
perphenazine
phenmetrazine
pilocarpine
prochlorperazine
promazine
promethazine

thioridazine
thiothixene
trifluoperazine
triflupromazine
trimeprazine

TABLE 5

Drugs That May Cause Blood Cell Dysfunction or Damage

All blood cells originate and mature in the bone marrow: red blood cells (erythrocytes), white blood cells (leukocytes), and blood platelets (thrombocytes). There are three kinds of white blood cells: granulocytes, monocytes (macrophages), and lymphocytes. Drugs that affect the formation or development of blood cells can (1) act on any stage of cell production; (2) impair the production of one cell line; (3) influence the production of all cell lines. Some medicines can adversely affect mature cells circulating in the bloodstream. Examples can be found in the tables that follow.

Drugs that cause inevitable (dose-dependent) *aplastic anemia* (see Glossary)

actinomycin D
azathioprine
busulfan
carboplatin
carmustine
chlorambucil
cisplatin
cyclophosphamide

cytarabine
doxorubicin
epirubicin
etoposide
fluorouracil
hydroxyurea
lomustine
melphalan

mercaptopurine
methotrexate
mitomycin
mitoxantrone
plicamycin
procarbazine
thioguanine
thiotepa

Drugs that may cause idiosyncratic (dose-independent) *aplastic anemia*

amodiaquine
benoxaprofen
carbimazole
chloramphenicol
chlorpromazine
gold
indomethacin

mepacrine
oxyphenbutazone
penicillamine
phenylbutazone
phenytoin
piroxicam
prothiaden

pyrimethamine
sulfonamides*
sulindac
thiouracils
trimethoprim/sulfamethox-
    azole

Drugs that may *impair red blood cell production* (only)

azathioprine
carbamazepine

chloramphenicol
chlorpropamide

dapsone
fenoprofen

*See Drug Class, Section Four.

Drugs that may *impair red blood cell production* (only) (cont.)

gold
halothane
isoniazid
methyldopa
penicillin
pentachlorophenol

phenobarbital
phenylbutazone
phenytoin
pyrimethamine
sulfasalazine
sulfathiazol

sulfonamides*
sulfonylureas*
thiamphenicol
tolbutamide
trimethoprim/sulfamethox-
    azole

Drugs that may significantly *reduce granulocyte cell counts* (various mechanisms)

acetaminophen
acetazolamide
allopurinol
amitriptyline
amodiaquine
benzodiazepines*
captopril
carbamazepine
carbimazole
cephalosporins*
chloramphenicol
chloroquine
chlorothiazide
chlorpromazine
chlorpropamide
chlorthalidone
cimetidine
clindamycin
dapsone
desipramine
disopyramide

ethacrynic acid
sulfadoxine/
    pyrimethamine
gentamicin
gold
hydralazine
hydrochlorothiazide
imipramine
indomethacin
isoniazid
levamisole
meprobamate
methimazole
methyldopa
oxyphenbutazone
penicillamine
penicillins*
pentazocine
phenacetin
phenothiazines*
phenylbutazone

phenytoin
procainamide
propranolol
propylthiouracil
pyrimethamine
quinidine
quinine
ranitidine
rifampin
sodium aminosalicylate
streptomycin
sulfadoxine
sulfonamides*
tetracyclines*
tocainide
tolbutamide
trimethoprim/sulfamethox-
    azole
vancomycin

Drugs that may significantly *reduce blood platelet counts*

acetazolamide
actinomycin
allopurinol
alpha-interferon
amiodarone
ampicillin
aspirin
carbamazepine
carbenicillin
cephalosporins*
chenodeoxycholic acid
chloroquine
chlorothiazide
chlorpheniramine
chlorpropamide
chlorthalidone
cimetidine
cyclophosphamide
danazol
desferrioxamine

diazepam
diazoxide
diclofenac
digoxin
diltiazem
furosemide
gentamicin
gold
hydrochlorothiazide
imipramine
isoniazid
isotretinoin
levamisole
meprobamate
methyldopa
mianserin
minoxidil
morphine
nitrofurantoin
oxprenolol

oxyphenbutazone
penicillamine
penicillin
phenylbutazone
phenytoin
piroxicam
procainamide
quinidine
quinine
ranitidine
rifampin
sodium aminosalicylate
sulfasalazine
sulfonamides*
thioguanine
trimethoprim/sulfamethox-
    azole
valproate
vancomycin

*See Drug Class, Section Four.

Drugs that cause *hemolytic anemia* due to glucose-6-phosphate dehydrogenase (G6PD) deficiency of red blood cells

acetanilid
methylene blue
nalidixic acid
naphthalene
niridazole
nitrofurantoin

pamaquine
phenazopyridine
phenylhydrazine
primaquine
sulfacetamide
sulfamethoxazole

sulfanilamide
sulfapyridine
thiazolsulfone
toluidine blue

Drugs that may cause *hemolytic anemia* by other mechanisms

antimony
chlorpropamide
cisplatin
mephenesin

methotrexate
para-aminosalicylic acid
penicillamine
phenazopyridine

quinidine
quinine
rifampin
sulfasalazine

Drugs that may cause *megaloblastic anemia*

acyclovir
alcohol
aminopterin
azathioprine
colchicine
cycloserine
cytarabine
floxuridine
fluorouracil
hydroxyurea
mercaptopurine

metformin
methotrexate
neomycin
nitrofurantoin
nitrous oxide
oral contraceptives
para-aminosalicylic acid
pentamidine
phenformin
phenobarbital
phenytoin

primidone
pyrimethamine
sulfasalazine
tetracycline
thioguanine
triamterene
trimethoprim
vinblastine
vitamin A
vitamin C (large doses)
zidovudine

Drugs that may cause *sideroblastic anemia*

alcohol
chloramphenicol
cycloserine

isoniazid
penicillamine
phenacetin

pyrazinamide

TABLE 6

Drugs That May Cause Heart Dysfunction or Damage

Drugs may adversely affect both function and structure of the heart. Heart problems themselves often determine the nature of adverse drug effects. Some are due to direct pharmacological actions of a drug on heart tissues, while other reactions are caused indirectly by altering chemical balances that diminish how well the heart works (as with the loss of potassium or magnesium due to diuretics).

Drugs that may cause or contribute to *abnormal heart rhythms* (arrhythmias)

aminophylline
amiodarone
amitriptyline
antiarrhythmic drugs*
bepridil
beta-adrenergic-blocking

drugs*
beta-adrenergic
   bronchodilators*
carbamazepine
chlorpromazine
cimetidine

digitoxin
digoxin
diltiazem
disopyramide
diuretics*
doxepin

*See Drug Class, Section Four.

Drugs that may cause or contribute to *abnormal heart rhythms* (cont.)

encainide
fentolterol
flecainide
isoproterenol
ketanserin
lidocaine
maprotiline
methyldopa

mexiletine
milrinone
phenothiazines*
prenylamine
procainamide
quinidine
ranitidine
sotalol

terbutaline
theophylline
thiazide diuretics*
thioridazine
trazodone
tricyclic antidepressants*
verapamil

Drugs that may *depress heart function* (reduce pumping efficiency)

beta-adrenergic-blocking
    drugs*
cocaine
daunorubicin
diltiazem

disopyramide
doxorubicin
epinephrine
flecainide
fluorouracil

isoproterenol
nifedipine
verapamil

Drugs that may *reduce coronary artery blood flow* (reduce oxygen supply to heart muscle)

amphetamines*
beta-adrenergic-blocking
    drugs* (abrupt
    withdrawal)
cocaine

ergotamine
fluorouracil
nifedipine
oral contraceptives
ritodrine

vasopressin
vinblastine
vincristine

Drugs that may *impair healing of heart muscle* following heart attack (myocardial infarction)

adrenocortical steroids*
nonsteroidal

anti-inflammatory drugs
    (NSAIDs)*

Drugs that may cause *heart valve damage*

dexfenfluramine (Redux)
ergotamine
fen-phen (fenfluramine-

phenteramine) (recently
    outlawed in some states)
methysergide

minocycline (blue-black
    pigmentation)

Drugs that may cause *pericardial disease*

actinomycin D
anthracyclines
bleomycin
cisplatin
cyclophosphamide

cytarabine
fluorouracil
hydralazine
methysergide
minoxidil

phenylbutazone
practolol
procainamide
sulfasalazine

TABLE 7

Drugs That May Cause Lung Dysfunction or Damage

Lung damage from medicines may be difficult to distinguish from natural diseases or disorders that involve lung function or structure. The lung is subject to: Type A—those due to known and expected pharmacological drug actions; Type B—those due to unex-

*See Drug Class, Section Four.

pected and unpredictable allergic or idiosyncratic reactions on the part of the drug user.

Drugs that may adversely affect *blood vessels of the lung*

Drugs that may cause thrombo-embolism

estrogens*
oral contraceptives
  (high-estrogen type)

Drugs that may cause pulmonary hypertension

amphetamines*	fenfluramine	tryptophan
dexfenfluramine (Redux)	oral contraceptives	

Drugs that may cause vasculitis (blood vessel damage) with or without hemorrhage

aminoglutethimide	febarbamate	phenytoin
amphotericin	nitrofurantoin	
cocaine	penicillamine	

Drugs that may cause adult respiratory distress syndrome (ARDS)

bleomycin	heroin	naloxone
codeine	hydrochlorothiazide	ritodrine
cyclophosphamide	methadone	terbutaline
dextropropoxyphene	mitomycin	vinblastine

Drugs that may adversely affect the *bronchial tubes*

Drugs that may cause bronchoconstriction (asthma)

acetaminophen	griseofulvin	anti-inflammatory
aspirin	maprotiline	drugs*
beta-adrenergic-blocking	methacholine	penicillins*
drugs*	methoxypsoralen	pilocarpine
carbachol	metoclopramide	propafenone
cephalosporins*	morphine	pyridostigmine
chloramphenicol	neomycin	streptomycin
deanol	neostigmine	tartrazine (coloring agent)
demeclocycline	nitrofurantoin	
erythromycin	nonsteroidal	

Drugs that may cause bronchiolitis (with permanent obstruction of small bronchioles)

penicillamine   sulfasalazine

Drugs that may *damage lung tissues*

Drugs that may cause acute allergic-type pneumonitis

ampicillin	chlorpropamide	mephenesin
bleomycin	gold	mercaptopurine
cephalexin	imipramine	metformin

*See Drug Class, Section Four.

Drugs that may cause acute allergic-type pneumonitis (cont.)

methotrexate
metronidazole
mitomycin
nalidixic acid
nitrofurantoin
nomifensine

nonsteroidal
  anti-inflammatory
  drugs*
para-aminosalicylic acid
penicillamine
penicillin

phenylbutazone
phenytoin
procarbazine
sulfonamides*
tetracycline
vinblastine

Drugs that may cause chronic pneumonitis and fibrosis (scarring)

amiodarone
bleomycin
bromocriptine
busulfan
carmustine
chlorambucil
cyclophosphamide

ergotamine
gold
hexamethonium
mecamylamine
melphalan
methysergide
nitrofurantoin

pentolinium
practolol
sulfasalazine
tocainide
tolfenamic acid

Drugs that may *damage the pleura*

bromocriptine

methysergide

practolol

TABLE 8

Drugs That May Cause Liver Dysfunction or Damage

The liver works to change drugs into forms that can be readily eliminated from the body. Medicines can hurt liver structure or function. The reactions range from mild and transient changes in liver function tests to complete liver failure and death. Many drugs may affect the liver in more than one way. Use of the following drugs requires careful liver monitoring.

Drugs that may cause *acute dose-dependent liver damage* (resembling acute viral hepatitis)

acetaminophen (overdose)
salicylates (doses over 2 g
  daily)

Drugs that may cause *acute dose-independent liver damage* (resembling acute viral hepatitis)

acebutolol
allopurinol
atenolol
carbamazepine
cimetidine
dantrolene
diclofenac
diltiazem
disulfiram
enflurane
ethambutol
ethionamide
halothane
ibuprofen

indomethacin
isoniazid
ketoconazole
labetalol
maprotiline
metoprolol
mianserin
naproxen
nifedipine
para-aminosalicylic acid
penicillins*
phenelzine
phenindione
phenobarbital

phenylbutazone
phenytoin
piroxicam
probenecid
pyrazinamide
quinidine
quinine
ranitidine
rifampin
sulfonamides*
sulindac
tricyclic antidepressants*
valproic acid
verapamil

*See Drug Class, Section Four.

Drugs that may cause *acute fatty infiltration of the liver*

adrenocortical steroids*
antithyroid drugs
isoniazid
methotrexate

phenothiazines*
phenytoin
salicylates*
sulfonamides*

tetracyclines*
valproic acid

Drugs that may cause *cholestatic jaundice*

actinomycin D
amoxicillin/clavulanate
azathioprine
captopril
carbamazepine
carbimazole
cephalosporins*
chlordiazepoxide
chlorpromazine
chlorpropamide
cloxacillin
cyclophosphamide
cyclosporine
danazol
diazepam
disopyramide
enalapril
erythromycin (estolate)

estradiol
flecainide
flurazepam
flutamide
glyburide
gold
griseofulvin
haloperidol
ketoconazole
mercaptopurine
methyltestosterone
nafcillin
nifedipine
nitrofurantoin
nonsteroidal
    anti-inflammatory
    drugs*
norethandrolone

oral contraceptives
oxacillin
penicillamine
phenothiazines*
phenytoin
propoxyphene
propylthiouracil
rifampin
sulfonamides*
tamoxifen
thiabendazole
tolbutamide
tricyclic antidepressants*
trimethoprim/sulfamethox-
    azole
troleandomycin
verapamil

Drugs that may cause *liver granulomas* (chronic inflammatory nodules)

allopurinol
aspirin
carbamazepine
chlorpromazine
chlorpropamide
diltiazem
disopyramide

gold
hydralazine
isoniazid
methyldopa
nitrofurantoin
penicillin
phenylbutazone

phenytoin
procainamide
quinidine
ranitidine
sulfonamides*
tolbutamide

Drugs that may cause *chronic liver disease*

Drugs that may cause active chronic hepatitis

acetaminophen (chronic
    use, large doses)
dantrolene

isoniazid
methyldopa
nitrofurantoin

trazodone

Drugs that may cause liver cirrhosis or fibrosis (scarring)

methotrexate
methyldopa

nicotinic acid

vitamin A

*See Drug Class, Section Four.

Drugs that may cause chronic cholestasis (resembling primary biliary cirrhosis)

chlorpromazine/valproic acid (combination)	ycin (combination)	phenytoin
chlorpropamide/erythrom-	imipramine	thiabendazole
	phenothiazines*	tolbutamide

Drugs that may cause *liver tumors* (benign and malignant)

anabolic steroids	oral contraceptives	thorotrast
danazol	testosterone	

Drugs that may cause *damage to liver blood vessels*

adriamycin	orine (combination)	mitomycin
anabolic steroids	dacarbazine	oral contraceptives
azathioprine	herbal teas, some	thioguanine
carmustine	mercaptopurine	vincristine
cyclophosphamide/cyclosp-	methotrexate	vitamin A (excessive doses)

TABLE 9

Drugs That May Cause Kidney Dysfunction or Damage

The kidneys perform two major drug functions: (1) alteration of the drug to help remove it; (2) elimination of the drug from the body in the urine. As with drug effects on the liver, many drugs may adversely affect the kidneys in several ways. The kidneys are quite sensitive to toxic effects of medicines. Careful monitoring is advisable when taking any of the drugs cited below.

Drugs that may primarily *impair kidney function* (without damage)

amphotericin	demeclocycline	nifedipine
angiotensin-converting enzyme inhibitors* (with renal artery stenosis; with congestive heart failure)	diuretics/NSAIDs* (avoid this combination)	nitroprusside
	glyburide	nonsteroidal anti-inflammatory drugs*
	isofosfamide	
	lithium/tricyclic antidepressants* (avoid this combination)	rifampin
beta-adrenergic-blocking drugs*		vinblastine
colchicine	methoxyflurane	

Drugs that may cause *acute kidney failure* (due to kidney damage)

Drugs that may damage the kidney filtration unit (the nephron)

acetaminophen (excessive dosage)	cisplatin	penicillamine
	cyclosporine	phenytoin
allopurinol	enalapril	quinidine
aminoglycoside antibiotics*	ergometrine	rifampin
	hydralazine	streptokinase
amphotericin	metronidazole	sulfonamides*
bismuth thiosulfate	mitomycin	thiazide diuretics*
carbamazepine	oral contraceptives	

*See Drug Class, Section Four.

Drugs that may cause *acute interstitial nephritis*

allopurinol
amoxicillin
ampicillin
aspirin
azathioprine
aztreonam
captopril
carbamazepine
carbenicillin
cefaclor
cefoxitin
cephalexin
cephalothin
cephapirin
cephradine
cimetidine
ciprofloxacin
clofibrate
cloxacillin
diazepam

diclofenac
diflunisal
fenoprofen
foscarnet
furosemide
gentamicin
glafenine
ibuprofen
indomethacin
ketoprofen
mefenamate
methicillin
methyldopa
mezlocillin
minocycline
nafcillin
naproxen
oxacillin
penicillamine
penicillin

phenindione
phenobarbital
phenylbutazone
phenytoin
piroxicam
pirprofen
pyrazinamide
rifampin
sodium valproate
sulfamethoxazole
sulfinpyrazone
sulfonamides*
sulindac
thiazide diuretics*
tolmetin
trimethoprim
vancomycin
warfarin

Drugs that may cause *muscle destruction and associated acute kidney failure*

adrenocortical steroids*
alcohol
amphetamines*
amphotericin
carbenoxolone
chlorthalidone
clofibrate

cocaine
cytarabine
fenofibrate
haloperidol
halothane
heroin
lovastatin

opioid analgesics*
pentamidine
phenothiazines*
streptokinase
suxamethonium

Drugs that may cause *kidney damage resembling glomerulonephritis or nephrosis*

captopril
fenoprofen
gold
ketoprofen

lithium
mesalamine
penicillamine
phenytoin

practolol
probcnecid
quinidine

Drugs that may cause *chronic interstitial nephritis and papillary necrosis* (analgesic kidney damage)

acetaminophen
aspirin

phenacetin (All with
    long-term use)

Drugs that may cause or contribute to *urinary tract crystal or stone formation*

acetazolamide
acyclovir
cytotoxic drugs
dihydroxyadenine
magnesium trisilicate
mercaptopurine
methotrexate

methoxyflurane
phenylbutazone
probenecid
salicylates*
sulfonamides*
thiazide diuretics*
triamterene

uricosuric drugs
vitamin A
vitamin C
vitamin D
warfarin
zoxazolamine

*See Drug Class, Section Four.

TABLE 10

Drugs That May Cause Nerve Dysfunction or Damage

Medicines may adversely affect any part of the nervous system from the brain to peripheral nerves. The extent of benefits or problems from drugs varies widely from person to person and results from inherited factors.

Drugs that may cause *significant headache*

amyl nitrate
bromocriptine
clonidine
ergotamine (prolonged use)
etretinate
hydralazine
ibuprofen

indomethacin
labetalol
naproxen
nifedipine
nitrofurantoin
nitroglycerin
perhexilene
propranolol

sulindac
terbutaline
tetracyclines*
theophylline
tolmetin
trimethoprim/sulfamethoxazole

Drugs that may cause *seizures* (convulsions)

ampicillin
atenolol
carbenicillin
cephalosporins*
chloroquine
cimetidine
ciprofloxacin
cycloserine
disopyramide

ether
halothane
indomethacin
isoniazid
lidocaine
lithium
mefenamic acid
nalidixic acid
oxacillin

penicillins* (synthetic)
phenothiazines*
pyrimethamine
terbutaline
theophylline
ticarcillin
tricyclic antidepressants*
vincristine

Drugs that may cause *stroke*

anabolic steroids
cocaine

oral contraceptives
phenylpropanolamine

Drugs that may cause features of *parkinsonism*

amitriptyline
amodiaquine
chloroquine
chlorprothixene
desipramine
diazoxide

diphenhydramine
droperidol
haloperidol
imipramine
levodopa
lithium

methyldopa
metoclopramide
phenothiazines*
reserpine
thiothixene
trifluperidol

Drugs that may cause *acute dystonias* (acute involuntary movement syndromes—AIMS)

carbamazepine
chlorzoxazone
haloperidol

metoclopramide
phenothiazines*
phenytoin

propranolol
tricyclic antidepressants*

Drugs that may cause *tardive dyskinesia* (see Glossary)

haloperidol

phenothiazines*

thiothixene

*See Drug Class, Section Four.

Drugs that may cause *neuroleptic malignant syndrome* (NMS)

See this term in the
  Glossary for a list of
  causative drugs.

Drugs that may cause *peripheral neuropathy* (see Glossary)

amiodarone
amitriptyline
amphetamines*
amphotericin
anticoagulants*
carbutamide
chlorambucil
chloramphenicol
chloroquine
chlorpropamide
cimetidine
clioquinol
clofibrate
colchicine
colistin
cytarabine
dapsone
disopyramide

disulfiram
ergotamine
ethambutol
glutethimide
gold
hydralazine
imipramine
indomethacin
isoniazid
methaqualone
methimazole
methysergide
metronidazole
nalidixic acid
nitrofurantoin
nitrofurazone
penicillamine
penicillin

perhexiline
phenelzine
phenylbutazone
phenytoin
podophyllin
procarbazine
propranolol
propylthiouracil
stavudine
streptomycin
sulfonamides*
sulfoxone
thalidomide
tolbutamide
vinblastine
vincristine

Drugs that may cause a *myasthenia gravis* syndrome

aminoglycoside
  antibiotics*
beta-adrenergic-blocking
  drugs*

penicillamine
phenytoin
polymyxin B
trihexyphenidyl

TABLE 11

Drugs That May Adversely Affect Sexuality

Many commonly prescribed drugs can cause both obvious or subtle effects on one or more aspects of sexual expression. Patients may be unaware that sexual changes can be related to medicines and are often reluctant to talk about it with their doctor. In some cases, sexual dysfunction may be a result of the disorder under treatment or an undetected disorder. Conditions such as diabetes, kidney failure, hypertension, depression, and alcoholism may reduce libido and cause failure of erection. Many of the drugs used to treat these conditions may worsen subclinical sexual dysfunction. Such situations require the closest cooperation between therapist and patient in order to correctly assess the possible cause-and-effect relationships and change therapy appropriately.

Possible Drug Effects on Male Sexuality

1. Increased libido
     androgens (replacement therapy in deficiency states)
     baclofen (Lioresal)
     chlordiazepoxide (Librium) (antianxiety effect)
     diazepam (Valium) (antianxiety effect)

*See Drug Class, Section Four.

haloperidol (Haldol)
levodopa (Larodopa, Sinemet) (may be an indirect effect due to improved sense
of well-being)

2. Decreased libido
antihistamines
barbiturates
chlordiazepoxide (Librium), sedative effect
chlorpromazine (Thorazine), 10 to 20% of users
cimetidine (Tagamet)
clofibrate (Atromid-S)
clonidine (Catapres), 10 to 20% of users
danazol (Danocrine)
diazepam (Valium), sedative effect
disulfiram (Antabuse)
estrogens (therapy for prostatic cancer)
fenfluramine (Pondimin)
finasteride (Propecia, Proscar)
heroin
licorice
medroxyprogesterone (Provera)
methyldopa (Aldomet), 10 to 15% of users
metoclopramide (Reglan), 80% of users
perhexilene (Pexid)
prazosin (Minipres), 15% of users
propranolol (Inderal), rarely
reserpine (Serpasil, Ser-Ap-Es)
spironolactone (Aldactone)
tricyclic antidepressants

3. Impaired erection (impotence)
anticholinergics
antihistamines
baclofen (Lioresal)
barbiturates (when abused)
beta-blockers (see Drug Classes, Section Four)
chlordiazepoxide (Librium) (in high dosage)
chlorpromazine (Thorazine)
cimetidine (Tagamet)
clofibrate (Atromid-S)
clonidine (Catapres), 10 to 20% of users
cocaine
diazepam (Valium) (in high dosage)
digitalis and its glycosides
disopyramide (Norpace)
disulfiram (Antabuse), uncertain
estrogens (therapy for prostatic cancer)
ethacrynic acid (Edecrin), 5% of users
ethionamide (Trecator-SC)
fenfluramine (Pondimin)
finasteride (Propecia, Proscar)
furosemide (Lasix), 5% of users
guanethidine (Ismelin)
haloperidol (Haldol), 10 to 20% of users
heroin
hydroxyprogesterone (therapy for prostatic cancer)
licorice
lithium (Lithonate)

marijuana
mesoridazine (Serentil)
methantheline (Banthine)
methyldopa (Aldomet), 10% to 15% of users
metoclopramide (Reglan), 60% of users
monoamine oxidase (MAO) type A inhibitors, 10 to 15% of users
perhexilene (Pexid)
prazosin (Minipres), infrequently
reserpine (Serpasil, Ser-Ap-Es)
spironolactone (Aldactone)
thiazide diuretics, 5% of users
thioridazine (Mellaril)
tricyclic antidepressants

4. Impaired ejaculation
anticholinergics
barbiturates (when abused)
chlorpromazine (Thorazine)
clonidine (Catapres)
estrogens (therapy for prostatic cancer)
guanethidine (Ismelin)
heroin
mesoridazine (Serentil)
methyldopa (Aldomet)
monoamine oxidase (MAO) type A inhibitors
phenoxybenzamine (Dibenzyline)
phentolamine (Regitine)
reserpine (Serpasil, Ser-Ap-Es)
thiazide diuretics
thioridazine (Mellaril)
tricyclic antidepressants

5. Decreased testosterone
adrenocorticotropic hormone (ACTH)
barbiturates
digoxin (Lanoxin)
haloperidol (Haldol)
—increased testosterone with low dosage
—decreased testosterone with high dosage
lithium (Lithonate)
marijuana
medroxyprogesterone (Provera)
monoamine oxidase (MAO) type A inhibitors
spironolactone (Aldactone)

6. Impaired spermatogenesis (reduced fertility)
adrenocorticosteroids (prednisone, etc.)
androgens (moderate to high dosage, extended use)
antimalarials
aspirin (abusive, chronic use)
chlorambucil (Leukeran)
cimetidine (Tagamet)
colchicine
cotrimoxazole (Bactrim, Septra)
cyclophosphamide (Cytoxan)
estrogens (therapy for prostatic cancer)
marijuana
medroxyprogesterone (Provera)
methotrexate

metoclopramide (Reglan)
monoamine oxidase (MAO) type A inhibitors
niridazole (Ambilhar)
nitrofurantoin (Furadantin)
spironolactone (Aldactone)
sulfasalazine (Azulfidine)
testosterone (moderate to high dosage, extended use)
vitamin C (doses of 1 g or more)

7. Testicular disorders
    Swelling
    —tricyclic antidepressants
    Inflammation
    —oxyphenbutazone (Tandearil)
    Atrophy
    —androgens (moderate to high dosage, extended use)
    —chlorpromazine (Thorazine)
    —cyclophosphamide (Cytoxan) (in prepubescent boys)
    —spironolactone (Aldactone)

8. Penile disorders
    Priapism (see Glossary)
    —anabolic steroids (male hormonelike drugs)
    —chlorpromazine (Thorazine)
    —clozapine (Clozaril)
    —cocaine
    —fluphenazine (Prolixin)
    —guanethidine (Ismelin)
    —haloperidol (Haldol)
    —heparin
    —hydralazine (Apresoline)
    —levodopa (Sinemet)
    —mesoridazine (Serentil)
    —molindone (Moban)
    —phenelzine (Nardil)
    —phenytoin (Dilantin)
    —prazosin (Minipres)
    —prochlorperazine (Compazine)
    —thioridazine (Mellaril)
    —trazodone (Desyrel)
    —trifluoperazine (Stelazine)
    —warfarin (Coumadin)
    Peyronie's disease (see Glossary)
    —beta-blocker drugs (see Drug Classes, Section Four)
    —phenytoin (Dilantin, etc.)

9. Gynecomastia (excessive development of the male breast)
    androgens (partial conversion to estrogen)
    busulfan (Myleran)
    carmustine (BiCNU)
    chlormadinone
    chlorpromazine (Thorazine)
    chlortetracycline (Aureomycin)
    cimetidine (Tagamet)
    clonidine (Catapres), infrequently
    diethylstilbestrol (DES)
    digitalis and its glycosides
    estrogens (therapy for prostatic cancer)
    ethionamide (Trecator-SC)

    finasteride (Propecia, Proscar)
    griseofulvin (Fulvicin, etc.)
    haloperidol (Haldol)
    heroin
    human chorionic gonadotropin
    isoniazid (INH, Nydrazid)
    marijuana
    mestranol
    methyldopa (Aldomet)
    metoclopramide (Reglan)
    phenelzine (Nardil)
    reserpine (Serpasil, Ser-Ap-Es)
    spironolactone (Aldactone)
    thioridazine (Mellaril)
    tricyclic antidepressants (TAD's)
    vincristine (Oncovin)

10. Feminization (loss of libido, impotence, gynecomastia, testicular atrophy)
    conjugated estrogens (Premarin, etc.)

11. Precocious puberty
    anabolic steroids
    androgens
    isoniazid (INH)

Possible Drug Effects on Female Sexuality

1. Increased libido
    androgens
    chlordiazepoxide (Librium) (antianxiety effect)
    diazepam (Valium) (antianxiety effect)
    mazindol (Sanorex)
    oral contraceptives (freedom from fear of pregnancy)

2. Decreased libido
    See list of drug effects on male sexuality. Some of these *may* have potential for reducing libido in the female. The literature is sparse on this subject.

3. Impaired arousal and orgasm
    anticholinergics
    clonidine (Catapres)
    methyldopa (Aldomet)
    monoamine oxidase (MAO) inhibitors
    tricyclic antidepressants

4. Breast enlargement
    penicillamine
    tricyclic antidepressants

5. Galactorrhea (spontaneous flow of milk)
    amphetamine
    chlorpromazine (Thorazine)
    cimetidine (Tagamet)
    haloperidol (Haldol)
    heroin
    methyldopa (Aldomet)
    metoclopramide (Reglan)
    oral contraceptives
    phenothiazines
    reserpine (Serpasil, Ser-Ap-Es)

        sulpiride (Equilid)
        tricyclic antidepressants

6. Ovarian failure (reduced fertility)
        anesthetic gases (operating room staff)
        cyclophosphamide (Cytoxan)
        cytostatic drugs
        danazol (Danocrine)
        medroxyprogesterone (Provera)

7. Altered menstruation (menstrual disorders)
        adrenocorticosteroids (prednisone, etc.)
        androgens
        barbiturates (when abused)
        chlorambucil (Leukeran)
        chlorpromazine (Thorazine)
        cyclophosphamide (Cytoxan)
        danazol (Danocrine)
        estrogens
        ethionamide (Trecator-SC)
        haloperidol (Haldol)
        heroin
        isoniazid (INH, Nydrazid)
        marijuana
        medroxyprogesterone (Provera)
        metoclopramide (Reglan)
        oral contraceptives
        phenothiazines
        progestins
        radioisotopes
        rifampin (Rifadin, Rifamate, Rimactane)
        spironolactone (Aldactone)
        testosterone
        thioridazine (Mellaril)
        vitamin A (in excessive dosage)

8. Virilization (acne, hirsutism, lowering of voice, enlargement of clitoris)
        anabolic drugs
        androgens
        haloperidol (Haldol)
        oral contraceptives (lowering of voice)

9. Precocious puberty
        estrogens (in hair lotions)
        isoniazid (INH, Nydrazid)

TABLE 12

Drugs That May Interact With Alcohol

Alcohol may interact with a wide variety of drugs. The most important (and most familiar) problem happens when the depressant action on the brain of sedatives, sleep-inducing drugs, tranquilizers, and narcotic drugs is intensified by alcohol. Alcohol may also reduce drug effectiveness or interact to produce toxic effects. Some drugs may increase the intoxicating effects of alcohol, producing further impairment of mental alertness, judgment, physical coordination, and reaction time.

Although drug interactions with alcohol are generally predictable, the intensity and significance can vary greatly from one person to another and from one occasion to another. This is because many factors influence what happens when drugs and alcohol interact. Factors include individual variations in sensitivity to drugs, the chemistry and quantity of the drug, the type and amount of alcohol consumed, and the sequence in which drug and alcohol are taken. If you need to use any of the drugs listed in the following table, you should ask your physician for help concerning alcohol use.

Drugs with which it is advisable to avoid alcohol completely

Drug name or class	Possible interaction with alcohol
amphetamines	excessive rise in blood pressure with alcoholic beverages containing tyramine**
antidepressants*	excessive sedation, increased intoxication
barbiturates*	excessive sedation
bromides	confusion, delirium, increased intoxication
calcium carbimide	disulfiramlike reaction**
carbamazepine	excessive sedation
chlorprothixene	excessive sedation
chlorzoxazone	excessive sedation
disulfiram	disulfiram reaction**
ergotamine	reduced effectiveness of ergotamine
fenfluramine	excessive stimulation of nervous system with some beers and wines
furazolidone	disulfiramlike reaction**
haloperidol	excessive sedation
MAO inhibitor drugs*	excessive rise in blood pressure with alcoholic beverages containing tyramine**
meperidine	excessive sedation
meprobamate	excessive sedation
methotrexate	increased liver toxicity and excessive sedation
metronidazole	disulfiramlike reaction**
narcotic drugs	excessive sedation
oxyphenbutazone	increased stomach irritation and/or bleeding
pentazocine	excessive sedation
pethidine	excessive sedation
phenothiazines*	excessive sedation
phenylbutazone	increased stomach irritation and/or bleeding
procarbazine	disulfiramlike reaction**
propoxyphene	excessive sedation
reserpine	excessive sedation, orthostatic hypotension**
sleep-inducing drugs (hypnotics)	excessive sedation
—carbromal	
—chloral hydrate	
—ethchlorvynol	
—ethinamate	
—glutethimide	
—flurazepam	
—methaqualone	

*See Drug Class, Section Four.
**See Glossary.

Drug name or class	Possible interaction with alcohol
—methyprylon	
—temazepam	
—triazolam	
thiothixene	excessive sedation
tricyclic antidepressants*	excessive sedation, increased intoxication
trimethobenzamide	excessive sedation

Drugs with which alcohol should be used only in small amounts (use cautiously until combined effects have been determined)

Drug name or class	Possible interaction with alcohol
acetaminophen (Tylenol, etc.)	increased liver toxicity
amantadine	excessive lowering of blood pressure
antiarthritic/anti-inflammatory drugs	increased stomach irritation and/or bleeding
anticoagulants (coumarins)*	increased anticoagulant effect
antidiabetic drugs (sulfonylureas)*	increased antidiabetic effect, excessive hypoglycemia**
antihistamines*	excessive sedation
antihypertensives*	excessive orthostatic hypotension**
aspirin (large doses or continuous use)	increased stomach irritation and/or bleeding
benzodiazepines*	excessive sedation
carisoprodol	increased alcoholic intoxication
diethylpropion	excessive nervous system stimulation with alcoholic beverages containing tyramine**
dihydroergotoxine	excessive lowering of blood pressure
diphenoxylate	excessive sedation
dipyridamole	excessive lowering of blood pressure
diuretics*	excessive orthostatic hypotension**
ethionamide	confusion, delirium, psychotic behavior
fenoprofen	increased stomach irritation and/or bleeding
griseofulvin	flushing and rapid heart action
ibuprofen	increased stomach irritation and/or bleeding
indomethacin	increased stomach irritation and/or bleeding
insulin	excessive hypoglycemia**
iron	excessive absorption of iron
isoniazid	decreased effectiveness of isoniazid, increased incidence of hepatitis
lithium	increased confusion and delirium (avoid all alcohol if any indication of lithium overdosage)
methocarbamol	excessive sedation
methotrimeprazine	excessive sedation
methylphenidate	excessive nervous system stimulation with alcoholic beverages containing tyramine**
metoprolol	excessive orthostatic hypotension**

*See Drug Class, Section Four.
**See Glossary.

Drug name or class	Possible interaction with alcohol
nalidixic acid	increased alcoholic intoxication
naproxen	increased stomach irritation and/or bleeding
nicotinic acid	possible orthostatic hypotension**
nitrates* (vasodilators)	possible orthostatic hypotension**
nylidrin	increased stomach irritation
orphenadrine	excessive sedation
phenelzine	increased alcoholic intoxication
phenoxybenzamine	possible orthostatic hypotension**
phentermine	excessive nervous system stimulation with alcoholic beverages containing tyramine**
phenytoin	decreased effect of phenytoin
pilocarpine	prolongation of alcohol effect
prazosin	excessive lowering of blood pressure
primidone	excessive sedation
propranolol	excessive orthostatic hypotension**
sulfonamides*	increased alcoholic intoxication
sulindac	increased stomach irritation and/or bleeding
tolmetin	increased stomach irritation and/or bleeding
tranquilizers (mild)	excessive sedation
—chlordiazepoxide	
—clorazepate	
—diazepam	
—hydroxyzine	
—meprobamate	
—oxazepam	
—phenaglycodol	
—tybamate	
tranylcypromine	increased alcoholic intoxication

Drugs capable of producing a disulfiramlike reaction** when used concurrently with alcohol

antidiabetic drugs (sulfonylureas)*	disulfiram	procarbazine
calcium carbimide	furazolidone	quinacrine
chloral hydrate	metronidazole	sulfonamides*
chloramphenicol	nifuroxime	tinidazole
	nitrofurantoin	tolazoline

TABLE 13

High-Potassium Foods

Diuretic drugs that cause loss of potassium are often used to treat conditions that also require a reduced intake of sodium. The high-potassium foods listed below have been selected for their compatibility with a sodium-restricted diet (500 to 1000 mg of sodium daily). Diuretics may also cause a loss of magnesium. Make sure this is tested, and the results discussed with your doctor.

*See Drug Class, Section Four.
**See Glossary.

Beverages

orange juice
prune juice

skim milk
tea

tomato juice
whole milk

Breads and Cereals

brown rice
cornbread
griddle cakes

muffins
oatmeal
shredded wheat

waffles

Fruits

apricot
avocado
banana

fig
honeydew melon
mango

orange
papaya
prune

Meats

beef
chicken
codfish
flounder

haddock
halibut
liver
pork

rockfish
salmon
turkey
veal

Vegetables

baked beans
lima beans
mushrooms
navy beans

parsnips
radishes
squash
sweet potato

tomato
white potato

TABLE 14
Your Personal Drug Profile

Knowing as much as possible about your body and your medicines can save your life. Please take the time to fill out this profile with the latest information. **Medicine never does you any good if you forget to take it.** Make time to copy the medication map and have your doctor or pharmacist fill it in and discuss it with you.

Name:

Age:

Weight in kilograms: (pounds divided by 2.2)

Height in inches:

Prescription drug allergies:

Non-prescription drug allergies:

Food allergies:

My kidneys* are: normal_____

mildly_____   moderately_____   severely_____   compromised.

My liver* is: normal_____

mildly_____   moderately_____   severely_____   compromised.

Conditions or diseases that I have or have had:

Prescription and non-prescription medications I take regularly:

*Make certain your dose is decreased if the drug is eliminated by an organ (such as the liver or kidneys) with which you have a problem. To determine which organs are involved, refer to the drug profile and "Conditions Requiring Dosing Adjustments" section for each medication you are taking.

Prescription and non-prescription medications I take periodically:

I find it very difficult_____

I find it very easy_____   to remember to take medicines.

I become constipated rarely_____   occasionally_____   never_____.

Urination is usually easy_____   rather difficult_____   difficult_____.

The phone number of the nearest Poison Control Center is _____.

I sleep well_____   OK_____   poorly_____   little_____   on most nights.

I have_____   have never_____   had blood problems in the past.

I am considering becoming_____   might be_____   am_____   pregnant.

I want the medications which offer the best balance of **price** and **outcomes** for my specific medical history and present conditions.

TABLE 15

The Medication Map

Today you are often given some brief information papers when you pick up your individual prescription medicines, but no one takes the time to map out all of the medicines you take during the day. I believe that this is a critical cause of drug interactions, irrational drug combinations, and noncompliance with medicines . . . all of which contribute to the 136 billion dollars spent each year on treatment problems. Use the map to talk with your doctor or pharmacist to schedule your prescription, nonprescription, or herbal medicines as you plan to take them. Make sure the timing and combinations are OK!

Midnight	Medicine and dose planned:	
1 A.M.	Medicine and dose planned:	
2 A.M.	Medicine and dose planned:	
3 A.M.	Medicine and dose planned:	
4 A.M.	Medicine and dose planned:	
5 A.M.	Medicine and dose planned:	
6 A.M.	Medicine and dose planned:	
7 A.M.	Medicine and dose planned:	*Morning Meal Time is*:
8 A.M.	Medicine and dose planned:	
9 A.M.	Medicine and dose planned:	
10 A.M.	Medicine and dose planned:	
11 A.M.	Medicine and dose planned:	
12 noon	Medicine and dose planned:	*Lunch or Brunch Time*:
1 P.M.	Medicine and dose planned:	
2 P.M.	Medicine and dose planned:	
3 P.M.	Medicine and dose planned:	
4 P.M.	Medicine and dose planned:	
5 P.M.	Medicine and dose planned:	
6 P.M.	Medicine and dose planned:	*Evening Meal Time*:
7 P.M.	Medicine and dose planned:	
8 P.M.	Medicine and dose planned:	
9 P.M.	Medicine and dose planned:	*Snack (if any)*:
10 P.M.	Medicine and dose planned:	
11 P.M.	Medicine and dose planned:	

Sources

The following sources were consulted in the compilation and revision of this book:

Abramowicz, M., ed. 1997. *Drugs of Choice: The Medical Letter on Drugs and Therapeutics.* New Rochelle, NY: The Medical Letter.

Ackerman, B. H., and N. Kasbekar. 1997. Disturbances of taste and smell induced by drugs. *Pharmacotherapy* 17(3):482–496.

Advances in Osteoporosis. 1996, 1997.

AIDS Clinical Care. Boston: Massachusetts Medical Society. 1996, 1997.

American Board of Internal Medicine. 1996. *Caring for the Dying.* American Board of Internal Medicine.

American Pain Society. 1996. *Principles of Analgesic Use in the Treatment of Acute Pain and Cancer Pain.* 3rd Ed. Glenview, IL: American Pain Society.

American Pharmaceutical Association. 1996. *Handbook of Nonprescription Drugs.* 11th Ed. Washington, DC: American Pharmaceutical Association.

American Psychiatric Association. 1997. *Practice Guideline for the Treatment of Patients with Alzheimer's Disease and Other Dementias of Late Life.* Washington, DC: American Psychiatric Association.

American Society for Pharmacology and Experimental Therapeutics. 1990. *Rational Drug Therapy and Pharmacology for Physicians.* Bethesda, MD: American Society for Pharmacology and Experimental Therapeutics.

Annals of Pharmacotherapy. 1996–1997.

Bartlett, J. 1996. *The Johns Hopkins Hospital 1996 Guide to Medical Care of Patients with HIV Infection.* Baltimore: Williams & Wilkins.

Bartlett, J. 1997. *Medical Management of HIV Infection: 1997 Edition.* Baltimore: Port City Press.

Berkow, R., ed. 1996. *The Merck Manual.* 15th Ed. Rahway, NJ: Merck Sharp & Dohme Research Laboratories.

Bonnick, S. L. 1994. *The Osteoporosis Handbook.* Dallas: Taylor Publishing.

Briggs, G. G., Bodendorfer, T. W., Freeman, R. K., and S. J. Yaffee. 1983. *Drugs in Pregnancy and Lactation.* Baltimore: Williams & Wilkins.

Brooke, M. H. 1986. *A Clinician's View of Neuromuscular Diseases.* 2nd Ed. Baltimore: Williams & Wilkins.

Canadian Pharmaceutical Association. 1991. *Compendium of Pharmaceuticals and Specialties.* 26th Ed. Ottawa: Canadian Pharmaceutical Association.

Canadian Pharmaceutical Association, St. Paul's Hospital British Columbia Center of Excellence for HIV–AIDS. Vancouver, BC: Canadian Pharmaceutical Association, 1997.

Cape, R. 1978. *Aging: Its Complex Management*. Hagerstown, MD: Harper & Row.

Classen, D. C., et al. 1997. Adverse drug events in hospitalized patients. *Journal of the American Medical Association* 277:301–306.

Clin-Alert. 1996–1997. Medford, NJ: Clin-Alert.

Clinisphere. 1997. Facts and Comparisons 1.0. Facts and Comparisons, St. Louis.

Cumming, R. G., et al. Use of inhaled corticosteroids and the risk of cataracts. *New England Journal of Medicine* 337(1):8–14, 1997.

Daniels, J. B., ed. 1997. *Infectious Disease in Clinical Practice*. Baltimore: Williams & Wilkins.

DiGregorio, J. G., et al. 1991. *Handbook of Pain Management*. Westchester, NY: Medical Surveillance.

Drug Information Journal. 1996–1997.

Drug Interactions Newsletter. 1997. Spokane, WA: Applied Therapeutics.

DrugLink. 1997. St. Louis: J. B. Lippincott, Facts and Comparisons.

Drug Newsletter. 1997. St. Louis: J. B. Lippincott, Facts and Comparisons.

Drug Therapy: Physicians Prescribing Update. 1992. Lawrenceville, NJ: Excerpta Medica.

Drugs and Therapy Perspectives. 1996–1997.

Dukes, M. N. G., ed. 1988. *Meyler's Side Effects of Drugs*. 11th Ed. Amsterdam: Excerpta Medica.

Electronic Library of Medicine, The. 1996. Boston: Little, Brown.

Farrell, B., and B. Farrell, eds. 1996. *Pain in the Elderly*. International Association for the Study of Pain Press.

Favus, M., ed. 1996. *Primer on the Metabolic Bone Diseases and Disorders of Mineral Metabolism*. 3rd Ed. Philadelphia, New York: Lippincott-Raven.

Fraunfelder, F. T. 1989. *Drug-Induced Ocular Side Effects and Drug Interactions*. 3rd ed. Philadelphia: Lea & Febiger.

Gleason, P. P., et al. 1997. Medical outcomes and antimicrobial costs with the use of the American Thoracic Society Guidelines for Outpatients with Community Acquired Pneumonia. *Journal of the American Medical Association* 278(1):32–39.

Goodman, L. S., and A. Gilman, eds. 1996. *The Pharmacological Basis of Therapeutics*. 9th ed. New York: Macmillan.

Graham, I. M., et al. 1997. Plasma homocysteine as a risk factor for vascular disease. *Journal of the American Medical Association* 277(22):1775–1781.

Griffiths, M. C., ed. 1988. *USAN 1989*. Rockville, MD: United States Pharmacopeial Convention.

Griffiths, M. C., ed. 1988. *The USP Dictionary of Drug Names*. Rockville, MD: United States Pharmacopeial Convention.

Handbook of Clinical Drug Data. 1993. Hamilton, IL: Drug Intelligence Publications.

Hansten, P. D. 1992. *Drug Interactions*. 6th Ed. Philadelphia: Lea & Febiger.

Heinonen, O. P., Slone, D., and S. Shapiro. 1977. *Birth Defects and Drugs in Pregnancy*. Littleton, MA: PSG Publishing.

Hollister, L. E. 1983. *Clinical Pharmacology of Psychotherapeutic Drugs*. 2nd Ed. New York: Churchill Livingstone.

Hospital Pharmacy. 32(5). 1997.

Huff, B. B., ed. 1997. *The Physicians' Desk Reference*. 47th Ed. Oradell, NJ: Medical Economics.

International Drug Therapy Newsletter. 1997. Baltimore: Ayd Medical Communications.

Jefferson, J. W., and J. H. Greist. 1977. *Primer of Lithium Therapy*. Baltimore: Williams & Wilkins.

Journal of Bone and Mineral Research. 1996–1997.

Journal of the American Medical Association. 1997.

Journal Watch. 1996–1997.

Journal Watch: Women's Health. 1996–1997.

Kaplan, N. M. 1995. *Management of Hypertension*. 6th Ed. Durant, OK: Essential Medical Information Systems.

Klippel, J. H., ed. 1997. Systemic Lupus Erythematosus demographics, prognosis and outcome. *J Rheumatol Suppl* 48:67–71.

Koda-Kimbal (Lloyd Yee Young). 1995. *Applied Therapeutics: The Clinical Use of Drugs*. 6th Ed. Vancouver, WA: Applied Therapeutics.

Koller, W. C., ed. 1987. *Handbook of Parkinson's Disease*. New York: Marcel Dekker.

Kolodny, R. C., Masters, W. H., and V. E. Johnson. 1979. *Textbook of Sexual Medicine*. Boston: Little, Brown.

Lawrence, R. A. 1980. *Breast-Feeding*. St. Louis: Mosby.

Lieberman, M. L. 1988. *The Sexual Pharmacy*. New York: New American Library.

Long, J. W. 1984. *Clinical Management of Prescription Drugs*. Philadelphia: Harper & Row.

Long, J. W. 1997. *The Essential Guide to Chronic Illness*. New York: HarperCollins.

Maddin, S., ed. 1982. *Current Dermatologic Therapy*. Philadelphia: W. B. Saunders.

Mayo Clinic Proceedings. 1996–1997.

McEvoy, G. K., ed. 1997. *American Hospital Formulary Service: Drug Information 1997*. Bethesda, MD: American Society of Hospital Pharmacists.

Medical Letter on Drugs and Therapeutics, The. 1997. New Rochelle, NY: The Medical Letter.

Melmon, K. L., and H. F. Morrelli. 1978. *Clinical Pharmacology*. 2nd Ed. New York: Macmillan.

Michelson, M. D., et al. 1996. Bone mineral density in women with depression. *New England Journal of Medicine*, 335(16):1176–1181.

Micromedex: Drugdex. 1997. Computerized Clinical Information System, Englewood, CO.

Mohler, S. R. 1982. *Medication and Flying: A Pilot's Guide*. Boston: Boston Publishing.

Murphy, J. E. 1993. *Clinical Pharmacokinetics*. Bethesda, MD: American Society of Hospital Pharmacists.

New England Journal of Medicine. 1997.

Olin, B. R., ed. 1992. *Patient Drug Facts*. St. Louis: J. B. Lippincott, Facts and Comparisons.

Olin, B. R., ed. 1997. *Facts and Comparisons*. St. Louis: J. B. Lippincott, Facts and Comparisons.

Pharmacotherapy: The Journal of Human Pharmacology and Drug Therapy. 1997.

Physician's GenRX. 1996. Version 96.1a. Mosby, St. Louis.

Physician's Therapeutics and Drug Alert, The. 1996–1997.

Postgraduate Medicine: The Journal of Applied Medicine for the Primary Care Physician. 1992.

Raj, P. P. 1986. *Practical Management of Pain*. Chicago: Year Book Medical Publishers.

Rakel, R. E., ed. 1992. *Conn's Current Therapy 1992*. Philadelphia: W. B. Saunders.

Reynolds, J. E. F., ed. 1997. *Martindale: The Extra Pharmacopoeia*. 29th Ed. London: The Pharmaceutical Press.

Rogers, C. S., and J. D. McCue, eds. 1987. *Managing Chronic Disease*. Oradell, NJ: Medical Economics Books.

Rybacki, J. J. 1997. Letter to the editor. *Journal of the American Medical Association* 277(17):1351.

Sanford, J., et al. 1996. *The Sanford Guide to HIV/AIDS Therapy*. 5th Ed. Antimicrobial Therapy, Inc. Vienna, VA: Lippincott-Raven.

Sauer, G. C. 1985. *Manual of Skin Diseases*. 5th Ed. Philadelphia: J. B. Lippincott.

Scan Newsletter. 1996–1997. Norwich, NY: Society for Clinical Densitometry.

Schardein, J. L. 1976. *Drugs as Teratogens*. Cleveland: CRC Press.

Scientific American Medicine. 1997. CD-ROM. Enigma Information Systems, New York.

Semla, T.P., et al. 1993. *Geriatric Dosage Handbook*. Cleveland: Lexi-comp.

Shepard, T. H. 1989. *Catalog of Teratogenic Agents*. 6th Ed. Baltimore: Johns Hopkins University Press.

Smith, L. H., and S. O. Thier. 1985. *Pathophysiology: The Biological Principles of Disease*. 2nd Ed. Philadelphia: W. B. Saunders.

Sorensen, S. J., and S. R. Abel. 1997. Comparison of the ocular beta-blockers. *Annals of Pharmacotherapy* 30:43–54.

Spath, P. L., ed. 1994. *Clinical Paths, Tools for Outcomes Management.* Chicago: The American Hospital Association.

Speight, T. M., and N. H. G. Holford, eds. 1997. *Avery's Drug Treatment.* 4th Ed. Auckland, NZ: Adis International.

Swash, M., and M. S. Schwartz. 1988. *Neuromuscular Diseases.* 2nd Ed. Berlin: Springer-Verlag.

Tatro, D. S., ed. 1997. *Drug Interaction Facts.* St. Louis: J. B. Lippincott, Facts and Comparisons.

Thordsen, D. J., and H. A. Barenholtz, eds. 1997. *Clinical Abstracts: Current Therapeutic Findings.* Cincinnati, OH: Harvey Whitney Books.

Tuchmann-Duplessis, H. 1975. *Drug Effects on the Fetus.* Sydney, Australia: ADIS Press.

United States Pharmacopeial Convention. 1997. *USP Dispensing Information 1997. Vol. 1: Drug Information for the Health Care Provider.* 12th Ed. Rockville, MD: United States Pharmacopeial Convention.

U.S. Department of Health and Human Services. 1993. *Depression in Primary Care. Volume 1: Detection and Diagnosis.* Washington, DC: U.S. Department of Health and Human Services.

U.S. Department of Health and Human Services. 1993. *Sickle Cell Disease: Screening, Diagnosis, Management and Counseling in Newborns and Infants.* Washington, DC: U.S. Department of Health and Human Services.

U.S. Department of Health and Human Services. 1996. *Morbidity and Mortality Weekly Report: Immunization of Adolescents,* 22 November. Washington, DC: U.S. Department of Health and Human Services.

U.S. Department of Health and Human Services. Food and Drug Administration. 1996–1997. *F.D.A. Drug Bulletin.* Rockville, MD: Department of Health and Human Services, Food and Drug Administration.

Utian, W. H. 1980. *Menopause in Modern Perspective.* New York: Appleton-Century-Crofts.

Wallach, J. B. 1996. *Interpretation of Diagnostic Tests.* 6th Ed. Boston: Little, Brown.

Wilcox, S. M., et al. 1994. Inappropriate drug prescribing for the community-dwelling elderly. *Journal of the American Medical Association* 272(4):292–296.

Worley, R. J., ed. 1981. Menopause. *Clinical Obstetrics and Gynecology* 24(1):163–164.

Young, D. S. 1991. *Effects of Drugs on Clinical Laboratory Tests.* 1991 supplement. Washington, DC: AACC Press.

Young, L. L., ed. 1996. *Nonprescription Products: Formulations and Features '96–97.* Washington, DC: American Pharmaceutical Association.

Index

This index contains all the brand and generic drug names included in Section Two.

Brand names of drugs appear in italic type and are capitalized.

Each brand name is followed by its generic name, the generic name is the name under which you'll find the drug profile in Section Two.

The symbol [CD] indicates that the brand name represents a combination drug that contains the generic drug components listed below it. To be fully familiar with any combination drug [CD], it is necessary to read the Drug Profile of each of the components listed. The brand name of a combination drug *may* or *may not* appear in the brand name list of each Drug Profile that is cited in the index as a component of a particular combination drug. The index listing of component drugs for any combination drug product represents the manufacturer's formulation of that brand at the time this information was compiled for publication.

The symbol ♣ before the brand name of a combination drug indicates that the brand name is used in both the United States and Canada, but that the ingredients in the combination product in each country differ. The Canadian drug is marked with the symbol ♣ to distinguish it from the American drug which has the same name.

A generic name with no page designation indicates an active component of a combination drug for which there is no Profile in Section Two. It is included to alert you to its presence, should you wish to consult your physician regarding its significance.

A & D with prednisolone [CD]:
   prednisolone, 0.5%, 791
   Vitamin A, 1,500 units/G*
   Vitamin D, 200 units/G*
A.B.C. compound with codeine
   [CD]:
   codeine, 222
Abitrexate, methotrexate, 594
acarbose, 27
AC & C [CD]:
   aspirin, 92
   codeine, 222
Accolate, zafirlukast, 88
Accopain, codeine, 222
Accupril, quinapril, 842
Accurbron, theophylline, 922
Accutane, isotretinoin, 504
acebutolol, 31
Acetaminophen-PM,
   diphenhydramine, 280
❀*Acet-Am*, theophylline, 922
❀*Acetazolam*, acetazolamide, 35
acetazolamide, 35
acetic acids, 39
acetylsalicylic acid. *See* aspirin, 98.
Aches-N-Pain, ibuprofen, 815
Achromycin, tetracycline, 918
Achromycin V, tetracycline, 918
❀*Acrocidin*, tetracycline, 918
Acroseb-Dex, dexamethasone, 251
Actagen-C [CD]:
   codeine, 222
   pseudoephedrine*
   triprolidine*
Actifed w/Codeine [CD]:
   codeine, 222
   pseudoephedrine*
   triprolidine*
❀*Actiprofen*, ibuprofen, 815
Actisite, tetracycline, 918
Actron, ketoprofen, 815
Acular, ketorolac ophthalmic, 39
acycloguanosin. *See* acyclovir,
   46.
acyclovir, 46
Adalat, nifedipine, 687
Adalat CC, nifedipine, 687
❀*Adalat FT*, nifedipine, 687
❀*Adalat P.A.*, nifedipine, 687
Adapin, doxepin, 299
Adrenaline, epinephrine, 312
Adreno-Mist, epinephrine, 312
Adsorbocarpine, pilocarpine, 774
Advil, ibuprofen, 815
Advil, Children's, ibuprofen, 815
A.E.A., theophylline, 922
Aerobid, flunisolide, 374
Aerobid-M, flunisolide, 374
Aerolate, theophylline, 922
Aeromax, salmeterol, 867
Afed-C [CD]:
   codeine, 222
   guifenesin*

pseudoephedrine*
triprolidine*
Akarpine, pilocarpine, 774
Ak-Chlor, chloramphenicol, 176
❀*Ak-Cide* [CD]:
   prednisolone, 791
   sulfacetamide*
❀*Ak-Dex*, dexamethasone, 251
AK-Mycin Ophthalmic,
   erythromycin, 566
Akne-Mycin, erythromycin, 566
❀*Ak-Pred*, prednisolone, 791
❀*Ak-Tate*, prednisolone, 791
Ak-Trol [CD]:
   dexamethasone, 251
   neomycin*
   polymixin B*
Ak-Zol, acetazolamide, 35
Alamine-C [CD]:
   chlorpheniramine*
   codeine, 222
   phenylpropanolamine*
Alamine Expectorant [CD]:
   codeine, 222
Alatone, spironolactone, 881
Alazine, hydralazine, 454
❀*Albert Furosemide*, 414
❀*Albert-Glyburide*, 434
albuterol, 50
alcohol. *See* ethanol, 329.
Aldactazide [CD]:
   hydrochlorothiazide, 928
   spironolactone, 881
Aldactone, spironolactone, 881
Aldochlor [CD]:
   chlorothiazide, 928
   methyldopa*
Aldoril–15/25 [CD]:
   hydrochlorothiazide, 928
   methyldopa*
Aldoril D30/50 [CD]:
   hydrochlorothiazide, 928
   methyldopa*
alendronate, 54
Aleve, naproxen, 815
Alka-Seltzer Effervescent Pain
   Reliever & Antacid [CD]:
   aspirin, 92
   citric acid*
   sodium bicarbonate*
Alka-Seltzer Night Time [CD]:
   aspirin, 92
Alka-Seltzer Plus [CD]:
   aspirin, 92
   chlorpheniramine*
   phenylpropanolamine*
Allay [CD]:
   acetaminophen*
   hydrocodone, 458
Allegra, fexofenadine, 627
Allerdryl, diphenhydramine, 280
Allergy capsules,
   diphenhydramine, 280

Allergy Formula,
   diphenhydramine, 280
Allergy Medication, Complete
   diphenhydramine, 280
Allergy Medicine, Valu-dryl,
   diphenhydramine, 280
Allermax, diphenhydramine, 280
❀*Alloprin*, allopurinol, 58
allopurinol, 58
Almocarpine, pilocarpine, 774
Alostil, minoxidil, 634
❀*Alpha-Tamoxifen*, 907
alprazolam, 62
Altace, ramipril, 851
Alubelap [CD]:
   aluminum hydroxide*
   belladonna*
   phenobarbital, 761
Alupent, metaproterenol, 586
Alzheimer's drugs, 84
amantadine, 66
Amaryl, glimepiride, 426
Ambenyl Expectorant [CD]:
   codeine, 222
   diphenhydramine, 280
Ambenyl Syrup [CD]:
   codeine, 222
   diphenhydramine, 280
Ambien, zolpidem, 1019
Amcill, ampicillin, 738
Amcort, triamcinolone, 963
Amen, medroxyprogesterone, 572
❀*Amersol*, ibuprofen, 815
A-Methapred,
   methylprednisolone, 602
amfebutamone, 139
amiloride, 67
Aminodrox-Forte [CD]:
   phenobarbital, 761
   theophylline, 922
Aminophyllin, aminophylline, 74
aminophylline, 74
5-aminosalicylic acid. *See*
   mesalamine, 583.
Amitril, amitriptyline, 74
amitriptyline, 74
amlodipine, 79
amoxapine, 83
amoxicillin, 738
Amoxil, amoxicillin, 738
ampicillin, 738
Ampicillin, Faspak, 738
❀*Ampicin*, ampicillin, 738
❀*Ampicin PRB* [CD]:
   ampicillin, 738
   probenecid, 802
❀*Ampilean*, ampicillin, 738
Anacin [CD]:
   aspirin, 92
   caffeine*
Anacin Maximum Strength [CD]:
   aspirin, 92
   caffeine*

*The symbol [CD] indicates that the brand name given is a combination drug consisting of generic drug components listed below it. If there is no page numbering following the name of the generic drug component, there is no Drug Profile for that ingredient in this book.

About the Authors

JAMES J. RYBACKI, Pharm. D., was born in Oneonta, New York. He received his prepharmacy education at Creighton University, and his Doctor of Pharmacy degree from the University of Nebraska Medical Center, College of Pharmacy, in Omaha. Over a quarter century of Dr. Rybacki's hospital and clinical experience includes early efforts in gas–liquid chromatography research characterizing human drug metabolites, and data collection for the College of American Pathologists to establish normal values for laboratory studies. He is a member of the clinical faculty at the University of Maryland School of Pharmacy and has provided clinical rounding and hospital experience for Pharm. D. and Bachelor students. He presently teaches a Drug Information rotation for Pharm. D. students at The Clearwater Group. He is board certified in pain management at the Diplomat level by the American Academy of Pain Management, and provides ongoing clinical pain management consulting nationwide. Dr. Rybacki is actively involved in the postmarketing monitoring of medicines via The Drug Surveillance Network, a nationwide association of clinical pharmacists, and he is an approved External New Drug Application reviewer for the Canadian Drug Ministry. He lives on the eastern shore of Maryland.

Dr. Rybacki's efforts in drug information and clinical pharmacy include many years of active practice, eight of which were at Dorchester General Hospital in Cambridge, Maryland, including infectious disease, pharmacokinetic, nutrition support, pain management, and pharmacological consultations. Through the Occupational Health Unit, he has offered independent pain management and pharmacological consultations nationwide. He has also advised the World Health Organization's Expert Committee regarding revisions as well as selection of drugs to be listed in the next edition of *The Use of Essential Drugs* and is an assistant editor for the Drugdex drug information system. His past role as Vice President Clinical Services has bought him added expertise in overseeing Occupational Health, Physical Medicines, Laboratory Services, Imaging, Cardiology, Respiratory Therapy, Cancer Programs, and Continuing Medical Education. He served as conference coordinator for the first and second annual Dorchester General Hospital Pain conferences, and seminar coordinator for the Eastern Shore of Maryland for the "Take Control" physician and public pain education programs with Johns Hopkins.

Dr. Rybacki is now president of The Clearwater Group, headquartered in Easton, Maryland, and provides drug information support and clinical pharmacy rounding to physician groups, consumers, and employers; holds seminars on medical cost containment, outcomes research, infectious disease, osteoporosis, pain management, and therapeutics; provides information support to insurance companies and HMOs; produces educational tapes on medicines; clinical program design; and conducts independent pharmacological evaluations. He was selected for full membership in the American College of Clinical Pharmacy, is a Certified Clinical Densitometrist (CCD) through the Society for Clinical Densitometry, and also holds board certification as a Forensic Examiner. He is a lifetime member of Who's Who in Global Business. Dr. Rybacki is also the director of clinical research, therapeutics, and outcomes at BoneSafe Osteoporosis Centers, a new and interdisciplinary osteoporosis testing, research, and consulting group.

Dr. Rybacki has been interviewed widely and is often a guest or guest host on numerous radio and television shows. He was featured on CNN's *Comcast Newsmakers* program as he spoke of the importance of taking medicines correctly. Recent interviews include *The Bill Miller Show*, *The Madison Show*, *Retail Pharmacy News*, and *The Wall Street Journal*. He also participates in numerous medical speakers bureaus, including Merck, Miles, Dupont Pharma, and Glaxo. He has been a member of the Bristol Myers Distinguished Speakers in HIV faculty since 1994 and lectures across the country. He has jointly authored several articles in professional journals on use of medicines in infectious diseases, critical care, therapeutics, and cost containment. His letter on medication use in the United States recently appeared in the *Journal of the American Medical Association* (JAMA). *The Essential Guide to Prescription Drugs*, first published in 1977, was co-authored by Dr. Rybacki since 1994, before he assumed full authorship in 1996. "The Medicine Man," a nationwide live radio show, was developed, written, produced, and hosted by Dr. Rybacki in 1995. He is the original writer and host of The American Pharmaceutical Association's *The Pharmacist Minute* radio program, sponsored by a grant from Johnson and Johnson Merck (Pepcid AC$^{(R)}$). This program—which is broadcast from more than 2,000 locations—was the largest launch of a radio program, and is now heard in 141 countries worldwide. Dr. Rybacki believes that the new art of prescribing medicines lies in cost containment without sacrifice of clinical outcomes. He has created a site on the World Wide Web at www.medicineinfo.com.

JAMES W. LONG, M.D., was born in Allentown, Pennsylvania. He received his premedical education from the University of Maryland and his medical degree from the George Washington University School of Medicine in Washington, D.C. For 20 years he was in private practice of internal medicine in the Washington, D.C., metropolitan area, and for over 35 years he was a member of the faculty of the George Washington University School of Medicine. He has served with the Food and Drug Administration, the National Library of Medicine, and the Bureau of Health Manpower of the National Institutes of Health. Prior to his retirement, Dr. Long was director of Health Services for the National Science Foundation in Washington. He lives in Oxford, Maryland.

Dr. Long's involvement in drug information activities includes service on the HEW Task Force on Prescription Drugs, on the FDA Task Force on Adverse Drug Reactions, as a delegate-at-large to the U.S. Pharmacopeial Convention, as editorial consultant for *Hospital Formulary*, as a director of the Drug Information Association, and as a member of the Toxicology Information Program Committee of the National Research Council/National Academy of Sciences. He was consultant to the Food and Drug Administration, serving as adviser to their staff on the development of patient package inserts. He is also the author of numerous articles in professional journals. *The Essential Guide to Prescription Drugs* is an outgrowth of his conviction that the general public needs and is entitled to practical drug information that is the equivalent of the professional "package insert." Dr. Long is the author of *The Essential Guide to Chronic Illness*, first published in 1997. He believes the patient can be reasonably certain of using medications with the least risk and greatest benefit only when the patient has all the relevant information about the drugs he or she is taking.

Controlled Drug Schedules

Schedule I: These medicines are those with a high abuse and dependence potential. Typically, the only use for these substances are for research purposes. Examples include LSD and heroin. A prescription cannot be legally written for these drugs for medicinal use.

Schedule II: These medicines have therapeutic uses and have the highest abuse and dependence potential for drugs with medicinal purposes. Examples include analgesics such as morphine (MS Contin) and meperidene (Demerol). A written prescription is required and refills are **not** allowed.

Schedule III: Medicines in this schedule have an abuse and dependence potential that is less than those in schedule II, but greater than those in schedule IV. These medicines have clear medicinal uses and include such medicines as hydrocodone, codeine, and paregoric in combination. Common names include Tylenol number three with codeine and Tenuate. A telephone prescription is permitted for medications in this class; however, it must be converted to a written form by a pharmacist. Prescriptions for these medicines may be refilled, but only five times in six months.

Schedule IV: This schedule contains medicines with less abuse and dependence potential than those in schedule III. Examples of medicines in this schedule include propoxyphene (Darvon), diazepam (Valium), and chlordiazepoxide (Librium). Prescriptions for these medicines may be refilled, but only five times in six months.

Schedule V: These medicines have the lowest abuse and dependence potential. Medicines in this class include diphenoxylate (Lomotil) and loperamide (Imodium). Drugs in this class which require a prescription are handled the same as any nonscheduled prescription medicine. Some drugs in this class do not require a prescription, and can be sold only with the approval of a pharmacist. The buyer is required to sign a log book when the drug is dispensed. Examples include codeine and hydrocodone in combination with other active nonnarcotic drugs sold in preparations that have limited quantities of codeine or hydrocodone for control of diarrhea or cough.

Pregnancy Risk Categories

Definitions of FDA Pregnancy Categories

Category A: Adequate and well-controlled studies in pregnant women are **negative** for fetal abnormalities. Risk to the fetus is remote.

Category B: Animal reproduction studies are **negative** for fetal abnormalities, and data from adequate and well-controlled studies in pregnant women are not available.

OR

Animal reproduction studies are **positive** for fetal abnormalities. Adequate and well-controlled studies in pregnant women are **negative** for fetal abnormalities, and fail to show a risk to the fetus.

Category C: Animal reproduction studies are **positive** for fetal abnormalities. Information from adequate and well-controlled studies in pregnant women is not available.

OR

Information from animal reproduction studies **and** from adequate and well-controlled studies in pregnant women is not available.

Category D: Studies in pregnant women and/or premarketing (investigational) or postmarketing uses show **positive** evidence of human fetal risk. The drug is only used in serious disease or in life-threatening situations where safer medicines will not work or cannot be used. These situations may make the medicine acceptable despite its risks.

Category X: Animal reproduction studies and/or human pregnancy studies are **positive** for fetal abnormalities.

OR

Studies in pregnant women and/or premarketing (investigational) or postmarketing (phase four) experience shows **positive** evidence of human fetal risk.

AND

Potential fetal risks outweigh possible benefits of the drug. These medicines **should never** be used in pregnancy.

The FDA is currently evaluating these pregnancy categories, and may opt to modify them.